a **LANGE** medical book

Clinical Cardiology

sixth edition

Melvin D. Cheitlin, MD
Professor of Medicine
Associate Member, Cardiovascular Research Institute
University of California, San Francisco
Chief of Cardiology, San Francisco General Hospital

Maurice Sokolow, MD
Professor of Medicine Emeritus
Senior Staff Member, Cardiovascular Research Institute
Formerly Chief of Cardiology and Program Director of
the USPHS Clinical Cardiology Training Program
University of California, San Francisco

Malcolm B. McIlroy, MD
Professor of Medicine
Senior Staff Member, Cardiovascular Research Institute
University of California, San Francisco

APPLETON & LANGE
Norwalk, Connecticut

0-8385-1093-0

Notice: The author and the publisher of this volume have taken care to
make certain that the doses of drugs and schedules of treatment are correct
and compatible with the standards generally accepted at the time of
publication. Nevertheless, as new information becomes available, changes in
treatment and in the use of drugs become necessary. The reader is advised to
carefully consult the instruction and information material included in the
package insert of each drug or therapeutic agent before administration.
This advice is especially important when using new or infrequently used drugs.
The publisher disclaims any liability, loss, injury, or damage incurred as
a consequence, directly or indirectly, of the use and application of any of
the contents of this volume.

Prentice Hall International (UK) Limited, *London*
Prentice Hall of Australia Pty. Limited, *Sydney*
Prentice Hall Canada, Inc., *Toronto*
Prentice Hall Hispanoamericana, S.A., *Mexico*
Prentice Hall of India Private Limited, *New Delhi*
Prentice Hall of Japan, Inc., *Tokyo*
Simon & Schuster Asia Pte. Ltd., *Singapore*
Editora Prentice Hall do Brasil Ltda., *Rio de Janerio*
Prentice Hall, *Englewood Cliffs, New Jersey*

ISBN: 0-8385-1093-0
ISBN: 0891-2092

Acquisitions Editor: Martin Wonsiewicz
Production Editor: Christine Langan

PRINTED IN THE UNITED STATES OF AMERICA

This book is dedicated to Hella Cheitlin; to Mollie and James
Cheitlin; to Margaret McIlroy; and to the memory of Ethel Sokolow

Table of Contents

Preface

No field in medicine has experienced an explosion in knowledge in such a brief period as has the field of cardiology in the past few years. Enormous strides in our understanding of the pathogenesis of cardiovascular disease and the development of new drugs, techniques, and technologies for the diagnosis and treatment of heart disease challenge the clinician's ability to include these advances in the daily management of patients.

In addition to established journals and books relevant to cardiologic practice, new journals, books, monographs, newspapers, and audio and video tapes appear almost weekly. It is a mammoth task to digest and monitor the flood of new information and impossible to instantaneously assess its value.

The sixth edition of *Clinical Cardiology* attempts to present a comprehensive but not encyclopedic account of the newer concepts in diagnosis and therapy of cardiovascular disease in a lucid, balanced manner. New information is documented rather than presented in dogmatic fashion. The approach always starts with the foundation of etiology, history, and physical examination—in other words, the bedside evaluation of the patient that is the bedrock of clinical evaluation upon which the clinician bases decisions about which studies are necessary for diagnosis and for planning patient management. Details of the bedside evaluation as well as the technical procedures are described so that the reader can integrate the two. Both are essential for the proper modern management of the patient with cardiovascular disease.

This book is written for medical students, medical house staff, cardiology trainees, internists, primary care physicians, and specialists in other fields who wish to "dip into" the book for specific information pertinent to their patients.

A significant change in authorship has occurred in the sixth edition. Dr Melvin Cheitlin, a coauthor of the fifth edition, has assumed responsibility as senior author. He has undertaken primary responsibility for updating the book in all matters pertaining to new advances in knowledge and changes in practice in the last three years. Dr Cheitlin is a clinician with 30 years of experience in the practice of cardiology. After 20 years in the United States Army Medical Department as Chief of Cardiology in the majority of the Army's medical centers, including Walter Reed Army Medical Center, he joined the University of California at San Francisco as Professor of Medicine and is currently Chief of the Cardiology Service at San Francisco General Hospital. Dr Sokolow, who was senior author of the first five editions, continues to be actively involved in the preparation of the book and has primary responsibility for the chapter on hypertension, which has now been totally rewritten. Dr McIlroy has rewritten parts of the chapter on physiology.

The considerable amount of new material has resulted in a modest increase in the size of the book, and new illustrations and references have replaced many of the older ones. Major new advances detailed in the book include extensive information on Doppler echocardiography, discussed throughout the book where appropriate, and new imaging techniques and agents for the diagnosis and treatment of coronary artery disease, valvular disease, endocarditis, pulmonary embolism, primary myocardial disease, and congenital heart disease.

New invasive and noninvasive techniques are discussed in some detail, and their value is assessed. Thrombolysis, antiplatelet agents, coronary angioplasty and its newer modifications such as mechanical and laser atherectomy, and angioscopy are described. Bypass coronary surgery and its indications, complications, and results are reviewed in detail. The rationale and indications for prevention and treatment of coronary disease, hypertension, cardiac failure, and transplantation are explored. More details related to the use of diagnostic and therapeutic modalities are presented for the assistance of the physician involved in patient care. An appreciation of the varieties of supraventricular arrhythmias and their treatment is provided. Ablative techniques to abolish aberrant pathways and prevent recurrent arrhythmias are detailed. The use of implanted antitachycardia defibrillation devices as well as attempts at ablation in the treatment of recurrent ventricular tachycardia and fibrillation are updated. The importance of beta-adrenergic-mediated ventricular tachycardia and right ventricular dysplasia in the genesis of ventricular tachycardia is discussed. The early use of angiotensin-converting enzyme inhibitors in heart failure is emphasized, and studies are cited supporting their use.

The chapters on hypertension, coronary artery disease, valvular heart disease, congestive heart failure, cardiomyopathy, and arrhythmias and conduction defects have all been largely or entirely rewritten. Extensive revisions have been made in most of the other chapters as well.

We welcome comments and suggestions from readers and reviewers and will respond to them appropriately with changes in the next edition.

Melvin D. Cheitlin, MD
Maurice Sokolow, MD
Malcolm B. McIlroy MD

Acknowledgments

We wish to thank our colleagues for providing illustrative material: Dr Elias Botvinick, Dr Bruce Brundage, Dr Eric Carlsson, Dr Roger Cooke, Dr Dai Ru-ping, Dr Gordon Gamsu, Dr Mervin Goldman, Dr Robert Grover, Dr Charles Higgins, Dr Arthur Hollman, Dr Martin Lipton, Dr Thomas Ports, Dr Nelson Schiller, Dr Norman Silverman, and Dr Paul Yock.

We are grateful for the excellent expert organizational and secretarial assistance of Mr Louis Henkenius, Ms Mary McLean, and Ms Judy Serrell.

Anatomy & Physiology of the Circulatory System

1

ANATOMY OF THE HEART

The cardiac muscle surrounding the chambers of the atria and the ventricles arises from and is attached to the fibrous skeleton of the heart, composed of the four fibrous valve rings, or annuli. The atrial muscle and arteries are attached superiorly and the ventricular muscle to the rings inferiorly. The only muscle connection between the atria and the ventricles is the specialized muscle of the conduction system, the His bundle, which perforates the confluence of the tricuspid, mitral, and aortic valve rings called the right fibrous trigone.

The ventricular muscle originates from the fibrous skeleton and in interdigitated layers passes spirally and circumferentially around the ventricle, inserting back on the annuli. With contraction of the muscles so arranged, the base of the ventricle moves toward the apex, and the diameters of the ventricles are shortened.

The normal heart lies within its pericardial sac in the middle of the thorax slightly to the left of the midline. The low-pressure right atrium and right ventricle occupy the anterior rightward portion of the heart and the higher-pressure left ventricle and atrium lie posteriorly leftward. The long axis of the heart, from the apex of the left ventricle to the root of the aorta, runs upward and backward at an angle of about 30 degrees from the horizontal plane and 45 degrees from the sagittal plane of the body. The apex of the heart rests on the upper surface of the diaphragm, which lies close to the posterior and inferior surfaces of the heart. The lie of the heart varies with the build of the patient and with respiration. It assumes a more vertical position during inspiration and in tall, thin persons, and a more horizontal position during expiration and in persons of heavier build.

THE PERICARDIAL SAC

The heart lies freely in the pericardial sac with attachments only at its venous and arterial ends. Embryologically, the heart invaginates the pericardial sac so that there is a visceral pericardium or epicardium on the surface of the heart and a parietal pericardium that forms the pericardial sac. This invagination results in pericardial reflections or attachments at the bifurcation of the main pulmonary artery and halfway up the ascending aorta. The attachments are also around the venae cavae and the pulmonary veins.

These pericardial reflections form two spaces within the pericardial sac. The reflections around the venae cavae and the four pulmonary veins form a horseshoe-shaped cul de sac with an inferior entrance, called the oblique sinus, and a space between the great arteries anteriorly and the superior pulmonary veins and superior vena cava posteriorly, called the transverse sinus.

EXTERNAL APPEARANCE

Anterior Aspect

As viewed from the front (Figure 1–1), the largest area of the surface of the heart is formed by the triangular right ventricle, with the pulmonary trunk arising from the apex of the triangle. Above and to the right of the right ventricle, one can see the right atrium—or, more specifically, the right atrial appendage—as an ear-shaped structure overlying the root of the aorta. The groove between the right atrium and the ventricle (coronary sulcus) is often filled with fat and is occupied by the right coronary artery. Above the right atrium, the superior vena cava is seen entering the right atrium through the pericardium. The inferior vena cava lies on the diaphragmatic surface of the heart and enters the right atrium from the back. The anterior aspect of the heart reveals only a small part of the left ventricle, lying to the left of the right ventricle and forming the apex of the heart. The anterior interventricular sulcus often contains fat and is occupied by the anterior descending branch of the left coronary artery. The only portion of the left atrium visible from the front is the left atrial appendage, which lies above the ventricle and curves around the left side of the origin of the pulmonary trunk. The lungs normally cover most of the anterior surface of the heart, especially during inspiration, leaving only a small area apposed to the back of the sternum and left ribs.

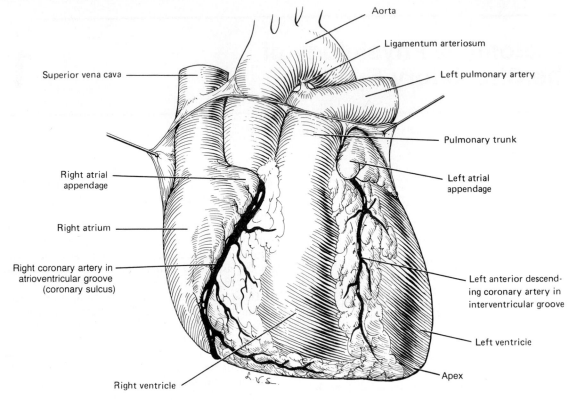

Figure 1–1. Anterior view of the heart.

Left-Sided Aspect

As viewed from the left side (Figure 1–2), the left ventricle and left atrium occupy most of the surface of the heart. The posterior interventricular groove separates the left ventricle above from the right ventricle below. The posterior descending branch of the right coronary artery lies in this groove. The atrioventricular groove runs almost vertically in this view, separating the left ventricle from the left atrium. The coronary sinus and the circumflex branch of the left coronary artery lie in this groove and complete the ring of blood vessels forming the base of the corona (crown) after which the blood vessels supplying the heart are named.

Posterior Aspect

The back of the heart mainly rests on the diaphragm and is largely occupied by the left atrium and ventricle plus portions of the right atrium and ventricle, as shown in Figure 1–3. The point at which all four chambers meet posteriorly is called the crux of the heart because of the cross-shaped pattern of blood vessels lying at the junction of the posterior interventricular groove and the atrioventricular groove. The vessels forming the cross are the coronary sinus and the posterior descending coronary artery. This latter vessel may be a branch of either the right or the

circumflex branch of the left coronary artery depending on whether the right or left coronary artery is the larger (dominant) vessel. In about 85% of hearts, the right coronary artery is dominant and gives origin to the posterior descending coronary artery. The pulmonary veins enter the back of the left atrium. The pattern may vary, but two right and two left pulmonary veins are normally present.

Right-Sided Aspect

When viewed from the right side, the right atrium and ventricle occupy most of the surface, as shown in Figure 1–4. The superior and inferior venae cavae enter the atrium at the back, and the aorta runs upward from the middle of the heart. The outflow tract of the right ventricle and the pulmonary trunk form the upper border of the heart in this view. The left atrium is posterior, and the left ventricle is not visible in this view.

The Great Vessels

The main **pulmonary artery** (pulmonary trunk) runs upward and to the left in front of the aorta and leaves the pericardial sac before dividing into its right and left branches. The left pulmonary artery continues to arch backward in the same line as the main trunk, while the right branch turns laterally behind the

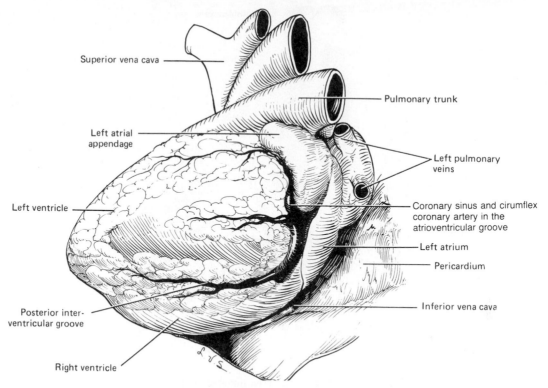

Figure 1–2. The heart viewed from the left side with the apex raised to show the back of the heart.

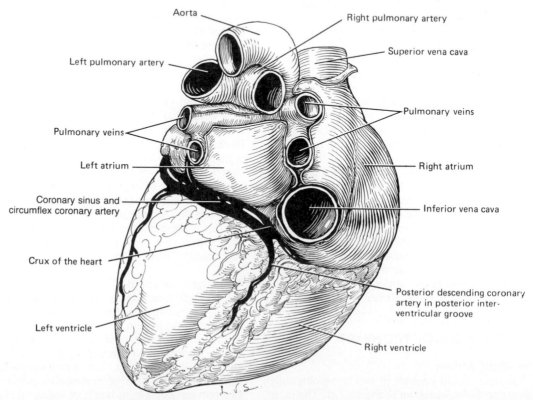

Figure 1–3. The heart viewed from below and behind.

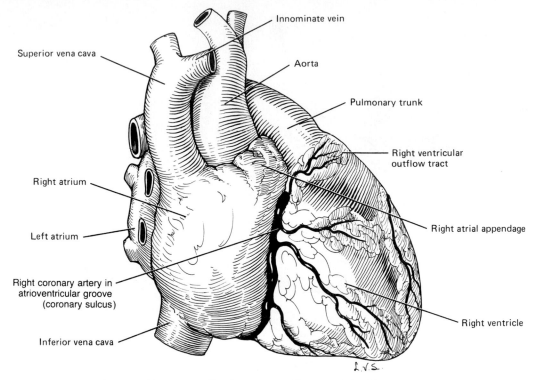

Figure 1–4. The heart viewed from the right side.

ascending aorta and the superior vena cava to reach the hilum of the right lung. The bifurcation of the pulmonary artery lies on the roof of the left atrium and above the left main bronchus.

The **aorta** arises deep within the heart, and its proximal portion is covered by the right atrial appendage. It runs upward beside the **superior vena cava** before giving off its first and largest (innominate) branch, which shortly divides into the right common carotid and right subclavian branches. The aortic arch passes backward and to the left, giving off its left common carotid and left subclavian branches before crossing the left pulmonary artery. There is a close relationship between the left pulmonary artery and the aorta. The ductus arteriosus, which connected these two structures during fetal development, persists as a remnant—the ligamentum arteriosum—in adults. The point at which it joins the aorta is termed the isthmus of the aorta, because there is sometimes a narrowing at this level. With trauma, stress is high at this point and also at the root of the ascending aorta, and it is at these places that tears usually occur.

THE CHAMBERS OF THE HEART

The Right Atrium

The right atrium consists of two embryologically distinct portions, as shown in Figure 1–5. The more posterior thin-walled portion into which the venae cavae and coronary sinus empty is formed from the sinus venosus and is composed of tissue similar to that of the great veins. Guarding the inferior vena cava orifice is a remnant valve, the eustachian valve, and a more defined valve guarding the coronary sinus ostium, the thebesian valve. The more anterior muscular portion includes the right atrial appendage and the tricuspid valve ring. Unlike the left atrium, the right atrium has thin columns of muscle in the more anterior portion called pectinate muscles. The fossa ovalis lies in the middle of the thin-walled portion and is the site of the fetal foramen ovale. This interatrial communication, which is present during fetal life, permits the flow of oxygenated placental blood from the inferior vena cava into the left heart. The foramen ovale remains open or potentially open in about 15% of normal subjects, but since it is a flap valve that only allows flow from right to left, it is normally functionally closed.

The Right Ventricle

The right ventricle is triangular in shape and forms a crescentic, shallow structure wrapped over the ventricular septum. It can be divided, as shown in Figure 1–6, into a proximal inflow portion, containing the tricuspid valve and its chordae tendineae, and a distal outflow tract, from which the pulmonary trunk arises. The line of demarcation between the two portions consists of bands of muscle formed by the crista supraventricularis, the parietal band, the

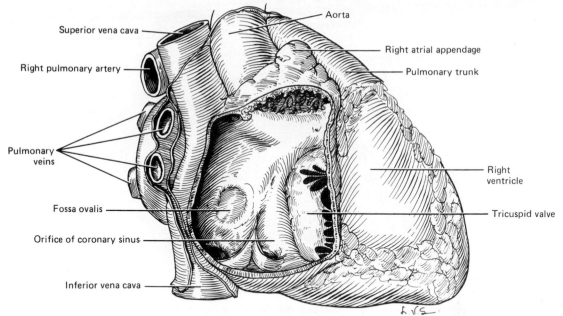

Figure 1–5. View of the right heart with the right wall reflected to show the right atrium.

septal band, and the moderator band. The outflow tract of the right ventricle is derived from the embryologically distinct bulbus cordis—in contrast to the inflow portion, which arises from ventricular tissue. The right ventricular wall is thinner than the wall of the left ventricle and has ridges and columns of muscles called trabeculae carneae. The septal surface is markedly trabeculated. There is a large anterior papillary muscle, a small papillary muscle of the conus from the septum, and a variable group of posterior papillary muscles from the diaphragmatic surface.

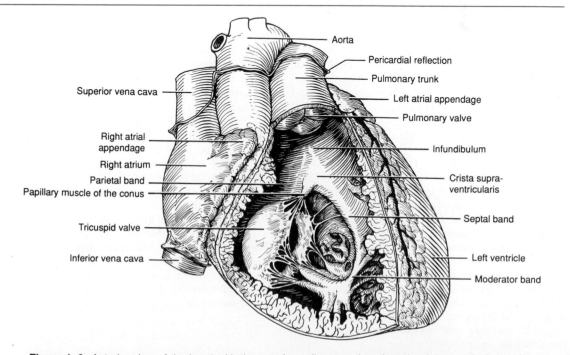

Figure 1–6. Anterior view of the heart with the anterior wall removed to show the right ventricular cavity.

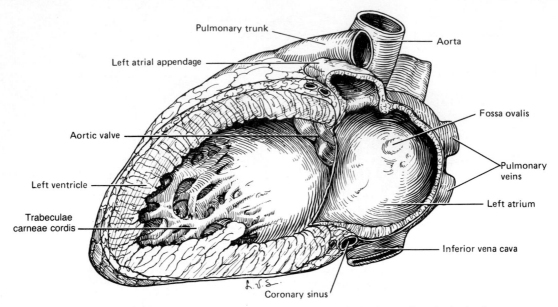

Figure 1–7. View of the left heart from the left side with the left ventricular free wall and mitral valve cut away.

The Left Atrium

The left atrium, like the right, is composed of a vein-like portion, into which the pulmonary veins drain, and a more muscular anterior portion, which includes the left atrial appendage. Its wall is slightly thicker than that of the right atrium, and the thinner area, corresponding to the fossa ovalis, can be seen on its right upper surface (Figure 1–7). Only the left atrial appendage has pectinate muscles.

The Left Ventricle

The left ventricular cavity is shaped like an egg. The base of the egg is formed by the mitral valve ring. The wall of the left ventricle is three to four times as thick as that of the right ventricle and accounts for about 75% of the mass of the heart. The aortic and mitral valve rings lie close to each other, with the larger anterior mobile cusp of the mitral valve adjacent to the left coronary and noncoronary cusps of the aortic valve. The posterior relatively immobile cusp of the mitral valve is shorter, and together with the anterior cusp, is tethered to the anterolateral and posteromedial papillary muscles in a parachute-like fashion by chordae tendineae, some of which are shared by the two cusps as shown in Figure 1–8. The interventricular septum, which forms the anterior aspect of the left ventricle, bulges into the right ventricle, making the cross section of the mid portion of the left ventricle circular in shape. The septal surface has flattened trabeculations in the mid and apical portions. At the top of the muscular septum, just below the right coronary and noncoronary cusps, is the membranous septum.

CARDIAC VALVES

The **tricuspid valve** is a thin, filmy tripartite structure with anterior, posterior, and medial or septal cusps. The septal leaflet meets the anterior leaflet across the right side of the membranous septum. The chordae tendineae anchor the leading edge of the tricuspid valve to the papillary muscles. The chordae branch once or twice before insertion on the leading edge and the ventricular surface of the valve. The **mitral valve,** which is thicker than the tricuspid valve, has two cusps and is shaped like a bishop's hat (miter) in which the anterior surface (anterior cusp) is longer and wider than the posterior surface. The chordae arise from the anteromedial and posteromedial papillary muscles and branch once or twice before attachment to the leading edge and the ventricular surface of the mitral valve. Fan-like branching of the chordae occurs at the commissures. The commissures are situated anterolaterally and posteromedially. The **pulmonary valve** is composed of three pocket-like cusps. Two of the cusps are situated anteriorly (right and left), and the third is posterior. It is constructed of thinner tissue than the aortic valve, which lies posterior, rightward, and inferior to the pulmonary valve. The aortic valve also has three cusps—the anterior (right coronary), the left posterior (left coronary), and the right posterior (noncoronary) cusps—associated with corresponding dilations of the aorta called the aortic sinuses or sinuses of Valsalva.

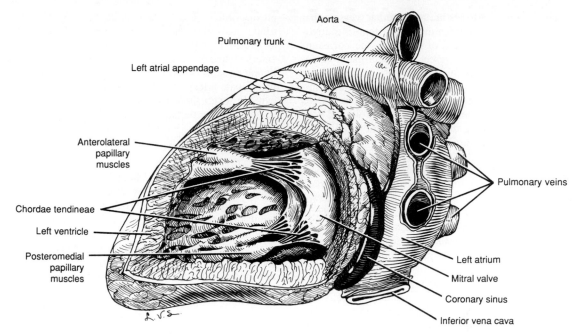

Figure 1–8. View of the left heart with the left ventricular wall turned back to show the mitral valve.

CORONARY CIRCULATION
(See also Figures 8–13 and 8–14.)

The coronary arteries are more variable in pattern than any other part of the cardiac anatomy. The two main coronary arteries—left and right—arise from the right and left aortic sinuses within the pockets of the aortic valve cusps. Although either vessel may predominate and supply the posteroinferior portion of the heart, in approximately 85% of persons the right coronary artery supplies the posterior descending coronary artery. In 70% of persons **the left coronary artery** is the larger of the two. The left coronary artery is likely to be dominant in patients with congenital aortic stenosis or bicuspid aortic valve. The left coronary artery runs behind the main pulmonary artery as a short main stem about 1 or 2 cm long before dividing into an anterior and a circumflex branch. The **anterior branch** usually has a **descending branch** that follows the interventricular groove. The anterior descending coronary artery gives rise to a large first septal perforating branch and a variable number of septal branches. Over the anterolateral left ventricle, there are one or two diagonal branches. The **circumflex branch** follows the left atrioventricular groove, curving around to the posterior surface of the heart. The area between these two vessels, each of which is defined by a course within a groove, is supplied by branches from one artery or the other. The left circumflex branches over the lateral left ventricle are called obtuse marginal branches. There may

be two to four or more such branches. Atrial branches arise from the circumflex coronary artery, and in about 45% of cases the left circumflex gives rise to a vessel supplying the sinus node. The left coronary artery consists of three branches, with the mid branch arising from the bifurcation of the more readily definable arteries. In this instance, the middle artery is called the intermediate coronary artery. The circumflex branch is larger in persons with a dominant left coronary pattern. In this case, the vessel may run as far as the crux of the heart and even give off the posterior descending branch, which runs in the posterior interventricular groove.

The right coronary artery runs in the right atrioventricular groove, downward and to the right, before curving around to the back of the heart to reach the crux, giving off a posterior descending interventricular branch. The right coronary may continue in the posterior atrioventricular groove, giving one or even two posterolateral branches. An anterior right atrial branch usually arises near the origin of the right coronary artery. It usually supplies a branch to the sinoatrial node. Also arising near the origin of the right coronary artery or even as a separate ostium from the anterior sinus of Valsalva is the conus artery supplying the outflow tract of the right ventricle. The atrioventricular node is also supplied in 90% of hearts by a branch of the right coronary artery that arises from the right coronary artery as it reaches the crux of the heart and makes a U-curve after giving off the left posterior descending coronary artery.

The coronary arteries are extracardiac vessels that are exposed to intrapericardial rather than intramyocardial pressure. Bridges of muscle tissue occasionally overlie a coronary vessel for a centimeter or so. They are seen both in the presence and in the absence of coronary artery disease and usually have no clinical significance. Occasionally, these muscle bridges can compress the coronary artery in systole and very occasionally may be the cause of myocardial ischemia and even myocardial infarctions.

The extent of collateral circulation in the coronary arterial bed is an important variable but almost impossible to assess. In the normal heart without coronary arterial obstructive disease, there are very few coronary collateral vessels visible or demonstrable by coronary artery injection. The extent of the collateral circulation both before and after the development of coronary disease probably plays an important role in prognosis.

Most of the coronary venous drainage is into the **coronary sinus.** The few veins that drain directly into the cardiac chambers are called thebesian veins. The main venous drainage of the left ventricle is via the great cardiac vein, which runs with the anterior descending branch of the left coronary artery, passing around the left atrioventricular sulcus to the posterior aspect of the heart, where it becomes the coronary sinus. The posterior cardiac vein joins the coronary sinus near its ostium in the right atrium.

CONDUCTION SYSTEM
(Figure 1–17)

The **sinoatrial node,** which initiates the normal cardiac impulse, lies at the junction of the superior vena cava and the right atrium. The **atrioventricular node** is located in the right posterior portion of the interatrial septum near the base of the tricuspid valve. The atrioventricular node is continuous with the **bundle of His,** which perforates the right fibrous trigone and divides into a left and a right bundle branch at the top of the interventricular septum. The right bundle branch passes subendocardially down the septum and then onto the moderator band of the right ventricle before branching into the Purkinje system. The left branch divides into anterior and posterior branches, which fan out and run subendocardially, close to the septum, before ramifying into the **Purkinje fibers,** which spread to all parts of the ventricular myocardium. The details of abnormal conduction pathways are given in Chapter 14.

LYMPHATICS

The lymphatics of the heart are arranged in three plexuses: subendocardial, myocardial, and subepicardial. The drainage is outward to the subepicardial plexus, where the vessels unite to form drainage trunks that follow the coronary arteries. They eventually form a single vessel that leaves the heart on the anterior surface of the pulmonary artery to reach a lymph node between the superior vena cava and the innominate artery. Cardiac transplantation, which inevitably severs the cardiac lymphatics, does not seem to produce any deleterious effect.

CARDIAC NERVES

The heart is innervated both by cholinergic fibers from the vagus nerve and by adrenergic fibers arising from the thoracolumbar sympathetic system and passing through the superior, middle, and inferior cervical ganglia. The efferent cholinergic supply is confined to the atria. Fibers from the right vagus nerve supply the sinoatrial node and serve to control the heart rate and the force of atrial contraction. Fibers from the left vagus nerve supply mainly the atrioventricular node, but there is usually some cross-innervation. The atria also receive sympathetic fibers, but most of the adrenergic nerves pass to the ventricles along with the coronary arteries, where they serve to increase the force of cardiac contraction. The heart also has an autonomic sensory innervation via small, mainly nonmedullated sympathetic fibers. These are thought to respond to nociceptive stimuli and to constitute the pathway through which cardiac pain is mediated. Like other visceral sensations, the pain of myocardial ischemia is poorly and variably localized. In addition, sensations originating in other intrathoracic structures such as the great vessels and pericardium can cause pain that is indistinguishable from it.

Vagally innervated receptors are also widely distributed in the atria and ventricles. The atrial receptors discharge into myelinated fibers and send impulses up the vagus nerve that reduce sympathetic output to the kidneys. Their effect is to cause an increase in urinary volume and sodium excretion. The ventricular receptors are served by nonmedullated fibers. The endings are thought to be mechanoreceptors that respond to changes in ventricular pressure and reinforce the effects of the carotid and aortic baroreceptors.

The efferent autonomic nerve supply to the coronary arteries is thought to play a role in the development of spasm of the coronary arteries. The mechanisms involved are poorly understood, but it seems likely that vasospasm can initiate myocardial ischemia and lead to the development of life-threatening ventricular arrhythmias culminating in sudden death.

MICROSCOPIC ANATOMY
OF THE HEART

The basic heart muscle cell forms part of a syncytium in which the individual cells are joined to-

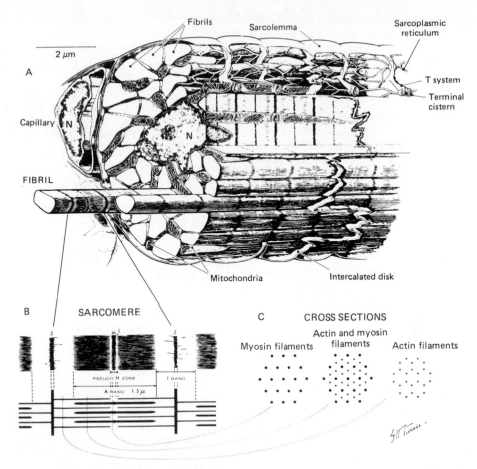

Figure 1–9. Diagram of cardiac muscle as seen under the electron microscope. **A:** A myocardial cell showing the arrangement of the multiple parallel fibrils. N, nucleus. **B:** An individual sarcomere from a myofibril. A representation of the arrangement of myofilaments that make up the sarcomere is shown below. **C:** Cross sections of the sarcomere, showing the specific lattice arrangement of the myofilaments. (Reproduced, with permission, from Braunwald E, Ross J Jr. Sonnenblick EH: Mechanisms of contraction of the normal and failing heart. N Engl J Med 1967;277:794).

gether in an irregular fashion in bands and spirals without the well-defined tendons and bony attachments characteristic of skeletal muscle. The heart muscle cell differs from the skeletal muscle cell also in that it possesses inherent rhythmicity. This property varies with different types of cardiac muscle; it is most marked in nodal tissue and least notable in peripheral muscle cells. The subcellular arrangement of cardiac muscle cells (Figure 1–9A) is similar to that of skeletal muscle. The cells are about 30 × 10 μm in size and contain about 20–50 fibrils. Each fibril is about 1μm in diameter and is composed of a series of sarcomeres, the basic muscle units. The cell contains a nucleus and numerous mitochondria. The limiting membrane is the sarcolemma, from which a sarcoplasmic reticulum invaginates the cell to form a complex tubular (T) system surrounding each fibril. The electrical activity triggering the contraction of each sarcomere passes through this complex membrane-like structure.

The Sarcomere

The structural unit of heart muscle—the sarcomere—is shown in Figure 1–9B. Its banded appearance results from overlapping of the two major muscle proteins—actin and myosin—which accounts for the striated appearance. The wide dark A bands are formed by overlapping of the thicker myosin elements with the thinner, lighter actin filaments. The thinner dark Z lines indicate the end of one sarcomere and the beginning of the next. The lighter I bands represent areas in which only actin filaments are present. The pattern of the sarcomere seen by electron microscopy varies with contraction and relaxation of the sarcomere. With contraction, the I band becomes shorter and the A band more dense. The Z lines come to lie closer together as the muscle contracts. When the muscle fibril is cut in cross section, a specific lattice pattern is seen (Figure 1–9C). In the zone in which the actin and myosin overlap, each thick myosin fiber is surrounded by six actin fibers. This hexagonal pattern is also seen in the lighter I band region. In the center of the sarcomere, where only myosin is present (M zone), the individual myosin filaments are arranged in a lattice pattern. A similar pattern is seen at the Z lines.

EMBRYOLOGY OF THE HEART

The embryology of the heart is as complex as that of any organ in the body. The heart develops mainly between the second and sixth weeks of gestation; thus, the factors responsible for the development of congenital heart lesions probably operate in most cases before the diagnosis of pregnancy is clinically certain.

Primitive Heart Tube

The heart is formed by the folding of the primitive vascular tube, which appears in the splanchnic mesodermal tissue near the pericardial cavity at about the start of the third week of gestation. At first the primitive heart tube is straight, but differential growth soon forms a cardiac loop bending toward the right or forming a D-loop, as shown in Figure 1–10. Three more or less distinct portions of the tube can be distinguished, and it is convenient to describe them separately even though their development proceeds in parallel. The three portions are (1) the sinus venosus, (2) the cardiac loop, and (3) the aortic and branchial arches.

The Sinus Venosus

The most caudad portion of the primitive heart tube gives rise to the sinus venosus. As shown in Figure 1–11, this is an independent chamber during the early stage of development of the heart. It originally consists of two horns, each receiving a duct of Cuvier.

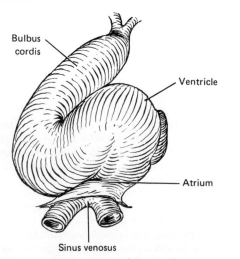

Figure 1–10. Formation of the cardiac loop.

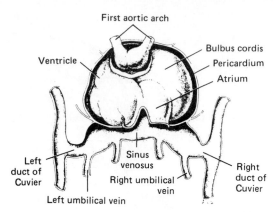

Figure 1–11. The sinus venosus, atrium, and ventricle as seen from the dorsal surface of an embryo at about the fourth week of gestation. (Modified and reproduced, with permission, from Davies J: *Human Development Anatomy.* Ronald Press, 1963.)

The umbilical veins are formed from this structure, which ultimately gives rise to the superior and inferior venae cavae, the pulmonary veins, the coronary sinus, and the posterior portions of the right and left atria.

The Cardiac Loop

The intermediate portion of the primitive heart tube bends to form the cardiac loop, which twists on itself to form three distinct portions: the primitive atrium, the ventricle, and, more distally, the bulbus cordis. In the process of twisting, the primitive heart comes to lie in close apposition to its surrounding pericardial sac, as shown in Figure 1–11. The cardiac chambers are at first single; septation to form separate right- and left-sided atria and ventricles occurs at a later stage.

Aortic (Branchial) Arches

The most distal portion of the primitive heart tube forms the aortic sac; distal to this sac, six paired aortic arches appear sequentially. Some disappear, but others persist to give rise to the great vessels. The original pattern of arches is shown in Figure 1–12, with the persisting vessels outlined. The third arch persists as the internal carotid artery; the left fourth arch forms the arch of the aorta; and the sixth arch gives rise to the pulmonary arteries and the ductus arteriosus.

Septation

The most complex stage of cardiac embryology is septation of the various parts of the heart (Figure 1–13). In the atrium, a septum extends downward and forward toward the center of the heart where the endocardial cushions are located and from which the atrioventricular valves subsequently develop. This is the septum primum. A second atrial septum—the septum secundum—grows on the right side of the

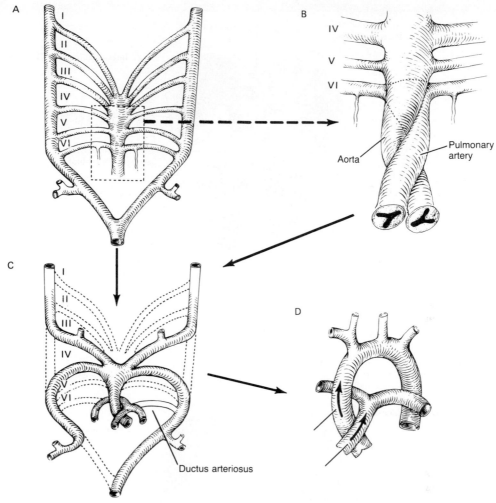

Figure 1–12. *A:* The primitive arches are shown as paired structures. *B:* Rotation and septation of the great vessels. *C:* The third, fourth, and sixth arches persist to form the adult pattern shown in *D*.

septum primum. A hole develops in the septum primum in the middle of the atrium, and atrial septation is never complete. The septum secundum does not extend all the way forward and downward to the endocardial cushions, and a persistent interatrial communication between the two atrial septa persists as the foramen ovale until birth.

Separation of the primitive ventricle into right and left chambers is accomplished by the development of an interventricular septum, which grows from the anterior wall of the common ventricle. Its free margin is aligned slightly to the right of the midline, toward the region of the endocardial cushions.

The most distal part of the primitive ventricle, the bulbus cordis, dilates to form the truncus arteriosus, which develops between the ventricles and the aortic arches. A spiral septum forms within the bulbus cordis and grows downward toward the center of the heart, where the endocardial cushions are forming the atrioventricular valves and meeting the ventricular

septum (Figure 1–13A). The upper (membranous) part of the ventricular septum is formed in this area from endocardial cushion tissue. The spiral bulbar septum separates the truncus arteriosus into right and left portions, forming the root of the aorta and the outflow tract of the right ventricle, respectively, along with their appropriate valves.

Abnormalities of septation account for a large number of congenital heart lesions. In the atrium, defects may occur in the septum primum or septum secundum, and associated abnormalities of the endocardial cushion (atrioventricular canal) area also occur. In the ventricle, the membranous portion of the septum is the site of most septal defects; and in the truncus arteriosus, abnormal septation accounts for transposition of the great vessels. The persistence of abnormal aortic arches gives rise to various lesions such as right-sided aortic arch and vascular anomalies of the aortic branches. Persistence of the normal fetal communications (ductus arteriosus and foramen

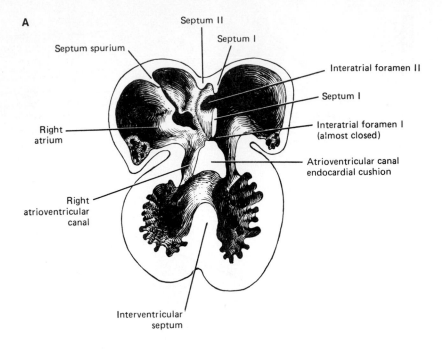

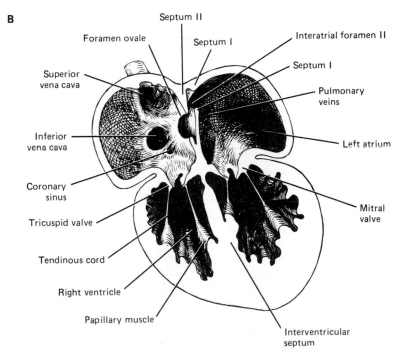

Figure 1–13. Early **(A)** and late **(B)** stages of atrial and ventricular septation.

ovale) also gives rise to congenital lesions, while developmental abnormalities of the sinus venosus account for anomalous pulmonary and systemic venous drainage patterns.

PHYSIOLOGIC FUNCTION OF THE CIRCULATION

OVERVIEW OF THE CIRCULATION

Normal Metabolic Needs & Their Variations

The mammalian cardiovascular system consists of the heart, great vessels, arteries, arterioles, capillaries, and veins, which function as a highly efficient integrated circulation to distribute amounts of blood adequate for the metabolic needs of the organs of the body during normal activity, at rest, and during periods of stress. Transport of oxygen—the most conveniently measured overall index of cardiovascular function—elimination of carbon dioxide, transport of nutrients, and control of body temperature are all vital functions of the circulation.

In the normal human adult, the resting metabolic rate, measured as oxygen consumption, is about 250 mL/min. This figure can increase more than 15-fold in normal subjects during strenuous muscular exercise, which is the most important physiologic stress to which the cardiovascular system can be subjected. Other normal and abnormal stresses—emotional stress, changes in external temperature or gravitational force (posture), sexual activity, pregnancy, changes in body weight, salt lack or excess, anemia, and fever—all cause increases in metabolic rate that seldom double resting values.

Evolutionary & Size Factors

The principal cardiovascular variable—the volume flow of blood in the aorta—varies widely in different mammalian species. Of its two components—aortic blood velocity and aortic cross-sectional area—the former shows much less variability with the size of the animal. Thus, while the aortic blood velocity in the mouse is of the same order of magnitude as that in the elephant, the cross-sectional area of the aorta is several orders of magnitude larger in the elephant. The other important variables—arterial pressure and heart rate—also show a range of variability with size that is much less than that of aortic cross-sectional area. In the present description of the mammalian circulation, the primary variables are considered to be aortic pressure and aortic blood velocity.

The mammalian cardiovascular system has evolved to deal with two conflicting problems: achieving maximal exercise performance and countering the effects of gravity. On the one hand, the system must provide enough blood flow to the muscles of locomotion to enable humans and other animals to survive by moving rapidly to catch prey or escape from predators. On the other hand, an economical resting metabolism is needed to conserve energy. Emergence from the ocean and development of the upright posture have called for a mean arterial blood pressure high enough to permit the appropriate distribution of blood to the brain at all times in the face of the force of gravity.

Component Parts of the Circulation

The heart provides the force that propels the blood through the body. The left ventricle generates an impulse of constant and short (about 0.1 s) duration. This short power stroke results from the rapid depolarization of the ventricle. The heart can increase its frequency of contraction (chronotropism), its force of contraction (inotropism), or both, but the duration of the ventricular power stroke (manifested by the QRS complex of the ECG) does not change with changes in the frequency or force of contraction. When output increases chronotropically, both systole and diastole shorten, but the duration of the impulse phase of rapid cardiac depolarization is unchanged. With inotropic stimulation, the force generated by each myocardial fiber increases, but the time for which the force is generated stays the same, and the duration of the QRS complex of the ECG is unchanged. The cardiac cycle is a transient event. The results of cardiac contraction depend on the forces encountered when the aortic valve opens and vary with beat to beat changes in heart rate or peripheral resistance.

The left ventricle pumps into a multibranched systemic circuit consisting of elastic arteries that contain a significant mass of blood. The compliance (analogue of electrical capacitance) of the elastic arteries and the inertia (analogue of electrical inductance) of the mass of blood within them combine to offer a special form of resistance (characteristic impedance) to the transmission of energy from the heart to the periphery. Characteristic impedance has the same units as conventional resistance and obeys Ohm's law, but its components (capacitance and inductance) involve no loss of energy and so can combine to offer a "lossless" form of resistance to blood flow. An important consequence of this form of impedance is that it introduces a significant time delay in the transmission of energy from the heart to the periphery. When the impedances are matched at branches in the arterial bed in accordance with Ohm's law, the cardiac impulse is transmitted in a delayed but undistorted manner to the peripheral arterioles where the "real" resistance is located.

The distribution of blood to the capillary bed of each organ is controlled at the level of the arterioles

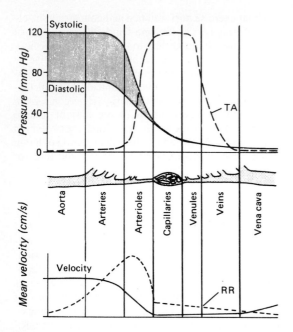

Figure 1–14. Diagram of the changes in pressure and velocity as blood flows through the systemic circulation. TA, total cross-sectional area of the vessels, which increases from 4.5 cm² in the aorta to 4500 cm² in the capillaries. RR, relative resistance, which is highest in the arterioles. (Reproduced, with permission, from Ganong WF: *Review of Medical Physiology,* 13th ed. Appleton & Lange, 1987.)

(Figure 1–14). The velocity of blood flow falls at this point, and the arterioles act as parallel resistance vessels controlling the distribution of flow to each capillary bed, where gas exchange takes place. The veins act both as return vessels to the heart and as capacitance vessels, whose large volume and high compliance provide an adequate reservoir of blood.

Control Mechanisms

Adaptation of the circulation to the varying needs of the body is achieved by the interplay of many complex—often interrelated—regulatory control mechanisms that reinforce one another and have different response times. Neural control mechanisms act rapidly and over a short interval, whereas humoral adjustments come into play more slowly and remain active for longer periods. The control systems support one another so effectively that reasonably satisfactory cardiovascular function can be maintained during exercise even after several important control mechanisms have been rendered inoperative.

PHYSIOLOGY OF THE HEART

The heart consists of a syncytium of striated muscle cells supported by fibrous tissue. Each muscle cell

is accompanied by a capillary vessel. The properties of cardiac muscle can be thought of as intermediate between those of skeletal muscle and smooth muscle: Cardiac muscle resembles skeletal muscle in being able to depolarize in about 2 ms to generate the large initial impulse of cardiac contraction, and it resembles smooth muscle in being able to maintain its contraction at slow heart rates for up to about 250 ms. It thus has a long refractory period. The duration of the phase of sustained depolarization decreases as the heart rate increases until at maximal heart rates sustained depolarization is virtually eliminated. Specialized muscle cells with a high degree of inherent rhythmicity are present in conduction tissue in the areas concerned with the generation and propagation of excitatory electrical activity.

The physiology of the heart involves molecular, electrical, mechanical, and metabolic factors.

1. THE MOLECULAR BASIS OF CARDIAC CONTRACTION

Mechanism of Contraction

The molecular basis of contraction of cardiac muscle is similar to that of other types of muscle throughout the animal kingdom. The muscle cell is composed of a number of muscle fibers that are in turn made up of muscle fibrils. The basic unit of the muscle fibril is the sarcomere, which is described above. The sarcomere consists of two main protein components—thick myosin filaments and thin actin filaments—that interdigitate with one another in parallel arrangement. A reaction between these two proteins at crossbridges generates mechanical force by mechanisms similar to those in skeletal muscle. The head of the myosin molecule is composed of heavy meromyosin, which can be split into two parts, whereas the tail consists of light meromyosin. Two separate proteins—tropomyosin and troponin—can be distinguished in association with the actin filament.

The sliding filament hypothesis, which is shown diagrammatically in Figure 1–15, is accepted as the most likely explanation of the phenomena associated with muscular contraction. The steps shown depict the influx of calcium as the action potential spreads via the transverse tubules. The actin filaments slide on the myosin filaments, and the Z lines move closer together. Calcium is then pumped back into the sarcoplasmic reticulum, and the muscle relaxes.

The interaction between the head of the myosin filament and the actin filament is depicted in Figure 1–16. In the relaxed state (Figure 1–16A), the myosin head is not attached to actin. When the muscle is activated by calcium ions interacting with troponin, adenosine triphosphate (ATP) is split, and the myosin head is thought to attach to a site on the actin (Figure 1–16B). The "power stroke" (Figure 1–16C) depends on the rate of switching between the two positions (B

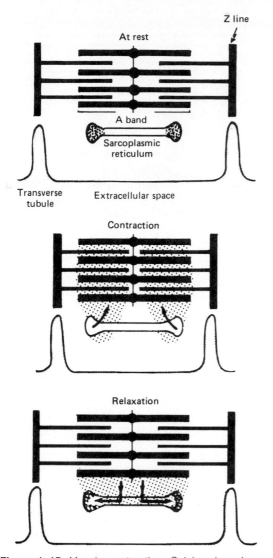

Figure 1–15. Muscle contraction. Calcium ions (represented by black dots) are normally stored in the cisterns of the sarcoplasmic reticulum. The action potential spreads via the transverse tubules and releases Ca²⁺. The actin filaments (thin lines) slide on the myosin filaments, and the Z lines move closer together. Ca²⁺ is then pumped into the sarcoplasmic reticulum and the muscle relaxes. (Modified and reproduced, with permission, from Layzer RB, Rowland LP: Cramps. N Engl J Med 1971;285:31.)

and C), which is thought to determine the force of contraction. With shortening, the cross-bridges move to the next attachment site. During isometric contraction, they continue to interact with the same site. Shortening occurs when the force of contraction exceeds the impedance to motion of the blood and continues after the period of active force generation.

2. ELECTRICAL ACTIVITY OF THE HEART

The Action Potential

The action potential is the electrical charge developed in a cell during activity. Cardiac muscle cells have the capability of generating and propagating electrical activity. All cardiac muscle cells show rhythmicity and fire when membrane potential reaches a certain threshold level. The threshold is reached earlier in nodal and conduction tissue.

At rest, the inside of the cardiac cell has a negative charge compared to the outside, so that the resting membrane potential is about –80 mV. Excitation produces a propagated charge that initiates contraction and causes the sequence of events shown as phases 0–4 in Figure 1–17. Depolarization (phase 0) is initially rapid and is constant in duration, lasting a few milliseconds. After an overshoot, there is a short period of repolarization (phase 1), followed by a plateau (phase 2) (corresponding to the ST segment on the ECG). Phase 3 of repolarization (corresponding to the T wave on the ECG) ends with the membrane potential returning to its resting value (phase 4). As in other excitable tissues, changes in K⁺ action concentration affect the duration of the potential, while changes in Na⁺ affect the intensity of the action potential. The initial rapid depolarization is due to a rapid increase in Na⁺ permeability, while the plateau phase is associated with a prolonged increase in Ca²⁺ permeability of the muscle cell membrane (Figure 1–18). Phase 3 is associated with a slow rise in K⁺ permeability. Repolarization time decreases as the heart rate increases, but the rapid depolarization phase remains constant in duration.

The Conduction System

Cells with increased rhythmicity that make up the specialized conduction tissue show an unstable membrane potential, with a gradual, slow depolarization toward the end of the cycle (phase 4). The rate of depolarization in phase 4 is more rapid in the sinoatrial node than in any other part of the conduction system (Figure 1–19). Thus, the threshold for firing is first reached at this site, and the electrical impulse that triggers the next impulse normally starts here.

Propagation of the Electrical Impulse

The cardiac cycle can be considered to start with sinoatrial firing, ie, the formation of an impulse in the sinoatrial node in the upper part of the right atrial muscle near the superior vena caval orifice (Figure 1–17). Mechanical events follow electrical events, and atrial contraction follows the P wave on the ECG and generates the atrial systolic activity (*a* wave). Activation proceeds in an orderly, repetitive fashion as the impulse spreads by several internodal pathways through both atria. When the impulse reaches the atrioventricular node, near the tricuspid valve, the

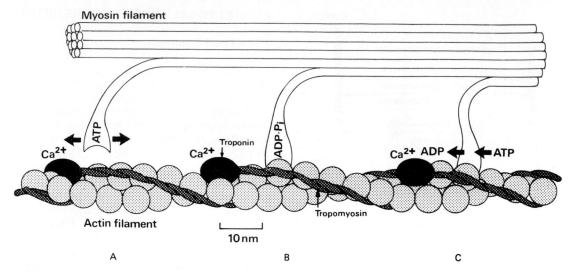

Figure 1–16. Diagram showing mechanism of contraction of striated muscle. For explanation, see text. (Courtesy of R Cooke.)

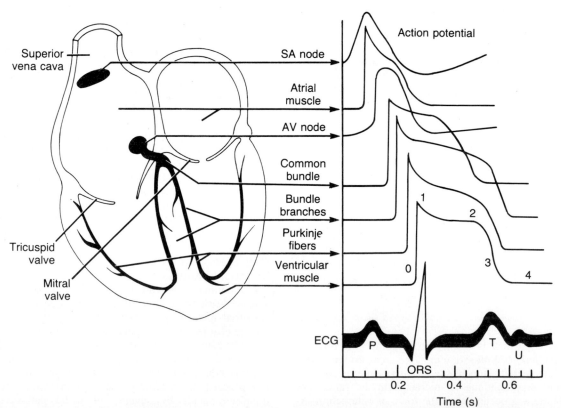

Figure 1–17. Schematic representation of the sequence of excitation in the heart. The relationship to the ECG is shown. (Modified and reproduced, with permission, from Noble MIM: *The Cardiac Cycle.* Blackwell, 1979.)

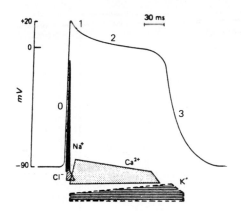

Figure 1–18. Phases of the action potential of a cardiac muscle fiber and the corresponding changes in ionic conductance across the muscle membrane. (0, depolarization; 1, rapid repolarization; 2, plateau phase; 3, late repolarization.) (Modified and reproduced, with permission, from Shepherd JT, Vanhoutte PM: *The Human Cardiovascular System: Facts and Concepts.* Raven Press, 1979.)

cells of the bundle of His are activated, and the impulse spreads via the Purkinje fibers to activate the ventricles, generating the Q, R, and S waves on the ECG. The impulse passes via the right and left bundle branches, the latter splitting into anterior and posterior divisions. Thus, there is a trifascicular ventricular conduction pathway through which the activating electrical impulse reaches each individual muscle cell at such a time that the result is an orderly sequence of ventricular contractions.

On the ECG, atrial and ventricular depolarization appear as P waves and QRS waves, respectively, and repolarization as ST–T waves. The shape and size of these waves do not vary with the force of cardiac contraction; in this respect, contracting cardiac muscle differs from contracting skeletal muscle, whose electromyographic tracings appear uncoordinated, asynchronous, and disorderly, varying as the force of contraction changes. In skeletal muscle, the number of fibers taking part in a contraction depends on the force required to carry out that task; recruitment of extra fibers causes increased electrical activity when the force of muscular contraction is increased. In contrast, all cardiac muscle cells contract with each heartbeat, and any increase in the force of contraction is achieved by modulating mechanisms that involve each individual muscle cell.

The configuration and duration of the QRS complex of the ECG are fixed. Neither changes in the force of contraction nor changes in heart rate affect the QRS complex. In contrast, the duration of repolarization (ST–T interval) decreases with increasing heart rate.

3. MECHANICAL EVENTS OF THE CARDIAC CYCLE

The mechanical events of the cardiac cycle are illustrated in Figure 1–20. The analysis presented here resembles the impulse theory of left ventricular action proposed by Rushmer (1964). It is based on studies in animals by Noble (1968) and in humans by Targett (1985), who used pulsed, range-gated Doppler ultrasound to study blood flow velocity in the aorta and systemic arterial system. This view of hemodynamics was further developed using a microcomputer model (McIlroy, 1986, 1988). It differs from conventional

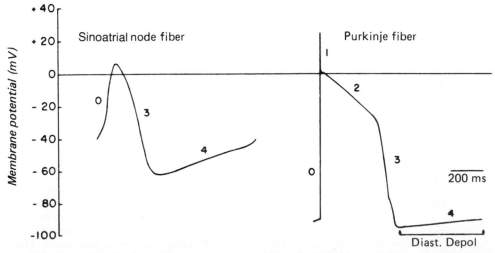

Figure 1–19. Action potential of sinoatrial node and Purkinje fibers. (0, rapid depolarization; 1, rapid repolarization; 2, plateau phase; 3, late repolarization; 4, slow diastolic depolarization.) (Modified and reproduced, with permission, from Levy MN, Vassalle M: *Excitation and Neural Control of the Heart.* American Physiological Society, 1982.)

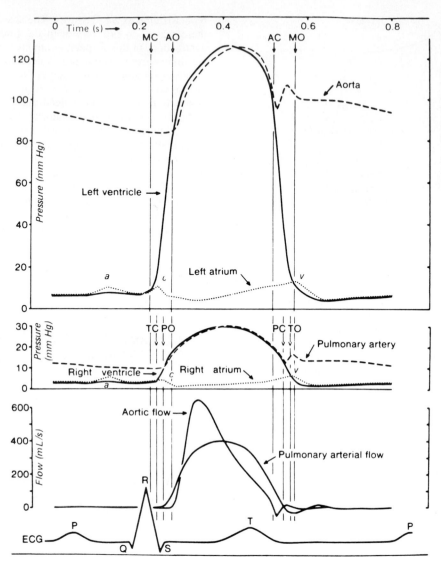

Figure 1–20. Diagram of events in the cardiac cycle. From top downward: pressure (mm Hg) in aorta, left ventricle, left atrium, pulmonary artery, right ventricle, right atrium; blood flow (mL/s) in ascending aorta and pulmonary artery; ECG. Abscissa, time in seconds. (Valvular opening and closing are indicated by AO and AC, respectively, for the aortic valve; MO and MC for the mitral valve; PO and PC for the pulmonary valve; TO and TC for the tricuspid valve.) (Modified and reproduced, with permission, from Milnor WR: The circulation. In: *Medical Physiology.* 2 vols. Mountcastle VB [editor]. Mosby, 1980.)

descriptions of the cardiac cycle in that ejection is divided into three phases: an early, active, impulse phase of constant duration; a later, more passive phase of sustained ventricular contraction that shortens with increasing heart rate; and a third phase of active ventricular relaxation.

Fourier Analysis

Most conventional studies of hemodynamics in the past have used Fourier analysis to describe the relationship of blood pressure to blood velocity in the frequency rather than in the time domain. Fourier analysis treats the pressure and velocity signals in the systemic circulation as a series of sine waves and uses complex algebra to calculate an impedance (effective resistance) in the circuit that varies with frequency (heart rate). Subjecting pressure and blood velocity signals to Fourier analysis does not contribute any new information. It merely expresses information in a different form—varying with the inverse of time (frequency) rather than with time itself. The form of analysis presented here differs in that it takes into account the specific form of the driving function generated by cardiac contraction and uses iterative computer analysis to generate pressure and blood velocity signals at different sites in the arterial system. The impedance to flow is treated as a factor that does not change with heart rate, and the cardiac cycle is treated as an event in which the overall patterns of ventricular pressure and blood flow vary with heart rate, while the power stroke of the ventricle remains of constant duration.

A. Phase 1—Early Active Ventricular Contraction: Contraction of the left ventricle generates an impulse of fixed duration that imparts a constant acceleration to the blood leaving the heart. The magnitude of the impulse varies with the force of cardiac contraction, but the time over which the force of contraction rises to its peak is constant. The contraction is initially isovolumetric (isovolumic), ie, there is an increase in tension and a change in shape, but no change in volume. Contraction follows the QRS complex of the ECG, and the force of contraction is determined during the development of the action potential (electrical activation) of ventricular muscle. Isovolumic contraction can be likened to the firing of a charge that expels a bullet from a gun. The velocity of the bullet depends on the force of the explosion, which occurs before the bullet starts to move. In cardiac contraction, the rate of motion of the blood depends on the force of the contraction, which is determined before ejection starts. The result of contraction depends on the time at which the valve opens and on the conditions encountered during ejection. The level of aortic pressure at the end of the previous diastole (afterload) is the prime determinant of the time of aortic valve opening and the most obvious measure of the load encountered by the ejecting ventricle.

Conditions distal to the aortic valve determine the time of onset of aortic blood flow. In one extreme case—aortic occlusion—maximal aortic pressure is developed, but there is no aortic flow. At the other extreme, when aortic resistance is zero, no pressure is developed, and flow is maximal. In practice, finite, submaximal pressure and aortic flow develop, and conditions in the aorta determine the time of aortic valve opening and the duration of aortic flow. If aortic diastolic pressure is low, eg, after an ectopic beat, flow starts early but acceleration is unchanged. If aortic diastolic pressure is high, flow starts later and systole is shortened.

The oxygen requirement for a contraction that is prevented from ejecting blood is the same as that for a contraction that ejects a normal volume of blood (Monroe, 1961). This indicates that ventricular contraction rather than aortic blood flow is the primary determinant of cardiac metabolism. During isovolumic contraction, the left ventricle changes shape as the pressure rises. The contraction is isovolumic, because blood is incompressible, but not isometric. Isovolumetric contraction ends when the aortic valve opens.

The impulse phase of ejection results from the force generated during phase 0 of the action potential. It lasts until the velocity of blood flow in the aorta reaches its peak after about 50 ms. During this time, the pressure in the ventricle exceeds that in the aorta (Figure 1–21) and the blood in the aorta gains momentum. The aortic blood velocity increases linearly with time during this phase (Figure 1–22). The magnitude of this constant acceleration of blood in cm/s^2 is the best and most convenient measure of the force of ventricular contraction.

The velocity profile across the aorta during the impulse phase of contraction is blunt, and all blood elements across the aorta move with the same velocity (Figure 1–23). This pattern results from the convective acceleration of blood passing from the relatively wide-open ventricle into the narrow confines of the aorta. This type of flow is known as "entry flow"

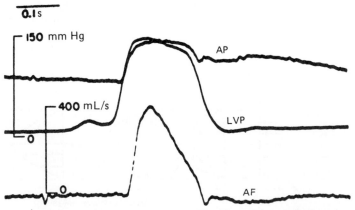

Figure 1–21. Aortic pressure (AP) and left ventricular pressure (LVP) recorded simultaneously, together with aortic flow (AF) via an electromagnetic flowmeter. LVP exceeds AP in the early part of systole. AP exceeds LVP in the latter part of systole. (Modified and reproduced, with permission of the American Heart Association, Inc., from Noble MIM: The contribution of blood momentum to left ventricular ejection in the dog. Circ Res 1968;23:663.)

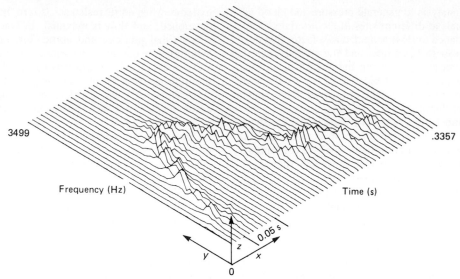

Figure 1–22. Three-dimensional plot of Doppler shift frequency (y axis), time (x axis), and intensity (z axis) during systole in the ascending aorta of a normal subject. The increase in frequency (proportionate to blood velocity) is close to linear in the first 0.05 s of ejection.

and tends with time to develop downstream into the classic Poiseuille flow, in which a parabolic velocity profile is seen, as in steady flow in rigid pipes.

B. Phase 2—Later Passive Sustained Contraction: The second phase of left ventricular contraction starts when the force of contraction reaches its peak and lasts until the ventricle starts to relax. This phase corresponds to the ST–T wave of the ECG. During this phase, the ventricle sustains its contraction but does not increase its force. The principal effect of the phase of sustained contraction is to keep a normal level of diastolic pressure in the arterial bed. The duration of the phase of sustained contraction varies with the heart rate, shortening with increase in rate, until this phase is virtually eliminated at maximal heart rate. The pressure in the ascending aorta in the phase of sustained contraction exceeds that in the ventricle (Figure 1–21), and momentum is responsible for blood flow.

Most of the decrease in left ventricular volume occurs in this phase, and the long axis of the ventricle shortens. The ventricle is supporting the aortic pressure at this time, maintaining rather than actively generating a force. The blood has enough momentum from the active phase to complete the normal ejection. The decrease in ventricular volume that occurs in this phase of the cardiac cycle is part of the mechanical work being done, but the oxygen consumption involved is negligible (Monroe, 1961). The duration of the second, more passive phase of ejection varies with the state of the arterial bed, as manifested by the aortic diastolic pressure. With vasodilation and a low aortic diastolic pressure, systole lasts longer and stroke volume is higher. With vasoconstriction and a high aortic diastolic pressure, systole is shorter and the stroke volume is lower. Thus, the overall stroke volume consists of a small, relatively constant volume that is actively ejected early in systole and a

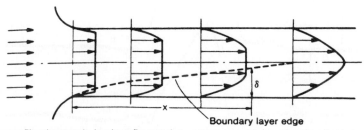

Figure 1–23. Velocity profiles in steady laminar flow at the entrance to a tube, showing the increasing width (δ) of the boundary layer, corresponding to the change from an initially flat profile in the entry region to a fully developed parabolic profile farther downstream. (Reproduced, with permission, from Caro CG et al: *The Mechanics of the Circulation.* Oxford Univ Press, 1978.)

larger, more variable volume that is passively ejected later in systole.

C. Phase 3—Active Ventricular Relaxation:
The phase of ventricular relaxation follows the phase of sustained contraction. The force and rate of ventricular relaxation are linked to the force of isovolumic contraction. Ventricular relaxation is an active process, and the pressure difference between the aorta and the ventricle increases as the ventricle relaxes. Relaxation does not change ventricular volume until ventricular pressure falls below atrial pressure and diastole starts. The pressure difference between the aorta and the left ventricle during this phase of the cardiac cycle provides the driving force for coronary flow and is greatest when relaxation is most rapid.

Ventricular Diastole

Ventricular diastole starts when aortic blood flow loses momentum, and the aortic valve closes. Ventricular filling starts when ventricular pressure falls below the level of atrial pressure. The velocity profiles at the mitral and tricuspid valves during diastole are normally blunt, as they are at the aortic and pulmonary valves early in systole. The acceleration of blood in response to active ventricular relaxation results in "entry flow" through the mitral and tricuspid valves. The diastolic pressure-volume relationship of the ventricle is not linear. The ventricle fills readily at first, with little increase in pressure. In the later phase of filling, pressure increases as the ventricle fills to near capacity, and atrial contraction boosts the ventricular pressure. The extent of filling plays an important role in determining the force of the next contraction, because the ventricular muscle responds to increased stretch with an increase in the force of its contraction.

Right Ventricular Dynamics

The right ventricle, like the left, imparts a constant acceleration to the blood ejected in early systole. The magnitude of the acceleration is less than that on the left side. The duration of the period of constant acceleration in the right ventricle is unaffected by heart rate, but it changes with age and with right ventricular hypertrophy. In newborn infants, in whom the right and left ventricles are similar in thickness, right ventricular events resemble those in the left ventricle. In adults, in whom the right ventricle is thin-walled and generates about tenfold lower pressures than the left, the constant acceleration phase lasts longer (100 ms or more). With increases in the force of cardiac contraction, right ventricular acceleration increases but the period over which acceleration remains constant does not change. With right ventricular hypertrophy, acceleration increases and acceleration time decreases. The velocity profile in the pulmonary artery is blunt, and, as in the left ventricle, ejection can be separated into an early active, impulse phase followed by sustained contraction and active relaxation.

Timing of Right & Left Ventricular Events

Right atrial systole precedes left atrial systole, but right ventricular contraction starts after left ventricular contraction. However, since pulmonary arterial pressure is lower than aortic pressure, right ventricular ejection starts before left ventricular ejection and lasts longer. Right-sided events are normally influenced by respiration, which alters venous return. During expiration, the aortic and pulmonary valves close at about the same time, but during inspiration, the aortic valve closes before the pulmonary valve. The later closure of the pulmonary valve is due to prolonged ejection of the increased venous return. When measured over time, the outputs of the two ventricles must be equal, but transient differences are seen with respiration.

Myocardial Work & Oxygen Consumption

The work of the heart—the integral of pressure with respect to volume—is not a true measure of the load on the heart. The heart uses more oxygen to produce a rise in pressure than to generate flow at a given level of pressure. This negates the usefulness of the measurement of cardiac work as an indication of cardiac performance (Table 1–1).

The most important indicator of the load on the heart is the oxygen consumption of the myocardium. This is difficult to measure, because it involves knowing both the total myocardial blood flow and the oxygen content difference between the blood in the aorta and that in the coronary venous drainage. Myocardial oxygen consumption is closely related to the "tension-time index"—the product of systolic pressure and heart rate. Myocardial oxygen consumption also depends on the mass of the heart muscle. Thus, when the heart hypertrophies in response to an increased mechanical load and the size of the individual muscle cells increases, oxygen consumption increases. Increased coronary flow is then required, and, if coronary flow cannot increase, myocardial ischemia will occur.

Myocardial Contractility

The term "contractility" is used somewhat loosely to denote the force of cardiac contraction. Measurement of the maximal rate of change of pressure during isovolumetric contraction (dP/dt) provides the best indicator of contractility. In order to make an

Table 1–1. The major determinants of myocardial oxygen demand.

- Left ventricular systolic pressure
- Left ventricular radius
- Heart rate
- Contractility
- Left Ventricular mass

A

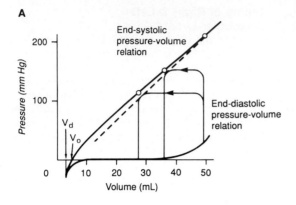

B

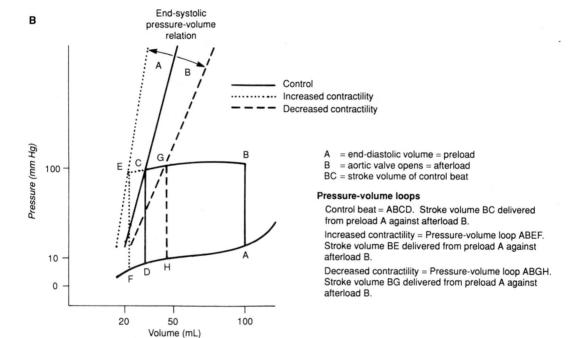

Figure 1–24. Schematic diagram of end-systolic pressure-volume relationship (ESPV) of the left ventricle. **A:** The three open circles on the solid line represent three isovolumetric peak pressures. The broken line represents the end-systolic pressure-volume relation from two ejecting beats. (Modified, redrawn, and reproduced, with permission of the American Heart Association, Inc., from Sagawa K: End-systolic pressure-volume relation of the ventricle: Definition, modifications and clinical use. [Editorial.] Circulation 1981;63:1223.) **B:** Note that with increased contractility the slope of the ESPV relationship becomes steeper and moves to the left. Therefore, from any given preload against any given afterload, a larger stroke volume is delivered. Since the end-systolic volume is decreased and there is no change in the end-diastolic volume, with a larger stroke volume the ejection fraction increases. With decreased contractility, the slope of the ESPV relationship becomes lower and moves to the right. Therefore, from any given preload against any given afterload, a smaller stroke volume is delivered. Since the end-systolic volume is increased and there is no change in the end-diastolic volume, with a smaller stroke volume the ejection fraction decreases.

accurate measurement of dP/dt, it is necessary to use a high-fidelity catheter-tip manometer, which detracts from the usefulness of the measurement. A more practical measure is the rate of change of aortic velocity (dv/dt) during the early, active phase of ventricular ejection. This can be measured noninvasively using an ultrasonic Doppler blood velocity meter.

Frank-Starling Law of the Heart

The Frank-Starling law states that the force of cardiac contraction increases in proportion to the degree of stretching of the cardiac muscle fibers during diastole. The law thus states a fundamental property of cardiac muscle that can be understood by reference to the sliding filament hypothesis described above. The same property is observed in skeletal muscle and reflects the length-tension relationships of muscle. The Frank-Starling law was established in animal studies in which a constant aortic pressure (afterload) and a constant contractility were maintained. In these circumstances, the heart behaves in a predictable manner, with stroke volume increasing with increased diastolic filling. Model studies (McIlroy, 1988) indicate that the Frank-Starling law does not apply when afterload or contractility are allowed to vary, as they inevitably do in clinical situations.

Sagawa has shown that when aortic resistance is fixed, the ratio of end-systolic volume to aortic pressure is constant (Figure 1–24A). When aortic resistance is high, stroke volume is small and aortic pressure increases. If aortic resistance is lowered, aortic pressure is reduced and stroke volume is larger. The position of the end-systolic pressure-volume line for a given ventricle is independent of preload and afterload. With an increase in contractility from a given end-diastolic volume against a given afterload, the ventricle will deliver a larger stroke volume. Therefore, the line will move to the left, and the slope will be steeper. With a decrease in contractility, the line will move to the right, and the slope will be decreased (Figure 1–24B). The end-systolic pressure-volume ratio has been proposed as a measure of contractility. Model studies indicate that the ratio changes with changes in afterload. The simpler measurement of the rate of change of aortic velocity (acceleration) is a more valid measure of "contractility."

Differences Between Skeletal & Cardiac Muscle

The action potentials in skeletal and cardiac muscle are different. There is a sharp initial spike of depolarization in both types of muscle, but repolarization is more rapid in skeletal muscle (being complete in 50 ms or less). In contrast, depolarization is sustained in cardiac muscle, lasting 350 ms or more at low heart rates. Its duration decreases with increasing heart rate as shown in Figure 1–25. With a rapid heart rate, depolarization lasts less than 200 ms, and the period of sustained ventricular contraction is correspon-

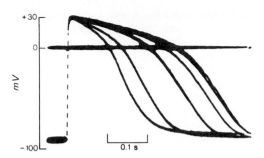

Figure 1–25. Superimposed action potential from a single fiber in an isolated ventricular trabecula obtained during an operation on a human heart. The record shows shortening of the action potential duration as stimulus frequency is raised in steps from 24/min to 162/min. The initial depolarization (phase 0) is unaffected by changes in rate. (Modified and reproduced, with permission of the American Heart Association, Inc., from Trautwein W et al: Electrophysiologic study of human heart muscle. Circ Res 1962;10:306.)

dingly reduced. The duration of the initial rapid depolarization (corresponding to the QRS complex of the ECG) is unaffected by changes in heart rate. This indicates that the duration of the initial phase of ventricular contraction is constant and uninfluenced by heart rate. In contrast, the ST–T interval, reflecting the period of sustained contraction, shortens as the heart rate increases.

A sustained contraction in skeletal muscle is achieved by repeated firing of different muscle fibers with relatively short refractory periods. In cardiac muscle, on the other hand, contraction involves the entire heart; and after the initial depolarization phase, tension is maintained for a much longer time. Because of these differences, calcium flux lasts much longer in cardiac muscle than in skeletal muscle, giving cardiac muscle a much longer refractory period. Calcium channel-blocking drugs, such as verapamil and nifedipine, are therefore more effective in cardiac than in skeletal muscle.

For years, studies of the length-tension relationships of skeletal muscle have been performed with use of supramaximal tetanizing stimuli for production of maximal muscular contraction. More recently, similar studies have been performed with ventricular papillary muscle. Because of its relatively long refractory period, cardiac muscle cannot be tetanized. Thus, although it can be shown that the force of contraction of isolated papillary muscle depends on the degree of stretch, both before (preload) and during the shortening (afterload), the quantitative results, especially the extrapolated values for the maximal speed of contraction during minimal loading, are open to question.

The length-tension relationships of cardiac muscle have been thought to depend on variations in the number of cross-bridges formed between the actin and myosin filaments at any given muscle length. Recent studies indicate that changes in permeability of the sarcoplasmic reticulum and cell membranes to calcium ions play a major part in determining the length-tension relationships in cardiac muscle. It appears that increasing the stretch of the muscle permits release of more calcium and that this, rather than changes in the amount of overlap of actin and myosin filaments, is responsible for the increased force of cardiac contraction (Sugi, 1979).

Length-Tension Relationships & Ventricular Pressure

The length-tension relationships of the individual sarcomeres must be viewed in light of the behavior of the whole heart. Tension must be converted into pressure and length into volume. The relationship between length, tension, and radius for a thin-walled, curved surface is stated by the law of Laplace. For a cylinder or a cone, the equation is as follows:

$$\text{Pressure} = 2 \times \frac{\text{Tension}}{\text{Radius}}$$

If the ventricle increases in size, the wall stress associated with a given pressure increases. These physical principles indicate that there is more mechanical advantage in applying a force to contract a small than a large ventricle. Thus, the larger and more dilated the ventricle, the larger is its radius and the greater the wall stress for a given ventricular pressure. Wall stress is also inversely related to wall thickness. Thus, a thinner ventricle is exposed to greater stress than a thicker one.

The second conversion, from a change in length of the individual sarcomere to a change in volume of the whole ventricle, involves assumptions about the shape of the ventricle. It is relatively easy to contrast two of the simple shapes that might be envisaged for the left ventricle, a sphere versus a cone. For a sphere in which volume (v) = $4/3 \ \pi r^3$, the rate of change of volume (dv/dt) would be $4\pi r^2$ and the acceleration would be $8\pi r$. In contrast, for a cone with radial shortening, volume = $\pi r^2 h$; the rate of change of volume is $\pi r h$; and the acceleration is πh. In a sphere, acceleration should be proportionate to the radius, whereas in a cone, acceleration should be constant—a finding compatible with the pattern of blood flow in the early active phase of ventricular ejection. According to this oversimplified analysis, the left ventricle acts in the same manner (linear circumferential shortening) as would a conical chamber, so blood is ejected with a constant acceleration during early systole.

Excitation-Contraction Coupling

Changes in force—not duration—modulate the active phase of cardiac contraction by an electrochemical interaction called excitation-contraction coupling.

In contrast to skeletal muscle, in which extra force is provided by recruitment of extra fibers, cardiac muscle relies on a modulating mechanism that increases the force generated by each individual fiber. It is best thought of as an increase in the rate of cross-bridge attachment and detachment at any given sarcomere length. Tropomyosin and troponin, the two cardiac muscle proteins that are found in association with the thin actin filament, play a regulatory role in actin-myosin interaction.

The increased force generation that occurs with enhanced excitation-contraction coupling is modulated by cyclic adenosine monophosphate (cyclic AMP, or cAMP). cAMP activates a protein kinase that increases the influx of calcium ions into the cytosol, and this increases the force of contraction. The activity of cAMP is in turn controlled by the sympathetic nervous system via beta receptors in the ventricle. Drugs such as isoproterenol and norepinephrine increase the force of cardiac contraction via this mechanism, as do glucagon, xanthines, and newer drugs such as amrinone and milrinone, which inhibit the breakdown of cAMP.

During maximal exercise, enhanced sympathetic nervous stimulation is both inotropic and chronotropic. Inotropic stimulation acts via changes in calcium flux in the transverse tubules and sarcoplasmic reticulum in a manner similar to that of the basic Frank-Starling mechanism; the two mechanisms are so closely linked that it is difficult to determine the effects of either alone during physiologic experiments.

Digitalis is thought to act via the excitation-contraction coupling mechanism. The drug has been shown to have no effect on cardiac output in persons with normal cardiac function, because the normal end-systolic volume is so close to the minimal end-systolic volume described by Sagawa that no increase in stroke volume can occur, although the rate of change of left ventricular pressure increases. In patients with diseased hearts in which end-systolic volume is abnormally large, the increased force of cardiac contraction resulting from digitalis therapy can increase stroke volume and improve cardiac output.

Another factor thought by some to increase the force of cardiac contraction is tachycardia. However, recent work has shown that oxygen consumption per beat is not increased when the heart rate is increased and that "contractility" is not enhanced unless there is associated inotropic stimulation.

Thyroid hormone also increases the force of cardiac contraction. The recent work of Morkin indicates that the synthesis of new isoenzymes of myosin with high ATPase activity is responsible for this effect.

Effect of Control Mechanisms

The circulatory control mechanisms respond to any change in cardiac output by the time approximately two heartbeats have occurred and act to modify cardiac performance and change the hemodynamic state.

It is thus difficult to determine the cause of changes in cardiac output corresponding with particular beats, and clear relationships between cardiac filling and stroke volume, which can be seen in isolated heart preparations with a constant afterload, tend to be masked in patients. It is possible, however, to recognize the direction of changes, and if an intervention causes an increase in cardiac output with a decrease in filling pressure, this can be seen to be beneficial, whether it results from the Frank-Starling mechanism, enhanced excitation-contraction coupling, or both.

4. METABOLIC BASIS OF CARDIAC CONTRACTION

The energy required for cardiac contraction is derived from the breakdown of high-energy phosphate compounds and is predominantly aerobic. The heart contains many mitochondria and is rich in myoglobin, a red pigment that releases oxygen at low oxygen tensions. Anaerobic myocardial metabolism can support cardiac contraction for only a short time, and an adequate supply of oxygenated blood is a prerequisite for normal contraction. The myocardium extracts the maximum amount of oxygen normally, and the coronary venous blood has the lowest oxygen content of any venous blood in the body. Therefore, any increase in myocardial oxygen demand must be met by an increase in myocardial blood flow. The heart can use virtually any substrate. Glucose, lactate, and free fatty acid can all act as fuel for cardiac metabolism. In the fasting state, free fatty acids provide the energy for contraction. Myocardial metabolism is increased when cardiac contraction is augmented via enhanced excitation-contraction coupling through mechanisms that increase supply of substrate.

FUNCTIONAL HEMODYNAMIC FACTORS & CARDIAC ANATOMY

The basic molecular mechanisms of cardiac muscle contraction must be viewed against the background of the functional anatomy of the heart as it beats within the chest. The change in shape of the heart during each cycle is complex, and using a sphere, cone, or ellipse to approximate the main bulk of the left ventricle is clearly an oversimplification, as is the description of its contraction by a change of one or two radii of curvature. Although an adequate description of the complex movements of the contracting left ventricle is not yet possible, a few important points can be made.

Change of Left Ventricular Axis With Contraction

The apex of the left ventricle remains relatively fixed during contraction, as does the ventricular septum. As shown in Figure 1–26, the left and posterior walls of the left ventricle thicken and move anteriorly and to the right during systole. The main axis of the ventricular cavity, which lies in a direct line below the mitral valve during diastolic filling, shifts in an anterior direction during systole, bringing its long axis to a position during ejection in which the ventricular cavity points directly into the ascending aorta.

Descent of the Base of the Heart

The base of the left ventricle, formed by the mitral and aortic valve rings, moves downward toward the apex of the heart during systole, as shown in Figure 1–27. The force of cardiac contraction expelling blood into the aorta produces an equal and opposite recoil that moves the heart in a caudad direction. These changes, which occur with ventricular filling and emptying, are preceded by isovolumetric relaxation and contraction phases, in which changes in

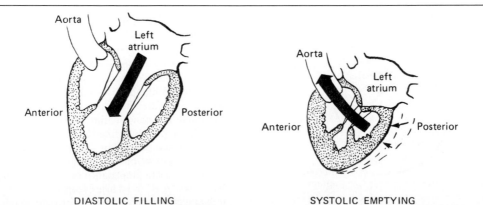

DIASTOLIC FILLING   SYSTOLIC EMPTYING

Figure 1–26. Diagram of the heart in the left anterior oblique view showing change in axis of the left ventricle between diastolic filling and systolic emptying.

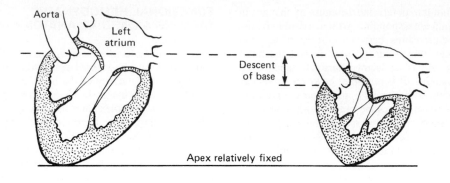

Figure 1–27. Diagram of the heart in the left anterior oblique view showing systolic descent of the base of the heart.

ventricular shape occur without any change in volume.

Right Ventricular Shape

The shape of the adult right ventricle is markedly different from that of the left. As shown in Figure 1–28, it has a narrow crescent-shaped cavity that lies on the anterior right-hand surface of the ventricular septum. The thin-walled right ventricle is more compliant and has a lower resting end-diastolic pressure than the left. Right ventricular volume is more likely to change because of changes in intrapericardial and intrathoracic pressure than is left ventricular volume.

Atrial Anatomy

The atrial musculature is even thinner than that of the right ventricle, and the atria are thus more compliant. The atrial musculature is thickest in the atrial appendages, which lie in the most anterior parts of the atria. The more posterior parts of the atria, around the sites of entry of the venae cavae, coronary sinus, and pulmonary veins, contain the least amount of cardiac muscle and resemble veins in structure. Since there

are no valves in the great veins on either side of the heart, the venae cavae on the right and the pulmonary veins on the left serve as reservoirs of blood for the ventricles. During ventricular diastole, as the base of the heart moves cephalad, the blood in the atria is transferred to the ventricles by the movement of the heart around it as well as by its own motion.

The atria are smaller than the ventricles. They act not only as reservoirs, filling during ventricular systole, but also as conduits during ventricular diastole, when venous blood flows directly through the atria to fill the ventricles.

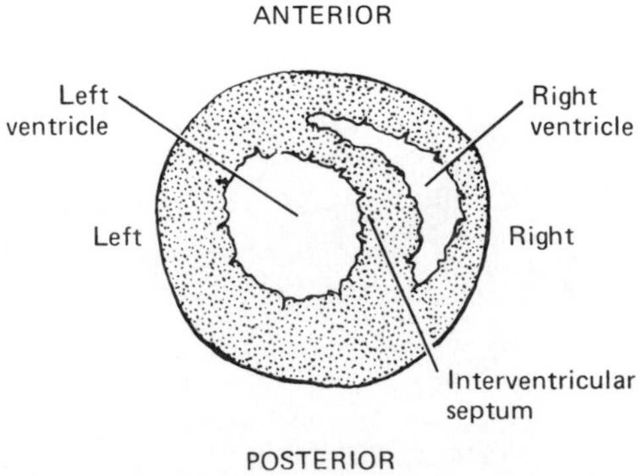

Ventricular Enlargement

When either ventricle enlarges, its cavity becomes more spherical. The septum tends to bulge at the expense of the smaller ventricle. Both ventricles eject about the same proportion of their contents with each systole. Approximately two-thirds of the end-diastolic volume of about 100 mL • m^{-2} is delivered per beat, but this figure varies with cardiac filling (preload) and aortic diastolic pressure (afterload) and is influenced by postural changes in venous return.

Hemodynamics of the Aorta & Arterial Circulation

A. Physical Principles: The pulsatile left ventricular ejection generates waves of pressure and blood velocity in the aorta and the systemic arteries. The aorta and systemic arteries offer a special form of resistance to blood flow—characteristic impedance—whose units are the same as those of conventional frictional resistance (mm Hg/cm/s). Characteristic impedance (Zo) is defined as the square root of inductance (inertia) divided by capacitance (compliance) of a given segment of the circulation.

Characteristic impedance obeys Ohm's law and behaves like "real" resistance except that its components—inductance and capacitance—involve no inherent loss of energy. If the characteristic impedance is matched in the different segments and at branch points in

Figure 1–28. Cross section of the heart showing relative positions of the left and right ventricles.

the circulation, the waves of pressure and blood velocity pass in a delayed but undistorted manner to the periphery.

The pressure and blood velocity waves reach the peripheral arteries after a delay that depends on the physical properties of the arterial tree. This delay is equal to the square root of the product of the inductance (inertia) and capacitance (compliance) of a given segment of the circulation. The waves travel at speeds of 5–10 m/s, taking about 0.15 s to reach the fingers and 0.25 s to reach the toes. In contrast, red blood cells travel in the resting subject at about 15 cm/s and take about 5 seconds to reach the fingers and 10 seconds to reach the toes.

The physical properties of the arterial bed are not homogeneous. The dilation at the root of the aorta, formed by the sinuses of Valsalva, offers a low-output resistance to the arterial bed that is normally adjusted to provide a critically damped input impedance. The central vessels are more compliant and contain more blood than the peripheral arteries. They thus offer more inertance and introduce more delay in the transmission of pressure and blood velocity waves. The peripheral vessels are less compliant and contain less blood. They thus offer less inertance and transmit pressure and blood velocity waves more rapidly. With the exception of the resistance at the aortic valve and the peripheral arteriolar resistance (Zt), the normal arterial bed offers no significant resistance to pressure and blood velocity waves. Since the inertial and compliant elements are conservative (involve no loss of energy), the normal arterial bed is effectively "lossless."

B. Wave Transmission and Reflection: The normal arterial bed should be thought of as consisting of a complex set of branching elements with characteristic impedances matched in series along the line of the vessel and in parallel at branches, according to Ohm's law. Impedance matching permits the pressure and blood velocity waves generated by the impulse phase of ventricular ejection to pass undistorted through the arterial bed without generating any reflections until they reach the arterioles.

When the pressure and blood velocity waves reach the peripheral arterioles, they encounter peripheral (terminal) resistance. If peripheral resistance is greater than the characteristic impedance of the line, as it normally is at rest, reflected waves are generated that pass back up the arteries, amplifying the pressure waves and attenuating the forward-traveling blood velocity waves. If the peripheral resistance is lower than the characteristic impedance of the line, the reflected waves attenuate the pressure waves and amplify the blood velocity waves.

The reflection coefficient ($Zt - Zc \div Zt + Zo$) gives a measure of the magnitude of the effects of reflections. The resting value of about 0.5 results from a terminal resistance three times the characteristic impedance. Wave reflections impair the transfer of power from the heart to the periphery. The efficiency of power transfer varies as the square of the reflection coefficient. Thus, both positive and negative reflection coefficients impair power transfer, and efficiency increases markedly as the absolute value of the reflection coefficient is reduced.

The high resting reflection coefficient serves to maintain a high level of aortic diastolic pressure. The magnitude of the local reflection coefficient plays an important role in determining the pressure and blood velocity in a given branch. Increases in local metabolic needs lead to vasodilation and a fall in reflection coefficient, which in turn increases flow to that area.

C. Secondary Reflections: One of the consequences of matching impedances to forward flow at arterial branch points is the generation of secondary reflections of retrograde-traveling pressure and flow waves. If the impedance to forward flow is matched at a branch point, the impedance must inevitably be mismatched for reflected waves traveling back up the vessel. This mismatch of the impedance to retrograde waves generates secondarily reflected waves that travel back toward the periphery, giving secondary and sometimes tertiary surges of pressure and velocity in peripheral vessels.

D. Optimal Power Transfer at Maximal Exercise: The most extreme and widespread vasodilation is that seen during maximal aerobic exercise. At the heart rate reached during maximal exercise, the level of peripheral resistance needed to maintain a normal diastolic arterial pressure falls to a level about equal to that of the characteristic impedance of the arterial bed. In this case, the impedance of the line comes close to matching that of the periphery, and virtually no reflections occur. An arterial bed in which the terminal impedance is matched to the characteristic impedance of the line transmits power in an optimal manner. Thus, while reflections result in submaximal power transfer at low heart rates at rest, power transfer becomes closer and closer to optimal as the level of exercise and the heart rate increase.

E. Interaction Between the Heart and the Periphery: An important consequence of the organization of the systemic arterial bed is isolation of the heart from the effects of its own contraction. The pressure and blood velocity waves generated by ventricular contraction normally take at least 0.2 s to travel to and return from the closest important reflection sites in the right arm and head. Matching impedance to forward flow permits the waves of pressure and blood velocity to pass in an undistorted manner for this period of time. The reflected waves, seen under resting conditions, returning to the central circulation, arrive at the aortic valve after the active, impulse phase of ejection is over. At this, time the heart is sustaining its contraction and not generating an increase in pressure. Thus, the heart is effectively isolated from the effects of reflections during its power stroke. With exercise and increases in heart rate, the peripheral resistance falls until, in severe exercise, it comes close to matching the characteristic impedance of the line and the circulation is maximally efficient.

F. Inotropic Stimuli: Inotropic stimuli increase the magnitude of the force generated by cardiac contraction without changing the time for which the force is applied. Model studies show that inotropic increase causes a proportionate increase in the pressure and flow at all points in the arterial system and does not alter the patterns of pressure and flow at any site. Thus, when the force of contraction increases by 50%, the pressure and flow at every point in each branch likewise increase by 50%. This means that the relative amounts of blood flow to different parts of the body, determined by the control mechanisms, are uninfluenced by inotropic change. Thus, the periphery is isolated from the effects of the pump, and changes in the force of cardiac contraction have an equal effect on distribution of pressure and flow to all parts of the periphery.

G. Overall Organization: This analysis of the hemodynamics of the heart and systemic arterial tree indicates that the mammalian systemic circulation is remarkably well adapted to its distributive function. The heart generates the force needed to propel the blood during a short power stroke of constant duration. The heart is effectively isolated from the effects of reflected waves of pressure and flow that result from its contraction. The ventricle has completed its power stroke by the time reflections return to the central circulation. The reflections that maintain aortic diastolic pressure at rest decrease with increasing heart rate until, under the stress of maximal exercise, the system transmits the force generated by the heart with maximal efficiency. Control of local blood flow is vested in local mechanisms, and the effects of inotropic agents are proportionately applied to all parts of the arterial tree. Interaction between the heart and the periphery sustains aortic diastolic pressure, and the system is highly sensitive to changes in afterload.

Right-Sided Hemodynamics

Contraction of the right ventricle, like that of the left, generates an impulse that sends waves of pressure and blood flow through the pulmonary arterial bed. Although the physical properties of the main pulmonary artery and its branches differ from those of the aorta, physiologic responses to the pressure and blood velocity waves are analogous. The compliance of the pulmonary artery is higher than that of the aorta, but the inertia of the mass of the blood is comparable. As a result, the impedance is lower but wave transmission is slower than in the aorta. Matching of the impedance at branch points permits the transmission of pressure and blood flow waves in an undistorted form during the active phase of right ventricular ejection. Because of the lower impedance, right ventricular ejection lasts longer than left, and acceler-

ation is lower. The lower impedance and lower peripheral resistance result in reflected waves that are similar to those in the systemic circulation. Pulmonary vascular resistance falls with exercise, and power is transferred to the pulmonary capillary bed in the same highly efficient manner during maximal stress as in the systemic circulation. The frictional resistance in the pulmonary arterial tree, while similar to that in the systemic circulation, constitutes a higher proportion of the overall impedance and so is not negligible. Model studies indicate that its value is about one-fourth the overall impedance at rest.

The effects of reflections are small in the normal adult pulmonary circulation. This is partly due to the low impedance and consequent low diastolic pressure. It is also due to the repeated branching pattern that sends reflected waves back to the periphery rather than allowing them to pass in a retrograde manner toward the heart.

CORONARY CIRCULATION

Coronary blood flow is an essential determinant of myocardial performance. It is precisely adjusted to the needs of myocardial metabolism by multiple mechanisms. Flow takes place at different times in the cardiac cycle in different parts of the coronary circulation. It is important to distinguish the timing of flow in the large coronary arteries that run on the surface of the heart from timing in the intramyocardial vessels and the coronary venous drainage.

Large Coronary Arteries

The coronary arteries that run in the atrioventricular grooves and on the surface of the heart are exposed to the relatively low intrapericardial pressure and act as storage vessels during ventricular systole. The high intramyocardial pressure during ventricular contraction prevents the flow of blood into the heart muscle during systole. Aortic pressure pumps blood into the relatively compliant superficial vessels during systole, and their elastic recoil provides a force to enhance perfusion of the myocardium during diastole. The magnitude of this flow into superficial vessels is greater in the distribution of the right coronary artery, because the pressure difference between the aorta and right ventricle is greater than that between the aorta and left ventricle and because the right coronary artery is usually larger than the left.

Intracardiac Coronary Vessels

The intramyocardial vessels are exposed to the force generated by cardiac contraction in a graded fashion, mostly in the subendocardial region and decreasingly toward the epicardial regions. The vessels are effectively collapsed during systole; as a result, virtually all myocardial perfusion (as opposed to coronary blood flow) occurs in diastole. Active ventriculai ielaxation at the start of diastole generates a pressure difference between the aorta and the intra-myocardial vessels that provides for rapid early diastolic flow to the myocardium. The magnitude of this pressure difference varies with the rate of ventricular relaxation which is, in turn, linked to the force of cardiac contraction. Thus, myocardial perfusion is linked to cardiac contractility.

Coronary Venous System

Coronary venous drainage is mainly via the coronary sinus to the right atrium; a small proportion of flow returns in thebesian veins directly to the atria. Because the coronary venous system contains no valves, blood is forced out of the intramyocardial vessels into the veins during systole. During diastole, it is possible for blood in the coronary venous system to flow back into the myocardium. The subendocardial veins are subject to compression by the left ventricular diastolic pressure, thus causing a resistance to venous flow in diastole. Since the left ventricular filling pressure is higher than the right, a "waterfall effect" is created such that the venous flow is not affected by changes in the right-sided diastolic pressure until it rises above the left-sided diastolic pressure. Attempts have recently been made to enhance retrograde flow by distending a balloon in the coronary sinus in time with diastole and pumping blood under pressure into the coronary sinus. This increases blood flow to the capillary bed and sustains myocardial oxygen supply in the presence of coronary artery obstruction. The efficacy of this has not been established.

Tissue Pressure

Coronary flow is regulated not by coronary venous pressure but by a higher level of pressure, presumably determined by extravascular tissue forces at the capillary level. The tissue pressure in the myocardium is an important factor modifying local blood flow. There is thus a gradient of vulnerability between the different layers of the myocardium: the subendocardial regions are more susceptible to ischemia than the superficial ones. When the coronary circulation is uniformly affected—for example, in aortic valve disease, severe anemia, rapid arrhythmias, shock, or acute hypoxia—diffuse subendocardial ischemia (with widespread ST-T changes on the ECG) is more likely to be found than transmural myocardial infarction (manifested by deep Q waves).

Blood Velocity Patterns

The pattern of blood velocity in the large coronary arteries varies with the distance from the aorta. Close to their origin, the coronary vessels show velocity patterns like those in the aorta. The farther down the vessels the measurements are made, the smaller the systolic component of flow and the larger the diastolic component. The velocity profile in the distal

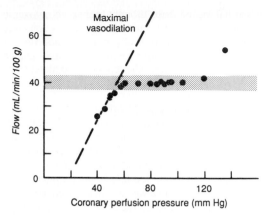

Figure 1–29. Pressure-flow relationships in the coronary circulation during maximal coronary dilation (broken line) and during normal coronary tone (solid circles). When normal tone is present, coronary flow remains relatively constant over a wide range of perfusion pressures. During maximal coronary dilation there is a steep relationship between coronary pressure and flow. (Modified and reproduced,with permission, from Marcus ML: *Coronary Circulation in Health and Disease.* McGraw-Hill, 1983.)

coronary arteries is parabolic, and velocity decreases nearly linearly during diastole. At a normal heart rate, peak velocity decreases from about 70 cm•s^{-1} at the start of diastole to 30 cm•s$^{-}_{1}$ at the end of diastole.

Coronary Flow Reserve

The velocity of diastolic blood flow in the large coronary arteries varies with the degree of tone in the intramyocardial vessels (Figure 1–29). Injection of vasodilator substances produces an increase in flow velocity that varies with the ability of the myocardial vessels to dilate. The injection of radiopaque contrast material to outline the coronary vessels at angiography produces a significant but submaximal dilation. Papaverine has been shown to be the most effective vasodilator drug in humans. In a dose of 12 mg for the left coronary artery and 8 mg for the right, it can be used to indicate how close to fully dilated a given coronary bed is at any time. The difference between the coronary blood flow at rest and after maximal vasodilation is known as the coronary flow reserve.

Effect of Aortic Pressure

The early diastolic pressure difference between the aorta and the relaxing left ventricle is a major factor in coronary perfusion, and myocardial ischemia may occur in any situation in which aortic diastolic pressure is reduced, especially in older patients with coronary atherosclerosis.

Autoregulation

Autoregulation is important in maintaining coronary flow, which tends to be kept constant by inherent myocardial mechanisms thought to involve myogenic responses in arteriolar smooth muscle. Autonomic nervous system regulation of coronary blood flow is not thought to be a major factor, but it may induce coronary arterial spasm (also called Prinzmetal's angina; see Chapter 8).

Local Chemical Regulation

Local chemical regulation via vasodilator substances is important, and adenosine, formed by the breakdown of adenosine phosphate compounds, has been shown to play an important role. This substance is so rapidly built back into its parent compounds that it persists in the tissues for less than 1 second.

The available evidence indicates that adenosine is by no means the only metabolic product capable of causing coronary vasodilation. Other vasodilating substances are adenine and guanine nucleotides, lactic acid, and prostaglandins. Hypoxia and increased CO_2, H^+, and K^+ also cause vasodilation.

Reactive Hyperemia

Reactive hyperemia of the type seen in all metabolizing tissues is readily produced in the heart. Interruptions of coronary blood flow, lasting for as short a time as 1 second, are followed by large increases in flow that more than compensate for the deficiency resulting from the original ischemia. Reactive hyperemia provides a mechanism for maintaining coronary flow in response to local needs and occurs so rapidly that it is difficult to see how neural or humoral factors can be responsible. It seems likely that local myogenic responses mediate this form of control. Thus, any fall in perfusion pressure reduces vascular tone and causes vasodilation, while a rise in perfusion pressure distends the vessel and evokes a vasoconstrictor response.

Anastomotic Vessels

Although the coronary arteries and arterioles anastomose freely with one another, in humans with unobstructed vessels these anastomoses are so small that in effect the coronary arteries act as end-arteries. With sudden occlusion, intense ischemia occurs, and infarction of the entire territory supplied by that artery occurs. With gradual obstruction—by atherosclerosis, for example—these anastomotic connections or collateral vessels enlarge and can carry flow sufficient to supply myocardial oxygen demand without ischemia. In this circumstance, it is possible for more than one major coronary vessel to be occluded without resulting in an infarct. The rate of development of the lesions seems to be an important variable; if they develop slowly, major lesions may persist for years before symptoms occur.

CONTROL OF THE CIRCULATION

The circulatory system is made up of a systemic circuit (Figure 1–30) composed of multiple (parallel)

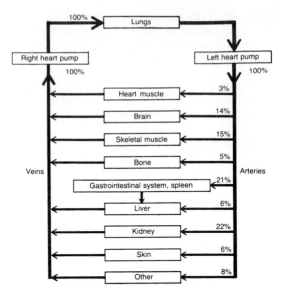

Figure 1–30. Diagram of the circulation showing percentages of cardiac output distributed to different organ systems. (Reproduced, with permission, from Heller LJ, Mohrman DE: *Cardiovascular Physiology.* McGraw-Hill, 1981.)

pathways, each with its own local control mechanisms, plus a pulmonary circulation that is essentially passive in the adult and almost entirely concerned with gas exchange in the lungs. The importance of each parallel pathway is determined by how long life can be maintained in a given tissue when its circulation is cut off. In descending order of vital importance, these circuits are the cerebral, coronary, renal, visceral, muscular, skin, and reproductive organ circulations.

Dominance of the Cerebral Circulation

Cerebral perfusion depends chiefly on the arterial blood pressure, and control of the circulation as a whole can be thought of as aimed primarily at providing the constant arterial pressure needed to maintain cerebral perfusion. The rigid cranium maintains perfusion of the brain. The pull of gravity on the flow of blood in the jugular veins performs a syphoning action that would not take place if the intracranial veins were not prevented from collapsing by the rigidity of the skull and the constancy of the volume of tissue within it.

Controlled Variables: Aortic Pressure & Circulating Blood Volume

The two main controlled variables in the circulatory system are the central aortic pressure and the circulating blood volume. The servomechanisms that control aortic pressure are reasonably well understood, and the mechanisms by which the blood volume is kept constant are becoming clearer. They involve atrial natriuretic factor (ANF), renin, angiotensin, aldosterone, vasopressin, and osmolality as well as purely physical factors.

Control of Arterial Pressure

A. Baroreceptor Mechanisms: Arterial pressure is kept constant by the baroreceptor servomechanism, which has multiple afferent sensory pathways and several efferent motor pathways. Arterial pressure is sensed via stretch receptors in the carotid sinuses near the bifurcations of the common carotid arteries in the neck (Figure 1–31) and by another set of stretch receptors in the arch of the aorta. Impulses from these receptors pass up the glossopharyngeal nerves to the medulla and provide a frequency-modulated input proportionate to the stretch of the vessel walls. Efferent impulses pass from the medullary centers via the vagus nerves to the sinoatrial (right vagus) and atrioventricular (left vagus) nodes. These impulses influence heart rate and modify the force of atrial contraction by inhibition of sympathetic activity. Other impulses pass via the sympathetic nerves to modify the level of arteriolar smooth muscle contraction in the limbs and in the visceral circulation via the thoracolumbar sympathetic outflow. The net effect of the system is to keep the mean arterial pressure almost constant. A rise in arterial pressure results in bradycardia, reduced force of atrial contraction, and release of peripheral arteriolar constriction. The active phase of the mechanism, which increases the frequency of impulses in the afferent nerves, is a rise in arterial pressure, and the response to a fall in pressure involves the inhibition of the reflex.

B. Speed of Response: The baroreceptor reflex represents a classic example of a short-term neural control mechanism. Heart rate changes take place within 1–2 seconds, whereas changes in vasomotor control take 5 or 6 seconds to act. Baroreceptor mechanisms are most readily brought into operation by changes in posture and also play a part in the increase in cardiac output that occurs in response to the start of exercise. They adapt to slow, prolonged changes in arterial pressure, and in systemic hypertension an abnormal level of blood pressure is kept constant on a short-term basis just as effectively as a normal level.

C. Effects of Disease: Normal baroreceptor function is impaired in disease affecting the autonomic nervous system; in conditions in which sensory input to the reflex is reduced, as in the prolonged weightlessness of space flight; and after the administration of sympatholytic drugs.

D. Baroreceptor Brake-Sympathetic Nervous System Accelerator: The baroreceptor reflex is best thought of as a brake inhibiting the heart through the action of the vagus nerves and protecting the cerebral circulation from excessive increases in perfusion pressure. Conversely, the sympathetic nervous system is thought of as an accelerator that reciprocally comes into play when the baroreceptor brake is removed. The vagally mediated aspects of the baroreceptor reflex have no direct action on the force of ventricular contraction, and ventricular function plays no direct part in the normal operation of the reflex. If arterial pressure falls because of impaired cardiac function, the reflex will come into play to increase heart rate and constrict the arterial bed even at the expense of further decreasing cardiac function. This type of response is seen after myocardial infarction.

E. Effects of Sympathetic Nervous System on Cardiac Contraction: The force of cardiac contraction is influenced by the sympathetic nerves to the heart. Short-term stimulation of cardiac action occurs reflexly in response to arousal, alarm, excitement, anticipation of exercise, and pain. Any sudden stimulus—usually auditory, visual, or tactile—can cause a sudden increase in cardiac output within a second or less. The subsequent changes in cardiac output depend on whether a true or a false alarm has sounded and are influenced by baroreceptor responses. The circulatory response to isometric exercise is similar to that of arousal. Active muscular contraction causes an increase in heart rate and a disproportionate increase in arterial pressure. Thus, straining, as in lifting heavy objects, causes an in-

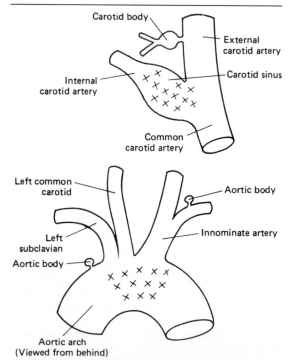

Figure 1–31. Baroreceptor areas in the carotid sinus and aortic arch. (Courtesy of JH Comroe Jr. Reproduced, with permission, from Ganong WF: *Review of Medical Physiology,* 14th ed. Appleton & Lange, 1989.)

crease in blood pressure; and since the response is not directly related to the stimulus, even simple clenching of a fist can cause significant hypertension. The heart also responds to traumatic events such as interference with its blood supply, sudden and intolerable increases in arterial pressure, or obstruction to its output. Such stimuli are thought to affect nonmedullated afferent fibers from endings in the coronary vessels and to result in poorly localized visceral sensations resembling angina pectoris and reflex bradycardia mediated through the vagus nerves, leading to hypotension.

F. Bezold Reflex: The Bezold reflex, discovered in the middle of the last century, involves vagally mediated bradycardia and hypotension after intracoronary administration of veratrum alkaloids. This "chemoreflex" has also been elicited following injection of more physiologically relevant compounds—namely, bradykinin and prostaglandin F_2. The receptors responsible for the Bezold reflex are thought to be stimulated during myocardial ischemia, producing bradycardia and hypotension in the early stages of inferior myocardial infarction. Similar hemodynamic changes often follow injection of contrast material into the right coronary artery. This reflex response is clearly vagally mediated, and atropine blocks the effect.

Control of Blood Volume

One of the most remarkable features of the mammalian circulation (Table 1–2) is the small size of the circulating blood volume (5 L) and the large proportion contained in the veins. Since the maximum cardiac output during exercise is normally 25 L/min or more, a volume of blood equal to the total contents of the circulation must pass through the aortic valve on an average of once every 12 seconds. Any change in

blood volume is likely to have a marked effect on venous return and hence on cardiac output.

A. Difficulty of Measurement: The measurement of blood volume, as either red cell or plasma volume, does not provide a clinically useful indication of the effective blood volume from a cardiovascular functional point of view. This is probably because mixing of the indicators used to measure blood volume with the contents of the circulation tends to be poor in the conditions in which disturbances of blood volume are important, eg, shock and heart failure.

B. Postural Change and Other Indirect Indications of Effective Blood Volume: Indirect evidence of the degree of filling of the circulation can be obtained by determining the effects of postural changes. When blood volume is large and the capacitance vessels are full, standing up has little or no effect on the heart, and the impedance of the arteries to the legs does not fall. The venous return does not decrease, because there is no room for pooling of blood in the lower body and the level of blood in the venous reservoirs does not decrease sufficiently to lower the cardiac output. An adequate systemic arterial pressure can thus be maintained, and no baroreceptor adjustments are necessary. When the effective blood volume is reduced and the capacitance vessels are relatively empty, standing up leads to lowering of the impedance of the arteries to the legs due to the effect of gravity. Pooling of blood in the veins of the legs reduces venous return, which in turn reduces cardiac output, and the arterial pressure falls acutely. Figure 1–32 shows a tracing of arterial pressure in a normal subject in whom venous return is decreased by applying negative pressure to the lower part of the body. Systolic blood pressure falls while diastolic pressure is maintained, and heart rate increases via the baroreceptor system. When the negative pressure is discontinued, blood pressure rises and baroreceptor responses come into play within a couple of beats and restore the arterial pressure level by causing bradycardia and peripheral vasodilation.

The simplest means of determining the adequacy of the circulating blood volume is to determine the effects of a simple change in posture on the patient's heart rate and blood pressure. The greater the increase in heart rate on standing, the smaller the effective blood volume. These changes have to be interpreted in light of the patient's build and the soundness of the autonomic control mechanisms. Tall persons are more subject to orthostatic changes, and any person in whom autonomic nervous paralysis is present will almost inevitably show a fall in blood pressure on standing.

C. Mechanisms of Control of Blood Volume: Control of the blood volume is determined by an interplay between osmolarity and thirst receptors working through antidiuretic hormone, aldosterone produced by the kidney, and renal clearance of sodium and water. Understanding of the mechanisms control-

Table 1–2. Characteristics of various types of blood vessels in humans.[1]

	Lumen Diameter	Wall Thickness	All Vessels of Each Type	
			Approximate Total Cross-sectional Area (cm²)	Percentage of Blood Volume Contained[2]
Aorta	2.5 cm	2 mm	4.5	2
Artery	0.4 cm	1 mm	20	8
Arteriole	30 μm	20 μm	400	1
Capillary	6 μm	1 μm	4500	5
Venule	20 μm	2 μm	4000	
Vein	0.5 cm	0.5 mm	40	54
Vena cava	3 cm	1.5 mm	18	

[1] Data from Gregg, in: *The Physiological Basis of Medical Practice,* 8th ed. Best CH, Taylor NB (editors). Williams & Wilkins, 1966.
[2] In systemic vessels. There is an additional 12% in the heart and 18% in the pulmonary circulation.

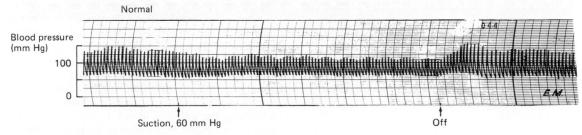

Figure 1–32. Brachial arterial blood pressure tracings in a normal subject. Venous return is reduced by applying suction to the lower half of the body. The baroreceptor reflexes maintain the mean level of arterial pressure, and there is overshoot of pressure when the venous return is restored.

ling blood volume has greatly increased since the discovery of the atrial natriuretic factor (ANF). This polypeptide hormone, which normally occurs in the atria, is secreted in response to atrial stretch, ordinarily caused by raised intra-atrial pressure. While granules containing ANF are normally found mainly in the atria, the cells of the ventricular myocardium come to contain the hormone when congestive heart failure is induced in experimental animals. The amino acid sequence of the hormone is known, and the active part of the molecule consists of 28 amino acids.

ANF promotes diuresis and natriuresis, thus counteracting the effects of blood volume expansion. ANF has widespread effects, including inhibition of aldosterone and cortisol secretion and decrease of renin and vasopressin secretion. It also has remote effects on the ciliary epithelium and the choroid plexus, decreasing intraocular pressure and the formation of cerebrospinal fluid. The highest levels in humans are found in congestive heart failure. Plasma levels are also raised in paroxysmal tachycardia, which explains the diuresis seen in that condition. The future therapeutic use of ANF or some related compound in the treatment of hypertension and congestive heart failure is still being investigated.

The biochemistry and molecular biology of this important cardiac hormone have developed with remarkable speed in the past few years, and numerous mysterious links, such as the diuretic and natriuretic effects of saline infusions and immersion in water have been explained by its actions.

DEVELOPMENT & AGING

The general physiologic principles set forth in the preceding pages are modified by growth and developmental influences from the fetal and neonatal period through adolescence and adult life up to the stage at which degenerative changes occur with aging. The special aspects of physiology of the fetus, infant, and growing child are outside the scope of this book, but aging is of increasing importance in cardiology in view of the increasing longevity of our population.

Age appears to increase the differences between "normal" individuals, and the definition of normal and the establishment of ranges of normality become increasingly difficult in older subjects.

Aging, which is most obvious in the skin, affects cell systems and tissue components such as collagen. Theories advanced to explain aging include random mutations in DNA that result in progressive abnormalities, the effects of oxygen-derived free radicals, and increased cross-linkages between macromolecules. Aging has been likened to an increase in entropy in which random errors in protein replication exert a cumulative effect. In addition, after the age of about 50, the maximal exercise heart rate decreases by approximately one beat per year. The effects of physical training on heart rate are seen at all ages, and elderly subjects can increase their maximal oxygen consumption by physical training to the same extent as younger subjects.

In the cardiovascular system, aging has its clearest effects on the compliance of systemic arteries. The vessels become stiffer and transmit pressure and velocity waves to the periphery more rapidly. The most obvious consequence is an increase in the amplification of the pulse pressure in the periphery, giving rise to systolic hypertension in brachial arterial recordings. This increased impedance to ejection by the left ventricle leads to left ventricular hypertrophy. This, together with other possible changes in the left ventricle, results in a decreasing compliance of the left ventricle and increasing diastolic dysfunction.

Other changes seen with aging are increasing fibrosis and calcification of the valvular annuli. There is also a loss of pacemaker cells in the sinoatrial node and conduction system disease in the elderly. The myocardial cell itself does not seem to exhibit decreased contractility with aging, though there is a progressive decrease in sensitivity to beta-adrenergic stimulation.

Degenerative Changes

Degenerative changes account for most cases of heart disease now seen in the Western world, and the inevitable aging processes seem to occur at widely differing rates in different people. Heart disease due to other causes does not protect patients from degenerative changes, and there is evidence that abnormally stressed tissues degenerate more rapidly than normally stressed ones. Patients with all forms of heart disease are coming to show more and more effects of the aging process as life expectancy increases and treatment to increase longevity becomes more effective.

SPECIAL CIRCULATIONS

Brain

The paramount importance of the cerebral circulation has already been mentioned. The blood supply to the brain is provided by an anastomosing system of arteries—the circle of Willis—and obstruction of a main vessel does not necessarily produce cerebral ischemia. As in the heart, it is not possible to be certain which cerebral or extracerebral vessel has been occluded in a patient in whom a particular part of the brain has been infarcted.

The principal factor influencing cerebral blood flow is the arterial CO_2 tension. Hyperventilation, by blowing off CO_2 in the lungs, decreases cerebral blood flow by causing arteriolar vasoconstriction. Conversely, CO_2 administration increases cerebral blood flow by causing vasodilation. Autonomic reflex control of the cerebral circulation is not well developed, and cerebral perfusion is primarily dependent on the systemic arterial pressure, which is maintained by baroreceptor activity. The cerebral venous system contains no valves, and since the cranial cavity is a closed space with rigid walls, the venous cerebral circulation acts as a siphon to maintain blood flow by physical means. The brain is well perfused in relation to its metabolism; thus, the cerebral venous blood is relatively high in oxygen.

Kidney

The renal circulation is under autonomic control, but mechanical and biochemical factors (probably bradykinin and prostaglandins) within the kidney play an important role in distributing flow preferentially to the cortex or medulla. The details of the intrinsic regulation of renal blood flow are not well understood. The arteriolar endothelium secretes a variety of vasoconstrictive and vasodilative substances that affect the relative preponderance of afferent as compared with efferent arteriolar constriction in the kidney. Imbalance may result in intraglomerular hyperperfusion, which in the presence of renal impairment—particularly diabetic nephropathy—accelerates the deterioration of renal function. In normal circumstances, sodium excretion is regulated to maintain a balance between intake and output; however, in conditions of stress, when renal blood flow is compromised, sodium retention occurs. When the cause of

inadequate renal perfusion is cardiac failure, the increased water retention that follows sodium retention increases blood volume and contributes to pulmonary and peripheral edema. The kidney is the most important organ influencing arterial pressure, and through the renin-angiotensin-aldosterone system influences blood pressure and body fluid volume. A decrease in the number of nephrons, perhaps genetic in origin, influences the kidney's ability to excrete a sodium load, which might be a factor in the pathogenesis of hypertension. The renal circulation, being concerned primarily with extraction of metabolites from the blood, has a perfusion rate that is high in relation to its metabolic rate. The renal venous blood is thus high in oxygen, and the kidney extracts relatively little oxygen from its arterial blood supply.

Other Viscera

Visceral blood flow is regulated by reflex hormonal and mechanical factors. The circulatory load imposed by visceral function is small and seldom compromises the general circulation. The viscera, being mainly involved in the transport of nutriments, have (like the kidneys) a low arteriovenous oxygen difference.

Muscle

The circulation to the muscles is potentially the largest in the body, and its regulation to meet the metabolic demands of muscular exercise is complex. The degree of local autonomy is great, and each group of muscles can provide the necessary stimuli to bring about a perfusion adequate to meet its own metabolic needs. Local vasodilation reduces the terminal (arteriolar) resistance, reducing the size of reflected waves and increasing the flow of blood to the exercising muscles. The overall cardiac output increases with muscular exercise as a result of sympathetic nervous activity. Any tendency for the blood pressure to fall as a result of the opening of muscle capillaries in response to muscular contraction causes release of the baroreceptor brake on the circulation and increases cardiac output. Increased muscular activity increases venous return to the heart, and this acts via the Frank-Starling mechanism to increase cardiac output. Local effects in the working muscles play an important role in the regulation of blood flow. Vasodilator substances—probably prostaglandins, bradykinin, endothelium-derived relaxing factor (EDRF), potassium ions, inorganic phosphate ions, and breakdown products of ATP—are responsible for much of the marked local vasodilation that occurs. The resistance to blood flow in the working muscles falls, and local muscular blood flow increases. It is probable that local neural stimuli from muscle spindles, mediated via nonmedullated fibers, pass to the medulla and help to stimulate increases in cardiac output and ventilation.

The muscular circulation, being concerned with

mechanical work, has a high metabolic rate in relation to its blood flow. The muscles extract more oxygen from their arterial blood supply than do other organs. The blood draining from exercising muscles, like that draining the heart, is thus low in oxygen. Muscular contraction raises the tissue tension and interferes with muscular perfusion. The situation is similar to that in the heart in that venous pressure does not regulate muscle blood flow.

Skin

The principal role of the skin circulation is temperature regulation. Since the mechanical efficiency of muscular work is only about 20–25%, large amounts of heat are generated during exercise. The skin acts as a radiator, and the evaporation of water from sweat acts as a means of cooling the blood perfusing the skin. This mechanism also comes into play in response to fever, with marked loss of heat occurring from the skin at times when the fever is subsiding. The converse occurs in response to low external temperatures and in periods when the body temperature is rising in febrile reactions. In this case, shivering and peripheral vasoconstriction act to generate and conserve heat. The demands of the skin circulation can become important in patients with severe heart disease when the cardiac reserves are seriously diminished.

The skin, being concerned primarily with temperature regulation, has the potential for a high perfusion rate in relation to its metabolic rate. The arteriovenous oxygen difference across the skin capillaries is thus small, especially when body temperature is raised and the skin is radiating heat.

Reproductive Organs

The circulation to reproductive organs is most important during pregnancy. The increased load of the placental circulation is sufficient to increase the resting cardiac output and blood volume. The peripheral resistance is lowered, and tachycardia and a wide pulse pressure can be noted as early as the middle of the second month of pregnancy. Since the change in cardiac output in pregnancy appears before there is sufficient low-resistance placental circulation to explain it, the earliest drop in peripheral resistance probably results from the hormonal changes seen in pregnancy.

Pulmonary Circulation

Whereas appropriate distribution of cardiac output is the most important factor in systemic circulatory dynamics, maximal blood flow with minimal perfusion pressure is what is required in the pulmonary circulation. With increasing right ventricular output, eg, during exercise, there is an increase in the area of the pulmonary capillary bed and little or no increase in pulmonary arterial pressure. The increased pulmonary blood flow occurs mainly by recruiting the capillary circulation of underperfused areas of the lung, so that flow increases without an increase in pulmonary artery pressure. Reflex control of the pulmonary bed is minimal when compared to the systemic circulation. For example, occlusion of one pulmonary artery in a normal adult man in the resting supine position causes no detectable change in the circulation, and release of the occlusion does not result in any increase in blood flow to the lung whose circulation was occluded. This lack of reactive hyperemia after pulmonary artery occlusion is in sharp contrast to the finding when systemic flow to any organ is cut off. However, reactive hyperemia in the pulmonary circulation probably does occur in human fetal and neonatal life.

The principal factor influencing pulmonary arterial pressure is alveolar hypoxia. A lowered alveolar oxygen tension produces pulmonary arteriolar vasoconstriction. This probably serves as a local mechanism to divert pulmonary blood flow away from areas of the lung in which ventilation is inadequate. Increased CO_2 tension and consequent increase in hydrogen ion concentration are important in enhancing the response to hypoxia.

DISTRIBUTION OF CARDIAC OUTPUT

All of the parallel systemic circulations compete for perfusion, and the total cardiac output reflects the sum of all their demands. The ratio of oxygen consumption to cardiac output represents the average systemic arteriovenous oxygen difference in milliliters of oxygen per liter of blood flow. The resting level of arteriovenous difference reflects the resting "mix" of perfusion of the brain, heart, kidneys, skin, and other viscera. Ordinarily, with normal cardiac function, enough blood flow is available for all circulations both at rest and during mild or moderate exercise. During severe exercise, however, the ability of other circulations to reduce their demands and thus free the maximal amount of blood for muscular perfusion is an important determinant of performance. When the cardiac output is inadequate because of heart disease, blood flow to less essential elements of the circulation (kidneys, viscera, and skin) is reduced, and the average systemic arteriovenous oxygen difference increases. This effect is sometimes interpreted as "an increase in oxygen extraction by the tissues" but in fact represents a redistribution of blood flow rather than a change in the behavior of any of the special circulations.

MUSCULAR EXERCISE

Muscular exercise constitutes the most severe physiologic stress to which the normal circulation is exposed. The systemic arterial circulation becomes more efficient with increasing exercise. The progressive fall in peripheral resistance leads to a decrease in the size of reflected waves, which in turn results in a progressively more efficient transfer of power from the heart to the periphery. The decrease in the size of reflected waves also reduces the amplitude of the arterial pressure in the periphery. In severe exercise, the aortic and peripheral arterial pressures are essentially equal. All forms of muscular activity are important—from feats of strength and short sprints to long-term endurance running—and the rate of recovery following exertion determines the level of performance that is possible after a short rest.

Isometric (Static) Exercise

Isometric exercise, involving lifting and straining, increases the systemic arterial pressure and heart rate and puts a "pressure load" on the circulation. The rise in blood pressure is partly reflex and partly mechanical. The reflex pathways are poorly understood, and the mechanical element stems from the increase in tissue pressure in the contracting muscles. Increased tissue pressure provides increased resistance, against which the left ventricle must eject blood. An individual's muscular strength bears no necessary relationship to the ability of the heart to increase its output during sustained exercise, and cardiac mechanisms mainly come into play when the muscles relax and perfusion is restored into a vasodilated muscular bed.

Short-Term Exercise

In short bursts of exercise, the muscles rely on fuel stored locally, and cardiopulmonary transport mechanisms are minimally involved. Thus, in a 100-meter dash, an accomplished athlete can take a deep breath before the start of a race and hold his or her breath during the few seconds needed to run the distance. Local substrates plus oxygen stored in the muscles and blood and the breakdown of muscle glycogen are used to provide the high-energy phosphate bonds needed for muscular contractions. These stores must be replenished during recovery.

Long-Term Exercise

In more prolonged intervals of exercise—minutes to hours—the cardiopulmonary transport of oxygen and removal of metabolic products become important considerations. The fuel stored in the muscles is not sufficient to provide the energy requirements, and increasing muscle blood flow leads to an increase in cardiac output and increased delivery of oxygen to the tissues. The sooner the cardiopulmonary transport mechanisms come into operation, the sooner the supply of oxygen can reach the level of the demand and a "steady state" of exercise be achieved. The arteriovenous oxygen difference increases as a larger proportion of the cardiac output is directed to the mus-

cles, and blood flow to the viscera tends to decrease as the level of exercise increases.

In more strenuous and protracted exercise, a steady state becomes progressively more difficult to maintain. Increased heat production by the exercising muscles leads to increased demands for skin perfusion to increase heat elimination, and ultimately, anaerobic metabolism, analogous to the use of energy stored in the muscle at the start of exercise, is superimposed on the steady state picture. The use of glycogen as a source of energy results in lactic acid production and makes available only a small proportion (about 10%) of the high-energy phosphate bonds provided by aerobic metabolism. Metabolic acidosis develops as lactic acid accumulates and escapes from the muscles into the blood. Increased ventilation and disproportionate tachycardia result, and the length of time that exercise can be continued at the same level of work becomes limited. Motivation becomes an important consideration, and all of the factors influencing oxygen transport—pulmonary ventilation, oxygen diffusion, stroke volume, and heart rate—reach their limits at about the same time in normal subjects.

Recovery From Long-Term Exercise

When exercise stops, the metabolic products that accumulated in the underperfused, contracting muscles cause a local vasodilation that imposes an important demand on the circulation. The initial stages of the return of the cardiovascular system toward normal following strenuous exercise are controlled by the baroreceptor reflexes. Muscular perfusion is limited by the need to maintain an adequate arterial pressure for cerebral perfusion. If circulatory function is good and a large cardiac output is available, muscular perfusion is well maintained during recovery, and the heart rate and cardiac output fall rapidly to normal as the load of metabolites that accumulated in the muscles during exercise is transferred to the rest of the circulation. If circulatory function is poor and there is little cardiac output to spare, the rate of recovery is slow, and the heart rate and cardiac output take longer to recover. In all cases, the rate of return of metabolism and heart rate toward normal follows an exponential pattern in the first few minutes of the recovery stage. In the longer term (first hour), recovery from exercise involves excretion of the metabolic products of exercise from the general circulation. Lactic acid and heat generated by muscular contraction are the most important factors in this phase of recovery, which also follows an exponential pattern but with a longer time constant (15 minutes or more).

Physical Training

Improving a person's physical condition by exercise training involves redistribution of systemic blood flow. In the untrained state, perfusion of visceral and skin circulations continues during exercise, and the cardiac output needed for a given level of submaximal work is increased. By exercise training, which involves habitually increasing the heart rate to moderately high levels (about 150/min) for an hour or so each day, blood flow is more efficiently distributed. Muscular perfusion is increased as blood is diverted from less essential parts of the circulation. The heart rate and cardiac output at submaximal loads are reduced, exercise performance is improved, and the rate of recovery from exercise is speeded up.

Athlete's Heart

Physical training results in an increase in cardiac muscle mass. The myocardial hypertrophy produced by athletic activity develops within weeks or months and can also regress when training stops. Both static (isometric) and dynamic (isotonic) training produce hypertrophy. Static training (eg, weight lifting) shows greater increases in wall thickness, whereas dynamic training (eg, cycling or running) produces greater increases in left ventricular dimensions. Athletes whose physical training starts earlier in life show greater changes, as do those who continue training into middle age. There is no clear evidence that the "physiologic" cardiac hypertrophy of athletes has any deleterious effect. Sudden death during athletic performance is usually due to identifiable disease.

LIMITATION OF CARDIAC PERFORMANCE

Performance during sustained activity in normal subjects is always limited by the capacity of the heart to meet the demands of the circulation. Cardiac capacity increases after birth, during the period of growth and development, up to a peak in early adult life. With disease and the degenerative changes associated with aging, the capacity of the heart to perform work decreases and the maximum cardiac output, the maximum oxygen consumption, and the maximal heart rate decrease. Both the maximal values and the rates at which the maximal values are reached decrease with age. When the capacity of the heart to do work falls to a level at which renal or cerebral perfu-

sion is compromised, a chain of events is initiated that leads to a vicious circle resulting finally in a clinical syndrome known as heart failure. This condition is easy to recognize but difficult to define. It is best viewed as a derangement of the normal circulatory control mechanisms mediated through the autonomic nervous system and will be discussed in Chapter 10.

Failure of the heart to maintain its own circulation at an adequate level also leads to a vicious circle that also results in what might just as well be called a form of heart failure but is in fact recognized as myocardial ischemia, discussed in Chapter 8.

The Heart as the Servant of the Circulation

The physiologic bases of these two forms of severe impairment of cardiac function—heart failure and myocardial ischemia—involve an understanding of the subservient role of the heart in relation to the overall circulation. The physiologic mechanisms involved in the maintenance of a normal blood pressure and blood volume so dominate the picture that when cardiac function is impaired, the autonomic nervous servomechanisms that ordinarily restore the status quo are activated even though the result is aggravation of the abnormal circulatory state.

Mechanisms of Heart Failure

"Inappropriate" physiologic mechanisms triggered by inadequate cardiac function are thus important in producing the vicious circles that result in the clinical syndromes of heart failure and myocardial ischemia.

To cite specific examples, if the heart cannot maintain an adequate blood pressure, vasoconstriction mediated via the sympathetic nervous system occurs; this increases the work of the heart, causing a vicious circle. If the heart cannot generate a blood pressure adequate to maintain renal perfusion, mechanisms physiologically appropriate for defense against loss of blood volume by dehydration, hemorrhage, or salt deprivation are set in motion. Retention of salt and water with blood volume expansion and restriction of urinary output then result in a vicious circle by overloading the already damaged circulation, causing heart failure.

REFERENCES

General

Becker AE, Anderson RH: *Cardiac Pathology.* Raven Press, 1983.

Campbell EJM, Dickinson CJ, Slater JDH (editors): *Clinical Physiology,* 4th ed. Lippincott, 1974.

Cohn PF: *Clinical Cardiovascular Physiology.* Saunders, 1985.

Eliot RS: *Stress and Heart Function.* Futura, 1988.

Fung YC: *Biodynamics: Circulation.* Springer, 1984.

Ganong WF: *Review of Medical Physiology,* 14th ed. Appleton & Lange, 1989.

Goerke J, Mines AH: *Cardiovascular Physiology.* Raven Press, 1988.

Green JF: *Fundamental Cardiovascular and Pulmonary Physiology,* 2nd ed. Lea & Febiger, 1987.

Heller LJ, Mohrman DE: *Cardiovascular Physiology.* McGraw-Hill, 1981.

Honig CR: *Cardiovascular Physiology.* Little, Brown, 1981.

Kitney RI, Rompelman O (editors): *The Beat-by-Beat Investigation of Cardiovascular Function.* Oxford Univ Press, 1987.

Maron BJ: Structural features of the athlete heart as defined by echocardiography. J Am Coll Cardiol 1986;7:190.

McDonald DA: *Blood Flow in Arteries,* 2nd ed. Williams & Wilkins, 1974.

McIlroy MB, Seitz WS, Targett RC: A transmission line model of the normal aorta and its branches. Cardiovasc Res 1986;20:581.

McIlroy MB, Targett RC: A model of the systemic arterial bed showing ventricular/systemic arterial coupling. Am J Physiol 1988;254:4609.

Milnor WR: *Hemodynamics.* Williams & Wilkins, 1982.

Wagner NK (editor): *Exercise and the Heart.* Davis, 1978.

Willerson JT, Sanders CA (editors): *Clinical Cardiology.* Grune & Stratton, 1977.

Anatomy of the Heart

Canale ED et al: *Cardiac Muscle.* Springer-Verlag, 1986.

Cheitlin MD, Finkbeiner WE: Cardiac anatomy. In: *Cardiology.* Parmley WW, Chatterjee K (editors). Lippincott, 1989.

Miller AJ: *The Lymphatics of the Heart.* Raven Press, 1982.

Walmsley R, Watson H: *Clinical Anatomy of the Heart.* Churchill Livingstone, 1978.

Cardiac Contraction

Huxley AF, Simmons RM: Proposed mechanisms for force generation in striated muscle. Nature 1971; 233:533.

Huxley HE: The mechanism of muscular contraction. Science 1969;164:1356.

Jewell BR: A re-examination of the influence of muscle length on myocardial performance. Circ Res 1977;40:221.

Monroe RG, French GN: Left ventricular pressure-volume relationships and myocardial oxygen consumption in the isolated heart. Circ Res 1961;9:362.

Noble MIM: *The Cardiac Cycle.* Blackwell, 1979.

Rushmer RF: Initial ventricular impulse: A potential key to cardiac evaluation. Circulation 1964;29:268.

Sagawa K: The end-systolic pressure-volume relation of the ventricle: Definitions, modifications and clinical use. (Editorial.) Circulation 1981;63:1223.

Sugi H, Pollack GH (editors): *Cross-Bridge Mechanisms in Muscle Contraction.* University Park Press, 1979.

Targett RC et al: Simultaneous Doppler blood velocity measurements from aorta and radial artery in normal human subjects. Cardiovasc Res 1985;19:394.

Trautwein W et al: Electrophysiologic study of human heart muscle. Circ Res 1962;10:306.

Cardiovascular Control

Brown E et al: Circulatory responses to simulated gravitational shifts of blood in man induced by exposure of the body below the iliac crests to subatmospheric pressure. J Physiol (Lond) 1966;183:607.

Cantin M, Genest J: The heart and the atrial natriuretic factor. Endocr Rev 1985;6:107.

Coleridge JCG, Coleridge HM: Chemoreflex regulation of the heart. Vol 1 in: *Handbook of Physiology.* American Physiological Society, 1979.

de Bold AJ: Atrial natriuretic factor: A hormone produced by the heart. Science 1985;230:767.

Donald DE, Shepherd JT: Cardiac receptors: Normal and disturbed function. Am J Cardiol 1979;44:873.

Levy MN, Vassalle M: *Excitation and Neural Control of the Heart.* American Physiological Society, 1982.

Mark AL: Implications of inhibitory reflexes originating in the heart. J Am Coll Cardiol 1983;1:90.

Rowell LB: *Human Circulation Regulation During Physical Stress.* Oxford Univ Press, 1986.

Shepherd JT: The heart as a sensory organ. J Am Coll Cardiol 1985;5(6 Suppl):83B.

Special Circulations

Bellamy RF: Diastolic coronary artery pressure-flow relations in the dog. Circ Res 1978;43:92.

Betz E: Cerebral blood flow: Its measurement and regulation. Physiol Rev 1972;52:595.

Cohen MV: *Coronary Collaterals: Clinical and Experimental Observations.* Futura, 1985.

Harris P, Heath D: *The Human Pulmonary Circulation,* 3rd ed. Churchill Livingstone, 1986.

Klocke FJ: Measurements of coronary flow reserve: Defining pathophysiology means making decisions about patient care. Circulation 1987;76:1183.

Knox FG (editor): *Textbook of Renal Pathophysiology.* Harper & Row, 1978.

Marcus HL: *The Coronary Circulation in Health and Disease.* McGraw-Hill, 1983.

Metcalfe J, Ueland K: Maternal cardiovascular adjustments to pregnancy. Prog Cardiovasc Dis 1974; 16:363.

Rouleau J et al: The role of auto-regulation and tissue diastolic pressures in the transmural distribution of left ventricular blood flow in anesthetized dogs. Circ Res 1979;45:804.

Zelis R (editor): *The Peripheral Circulations.* Grune & Stratton, 1975.

History Taking

A medical history carefully elicited by an understanding and competent clinician is usually the most important factor in the evaluation of the patient with cardiovascular disease. Skill in history taking is the principal aspect of clinical cardiology that the physician can continue to refine almost indefinitely. Experience and practice are vital to this art. The physician should not allow technologic developments in the investigation of patients to detract from the importance of history taking.

Because of the great fear of heart disease by most patients, the physician's questioning should be unhurried and nonthreatening but nonetheless thorough. Skillful interrogation, appropriate to the urgency of the situation, must be matched by thoughtful listening. Questions should be as free as possible of the force of suggestion. The patient must be permitted to raise questions at appropriate times. The history is the starting point in the diagnostic process and to a large extent determines the direction and extent (and delays, costs, and inconveniences) of further studies.

Artful history taking brings the patient and physician close together. In many respects, the history, taken properly, is therapeutic in itself. For this reason, it is a critical factor not only in establishing the diagnosis but also in determining the outcome of subsequent therapy.

Subclinical Disease; Asymptomatic Patients

The modern tendency for patients with no symptoms to consult physicians for routine "checkup" examinations has increased the possibility that doctors might cause unnecessary anxiety in their patients even though the intent of such examinations is to discover latent or developing illness. Since symptoms of disease are often exaggerations of normal findings (eg, dyspnea, fatigue), the borderline between normality and disease is often ill-defined. The problem becomes greater as the patient becomes older, because the range of normality widens with advancing years. Some patients deny the existence of symptoms, fearing to be told that they are ill and may die; and some may exaggerate symptoms for secondary gain. Decreasing activity, failing memory, and wishful thinking may lead people to defer seeking advice until disease is far-advanced. Persons with no complaints are technically not "patients," and a distinction should be maintained between conditions discovered during routine examinations and the diseases of patients with true symptoms. Experience in dealing with clinical and laboratory information obtained from checkup examinations is relatively small, and physicians tend to forget that under such circumstances they are dealing with a presymptomatic phase of disease.

DYSPNEA

The problem of interpreting a symptom that may also be a normal physiologic response is perhaps most strikingly demonstrated in the case of the cardinal symptom of heart disease—dyspnea, or shortness of breath. Shortness of breath on exertion is a normal phenomenon. In most cases, exercise performance is limited by shortness of breath rather than by fatigue, chest pain, leg pain, dizziness, or syncope. Dyspnea on progressively less severe exertion is also a normal accompaniment of the common modern combination of a sedentary life, increasing weight, and advancing age. It may therefore be more difficult to determine whether heart disease is present with dyspnea than if there are more obvious symptoms such as hemoptysis or severe chest pain.

"The unpleasant sensation of the need for increased ventilation" is the best description of dyspnea. It is a cortical sensation involving consciousness and must be distinguished from hyperpnea (increased ventilation), which may occur without discomfort or distress and which may be seen in unconscious patients.

Types of Dyspnea

The mechanism of dyspnea in normal and abnormal conditions is not always clear. Two main varieties have been distinguished. With the first variety, the patient feels that extra work on the part of the respiratory muscles is required to achieve adequate ventilation. With the second type, the patient is aware of a feeling of smothering and feels an urgent need to take another breath; the smothering sensation is akin to that associated with breath-holding.

Dyspnea in Normal Subjects

Dyspnea normally limits exercise performance in almost everyone. The ease with which dyspnea is provoked varies with the amount of ventilation required for that task. This in turn depends on a person's physical condition, weight, age, and life-style. A person also becomes conditioned to a certain level of discomfort arising from some particular task, such as walking up a familiar hill. In sedentary persons, the ability of the circulation to distribute maximum blood flow to the exercising muscles while decreasing perfusion of relatively nonessential vascular beds (eg, adipose tissue, skin, and viscera) is impaired.

Dyspnea in Heart Disease

The dyspnea of patients with heart disease most closely resembles the dyspnea of normal exertion and is characteristically directly related to the degree of exertion. The patient complains that some effort that previously did not result in awareness of breathing now causes an unpleasant gasping sensation. The feeling of discomfort is in the chest but is not well localized to any single structure such as the diaphragm or the intercostal muscles.

In contradistinction to cardiac dyspnea, shortness of breath at rest is more common in lung diseases such as asthmatic attacks, bronchitis, pneumonia, or pneumothorax, but not in emphysema.

A. Dyspnea Associated With Low Cardiac Output: When cardiac output is inadequate to meet the metabolic needs of the body, hyperventilation and subsequent dyspnea occur. Nonmedullated sensory fibers arising from stretch receptors in muscle spindles monitor local metabolic conditions and cause reflex medullary ventilatory stimulation when flow to the exercising muscle is inadequate to meet metabolic needs. These nervous mechanisms involve primitive visceral sensory fibers that are highly resistant to blocking agents. In this form of dyspnea, oxygen inhalation has little effect, because the extra oxygen carried in solution in the plasma is not sufficient to relieve the symptoms. Pulmonary congestion need not be present, although the dyspnea is similar to that occurring in pulmonary congestion and, as in pulmonary congestion, is quantitatively related to exertion.

B. Dyspnea Due to Pulmonary Congestion: Dyspnea on exertion is the cardinal symptom of pulmonary congestion. It results from a rise in left ventricular end-diastolic pressure or, in mitral valve disease, a raised left atrial pressure with a normal left ventricle. In both cases, increased pulmonary venous and pulmonary capillary pressures increase the stiffness of the lungs and the work of breathing by decreasing the compliance of the lungs, mainly by causing interstitial pulmonary edema. In addition to the mechanical changes, there is also a reflex autonomic visceral sensation, probably mediated through nonmedullated sensory fibers in the lungs and passing up the vagus nerves to the medulla, which contributes to dyspnea by direct autonomic sensory stimulation.

In the early stages of heart disease, dyspnea only occurs with severe exertion, but as pulmonary congestion becomes more severe, permanent changes in the lungs occur: resting lung compliance is reduced, and increased lymphatic drainage, thickening of inter-

stitial tissues, and other compensatory changes occur. Such changes reduce the chances of acute pulmonary edema and enable the body to tolerate high pulmonary capillary pressures because of thickened barriers between the blood in the capillaries and the gas in the alveoli.

In acute pulmonary congestion in bedridden patients, the least exertion, such as eating, use of a bedpan or commode, washing, or the minor excitement of a visitor, may provoke an episode of dyspnea. The dyspnea of acute pulmonary congestion, if not relieved, will progress to acute pulmonary edema, which can cause circulatory collapse, with restlessness, anxiety, apprehension, sweating, tachycardia, tachypnea, and acute respiratory distress.

C. Dyspnea in Acute Pulmonary Edema: When pulmonary congestion is acute and severe, dyspnea occurs with minimal exertion. The mechanism of the dyspnea and tachypnea with acute pulmonary edema includes the development of hypoxia and CO_2 retention, both powerful stimulators of the respiratory center. Dyspnea resulting from pulmonary edema and impaired gas exchange is often relieved by inhalation of oxygen, which increases the oxygen saturation of blood leaving the lungs.

D. Dyspnea Associated With Other Forms of Heart Disease: Dyspnea occurs in forms of heart disease other than those involving pulmonary congestion and low cardiac output. In cyanotic congenital heart disease, shunting of venous blood into the systemic circulation lowers arterial oxygen tension and contributes to dyspnea by stimulating the carotid bodies and increasing the ventilation needed for a given work load. In pulmonary embolism and pulmonary infarction, dyspnea may result from reflex stimulation of medullary centers by impulses from vagal nerve endings in the lungs and pulmonary arteries. Dyspnea due to such causes may be in addition to that due to inadequate cardiac output.

Dyspnea Resulting From Chemical Stimuli

Other mechanisms involved in dyspnea include chemical stimuli to ventilation mediated through hypoxia, as seen at high altitude; increase in CO_2 (hypercapnia); and metabolic acidosis. The chemoreceptor cells of the carotid and aortic bodies respond primarily to hypoxia and secondarily to increased CO_2. The central chemosensitive areas in the medulla stimulate respiration primarily in response to acidosis resulting from CO_2 and only secondarily in response to hypoxia. Chemically mediated stimuli to ventilation provide slowly responding and long-lasting control mechanisms and are chiefly involved in controlling depth and rate of breathing rather than causing dyspnea.

Hypoxia, as demonstrated by a lowered arterial oxygen tension while the patient is breathing air at rest or during exercise ($PO_2 < 70$ mm Hg), is not generally found in dyspneic cardiac patients. Hyperventilation with low PCO_2, low pH, and a normal or raised PO_2 is the usual finding. This is caused in cardiac patients by the release of acid metabolites from inadequately perfused tissues rather than by anxiety.

Dyspnea also results from acute changes in the permeability of the pulmonary capillaries, as when pulmonary edema develops in heroin overdose, or on exposure to toxic fumes such as chlorine, phosgene, or other noxious gases.

Episodic Dyspnea

Episodic dyspnea and dyspnea in the supine position that is relieved by sitting up (orthopnea) are important indicators of severe disease. The mechanism of orthopnea involves an increase in pulmonary capillary pressure and a decrease in lung volume when in the supine position. Lung compliance decreases and respiratory resistance increases to cause an acute increase in the work of breathing. *Paroxysmal dyspnea* classically occurs at night, often after a strenuous day or an evening out dancing or after excessive salt or fluid intake. It characteristically wakes the patient up around 2:00 AM and is so clearly relieved by sitting or standing and made worse by lying flat that many patients who have once experienced this symptom will never sleep flat in bed again.

When dyspnea is relieved by postural change other than sitting or standing, the possibility of pressure on intrathoracic structures by a tumor or aneurysm should be suspected. In pericardial disease, kneeling face down may relieve pressure on the heart and alleviate distress.

Dyspnea Associated With High-Altitude Pulmonary Edema

Dyspnea on exertion is normally seen at high altitude. Dyspnea at rest due to pulmonary edema may occur in persons acutely exposed to hypoxia at altitudes of 2000 m or more. The breathlessness usually comes on in the evening or during the night of the first day at high altitude. The patient often gives a history of unaccustomed exertion during the day. Even previously acclimatized persons returning to high altitude after a stay at sea level may be affected. Dyspnea, cough, frothy pink sputum, and circulatory collapse may develop if treatment is not forthcoming, and mountain climbers have died from the condition. Oxygen inhalation and returning to lower altitude provide relief. The causative mechanism is almost certainly increased permeability of the alveolocapillary membrane of the lungs. Pulmonary edema is more likely to occur in persons who show a marked pulmonary hypertensive response to alveolar hypoxia. Left atrial pressure has been shown to be normal in at least one person with the condition, and left heart failure is not the primary cause. The chest x-ray shows diffuse patchy opacities that disappear rapidly with treatment.

Dyspnea Due to Anxiety

Dyspnea at rest commonly accompanies anxiety. The patient complains that normal breathing is not satisfactory, and it is only by taking deep sighing breaths that relief is obtained. This form of dyspnea is not generally provoked by exertion and is associated with symptoms due to hyperventilation (see Chapter 21).

CHEST PAIN

Chest pain occurs in many varieties of heart disease and also in noncardiac diseases, and it is occasionally almost impossible to interpret.

Ischemic Cardiac Pain (Angina Pectoris) (See also Chapter 8.)

Classic ischemic pain (angina pectoris) can be either so obvious that it is easily recognizable or (uncommonly) so atypical that even after complete investigation, significant doubt exists about the nature of the pain. The basic mechanism of ischemic pain is an increase in the demand for both coronary blood flow and oxygen delivery that exceeds the available supply (Sampson, 1971).

The mechanism producing cardiac pain is not clearly understood. Nonmedullated small sympathetic nerve fibers paralleling the coronary vessels are thought to provide the afferent pathway. The pain, like other forms of visceral sensation, is referred to the equivalent spinal segments C8 and T1–5. Relief of angina following nonspecific surgical procedures such as thoracotomy is well recognized but not consistent. Although it is thought to be a placebo effect, the severing of afferent autonomic nerves may play a role in relieving pain.

A. Angina of Effort:

1. Character and duration— The original subjective description in the late 18th century by William Heberden of his own angina of effort has not been surpassed. He wrote that ". . . they who are afflicted with it, are seized while they are walking (more especially if it be uphill, and soon after eating) with a painful and most disagreeable sensation in the breast, which seems as if it would extinguish life, if it were to increase or to continue; but the moment they stand still, all this uneasiness vanishes. In all other respects, the patients are, at the beginning of this disorder, perfectly well, and in particular have no shortness of breath, from which it is totally different. The pain is sometimes situated in the upper part, sometimes in the middle, sometimes at the bottom of the sternum, and more often inclined to the left than to the right side. It likewise very frequently extends from the breast to the middle of the left arm. Males are most liable to this disease, especially such as have passed their fiftieth year." The pain is described as crushing, squeezing, vise-like, and resembling a weight on the chest but not as shooting or jabbing. It is a steady, constant pain that does not wax and wane. Occasionally, the patient describes only transient dyspnea rather than chest discomfort, reflecting the diastolic dysfunction that occurs with ischemia, resulting in an increase in pulmonary capillary pressure. This has been called an "anginal equivalent." Angina pectoris normally subsides rapidly, especially when it is provoked by effort. It usually lasts for minutes rather than seconds and seldom for hours or days. Long-lasting cardiac pain implies myocardial infarction or unstable angina.

2. Site and radiation– Anginal pain is ordinarily substernal or felt slightly to the left of the midline, beside or partly under the sternum. It is not felt solely at the cardiac apex in the inframammary region. It tends to radiate bilaterally across the chest, into the arms (left more than right), and into the neck and lower jaw. Occasionally, it radiates to the left scapular and shoulder area. It does not radiate into the upper jaw, the lower back, or below the umbilicus and is rarely felt in the abdomen alone. In the arms, the pain passes down the ulnar and volar surface to the wrist and then only into the ulnar fingers, never into the thumb or down the outer (extensor) surface of the arm. Pain may occasionally be felt only in the arm or may start in the arm and radiate to the chest.

3. Provocation and relief– Angina of effort represents the commonest form of cardiac pain. The pain or discomfort is provoked by any effort that raises the metabolic demand for coronary flow above the available supply. The pain is quantitatively related to exertion, and the patient often learns to identify the level of exercise that will bring on pain, and by avoiding that level, may obtain relief of symptoms. Attacks are precipitated by walking uphill or upstairs. Pain is more likely to occur when the patient is outdoors, especially when the temperature is high or low or when the patient is walking against the wind with face unprotected; after the patient has eaten a heavy meal; or when the patient is excited, angry, or tense. Pain sometimes comes on more readily with arm exercise or carrying heavy objects. Hot or cold showers or baths may precipitate pain, as may brisk toweling afterward. The sensory effects of temperature are mediated through the fifth nerve and cause reflex autonomic changes in blood pressure and heart rate. Cold showers raise blood pressure and heart rate; hot showers result in increased cardiac output in response to vasodilation.

Angina of effort is normally relieved by rest, with or without the help of vasodilator drugs such as nitroglycerin. Failure to obtain relief suggests another cause of pain or actual or impending myocardial in-

farction. In some instances, belching may relieve pain; this does not necessarily indicate a gastrointestinal source of pain. Patients sometimes find that continuing exercise (in some cases at a slower pace) leads to relief of pain ("walk-through angina"). This suggests either relief of vasospasm or an increase in the delivery of substrate to the myocardium.

B. Rest Pain: Anginal pain may be so readily provoked that it occurs at rest *(angina decubitus)*. Excitement, mental activity, and physical tension (eg, even simple clenching of a fist) raise arterial pressure and heart rate and increase myocardial oxygen consumption. Rest pain is likely to occur at night and may wake the patient. Increases in blood pressure and cardiac output during dreams may be sufficient to induce ischemia. When the coronary circulation is severely diseased, even minor circulatory changes may provoke pain. Anginal pain comes on more readily in the presence of fever, anemia, or arrhythmia (both bradycardia and tachycardia).

C. Variant (Prinzmetal) Angina: A paradoxic form of angina occurs in some patients as a result of coronary arterial spasm. The pain is like that of classic angina but occurs at rest, frequently at night, rather than on effort. In some cases, the pain is relieved, rather than brought on, by exercise. Variant angina is likely to be associated with ST segment elevation rather than depression on the ECG. This form of angina may occur either in patients with normal coronary arteries at angiography or in those with significant coronary atherosclerosis.

D. Coronary Arterial Spasm: While all variant (Prinzmetal) angina is probably due to coronary spasm, not all forms of coronary spasm produce variant angina. Coronary spasm may be provoked by vasoconstrictive drugs, such as ergotamine used for the control of migraine. Coronary spasm is commoner in women and may be associated with increased reactivity in other vascular beds (eg, Raynaud's disease or scleroderma). The pain associated with coronary spasm may be atypical and is not usually accompanied by tachycardia or a rise in arterial pressure. Electrocardiography may show ST segment depression or arrhythmia; it is important to obtain an ECG while the patient is experiencing pain.

E. Unstable Angina: The pain of unstable angina is like that of other forms of myocardial ischemia, but the circumstances in which the pain occurs are different. A diagnosis of unstable angina is suggested when a lower level of exercise is needed to provoke angina, by pain of different duration, by rest pain, or by failure to obtain relief with nitroglycerin. The mechanism of unstable angina is frequently the development of an increase in coronary arterial obstruction due to rupture of an atherosclerotic plaque and platelet aggregation leading to fibrin deposition and thrombus formation. Relatively minor changes in symptoms may indicate impending myocardial infarction. Retrospective analysis of patients with established infarction often reveals one or more premonitory episodes that either the physician or the patient did not consider severe enough to heed.

F. Pain of Myocardial Infarction: The pain of myocardial infarction is similar in character, site, and radiation to that of angina pectoris, but it is more severe and longer-lasting and associated at times with a feeling of impending death (**angor animi**) and also with circulatory collapse and shock. The patient may be short of breath, but pain is usually the dominant symptom. The patient is restless and often seeks, but cannot find, a comfortable position in which the pain is relieved. In myocardial infarction, the pain ordinarily lasts until the patient is given an analgesic such as morphine or meperidine. If such relief is unobtainable, the pain can last for several days.

G. Silent Myocardial Ischemia: Not all persons with myocardial ischemia experience pain. The finding of clear evidence of previous myocardial infarction on the ECG in completely asymptomatic patients and the occurrence of obvious ST depression on Holter monitoring or exercise electrocardiography without pain leave no doubt that "silent" ischemia can exist. In some cases, diabetic autonomic neuropathy can account for the finding. In others, the reasons for silent ischemia are obscure. The question whether or not to treat such patients is controversial.

Extracardiac Chest Pain

A. Pain in Acute Thoracic Disease: Pain similar to that of myocardial infarction also occurs with other acute intrathoracic disorders. **Aortic dissection** can cause severe chest pain. This frequently starts in the back or radiates to it. **Acute pulmonary embolism** also causes acute chest pain and shock that may be indistinguishable from that due to myocardial infarction. The cause is thought to be sudden acute right ventricular distention that stimulates ventricular receptors whose sensory representation resembles that of the left ventricle. Spontaneous pneumothorax and acute pleurisy, especially at the onset of lobar pneumonia, also cause chest pain and must be distinguished from pericardial disease, which causes a pain similar in distribution to other cardiac pains but more related to posture. Like pleural pain, pericardial pain is often worse with respiration, but relief obtained from sitting up and leaning forward or even from crouching on all fours face down is particularly suggestive of pericardial pain. Such maneuvers presumably alter tension on the pericardial sac. Like pleural pain, pericardial pain is often relieved when effusion develops.

B. Pain Associated With Anxiety States: The most troublesome pain to explain is the noncardiac pain of anxiety states and effort syndrome. The pain is stabbing, felt at the apex of the heart in the left inframammary region, and associated with a feeling of anxiety, breathlessness, and inability to take a satisfying deep breath (Da Costa's syndrome). It seems to be related to the sympathetic nervous system responses of fright. The more knowledge the patient has of heart disease, the more difficult it may be to interpret such pain, because the description may be unconsciously molded to emphasize or minimize a possible illness.

C. Pain Associated With Herpes Zoster: The pain of herpes zoster classically precedes the rash, and this diagnosis should be borne in mind, especially in older persons. The pain is radicular in nature, gripping, tight, constricting, and sometimes burning, and it may be severe. The diagnosis, which may be suspected when hyperesthesia is found in the affected area, becomes obvious when the eruption develops in a few days.

D. Musculoskeletal Pain: Musculoskeletal pain due to cervical or thoracic spinal bone or joint disease is readily confused with cardiac pain. Dorsal root pain (girdle pain) tends to be gripping and constricting and causes tightness. It is often associated with local tenderness, whereas angina is not. The presence of degenerative changes in spinal radiograms is no positive evidence of a musculoskeletal origin of the pain, any more than ST and T wave changes on the ECG indicate a cardiac origin. Provocation of the pain by movement, jarring, coughing, and sneezing and relief of pain by means of massage, heat, and manipulation are useful in suggesting a musculoskeletal origin. Tenderness of the anterior rib cage suggests costochondritis (Tietze's syndrome).

E. Abdominal Pain: Abdominal pain sometimes occurs in patients with heart disease, especially in acute, severe right-sided failure. Hepatic distention is usually invoked as the causative mechanism. Abdominal pain, usually in the epigastrium, also occurs in angina and in myocardial infarction, but the pain is never solely abdominal.

Esophageal spasm and pain associated with esophageal reflux can mimic angina exactly, including precipitation by exercise. Furthermore, esophageal reflux occurs not infrequently in patients with coronary artery disease, and so the patient may have symptoms from both conditions. The esophagus and the stomach are innervated by the autonomic nervous system and are capable of causing visceral pain having the same area of radiation as the heart. Any disease of the epigastric viscera can cause chest pain, which can be confused with cardiac pain. The pain of gallbladder disease is also difficult to distinguish from cardiac pain, since gallbladder disease and coronary disease often coexist.

PALPITATIONS

Awareness of the beating of the heart varies with the sensitivity of the patient and the severity of any disturbance of the force or rhythm of the heartbeat. The variation in these factors is great. Awareness of each ectopic beat or even of normal sinus rhythm may be extremely troublesome to some patients. Others may have an extremely forceful heartbeat owing to free aortic incompetence, or they may be subject to episodes of ventricular or supraventricular tachycardia with heart rates of over 180 beats/min without noticing anything. One must therefore differentiate between awareness of forceful heart action and an arrhythmia when the patient complains of palpitations. Most patients notice irregular rhythms more than they do regular tachycardia, but the more rapid the heartbeat, the more likely the patient is to notice an abnormality. In some cases, arrhythmia is only noticed during exercise when the heart rate is rapid.

Associated Symptoms

An important question is whether the palpitations are accompanied by any other symptoms such as dizziness, chest pain, or dyspnea. The functional effect of an arrhythmia may sometimes be a clue to its cause, as for example in mitral stenosis, in which dyspnea is almost always provoked when the arrhythmia occurs.

Examination & Recording of an ECG During an Attack

It is imperative to examine any patient with palpitations and record an ECG during an episode of palpitation. Until this has been done, it is essential to keep an open mind concerning the diagnosis. Palpitations often begin abruptly and cease gradually, and because the sinus tachycardia resulting from anxiety caused by the arrhythmia subsides only gradually, the patient may not be aware that the arrhythmia itself has stopped. The functional consequences of an episode of palpitations depend on the duration, the rapidity of the heart rate, and the state of the heart before the episode started. A paroxysm of tachycardia at a rate of about 140 beats/min may be well tolerated for a day or two, but any rapid arrhythmia with an acute onset and a duration of more than a week to 10 days is likely to provoke heart failure, even in healthy young persons. In older, sicker patients, especially those with anemia or hypoxia, a shorter time elapses before serious heart failure develops.

DIZZINESS & SYNCOPE

Dizziness and syncope are difficult symptoms to interpret if the patient's consciousness has been impaired and recollection of the events surrounding the attack is hazy. The effects of alcohol or drugs cloud the patient's consciousness and interfere with interpretation of events. Dizziness and syncope both occur more commonly as benign manifestations than as symptoms of serious disease. They are most commonly due to noncardiac causes such as epileptic seizures, transient ischemic attacks due to cerebral or

carotid vascular disease, and cerebrovascular accidents and vertigo due to vestibular disease rather than cardiac disease. A description of the episode from witnesses is of great value, but much can be learned from the circumstances surrounding the episode, as related by the patient. Dizziness is a frequent but not a necessary precursor of syncope, and one or both occur in three main types of conditions involving the cardiovascular system. The commonest form of cardiac syncope is simple vasovagal fainting resulting from certain autonomic nervous system effects. This is described in the chapter on hypotension (Chapter 21). The next most common is cardiac syncope due to arrhythmia or cardiac standstill, in which the heartbeat does not maintain adequate blood flow to the brain. The least common is syncope on unaccustomed effort, in which the demand for systemic perfusion exceeds the supply during severe stress, and cerebral ischemia ensues. Cardiac syncope is described in the chapter on arrhythmias (Chapter 15), and effort syncope is described under the heading of aortic stenosis (see Chapter 13). Effort syncope can also occur in severe pulmonary stenosis and in primary pulmonary hypertension.

Fainting Attacks in Tetralogy of Fallot

A specific form of syncope occurs in patients with tetralogy of Fallot in whom infundibular obstruction is present. One suggested mechanism for the development of syncope is spasm of the outflow tract of the right ventricle, resulting in an acute decrease in pulmonary blood flow. Right-to-left shunting of blood through the ventricular septal defect into the aorta increases as a result, and acute severe arterial hypoxemia occurs, leading to loss of consciousness. The factors precipitating the infundibular spasm are not known. Another possible mechanism may be related to a drop in systemic vascular resistance, which leads to an increase in right-to-left shunting, a further increase in arterial hypoxia due to the shunt, and further decrease in pulmonary blood flow, resulting in syncope.

Carotid Sinus Syncope

Another rare cause of syncope is excessive sensitivity of the carotid sinus baroreceptor mechanism. Extreme bradycardia and peripheral vasodilation may occur in response to minor mechanical stimulation of the neck, as in sharp turning of the head or pressure on the neck from too tight a collar. The condition is generally seen in older atherosclerotic men.

Cough Syncope

Syncope sometimes follows a bout of coughing. In this case, the repeated large ($>$ 100 mm Hg) increases in intrathoracic pressure reduce systemic venous return enough to lower the systemic arterial pressure to levels of 50 mm Hg or less. Syncope results from inadequate cerebral perfusion. Either continuous or intermittent coughing spasms may cause these effects, which are commonest in middle-aged male smokers.

OTHER SYMPTOMS OF HEART DISEASE

Cough & Hemoptysis

Hemoptysis may occasionally be the first symptom of heart disease, and since there can be no hemoptysis without cough, cough is technically the presenting symptom. Mitral valve stenosis is the commonest cardiac condition in which hemoptysis is the presenting manifestation, and pulmonary congestion, frank pulmonary hemorrhage due to a ruptured bronchial vein, and pulmonary infarction account for almost all cases. Cough without hemoptysis also occurs in any condition causing pulmonary congestion, and cough on exercise is sometimes seen in patients with mitral stenosis. Dry, nonproductive cough is usually the earliest manifestation of impending pulmonary edema and precedes the profuse, watery, frothy pink sputum seen in the fully developed picture of acute pulmonary edema.

Cough may also occur as a manifestation of pressure on the bronchial tree in patients with cardiovascular disease. Left atrial enlargement may compress the left main bronchus in patients with mitral valve disease, and it may irritate the recurrent laryngeal nerve on the left side as it hooks under the aorta at the ligamentum arteosum. Enlarging aortic aneurysms involving the aortic arch and tumors involving the heart may also cause cough when they compress mediastinal structures. Cough that occurs when the patient lies flat and is relieved when the patients sits up is particularly suggestive of pressure on the bronchial tree.

Fatigue

Fatigue is the most difficult cardiac symptom to evaluate. Whereas other symptoms of heart disease have associated outward manifestations, fatigue is entirely subjective. Although it is sometimes due to heart disease, fatigue is far more frequently due to noncardiac causes. Fatigue as a cardiac symptom is almost never of diagnostic value except as an indication of low cardiac output. It is rarely the first or the only symptom of significant organic heart disease, although it is a prominent symptom of neurocirculatory asthenia (Da Costa's syndrome; see Chapter 21). It commonly accompanies severe long-standing heart disease, especially chronic valvular disease with persistent right heart failure and low cardiac output. It is seen in patients with severe coronary artery disease after myocardial infarction, in mitral stenosis with marked increase in pulmonary vascular resistance, and in primary pulmonary hypertension. Dehydration due to excessive diuretic therapy and potassium depletion are two additional contributing factors.

Nocturia & Polyuria

Nocturia is occasionally the earliest symptom of raised left atrial pressure in left ventricular failure or mitral stenosis. Transfer of fluid from the legs to the trunk when the patient lies down may play a part. Raised atrial pressure in the recumbent position provokes the release of atrial natriuretic factor (ANF) from granules in the atrial myocytes. Reflex connections have been demonstrated between left atrial receptors and the central nervous system, and the efferent pathway is known to involve the kidneys. Nocturia implies the passage of an abnormally large amount of urine at night, rather than an increased frequency of micturition at night, as occurs in prostatic disease. In the healthy state, the cardiac output is sufficient to provide adequate renal blood flow during the day, and urine flow at night is therefore conveniently reduced to a minimum. It may be that in early heart failure this mechanism breaks down because of inadequate cardiac output. There is also a connection between cardiac function and urinary output in patients with paroxysmal tachycardia due to any cause. Some patients note an increased urinary volume within 15–30 minutes of the start of tachycardia. The urine is of low specific gravity. The cause of this type of diuresis is thought to be the release of atrial natriuretic factor following atrial distention.

Relief of Dyspnea on Squatting

Exertional dyspnea that is relieved by squatting during recovery from exercise strongly suggests the diagnosis of tetralogy of Fallot. The central blood volume and pulmonary blood flow are both increased by squatting. It has been shown that it is the change in the amount of venous return and not the change in posture that is important, because squatting in water has no hemodynamic effect. Thus, in tetralogy of Fallot, squatting increases venus return, and increases the systems resistance, and arterial pressure, providing more blood flow to the lungs by deccreasing the right-to-left shunt across the ventricular defect. A similar result can be obtained by lying down, but children find it easier to squat after exertion. It is the pooling of blood in the legs in the upright position after stopping exercise that is the primary problem; if this does not occur, as in patients with large pulmonary blood volume, the benefit from squatting is not seen. A tracing showing the time course of the changes in arterial pressure and arterial saturation on standing and aquatting in a pateint with tetralogy of Fallot is seen in Figure 2–1.

Hoarseness

Hoarseness as a manifestation of heart disease is seldom, if ever, a presenting symptom. It occurs in cardiac patients with gross left atrial enlargement in mitral valve disease, in giant left atrium, and in aortic aneurysm with or without dissection. All of these conditions cause pressure on the left recurrent laryngeal nerve and result in hoarseness. Hoarseness is

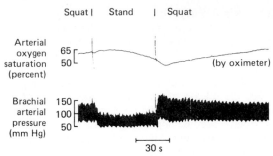

Figure 2–1. Changes in arterial oxygen saturation and blood pressure on standing and squatting in a patient with tetralogy of Fallot.

also seen in patients with myxedema, in whom it may be the first clue to diagnosis.

Edema

Edema due to cardiac disease is a result of right heart failure and is seldom seen early, because right heart failure is a late development in heart disease. A complaint of edema as a primary symptom implies a noncardiac cause such as venous stasis, thrombophlebitis, nephrotic syndrome, lymphedema, or idiopathic edema. Right heart failure can be surprisingly severe, with hepatic enlargement, ascites, and a raised venous pressure, but no significant pitting edema of the ankles.

Cyanosis

Patients occasionally complain of blueness of the extremities, face, and lips. Cyanosis may be peripheral and associated with a low cardiac output, peripheral vasoconstriction, and a feeling of coldness. In this case, the blueness is due to a high concentration of reduced hemoglobin in the blood in the veins of the skin, and arterial saturation is normal. In true central cyanosis, the arterial oxygen saturation is reduced because of right-to-left shunting or lung disease. In this case, the patient's extremities are often warm, or if they are made warm, the blue color does not disappear.

Loss of Weight (Cardiac Cachexia)

Loss of weight is not a presenting symptom of heart disease, but it does occur in chronically ill cardiac patients, especially when the cardiac output is low. It is probably related to secondary anorexia; however, production of cytokines such as tumor necrosis factor (TNF) in severe heart failure may be responsible for the cachexia. The patient characteristically loses weight from the limbs and accumulates fluid in the abdomen. It is difficult to establish the true extent of the cachexia, because the accumulation of fluid tends to maintain total body weight.

FUNCTIONAL & THERAPEUTIC CLASSIFICATION OF HEART DISEASE

Overall Functional Capacity

The patient's overall disability is conventionally expressed in terms of the New York Heart Association's criteria for functional capacity.

Class I: No limitation of physical activity. Ordinary physical activity does not cause undue fatigue, palpitation, dyspnea, or anginal pain.

Class II: Slight limitation of physical activity. Comfortable at rest, but ordinary physical activity results in fatigue, palpitation, dyspnea, or anginal pain.

Class III: Marked limitation of physical activity. Comfortable at rest, but less than ordinary activity causes fatigue, palpitation, dyspnea, or anginal pain.

Class IV: Unable to carry on any physical activity without discomfort. Symptoms of cardiac insufficiency or of the anginal syndrome may be present even at rest. If any physical activity is undertaken, discomfort is increased.

While this classification gives a good overall indication of the patient's status, many physicians prefer to subdivide class II into classes IIa and IIb. In class IIa, the patient can keep up with others walking on the flat but has limitation on more severe exercise such as climbing stairs. In class IIb, the patient has slight limitation on all forms of physical activity.

Functional Capacity in Angina

The Canadian Cardiovascular Society has put forward the following functional classification of the severity of angina. It resembles the New York Heart Association's classification of overall disability.

Class I: Ordinary physical activity—walking and climbing stairs—does not cause angina. Angina with strenuous, rapid, or prolonged exertion at work or recreation.

Class II: Slight limitation of ordinary activity—walking or climbing stairs rapidly; walking uphill; walking or climbing stairs after meals, in cold, in wind, under emotional stress, or during the few hours after awakening. Walking more than two blocks on the level and climbing more than one flight of ordinary stairs at a normal pace under normal conditions.

Class III: Marked limitation of ordinary physical activity—walking one or two blocks on the level or climbing one flight of stairs at a normal pace under normal conditions.

Class IV: Inability to carry out any physical activity without discomfort. Anginal syndrome may be present at rest.

REFERENCES

Almquist A et al: Carotid sinus hypersensitivity: Evaluation of the vasodepressor component. Circulation 1985;71:927.

Boucher IAD, Morris JS: *Clinical Skills.* Saunders, 1982.

Fasules JW, Wiggins JW, Wolfe RR: Increased lung vasoreactivity in children from Leadville, Colorado, after recovery from high-altitude pulmonary edema. Circulation 1985;72:957.

Frank MJ, Alvarez-Mena SC, Abdulla AM: *Cardiovascular Physical Diagnosis,* 2nd ed. Year Book, 1983.

Gottlieb SO et al: Silent ischemia as a marker for early unfavorable outcomes in patients with unstable angina. N Engl J Med 1986;314:1214.

Heberden W: *Commentaries on the History and Cure of Diseases.* London, 1802.

Herrick JB: Clinical features of sudden obstruction of the coronary arteries. JAMA 1912;59:2015.

Horwitz LD, Groves BM: *Signs and Symptoms in Cardiology.* Lippincott, 1984.

Levine H: Difficult problems in the diagnosis of chest pain. Am Heart J 1980;100:108.

Lewis HP: *The History and the Physical Examination.* Appleton-Century-Crofts, 1979.

McIlroy MB: Breathlessness in cardiovascular disease. In: *Manchester Symposium on Breathlessness.* Blackwell, 1966.

Mendel D: *Proper Doctoring.* Springer-Verlag, 1984.

Nicklas JM et al: Plasma levels of immunoreactive atrial natriuretic factor increase during supraventricular tachycardia. Am Heart J 1986;112:923.

O'Donnell TV, McIlroy MB: The circulatory effects of squatting. Am Heart J 1962;64:347.

Parry CH: *An Inquiry Into the Symptoms and Causes of the Syncope Anginosa, Commonly Called Angina Pectoris: Illustrated by Dissections.* London, 1799.

Prinzmetal M et al: Angina pectoris. 1. A variant form of angina pectoris. Am J Med 1959;26:375.

Sampson JJ, Cheitlin MD: Pathophysiology and differential diagnosis of cardiac pain. Prog Cardiovasc Dis 1971;13:507.

Sharpey-Schafer EP: The mechanism of syncope after coughing. Br Med J 1953;2:860.

Silverman ME: *Examination of the Heart.* Part 1: *The Clinical History.* American Heart Association, 1975.

Stern S, Tzivoni D: Early detection of silent ischaemic heart disease by 24-hour electrocardiographic monitoring of active subjects. Br Heart J 1974;36:481.

Sugrue DD et al: Symptomatic "isolated" carotid sinus hypersensitivity: Natural history and results of treatment with anticholinergic drugs or pacemaker. J Am Coll Cardiol 1986;7:158.

Swartz MH: *Textbook of Physical Diagnosis: History and Examination.* Saunders, 1989.

Wood P: Polyuria in paroxysmal tachycardia and paroxysmal atrial flutter and fibrillation. Br Heart J 1963;25:273.

Physical Examination

This chapter deals with only the more general or introductory aspects of the physical examination of the patient with heart disease. Details of the physical manifestations of cardiac disease appear under the description of each disease.

It is important to emphasize that examination of the cardiac patient is not confined to those parts of the body in which manifestations of cardiac disease are most commonly seen. Physicians should remember that cardiac disease can be associated with any disease from acromegaly to Zollinger-Ellison syndrome and that clues to the existence of noncardiac disorders which simulate, complicate, or merely coexist with heart disease may be apparent on methodical physical examination.

Approach to the Physical Examination

The general appearance and behavior of the patient are noted as the medical history is recorded. Similarly, the history-taking process may continue during the physical examination. The patient may be questioned about any findings and asked about awareness of signs and their duration.

Examination of the patient usually starts from the head and proceeds downward. Inspection precedes palpation, percussion, and auscultation. The cardiologist traditionally feels the patient's pulse while carrying out the preliminary inspection, and many physicians start by recording the vital signs—pulse, temperature, and respiration—and blood pressure.

PULSES

The Radial Arterial Pulse

Palpation of the pulse wave that results from transmission of the pressure wave down the artery is usually performed on the patient's right wrist, with the examiner using the first three fingers of the right hand. The frequency, regularity, amplitude, rate of upstroke, and volume of the radial pulse require only one finger for their evaluation, but the rate of propagation of the wave and the thickness of the artery can only be properly examined with three fingers. The amplitude of the pulse (small or large) depends mainly on the *pulse pressure* (the difference between systolic and diastolic pressure) and gives a rough indication of stroke volume. Thus the "small" pulse of severe mitral stenosis contrasts with the "large," jerky

pulse seen in patients with mitral incompetence. In aortic stenosis, the rate of travel of the wave is slow; the "pulsus tardus" in this condition means that the pulse takes longer to pass under the examiner's fingers. The ease with which the pulse can be obliterated is felt by compressing the artery with the proximal finger and palpating with the other two in order to ascertain when the wave has disappeared. This is a rough indication of the systolic arterial pressure and is considerably less accurate than the measurement obtained by sphygmomanometry. The thickness of the undistended arterial wall can be felt using the middle finger to palpate while the proximal and distal fingers simultaneously occlude the vessel. This gives an indication of the degree of arteriosclerosis.

A. Sinus Arrhythmia: In sinus arrhythmia, the heart rate varies with the phase of respiration. Inspiration increases and expiration decreases the rate via vagally mediated reflexes. Expiration decreases the rate because it favors left ventricular filling by increasing the return to the left heart of blood that was stored in the lungs during inspiration. In accordance with **Frank-Starling's law,** increased filling increases stroke volume, and the consequent increase in arterial pressure provokes reflex bradycardia. Sinus arrhythmia is commoner in young, healthy athletes. It is not seen in patients with heart failure or large left-to-right shunts and is less marked in sick sinus syndrome.

B. Atrial Fibrillation: In atrial fibrillation, the heartbeat is irregular in rate and in force. The irregular beats occur in an irregular pattern, and the force of cardiac contraction varies from beat to beat. The irregularity is usually more obvious during exercise.

C. Ectopic Beats: In ectopic beats, the heart rate is irregular but the pattern is often regular. Beats may occur in pairs **(pulsus bigeminus)** or in runs of three or more. Ectopic beats in persons with normal cardiovascular function often disappear on exercise.

Other Arterial Pulses (See also Neck, below.)

It is important to feel the pulse bilaterally to check for differences in timing and intensity. Brachial, radial, carotid, femoral, popliteal, and posterior tibial pulses are usually examined routinely. By this means, the physician may obtain clues about peripheral vascular disease, aortic dissection, and coarctation of the aorta. The closer the vessel lies to the heart, the more reliable the pulse is as an indicator of aortic pressure wave characteristics. Thus, the carotid arterial pulse is best for assessment of aortic valve disease. If there is a prominent pulse in the neck or if coarctation of the aorta is suspected for any other reason, it is important to feel the radial and femoral pulses simultaneously. In normal subjects, the two pulses are synchronous, whereas in coarctation of the aorta the femoral pulse is absent or diminished and felt up to 0.15 s after the radial.

BLOOD PRESSURE

Measurement of Blood Pressure

A. Measurement in the Arms: Indirect measurement of the systemic arterial pressure is conventionally performed using a sphygmomanometer on the right arm. A 12.5 cm cuff is wrapped around the upper arm and connected to a mercury or aneroid manometer. The patient should not have smoked or ingested caffeine for 30 minutes and should have rested for at least 5 minutes before the measurement is made. The patient should sit with the arm at heart level, and the rubber bladder of the cuff should encircle at least two-thirds of the upper arm. The cuff is inflated to a level above the systolic pressure. The absence of a radial pulse is checked at the wrist. The cuff is slowly deflated (around 2 mm/beat) while the examiner feels the radial pulse. The pressure level at which the pulse is first felt is noted, and the cuff is reinflated. The cuff is then deflated a second time, with the examiner listening over the brachial artery with the stethoscope. The pressure level at which a

sound is first heard over the artery is recorded as the systolic pressure. As deflation of the cuff continues, the sound arising from the vessel wall increases in intensity, decreases, becomes muffled, and finally disappears. The pressure at which the sound becomes muffled is usually within 2–4 mm Hg of the pressure at which the sound disappears. The pressure at which the sound disappears is the diastolic pressure. Correlation between direct arterial pressure measurement and sphygmomanometry has shown reasonable agreement between the two methods, especially in normal subjects, but the differences are sometimes marked in individual cases.

Blood pressure should be measured in the standing and supine positions in patients who might have hypotension or hypertension, and the pulse rate should always be measured and recorded along with the pressure. Blood pressure should be measured in both arms when the patient is first seen. On subsequent visits, it is taken in the right arm, except when the pulse in that arm is significantly reduced, as, for example, after a Blalock-Taussig operation for tetralogy of Fallot. The site of the measurement and position of the patient should be recorded.

Artifacts in measurement. Artifacts in indirect measurement occur when the arm is large in relation to the cuff (Figure 3–1); when a patient has aortic incompetence, in which the indirectly measured diastolic pressure is usually falsely low; and when the patient is in shock. With aortic incompetence, the pressure at which the sound is muffled is closest to the true diastolic blood pressure. An erroneously low systolic pressure may be obtained in some hyperten-

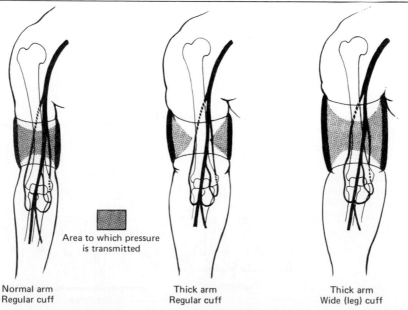

Area to which pressure is transmitted

Normal arm   Thick arm   Thick arm
Regular cuff   Regular cuff   Wide (leg) cuff

Figure 3–1. Diagram showing that pressure is not transmitted to the brachial artery when a regular cuff is used to measure blood pressure in a thick arm.

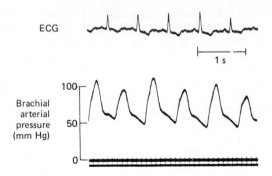

ECG

1 s

100

Brachial
arterial
pressure
(mm Hg)

50

0

Figure 3–2. ECG and brachial arterial pulse pressure showing pulsus alternans in a patient with aortic stenosis.

sive patients in whom the systolic pressure is not checked by palpation. An "auscultatory gap" may be present in such patients and in those with aortic stenosis and localized arteriosclerosis. The auscultatory gap is a range of pressures over which arterial sounds are absent even though a pulse is present.

B. Measurement in the Legs: The measurement of arterial pressure in both arms and both legs is advocated by some as a routine measure. If the leg pressure is to be measured, a special wide (20 cm) cuff is used; such a cuff is also needed for patients with thick or fat arms.

Pulsus Alternans & Pulsus Paradoxus

A. Pulsus Alternans: Pulsus alternans and pulsus paradoxus should be sought when the blood pressure is measured. Pulsus alternans, the alternation of small- and large-amplitude beats with a regular rhythm, can be detected by palpation of the pulse.

Minimal pressure on the pulse should be exerted for greatest sensitivity in detecting pulsus alternans. The mechanism is unknown although many theories have been proposed, and the finding, which is seen in left ventricular failure, carries a poor prognosis, especially if the heart rate is slow. Figure 3–2 shows an example of pulsus alternans in a brachial arterial pressure tracing in a patient with aortic stenosis.

A similar form of alternation in the force of cardiac contraction occurs in the right heart in response to right heart failure. Pulsus alternans sometimes starts after an ectopic beat and lasts for several beats. It may occur when the patient stands or starts to exercise. The more constant the pulsus alternans, the worse the prognosis.

B. Pulsus Paradoxus: This abnormality (Figure 3–3) consists of an exaggeration of the normal respiratory fluctuation in systolic pressure (decrease in the strength of the pulse during inspiration). The arterial pressure (systolic, diastolic, and mean) normally falls by a few mm Hg when intrathoracic negative pressure increases during inspiration. If the systolic fall amounts to greater than 10 mm Hg (or more than 10% of the systolic pressure), pulsus paradoxus is present.

The phenomenon can be due to an increase in the amplitude of intrathoracic pressure fluctuations resulting from changes in the mechanical properties of the lungs, as occurs in large pneumothorax, pleural effusion, or obstructive lung disease. It is more commonly due to pericardial disease, especially cardiac tamponade, in which cardiac filling is compromised. As fluid accumulates in the pericardial cavity in the course of pericardial effusion, the intrapericardial pressure rises. If the fluid is formed more rapidly than the pericardium can stretch, the rise in pressure may be sufficient to compress the heart in diastole. Cardiac tamponade occurs when the pericardial pressure reaches the level of the diastolic pressure in the heart.

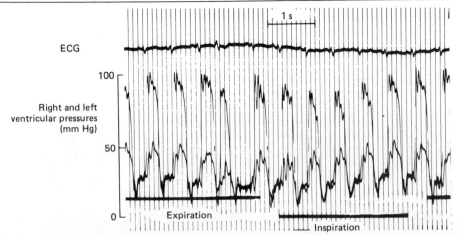

ECG

100

Right and left
ventricular pressures
(mm Hg)

50

0

Expiration

Inspiration

1 s

Figure 3–3. Pulsus paradoxus in right and left ventricular pressure tracings in a patient with chronic constrictive pericarditis.

Since the right-sided pressures are lower than those of the left, the right heart is the first to be compressed. If pericardial fluid is formed slowly, as in myxedema, the pericardium often has time to stretch, and cardiac tamponade may not occur.

In tamponade, the maintenance of cardiac volume and output depend on the level of the venous pressure (right- and left-sided), and the two ventricles compete for blood with which to fill in diastole. Respiration has a marked effect on hemodynamics, with inspiration favoring the right ventricle both by increasing its filling, volume, and output and also by pooling blood in the lungs, decreasing left-sided venous return and occasionally displacing the ventricular septum in severe cases. Conversely, expiration favors the left ventricle, and the extra blood passes from the lungs to the left ventricle as the right ventricle is compressed and left-sided output enhanced. Pulsus paradoxus is the most obvious clinical sign of this process. It does not occur in cardiac tamponade until the pericardial pressure has risen to the level of the right atrial pressure, and it disappears when sufficient fluid is withdrawn to make the pericardial pressure lower than the atrial pressure. The pericardial pressure must rise to equal or exceed that in both the left and the right ventricles before pulsus paradoxus occurs. If the left ventricle is hypertrophied, as in hypertension associated with chronic renal disease, it is less readily compressed by pericardial effusion, and right ventricular tamponade can occur before left ventricular tamponade and pulsus paradoxus appear. Pulsus paradoxus does not occur until filling of both ventricles is impaired, because the reciprocal effect of respiration is an essential part of the mechanism in pericardial tamponade.

EXTRACARDIAC MANIFESTATIONS OF HEART DISEASE

Examination of organs of the body other than the heart can provide important clues in the diagnosis of heart disease.

SKIN & MUCOUS MEMBRANES

The state of the peripheral circulation can be determined by inspection and palpation of the skin. If there is vasoconstriction, the skin will be pale, blue, and cold, with diminished flow in the superficial veins. There may be cold, clammy perspiration in low-output states. If there is widespread vasodilation, as seen in high-output states (Chapter 20) or aortic incompetence, the skin is warm, pink, and moist. The forearm veins are usually distended, and venous flow

is high. Pallor of the skin and mucous membranes suggests anemia, and coarse, dry, scaly skin is seen in myxedema. In scleroderma, the skin is tight, smooth, and shiny. These changes are best seen in the fingers and backs of the hands and in the face over the nose.

Cyanosis

The color of the skin and mucous membranes can reflect the oxygen saturation of the blood. Bluish, cyanotic skin may be due to increased concentration of reduced hemoglobin in the arterial blood, indicating arterial anoxemia, or to reduced blood flow in the skin, leading to pooling of blood in the skin (peripheral cyanosis). The detection of cyanosis and the distinction between central (arterial) and peripheral (venous) cyanosis should be based on measurements of arterial oxygen levels.

With reversed (right-to-left) shunting through a patent ductus arteriosus, mixed venous blood is shunted to the legs, while arterial blood reaches the arms through the left side of the heart. There may be cyanosis and perhaps clubbing of the toes but normal color in the hands and no clubbing of the fingers. This characteristic abnormality is more easily recognized if the arms and legs are compared after a hot bath.

Nodes & Other Skin Lesions

A. Rheumatic Nodules: Rheumatic nodules are seen around the joints in both rheumatic fever and rheumatoid arthritis. They are painless, mobile, subcutaneous lesions measuring up to about 1 cm in diameter, occurring around the elbows, knees, and knuckles and also in the occipital region.

B. Osler's Nodes: Osler's nodes are small, tender, red lesions that should be looked for in the pulp of the fingers and toes and on the palms and soles. They are transient embolic lesions characteristic of infective endocarditis (Chapter 16). They last for 4–5 days and gradually darken before fading and becoming painless. Such lesions seldom, if ever, suppurate.

C. Erythema Nodosum: Erythema nodosum causes pinkish-red, raised, tender lesions on the shins or forearms that represent a nonspecific allergic response to antigens, including streptococcal infections associated with rheumatic fever, coccidioidomycosis, and sarcoidosis.

D. Xanthoma Tuberosum: Xanthoma tuberosum causes pale, yellowish skin lesions that are often superficial extensions of tendinous xanthomas. The lesions are seen on the hands and feet and around the elbows and knees and represent deposits of lipid material in familial hypercholesterolemia.

E. Lesions Associated With Osler's Disease: The lesions of Osler's disease (hereditary hemorrhagic telangiectasia) are also seen on the skin. They are multiple dark-red lesions 1 or 2 mm in diameter that often occur on mucous membranes in the nose and mouth. They may also occur in the viscera and cause hemorrhage. Pulmonary arteriovenous fistulas

(Chapter 19) may occur in association with this condition.

F. Petechiae: Petechiae are due to minute hemorrhages into the skin, resulting from increased capillary fragility. They tend to occur in crops and fade over several days, in contrast to telangiectases, which are permanent.

G. Spider Nevi: Spider nevi, seen in liver disease, are also permanent telangiectatic lesions. They are seen on the skin over the upper part of the body. As their name implies, there is a central body with radiating vascular channels.

EYES

Examination of the conjunctival membranes may detect petechial hemorrhages. An abnormal pupillary reflex in which the reaction to light is lost but the accommodation reaction is retained (**Argyll-Robertson pupil**) is strong evidence for the presence of syphilis, which may involve the cardiovascular system. The presence of a hazy gray ring about 2 mm in width in the cornea (**arcus senilis**) is, as its name implies, commonly seen in older persons. It is of no clinical significance. Direct visual examination of small arteries and arterioles in the fundus offers an important opportunity to assess the condition of the blood vessels, the retina, and the optic disk. The findings and their classification are discussed in Chapter 9. Hemorrhages and embolic phenomena (Roth spots) can also be seen in the retinas of patients with infective endocarditis.

EARS

Inspection of the earlobe may reveal a deep crease at the site shown in Figure 3–4. Ear creases are associated with age and are present in most people in the USA over age 60. However, their occurrence in younger people is associated with a high incidence of premature atherosclerotic changes involving the cerebral, coronary, or aortoiliac vessels. Ear creases are more common in males and are rare in Asians or American Indians of all ages.

NECK

The neck is examined for the nature of the jugular venous pulse and pressure, the timing of the jugular venous pulse in relation to the carotid pulse, and the presence of a goiter. Thyroid swellings are best detected by the examiner standing behind the seated patient, with both hands around the neck. The upward movement of the gland with swallowing is the most important means of identifying a thyroid origin for a palpable mass.

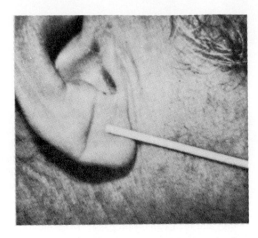

Figure 3–4. The earlobe sign—a deep crease in the lobular portion of the auricle. (Reproduced, with permission, from Frank ST: Aural sign of coronary-artery disease. N Engl J Med 1973;289:327.)

A benign, marked pulsation in the base of the neck on the right side is seen in elderly atherosclerotic patients, more commonly women. It is due to kinking of the right carotid artery resulting from dilation of the aortic arch, which causes the aorta to occupy a higher position in the mediastinum.

Jugular Venous Pulse & Pressure

The level of the venous pressure and the nature of the venous pulse are perhaps the most important observations to be made in the examination of the neck. The internal jugular vein should be examined because it lies deep to the sternocleidomastoid muscle and is in free communication with the right atrium. (The external jugular vein is often easier to see, but it may be constricted as it passes through the fascial planes of the neck and may give an inaccurate assessment of venous events.)

Direct bedside assessment of right atrial pressure requires skill and practice, but it can obviate the need for central venous pressure measurement, which requires use of a catheter. The level of the venous pressure is most important in distinguishing cardiac failure with edema and ascites from hepatic or renal disease with similar findings. Unfortunately, it is often in those patients with highest venous pressures that the examiner fails to note the raised pressure.

The positioning of the patient is most important in examining the veins in the neck. The angle at which the patient is supported in the bed should be adjusted to bring the meniscus of blood in the vein to a level between the clavicles and the angle of the jaw (Figure 3–5). The higher the venous pressure, the more erect the patient should be; patients with severe venous congestion may have to stand up and breathe in deeply in order to bring the level of the meniscus into view. The head should be comfortably supported in

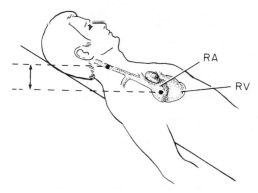

Figure 3–5. Examination of jugular venous pulse and estimation of venous pressure. RA, right atrium; RV, right ventricle. In any body position the sternal angle is 5 cm above the right atrium.

order to relax the neck muscles. Distinguishing arterial from venous pulses in the neck can be difficult. Venous pulses can be palpable; they are diffusely expansile and influenced by respiration. Any movement of the earlobes should be noted, because this is almost always due to venous rather than arterial pulsation. Timing of the venous waves against the carotid pulse is carried out by feeling the artery on the opposite side of the neck or by listening to the heart, and not by feeling the radial pulse. Interpretation of the pulse wave pattern is sometimes facilitated by observing when the venous pressure falls. The first venous trough, the *x* descent, coincides with the carotid arterial pulse. Figure 3–5 illustrates a method of roughly calculating the venous pressure; normally, the pressure is below 10 mm Hg by this method.

Some authorities advocate exerting pressure over the abdomen to distend the neck veins, maintaining that the magnitude of the resulting venous distention (hepatojugular reflux) reflects the level of venous

pulmonary congestion. The results of this techique are shown in Figure 3–6. We believe that although hepatojugular reflux is especially marked in right heart failure, it can also be seen in normal subjects, and that proper positioning of the patient, relaxation with the mouth open, and quiet normal breathing are more important factors in evaluating venous pressure.

A. Normal Venous Pulse: The normal waves seen in the venous pulse in the neck are shown in the first and fourth beats in the tracing in Figure 3–7. The positive waves are *a, c,* and *v,* and the troughs are x_1, x_2, and *y.* The *a* wave is due to atrial contraction. It follows the P wave of the ECG and is absent in atrial fibrillation. The origin of the *c* wave is more controversial. It was originally noted in tracings of the venous pressure in the neck and attributed to the effects of carotid arterial pulsation. When it was also observed in right atrial pressure tracings, however, this explanation became untenable. It is now thought to be due to bulging of the tricuspid valve back into the atrium at the start of ventricular systole. The *v* wave is associated with atrial filling; pressure in the atrium rises to the v peak and falls as the tricuspid valve opens and the atrium empties into the ventricle. The x_1 and x_2 troughs are attributed to descent of the base of the heart during ventricular systole. The backward bulging of the valve interrupts this process to produce the *c* wave. The *c* wave is not always seen. When it is absent, there is a single *x* descent. The *y* descent to the *y* trough is due to atrial emptying, and its rate is influenced by stenosis or insufficiency of the atrioventricular valve.

B. Abnormal or Exaggerated Venous Pulse:
1. Cannon waves– The magnitude of the *a* wave resulting from atrial contraction varies with the PR interval. In the tracing shown in Figure 3–7, all but beats 1 and 4 are ectopic, with the P wave occurring at the start of the QRS complex. The *a* waves associ-

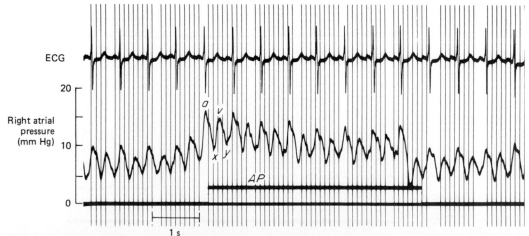

Figure 3–6. ECG and right atrial pressure in a normal subject showing the response to external abdominal compression (AP).

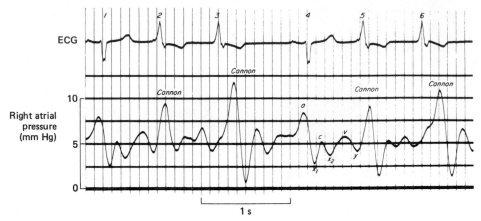

Figure 3–7. Right atrial pressure tracing in a patient with junctional ectopic beats. Beats 1 and 4 are sinus beats and produce normal venous pressure pulses. The other beats are junctional and give rise to cannon waves of varying sizes.

ated with these beats are larger and are referred to as cannon waves because of their explosive appearance when seen in the neck. The largest cannon waves are seen when atrial contraction occurs at a time when the tricuspid valve is closed, as in beats 3 and 6 in the tracing. Here the P wave is buried in the QRS complex, and large cannon waves can be seen. Irregular cannon waves of this type are also seen in complete atrioventricular block with atrioventricular dissociation. Regular cannon waves are seen in junctional (nodal) tachycardia, in which atrial contraction occurs late via an impulse passing in a retrograde manner from the atrioventricular node.

2. Giant a wave– The *a* wave is increased in force and amplitude in the presence of right ventricular hypertrophy. It is best seen as the "giant *a* wave" of pulmonary stenosis, shown in Figure 3–8, which is a short, sharp, flicking wave occurring just before ventricular systole. A large *a* wave is also seen in pul-

monary hypertension and in tricuspid valve disease with stenosis.

3. Giant v wave– A large *v* wave is seen in patients with tricuspid incompetence, especially when atrial fibrillation is present, as in the tracing in Figure 3–9. Tricuspid incompetence is seldom seen in patients with sinus rhythm, but when it occurs, *a, x, v,* and *y* peaks and troughs are present. The *x* descent is usually absent in patients with either tricuspid incompetence or pericardial constriction, and the *y* descent may be the principal event in the venous pulse.

4. Effect of inspiration– Inspiration increases venous return and may stretch the tricuspid valve and make it incompetent, thus increasing the height of the *v* wave and the depth of the *y* trough, as shown in Figure 3–9. When right heart filling is severely impaired, inspiration causes a rise in venous pressure, as shown in Figure 3–10. This rise is known as Kussmaul's sign, and it is seen in pericardial constric-

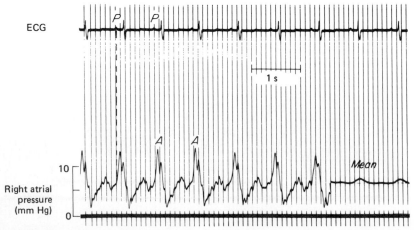

Figure 3–8. Right atrial pressure tracing showing giant *a* wave (A) in a patient with severe pulmonary stenosis. The *a* wave follows the P wave of the ECG.

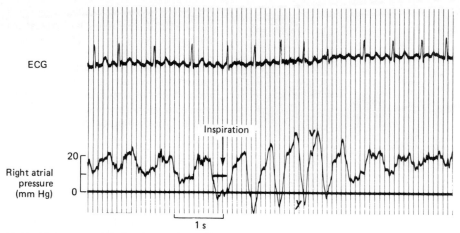

Figure 3–9. Right atrial pressure tracing in a patient with tricuspid incompetence and atrial fibrillation. The *v* peak and the *y* trough are exaggerated during inspiration.

tion and severe right heart failure. The overfilled right heart cannot accommodate the increased venous return associated with the inspiratory fall in intrathoracic pressure. The venous pressure therefore shows a rise with inspiration, instead of the normal fall. In tricuspid incompetence, it is the amplitude of the pulsations that tends to increase (Figure 3–9) rather than the mean pressure, as in pericardial disease (Figure 3–10).

ARMS

Brachial and radial pulses should be compared between the two arms, and they should also be compared with the femoral pulses. The fingers, nails, and palms should be examined for evidence of embolism.

FINGERS

Clubbing of the fingers and nail beds (Figure 3–11) is seen in cyanotic congenital heart lesions, infective endocarditis, cor pulmonale, and occasionally in left atrial myxoma. Clubbing of the fingers is also seen in chronic pulmonary infections, cirrhosis of the liver, and bronchial carcinoma. In the latter, severe clubbing with hypertrophic osteoarthropathy may occur; clubbing is sometimes unilateral and may disappear after resection of the tumor.

Splinter hemorrhages in the nail beds should be sought as an indication of endocarditis, although it should be noted that similar findings may sometimes be seen in normal people. Other finger abnormalities associated with congenital heart disease include arachnodactyly, in which the fingers are long and

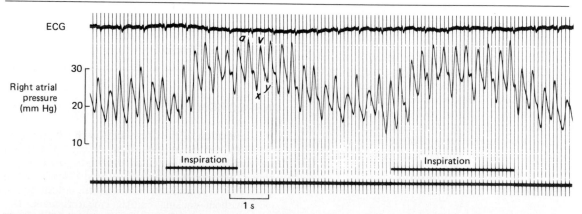

Figure 3–10. ECG and right atrial pressure tracings in a patient with constrictive pericarditis, showing inspiratory increase in pressure (Kussmaul's sign).

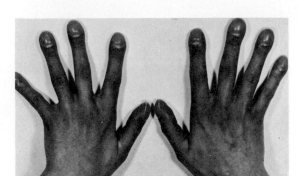

Figure 3–11. Clubbing of the fingers in a patient with congenital heart disease.

spidery. This is seen in Marfan's syndrome and in some patients with atrial septal defect. Supernumerary digits and skeletal forearm anomalies are seen in Holt-Oram syndrome with atrial septal defects.

LUNGS

Examination of the lungs in patients with heart disease focuses on the detection of pleural fluid and a search for rales or crackles and crepitations, especially at the base of the lungs posteriorly. Such findings reflect raised pulmonary venous pressure. Added sounds are noted when there is fluid in the alveoli, but the signs are not specific, and they may be absent in some cases of obvious pulmonary edema. They are often due to other causes. Pleural effusion due to heart failure is usually bilateral; in unilateral cases, it is commoner on the side on which the subject habitually lies. Evidence of collapse of the left lower lobe should be sought in patients with marked left atrial enlargement.

BACK

Some cardiac murmurs are heard well in the back. The best examples are the murmurs of coarctation of the aorta, increased bronchial collateral flow, and peripheral pulmonary artery stenosis; the last is often heard well in the axilla as well. Evidence of systemic collateral vessels in coarctation of the aorta is also well seen and felt in the back. Large, pulsating vessels can be detected near the angles of the scapulas. Edema of the lumbar region and sacrum is also sought while the physician examines the patient's back.

ABDOMEN

In examining the abdomen, enlargement and tenderness of the liver and spleen should be sought as evidence of systemic venous congestion. With light palpation and sometimes with visual inspection, venous pulsation of the liver can be seen with severe tricuspid insufficiency. In infective endocarditis, the spleen may also be enlarged and be the site of a friction rub. Ascites and pitting edema of the ankles are evidence of congestive heart failure. Disproportionate ascites with minimal leg edema suggests pericardial constriction or prolonged diuretic therapy.

LOWER EXTREMITIES

In examining the lower extremities, the physician palpates the femoral pulse; if its palpability is in question or if the patient is hypertensive, it is useful to palpate the right radial artery and the femoral artery together and look for delay between the radial and femoral pulse. A decrease in the femoral artery pulse compared with the radial artery pulse can be seen in coarctation of the aorta. Absence of femoral pulsations and inequality between the two sides may suggest embolic disease or aortic dissection. Calf tenderness and pain on dorsiflexion of the foot (**Homans' sign**) suggest venous thrombosis. Clubbing of the toes is seen in cyanotic congenital heart disease. In addition to looking for edema of the sacrum, the examiner should check for edema in the flanks and medial aspects of the thighs in bedridden patients.

URINE

Examination of the urine is an important adjunct to the physical examination. Proteinuria should be sought in heart failure, in hypertensive patients, and in primary renal disease. Hematuria suggests renal infarction; if microscopic, infective endocarditis. Specific gravity should be recorded and the urinary sediment examined for casts and other abnormalities.

EXAMINATION OF THE HEART & CHEST

INSPECTION

Examination of the chest starts with inspection of the shape and movements of the thorax and a search for visible pulsations. Chest deformities such as kyphosis and scoliosis may cause heart disease, but in general, it is remarkable how a severe deformity can exist without causing cardiac embarrassment. Depressed sternum with pectus excavatum is obvious on inspection, and although it is often associated with mitral valve prolapse, it is seldom of more than cosmetic importance. The left parasternal area sometimes bulges in patients who have had heart disease since early in life. Ventricular septal defect is the commonest lesion causing this sign.

Visible Pulsations

The cardiac impulse can sometimes be seen in normal subjects either in the area of the left nipple or in the epigastrium. Pulsation in the second or third left interspace over the right ventricular outflow tract can be seen in normal thin persons, but it can also suggest pulmonary hypertension or increased pulmonary blood flow. Pulsation to the right of the sternum is always abnormal, and when seen in the second or third interspace, it indicates aneurysmal dilation of the ascending aorta.

Periodic Breathing

Abnormalities of respiratory rhythm should be noted during inspection of the chest. The commonest abnormality is periodic breathing (**Cheyne-Stokes breathing**). This can occur in normal subjects at high altitude and may also be seen after head injuries. When it is due to heart disease, the cycle of hyperventilation followed by hypoventilation and apnea with subsequent gradual increase of ventilation lasts 40–120 seconds. The phenomenon results from oscillation of the feedback control mechanisms regulating respiration. In a patient with severe ventricular failure, there is an abnormal lag between the timing of the neurologic stimulus to breathe and the arrival back at the control center in the brain of the humoral signal resulting from respiratory changes in blood gases following the breath. This lag is thought to play an important part in the mechanism of periodic breathing. The length of the lung-to-brain circulation time determines the length of the period of one cycle. By following this measurement, the examiner can note the progress of left ventricular failure.

Periodic breathing is usually a manifestation of hyper- rather than hypoventilation and is generally abolished by giving oxygen, CO_2, or aminophylline. It tends to occur at night when sensory input is low and to disappear when a mouthpiece and nose clip are used to obtain spirometric tracings.

In the classic description of Cheyne-Stokes breathing, apnea was present, but this feature is not necessarily a component.

PALPATION

Palpation of the chest is used to confirm the presence of pulsations that have been noted on inspection. The cardiac impulse is routinely sought and can be elicited by having the patient roll over to the left side. The examiner should note the nature of the impulse and distinguish between the feel of a large left ventri-

cle and a right ventricle. The right ventricular impulse is more lifting than the left, is perceived as being farther from the hand, and less readily moves the examining fingers.

The feel of a ventricle with a large stroke volume should be distinguished from the feel of a hypertrophied ventricle. Hypertrophy imparts a forceful sustained thrust (heave) with relatively little movement of the examiner's hand, whereas increased stroke volume gives a more dynamic movement of greater amplitude. A "tapping" impulse is found in patients with mitral valve disease. This reflects the palpable vibrations of a loud first heart sound felt at the apex. The point of maximal apical impulse and the carotid artery should be palpated simultaneously. Normally, the apex beat collapses before the carotid pulse. If the apex beat is sustained beyond the carotid pulse, left ventricular hypertrophy is probably present.

Position of Apex Beat

The position of the apex beat is the point farthest downward and outward at which the cardiac impulse can be clearly felt. It should always be located by palpation. Before the determination of cardiac size by chest radiography became routine, the position of the apex beat in the absence of lung disease was the most important measure of heart size. Its position should be described in relation to the intercostal space and to the distance from the midline, the nipple, or the midclavicular, anterior axillary, or midaxillary lines. Palpation of the base of the heart may detect an impulse caused by closure of the aortic or pulmonary valves or arising from an aneurysm. The findings should be interpreted in light of the patient's build.

Thrills

Thrills are palpable, sustained, high-frequency vibrations associated with the same disturbances of flow that cause heart murmurs. The significance of palpable thrills is similar to that of cardiac murmurs and is discussed below (see Auscultation). A murmur that is associated with a thrill is likely to have an organic cause.

Palpable Impulses

Palpable impulses over the precordium must be interpreted in light of their associated findings; it is not always possible to be certain of their origin. In a patient with mitral incompetence, a substernal impulse may be due to systolic expansion of the left atrium rather than to right ventricular overactivity. Epigastric pulsations may arise from the abdominal aorta or the right ventricle or be transmitted from the right atrium to an enlarged liver in tricuspid incompetence.

Paradoxic rocking impulses can sometimes be felt after myocardial infarction, especially when a left ventricular aneurysm is present. When the aneurysm involves the free ventricular wall, the outward motion of the aneurysmal sac can sometimes be felt in early systole.

Palpable Gallops

The vibrations produced by loud third and fourth heart sounds can often be felt. If the sounds are of very low pitch, the gallop may be easier to appreciate on palpation than on auscultation. In most cases in which a gallop is palpable, it is also audible.

PERCUSSION

Percussion of the heart has virtually no place in physical examination today because it is open to error and because the size of the heart is better determined by chest radiography.

AUSCULTATION

Auscultation of the heart is performed with a properly fitting stethoscope that uses either an open bell or a closed diaphragm as the means of coupling the examiner's ear to the patient's chest. The diaphragm transmits more sound and is better for listening to high-pitched sounds (such as the second heart sound) and murmurs. The bell is better for low-pitched noises, and variation of the pressure of the bell on the skin can be used to alter the intensity of the sounds and murmurs heard. Auscultation focuses more on the timing of events within the cardiac cycle than on their intensity or the site at which they are heard best. It is important to move the chest piece of the stethoscope to sites where specific sounds can best be heard. Do not restrict examination to the classic "valvular" areas described in older textbooks. Listen selectively (eg, to heart sounds or murmurs, but not both at once).

Heart Sounds

The timing of the different heart sounds is diagrammatically shown in Figure 3–12. First and second heart sounds are normally audible, and an early (diastolic gallop) third sound is often present in children and young adults. In addition, a fourth (atrial) sound can sometimes be recorded by phonocardiography.

A. First Heart Sound: The first heart sound (S_1) is attributed to tensing of the mitral and tricuspid valves at the start of ventricular systole. The two components can sometimes be clearly distinguished, and although the right atrial contraction precedes the left, the mitral valve tenses before the tricuspid, and the first component of the first heart sound is mitral in origin. The position of the valve leaflets at the time of the start of systole influences the loudness of the first sound. As heard at the apex, the first heart sound is generally louder, longer, and lower pitched than the

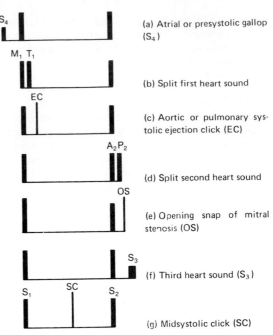

Figure 3–12. Timing of the different heart sounds and added sounds. (Modified and reproduced, with permission, from Wood P: *Diseases of the Heart and Circulation,* 3rd ed. Lippincott, 1968.)

second heart sound. In normal resting subjects, the atrioventricular valve leaflets have drifted into an almost closed position by the time systole starts, because diastolic flow is more or less complete by late diastole. Atrial contraction tends to reopen the valves. Consequently, the length of the PR interval affects the loudness of the first sound. When flow across an atrioventricular valve is increased for any reason or lasts longer than normal, the valve tends to shut from a more open position and produces more noise. The situation is similar to that encountered in closing an open door: the wider the door stands open before it is slammed shut, the louder the resulting noise. Thus, a loud first sound is heard in patients who are exercising, in patients with mitral stenosis in whom flow lasts throughout the whole of diastole, and in patients with left-to-right shunts and increased atrioventricular flow, eg, atrial septal defect. In complete atrioventricular block in which the PR interval varies, the loudness of the first sound varies, being loudest when the PR interval is slightly shortened to about 0.1 s, as shown in Figure 3–13.

B. Second Heart Sound: The second heart sound (S_2) is due to closure of the aortic and pulmonary valves and normally consists of two components (Figure 3–14). The earlier component (A_2) is normally aortic in origin; the later one arises from the pulmonary valve (P_2). The location at which the second heart sound is best heard varies. It is normally heard well at the base of the heart and is almost always

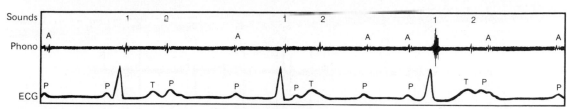

Figure 3–13. Phonocardiogram and ECG showing intensity of first sound varying with position of P wave on the ECG and atrial sound in complete atrioventricular block. Extreme shortening of the PR interval is not associated with a loud first heart sound. (Courtesy of Roche Laboratories Division of Hoffman-La Roche, Inc.)

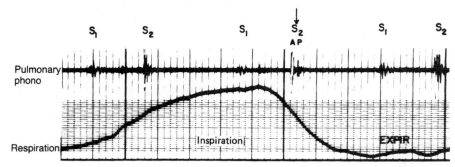

Figure 3–14. Phonocardiogram taken from the pulmonary area in a healthy 28-year-old man. It shows that splitting of the second sound becomes distinct after inspiration. The curve of respiration moves upward during inspiration. (Reproduced, with permission, from Dressler W: *Clinical Aids in Cardiac Diagnosis.* Grune & Stratton, 1970.)

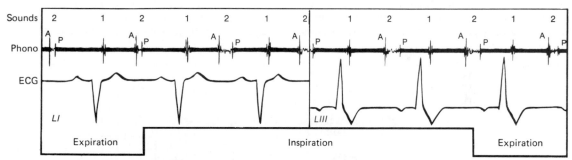

Figure 3–15. Phonocardiogram showing widely split second sound in right bundle branch block with P_2 even later on inspiration. (Courtesy of Roche Laboratories Division of Hoffman-La Roche, Inc.)

louder than the first sound in that area. It is sometimes necessary to listen at the apex or even in the epigastrium. Hearing the pulmonary valve closure sound at the apex suggests the presence of pulmonary hypertension.

1. Splitting of the second heart sound– Right and left ventricular stroke volumes vary reciprocally with quiet respiration when there is adequate venous return. Inspiration favors right ventricular output, and expiration favors left ventricular output. Thus, in normal subjects resting quietly and breathing easily, the time of pulmonary valve closure with inspiration can be shown to move later in the cardiac cycle by 0.02–0.04 s, as seen in Figure 3–15. Increased filling of the right heart is associated with a more negative

pressure within the thorax during inspiration, which increases right ventricular output in accordance with the Frank-Starling mechanism. The extra output has a longer ejection time; consequently, the pulmonary valve closure sound is delayed. The opposite occurs with aortic valve closure during expiration, but the magnitude of the changes is less. Thus, although both the aortic and pulmonary components of the second heart sound move, the pulmonary component moves more. The net effect is that the interval between the two components of the second sound increases with inspiration and then decreases until the interval between the two sounds is not appreciable during expiration. The process is conventionally referred to as **physiologic splitting of the second heart sound.**

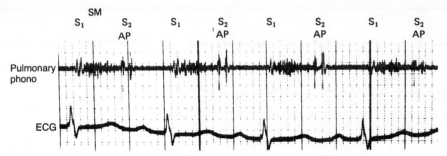

Figure 3–16. Phonocardiogram from the pulmonary area in a patient with ostium secundum atrial septal defect showing wide splitting of the second heart sound that remained constant although normal breathing was not interrupted while the phonocardiogram was obtained. (SM, systolic murmur.) (Reproduced, with permission,from Dressler W: *Clinical Aids in Cardiac Diagnosis.* Grune & Stratton, 1970.)

When right ventricular systole is prolonged because of right bundle branch block, pulmonary valve closure is delayed. In this case, both the first and the second heart sounds tend to be split throughout the respiratory cycle, with the split widening further with inspiration (Figure 3–15).

When right ventricular stroke volume is increased and venous return is high, as in atrial septal defect with large pulmonary blood flow, respiration has relatively little effect on right ventricular output. In this case, pulmonary valve closure is greatly delayed and the second sound is widely split; respiration has no effect, and the split is "fixed" even during expiration (Figure 3–16). Splitting of the second heart sound is almost always found in atrial septal defect with left-to-right shunt, but the finding of a **fixed split** is indicative of a significant left-to-right shunt. If the venous return is reduced when the patient stands up, the splitting of the second sound will become more normal, becoming either movable with respiration or less widely split.

2. Paradoxic splitting of the second sound– When left ventricular contraction is prolonged (eg, poor contractility, aortic stenosis), aortic valve closure is delayed and occurs after pulmonary closure. Aortic valve closure can be identified by timing it against the dicrotic notch of the carotid artery tracing (Figure 3–17). In paradoxic splitting, aortic and pul-

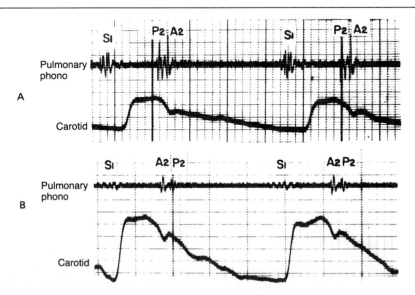

Figure 3–17. Paradoxic splitting of S_2 in a 55-year-old patient with Stokes-Adams syndrome with artificial pacing. **A:** The electrical pacemaker is in the right ventricle. The phonocardiogram shows splitting of the second sound. Comparison with the carotid pulse shows that the aortic element, which occurs 0.03 s prior to the dicrotic notch, follows the pulmonary component. **B:** The electrical pacemaker is in the left ventricle. The aortic element now precedes the pulmonary component of the second sound. (Reproduced, with permission, from Dressler W: *Clinical Aids in Cardiac Diagnosis.* Grune & Stratton, 1970.)

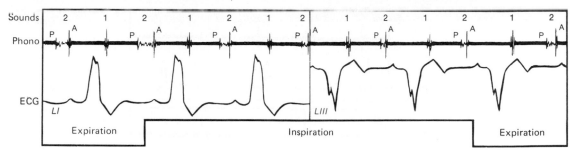

Figure 3–18. Phonocardiogram showing paradoxic splitting (split on expiration, narrower on inspiration) in left bundle branch block. (Courtesy of Roche Laboratories Division of Hoffman-La Roche, Inc.)

monary valve closure sounds coincide toward the end of inspiration, and splitting is greatest during expiration. This is also referred to as "reversed" splitting of the second sound and is found in patients with left bundle branch block, in aortic stenosis, in hypertrophic cardiomyopathy, and in any other condition that greatly overloads the left ventricle. The effect of respiration on the second heart sound in paradoxic splitting is shown in Figure 3–18.

3. Intensity– Aortic valve closure tends to be delayed and diminished in aortic stenosis and may be absent when the lesion is severe. The second heart sound is also important in patients with pulmonary stenosis. Here the timing and intensity of the sound vary with the severity of the stenosis. In mild cases, the second sound is normal. In cases with more severe stenosis, the second sound is delayed and diminished because pulmonary blood flow is less (Figure 3–19). Thus, in severe cases the sound of pulmonary valve closure is inaudible. However, it can usually be detected by phonocardiography and is shown to occur up to 0.12 s after aortic valve closure.

The loudness of each component of the second sound varies with the pressure in the corresponding vessel. Thus, a loud aortic valve closure sound is heard in systemic hypertension, and a loud pulmonary second sound in pulmonary hypertension (Figure

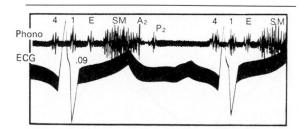

Figure 3–19. Phonocardiogram from a patient with pulmonary stenosis showing the typical presystolic gallop (4), ejection click (E), systolic murmur (SM), and delayed pulmonary valve closure sound (P_2). Recorded at left sternal border. (Courtesy of Roche Laboratories Division of Hoffman-La Roche, Inc.)

3–20). Loudness of the components of the second sound is not an accurate indicator of pressure, which should be directly measured in doubtful cases.

The character of the aortic valve closure sound is altered in patients with aortic disease. In patients with syphilitic aortitis and other diseases that dilate the root of the aorta, aortic valve closure has a high-pitched, drum-like, "tambour" quality. The reason for this is not known. In systemic hypertension, the aortic valve closure sound is not only loud but also clear and ringing.

C. Third Heart Sound: The third heart sound (S_3) shown in Figure 3–21 is associated with ventricular filling. It is a dull, low-pitched, localized sound occurring about 0.12–0.16 s after the second sound. If the sound arises from the right heart, it increases in intensity during inspiration and is heard at the lower sternal edge. Conversely, a left-sided third sound increases on expiration. It is not clear why this sound is normally present in young persons and disappears with age. An audible third heart sound is also found when there is an abnormally large diastolic flow into a normal ventricle or a normal flow into an abnormal ventricle. The former occurs in patients with left-to-right shunt and also occurs in mitral or tricuspid incompetence. The latter is seen in patients with left or, less commonly, right ventricular disease.

D. Fourth Heart Sound: The fourth heart sound (S_4) results from atrial contraction and is thought to be a filling sound arising within the ventricle. Although it can often be recorded by phonocardiography, it is not normally audible. A fourth heart sound is heard shortly before the first heart sound in any condition in which the force of either the right or the left atrial contraction is increased. This means that atrial sounds are heard in conditions in which the ventricle is working against high pressure and the atria are contracting against increased resistance, as shown in Figure 3–22. Thus, pulmonary or aortic stenosis and pulmonary or systemic hypertension are the commonest causes of a fourth heart sound. A fourth heart sound is also often audible during an episode of angina pectoris. Here, too, the ventricular compliance is reduced, and the left atrium contracts

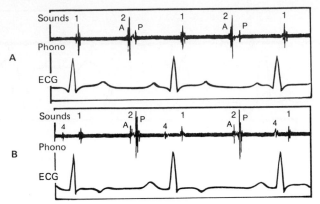

Figure 3–20. **A:** Phonocardiogram demonstrating loud aortic valve closure sound (A_2) in systemic hypertension. **B:** Phonocardiogram demonstrating loud pulmonary valve closure sound (P2) in pulmonary hypertension. (Courtesy of Roche Laboratories Division of Hoffman-La Roche, Inc.)

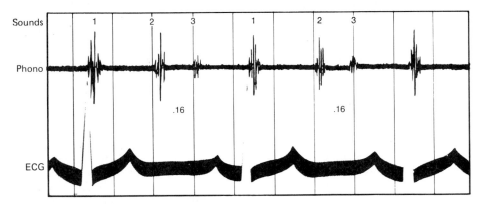

Figure 3–21. Phonocardiogram showing typical third heart sound (S_3). It follows the second sound (S_2) by 0.16 s. (Courtesy of Roche Laboratories Division of Hoffman-La Roche, Inc.)

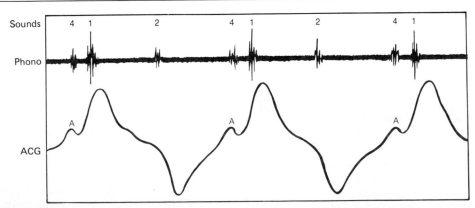

Figure 3–22. Phonocardiogram showing a fourth heart sound (S_4) and its relation to first sound (S_1). Below, an apexcardiogram (ACG) shows the occurrence of the wave of atrial contraction together with the presystolic gallop sound. (Courtesy of Roche Laboratories Division of Hoffman-La Roche, Inc.)

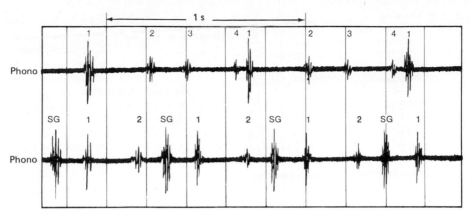

Figure 3–23. The phonocardiographic strip above shows separate presystolic and diastolic gallop; the strip below shows their fusion, which results in a summation gallop (SG). (Courtesy of Roche Laboratories Division of Hoffman-La Roche, Inc.)

against increased resistance. Right and left atrial sounds can often be distinguished on the basis of their response to respiration and the site where they are most clearly heard.

E. Gallop Rhythm: When a third or a fourth heart sound is present, the extra heart sounds give rise to a gallop, or triple, rhythm. When the extra sound is presystolic, it is difficult to distinguish the rhythm from that of a split first sound or even an ejection click following the first sound. The presystolic gallop is said to have the cadence of the word "Tennessee," whereas diastolic gallop has been likened to "Kentucky." In some cases, both third and fourth heart sounds can be heard. If the heart rate is rapid—about 120/min—the third and fourth sounds may be superimposed, giving rise to summation gallop (Figure 3–23). In this case, two inaudible sounds may combine to give an audible sound. It is possible to slow the heart rate by carotid sinus massage (see below) and listen to hear whether the gallop disappears or whether either the third or the fourth sound or both can be distinguished; this causes a quadruple rhythm.

A prominent filling sound is also heard in patients with impaired ventricular filling in pericardial constriction. This can be as loud a sound as the second heart sound and is sometimes called a "pericardial knock." It is thought to be caused by the sudden cessation of right ventricular filling.

A loud early diastolic sound is sometimes heard in left atrial myxoma. It is attributed to a pedunculated tumor falling into the mitral orifice as cardiac filling starts. The sudden change in rate of filling of the ventricle due to the tumor's obstruction creates the sound. This sound has been called "tumor plop."

F. Opening Snap: The opening snap of the mitral valve heard in patients with rheumatic mitral stenosis is also considered as a heart sound. It is heard 0.06–0.12 s after the second heart sound and is shown in Figure 3–24. It may be the loudest and most widely heard sound in the cardiac cycle and is heard best in the third or fourth left interspace just inside the apex in most cases.

The interval between the second heart sound and the opening snap can vary with posture, decreasing

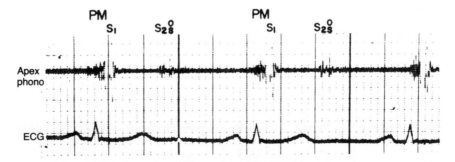

Figure 3–24. From a 24-year-old woman with mitral stenosis and sinus rhythm. The first sound (S_1) shows high-amplitude vibrations that merge with a presystolic murmur (PM). There is also a mitral opening snap (OS). The opening snap occurs about 0.06 s after the onset of S_2. (Reproduced, with permission, from Dressler W: *Clinical Aids in Cardiac Diagnosis.* Grune & Stratton, 1970.)

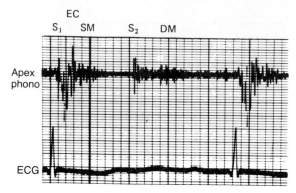

Figure 3–25. Systolic ejection click and murmur in a patient with rheumatic aortic regurgitation. The diastolic murmur is most distinct in the apical area. A phonocardiogram taken from that region shows a first sound of marked intensity. It is closely followed by a systolic murmur (SM) that starts with an ejection click (EC). The systolic murmur occupies the first half of systole. The second sound is immediately followed by a diastolic murmur that extends over the entire diastolic phase. (Reproduced, with permission, from Dressler W: *Clinical Aids in Cardiac Diagnosis.* Grune & Stratton, 1970.)

when the patient stands up and the left atrial pressure falls. It also varies with the severity of mitral stenosis. The higher the left atrial pressure when the mitral valve opens, the closer the opening snap to the aortic sound (A_2) and the shorter the A_2 to the opening-snap interval.

G. Systolic Clicks: Extra intracardiac sounds are also heard during systole. These, like the opening snap, arise from valves. The sound is probably generated by sudden resistance of the valve to further opening, thus suddenly decreasing the velocity of blood moving through the valve and causing the entire cardiohemic system to vibrate. The commonest is the systolic ejection click, which can arise from either the aortic or the pulmonary valve. The click occurs early in systole, about 0.02 s after the first sound. It usually ushers in a systolic ejection murmur, as shown in Figure 3–25. Ejection clicks commonly occur when dilation of the great vessel (aorta or pulmonary artery) with which they are associated is combined with normal or increased flow through the vessel. A pulmo-

nary ejection click is louder during expiration because tension in the valve structures is less when intrathoracic pressure is less negative. Ejection clicks are sometimes heard in normal subjects but are most common in patients with insignificant or mild stenosis of the valve. A different variety of systolic click is heard in patients with insignificant mitral disease, as shown in Figure 3–26. The clicks, which may be multiple, occur in mid or even late systole and may precede, follow, or accompany the late systolic murmur heard in this lesion (**click-murmur syndrome).** In some cases, the click occurs without any murmur. The basic lesion is prolapse of the mitral valve cusp, and although the sound is thought to originate in the valve, the exact mechanism of its production is not known.

Heart Murmurs

Cardiac murmurs are thought to result from disturbances of normal blood flow patterns in the heart and great vessels. They are classified on the basis of their timing as systolic, diastolic, and continuous murmurs. The timing of the principal heart murmurs is shown diagrammatically in Figure 3–27.

A. Systolic Murmurs: Systolic murmurs are generally less significant than diastolic murmurs and may occur in patients in whom no evidence of heart disease can be found.

1. Ejection murmurs– An ejection murmur begins when flow starts in one of the great vessels and finishes before the time of valve closure. It thus starts after the first heart sound and ends before the second heart sound. Murmurs of this type do not necessarily indicate the presence of heart disease and may be "innocent." An abnormally large flow through a normal valve may cause a systolic ejection murmur. Trained athletes with slow heart rates may have systolic murmurs, especially when they are examined while supine. The murmur usually disappears when the heart rate increases as the subject stands up or exercises. However, care must be taken in interpreting new murmurs in adults as "innocent," because the murmur may signify early aortic stenosis. Systolic ejection murmurs can be heard in high-output states such as anemia, pregnancy, or thyrotoxicosis and also in patients with dilated aortic root due to athero-

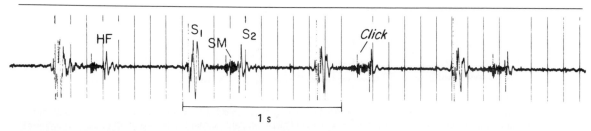

Figure 3–26. Apical high-frequency (HF) phonocardiogram showing late systolic click and murmur (SM) in a patient with hemodynamically insignificant mitral incompetence.

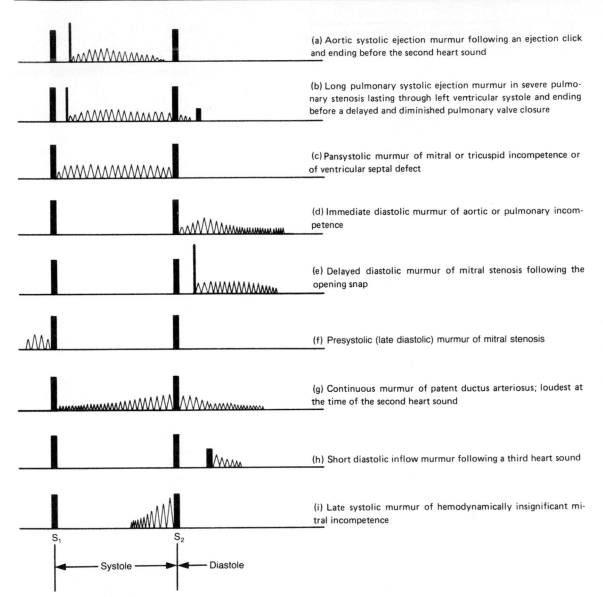

(a) Aortic systolic ejection murmur following an ejection click and ending before the second heart sound

(b) Long pulmonary systolic ejection murmur in severe pulmonary stenosis lasting through left ventricular systole and ending before a delayed and diminished pulmonary valve closure

(c) Pansystolic murmur of mitral or tricuspid incompetence or of ventricular septal defect

(d) Immediate diastolic murmur of aortic or pulmonary incompetence

(e) Delayed diastolic murmur of mitral stenosis following the opening snap

(f) Presystolic (late diastolic) murmur of mitral stenosis

(g) Continuous murmur of patent ductus arteriosus; loudest at the time of the second heart sound

(h) Short diastolic inflow murmur following a third heart sound

(i) Late systolic murmur of hemodynamically insignificant mitral incompetence

S_1 S_2

Systole — Diastole

Figure 3–27. The timing of the principal cardiac murmurs. (Modified and reproduced, with permission, from Wood P: *Diseases of the Heart and Circulation,* 3rd ed. Lippincott, 1968.)

sclerosis, hypertension, syphilis, or other forms of aortitis. They occur when there is a high stroke volume, as in complete atrioventricular block with bradycardia. Increased flow through the pulmonary valve occurs in patients with left-to-right shunts, especially in atrial septal defect, and a systolic ejection murmur is virtually always found in such conditions (Figure 3–28).

The most important causes of systolic ejection murmurs are aortic and pulmonary stenoses at a valvular level. The intensity and duration of such murmurs vary with the severity of the stenosis and with the stroke volume. When the stroke volume is low, the murmur may be of low intensity, and it does not last as long as it does when there is normal flow. Because a systolic ejection murmur can also occur when the stenosis is mild and the valve is merely thickened, it is unwise to base any assessment of the severity of the stenosis on the intensity of the murmur.

2. Pansystolic murmurs– Pansystolic (holosystolic) murmurs start with the first sound and continue up to the second sound, as shown in Figure 3–29. They are commonly due to incompetence of the mitral or tricuspid valve. The valve leaks throughout systole, and the relatively high pressure difference across the valve accounts for the murmur. The mur-

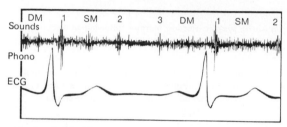

Figure 3–28. Phonocardiogram in atrial septal defect showing a systolic ejection murmur (SM), split second sound, and tricuspid diastolic murmur (DM). (Courtesy of Roche Laboratories Division of Hoffman-La Roche, Inc.)

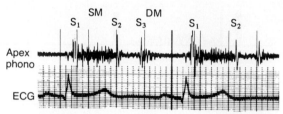

Figure 3–30. Pansystolic murmur (SM) and third heart sound (3) recorded at left sternal border in a patient with ventricular septal defect. (Courtesy of Roche Laboratories Division of Hoffman-La Roche, Inc.)

mur is high-pitched and more musical (of purer tone) than an ejection murmur. A similar murmur is heard when there is flow across a ventricular septal defect with a large pressure difference between the two ventricles (Figure 3–30).

3. Late systolic murmurs– Mitral incompetence can also result in a late systolic murmur that increases in intensity up to the second sound, as shown in Figure 3–26. The murmur does not begin until enough prolapse of the mitral leaflet has occurred to lose coaptation with the other leaflet and form a regurgitant orifice. This murmur has a peculiar quality, and inexperienced observers may find it difficult to time. Once recognized, it is never forgotten. This late systolic murmur may become pansystolic when the degree of incompetence increases, eg, when peripheral resistance is increased during the overshoot that occurs following Valsalva's maneuver.

4. Other systolic murmurs– Although in theory it is easy to classify murmurs as ejection or pansystolic, it may be difficult to make this distinction in practice. In some cases, the murmur exhibits features of both varieties, and it varies in timing at different sites. In infundibular stenosis involving the outflow tract of the right ventricle or in hypertrophic obstructive cardiomyopathy, which produces a rather similar lesion in the left ventricle, there is usually a harsh murmur that lasts throughout systole but peaks in intensity in the middle of systole, when flow is greatest

(Figure 3–31). Similarly, when pulmonary stenosis and ventricular septal defect coexist, the murmur has characteristics of both pansystolic and ejection murmurs.

A special type of systolic murmur may occur in coarctation of the aorta or peripheral pulmonary arterial stenosis. In these conditions, there may be a murmur late in systole owing to the late peaking of flow across the narrowing in the vessel. In coarctation, there may also be a systolic murmur that lasts longer and is due to flow through collateral vessels in the chest wall that have developed in response to the lesion. This murmur is similar to that of bronchial collateral flow, which is heard in patients who have markedly reduced flow to the lungs via the pulmonary artery, as in pulmonary atresia. This systolic murmur also resembles the bruit heard over an arteriovenous fistula or over an extremely active toxic goiter. Systolic bruits are also heard over stenotic lesions in peripheral vessels. Carotid arterial and renal arterial stenotic lesions are the most important examples. These murmurs can be systolic or may extend into diastole in timing and are ejection in character. They tend to occur late in the cardiac cycle.

B. Diastolic Murmurs: Diastolic murmurs are almost always due to significant lesions, though they can rarely occur in severe anemia. They are either **immediate,** caused by incompetence of the aortic or pulmonary valve, or **delayed,** caused by actual or

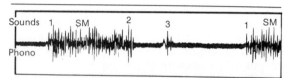

Figure 3–29. Pansystolic murmur in a 25-year-old woman with a rheumatic lesion of the mitral valve. Mitral incompetence is dominant. The phonocardiogram shows a pansystolic murmur (SM) and a third heart sound (S_3) that is followed by a short diastolic murmur (DM). (Reproduced, with permission, from Dressler W: *Clinical Aids in Cardiac Diagnosis.* Grune & Stratton, 1970.)

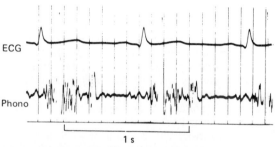

Figure 3–31. Long pansystolic ejection murmur in hypertrophic obstructive cardiomyopathy.

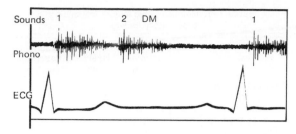

Figure 3–32. Phonocardiogram showing typical diastolic murmur in aortic incompetence and, in this instance, a systolic murmur although no aortic stenosis is present. (Courtesy of Roche Laboratories Division of Hoffman-La Roche, Inc.)

relative mitral or tricuspid stenosis. A special form of diastolic murmur that is commonest in mitral stenosis is the **atrial systolic (presystolic) murmur.**

1. Immediate (early diastolic) murmurs– Immediate, or early, diastolic murmurs start immediately after the time of closure of the valve, as shown in Figure 3–32. They decrease in intensity during diastole and are high-pitched and difficult to hear. They are heard best using the diaphragm of the stethoscope, with the subject sitting up and leaning forward and the breath held in expiration. These murmurs are heard on either side of the sternum in the third, fourth, and fifth interspaces. Their duration is roughly related to the degree of aortic or pulmonary valvular incompetence. Similar murmurs are heard when there is diastolic flow from the aorta into any low-pressure chamber, eg, the right ventricle or an atrium.

2. Delayed (middiastolic) murmurs– The delayed, or middiastolic, murmur does not start until the ventricular pressure has fallen below the level of the atrial pressure. There is thus a sound-free interval between the second heart sound and the start of the murmur, as shown in Figure 3–29. The murmur is low-pitched and rumbling, and its duration is related

to the severity of the stenosis and the size of the stroke volume. Mitral stenosis is the commonest cause of such a murmur; patent ductus arteriosus and ventricular septal defect on the left side and atrial septal defect and tricuspid stenosis on the right side are other causes. An example of a tricuspid flow murmur in a patient with atrial defect is shown in Figure 3–28. Pure tricuspid stenosis is extremely rare, but mixed incompetence and stenosis occasionally gives rise to a delayed diastolic murmur. The right-sided murmurs increase with inspiration and are heard near the sternum. The left-sided murmurs are best heard with the patient lying in the left lateral position and the stethoscope applied directly over the point of maximal cardiac impulse.

3. Presystolic murmurs– Presystolic accentuation of a delayed diastolic murmur is characteristic of mitral stenosis. In some cases, the presystolic murmur is all that can be heard with the patient supine and at rest, as in Figure 3–24. The delayed diastolic murmur is often elicited by having the patient exercise and then lie on the left side. Presystolic accentuation of a murmur is also encountered in patients with severe aortic incompetence (**Austin Flint murmur**). Austin Flint described this as a "blubbering murmur" that may appear or become louder at the time of atrial systole and thus be confused with the murmur of mitral stenosis (Landzberg, 1992). In practice, the two lesions—mitral stenosis and aortic incompetence—are readily distinguished, and it is only when the lesions are thought to coexist that difficulties in diagnosis arise (see Chapter 13).

C. Continuous Murmurs: Continuous murmurs arise when there is a pressure difference between two communicating vessels or chambers at all times in the cardiac cycle. The commonest example is that found in patent ductus arteriosus with left-to-right shunt (Figure 3–33). This lesion gives rise to a continuous "machinery" murmur. The characteristic feature of the murmur is that it is loudest at the time of the second heart sound. At this time, right ventricular ejection is coming to an end and pulmonary arterial

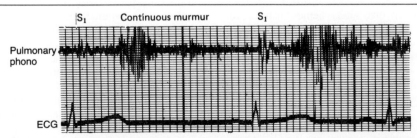

Figure 3–33. Patent ductus arteriosus characterized by a continuous murmur. The phonocardiogram, taken from the pulmonary area, shows a murmur that occupies the entire length of the cardiac cycle. It waxes at the end of systole and during early diastole, reaching at that point its highest frequency and intensity and enveloping the second sound. Only the first sound is distinctly visible. (Reproduced, with permission, from Dressler W: *Clinical Aids in Cardiac Diagnosis.* Grune & Stratton, 1970.)

pressure is falling, while aortic pressure is remaining high. Similar continuous murmurs are heard with aortopulmonary fistulas and after surgical creation of a shunt for the relief of tetralogy of Fallot (Blalock's operation).

D. Differential Diagnosis: Murmurs that come close to being continuous can be readily confused with the "machinery" murmur if their relationship to the second heart sound is not taken into account. In mixed aortic stenosis and incompetence, there is a to-and-fro systolic and diastolic murmur that can appear almost continuous. There is, however, a gap at the time of the second heart sound. Similarly, in patients with ventricular septal defect and aortic incompetence, the murmur may appear continuous. Coronary arteriovenous fistula and anomalous drainage of a coronary vessel into the pulmonary artery also give continuous murmurs, and in cases of rupture of a sinus of Valsalva aneurysm into a chamber with a lower pressure, the murmur is continuous or near continuous. The murmur of a patent ductus may only be heard high in the left chest below the left clavicle. In some patients, it may be confused with a venous hum. This is a sound that may be continuous and results from high venous flow past a narrowing of a large vein, such as the internal jugular vein. The internal jugular vein may be partially collapsed as it passes through the thoracocervial fascia into the thorax. Such a bruit is abolished by pressure over the root of the neck or by a change in the patient's position. The hum is never loudest at the time of the second heart sound.

E. Transmission of Murmurs: The interpretation of the origin of murmurs can be assisted by determining the direction of transmission of the murmur. The stethoscope is moved over various areas of the precordium to determine where the murmur can still be heard. Murmurs arising from the mitral valve are transmitted toward the axilla. Aortic and pulmonary diastolic murmurs are transmitted down the sides of the sternum. Aortic stenotic murmurs are usually but not always transmitted into the neck. The information obtained from determining the direction of transmission of murmurs is only of secondary value, however.

F. Hemodynamic Factors Influencing Murmurs: Any factor that alters hemodynamics can change the auscultatory findings and may on occasion be useful in diagnosis (Table 3–1).

1. Inspiration and expiration– Inspiration increases venous return to the right heart and tends to accentuate right-sided murmurs. This effect is of more significance than any tendency for a left-sided murmur to be louder during expiration. All intrathoracic sounds tend to become less loud with inspiration, simply because the stethoscope moves farther away from the origin of the sound and because lung tissue is likely to be interposed and decreases sound transmission. Thus, exaggeration of a murmur with

Table 3–1. Hemodynamic factors influencing auscultatory findings.

	Stroke Volume	Heart Rate	Systemic Vascular Resistance
Physical factors			
Respiration			
Inspiration	−	+	+
Expiration	+	+	−
Posture			
Standing	−	+	+
Squatting	+	−	−
Exercise			
Upright	+	+	+
Supine	+ or −	+	+
Isometric			
Handgrip	+ or −	+	+
Carotid sinus			
massage	−	−	−
Valsalva's maneuver		See Chapter 4.	
Cold pressor test	+ or −	+	+
Pharmacologic factors			
Vasodilators (nitrites)	+	+	−
Beta blockers	−	−	+ or −
Beta agonists	+	+	−
Alpha agonists	−	+	+

Key:
+ = Increases
− = Decreases
+ or − = Variable

inspiration is of greater significance than exaggeration with expiration.

2. Posture– Although examination of the heart is ordinarily performed with the subject supine, it is also useful to have the patient assume the left lateral decubitus position, so that mitral murmurs can be heard, especially after the patient has done several sit-ups to increase cardiac output. Having the patient sit up, lean forward, and breathe out can make an aortic diastolic murmur more readily audible. Examining the patient when standing tends to increase the systemic vascular resistance, as pooling of blood in the legs causes a fall in arterial pressure that triggers peripheral vasoconstriction via the baroreceptor reflexes. By decreasing heart size, standing may thus increase mitral incompetence and convert a late systolic murmer in a patient with click-murmur syndrome to a pansystolic murmur. Squatting, like lying down, increases venous return and shifts blood into the central circulation, increasing pulmonary and left heart blood volumes. This, squatting tends to increase left ventricular volume and reduce or abolish the murmur of hypertrophic obstructive cardiomyopathy. Standing after squatting decreases venous return, decreases left ventricular volume, and increases the murmur in this disease.

The effects of postural change on murmurs must be interpreted in the light of associated circulatory changes. If the heart rate does not slow on squatting and quicken on standing, postural effects on murmurs should be discounted. In general, the absence of change in a murmur with posture is not of significance.

3. Isometric handgrip; cold pressor test– An isometric handgrip and the cold pressor test (immersion of a hand in ice water for 1 minute) produce a relatively pure increase in systemic vascular resistance and arterial pressure. This increases the intensity of aortic diastolic and mitral systolic murmurs and also tends to reduce the intensity of aortic systolic murmurs.

4. Carotid sinus massage– Carotid sinus massage, which slows the heart rate and may facilitate auscultation, should be used with caution and only in a supine patient, preferably with electrocardiographic control. It should never be performed bilaterally and is contraindicated when there is a carotid bruit. The patient should turn the head to one side, and the area of the carotid sinus, below the angle of the jaw, should be gently massaged (not occluded) for no more than 5 seconds, in order to determine if bradycardia is present. The maneuver can be useful in separating the sounds of summation gallop.

5. Valsalva's maneuver– Listening during the period of strain in Valsalva's maneuver or during the overshoot after the release of strain can help in diagnosis. Right-sided murmurs disappear or diminish early during strain and return early after release of pressure in Valsalva's maneuver. While the Valsalva maneuver is held, venous return progressively decreases, as does ventricular volume; this causes an increase in loudness of the murmur observed with hypertrophic obstructive cardiomyopathy. The increase in pressure during the period of overshoot tends to accentuate the murmur of mitral incompetence and decrease the intensity of murmurs in aortic stenosis and hypertrophic obstructive cardiomyopathy.

6. Drugs– Vasodilator drugs such as amyl nitrite by inhalation and sublingual nitroglycerin reduce systemic resistance and increase cardiac output. This accentuates the murmurs of aortic stenosis and obstructive cardiomyopathy and decreases the murmur of mitral incompetence. The actions of alpha-adrenergic and beta-adrenergic blockade and stimulation can be inferred from their effects on the systemic circulation.

Pericardial Friction Rubs

Pericardial friction rubs are heard over the precordium as harsh, grating sounds related to the cardiac cycle and having a systolic component. When they have several components—most typically they have three—they may be confused with murmurs. They tend to vary with time, posture, and the phase of respiration. Their intensity tends to vary with the degree of pressure of the bell of the stethoscope on the chest, and they sound superficial, like the noise of hair rubbing against the diaphragm of the stethoscope.

REFERENCES

Constant J: *Essentials of Bedside Cardiology.* Little, Brown, 1989.

Curtiss EI et al: Pulsus paradoxus: Definition and relation to the severity of cardiac tamponade. Am Heart J 1988;115:391.

Dressler W: *Clinical Aids in Cardiac Diagnosis.* Grune & Stratton, 1970.

Elliott WJ: Earlobe crease and coronary artery disease: 1000 patients and review of the literature. Am J Med 1983;75:1024.

Fowler NO: *Inspection and Palpation of Venous and Arterial Pulses.* Part 2 of *Examination of the Heart.* American Heart Association, 1972.

Hada Y, Wolfe C, Craigie E: Pulsus alternans determined by biventricular simultaneous systolic time intervals. Circulation 1982;65:617.

Horwitz LD, Groves BM: *Signs and Symptoms in Cardiology.* Lippincott, 1984.

Hurst JW, Schlant RC: *Inspection and Palpation of the Anterior Chest.* Part 3 of *Examination of the Heart.* American Heart Association, 1972.

Landzberg JS et al: Etiology of the Austin Flint murmur. J Am Coll Cardiol 1992;20:408.

Lange RL, Hecht HH: The mechanism of Cheyne-Stokes respiration. J Clin Invest 1962;41:42.

Leatham A: *An Introduction to the Examination of the Cardiovascular System,* 2nd ed. Oxford Univ Press, 1979.

Leech G et al: Mechanism of influence of PR interval on loudness of first heart sound. Br Heart J 1980;43:138.

Leonard JJ, Kroetz FW: *Auscultation.* Part 4 of *Examination of the Heart.* American Heart Association, 1967.

1988 Joint National Committee. The 1988 report of the Joint National Committee on Detection, Evaluation, And Treatment Of High Blood Pressure. Arch Intern Med 1988;148:1023.

Nitta M, Ihenacho D, Hultgren HN: Prevalence and characteristics of the aortic ejection sound in adults. Am J Cardiol 1988;61:142.

Perloff JK: The physiologic mechanisms of cardiac and vascular physical signs. J Am Coll Cardiol 1983;1:184.

Stein PD: *A Physical and Physiological Basis for the Interpretation of Cardiac Auscultation.* Futura, 1981.

Swartz MH: *Textbook of Physical Diagnosis: History and Examination.* Saunders, 1989.

Teavel ME (editor): *Dynamic Auscultation and Phonocardiography: The Contribution of Vasoactive Drugs to the Diagnosis of Heart Disease.* Charles Press, 1979.

Thompson R: *An Introduction to Physical Signs.* Blackwell, 1980.

4

Clinical Physiology

Knowledge of the pathophysiologic changes that occur in heart disease is essential for understanding and interpreting the results of diagnostic investigations in clinical cardiology and for assessing the results of treatment. An introductory discussion of the function and control of the normal cardiovascular system has been given in Chapter 1.

Clinical physiology is additionally concerned with two different but interrelated sets of measurements. The first set of measurements relates to overall circulatory function, more particularly to the transport systems for oxygen and CO_2. The second set comprises purely cardiac measurements such as cardiac output, intracardiac pressures, cardiac volumes, assessment of valvular stenosis and incompetence, intracardiac shunts, coronary blood flow, and assessment of cardiac function. Both applied physiology and normal basic physiology must be understood before the physician can develop a rational approach toward the special investigations undertaken for some patients and toward the interpretation of data obtained at the bedside or in the clinical laboratory. Practical experience in applying the clinical techniques to patients is invaluable.

OXYGEN & CARBON DIOXIDE TRANSPORT

The basic mechanisms involved in cardiopulmonary function are oxygen uptake in the lungs, O_2-CO_2 exchange in the tissues, and elimination of CO_2 in the lungs.

Gas Tension

A. Partial Pressure: It is the partial pressure, or tension, of each gas that provides the force which determines how the gas will pass across the various membranes involved in gas transfer. The partial pressure of any gas in a mixture of gases is equal to the total pressure (barometric pressure) multiplied by the fraction of that gas in the mixture. Thus, since there is 20.9% oxygen in the atmosphere, the partial pressure of oxygen (Po_2) in the atmosphere at normal barometric pressure (760 mm Hg) is (20.9/100) × 760, or 159 mm Hg. If the barometric pressure is reduced, as at high altitude, the same fraction of oxygen in the atmosphere (20.9%) exerts a lower partial pressure because the total pressure is lower. Thus, at 3000 m the barometric pressure is about 525 mm Hg, and the

partial pressure of oxygen is reduced to 110 mm Hg. Similarly, a gas mixture of higher oxygen content (50%) exerts a higher Po_2 at sea level: (50/100) × 760, or 380 mm Hg.

If any liquid, such as blood, is allowed to equilibrate with a gas, the partial pressure of the gas in the liquid will come to equal that in the gas. The amount of gas entering the liquid will depend on the solubility of the gas in the liquid and on any chemical reaction occurring between the gas and the liquid.

B. Oxygen Tension, Saturation, and Content: Hemoglobin, the respiratory pigment of blood, has an affinity for oxygen and combines reversibly with it. Hemoglobin exists in two forms, a red (oxygenated) form and a blue (reduced) form, depending on the oxygen content of the blood. The proportion of oxygenated blood can vary from nil to 100%; this is the oxygen saturation of blood. Arterial oxygen saturation is reduced in cyanotic congenital heart disease and hypoxic patients. The complex relationship between oxygen tension and oxygen saturation is illustrated by the dissociation curve of hemoglobin shown in Figure 4–1. The curve shifts to the right with increasing temperature and acidity (lower pH) of the blood. The hemoglobin concentration in blood varies with the degree of anemia or polycythemia, and the oxygen-carrying capacity is directly related to hemoglobin concentration. One gram of hemoglobin when fully saturated can carry 1.34 mL of oxygen. Thus, a normal person with 149 g of hemoglobin per liter of blood has an oxygen capacity of 149 × 1.34, or 200 mL oxygen per liter of blood. Hemoglobin becomes effectively fully saturated with oxygen at a Po_2 of 150–200 mm Hg. At this Po_2 there is also a small amount (5–6 mL/L) of oxygen in solution in the plasma.

At a normal arterial Po_2 of 70–100 mm Hg, hemoglobin is about 97% saturated. Further increase in Po_2 to about 200 mm Hg will almost completely saturate hemoglobin and also result in an increase in the amount of oxygen in solution. Thus, on exposure to 100% oxygen, blood is fully saturated with oxygen and, in addition, contains about 21 mL/L of oxygen in solution, since solution of the gas in blood is directly proportionate to Po_2.

It is important to distinguish between Po_2, oxygen saturation, and oxygen content. Po_2 is the force driving oxygen across cellular membranes; oxygen saturation represents the relative proportions of reduced and oxygenated hemoglobin in the blood; and oxygen

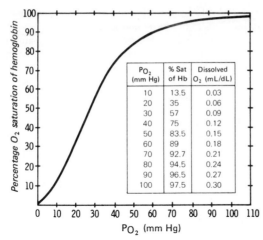

Figure 4–1. Oxygen hemoglobin dissociation curve. pH 7.40, temperature 38 °C. (Redrawn and reproduced, with permission, from Comroe JH et al: *The Lung: Clinical Physiology and Pulmonary Function Tests,* 2nd ed. Year Book, 1962.)

content is the volume of oxygen in the blood. The last measurement is most relevant to the cardiopulmonary transport of oxygen.

Oxygen content depends on hemoglobin level and is influenced by oxygen in solution, especially during oxygen breathing. Blood pH, temperature, and hemoglobin level must be known if oxygen content is to be accurately calculated from arterial P_{O_2}. The Severinghaus slide rule provides a convenient means of making this calculation.

CO_2 Transport

CO_2 production, which results from metabolism of substrates in the tissues, is the other aspect of gas exchange that equals oxygen consumption in importance. In addition, the regulation of the level of CO_2 in the blood plays a major role in determining the acid-base balance of the blood and of the body as a whole. It also sets the level of arterial pH (negative logarithm of the H + ion concentration). CO_2 is carried in the blood in three different ways. Like oxygen it dissolves in blood, but to a much greater degree (25 times greater, or about 27 mL/L at a normal P_{CO_2} of 40 mm Hg in arterial blood). CO_2 is also carried as bicarbonate in the buffering system of the blood and in combination with hemoglobin as a carbamino compound. Arterial CO_2 tension is the most closely controlled variable in the respiratory system. The normal value of 40 mm Hg is equivalent to $(40/760) \times 100$, or 5.25% CO_2 in the alveolar gas, and free equilibration takes place across the pulmonary membrane. Pulmonary ventilation is the most important determinant of arterial P_{CO_2}; hypoventilation raises the P_{CO_2} level. The level of ventilation is normally closely controlled by servomechanisms, and the arterial P_{CO_2}

is maintained within a few mm of 40 mm Hg. The level of metabolism and the adequacy of tissue perfusion determine the pH and P_{CO_2} of venous blood returning to the lungs, and the adequacy of ventilation determines the extent to which the products of metabolism are cleared from the blood by the lungs. Abnormalities of the arterial P_{CO_2} result both from abnormalities of ventilation and from disturbances of acid-base balance.

Relationship Between P_{CO_2} & pH

Alterations in the relationship between arterial P_{CO_2} and pH may be grouped into four categories, two of which are respiratory and two of which are metabolic (Table 4–1).

Ventilation is the most important means of influencing P_{CO_2} and pH. (1) With hypoventilation, arterial pH falls and P_{CO_2} rises as CO_2 accumulates in the blood (respiratory acidosis). (2) With hyperventilation, arterial pH rises and P_{CO_2} falls as CO_2 is washed out of the blood (respiratory alkalosis).

Metabolism influences P_{CO_2} in the reverse direction. (1) In metabolic acidosis, although blood pH falls, the increased acidity of the blood stimulates ventilation so that arterial P_{CO_2} also falls. A low pH associated with a low P_{CO_2} is common in cardiac failure, because inadequate tissue perfusion results in excessive anaerobic metabolism and lactic acid accumulation. (2) In metabolic alkalosis, the arterial pH and P_{CO_2} are both elevated. This is by far the least common disturbance of the group and may occur as a result of alkali ingestion or following prolonged vomiting with loss of acid gastric contents.

Assessment of Acid-Base Balance

Unless calculations are performed, it is not always easy to see the accommodation of pH level to changes in P_{CO_2}, both because renal compensatory forces may come into operation and because pH involves a logarithmic scale. The Severinghaus slide rule, which takes into account the buffering properties of hemoglobin, is particularly helpful in calculating a value for base deficit or base excess from arterial P_{CO_2} and pH. It enables the clinician to accurately determine the acid-base balance of acutely ill patients and to

Table 4–1. Alterations in relationships between arterial P_{CO_2} and pH.

Alteration	pH	P_{CO_2}
Respiratory		
Acidosis (hypoventilation)	Falls	Rises
Alkalosis (hyperventilation)	Rises	Falls
Metabolic		
Acidosis	Falls	Falls
Alkalosis	Rises	Rises

plan appropriate therapy for acid-base disturbances. Interpretation of the various disturbances of blood gas tensions commonly requires measurements of the P_{O_2}, P_{CO_2}, and pH of arterial blood. These measurements are indicated in almost all acutely ill patients with cardiopulmonary disease and also in postoperative care of patients after major surgery, especially after cardiac surgery. They are routinely available in most intensive care and coronary care units, where specially trained nurses and technicians can perform the analyses on the spot, without sending the specimen to a laboratory, and the information is available at any time.

MEASUREMENT OF BLOOD FLOW

Cardiac Output

A. Fick Principle: Cardiac output is most commonly measured by the Fick principle. An equation based on this principle states that in a steady state the flow of blood through an organ (eg, the lungs) is equal to the amount of a substance (eg, oxygen) absorbed by the blood flowing through the organ, divided by the difference in oxygen concentration between the blood entering and blood leaving the organ. Thus, pulmonary blood flow is the oxygen consumption in milliliters per minute divided by the arteriovenous difference across the lungs (pulmonary venous oxygen content minus pulmonary arterial oxygen content in milliliters per liter):

$$\text{Pulmonary flow} = \frac{\text{Oxygen uptake (mL/min)}}{\substack{\text{Pulmonary venous} - \text{Pulmonary arterial} \\ \text{oxygen content (mL/L)}}}$$
(L/min)

The same principle applies to the systemic capillary beds of the entire systemic circulation. Thus, systemic blood flow is equal to the oxygen consumption of the body (equal in the steady state to the uptake in the lungs) divided by the difference in oxygen content between arterial blood going to the tissues and mixed venous blood (pulmonary arterial blood) returning to the lungs for oxygenation:

$$\text{Systemic flow} = \frac{\text{Oxygen consumption (mL/min)}}{\substack{\text{Arterial} - \text{Mixed venous} \\ \text{oxygen content (mL/L)}}}$$
(L/min)

In normal subjects, blood flow through the lungs is virtually equal to blood flow to the body, since no substantial right-to-left or left-to-right shunt is present.

In a normal subject the oxygen consumption is about 250 mL/min. The arterial oxygen content is about 200 mL/L, and the mixed venous (pulmonary arterial blood) content is about 150 mL/L. Thus, the cardiac output is 250/50, or 5 L/min. This value in liters per minute is often adjusted to the size of the subject by dividing it by the body surface area derived from standard tables and expressed in m^2. The adjusted value is called the cardiac index; the normal value is about 4 L/min/m^2.

B. Indicator Dilution Method: The Fick principle also forms the basis for the indicator dilution method of measuring cardiac output, which uses green dye (indocyanine green), a radioactive isotope, or cold saline (thermodilution) injected into one place in the circulation and measured in another. A known amount of indicator is injected, usually into the right atrium, and the concentration of the indicator is subsequently measured at a downstream site after the indicator has thoroughly mixed with the blood. If cold saline is used, the temperature of blood in the pulmonary artery is measured continuously with a thermistor at the tip of a catheter (Swan-Ganz catheter). If green dye is used, the concentration is measured in systemic arterial blood by drawing a sample continuously through a photoelectric instrument (cuvette densitometer) that measures the optical density of blood at an appropriate wavelength. If a radioisotope is used, a counter is positioned over the heart or lungs.

The cardiac output equals the amount of indicator injected, divided by its average concentration during its passage past the sampling site (Figure 4–2). The indicator must not leave the circulation between the injection and the sampling sites, nor can it cause harmful effects or those that alter hemodynamic status. In practice, when green dye is used, the logarithm of the concentration of dye is plotted against time as the concentration rises to a peak, falls, and then rises again as recirculation of dye occurs. With thermodilution, recirculation is negligible, and the disappearance follows an exponential pattern (straight line on a semilog plot). With dye, the exponential disappearance is interrupted by recirculation of dye, as shown in Figure 4–2, and the initial linear portion of the curve must be extrapolated to zero concentration to define the time-concentration curve during the first passage of the dye. Cardiac output is then calculated as shown in Figure 4–2. In practice, computers are used to extrapolate the curves and calculate cardiac output.

Flowmeter Techniques

Electromagnetic and ultrasonic Doppler flowmeters are used to measure the instantaneous (every 5 ms) velocity of blood flow in different parts of the circulation.

A. Electromagnetic Flowmeter: The electromagnetic flowmeter is mounted at the tip of a catheter and introduced into the circulation via an artery or a vein. The accuracy of the technique has been vali-

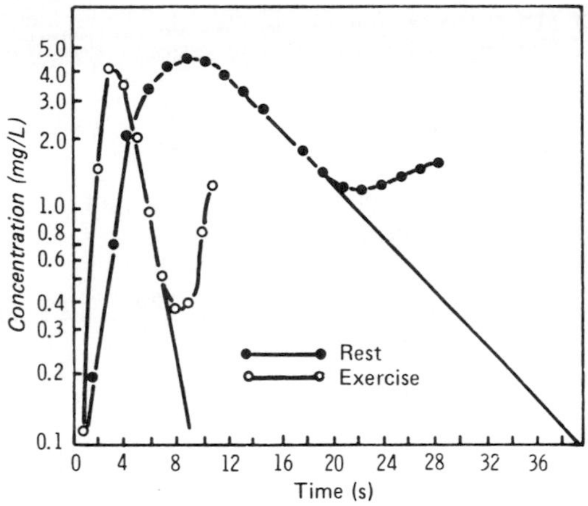

$$F = \frac{E}{\int_0^\infty Cdt}$$

F = flow
E = amount of indicator injected
C = instantaneous concentration of indicator in arterial blood

In the *rest* example above,

$$\frac{\text{Flow in 39 s}}{\text{(time of first passage)}} = \frac{\text{5-mg injection}}{\frac{\text{1.6 mg/L}}{\text{(avg concentration)}}}$$

Flow = 3.1 L in 39 s

$$\text{Flow (cardiac output)/min} = 3.1 \times \frac{60}{39} = 4.7 \text{ L}$$

For the *exercise* example,

$$\text{Flow in 9 s} = \frac{5 \text{ mg}}{1.51 \text{ mg/L}} = 3.3 \text{ L}$$

$$\text{Flow/min} = 3.3 \times \frac{60}{9} = 22.0 \text{ L}$$

Figure 4–2. Determination of cardiac output by indicator (dye) dilution. (Data and graph from Asmussen E, Nielsen M: The cardiac output in rest and work determined by the acetylene and the dye injection methods. Acta Physiol Scand 1952;27:217.)

dated in studies in animals. However, the catheters are so fragile and expensive that the technique is used almost exclusively in research studies.

B. Doppler Ultrasound: Transcutaneous ultrasonic Doppler blood velocity measurements (see also Chapter 5) can be made with pulsed, range-gated transducers aimed as closely as possible along the axis of flow in the vessel under study. The accuracy of Doppler measurements using spectral analysis to calculate instantaneous mean velocity has been checked by comparison with electromagnetic flowmeter measurements. Provided that the angle between the ultrasound beam and the flowing blood is close to zero, the signals accurately reflect blood flow velocity. The transducer can be aimed from the suprasternal notch in the axis of flow in the ascending or descending aorta and from the second or third left intercostal space in the axis of the main pulmonary artery. In the carotid, radial, brachial, femoral, and tibial vessels, the aim cannot be axial. Special dual Doppler transducers with two piezoelectric crystals set at a known angle can be used to obtain accurate measurements from the side of a vessel.

In Doppler studies, the velocity of blood flow is proportionate to the frequency shift of ultrasound reflected from red cells. The process is governed by the Doppler equation:

$$\Delta f = \frac{2 \times f \times v \times \cos\theta}{c}$$

where Δf is the shift in frequency, f the transmitted frequency, v the velocity of the moving target, θ the angle between the ultrasound beam and the target, and c the speed of sound in the tissues. The mean velocity of blood flow and evidence about the flow profile can be obtained from spectral analysis of the Doppler signals. This analytic technique (see Chapter 5) employs Fourier analysis to convert the audio Doppler signal into its frequency components at discrete intervals of 5–10 ms during the cardiac cycle.

Cardiac output measurements by the Doppler technique are only valid in subjects with no evidence of valve lesions or shunts. The method involves aiming a small, hand-held transducer in the axis of flow. A pulsed, range-gated Doppler instrument must be used, and it is necessary to know the cross-sectional area of the vessel under study. This can be estimated roughly by echocardiography from the left parasternal (aorta) or second or third intercostal space (pulmonary artery) (see Chapter 5). The angle between the ultrasound beam and the axis of flow in the vessel can be close enough to axial to reduce the error in the estimation of cos θ to less than 5%. The transducer is aimed to give the highest frequency audio signals as judged by the operator's ear, and the range gate is adjusted in a similar manner.

Doppler-based measurements of flow made in the ascending aorta have been compared with simultaneously measured thermodilution studies. The agreement has been good (correlation coefficient about 0.93) in studies in patients in intensive care units. The validity of similar measurements made using continuous wave (rather than pulsed) Doppler instruments is open to question.

Cardiac Shunts

A. Use of Fick Principle to Estimate Shunts: Methods based on the Fick principle can be used to estimate and investigate intracardiac and intrapulmonary shunts seen in congenital heart disease in which blood passes from one side of the circulation to another without traversing a capillary bed.

B. Right-to-Left Shunts: The characteristic feature of a right-to-left shunt is a reduction in systemic arterial saturation resulting from mixing of venous blood with oxygenated blood returning from the lungs. The right-to-left shunt can be calculated by applying the Fick equation to both the pulmonary and systemic circuits and subtracting the pulmonary flow from the systemic. As an example, in a patient with Fallot's tetralogy with mild polycythemia (hemoglobin 18.6 g/dL; oxygen capacity 250 mL/L; $\dot{V}O_2$ 200 mL/min), pulmonary arterial (mixed venous) saturation might be 70% (oxygen content [70/100] $\times$ 250, or 175 mL/L); systemic arterial saturation 85% (oxygen content 212.5 mL/L); and end-pulmonary capillary saturation 97% (oxygen content 242.5 mL/L). The Fick principle can be used to calculate systemic flow ($\dot{Q}$s):

$$\text{Systemic flow} = \frac{200}{(212.5 - 175)} = \frac{200}{37.5} = 5.3 \text{ L/min}$$

The Fick principle can also be used to calculate pulmonary flow ($\dot{Q}$p):

$$\text{Pulmonary flow} = \frac{200}{(242.5 - 175)} = \frac{200}{67.5} = 3 \text{ L/min}$$

In this example, the right-to-left shunt is $5.3 - 3.0$, or 2.3 L/min.

C. Left-to-Right Shunts: The characteristic feature of left-to-right shunts is an increase in oxygen content and saturation in the chamber into which the shunt flows. In other words, the oxygen content is higher than in the immediately preceding cardiac chamber. The magnitude of left-to-right shunts can be conveniently calculated by applying the Fick equation to both the pulmonary and systemic circuits as illustrated above for right-to-left shunts.

For example, in a patient with an atrial septal defect, samples from the right heart chambers might show 85% saturation in the pulmonary arterial blood, 86% in the right ventricle, 83% in the right atrium, 67% in the superior vena cava, and 73% in the inferior vena cava. Arterial saturation and pulmonary venous saturation are 97% each. The oxygen capacity is 200 mL/L and the oxygen consumption 225 mL/min. The increase in this example occurs between the venae cavae and the right atrium; the venae cavae samples represent venous blood returning from the tissues, whereas the right atrial blood is of higher saturation because the blood shunted across the atrial defect is mixed with it. Assuming that the inferior vena cava drains two-thirds of the body and the superior vena cava one-third, the mixed venous saturation can therefore be calculated as:

$$\frac{67 + (2 \times 73)\%}{3}$$

or 71% (oxygen content 142 mL/L). The Fick equation can be applied to calculate systemic flow ($\dot{Q}$s):

$$\text{Systemic flow} = \frac{225}{(194 - 142)} = \frac{225}{52} = 4.3 \text{ L/min}$$

The Fick principle can be similarly used to calculate pulmonary flow ($\dot{Q}$p):

$$\text{Pulmonary flow} = \frac{225}{(194 - 170)} = \frac{225}{24} = 9.4 \text{ L/min}$$

In this example, the left-to-right shunt is $9.4 - 4.3$, or 5.1 L/min.

D. Pulmonary to Systemic Flow Ratio: The size of left-to-right shunts is often expressed in terms of the ratio of pulmonary to systemic flows. In the example above, the ratio is 9.4/4.3, or 2.2:1. This is a small flow ratio, and values of 3:1 or 4:1 are not uncommon.

E. Accuracy of Shunt Estimations: The accuracy of shunt flow calculations based on intracardiac samples is not high. Bloodstreams tend not to mix fully in the right heart chambers, and if there is valvular incompetence, blood from a more distal chamber can contaminate the next most proximal one. As the pulmonary arteriovenous oxygen difference becomes smaller in patients with large left-to-right shunts, the magnitude of the calculated pulmonary blood flow comes to vary widely in response to small differences in pulmonary arterial oxygen content. Blood oxygen content measurements are usually accurate to within $\pm$ 2 mL/L, and when the pulmonary arterial oxygen saturation is 90% or more, the pulmonary arteriovenous oxygen difference may be as low as 14 mL/L. Measurement errors then have a marked effect.

F. Bidirectional Shunts: The calculation of blood flow in bidirectional shunts in congenital heart disease is even more inaccurate than that in left-to-right shunts. The most satisfactory method of calculation is the measurement of "effective" blood flow. The concept of "effectiveness" of flow implies that any blood flow that fails to traverse a capillary bed is "ineffective." Thus, left-to-right shunt constitutes ineffective pulmonary flow and right-to-left shunt ineffective systemic flow. Effective flow ($\dot{Q}$eff) is calculated from the Fick equation as:

$$\text{Effective cardiac output} = \frac{\text{Oxygen consumption in mL/min}}{\text{Pulmonary venous} - \text{Mixed venous oxygen content in mL/L}}$$

In a patient with Eisenmenger's syndrome and a bidirectional shunt at ventricular level, samples from the right heart might show a pulmonary arterial saturation of 80%, right ventricle 78%, right atrium 65%, superior vena cava 63%, and inferior vena cava 67%.

With oxygen consumption at 250 mL/min, oxygen capacity 210 mL/L, end-pulmonary capillary saturation 97%, and arterial saturation 92%, the systemic flow is calculated from the arterial and mixed venous (right atrial) samples as follows:

$$\text{Systemic flow} = \frac{250}{(193.2 - 136.5)} = \frac{250}{56.7} = 4.4 \text{ L/min}$$

Pulmonary flow is calculated from end-pulmonary capillary and pulmonary arterial blood:

$$\text{Pulmonary flow} = \frac{250}{(203.7 - 168)} = \frac{250}{35.7} = 7 \text{ L/min}$$

Effective flow is calculated from end-pulmonary capillary and mixed venous blood:

$$\text{Effective flow} = \frac{250}{(203.7 - 136.5)} = \frac{250}{67.2} = 3.7 \text{ L/min}$$

The left-to-right shunt equals the difference between the pulmonary and effective flows (7 – 3.7), or 3.3 L/min, and the right-to-left shunt equals the difference between the systemic and effective flows (4.4 – 3.7), or 0.7 L/min. It is easy to see that these calculations may be subject to error when the arteriovenous difference becomes small and when mixing may be incomplete. It is important to realize that all shunt calculations must be regarded as approximate only.

G. End-Pulmonary Capillary Oxygen Saturation: The clinician must realize the importance of the value selected for end-pulmonary capillary saturation .in all the calculations noted above. Pulmonary venous samples are seldom available, and arterial samples are not relevant if a right-to-left shunt is present. Therefore, the clinician must arbitrarily select a value for end-capillary saturation, and it is necessary to decide whether the conventional value of 97% is appropriate in any given case.

If the arterial oxygen saturation is normal, the conventional value is appropriate. If arterial saturation is low, the effect of oxygen breathing can be used to make the distinction between arterial hypoxia due to right-to-left shunt and arterial hypoxia due to abnormal pulmonary function.

H. Effect of Oxygen Breathing: Breathing 100% oxygen eliminates oxygen exchange problems in the lungs and raises end-pulmonary capillary content to supernormal levels. If arterial hypoxia is due to lung disease, arterial oxygen content rises markedly with oxygen breathing. In patients with arterial hypoxia due to right-to-left shunt, end-pulmonary capillary saturation is normal, and oxygen breathing has only a small and predictable effect on arterial oxygen content.

Breathing 100% oxygen raises end-pulmonary cap-

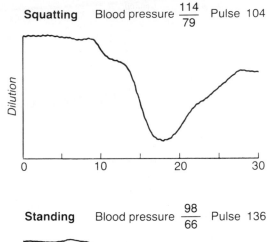

Squatting   Blood pressure $\frac{114}{79}$ Pulse 104

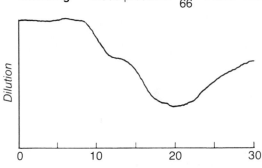

Standing   Blood pressure $\frac{98}{66}$ Pulse 136

Time (s) after injection

Figure 4–3. Indicator dilution curves showing early appearance at the ear of Cardio-Green dye injected into the right atrium in a patient with Fallot's tetralogy. The initial due to right-to-left shunt is in the standing position.

illary oxygen content by increasing the amount of oxygen carried in solution in the blood. An increase of 18 mL/L in end-pulmonary capillary blood occurs if alveolar P_{O_2} changes from 100 mm Hg to 700 mm Hg. As long as the hemodynamic status of the patient remains unchanged, an equal increase of 18 mL/L in oxygen content will occur in all sites of the body. The rise of 18 mL/L corresponds to an increase in saturation of 9% if the oxygen capacity is 200 mL/L. If the oxygen capacity is higher than 200 mL/L, the percentage change in saturation is lower, and vice versa.

I. Qualitative Estimation of Shunts by Indicator Dilution Methods: Indicator dilution curves using dye or radioactive isotope provide qualitative information about shunts. In right-to-left shunts, a portion of the injected dose of indicator—which passes from an injection site in the right heart through the shunt—traverses a shorter path through the circulation than does the main bolus, as shown in Figure 4–3. It thus appears earlier as a hump on the build-up phase of dye curve recorded in the arterial tree. In left-to-right shunts, blood containing indicator recir-

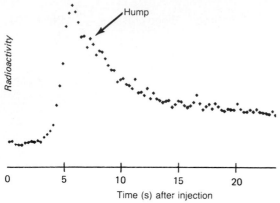

Figure 4–4. Indicator dilution curve showing early appearance at the ear of radioactive isotope injected into the right atrium in a patient with left-to-right shunt due to atrial septal defect (pulmonary/systemic flow ratio 2:1). The hump on the disappearance curve results from early recirculation of shunted blood. (Courtesy of E Botvinick.)

culates abnormally early and produces a hump on the disappearance curve (Figure 4–4).

J. Detection of Small Shunts: A number of methods are available for the detection of shunts that are too small to be detected from differences in the oxygen content of blood samples. These techniques generally involve sampling blood from the right side of the heart after the patient has inhaled gaseous indicators such as hydrogen, nitrous oxide, or radioactive krypton that enter the pulmonary capillary blood. Hydrogen has the advantage that it can be detected with a platinum electrode at the tip of a catheter, thus eliminating the need for blood sampling. In practice, the detection of small shunts that are not discovered by means of right heart sampling of oxygen content or angiocardiography is of little clinical significance.

Coronary Blood Flow

None of the methods available for the measurement of coronary blood flow in humans gives a direct measure of volume flow in milliliters per minute.

A. Clearance Methods: Inert gas clearance methods for the measurement of coronary blood flow are based on the approach of Kety and Schmidt (1948). Originally applied to the cerebral circulation, it involves introducing an inert gas into the circulation via the lungs and following the progressive saturation of cardiac tissue. The increases in the systemic arterial and coronary sinus concentrations of indicator are measured over the time that it takes for the arteriovenous difference to reach zero. The reciprocal of the time taken for equilibrium to be reached reflects the blood flow in milliliters per minute per 100 g of tissue. Nitrous oxide was the first gas to be used for this purpose; subsequently, helium, hydrogen, and argon have proved equally useful. The method is slow and entails coronary sinus catheterization and sam-

pling. A single measurement takes 5–30 minutes, during which a steady state must be assumed to be present.

A more invasive method involving coronary arterial catheterization also measures the rate of indicator clearance. The indicator, radioactive xenon (^{133}Xe) dissolved in saline, is injected into a coronary artery, and the rate of decay of radioactivity is measured over the precordium with a gamma camera. The reciprocal of the clearance time gives a value related to the coronary blood flow.

B. Thermodilution: Another method based on a different form of indicator dilution has been used to measure coronary sinus flow by Ganz et al (1971). A special catheter is passed into the coronary sinus and a continuous infusion of cold saline made through a lumen near the tip at a constant rate of 35–55 mL/min for up to 20 seconds. The temperature of the blood at a site several centimeters back from the tip of the catheter is measured with a thermistor. The method uses the form of the Fick equation dealing with continuous (rather than bolus) infusion of indicator:

$$Q = I \div C$$

where $\dot{Q}$ is the blood flow in mL/min, I the rate of infusion of indicator, and C the steady level of indicator (temperature difference) resulting from the infusion. The method has the advantage of measuring flow in milliliters per minute rather than relative flow per 100 g of tissue. It assumes adequate mixing of the cold saline with blood over the short distance between the injection and sampling sites in the coronary sinus. The method can provide measurements every few minutes but is probably only valid in subjects without coronary disease. The flow to the right ventricle that does not drain via the coronary sinus is excluded, and stable positioning of the coronary sinus catheter cannot always be achieved.

C. Densitometry: Measurement of the transit time of radiopaque material along a vessel can give an indication of coronary flow. The method is best suited to measurement of flow in aortocoronary saphenous vein grafts that follow a straight course for 10 cm or more without branching. Computerized tomography and digital subtraction angiography (see Chapter 5) can be used to enhance the images. The contrast material used to provide the images produces a submaximal coronary arterial vasodilation, and the values obtained are intermediate between resting and maximally dilated values.

D. Flowmeter Techniques: More direct methods for measurement of the velocity of blood flow include electromagnetic and Doppler blood velocity flowmeters. Electromagnetic flowmeters that surround the vessel have been widely used in animals, implanted at surgery. The fat in the atrioventricular groove must be dissected free to permit the placement of the flowmeter around the vessel, and several days must be allowed for the position of the flowmeter to stabilize. Chronic implantation is clearly not feasible in humans. Electromagnetic and Doppler flowmeters have been used at surgery, where they are best suited for measurement of the flow in vein grafts. The native coronary vessels should never be dissected for the sole purpose of placing a flowmeter. It is difficult to achieve the stable, close contact between flowmeter and vessel that is needed to provide accurate tracings, and calibration is a problem.

E. Catheter-Tip Flowmeters: Catheter-tip Doppler flowmeters small enough to enter the coronary vessels without obstructing flow have been used to measure blood velocity, but problems arise in calibrating in terms of volume flow and finding a stable position for the catheter away from the wall of the vessel. A more recent development is to use laser Doppler probes small enough to record from intramyocardial vessels. This is the only technique that can potentially measure flow velocity in intramyocardial vessels.

MEASUREMENT OF BLOOD VOLUME

The circulating blood volume can be determined either from measurements of red cell volume or from plasma volume plus hematocrit. The values are subject to considerable variation, and the range of normal values is wide. A tracer material is injected that mixes with the total blood volume before it is excreted. The degree of dilution of the tracer is measured in a sample of blood drawn after mixing is complete. Commonly used tracers are radioactive chromium-labeled red cells, which measure red cell volume, or iodine-labeled albumin, which measures plasma volume. The total blood volume is calculated from the hematocrit:

$$\frac{\text{Red cell volume}}{\text{Red cell volume} + \text{Plasma volume}}$$

Thus, total blood volume equals

$$\text{Red cell volume} \times \frac{1}{\text{Hematocrit}}$$

or:

$$\text{Plasma volume} \times \frac{1}{1 - \text{Hematocrit}}$$

In practice, mixing of the indicator is not always complete before the indicator begins to be excreted, and incomplete mixing of indicator often gives falsely low values, especially in patients with heart disease in whom the cardiac output is low.

Regional Blood Volume

Indicator dilution techniques can be used to measure the volume of blood in a specific part of the circulation. The volume of blood in the heart and lungs (**central blood volume**) is the most commonly measured value. The mean transit time of indicator is measured between an injection site (usually the right atrium) and a sampling site (the aorta or a systemic artery). Multiplying the mean transit time by the cardiac output measured during the same injection gives a value that represents the volume between the two sites (needle-to-needle). Volumes determined by this method are only roughly related to the corresponding anatomic volumes.

Ventricular Volume

A. Left Ventricular Volume: Left ventricular volume is most commonly measured from cineangiograms recorded following the injection of iodine-containing contrast material into the ventricle during left heart catheterization. It is calculated from the dimensions of opacified areas of individual films or cine frames exposed at the end of systole and the end of diastole.

The angiographic image of the left ventricle may be recorded in a single plane (usually the right anterior oblique) or in two planes: posteroanterior (shown in Figure 4–5) and lateral or two obliques. The examiner must make some assumption about the shape of the ventricle in the axis of revolution about the plane or planes in which measurements are made. The simplest assumption is to consider the left ventricle as a sphere, but the slightly more complex figure of a prolate ellipse is frequently used. Computer programs

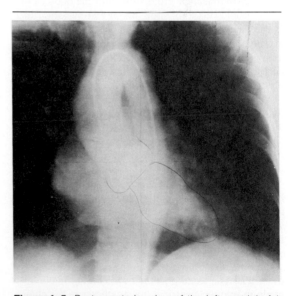

Figure 4–5. Posteroanterior view of the left ventricle following injection of contrast material. The outline of the ventricle from which volume was calculated is drawn on the x-ray.

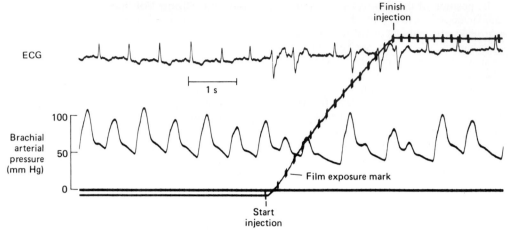

Figure 4–6. ECG and brachial arterial pressure tracing obtained during an injection of contrast material into the left ventricle in a patient with aortic stenosis. The timing of the angiographic film exposures is indicated. Pulsus alternans is present, and ectopic beats are seen during the injection.

are commonly used to calculate left ventricular volume from a small number of specific angiographic measurements. A more accurate method for calculating ventricular volumes is by the Simpson's rule method. This involves dividing the ventricle into a series of sections 1 cm thick, calculating the volume of each section, and summing the volumes. This method is more accurate for volumes of irregular geometry, as is frequently the case with the end-systolic volumes.

B. Errors of Method: The process of defining the edge of the ventricular shadow is often subjective. Blood trapped between the trabeculae carneae cordis, which form muscular projections into the body of the left ventricle, may not show up on end-systolic films as an opacity. The assumption made about a particular geometric shape for the ventricle introduces an unknown error. The end-diastolic volumes are more accurate than the end-systolic values, which are probably too small.

Ventricular volume can also be estimated from two-dimensional echographic images. Several geometric approaches have been used, and most give smaller volumes than angiography. The reason for this discrepancy is not clear, and errors are possible with both techniques.

C. Ejection Fraction: The ratio of stroke volume (end-diastolic minus end-systolic volume) to end-diastolic volume (the ejection fraction) has become a widely accepted measure of left ventricular function. It is a ratio that expresses the percentage of blood in the ventricle that is ejected per beat. The normal value obtained from a measurement in two planes is 67 ± 9%. The usual practice of injecting the contrast medium into the ventricle via a catheter in the chamber often provokes ectopic beats (Figure 4–6). Less invasive methods using intravenous radioactive indicators or right-sided injections of contrast media are sometimes employed. A false idea of ejection fraction can also be obtained from the abnormally forceful left ventricular contraction that usually follows a run of ectopic beats. (See below and Chapter 5 for other measures of left ventricular function.)

Ejection fraction can also be measured from two-dimensional echocardiograms. The measurement is greatly facilitated if a "light pen" is used to outline the ventricle and calculations are performed by computer (Figure 4–7).

Right ventricular ejection fraction is best measured by gated equilibrium radionuclide angiography. This method has the advantage that it does not assume that the ventricle has any specific shape.

D. Effects of Contrast Material: The contrast material itself also influences left ventricular function, mainly because of its hyperosmolarity. This factor is thought to be unimportant in the first seven beats following injection, however, and it generally influences left ventricular end-diastolic pressure rather than ejection fraction. Left ventricular ejection fraction has proved to be a useful functional measurement that is greatly preferred to a visual impression of the force of contraction, which can be misleading. The right ventricle is of a completely different shape from the left and varies more in shape in disease. It is inappropriate to apply methods developed for computing left ventricular volume to the right side of the heart.

E. Wall Motion Abnormalities: Localized abnormalities of the motion of the heart can be detected from angiograms. These abnormalities almost always involve the left ventricle and are usually due to coronary artery disease. Changes in the shape of the left ventricle as seen on angiography also give clues to the site of ischemic areas of the left ventricular myocardium. It is difficult to obtain quantitative measurements of regional ventricular function, but a qualita-

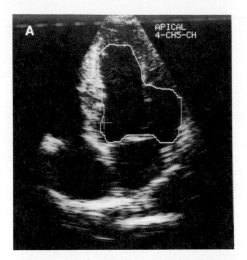 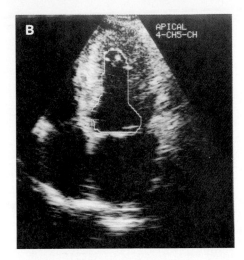

Figure 4–7. End-diastolic (A) and end-systolic (B) two-dimensional echographic images of the left ventricle with the cavity outlined with a "light pen." Ejection fraction is calculated from the ratio of the areas at end-systole and end-diastole. (Courtesy of Elscint Inc.)

tive impression of the site of noncontracting or poorly contracting areas can be readily obtained.

Similar information is available from echocardiographic studies, especially those using two-dimensional sector scanning. Although nuclear medical techniques are also being used for this purpose, radiography provides the clearest image. The errors inherent in calculations based on angiography are even more of a problem in echocardiographic and nuclear medical techniques, whose level of resolution is relatively low.

Using radioisotope blood volume multigated radio nuclide angiographic studies, ventricular volumes and ejection fractions can be calculated. From a collimated image of the ventricle in diastole and systole, the number of total counts can be obtained which, when corrected for background counts, will reflect the volume of blood in the ventricle. From the difference in counts between the left ventricle in diastole and systole, the left ventricular stroke volume can be calculated and therefore the ejection fraction. If a blood sample is taken at the time of complete mixing, the counts per milliliter of blood can be measured and the absolute volume of blood in the left ventricle in systole and diastole can be calculated; this technique has the advantage of not being dependent on any particular geometric form.

Measurement of Valvular Incompetence

Angiographic measurements of stroke volume include all the blood pumped by the ventricle, whereas methods based on the Fick principle measure only the blood that flows forward to the systemic arterial bed. It is thus possible by combining the two methods to measure the volume of blood returning to the ventricle or atrium through the incompetent aortic or mitral valve. The angiographic stroke volume minus the forward (Fick) stroke volume gives a measure of the amount of backflow, which is usually expressed as the "regurgitant fraction," the proportion of the angiographic stroke volume flowing back per beat:

$$\text{Regurgitant fraction} = \frac{\substack{\text{Total (angiographic)} \\ \text{stroke volume} - \text{Forward (Fick)} \\ \text{stroke volume}}}{\text{Total stroke volume}}$$

A value of 50% or more indicates severe valvular incompetence.

MEASUREMENT OF BLOOD PRESSURE

Systemic Arterial Pressure

Systemic arterial pressure is the most important pressure, because it is the most closely controlled. Control is established mainly by the action of the baroreceptor system. The normal arterial wave form is shown in Figure 4–8. Peak arterial pressure roughly coincides with the T wave of the ECG. There is often a prominent (dicrotic) notch on the downstroke associated with aortic valve closure. The normal values (110–120 mm Hg peak systolic and 70–80 mm Hg minimal diastolic pressure) change in response to physiologic stimuli such as exercise, excitement, mental stress, sleep, external temperature, posture, pregnancy, growth and development, and age. The range of normal values is wide and increases with age. The pulse pressure (the difference between systolic and diastolic pressure) is usually about 40 mm Hg and mirrors stroke volume, changing magnitude in the same direction as stroke volume in exercise, shock, or heart failure.

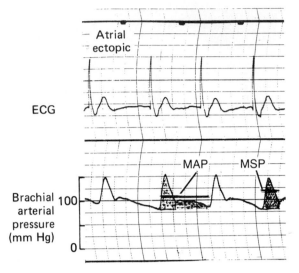

Figure 4–8. ECG and brachial arterial pressure in a normal subject. Mean arterial pressure (MAP) and mean systolic pressure (MSP) are indicated. One atrial ectopic beat is shown.

Mean arterial pressure is usually recorded by electrically integrating the pressures recorded during the cardiac cycle. It is roughly equal to the diastolic pressure plus one-third of the pulse pressure. The systemic arterial bed senses the mean arterial pressure as the force pressing against the walls of the blood vessels and influencing the rate of wear and tear on vascular tissues.

Mean systolic pressure (the average pressure during ventricular systole) can be measured by planimetry of an arterial pressure tracing, as shown in Figure 4–8. It gives an indication of the force against which the left ventricle must eject blood. Mean systolic

pressure is higher than mean arterial pressure, which averages the whole cardiac cycle. In atrial fibrillation, especially in association with mitral valve disease, the systolic arterial pressure varies with the RR interval, being lower after a short pause and higher after a long pause, as shown in Figure 4–9. This reflects the effect of ventricular filling on the subsequent ventricular systole in accordance with the Frank-Starling mechanism. A similar effect is seen with an ectopic beat, even if it is atrial, as shown in Figure 4–8, in which the level of systolic arterial pressure in the beat after the pause following the ectopic beat is higher. When the ectopic beat is ventricular, the arterial pressure is increased by another mechanism, **postectopic potentiation,** which involves the excitation-contraction coupling mechanism. It is seen in Figure 4–9, in which the beat following the ventricular ectopic beat shows the highest systolic arterial pressure in the strip. If regular ectopic beats are produced by pacing the heart after each normal beat (paired pacing), cardiac output increases, as does myocardial oxygen consumption.

Pressures in the Heart & Great Vessels

A. Technique: Measurements of pressures in the heart and great vessels are almost always made through long, small-bore catheters connected to electromanometers of the strain-gauge type. Obtaining accurate pressure recordings presents significant problems, especially when the catheter is subject to motion because of the action of the heart. The only satisfactory solution is to use catheter-tip manometers. Unfortunately, these are so expensive that their use outside research laboratories has not yet become practical. Experience and comparison of conventional and catheter-tip manometer tracings have made it possible to recognize high-quality pressure tracings and

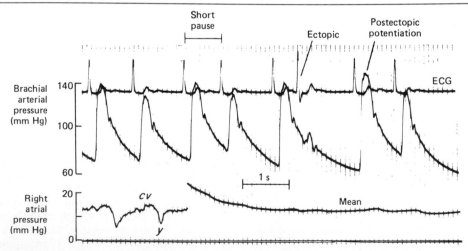

Figure 4–9. Brachial arterial and right atrial pressure tracings in a patient with mitral valve disease in atrial fibrillation. The effect of varying cycle lengths and an ectopic beat on arterial pressure are shown.

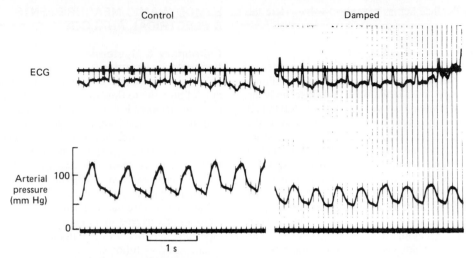

Figure 4–10. Control and damped brachial arterial pressure tracings obtained several minutes apart from a patient with aortic stenosis. Both the amplitude and the mean pressures decreased as the pressure was damped.

know when serious artifacts are present. Excessive damping of pressure tracings resulting from leaky stopcocks, bubbles of air in the catheter or manometer, or blockage of the catheter should be easily recognized, as shown in Figure 4–10. Excessive overswing due to catheter fling in hyperdynamic hearts is more difficult to deal with. The problems in this case mainly relate to inertia and depend on the magnitude of the accelerative forces involved; they are thus greatest with rapidly changing pressure signals. Electrical and mechanical damping systems are of some help but are still not entirely satisfactory. Obtaining acceptable readings of intravascular pressure depends more on skill and experience in positioning the catheter than on any objective knowledge of the scientific principles involved in damping. Part of the expertise of cardiac catheterization is recognizing an adequate tracing.

The pressures in each cardiac chamber are different. Examples are found in the sections on different diseases.

B. Pressure Gradients: The pressure difference between different chambers or across valves is important clinically. The difference between the peak left ventricular systolic pressure and the peak aortic systolic pressure is called the **peak gradient across the aortic valve.** Similarly, the difference between the left atrial diastolic (wedge) pressure and the left ventricular diastolic pressure is the **peak gradient across the mitral valve.** The gradient is often used as an indication of the severity of stenosis of the affected valve.

The area between the superimposed, preferably simultaneously recorded ventricular and aortic pressure tracings during systole, divided by the time for which a pressure difference is present, gives a measure of the mean gradient across the aortic valve. The equivalent diastolic values recorded at the mitral valve give the mean mitral valve gradient.

The pressure difference across stenotic valves varies with the flow across the valve, and the relationship is nonlinear. Doubling the blood flow does not merely double the pressure difference but produces closer to a fourfold increase. This consideration is most important in patients with mitral and aortic stenosis, since it affects calculations concerning the severity of the stenosis. The situation in patients with stenosis is further complicated by changes in heart rate that alter the relative lengths of systole and diastole. Whenever possible, cardiac output and the difference in pressure between two chambers should be measured simultaneously. In some cases this is not possible, and withdrawal tracings are obtained as the catheter is pulled from one chamber to another. Such tracings have the advantage that errors in calibrating two strain gauges are avoided, since only one gauge is used. It is important to record the heart rate at the time that each pressure measurement is made, as a rough indication that the hemodynamic status of the patient has not changed significantly.

Measurement of peak gradient by continuous wave Doppler ultra-sound. A simplified equation based on the Bernoulli principle has been used for the indirect measurement of peak pressure gradients across stenotic valves using continuous wave Doppler ultrasound (see Chapter 5). The peak velocity in a jet of blood passing through a stenosed valve bears a significant relationship to the pressure difference across the valve. The simplified form of the Bernoulli equation is:

$$P = 4 \times V^2$$

where P is the peak pressure gradient in millimeters of mercury and V the maximal velocity in meters per second. An equivalent method has been applied to the pressure difference across the mitral valve. Here the relationship has been expressed as:

$$P = 220 \div t$$

where P is the peak pressure of gradient in millimeters of mercury and t is the time in milliseconds the diastolic mitral valve flow velocity takes to fall to half its maximal value. This has been referred to as the mitral valve pressure gradient half-time. The pressure half-time is relatively independent of flow and is therefore a more accurate measure of mitral valve area when there is mitral insufficiency than is the Gorlin equation. The pressure gradients measured by these techniques have been compared with directly measured values, and reasonable agreement has been demonstrated (Stamm and Martin, 1983). The methods have the advantage of being noninvasive, but it is important to take into account the blood flow at the time that pressure measurements are being made.

C. Measurements of Valve Area: Hydraulic formulas have been adapted for use in estimating valve area based on pressure differences and flows across valves. The formulas are most commonly applied to stenotic lesions of the mitral and aortic valves. They are based on steady turbulent flow under stable conditions in smooth, cylindric pipes and should not be used when there is valvular incompetence unless the extra forward flow resulting from the incompetence can somehow be incorporated in the calculations. Although the assumptions underlying the formulas clearly do not apply to flow across cardiac valves, these valve area calculations represent the best available means of obtaining numerical estimates of valve orifice size and do take into account both pressure and flow.

The formula for mitral valve area (MVA) is:

$$\text{MVA in cm}^2 = \frac{\text{Diastolic mitral flow in mL/s}}{31 \times \sqrt{\Delta P} \text{ in mm Hg}}$$

where ΔP is the average pressure difference in mm Hg between the left atrium and the left ventricle during the period of diastolic flow. The value of 31 represents an arbitrary constant required to adjust the units appropriately.

The formula for aortic valve area (AVA) is:

$$\text{AVA in cm}^2 = \frac{\text{Systolic flow in mL/s}}{44.5 \times \sqrt{\Delta P} \text{ in mm Hg}}$$

where ΔP is the mean pressure difference across the valve during the time of systolic flow and 44.5 is the arbitrary constant.

HEMODYNAMIC MEASUREMENTS & ELECTRICAL ANALOGS

Pulmonary & Systemic Vascular Resistance

Vascular resistance is customarily defined as the ratio of pressure to flow in the circulation. Its reciprocal, conductance, is the ratio of flow to pressure. This is a simplistic application of Ohm's law, and it assumes that the circuits involved are linear and that there is no phase difference between pressure and flow. In spite of these inaccuracies, pulmonary and systemic resistances are useful clinical measurements if their limitations are kept in mind.

Pulmonary vascular resistance (PVR) is a useful index of the degree of pulmonary vasoconstriction, especially in patients with pulmonary hypertension. It is calculated as follows:

$$\text{PVR in mm Hg/ L/min} = \frac{\text{Mean pulmonary arterial pressure} - \text{Mean atrial pressure}}{\text{Pulmonary blood flow}}$$

If pressure is expressed as dynes/cm² and flow in cm³/s, the units can be expressed as dyne•s•cm⁻⁵. However, these units do not show how the measurement is derived, and the equivalent units of mm Hg/L/min (Wood units) are preferable. One can convert mm Hg/L/min to dyne•s•cm⁻⁵ by multiplying by 80. Systemic vascular resistance (SVR) is the analogous measurement in the systemic circulation. It is calculated as:

$$\text{SVR in mm Hg/ L/min} = \frac{\text{Mean arterial pressure} - \text{Mean right atrial pressure}}{\text{Systemic blood flow}}$$

Vascular Compliance

Compliance is the term used in clinical physiology to describe the elastic behavior of elements involved in cardiovascular phenomena. It also refers to the storing of energy in a system, as in a spring. Like the term resistance, it is borrowed from the nomenclature of electrical theory, in which its analog is capacitance. Compliance is the ratio of volume change to pressure change and is measured in terms of units of volume change per unit of pressure change. Decreased compliance involves increased stiffness, which is the inverse of compliance. The word compliance first came into use in pulmonary physiology as a ratio expressing the volume of lung distention resulting from a given inflating transpulmonary pressure change.

Applied to the atria and ventricles, compliance refers to a change in pressure proportionate to a given amount of diastolic filling. If a chamber is compliant, it can accept a large volume with little rise in pressure. The term compliance is also used to describe the elastic behavior of the pulmonary and systemic arterial beds. A compliant bed can distend more with a given pressure change. The venous bed is referred to as a high compliance or high capacitance part of the circulation.

The use of a single value to express the compliance of a structure implies a linear relationship between volume and pressure. However, the left ventricle is more compliant at low volumes and becomes less compliant as it is distended. Thus, diastolic pressure tends to remain low until greater levels of distention occur, after which pressure rises more steeply. In general, the diastolic ventricular pressures seen in patients with acute heart failure are higher than those in patients with chronic heart failure. An indirect indication of ventricular compliance is given by the height of the *a* wave. If the ventricle is stiff and noncompliant, atrial contraction results in a larger pressure wave per given force of atrial contraction.

Time Constant

As a further extension of the electrical analogy it is possible to think in terms of the product of resistance and compliance. The units of this product are:

$$\text{Time in min} = \frac{\text{mm Hg}}{\text{L/min}} \times \frac{\text{L}}{\text{mm Hg}}$$

The time constant is used in describing the exponential fall in left atrial pressure during diastole in a patient with mitral valve disease. In this case, the rate of left atrial pressure fall depends on both the resistance to flow across the mitral valve and the compliance (stiffness) of the left atrium. Either a high resistance to mitral valve flow (stenosis) or a large overdistended compliant atrium can increase the time constant of left atrial emptying. The time constant is the time taken for the pressure to fall to $1/e$ times (37%) the original value, where e is the base of natural logarithms (2.718). The time constants of the systemic and pulmonary circulations can also be determined from the diastolic fall of pressure in the system.

ASSESSMENT OF CARDIAC FUNCTION: "CONTRACTILITY"

One of the most important aspects of clinical cardiac physiology is the assessment of cardiac function. The reserve capacity of the heart is so large that disease must generally be far advanced before resting cardiac function is detectably impaired. Cardiac function normally deteriorates with age and is poor in sedentary people, and these factors contribute to the mixed load on the heart in patients with cardiac symptoms. In addition to structural and mechanical problems there may be a functional myocardial factor and also an element of poor function owing to disuse.

Assessment of cardiac function involves identifying each of these components in the patient. It is most commonly required when surgical correction of an anatomic defect is under consideration.

There are many measurements and indices available to assess cardiac dysfunction, but none is entirely satisfactory, and it is not possible to predict with certainty how a given patient's heart will function when a mechanical load such as valvular stenosis or incompetence is relieved. A number of measurements give an indication of ventricular function involving different levels of invasiveness. Although they are of value in prognosis, their results are almost never a complete contraindication to attempts to correct severe valvular lesions such as aortic stenosis.

Valsalva's Maneuver

One of the most readily performed tests of cardiac function determines the patient's response to straining (Valsalva's maneuver). The patient blows against a mercury manometer to raise the intrapulmonary pressure. The height of the pressure and the duration of the period of strain can be varied, but 40 mm Hg and 10 seconds are conventional. The subject should not inhale deeply before straining; a small leak in the system forces the subject to use the thoracic and abdominal muscles (rather than the cheeks) to generate the pressure. The sudden strain of the maneuver causes a complex sequence of mechanical and reflex changes in the circulation that depend on two factors: (1) the level of cardiac function and effective central blood volume and (2) the speed and magnitude of the baroreceptor responses to a change in arterial pressure. The maneuver is best performed with a continuous recording of arterial pressure and is shown in Figure 4–11.

A. Normal Response: The first effect is a rise in arterial pressure owing to the transmission of applied pressure to the intrathoracic structures (heart and great vessels). The magnitude and speed of the rise depend on the suddenness and force of the strain. The arterial pressure then starts to fall, the pulse pressure narrows because the venous return is cut off, and the normal heart responds to a decrease in filling with a fall in output. The rate and magnitude of the fall during this period of strain reflect the size of the central blood volume. The reflex changes of Valsalva's maneuver depend on baroreceptor activity. In a normal response to Valsalva's maneuver, the falls in blood pressure and pulse pressure trigger reflex tachycardia within about 5–7 seconds and a rise in peripheral resistance a few seconds later. Thus, the arterial pressure stops falling and starts to rise toward the end of the period of strain. When the strain ends, the blood pressure falls and venous return is restored. The cardiac output increases and the blood pressure rises. The peripheral resistance is still raised in response to the previously low pressure, and the surge of blood into constricted vessels causes an overshoot

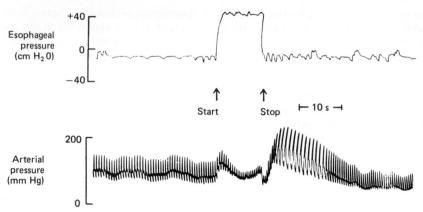

Figure 4–11. Tracing of the normal blood pressure and pulse response to straining (Valsalva's maneuver) in a normal man, recorded with a needle in the brachial artery.

of pressure. This overshoot in turn causes vagally mediated reflex bradycardia within 3–5 seconds and is followed by vasodilation, which restores the pressure to normal.

The response to Valsalva's maneuver also offers a convenient means of testing the reactivity of the baroreceptor reflex arc. It is primarily used in the investigation of patients with disease of the autonomic nervous system (Chapter 21). The intense vagal stimulation associated with the overshoot after Valsalva's maneuver may be sufficient to stop paroxysmal atrial tachycardia, and the maneuver may be useful therapeutically.

B. Square Wave Response: In the case of a large central blood volume due to pulmonary congestion or a large left-to-right shunt, there is sufficient blood in the central circulation to maintain a constant pressure throughout the period of strain. This type of response is termed a square wave response and has in the past been incorrectly termed the heart failure response. It is seen in congestive heart failure but is also found in overhydrated normal subjects and in symptom-free patients with large left-to-right shunts, especially those with atrial septal defects. Figure 4–12 shows an example from a patient with atrial

septal defect. The rate at which the heart empties during the period of straining depends on cardiac output. In congestive heart failure, the central circulation is overloaded and the cardiac output is low, so that the heart does not empty; thus, a square wave response is due to a combination of factors.

Left Ventricular Function

A. Maximum dp/dt: The maximum rate of change of left ventricular pressure (dp/dt_{max}) during the phase of isovolumetric contraction is probably the purest indicator of ventricular function (Figure 4–13). The measurement is valid only if a catheter-tip manometer is used.

B. Aortic Acceleration: The best noninvasive indication of ventricular function is given by the rate of ejection in early systole. This can be measured by Doppler ultrasound as the average rate of increase in the mean aortic or pulmonary blood velocity over the first 45 ms of ventricular ejection (see Chapter 5). This represents the linear acceleration in $cm \bullet s^{-2}$ imparted to the blood in the aorta or pulmonary artery in the early ejection phase of systole. The normal value in resting adults is about 900–1200 $cm \bullet s^{-2}$ for the left and about 400–600 $cm \bullet s^{-2}$ for the right ventri-

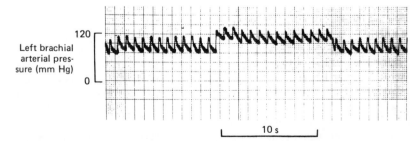

Figure 4–12. Arterial pressure tracing showing the response to Valsalva's maneuver in a patient with atrial septal defect and a large pulmonary blood flow. The pulse pressure is maintained during the period of strain, and there is no overshoot on release of the strain.

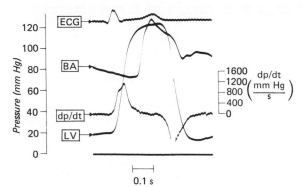

Figure 4–13. Pressure tracings and ECG showing the rate of change of left ventricular pressure. BA, brachial artery pressure; dp/dt, first derivative of left ventricular pressure; LV, high-fidelity left ventricular pressure. (Reproduced, with permission of the American Heart Association, Inc., from Kreulen TH et al: The evaluation of left ventricular function in man: A comparison of methods. Circulation 1975;51:677.)

cle. It depends in part on the quality of the match of aortic impedance (afterload) to the force of cardiac contraction.

Other indicators of ventricular function can be assessed by angiography, M mode or two-dimensional echocardiography, and radionuclear techniques. The size of the left ventricle and its ejection fraction, although well established as indicators of cardiac function, are not strictly measures of "contractility," because both are influenced by afterload. The time resolution of all these methods is unsatisfactory, because measurements can only be made 30–60 times a second by all but M mode echocardiography, and it gives only a one-dimensional view. The period of constant acceleration of blood flow out of the left ventricle lasts for only about 50 ms, so that only one or two frames of a left ventricular angiogram will be exposed during the rapid phase of ejection, and acceleration cannot be accurately assessed from two frames. Similar problems arise with two-dimensional echocardiography and radionuclear measurements, but they have the advantage of being applicable during exercise.

It is important to remember that several crucial assumptions are made whenever left ventricular volumes are calculated. For example, the measurement of ventricular volume is likely to involve an assumption about the shape of the ventricle (spherical, conical, or elliptical), and if the measurement uses M mode echocardiography, a single dimension is ordinarily measured and the radius cubed to give a volume measurement. Only measurement of volume by radionuclide angiography is independent of geometric shape. Measurements such as the rate of circumferential shortening involve similar assumptions that must not be forgotten by those interpreting the studies.

It seems clear that no assessment of ventricular

function can predict how the heart will behave after a mechanical load is removed. Even retrospective analysis of preoperative studies cannot distinguish between those who will survive and those who will succumb to an operation. There is thus no alternative to accepting patients for surgical treatment even though operative risks may be high. Statistical analysis has shown that left ventricular function measurements are significant indicators of the prognosis, but they should not be used to make absolute predictions or to make the decision in individual cases. The most logical approach—although it is not easy to achieve—is to follow patients as closely as possible, recognize surgically treatable lesions at an early stage, and operate before severe myocardial damage occurs.

NORMAL VALUES

At Rest

Equations and normal values for pressures, flows, and resistances are shown inside the back cover.

The normal resting cardiac output of about 6 L/min (cardiac index about 4.1 L/min/m²) varies from about 3.5 L/min to 7.5 L/min, or a cardiac index of 2.5–3.5 L/min/m².

The normal blood volume of about 5 L is composed of about 2.75 L of plasma and 2.25 L of red cells to give a hematocrit of 2.25 ÷ 5, or 45%. The volume of blood in the heart and lungs (central blood volume) totals about 1.5 L. About 0.9 L is contained in the pulmonary arteries, capillaries, and veins, but only about 75 mL is in the pulmonary capillaries at any instant. The total volume of blood in the heart is about 0.6 L. Left ventricular volume at the end of diastole is about 150 mL; with a stroke volume of 100 mL and an ejection fraction of 67%, the end-systolic volume is 50 mL. The conventional normal values for arterial pressure of 120 mm Hg systolic and 80 mm Hg diastolic should be thought of as normal for young adults. Arterial pressure varies with age. (See Chapter 9 regarding the upper limit of normal.) Mean arterial pressure changes little with posture; systolic pressure may fall when the patient stands up after having been supine. Depending on the effective blood volume, diastolic pressure rises, pulse pressure decreases, and heart rate increases.

The normal mitral valve area is greater than 3 cm². Values of about 1.5 cm² indicate slight stenosis, and 1 cm² or less indicates significant stenosis. Aortic valve area is greater than 2 cm². Values of about 1 cm² indicate mild stenosis and 0.7 cm² or less, significant stenosis. The normal pulmonary vascular resistance is less than 2 mm Hg/L/min, or less than 160 dyne•s•cm⁻⁵. The normal systemic resistance is less than 20 mm Hg/L/min, or less than 1600 dyne•s•cm⁻⁵.

The maximal rate of change of left ventricular

pressure is about 1200 mm Hg/s, and the corresponding figure for the right ventricle is about 250 mm Hg/s.

The normal resting ventilation is about 5 L/min. Normal arterial PO_2 is between 70 and 100 mm Hg, PCO_2 is 37–42 mm Hg, and pH is 7.36–7.43.

With Exercise

During moderate exercise (sufficient to increase heart rate to about 120/min), oxygen consumption increases from about 250–300 mL/min to 1200–1500 mL/min. Arteriovenous oxygen difference increases from 50 mL/L to about 100 mL/L; and cardiac output to about 15 L/min. Blood gas tensions and pH do not change significantly. Ventilation increases to 30–40 L/min. Stroke volume increases to about 125 mL and arterial pulse pressure to about 60 mm Hg, with a systolic pressure of 130 mm Hg and a diastolic pressure of 70 mm Hg. With more severe exercise (oxygen consumption about 2500 mL/min), most untrained normal subjects show evidence of metabolic acidosis, with an increase in arterial lactate, a fall in pH, and a fall in arterial PCO_2 to about 35 mm Hg. The maximal heart rate in young adults of about 195/min falls to about 170 at the age of 60 years. Most patients with heart disease do not complain of dyspnea until their maximal oxygen consumption falls to less than 1200–1500 mL/min. By the time they are seriously disabled, their maximal cardiac output is about 10 L/min.

REFERENCES

AHA Committee Report: Recommendations for human blood pressure determination by sphygmomanometers: Circulation 1980;62:1145A.

Antman EM et al: Blood oxygen measurement in the assessment of intracardiac left to right shunts: A critical appraisal of methodology. Am J Cardiol 1980;46:265.

Bennett ED et al: Ascending aortic blood velocity and acceleration using Doppler ultrasound in the assessment of left ventricular function. Cardiovasc Res 1984;18:632.

Bryg RJ et al: Effect of coronary artery disease on Doppler-derived parameters of aortic flow during upright exercise. Am J Cardiol 1986;58:14.

Cohn PF: *Clinical Cardiovascular Physiology.* Saunders, 1985.

Currie PJ et al: Continuous wave Doppler echocardiographic assessment of severity of calcific aortic stenosis: A simultaneous Doppler-catheter correlative study in 100 adult patients. Circulation 1985;71:1162.

De Zuttere D et al: Doppler echocardiographic measurement of mitral flow volume: Validation of a new method in adult patients. J Am Coll Cardiol 1988;11:343.

Dodge HT, Sheehan FH: Quantitative contrast angiography for assessment of ventricular performance in heart disease. J Am Coll Cardiol 1983;1:73.

Ganz W, Swan HJC: Measurement of blood flow by thermodilution. Am J Cardiol 1972;29:241.

Ganz W et al: Measurement of coronary sinus blood flow by continuous thermodilution in man. Circulation 1971;44:181.

Gorlin R, Gorlin SG: Hydraulic formula for calculation of the area of the stenotic mitral valve, other cardiac valves, and central circulatory shunts. Am Heart J 1951;41:1.

Hatle L: Doppler echocardiographic evaluation of mitral stenosis. Cardiol Clin 1990;8:233.

Hatle L, Angelsen BA, Tromsdol A: Noninvasive assessment of aortic stenosis by Doppler ultrasound. Br Heart J 1980;43:284.

Hoosack KF et al: Maximal cardiac output during upright exercise: Approximate normal standards and variations with coronary disease. Am J Cardiol 1980;46:204.

Judge KW, Otto CM: Doppler echocardiographic evaluation of aortic stenosis. Cardiol Clin 1990;8:203.

Kety SS, Schmidt CF: The nitrous oxide method for the quantitative determination of cerebral blood flow in man: Theory, procedure and normal values. J Clin Invest 1948;27:476.

Klocke FJ: Measurements of coronary blood flow and degree of stenosis: Current clinical implications and continuing uncertainties. J Am Coll Cardiol 1983;1:31.

Levy BI et al: Non-invasive ultrasonic cardiac output measurement in intensive care unit. Ultrasound Med Biol 1985;11:841.

Levy B et al: Quantitative ascending aortic Doppler blood velocity in normal human subjects. Cardiovasc Res 1985;19:383.

Marcus ML, Wilson RF, White CW: Methods of measurement of myocardial blood flow in patients: A critical review. Circulation 1987;76:245.

Mehta N et al: Usefulness of noninvasive Doppler measurement of ascending aortic blood velocity and acceleration in detecting impairment of the left ventricular functional response to exercise three weeks after acute myocardial infarction. Am J Cardiol 1986;58:879.

Millar HD, Baker LE: A stable ultra-miniature catheter-tip pressure transducer. Med Biol Eng 1973;11:86.

Mills CJ: A catheter-tip electromagnetic velocity probe. Phys Med Biol 1966;11:323.

Murray JF: The Normal Lung: *The Basis for Diagnosis and Treatment of Pulmonary Disease,* 2nd ed. Saunders, 1986.

Narins RE, Emmett M: Simple and mixed acid-based disorders: A practical approach. Medicine 1980;59:161.

Popp RL: Echocardiography. (Two parts.) N Engl J Med 1990;323:101, 165.

Ross JJ: Cardiac function and myocardial contractility: A perspective. J Am Coll Cardiol 1983;1:52.

Severinghaus JW: Blood gas calculator. J Appl Physiol 1966;20:1108.

Sharpey-Schafer EP: Effects of Valsalva's manoeuver on

normal and failing circulation. Br Med J 1955;1:693.

Stamm RB, Martin RP: Quantification of pressure gradients across stenotic valves by Doppler ultrasound. J Am Coll Cardiol 1983;2:707.

Swan HJC: Indicator-dilution methods in the diagnosis of congenital heart disease. Prog Cardiovasc Dis 1959;2:143.

Wilson RF et al: Transluminal, subselective measurement of coronary artery blood flow velocity and vasodilator reserve in man. Circulation 1985;72:82.

5

Special Investigations: Noninvasive

INTRODUCTION

Special cardiologic investigations are dealt with under the headings of noninvasive and invasive studies. This distinction is maintained in the subsequent chapters dealing with individual diseases. The descriptions of special investigations given here and in Chapter 6 deal in general terms with the principles involved in the various studies. They are intended not to provide sufficient technical details to enable a person to carry out the procedures but rather to aid in the understanding and interpretation of the various tests.

Routine Cardiologic Investigations

The clinical examination of all cardiac patients is incomplete without the recording of a 12-lead ECG and a chest x-ray. The physician should interpret the ECG and chest x-rays independently before reading the opinions of the radiologist or electrocardiographer who may have provided a written interpretation of the findings. Both investigations are so important to clinical evaluation that a valid opinion about a patient's condition cannot be given until both have been seen by the physician.

Special Investigations

All investigations other than chest x-rays and ECG are considered to be special studies indicated by some clinical finding. Standard laboratory tests of blood, urine, feces, sputum, bone marrow, and cerebrospinal fluid may be required in the diagnostic investigation of the patient with cardiovascular disease. The laboratory findings in each type of cardiac disease are covered in the chapters dealing with that disease.

Special Cardiovascular Studies

Two main types of information are sought by cardiologic studies: anatomic (structural) and physiologic (functional). Although the relationship between structure and function is usually close, it is important to keep clearly in mind what specific information is being sought in any study. In many types of investigations (eg, cardiac catheterization) both structural and functional information is provided. In general, ana-

tomic abnormalities relate to a specific diagnosis, whereas physiologic findings are more pertinent to degrees of functional impairment.

Most forms of cardiac investigation start as research procedures. Whether any new procedure will ultimately be accepted by the medical community is not usually decided for several years. The decisive factors include the clinical usefulness of the procedure, the prevalence of the conditions for which it is indicated, and economic factors such as cost of equipment that are outside the scope of this book. Not surprisingly, the current cardiologic literature is largely preoccupied with new forms of investigation that are still in the uncertain stage between research studies and standard procedures.

In all forms of investigation, it is important for the physician to bear in mind the cost to the patient in danger, discomfort, and expense and to distinguish clearly between clinically indicated studies and ancillary confirmatory procedures. Accurate diagnosis is always required and is essential in every case in which cardiac surgery is contemplated. Because being right 85–90% of the time is not enough, studies must sometimes be done for confirmatory purposes even though the diagnosis is clinically almost certain.

Interpretation of Results

The greatly increased use of noninvasive tests to diagnose disease, especially in its early, presymptomatic stages, has led to problems in the interpretation of test results. The importance of the result of a given test is difficult to determine accurately. The results of any test must be considered in the context of the patient as a whole, including the history and physical examination. At present, decisions for and against surgical intervention are heavily dependent on the patient's symptoms and the degree of interference in the patient's life which has occurred because of the disease. In making this evaluation, there is no better "test" than a good, probing history.

A. Sensitivity and Specificity: The significance of a "positive test" is reflected in the sensitivity of the test, which expresses its ability to detect "the disease" in patients in whom it is present. Sensitivity is defined as—

$$\frac{\text{True positive}}{\text{True positive + False negative}} = \text{Tests \%}$$

The significance of a negative test is reflected in the specificity of the test, which expresses its ability to exclude "the disease." Specificity is defined as—

$$\frac{\text{True negative}}{\text{True negative + False positive}} = \text{Tests \%}$$

The concept of "false-positive" and "false-negative" tests implies a "gold standard" or accurate means of deciding whether a given disease is present or not, but disease is not an all-or-none phenomenon, especially in its early stages, and "gold standards" of diagnosis are necessarily fallible and subject to change. The prevalence of "the disease" in the population under study is also an important variable that influences the probability of finding a given test positive or negative. (See also Chapter 8.) In practice, especially in patients with coronary artery disease, the finding of agreement (for or against the diagnosis) in several elements in the diagnosis—history, ECG, exercise test, or radionuclide study—is the most important evidence for or against.

B. Results of Tests in Asymptomatic Persons: The problem of dealing with asymptomatic persons is difficult. Most cardiac diseases cannot be defined in terms of a single specific abnormality but consist of constellations of findings. Diagnoses of conditions such as coronary artery disease, mitral valve prolapse (click-murmur syndrome), and hypertrophic cardiomyopathy should be regarded with caution when made on the basis of abnormalities discovered on a single test in an asymptomatic, otherwise normal person. The overenthusiastic use of a particular test to find persons with subclinical disease is of doubtful value unless specific treatment is indicated.

RECORDING OF THE ECG

Technique

The simplest diagnostic procedure with which every physician must be familiar is the taking of a standard 12-lead electrocardiogram (ECG). Modern electrocardiographs have become simple to use, and problems are most likely to be related to matching wall plugs, connecting the cables to the electrodes properly, and eliminating electrical interference. With any type of electrode, providing adequate localized skin contact with the right amount of electrode paste is important. Correct and consistent precordial electrode placement is important, especially when serial records are needed. Interference from other electrical equipment, eg, electric blankets in domiciliary practice, should be suspected when 60-cycle noise is encountered. Increased electronic filtering should not be used to eliminate this, as it will almost certainly decrease the frequency response of the equipment and give a damped and inaccurate ECG.

Each lead of the ECG should be properly calibrated.

Safety

The examiner should remain alert to the possibility of ground loops, which present a risk of electrocution when more than one electrical device is attached to the patient. Patients with temporary artificial pacemakers are particularly vulnerable, because currents as low as 10 μA applied directly to the endocardium via the pacemaker catheter can cause ventricular fibrillation.

Electrocardiographic Interpretation

The details of electrocardiographic interpretation per se are not presented in this book. The electrocardiographic findings are discussed in the chapters dealing with individual diseases. For further information on the theory and practice of electrocardiographic interpretation, the reader is referred to Goldschlager N, Goldman MJ: *Principles of Clinical Electrocardiography,* 13th ed. Appleton & Lange, 1989.

Computer-Assisted Electrocardiography

Computer analysis of ECGs has been available for more than 2 decades. The development of self-contained microprocessor-based analysis systems small enough to fit on a small mobile cart has improved the availability and accuracy of electrocardiographic interpretation. It is estimated that more than a third of ECGs now recorded in the USA are interpreted by computer. Computer interpretation is most accurate in identifying normal ECGs and most likely to be inaccurate in properly identifying arrhythmias and in the qualitative evaluation of ST segment changes. The current optimal approach is immediate interpretation by computer analysis that is later confirmed or revised by a cardiologist (Schlant, 1992).

Reporting Results; Display of Tracings

The tracing should be examined, mounted, and reported and the results returned to the patient's chart as soon as possible (within 24 hours). Care must be taken to correctly identify the ECG with the patient's name and hospital number. The interpretation should include the rhythm; rate; axis; duration of the PR, QRS, and QT_c intervals; and description of P, QRS, and ST–T abnormalities in each lead, followed by an estimate of the significance of the findings.

Serial records or comparisons with previous tracings are often necessary for proper interpretation.

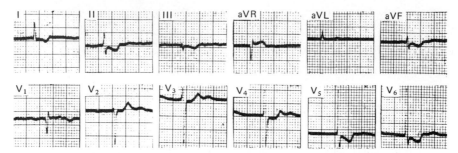

Figure 5–1. Effect of digitalis: The rhythm is atrial fibrillation. Note the ST segment depression. This produces an oblique downward configuration of the first portion of the ST in leads I, II, III, aVF, and V_{5-6}. There is a rounded ST segment depression in V_{3-4}. As a result, the T waves are "dragged" downward. There is reciprocal ST elevation in aVR. The above changes are indicative of digitalis effect but do not indicate digitalis toxicity. (Reproduced, with permission, from Goldschlager N, Goldman MJ: *Principles of Clinical Electrocardiography,* 13th ed. Appleton & Lange, 1989.)

Records obtained over 1–5 minutes or 4- to 24-hour monitoring or those obtained during or after exercise or interventions such as carotid sinus massage may clarify the relationship between symptoms and electrocardiographic abnormalities. The role of medications and metabolic or electrolyte state must be considered in interpretation. For example, digitalis or quinidine therapy, hyperkalemia, or hypokalemia can often be confused with primary myocardial disease (Figures 5–1 to 5–4).

Signal-Averaged Electrocardiography (See Chapter 15.)

A recent development in electrocardiography has been the introduction of the signal-averaged ECG. In this technique, the ECG is recorded as high speed (200 mm/s) and high sensitivity (1.00 mm/μV). The signal is signal-averaged to filter out baseline noise and filtered usually at 40–250 Hz. Abnormal low-frequency late potentials in the last 40 ms of the QRS can be detected which correlate with afterdepolarizations seen in patients who develop malignant ventricular tachyarrhythmias. The absence of these late low-frequency potentials predicts the inability to induce sustained ventricular tachycardia at invasive electrophysiologic study (Breithardt, 1991).

CHEST X-RAYS

Size of Heart Shadow

The posteroanterior chest x-ray is used for overall assessment of heart size. It should be taken with the x-ray tube 6 feet from the x-ray so that distortion of heart size is avoided. As a rough guide, the widest part of the heart should be less than half the diameter of the thorax. The Ungerleider tables, which relate the transverse diameter of the heart to the patient's height and weight, are probably more reliable than the simple measurement.

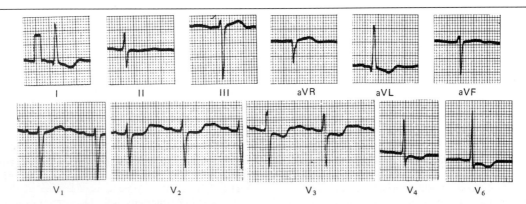

Figure 5–2. Effect of quinidine. The rhythm is regular sinus; PR = 0.2 s. The R in aVL = 14 mm. There is ST depression and T wave inversion in I, aVL, and V_{2-6}. The measured QT interval (see V_{2-3}) = 0.6 s (QT_c = 0.65 s). ***Clinical diagnosis:*** Aortic stenosis; quinidine therapy for previous ventricular arrhythmias. The R voltage in aVL and some of the ST–T changes are due to left ventricular hypertrophy. The long QT interval is due to quinidine. (Reproduced, with permission, from Goldschlager N, Goldman MJ: *Principles of Clinical Electrocardiography,* 13th ed. Appleton & Lange, 1989.)

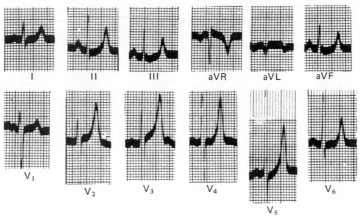

Figure 5–3. Hyperkalemia (chronic glomerulonephritis with uremia). Tall slender T waves are seen in I, II, III, aVF, and V_{2-6}. The rhythm is regular sinus; QRS interval = 0.09 s. Serum potassium = 7.2 meq/L. (Reproduced, with permission, from Goldschlager N, Goldman MJ: *Principles of Clinical Electrocardiography,* 13th ed. Appleton & Lange, 1989.)

Shape of the Heart

A. Posteroanterior View: (Figure 5–5A.) From above downward one sees the aortic knob or knuckle, the pulmonary artery, the left atrial appendage, and the rounded shadow of the left ventricle. The left atrial appendage is not normally visible as a bulge. The right border of the heart is formed by the superior vena cava or aorta above and by the right atrium below, and it is difficult to be sure whether the atrium is enlarged or displaced when the heart shadow is large. **Note:** Differentiation between the left and right ventricle cannot always be made accurately on chest radiography; the echocardiogram is more accurate than the chest radiograph in identifying individual chamber size. The ECG reflects hypertrophy, whereas the chest film reflects dilation.

B. Lateral View: (Figure 5–5B.) The lateral chest x-ray is useful in assessing left ventricular and left atrial size. These two structures form the posterior wall of the heart, and marked posterior displacement

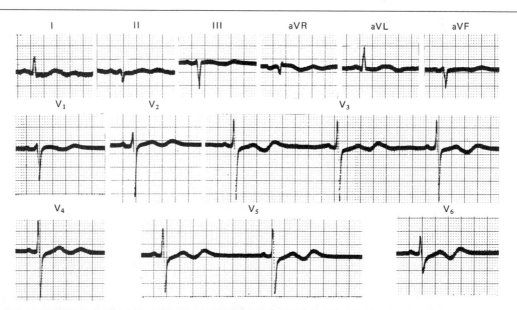

Figure 5–4. Hypokalemia (Cushing's syndrome). Regular sinus rhythm; PR = 0.16 s; QRS = 0.1 s. The frontal plane QRS axis = –40 degrees. There is ST depression in leads I, aVL, and V_{3-6}. Prominent U waves are seen in all precordial leads. The measured QT interval = 0.51 s, but when corrected for a heart rate of 37, the QT_c = 0.39 s. Serum potassium = 2.5 meq/L. (Reproduced, with permission, from Goldschlager N, Goldman MJ: *Principles of Clinical Electrocardiography,* 13th ed. Appleton & Lange, 1989).

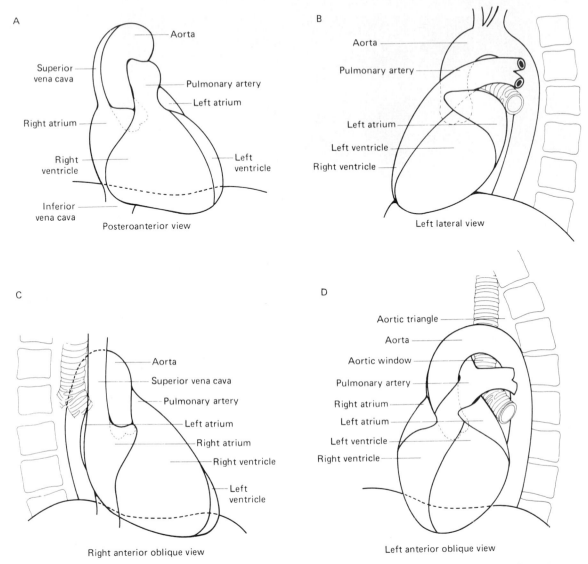

Figure 5–5. Diagrams showing radiologic features in a normal cardiac series. **A:** posteroanterior view; **B:** left lateral view; **C:** right anterior oblique view; **D:** left anterior oblique view.

of the cardiac shadow is usually seen best when the esophagus has been filled with barium. The downward sweep of the posterior part of the left ventricle passes below and behind the inferior vena cava when the left ventricle is enlarged. The right ventricle tends to lie close to the sternum when it enlarges. This sign is not specific, however, and displacement as well as enlargement may be responsible.

C. Right Anterior Oblique View: (Figure 5–5C.) The right anterior oblique view of the cardiac silhouette is most valuable in the assessment of enlargement of the right ventricular outflow tract and main pulmonary artery. These structures form the anterior border of the heart in this view, and absence or decrease in the size of the outflow tract, as in Fallot's tetralogy and pulmonary atresia, is also discernible.

D. Left Anterior Oblique View: (Figure 5–5D.) The left anterior oblique view is most valuable in left-sided lesions. The left atrium and left ventricle form the posterior edge of the cardiac shadow in this view, and the aortic arch is seen in its widest aspect, arching from front to back above the cardiac shadow. Two landmarks in this view are the aortic triangle above and the aortic window below the arch. Their boundaries are indicated in Figure 5–5D. Coarctation of the aorta is best seen in this view, which is also best for demonstrating dilation of the ascending aorta. The degree of penetration which is optimal for cardiac x-rays is greater than that for pulmonary x-rays. Overpenetrating x-rays are sometimes useful, especially to demonstrate the size of the left atrium.

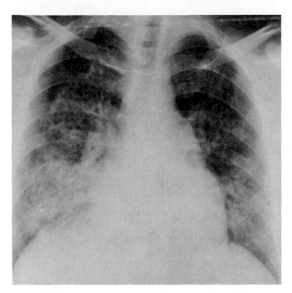

Figure 5–6. Chest x-ray of a patient with pulmonary edema showing perihilar ("bat's wing") distribution, especially on the right side. The lung periphery is relatively free of infiltrate.

Lung Fields

Interpretation of the chest x-ray also involves examination of the lung fields for evidence of pulmonary congestion, redistribution of blood flow to the upper lung fields, pulmonary plethora in left-to-right shunts, and pulmonary oligemia with reduced pulmonary blood flow. Pulmonary edema tends to be central in origin and to spread out from the root of the lung. It is not infrequently asymmetric, perhaps because the patient lies on one side or the other. An example is shown in Figure 5–6.

ULTRASONOGRAPHY, ECHOCARDIOGRAPHY & DOPPLER ECHOCARDIOGRAPHY

Ultrasonography has developed rapidly as an important form of noninvasive cardiac investigation. Ultrasonic energy within the range of frequencies used in clinical studies has proved to be harmless in more than a decade of use. The standard ultrasound transducer consists of a piezoelectric crystal that is excited electronically to transmit sound waves at frequencies between 2 and 13 MHz. The beam of sound waves penetrates soft tissues and is reflected at interfaces, eg, between blood and heart muscle or heart valves. The ultrasound reflected from cardiac tissues is received at the transducer and electronically processed to provide images of the heart. The penetration of tissues by ultrasound depends on the frequency of the ultrasound. High frequencies (10 MHz) penetrate

poorly and can only be used for tissues within a few millimeters of the surface. Low frequencies (2 MHz) penetrate more deeply (up to 20 cm) and can reach all intracardiac structures.

Blood is a poorer reflector than tissue, but as it moves, it causes a shift in the frequency of reflected ultrasound that can be detected and used to measure flow in the circulation using the Doppler principle (see Chapter 4). Ultrasound does not penetrate bone or air-containing lung tissue, because it is strongly reflected at interfaces where there is a large acoustic impedance mismatch. Thus, in adults, access from the skin to the heart is limited to areas where the heart abuts against the intercostal spaces and to suprasternal and subcostal approaches. A newer technique that places an ultrasonic crystal on the end of a gastroscope allows echocardiographic access to the heart from the esophagus, thus coming closest to the heart and offering the further advantage of having no air interspersed between the ultrasound crystal and the heart. An aqueous gel is used to couple the transducer to the skin, and the transducers are usually focused at a depth of 5–10 cm. The several modes available for the display of the ultrasonic signals are illustrated in Figure 5–7.

The time required for the reflected sound signals to return to the transducer varies with the distance traveled and provides a form of echo ranging. The transducer is switched to receive when it is not transmitting and puts out an electronic signal proportionate to the intensity of the echoes.

A Mode

In an A mode echo system, the intensity of the returning echoes is displayed on one axis of an oscilloscope (horizontal axis in Figure 5–7), and the time required for the transmitted wave to travel from the transducer to the target and back is displayed on the other axis (vertical axis in Figure 5–7).

B Mode

In B mode echocardiography, the intensity of the echo signal is displayed as the brightness of the signal on the oscilloscope screen, and the distance from the transducer appears on the y axis.

M Mode

In M mode (motion) echocardiography, a B mode echo signal is recorded on the vertical axis, with time on the horizontal axis, either by sweeping the oscilloscope screen or by photographing the oscilloscope face on moving paper. Thus, the conventional M mode display shows time on the horizontal axis, distance on the vertical axis, and intensity of the echo by brightness. An ECG is recorded for timing, and the movement of the structures within the beam is displayed during the cardiac cycle. In M mode echocardiography, the transducer is excited at 2–7 MHz with 1000 pulses per second (repetition rate 1 kHz). The

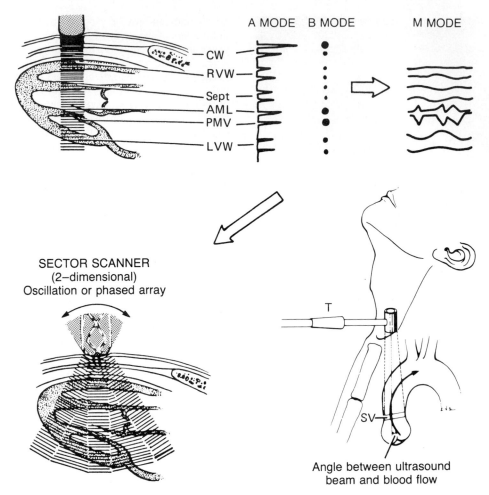

Figure 5–7. Different modes of display of ultrasonic information. The structures displayed in A mode, B mode, M mode, and sector scanning, from front to back, are the chest wall (CW), the right ventricular wall (RVW), the interventricular septum (Sept), the anterior mitral valve leaflet (AML), the posterior mitral valve leaflet (PMV), and the posterior wall of the left ventricle (LVW). The Doppler transducer (T) is depicted in the suprasternal notch with its sample volume (SV) in the ascending aorta. (Courtesy of NH Silverman and NB Schiller.)

image is thus updated every 1 ms, giving a signal with an excellent frequency response.

M mode echocardiography is now used in conjunction with two-dimensional echocardiography mainly to make accurate measurements of wall thickness and chamber diameter. It is also the best way to see early closure of the mitral valve in acute aortic regurgitation and systolic anterior motion of the mitral valve in hypertrophic cardiomyopathy.

Two-Dimensional (2-D) Echocardiography

A more complicated and expensive two-dimensional scanning technique is now universally used. In these studies, a B mode echographic tracing is rapidly and sequentially scanned across a sector field at a rate sufficient to provide a continuous image to the unaided eye (frequency 20–30 Hz). The scanning pro-

cess, depicted in Figure 5–7, can be either mechanical, with rapid oscillation of the transducer, or, as is most common, electronic, with an array of crystals being sequentially and repeatedly excited to provide a similar form of scan (phased array). The sector scanner provides a pie-shaped image within which the reflective cardiac structures move in two dimensions. By placing the transducer appropriately, transverse, sagittal, or coronal sections can be displayed and the scope of the ultrasonic examination greatly increased. The frequency response of sector scanners is inferior to that of M mode echocardiography and is comparable to that of x-ray angiography. However, the advantages of seeing the motion of the heart in two dimensions in real time far outweigh any loss of resolution resulting from the use of two-dimensional instruments. It is not possible to do justice to the technique with single-frame pictures, and it is not surprising that two-dimensional echocardiography is the primary form of ultrasonic investigation, with M mode being relegated to an ancillary role.

Doppler Ultrasound

In Doppler studies, the velocity of blood flow is detected via the frequency shift of reflected ultrasound. The process is governed by the Doppler equation (see Chapter 4).

A. Continuous Wave and Pulsed, Range-Gated Doppler: Two forms of Doppler ultrasonic instrument are used: continuous wave Doppler and pulsed, range-gated Doppler. In the simpler, continuous wave instruments, separate transmitting and receiving crystals are continuously active, and reflected signals are obtained from all structures within the ultrasound beam. In pulsed, range-gated instruments, a single crystal is used to transmit pulses at a rate of 7–10 kHz. Between transmitted bursts, the transducer is switched to receive signals from moving targets. The longer the time between the burst (pulse) of ultrasound and the time of reception of reflected signals, the farther the target is from the transducer. By opening the "gate" at specific times and receiving reflected signals at varying intervals after transmission, it is possible to restrict the received signals to structures at specific distances from the surface of the chest. Pulsed, range-gated Doppler instruments can thus detect blood flow in specific blood vessels (aorta or pulmonary artery) and cardiac chambers.

Compared with continuous wave Doppler instruments, pulsed, range-gated instruments are limited in the range of frequencies (velocities) they can record, because of factors related to the repetition rate. By increasing the repetition rate, it is possible to increase the range of frequencies recorded, but this technique is less satisfactory than the use of simpler, less expensive continuous wave instruments, whose main advantage is that there is no limit to the range of frequencies they can record. The main disadvantage of continuous wave instruments is that information is obtained without regard to the site of origin of the signal. Conversely, pulsed instruments can record accurate signals only over a limited range of frequencies but can restrict the received information to structures located at specific distances from the transducer.

B. Doppler Combined With Echocardiography: When Doppler techniques are combined with echocardiography (two-dimensional or M mode), it is possible to obtain a combination of anatomic and physiologic information and correlate structure with function. Doppler techniques have been combined with echocardiography in the assessment of valvular lesions, which alter the pattern of blood flow. Disturbed flow associated with stenosis, incompetence, and shunt lesions (eg, ventricular septal defect, patent ductus arteriosus) can be recognized using this technique.

Quantitative measurements with simultaneous echo and Doppler recordings are difficult because the optimal angle for echographic investigations is not generally compatible with that for Doppler studies. The best definition of echographic signals is obtained when the ultrasound beam intersects its target at right angles. With this aim, the shift in frequency is, in theory, zero, since the value of cos Θ in the Doppler equation should be zero. Doppler signals are best recorded with transducers aimed nearly axially. Intracardiac recordings present less of a problem. Using an apical four-chamber view of the heart, it is possible to aim the transducer in the axis of flow through either the mitral or the aortic valve and obtain satisfactory Doppler and echographic signals with the same transducer position.

C. Assessment of Left Ventricular Function: Measurement of the rate of increase in blood velocity in the ascending aorta during early ejection provides evidence about left ventricular function. This measure of acceleration in $cm \bullet s^{-2}$ can be made during exercise. It is important to measure the mean velocity rather than the highest velocity in the signals.

D. Assessment of Pulmonary Vascular Resistance: The equivalent measurement of the acceleration of blood in the pulmonary artery provides an indication of pulmonary vascular resistance as well as right ventricular function. The time to peak velocity provides a simple index of pulmonary vascular resistance that has been used to follow changes in the pulmonary circulation during growth and development from infancy to adulthood. The main pulmonary artery is much more readily accessible in children. With aging and the development of lung disease, the pulmonary artery becomes harder to find.

Measurement of Pressure Gradients

The use of measurements of the peak velocity of blood flow in a jet of blood passing through a stenosed valve to calculate the pressure gradient across the valve has already been described (see Chapter 4). The method, which uses a continuous wave instrument, has been validated in patients with aortic, pulmonary, and mitral stenosis.

Contrast Echocardiography

Ultrasound is particularly sensitive to the presence of microscopic bubbles in the circulation. The interface between the gas in the bubble and the blood reflects ultrasound strongly. Any freshly made solution or forceful injection of liquid contains or generates sufficient intravascular bubbles to be detectable in either echocardiographic or Doppler recordings from the heart. These effects have been used to carry out the equivalent of indicator dilution curve studies, identifying intracardiac shunts by means of ultrasound and establishing connections between different areas of the heart and great vessels. The techniques are qualitative rather than quantitative and are harmless. Recent work has been directed toward the preparation of particles that will generate bubbles small enough to pass through the pulmonary capillary bed and enhance ultrasonic contrast in the left heart. The use of such a contrast agent should also permit the ultrasonic assessment of myocardial perfusion following intracoronary injection. Starting with handshaken or sonicated saline or dilute radiopaque contrast material, various techniques have been used to develop a satisfactory ultrasonic contrast material. Achieving a stable, uniform particle size approximating that of a red cell is an important problem. The possibility has also been raised of determining intracardiac pressure noninvasively by detecting the resonant frequency of bubbles excited by ultrasound.

Transesophageal Echocardiography (TEE)

Miniature phased-array transducers mounted at the end of a gastroscope have been developed to image the heart anteriorly and the descending aorta posteriorly through the esophageal wall. The transesophageal echo probe is passed—after local anesthesia is achieved to eliminate the gag reflex—down the esophagus, visualizing different levels of the heart and great vessels. At first, the level of the aortic arch is seen, then the ascending and descending aorta. Passing caudally, the left atrium, left ventricle, and right ventricular outflow tract can be seen. Farther down, the mitral valve with leaflets and chordae tendineae can be visualized, and lower down the papillary muscles all can be visualized with exquisite clarity. Transesophageal echocardiography has importance because the transducer is near the areas of interest without interposing lung. The images are magnified and very detailed. The procedure is extremely useful for visualizing the anatomy of the aortic and mitral valves and valve rings, the ascending aorta and the entire descending aorta up to the arch, and the left ventricle in cross-section. During surgery, cardiac anesthesiologists have come to rely on Transesophageal echocardiography to monitor cardiac function. With this technique, the cross-sectional view of the left ventricle can be constantly imaged and the wall motion analyzed moment-to-moment. With ischemia, there are immediate changes in diastolic and then systolic function.

Color Doppler can also be used with this technique, making it especially valuable in assessing the severity of mitral and aortic valve regurgitation and stenosis. This is especially important in evaluating the mitral valve for repair rather than replacement and judging the competence of the valve after repair. It is also valuable in detecting the intimal flap in dissection of the aorta, because both the ascending aorta and the entire descending aorta can be visualized. With infective endocarditis, mitral and aortic ring abscesses can be seen that are entirely missed by transthoracic echocardiography. Transesophageal echocardiography is especially helpful in evaluating prosthetic valves.

Color Flow Doppler Echocardiography

Color flow Doppler mapping is an important new development in the field of ultrasound. A wide-angle, phased-array transducer samples the Doppler shift frequency at multiple levels along each radial line of ultrasound, while a two-dimensional echocardiographic image is recorded. The multiple Doppler signals are separated according to their direction toward or away from the transducer and transmitted to an autocorrelator and then to a color convertor. The degree of spectral broadening is detected and color-coded as a green mixed with the red and blue that are conventionally used to code flow respectively toward and away from the transducer. The brightness of the red and blue signals is proportionate to the velocity of the target. When the velocity of blood flow exceeds the range of the pulsed Doppler instrument, an apparent reversal of the direction of flow occurs. This phenomenon, called **aliasing,** causes high-velocity blue jets to develop a red central zone and red jets to develop a blue central zone.

This new and expensive technique provides color patterns that are relatively easy to recognize. It greatly helps in interpreting studies of patients with congenital heart disease. In valvular disease, it is valuable in identifying jets related to stenotic or incompetent valves. The technique makes it easier to localize jet lesions and position the sample volume in the axis of the jet. This improves the accuracy of pressure gradient measurements. Because the angle between the ultrasound beam and the flowing blood varies in different parts of the image, quantitative measurements cannot be made; however, the method provides information that is as useful in the diagnosis of congenital heart disease as that provided by conventional angiocardiography.

Normal M Mode Findings

The structures that can be observed in what has come to be the basic echocardiographic scanning maneuver are shown in Figure 5–8.

A. Mitral Valve: With the transducer (T) in constant contact with the patient's skin through a layer of coupling jelly, the beam is aimed posteriorly through the fourth left intercostal space to the left of the sternum. In position 1 (Figure 5–8), the mitral valve leaflet echo is readily picked up. The beam intersects the right ventricular cavity, the interventricular septum, and the left ventricular cavity before passing through the mitral valve to reach the posterior wall of the left ventricle. In the example shown in Figure 5–8, there is an echo-free space anterior to the right ventricle and behind the left ventricle owing to pericardial effusion. Clearer pictures can usually be obtained when the heart is surrounded by fluid, which

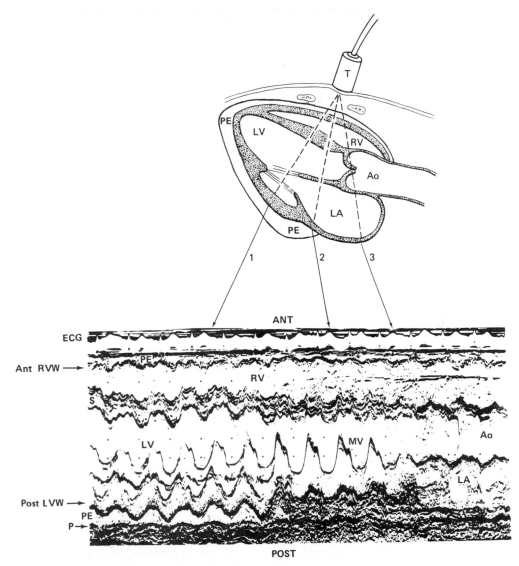

Figure 5–8. M mode echocardiogram showing normal intracardiac structures in a patient with pericardial effusion. The transducer (T) was moved from position 1 to position 3 during the recording. ANT, anterior; RV, right ventricular cavity; LV, left ventricular cavity; S,septum; MV, mitral valve; Ao, aorta; LA, left atrium; PE, pericardial effusion; POST, posterior; Ant RVW, anterior right ventricular wall; Post LVW, posterior left ventricular wall; P, pericardium. (Courtesy of NB Schiller.)

acts like aqueous coupling jelly to improve the quality of the signals. During systole, the anterior leaflet lies close to the posterior leaflet. Diastole starts from point D, and the anterior leaflet moves forward toward the septum, reaching point E. As flow falls off in mid diastole, the anterior leaflet moves backward to a minimum point (F) before moving forward again as a result of atrial contraction to a new point A. Throughout the whole of diastole, the posterior leaflet remains close to the posterior wall of the left ventricle.

B. Left Ventricle: By tilting the transducer in the direction of the feet, a picture of the left ventricular cavity is obtained.

C. Aortic Valve: Tilting the transducer upward and slightly medially through position 2 to position 3 in Figure 5–8 brings the aortic valve into view. Behind the aortic root, the left atrium can be visualized.

Normal Two-Dimensional Findings

The three standard orthogonal imaging planes used in two-dimensional echocardiography are illustrated in Figure 5–9. In the long-axis view, the transducer is placed in the third or fourth left intercostal space, beside the sternum. The scanner sweeps in a sagittal plane, intersecting the aortic and mitral valves, both ventricles, and the left atrium. The apex of the pie-

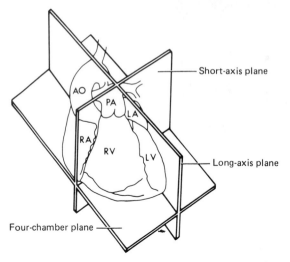

Figure 5–9. Diagram of the three orthogonal imaging planes used to visualize the heart with two-dimensional echocardiography. (Ao, aorta; LA, left atrium; LV, left ventricle; PA pulmonary artery; RA, right atrium; and RV, right ventricle.) (Reproduced, with permission of the American Heart Association, Inc., from Henry WL et al [editors]: Report of the American Society of Echocardiography Committee on Nomenclature and Standards in Two-Dimensional Echocardiography. Circulation 1980; 62: 212.)

shaped display is closest to the outflow tract of the right ventricle. The actions of the aortic and mitral valves are well seen in this view.

The short-axis view is obtained from the same position on the chest but with the axis of the scanner turned through 90 degrees, as shown in Figure 5–9. In this view, the body of the left ventricle occupies most of the field, with the right ventricle in front and to the left side of the image. Two dimensional images in the short-axis (coronal) plane are conventionally displayed as if they were seen from the feet of the subject, with the left ventricle on the right and vice versa.

The four-chamber view is obtained from the apex of the heart, with the scanner being aimed in a plane that is close to frontal. The left ventricle and atrium are on the right in this view, which intersects both the tricuspid and the mitral valves. Figure 5–10 shows the structures that can be seen in the three standard planes (long-axis, short-axis, and four-chamber).

Clinical Uses of Echocardiography

A. M Mode: The clinical value of M mode echocardiography is now clearly established, but the development of two-dimensional echocardiography has made M-mode imaging much less important. The findings in individual diseases are described in the appropriate chapters.

B. Two-Dimensional Echocardiography: Two-dimensional echocardiographic scanning can be used to display all the features that can be seen with M mode techniques. The extra dimension adds greatly to the flexibility of the study, and it is difficult with still photographs to give an adequate idea of the advantages of this technique. It has now superseded M mode echocardiography in the routine investigation of almost all forms of heart disease. Images from normal hearts are provided, showing the six conventional views: long-axis, Figure 5–11; short-axis, Figure 5–12; apical four-chamber, Figure 5–13; apical two-chamber, Figure 5–14; subcostal (inferior vena cava), Figure 5–15; and suprasternal, Figure 5–16.

C. Left Ventricular Function: Both M mode and two-dimensional echocardiography have been used to investigate left ventricular function.

1. Ventricular volume and ejection fraction– M mode echocardiography provides only a single measurement from which to calculate ventricular volume. The errors inherent in this approach preclude its use for this purpose.

Two-dimensional signals provide much superior images of the ventricle in long-axis and short-axis views. Their use for the calculation of left ventricular volume and ejection fraction is described in Chapter 4, and examples of end-systolic and end-diastolic views with the ventricular cavity outlined are shown in Figure 4–7.

2. Left ventricular mass– The thickness of the septal and posterolateral walls of the left ventricle can be readily estimated by echocardiography. Using assumptions about ventricular shape, it is possible to calculate a value for left ventricular mass that has been shown to correlate well with measurements made at autopsy. When left ventricular hypertrophy is developing, the increase in mass precedes electrocardiographic changes and is a more reliable indicator of the hypertrophic process.

3. Velocity and extent of shortening– Attempts have been made to assess ventricular "contractility" from measurement of the rate of change of position of echographic images. Such measurements should probably not be made using two-dimensional techniques, because the rate of imaging (20–30 Hz) is too slow for adequate temporal resolution. M mode signals have a better frequency response (1000 Hz), but the assumptions involved make the calculation of shortening rates only marginally acceptable.

4. Wall motion– The movement of the left ventricular wall can be readily investigated using two-dimensional scanners. An accurate visual impression of the extent and timing of the motion of different areas can be obtained that is clinically valuable, but translating this into numerical terms presents significant difficulties.

Limitations of Echocardiography

The principal limitation of ultrasonic examinations, as compared to conventional radiography, is

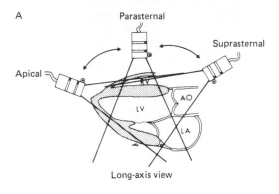

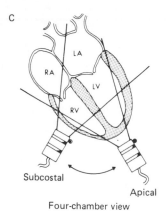

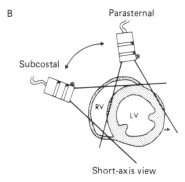

Figure 5–10. Diagram of the transducer orientations used to obtain long-axis views **(A),** short-axis views **(B),** and four–chamber views **(C)** of the heart. Note that the transducer index mark is always pointed either in the direction of the patient's head or the patient's left side. Abbreviations are as in Figure 5–12. (Reproduced, with permission of the American Heart Association, Inc., from Henry WL et al [editors]: Report of the American Society of Echocardiography Committee on Nomenclature and Standards in Two-Dimensional Echocardiography. Circulation 1980;62: 212.)

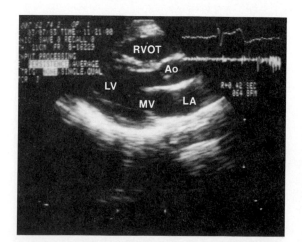

Figure 5–11. Normal two-dimensional echocardiogram, long-axis, parasternal view. (LV, left ventricle; MV, mitral valve; LA, left atrium; RVOT, right ventricular outflow tract; Ao, aorta.) Compare with Figure 5–11A. (Courtesy of NB Schiller.)

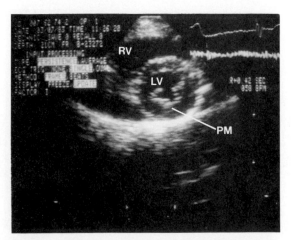

Figure 5–12. Normal two-dimensional echocardiogram, short-axis, parasternal view at ventricular level. (LV, left ventricle; RV, right ventricle; PM, papillary muscles. Compare with Figure 5–11B.) (Courtesy of NB Schiller.)

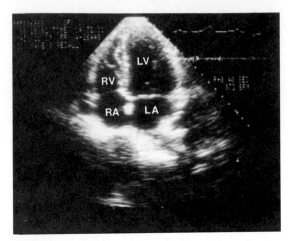

Figure 5–13. Normal two-dimensional echocardiogram, apical four-chamber view. (LV, left ventricle; RV, right ventricle; LA, left atrium; RA, right atrium.) (Courtesy of NB Schiller.)

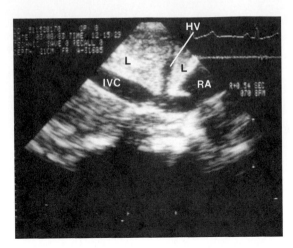

Figure 5–15. Normal two-dimensional echocardiogram, subcostal view. (L, liver; IVC, inferior vena cava; HV, hepatic vein; RA, right atrium.) (Courtesy of NB Schiller.)

that sound waves travel more slowly through tissue (about 1.5 km/s) than do x-rays (2.99×10^5 km/s). The longer wave length of the more slowly moving sound waves limits the resolution of ultrasonic examinations. Ultrasound is, however, much less damaging to tissues than x-rays, and there is as yet no clinical evidence of ill effects despite extensive use of the technique over more than 2 decades.

Skill, experience, and judgment are involved in the performance and interpretation of echocardiographic studies. The variability and the effects of observer error on the interpretation of echocardiography are now becoming apparent. The measurements made are valid in that they are made in millimeters. There is,

however, a certain element of subjectivity in setting the controls that determine the intensity of the signal, and it is possible to have structures drop out or to introduce artifacts.

PHONOCARDIOGRAPHY

Phonocardiography, the recording of heart sounds, is a standard (but not routine) study that is perhaps the most difficult and subjective of all noninvasive investigations. The apparatus is no longer available in most hospitals. Although modern bedside auscultation owes an enormous debt to phonocardiography, a re-

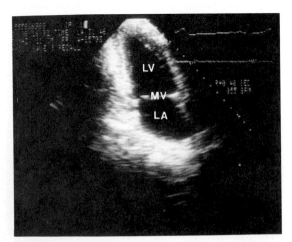

Figure 5–14. Normal two-dimensional echocardiogram, apical two-chamber view. (LV, left ventricle; LA, left atrium; MV, mitral valve.) Compare with Figure 5–11A. (Courtesy of NB Schiller.)

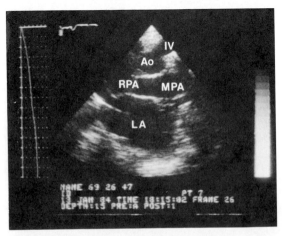

Figure 5–16. Normal two-dimensional echocardiogram, suprasternal view. (Ao, aorta; MPA, main pulmonary artery; RPA, right pulmonary artery; IV, innominate vein; LA, left atrium.) (Courtesy of NB Schiller.)

cording of heart sounds is seldom of clinical importance. Phonocardiography is most valuable in conjunction with echocardiography as a means of timing the events of the cardiac cycle and demonstrating their relationship to indirectly recorded pressure tracings such as the apexcardiogram, indirect carotid pulse tracings, external phlebograms, and stethographic recordings of respiration. It is of little value in analyzing the sound content of murmurs and heart sounds because the harmonic content of the recordings obtained is so dependent on the electrical filters used, the placing of the microphones, and the position of the patient. In consequence, phonocardiography is of most practical value in teaching auscultation and in settling differences of opinion. Its value in confirming the auscultatory findings is well established. Most people find it easier to appreciate sensory information when it is received simultaneously by two senses. Thus, listening to a patient's heart with a stethoscope and watching an oscilloscopic recording of the sounds at the same time is most valuable in teaching.

SPECIAL ELECTROCARDIOGRAPHIC INVESTIGATIONS

1. VECTORCARDIOGRAPHY

Vectorcardiography is a well-established electrocardiographic technique that has never achieved great popularity and is now rarely used. The apparatus required is not expensive but differs from that needed for routine scalar electrocardiography. The electrical potentials generated by the heart during the cardiac cycle are displayed in a form that emphasizes their spatial orientation as vectors in the three conventional planes of the body: horizontal, sagittal, and frontal. Various lead systems are available, but the Frank lead system is the most popular. The electrocardiographic signals are displayed on the x and y axes of an oscilloscope, and the dimension of time is indicated by interrupting the ECG signal every 2 ms. The ECG signal traces out loops on the screen during the P, QRS, and T phases of the cardiac cycle, which can be displayed in the frontal, sagittal, and horizontal views. The standard 12-lead ECG was so well established by the time vector cardiography became available that the dominant position of the ECG as an empiric pattern recognition system has never been seriously challenged.

2. CONTINUOUS ELECTROCARDIOGRAPHIC MONITORING

Continuous electrocardiographic monitoring outside a laboratory has become a standard means of identifying arrhythmias, ischemic changes, and conduction defects; this technique should be considered in any patient in whom an exact diagnosis of an arrhythmia or conduction defect has not yet been established and in recognizing silent ischemia. The apparatus required, which is moderately expensive, is available in most large hospitals. It is also routinely used in coronary care units to obtain the earliest possible indication of the onset of arrhythmia or conduction defect or to monitor the frequency of premature beats.

Monitoring for up to 24 hours can readily be carried out in patients going about their normal business. One lead of an ECG is usually recorded on a tape recorder that is strapped around the patient's waist. The tape recording of the ECG is played back at speeds of 10–100 times the recording speed and scanned for abnormalities, either visually or using a special computer program. These areas of interest are then recorded at standard speed for analysis. Both arrhythmias and ST–T wave changes of ischemia can be detected in this way and the time of their occurrence correlated with events in the patient's life.

Patient-Activated Electrocardiographic Recordings

To detect arrhythmias or record the ECG during the development of intermittent symptoms such as presyncope or palpitations, patient-controlled electrocardiographic recordings have been developed that can be transmitted over the telephone to a receiver that reproduces the ECG. There are devices with intermittent memory loops which can be patient-activated at the time of symptoms such as presyncope or palpitations and which have recorded 1 to several minutes of ECG before and after the time of activation. This taped rhythm can then be either decoded by the physician or transtelephonically transmitted to a receiver that prints out the rhythm for interpretation (Cumbee, 1990; Brown, 1987).

In the Coronary Care Unit

In continuous monitoring in a coronary care unit, the ECG is usually continuously displayed on an oscilloscope and can be recorded on chart paper by simply pressing a button. Alarms are often arranged to provide a signal when the patient's heart rate falls outside a prescribed range. These are not always desirable, because displacement of electrocardiographic electrodes and disconnection of leads tend to trigger the alarm systems inappropriately. It is especially valuable to use a system that includes a memory loop. In this case, the immediate past portion (say the last 20 seconds) of the patient's electrocardiographic signal is continuously stored in a memory, which is continuously erased after 20 seconds. When some untoward event occurs, it is then possible to stop erasing the memory and examine the ECG during the period immediately preceding the untoward event.

3. EXERCISE ELECTROCARDIOGRAPHY (See also Chapter 8.)

Exercise electrocardiography is a standard procedure for investigation of patients in whom a diagnosis of angina pectoris is being considered as well as in the follow-up of patients who have had a myocardial infarction or thrombolytic therapy. The apparatus required is not expensive, and the test is available in many doctors' offices. The aim of an exercise test is to induce the symptoms of which the patient is complaining in the laboratory, in the presence of a physician, and with an ECG running continuously.

Safety Precautions

There is a small but significant (1:10,000) risk in exercising patients with angina until they develop pain or have to stop because of fatigue or severe shortness of breath. The risk mainly stems from the possibility that the patient may have developed a myocardial infarction since last seen, but ventricular arrhythmias, myocardial infarction, collapse, and sudden death may occur during the test. Care must be taken prior to testing to make sure that the patient's symptoms have not changed, and a 12-lead ECG is taken at rest in the supine and upright positions and compared with the most recent previous ECG. *An exercise test should never be done without a doctor present and resuscitation equipment available.* The physician in charge must strike a balance between failing to stress the patient enough to bring out symptoms and encouraging excessive and dangerous overexertion. It is, however, safer for patients with angina to bring on their pain in a laboratory than in the course of their daily activities.

Technique

The exercise stress consists of walking on a motor-driven treadmill or pedaling a cycle ergometer. Several patterns of graded exercise are in common use. The commonest is the Bruce protocol, in which the test is divided into four stages, each lasting 3 minutes. In stage I, the patient walks at 1.7 mph at a 10% grade; in stage II, the speed is increased to 2.5 mph at a 12% grade; in stage III, the speed is 3.4 mph and the grade 14%; and in stage IV, the speed is 4.2 mph and the grade 16%. Comparable protocols are used for cycle ergometer exercise. Other protocols are available for more gradual increase in workload.

Blood pressure is often measured by sphygmomanometry during the test, but the values obtained tend to be unreliable because of the motion of the patient and the noise of the treadmill.

The patient is instructed to stop exercise when anginal discomfort would ordinarily cause him or her to stop, or when shortness of breath or fatigue requires cessation of exercise. This is called a "symptom-limited" stress test. The physician stops the test if arrhythmia develops or the patient shows obvious signs of distress. Marked (> 3 mm) ST depression or a falling blood pressure is also an indication to stop.

The heart rate is monitored and the ECG continuously observed during the test. A significant increase in heart rate is sought. Since the maximal heart rate that can be achieved during exercise by normal subjects decreases with age, the expected heart rate for a given patient is obtained from tables, and about 85% of this value used as a target. A rough guide to the maximal heart rate is 220 beats/min minus the patient's age in years. In practice, most patients with angina of effort develop chest pain at heart rates below 130/min. The ECG is recorded during the first 3 minutes of recovery, since ST–T wave changes sometimes do not develop until after exercise. Exercise electrocardiography is often combined with thallium-201 imaging. The radionuclide is injected at the height of exercise and the images obtained after recovery. If the patient is unable to exercise, thallium imaging can be combined with a drug that increases coronary blood flow, such as dipyridamole, adenosine, or increases myocardial oxygen demand, such as dobutamine.

It is possible to obtain stable tracings even during severe exercise on a cycle ergometer or treadmill. Although various lead systems have been used, a single unipolar lead or a bipolar lead from the right subclavicular region to the apex beat, with an indifferent electrode on the head or left shoulder, will detect ischemic changes in the ECG during exercise almost as effectively as more complicated lead systems. In practice, three leads are monitored continuously, usually I, II, and V_5, and every 3 minutes all 12 leads are recorded.

Results

The changes of myocardial ischemia occur during exercise and are virtually always visible in the left ventricular leads (V_5 is probably the best). They consist of flat or downsloping ST–T wave depression with T wave inversion. Junctional depression and upsloping ST segments are not significant, although ST depression of 2 mm and a duration of 0.08 s are considered definite positive findings indicating ischemia. ST depression of 1–2 mm is deemed equivocal.

There is some relationship between the ease with which electrocardiographic changes can be provoked, their magnitude, the length of time they last, and the severity and prognosis of the coronary lesions. Patients with significant left main coronary artery lesions often show marked ST depression with minimal exercise.

Interpretation

The significance of electrocardiographic changes during exercise is greatest in patients with a normal resting tracing who develop "their pain" during the test. Digitalis therapy and the presence in the body of beta-adrenergic blocking agents make interpretation difficult. Digitalis produces ST–T wave changes that may mimic ischemia, and propranolol reduces the heart rate and makes pain less likely to be the limiting factor during exercise. Exercise testing may establish a diagnosis of ischemic heart disease, but the significance of the results is not easy to determine.

A. "False-Positive" Results: Results are generally interpreted as "false-positive" if changes occur in the ECG in patients whose coronary arteries are found to be normal at angiography. False-positive exercise results may be due to misinterpretation of the coronary angiograms. Atherosclerotic changes may be missed because of overlapping vessels or inadequate or technically unsatisfactory views. Typical angina with a normal coronary angiogram does, however, undoubtedly occur, especially in young women. There is increasing evidence that "ischemic" ST depression can result from a failure of coronary arterioles to properly vasodilate with exercise, a loss of coronary vascular reserve. ST–T wave changes can also result from autonomic nervous system influence. The results of exercise tests are less reliable in patients with abnormal resting ECGs and in those in whom pain does not develop. The magnitude of the ST depression is also related to the significance of the test, both regarding severity of coronary arterial obstruction and prognosis.

B. "False-Negative" Results: "False-negative" results are assumed if coronary disease is seen on angiography in patients in whom no changes occurred in the ECG during exercise. False-negative results are common, especially in patients who do not develop pain or a high enough heart rate or in asymptomatic persons. If the coronary arteriograms are taken as the "gold standard" for diagnosis, this result is not surprising. There is no necessary or inevitable relationship between the presence of obstructive lesions in the coronary circulation and the presence of ischemic pain or changes on an ECG, but significant lesions are usually present when angina and electrocardiographic changes are found on exercise. Coronary artery disease is undoubtedly present in a presymptomatic (latent) form in many "normal" persons past middle age. "False-negative" results are most common when only one coronary vessel is significantly obstructed, especially in the presence of isolated circumflex vessel disease.

C. Interpretation in Other Uses: Exercise tests are also used to assess the fitness of normal persons in particular occupations, eg, airline pilots. The interpretation of changes in the ECG induced by exercise in such cases is less reliable than in patients with chest pain.

In recent years, exercise tests have been commonly used as a means of assessing patients with recent myocardial infarction. If the patient develops chest pain or changes in the ECG during the test, the prognosis is worse, and if ST segment depression is 2 mm or greater or if it occurs at low double-product (heart rate × systolic blood pressure), coronary arteriography is indicated. The time after an infarction at which it is safe to do an exercise test is an open question. In many institutions, heart rate-limited stress tests (limited to a heart rate of 120/min) are done before the patient leaves the hospital to identify patients with severe ischemia. It is probably just as well in patients without heart failure or angina on minimal activity to wait until 3 weeks after the infarction and then do a symptom-limited stress test to risk-stratify the patient.

4. STRESS ECHOCARDIOGRAPHY

A recent advance in stress testing has been the detection of changes in wall motion by two-dimensional echocardiography brought about by exercise or infusion of dobutamine. Imaging is done immediately after exercise on the treadmill or bicycle, with the patient supine or with the left side down. Imaging is done during infusion of increasing amounts of dobutamine: 5, 10, 20, and 30 μg/kg/min. In normal patients, there is an increase in contractility of all ventricular walls, resulting in hyperkinesis brought about by sympathetic and catecholamine stimulation. In patients with significant obstructive coronary artery disease, exercise or dobutamine precipitates myocardial ischemia in those segments supplied by the obstructed coronary arteries, resulting in failure to increase wall motion or the development of hypokinesis or akinesis of those segments.

The specificity and sensitivity of both exercise and dobutamine stress echocardiography are equivalent to or better than those of exercise electrocardiography (Marcovitz, 1992). The specificity of stress echocardiography decreases when there is resting abnormal wall motion by echocardiography.

5. MYOCARDIAL ST SEGMENT MAPPING

This procedure, still in the research phase, is another form of investigation designed to follow the progress and assess the size of myocardial infarctions. It is moderately expensive and involves multiple ECGs recorded from different sites of the precordium. In patients with anterior infarcts, the extent of the area over which ST elevation can be detected bears a relationship to the size of the infarcted area. By summing the total extent of ST elevation in 30 or so electrocardiographic leads placed in standard positions on the surface of the left chest, it is possible to obtain a numerical assessment that bears a relationship to infarct size. Unfortunately, changes in position of the heart and thickness of the chest wall vary greatly from patient to patient, and this detracts from the general usefulness of the technique.

MYOCARDIAL ENZYME DETERMINATIONS

A number of enzymes (eg, glutamic-oxaloacetic transaminase [GOT], lactate dehydrogenase [LDH], creatine phosphokinase [CPK]) are released into the blood following myocardial infarction. Necrosis of tissue with rupture of cell membranes and release of intracellular components must occur before the increased levels of enzyme are found. More specific enzymatic fractions have now been identified, and the MB ("myocardial band") fraction of creatine phosphokinase isoenzyme has become the standard test used to confirm that myocardial infarction has occurred. The level of this enzyme gives more specific information about myocardial necrosis than any other available at the moment. Attempts have been made to relate serial measurements of enzyme levels to the size of the infarction and the patient's clinical progress, with the examiner seeking evidence of healing on the one hand or extension with increasing enzyme levels on the other. Since the enzyme mixes with a large and potentially variable blood volume at an undetermined rate, such measurements tend to be relatively insensitive.

Creatine kinase is released into the serum soon after a myocardial infarction. There are isoforms of CK-MM and CK-MB which are distinguished by differing isoelectric points on electrophoresis. All three isoforms of CK-MM can be distinguished. When first released into the plasma, it is in the form of $CK-MM_3$ and is rapidly degraded into MM_2 and MM_1. Within 1 hour after infarction, the percentage of MM_3 in the serum rises, and MM_2 falls. It is possible to diagnose myocardial infarction early and, by observing the ratio of MM_3 to MM_2, to time the onset of the myocardial infarction (Abendschein, 1988).

Other macromolecules are released after a myocardial infarction and have been used in diagnosis. Myoglobin, a smaller molecule than CK-MB, is released into the plasma rapidly with reperfusion and cleared from the circulation rapidly. It rises within 2 hours of reperfusion after the myocardial infarction and has been used to make a rapid diagnosis (Ellis, 1989).

SPECIAL RADIOLOGIC INVESTIGATIONS

1. CINEFLUOROSCOPY

Cinefluoroscopy is of greatest value in establishing the presence of calcification in the heart valves, the myocardium, the coronary arteries, or the pericardium or in recognizing paradoxic motion of a left ventricular aneurysm. It is also valuable in patients with prosthetic heart valves in whom the question of valve dehiscence is raised. A permanent postopera-tive record of artificial valve movement should therefore be obtained in all patients subjected to valve replacement for comparison with later studies if trouble arises. This function has been largely replaced by two-dimensional echocardiography.

2. COMPUTER-ENHANCED DIGITAL ANGIOGRAPHY

Recent advances in computer technology have led to the development of this new radiologic technique. An analog-to-digital converting system is used to transform the information in a fluoroscopic x-ray image or a television (video) image into a set of numbers (commonly 512×512 picture elements; "pixels"). Once entered into the computer, the information in the stored images can be manipulated in a number of ways, being amplified linearly or logarithmically or subtracted. One technique (temporal subtraction angiography) subtracts a "blank" or "mask" image, recorded without contrast injection and stored in the computer, from a second image recorded while intravenously injected contrast material is passing through the circulation. The patient must be in exactly the same position for the two images and must have a similar level of lung inflation. A more complex type of imaging employs "energy subtraction." In this case, the energy of the x-ray generator is changed rapidly to provide two different types of image, one favoring the "blank" or "mask" image and the other the image with contrast material in the heart and vessels. In this form of imaging, the time between the recording of the two images is shorter, and movement of the patient is less of a problem.

The spatial resolution of the images recorded with digital angiography is not yet up to the standard of conventional angiography, but satisfactory images of major blood vessels and cardiac chambers can be obtained with peripheral venous injections of relatively small amounts of contrast material. The technique has proved valuable for demonstrating the patency of coronary bypass grafts and for ventricular ejection fraction measurements. Selective injections through arterial catheters can be avoided and studies performed on outpatients. The technique, which has been used to measure coronary flow reserve, has potential for further development. Among its advantages are the possibilities for storage and transmission of angiographic information in digital form and elimination of film records. At its present stage of development, digital subtraction angiography cannot compete successfully with conventional selective coronary angiography.

3. COMPUTER-BASED X-RAY TOMOGRAPHY

Computer-based x-ray tomography is coming to be more widely used in specialized centers for cardi-

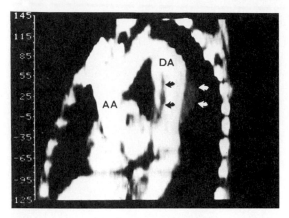

Figure 5–17. Oblique reconstruction of a series of transverse computer-based x-ray tomographic scans obtained during contrast drip infusion demonstrating aortic dissection. The intimal flap (black arrows) and an associated hematoma (white arrows) are shown. (AA, ascending aorta; DA, descending aorta.) (Reproduced, with permission, from Brundage BH, Lipton MJ: The emergence of computed tomography as a cardiovascular diagnostic technique. Am Heart J 1982;103:313).

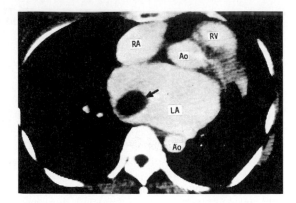

Figure 5–18. Computer-based x-ray tomographic scan of the thorax showing thrombus in the left atrium (black arrow) of a patient with mitral valve disease. (RA, right atrium; LA, left atrium; Ao, aorta; RV, right ventricle.) (Reproduced, with permission, from Tomoda H et al: Evaluation of left atrial thrombus with computed tomography. Am Heart J 1980;100:306.)

ologic investigation. The equipment used is extremely expensive; significant amounts of ionizing radiation are employed; and the imaging of moving structures such as the heart and blood vessels presents serious problems. The technique relies on variations in tissue density to distinguish between different structures in the line of an x-ray beam sequentially aimed in a radial direction through cross sections of the body. The reconstruction of an image from the basic density data depends on complicated computer methods. The "scan time" for the present generation of instruments has been reduced to 0.05 seconds, which permits the development of cine CT scanning. The three modes in which ultrafast CT scanning can be used are: (1) electrocardiographically triggered scanning at a rate of 17 images per second; (2) a "flow mode," in which a bolus of contrast is followed as it passes through the heart; and (3) a "volume mode," in which the "target ring" is automatically moved to cover up to 80 adjacent slices sequentially, with or without contrast enhancement. The patient is expected to keep still and not breathe during scanning. Intravenous injections of radiopaque contrast material are generally used to enhance the density differences between circulating blood and cardiac tissue. The cross-sectional images can be computer "stacked" to form a three-dimensional structure, and the computer can be asked to "cut" this structure in any plane, thus obtaining coronal, frontal, and sagittal sections of the cardiovascular structures.

The technique can accurately determine the patency of aortocoronary artery bypass grafts. It can detect many anterior (fewer posterior) myocardial infarctions and outline aortic dissections, as shown in

Figure 5–17. It is well suited to the detection of calcification in coronary arteries or in the pericardium and can also delineate intracardiac tumor or thrombus, as shown in Figure 5–18. The resolution with this technique is inevitably inferior to that with conventional angiography, both in space and in time. Its major advantage is that it is noninvasive.

NUCLEAR MEDICAL INVESTIGATIONS

The various techniques used in radionuclear investigations involve the injection of specially prepared radioactive materials that can be detected either in the bloodstream or in the tissues. Radioactivity is detected with a nuclear (gamma) camera. Radioactivity is converted into light energy in the crystals of the camera. This is in turn converted to electrical signals by photomultiplier tubes. The x, y coordinates of the energy from each part of the crystal are stored in an x, y matrix of a computer and converted into a "time activity" curve for the areas covered by the camera. The apparatus required for recording the patterns of radioactivity is expensive. The images lack the definition seen in other imaging techniques, but the studies can frequently be done at the bedside and, with the exception of the injection of radioisotopes, are noninvasive. The major use of these techniques is to provide functional information concerning the uniformity of lung and myocardial perfusion, information not readily obtainable by other means.

Lung Scanning

A gamma camera can be used to determine the distribution of radioactivity in the lungs following intravenous injection of 99m technetium (^{99m}Tc)-

labeled albumin particles. This technique has proved valuable in localizing pulmonary arterial emboli and is most specific in patients with a normal chest x-ray (see Chapter 19). The technique is available in many large hospitals and is useful in pulmonary as well as cardiac disease.

Myocardial Imaging

A. Perfused Areas: Scanning of the precordium after the intravenous injection of thallium-201 (^{201}Tl) outlines perfused areas of the heart with the concentration of the radioisotope proportionate to the myocardial blood flow. Imaging can start 5–10 minutes after injection of the isotope through a short intravenous catheter. The advantage of this technique is that the injection can be made within a few seconds of the end of a maximal exercise test, and the scanning can be carried out with the subject at rest after recovery. Images are produced by a gamma camera in anteroposterior, left anterior oblique, and left lateral views. Imaging can also be done tomographically. If the study is technically satisfactory and no defect is seen in the image, ischemia can be excluded with about 90% accuracy. If an area of abnormality ("cold spot") is seen, a further image is obtained 3–24 hours later to distinguish between reversible ischemia in which the defect disappears and permanent impairment of blood supply to the region, such as scarring from a previous infarct, or some other cause of myocardial fibrosis. No further injection is needed for the second scan. Alternatively, a resting image can be obtained, but this requires a second injection of radionuclide after a delay to allow the isotope to clear from the heart. An example of this type of study is shown in Figure 5–19. It is also possible to digitalize the counts accumulated in each pixel and display this information as counts per pixel. The information may be presented as counts from all pixels in each region of the myocardial image, with the image displayed linearly from some arbitrary 0 degree axis proceeding clockwise 360 degrees around the image. Relative intensities of activity can be easily visualized, and areas of relative decrease in activity can be identified.

This form of scanning is useful for the detection of ischemia in groups of patients with a low prevalence of coronary disease, eg, patients with atypical pain or airline pilots with equivocal electrocardiographic changes and no symptoms. A normal test can exclude significant ischemia with a high degree of confidence and make coronary angiography unnecessary. The test can also be used to assess the significance of minor abnormalities found on coronary angiography or electrocardiographic studies, either at rest or during exercise, by determining whether the myocardium in the territory supplied by a given artery does or does not become ischemic on exercise. The effect of surgical treatment can also be assessed by establishing whether an ischemic area, present before operation, is adequately perfused postoperatively. To-

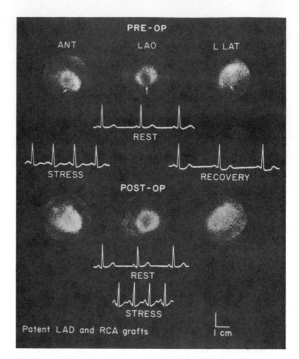

Figure 5–19. Pre- and postoperative thallium-201 stress scintigrams and ECGs obtained before and after placement of right coronary (RCA) and left anterior descending (LAD) grafts for treatment of angina pectoris. The preoperative study revealed an inferior wall perfusion abnormality (arrows). Perfusion is normal in the postoperative stress scintigram, and the patient was symptom-free. (ANT, anterior; LAO, left anterior oblique; LLAT, left lateral.) (Reproduced, with permission, from Greenberg BH et al: Thallium-201 myocardial perfusion scintigraphy to evaluate patients after coronary bypass surgery. Am J Cardiol 1978;42:167.)

mographic images of the heart obtained with this technique increase the chance of detecting a lesion. An example of this type of study is shown in Figure 5–20. Imaging with thallium (^{201}Tl) detects ischemia, not obstruction of coronary arteries. The test thus detects the effects of coronary disease on myocardial perfusion and not coronary lesions per se. Radionuclear studies are also useful in patients with equivocal findings, eg, if the ECG shows bundle branch block or permanent abnormalities due to previous myocardial infarction.

New perfusion tracers have recently become available that do not redistribute and have a better energy spectrum for imaging than thallium-201. These isonitrile compounds (methoxy-isobutyl-isonitrile, or MIBI), labeled with technetium-99m as perfusion tracers, called sestamibi, distribute proportionately to the regional myocardial blood flow, require living myocardial cells for uptake, have minimal washout, and have no redistribution. The perfusion scan is therefore representative of myocardial blood flow as

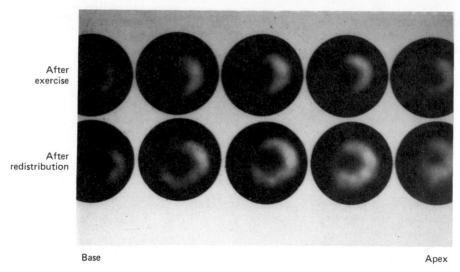

Figure 5–20. Tomographic thallium (^{201}Tl) scintigraphic images in the left anterior oblique position after exercise (above) and redistribution (below). The tomographic slices are from base (left) to apex (right). The septal area is ischemic during exercise and well perfused after recovery. (Courtesy of EH Botvinick.)

it existed during injection of the isonitrile compound. With several injections, it is possible to image the extent of myocardial blood flow both before and after reperfusion, thus theoretically estimating the amount of myocardial salvage (Figure 5–21).

B. Infarcted Areas: The injection of radionuclear materials that localize in necrotic tissue ("hot spot imaging") can be used to detect myocardial infarctions. In this type of study, technetium (^{99m}Tc)-labeled pyrophosphate is injected intravenously, and imaging is done with a gamma camera about 2 hours later. The isotope is concentrated about 11-fold in infarcted heart muscle, and the image becomes visible 10–12 hours after the infarction occurs. The intensity of the image is greatest at about 72 hours, and, while it usually fades in about a week, it may persist for months. Anterior myocardial infarcts produce better images than posterior infarcts, and if the first image is negative, a later scan after another 24–48 hours may be positive. More than 95% of patients with transmural infarcts imaged within 6 days of the onset of infarction give positive scans. The technique gives a valuable indication of the extent of myocardial infarction. The detection of subendocardial infarcts is less reliable. False-positive results occur in 1–2% of cases due to rib fractures related to resuscitative measures or breast or chest wall lesions.

This form of imaging is useful in patients who are not seen until a week or so after the onset of symptoms. At this point, the electrocardiographic and enzyme changes may have cleared, but radionuclear examination may establish the diagnosis of infarction. Perioperative infarcts can be detected when nonspecific electrocardiographic changes and trauma-related enzyme elevation cause confusion. Traumatic myocardial contusion produces a positive test, usually without specific electrocardiographic changes. An example of a positive scan is shown in Figure 5–22. The radioisotope is concentrated in the sternum and ribs, in addition to the infarcted area in the heart.

C. Radionuclide Angiography: Radionuclide angiography has developed to a stage at which it can provide significant structural and functional information. It is best thought of as a noninvasive equivalent of cineangiography in which resolution is comparatively low. It relies heavily on expensive equipment and computer-based analyses, but it has a major advantage in that it can be done at the bedside and can be applied during exercise. Two types of study are used: first-pass and gated equilibrium techniques.

1. First-pass technique– A bolus of sodium pertechnetate (^{99m}Tc) is injected intravenously and followed through the right and left heart chambers. The examination is carried out in the 30 degree right anterior oblique position in order to separate the atrial and ventricular images. The right and left sides of the heart overlap in this view, but radioactivity has normally cleared from the right heart by the time the left heart is imaged. The technique provides a quick, relatively simple means of outlining the cardiac chambers. Appropriate positioning of the patient is important, and serial studies require repeated injections. Two injections ordinarily constitute a full dose of radioactivity. This method provides the best estimate of right ventricular ejection fraction, especially when the ECG is recorded and used to identify end systolic and end-diastolic images. The ratio of the number of counts in the area of interest at end-systole and end-diastole provides a measure of ejection fraction that depends not on the assumption of a specific geometric

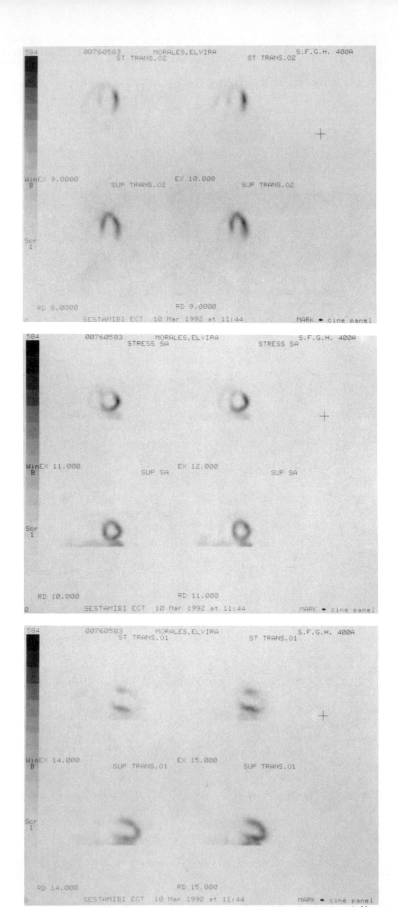

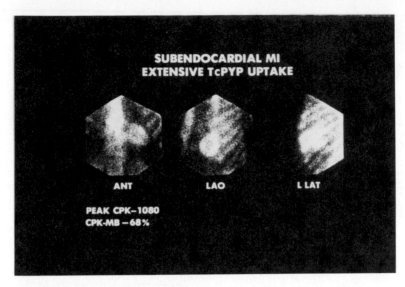

Figure 5–22. Anterior (ANT), left anterior oblique (LAO), and left lateral (LLAT) views of the left chest showing technetium ^{99m}Tc-labeled pyrophosphate taken up by infarcted cardiac tissue in a patient with extensive subendocardial infarction. (Courtesy of EH Botvinick.)

shape for the ventricle but rather on delineating the borders of the ventricular image. Computer assistance with this task is often sought.

2. Gated equilibrium technique– In this method, the radionuclide (usually ^{99m}Tc-labeled red cells) is injected intravenously and allowed to equilibrate with the blood volume for 5–10 minutes before imaging starts. Imaging can continue for up to 6 hours, and the patient's position or circulatory state can be altered between images. This technique is particularly applicable to exercise studies. The images are "gated" to the ECG, so that imaging is restricted to certain times during the cardiac cycle. Gating to end-systole and end-diastole, shown in Figure 5–23, is used in ejection fraction measurements, and data from several hundred beats are stored in a computer to obtain signals of adequate intensity. The start of imaging is linked to the R wave, and the subsequent images are recorded at regular intervals during the cardiac cycle.

Both this technique and the first-pass method have the potential for identifying wall motion abnormalities in the left ventricle. Images are usually obtained in the left anterior oblique position to minimize overlap between the right and left ventricles. Computer-assisted "region of interest" delineation is commonly used to outline the edges of the left ventricular image in ejection fraction measurements. The values for ejection fraction by this method correlate well (correlation coefficient about 0.9) with angiocardiographic measurements. The radionuclear studies can be done during exercise on a cycle ergometer, but loss of resolution due to patient movement is inevitable. With all radionuclear techniques, the visual impact of the images is not outstanding, and spatial and temporal resolution are poor compared to radiologic and ultrasonic techniques. Computer assistance with data analysis is almost essential, and color coding helps in the display of data. Operator bias may distort results. "Computer enhancement" of images and edge detection are subjective activities, and care must be taken to obtain an unbiased measurement.

D. Phase Image Analysis: The pattern of ventricular activation can be determined by phase image analysis. In this technique, the time that radioactivity is detected in different areas of the heart is coded in terms of a gray scale. By this means, the sequence of contraction of different areas (eg, left versus right ventricle) can be demonstrated. The technique may be valuable in the analysis of complex arrhythmias, detecting the focus in the myocardium where contraction first begins and the sequence of spread of the myocardial contraction.

Positron Emission Tomography (PET)

Positron emission tomography is an expensive radionuclide-based imaging technique that has poten-

Figure 5–21. SPECT sestamibi ^{99m}Tc tomographic images. Selected frames. Top: exercise images. Bottom: rest images. **A:** Horizontal tomograms. Note defect on exercise images in the apical-septal areas which fills in with rest injection. **B:** Short-axis tomogram. Note anteroseptal defect on exercise image which fills in with the rest injection. **C:** Frontal tomogram. Note the anteroapical defect on the exercise image which fills in with the rest infection.

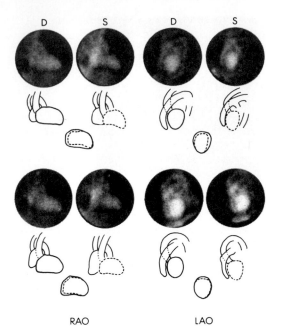

RAO   LAO

Figure 5–23. Diastolic (D) and systolic (S) frames from an equilibrium multiple-gated blood pool scintigram in the right anterior oblique (RAO) and left anterior oblique (LAO) positions. The upper images were obtained on the second day after the patient suffered a myocardial infarction. Left ventricular function was better on this occasion than in the study illustrated below, obtained 3 weeks later when left ventricular failure had developed. (Reproduced, with permission, from Botvinick EH, Shames DM: *Nuclear Cardiology: Clinical Applications.* Williams & Wilkins, 1979.)

tial for the quantitative analysis of metabolic processes. It uses physiologically relevant radioisotopes of common elements (^{15}O, ^{13}N, ^{11}C, or ^{18}F) with such short half-lives (2 minutes to 2 hours) that a cyclotron or its equivalent must ordinarily be located in the building in which the studies are performed.

The radioisotopes are incorporated into biochemically relevant compounds—eg, ^{11}C palmitate or FDG (^{18}F-2-fluoro-2-deoxy glucose)—and their radioactivity followed in cardiac tissue. The tomographic technique depends on the emission of positrons ("anti-electrons") that combine with electrons in the tissue, emitting two photons that travel in opposite directions (180 degrees apart). These photons readily pass through the tissues and are simultaneously detected by counters placed on opposite sides of the body. The process is called "annihilation coincidence detection" and has a better signal-to-noise ratio than conventional gamma counting.

This type of imaging is particularly well suited to tomography. Computer-based reconstruction techniques analogous to those used in x-ray tomography are used to generate images of the tissues under study. The spatial resolution of the images (about 18 mm) is

similar to that of conventional radionuclear techniques and inferior to those of x-ray tomography imaging or magnetic resonance imaging. The absorption of radioactivity by the tissues is not as great as—and more constant than—that with gamma-emitting compounds, and the potential for accurate metabolic studies is clear. The technique has been used to distinguish between old and new myocardial infarctions and to study ^{11}C palmitate metabolism in the heart. It can also be used to distinguish between ischemic but viable (metabolizing) heart muscle and dead myocardium in which metabolism has ceased. The wide range of substrates that the heart can metabolize is a complicating factor, and large differences between fed and fasted subjects have been seen. Imaging following the injection of two isotopes (^{13}N ammonia for blood labeling and FDG for heart muscle) has been reported (Marshall, 1983). The time between the two injections must be at least 45 minutes, and several minutes are needed for the acquisition of each image.

Single Photon Emission Computed Tomography (SPECT)

This less expensive and less accurate technique employs conventional, single-photon, gamma-emitting radionuclides such as technetium 99 (^{99}Tc) and thallium-201 (^{201}Tl) and does not require the proximity of a cyclotron. As in PET scanning, a computer-based reconstruction is used to generate an image which is affected by variable attenuation of the radiation by the tissues. SPECT provides radionuclear images of a quality intermediate between those of PET and conventional scans. The images are presented as tomographic slices in each plane, cross-sectioned from apex to base, horizontal long-axis slices and vertical long-axis slices.

MAGNETIC RESONANCE IMAGING (MRI)

Magnetic resonance detection is a complicated analytical technique that has been used to perform spectroscopy of biologic materials in biochemistry laboratories for more than a decade. The new application that has great potential for clinical use requires computer-based reconstruction of images derived from measurements involving proton density in the tissues. While the nuclei of many compounds exhibit the phenomenon of magnetic resonance, the proton (^1H) is the element that can be used most effectively for imaging. The next most suitable element, phosphorus (^{31}P), is five orders of magnitude less effective.

The apparatus used is large and expensive, principally because of the size and power of the permanent magnets needed for imaging the heart. The principle of MRI depends on the ability of external radiofrequency fields of appropriate frequency to induce resonance in protons lined up in a powerful magnetic field. The protons behave as tiny bar magnets that spin like tops. When an external pulse of appropriate radio frequency is applied at 90 degrees to the alignment of the protons by means of an external coil, the protons rotate from the longitudinal to the transverse plane. When the pulse is turned off, the magnetized protons swing back in an exponential manner to their original position. A receiver coil, surrounding the patient, detects an electrical signal during the "magnetic relaxation time," and this forms the basis of the imaging technique.

Four factors determine the intensity of the signal detected by the receiver coil: (1) the proton density in the tissue; (2) and (3) the magnetic relaxation time constants—τ_1 for the return of the proton in its long axis to its rest position (spin-lattice relaxation) and τ_2 for the return of the proton in its transverse axis (spin-spin relaxation); and (4) blood flow, based on the entry of blood, containing undisturbed protons, into the field. The values for τ_1 and τ_2 vary from tissue to tissue, so that by varying the sequence and duration of the distorting radio-frequency pulse in the coil and the time of data collection, it is possible to alter the intensity of the signals obtained from different tissues. Signal collection takes about 10–30 ms, using a 512×512 matrix, and serial images are obtained at about 1-second intervals. The patient must lie still in the scanner for several minutes. Gating of the signals to the ECG has been achieved by using fiberoptic techniques to conduct the electrocardiographic signals through the strong electromagnetic fields surrounding the patient. With rapid acquisition, cine-loops can be made and displayed as moving images in any plane. With this display, turbulent flow is seen as image dropout, so that regurgitant or high-velocity jets can be visualized much in the same way the color Doppler visualizes those areas of increased velocity and turbulent flow (Figures 5–24 and 5–25). The technique cannot be applied to patients with magnetizable material in their bodies, eg, pacemakers, artificial valves, prosthetic joints, or metal clips. Care must be taken to keep metal objects and magnetized materials (watches, keys, floppy disks, etc) away from the powerful magnets needed for this form of investigation. The technique is valuable in the diagnosis of aortic dissection and for distinguishing between constrictive pericarditis and restrictive cardiomyopathy (see Chapter 18). MRI displays cardiac activity very well, and the diagnosis of most congenital heart lesions, vascular ring abnormalities, and diseases of the aorta and great vessels can be accurately made.

MAGNETIC RESONANCE SPECTROSCOPY

Magnetic resonance spectroscopy based on phosphorus 31 is coming to be applied to the study of heart muscle. The phosphorus magnetic resonance spectrum of cardiac muscle (Figure 5–26) shows separate peaks that correspond to the concentrations of different phosphorus-containing compounds. Inorganic phosphorus (P_i), phosphocreatine (P_{Cr}), and the three phosphorus elements in ATP are represented in a spectrum that resembles that of skeletal muscle. The relative positions of the P_i and P_{Cr} peaks are determined by the level of intracellular pH. The development of larger, more powerful, supercooled magnets has made it possible to examine intact human tissues (eg, the forearm), and attempts are being made to measure spectra via surface coils over the precordium. The technique has the potential for the repetitive, noninvasive, nondestructive analysis of the levels of phosphorus-containing compounds (eg, ATP, P_{Cr}) that are of fundamental importance in the energetics of cardiac contraction.

COST EFFECTIVENESS & EVALUATION OF DIFFERENT TECHNIQUES

The technologic explosion of the last decade has led to the development of a large number of expensive instruments costing from $100,000 up to $1,000,000 or more. The proponents of each technique tend to imply that their method is better than its competitors, and it is difficult for the cardiologist to form a clear opinion of the relative merits of different

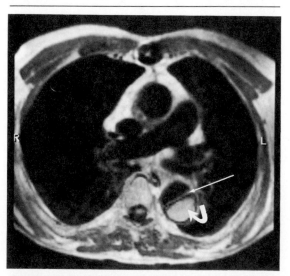

Figure 5–24. Magnetic resonance image of cross-section of the thorax in a patient with aortic dissection. The intimal tear (thin arrow) and the sluggish blood flow (thick arrow) in the false lumen can be seen. (Courtesy of C Higgins.)

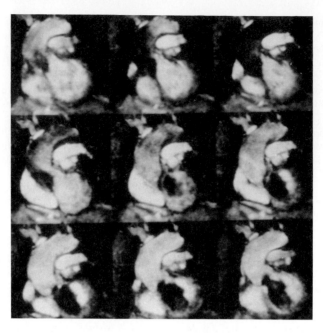

Figure 5–25. Rapid-sequence gated MRI in a patient with severe chronic aortic regurgitation. Frontal plane. Sequences from systole in the upper left-hand panel to diastole in the middle and lower panels. Note the development of a signal-free area in the left ventricle which becomes larger, occupying most of the left ventricular cavity by the lower three panels. This represents the turbulence resulting from the aortic regurgitation jet in diastole.

approaches. Few institutions can buy a color Doppler instrument, an MRI system, an ultrafast CT scanner, a magnetic resonance spectroscope, a digital subtraction angiographic system, a single photon emission computed tomographic instrument, and a positron emission tomographic apparatus with its concomitant on-site cyclotron. In addition, any instrument that the institution acquires is likely to be out of date by the time it is installed. It is important to keep an open mind and resist the modern assumptions that new is necessarily good and bigger necessarily better. One should ask what specific piece of information each instrument provides and how it contributes to the diagnosis and management of each patient in whom it is used.

CARDIOPULMONARY FUNCTION TESTING

Pulmonary function testing of varying degrees of complexity is available in most hospitals of moderate size. It is used mainly for the study of patients with lung disease, but since pulmonary function is likely to be impaired in patients with heart disease, tests of pulmonary function are often needed in the assessment of cardiac patients. The three main elements of pulmonary function—ventilation, diffusion, and pulmonary blood flow—and the relationships between them need to be tested, both at rest and during exercise. The conventional measurements of vital capacity and maximum expiratory flow rate give an indication of the maximal ventilation the patient can achieve voluntarily; but maximal exercise ventilation may be a more relevant measurement, since it tests the response to natural stimuli rather than the ability to perform a respiratory maneuver.

Diffusion of oxygen across the alveolar membrane

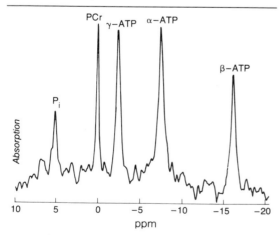

Figure 5–26. Magnetic resonance spectroscopy ^{31}P tracing of normal heart muscle. (ATP, adenosine triphosphate; PCr, phosphocreatine; P_i, inorganic phosphate.) (Courtesy of C Higgins.)

is assessed by measuring the transfer of carbon monoxide into the blood. This process may be impaired in severe pulmonary congestion with edema.

Information about the adequacy of ventilation, its distribution, and its relationship to perfusion can be gained by measuring concentrations of physiologically relevant gases (oxygen and CO_2) or inert gases (usually helium) in the respired air at the mouth. Specific gas analyzers and flowmeters are now available with which to make appropriate measurements of cardiopulmonary function in patients at rest and during exercise.

The mechanical properties of the lungs can be tested by measuring the force applied to the lungs (intrathoracic pressure) from esophageal pressure records using an air-filled balloon connected to a pressure transducer by a plastic tube. The compliance (stiffness) of the lungs and the resistance to air flow in the bronchial tree can be calculated.

Arterial oxygen saturation can be measured noninvasively with an ear or finger oximeter. The absorption of light transmitted through the illuminated ear or fingernail bed is recorded at different wavelengths, and the concentration ratio of oxygenated and reduced hemoglobin is calculated. Arterial desaturation is more commonly found in lung disease but occurs in pulmonary edema and in patients with cyanotic congenital heart disease. Arterial oxygen and CO_2 tensions can also be measured via the heated skin by using electrodes.

EXERCISE TESTING

Muscular exercise is the most significant, repeatable, and physiologically relevant stress to which a patient can be subjected. Exercise tests provide objective evidence of the patient's work capacity and record work load, heart rate, changes in the ECG, and blood pressure. They are most helpful in following individual patients and assessing the effects of therapy and the progress of disease.

The apparatus involved varies in complexity and in cost. The information obtained by exercise testing is almost entirely functional. The patient can conveniently perform the exercise on either a cycle ergometer or a motor-driven treadmill. *An ECG must always be recorded, and resuscitation equipment must be available.*

Additional measurements such as ventilation, oxygen consumption, respiratory exchange ratio, cardiac output, and lung-to-ear circulation time by oximetry can be added to give additional physiologic information using noninvasive methods. Many noninvasive tests can be applied during exercise, the most common being echocardiography, thallium (^{201}Tl) imaging and radionuclide angiography. However, the inevitable increased motion of the subject and thoracic movement due to increased ventilation often interfere with the tests.

Other Forms of Stress

Many patients are incapable of walking on a treadmill or pedaling a cycle ergometer. Orthopedic problems and intermittent claudication in the legs are the commonest reasons for failure to achieve an adequate level of exercise. Static graded handgrip or arm exercise can be used in some patients, but pharmacologic stress is often more satisfactory in the assessment of patients with ischemic heart disease. Two-dimensional echocardiography or thallium scintigraphy is performed at rest and then repeated during the infusion of some compound that increases coronary blood flow. Dipyridamole, the most commonly used vasodilator, is given by intravenous infusion in the relatively high dose of 0.5–1 mg/kg over about 5 minutes. Dipyridamole blocks the enzyme that degrades adenosine and therefore increases its availability to the vascular smooth muscle, which results in coronary arteriolar vasodilation and increase in coronary blood flow. Electrocardiographic and blood pressure monitoring are carried out, and development of symptoms is noted. Cardiac pain may be precipitated, and dizziness and faintness may occur. Aminophylline must be available as an antidote and will also relieve any bronchospasm that may develop. Adenosine, itself a vasodilator that has a very short half-life, has recently become available for use in this test. It is given intravenously in a dose of 0.14 mg/kg/min over 6 minutes. The infusion usually produces a three- to fourfold increase in coronary flow, and significant changes in response to the drug are interpreted in the same way as exercise test results. Recently, adenosine, itself a vasodilator that has a very short half-life, has become available for use in this test. It is given intravenously in a dose of 0.14 mg/kg/min over 6 minutes. The fact that the patient can keep still facilitates the studies, but dynamic exercise involving large muscle groups is the preferred form of stress.

REFERENCES

General

Come PC: *Diagnostic Cardiology: Noninvasive Imaging Techniques.* Lippincott, 1985.

Hammond HK, Kelly TL, Froelicher VF: Noninvasive testing in the evaluation of myocardial ischemia: Agreement among tests. J Am Coll Cardiol 1985;5:59.

Hlatky MA et al: Rethinking sensitivity and specificity. Am J Cardiol 1987;59:1195.

Miller DD (editor): *Clinical Cardiac Imaging*. McGraw-Hill, 1987.

Electrocardiography

Breithardt G: Standards for analysis of ventricular late potentials using high-resolution or signal-averaged electrocardiography. Circulation 1991;83:1481.

Brown AP et al: Detection of arrhythmias: Use of a patient-activated ambulatory electrocardiogram device with a solid-state memory loop. Br Heart J 1987;58:251.

Camici PG et al: Coronary reserve and exercise ECG in patients with chest pain and normal coronary angiograms. Circulation 1992;86:179.

Cumbee SR et al: Cardiac loop ECG recording: A new noninvasive diagnostic test in recurrent syncope. South Med J 1990;83:39.

Dunn RF et al: Exercise-induced ST-segment elevation: Correlation of thallium-201 myocardial perfusion scanning and coronary arteriography. Circulation 1980;61:989.

Famularo MA, Kennedy HL: Ambulatory electrocardiography in the assessment of pacemaker function. Am Heart J 1982;104:1086.

Goldschlager N, Goldman MJ: *Principles of Clinical Electrocardiography*, 13th ed. Appleton & Lange, 1989.

Mitchell LB et al: Electrocardiographic body surface mapping in patients with ventricular tachycardia: Assessment of utility in the identification of effective pharmacologic therapy. Circulation 1992;86:383.

Muller JE, Maroko PR, Braunwald E: Precordial electrocardiographic mapping: A technique to assess the efficacy of interventions designed to limit infarct size. Circulation 1978;57:1.

Schlant RC et al: Guidelines for electrocardiography: A report of the American College of Cardiology/American Heart Association Task Force on Assessment of Diagnostic and Therapeutic Cardiovascular Procedures. (Committee on Electrocardiography.) Circulation 1992;85:1221.

Sheffield LT: Computer-aided electrocardiography. J Am Coll Cardiol 1987;10:448.

Simson MB: Non-invasive identification of patients at high risk for sudden cardiac death: Signal-averaged electrocardiography. Circulation 1992;85(1 Suppl): I145.

X-Ray Investigations

Bateman TM et al: Prospective evaluation of ultrafast cardiac computed tomography for determination of coronary bypass graft patency. Circulation 1987;75:1018.

Booth DC, Nissen SE, DeMaria AN: Assessment of the severity of valvular regurgitation by digital subtraction angiography compared to cineangiography. Am Heart J 1985;110:409.

Booth DC, Nissen SE, DeMaria AN: The promise of digital cardiac angiography. J Am Coll Cardiol 1986;8:817.

Brundage BH, Spigos D: The future of computed tomography for the evaluation of ischemic heart disease. Int J Cardiol 1985;7:187.

Cooley RN, Schreiber MH: *Radiology of the Heart and Great Vessels*, 3rd ed. Williams & Wilkins, 1978.

Detrano R et al: Videodensitometric ejection fraction from digital subtraction right ventriculograms: Correlation with first pass radionuclide ejection fraction. J Am Coll Cardiol 1985;5:1377.

Foster CJ et al: Computed tomographic assessment of coronary artery bypass grafts. Br Heart J 1984;52:24.

Goldberg HL et al: Digital subtraction intravenous left ventricular angiography: Comparison with conventional intraventricular angiography. J Am Coll Cardiol 1983;1:858.

Legrand V et al: Abnormal coronary flow reserve and abnormal radionuclide exercise test results in patients with normal coronary angiograms. J Am Coll Cardiol 1985;6:1245.

Mehlman DJ, Resnekov L: A guide to the radiographic identification of prosthetic heart valves. Circulation 1978;57:613.

Sethna DH et al: Comprehensive and quantitative cardiac assessment using cine-CT: Description of a new clinical diagnostic modality. Am J Cardiac Imag 1987;1:18.

Skioldebrand CG et al: Assessment of ventricular wall thickness in vivo by computed transmission tomography. Circulation 1980;61:960.

Stein PD et al: Relation of plain chest radiographic findings to pulmonary arterial pressure and arterial blood oxygen levels in patients with acute pulmonary embolism. Am J Cardiol 1992;69:394.

Tobis J et al: Videodensitometric determination of minimum coronary artery luminal diameter before and after angioplasty. Am J Cardiol 1987;59:38.

Ultrasonography

Bansal RC et al: Feasibility of detailed two-dimensional echocardiographic examination in adults: Prospective study of 200 patients. Mayo Clin Proc 1980;55:291.

Crouse LJ et al: Exercise echocardiography as a screening test for coronary artery disease and correlation with coronary arteriography. Am J Cardiol 1991;67:1213.

Duncan WJ: *Color Doppler in Clinical Cardiology*. Saunders, 1988.

Feigenbaum H: *Echocardiography*, 4th ed. Lea & Febiger, 1986.

Feinstein SB et al: Contrast echocardiography during coronary arteriography in humans: Perfusion and anatomic studies. J Am Coll Cardiol 1988;11:59.

Gibbs JL et al: Diastolic forward flow in the pulmonary artery detected by Doppler echocardiography. J Am Coll Cardiol 1985;6:1322.

Goldberg SJ et al: Evaluation of pulmonary and systemic blood flow by two-dimensional Doppler echocardiography using fast Fourier transform spectral analysis. Am J Cardiol 1982;50:1394.

Gould KL: Noninvasive assessment of coronary stenoses by myocardial perfusion imaging during pharmacologic coronary vasodilation. 1. Physiologic basis and experimental validation. Am J Cardiol 1978;41:267.

Gupta NC et al: Comparison of adenosine and exercise thallium-201 single photon emission computed tomography (SPECT) myocardial perfusion imaging. J Am Coll Cardiol 1992;19:248.

Gussenhoven EJ et al: Transesophageal two-dimensional echocardiography: Its role in solving clinical problems. J Am Coll Cardiol 1986;8:975.

Harrigan P: *Principles of Interpretation in Echocardiography.* Wiley, 1985.

Hatle L, Angelsen B: *Doppler Ultrasound in Cardiology,* 2nd ed. Lea & Febiger, 1985.

Huang HK et al: Advances in medical imaging. Ann Intern Med 1990;112:203.

Kostucki W et al: Pulsed Doppler regurgitant flow patterns of normal valves. Am J Cardiol 1986;58:309.

Labovitz AJ, Williams GA: *Doppler Echocardiography: The Quantitative Approach,* 2nd ed. Lea & Febiger, 1988.

Marcovitz PA, Armstrong WF: Accuracy of dobutamine stress echocardiography in detecting coronary artery disease. Am J Cardiol 1992;69:1269.

Marwick TH et al: Accuracy and limitations of exercise echocardiography in a routine clinical setting. J Am Coll Cardiol 1992;19:79.

Meltzer RS, Klig V, Teichholz LE: Generating precision microbubbles for use as an echocardiographic contrast agent. J Am Coll Cardiol 1985;5:978.

Miyatake K et al: Clinical applications of a new type of real-time two-dimensional Doppler flow imaging system. Am J Cardiol 1984;54:857.

Miyatake K et al: Semiquantitative grading of severity of mitral regurgitation by real-time two-dimensional Doppler flow imaging technique. J Am Coll Cardiol 1986;7:82.

Oesterle S et al: A new method for assessing right-sided heart pressures using encapsulated microbubbles: A preliminary report. West J Med 1985;143:463.

Picano E et al: Dipyridamole-echocardiography test in effort angina pectoris. Am J Cardiol 1985;56:452.

Popp RL et al: Optimal resources for ultrasonic examination of the heart: Echocardiography study group. Circulation 1982;65:423A.

Quinones MA et al: Exercise echocardiography versus ^{201}Tl single-photon emission computed tomography in evaluation of coronary artery disease: Analysis of 292 patients. Circulation 1992;85:1026.

Santoso T et al: Myocardial perfusion imaging in humans by contrast echocardiography using polygelin colloid solution. J Am Coll Cardiol 1985;6:612.

Seward JB: Transesophageal echocardiography: ACC Position Statement. J Am Coll Cardiol 1992;20:506.

Silverman NH, Schiller NB: Apex echocardiography: A two-dimensional technique for evaluating congenital heart disease. Circulation 1978;57:503.

Smith JS et al: Intraoperative detection of myocardial ischemia in high-risk patients: Electrocardiography versus two-dimensional transesophageal echocardiography. Circulation 1985;72:1015.

Stewart WJ et al: Comparison of high pulse repetition frequency and continuous wave Doppler echocardiography in the assessment of high flow velocity in patients with valvular stenosis and regurgitation. J Am Coll Cardiol 1985;6:565.

Switzer DF, Nanda NC: Doppler color flow mapping. Ultrasound Med Biol 1985;11:403.

Tajik AJ et al: Two-dimensional real-time ultrasonic imaging of the heart and great vessels. Mayo Clin Proc 1978;53:271.

Valdes-Cruz LM, Sahn DJ: Two dimensional echo Doppler for non-invasive quantitation of cardiac flow: A status report. Mod Concepts Cardiovasc Dis 1982;51:123.

Radionuclide Investigations

Bodenheimer MM, Banka VS, Helfant RH: Nuclear cardiology. 1. Radionuclide angiographic assessment of left ventricular contraction: Uses, limitations and future directions. Am J Cardiol 1980;45:661.

Botvinick EH, Shames DM: *Nuclear Cardiology: Clinical Applications.* Williams & Wilkins, 1979.

Botvinick EH et al: Phase image evaluation of patients with ventricular pre-excitation syndromes. J Am Coll Cardiol 1984;3:799.

Boucher CA et al: Determination of cardiac risk by dipyridamole-thallium imaging before peripheral vascular surgery. N Engl J Med 1985;312:389.

Brunken R et al: Regional perfusion, glucose metabolism, and wall motion in patients with chronic electrocardiographic Q wave infarctions: Evidence for persistence of viable tissue in some infarct regions by positron emission tomography. Circulation 1986;73:951.

Eagle KA et al: Dipyridamole-thallium scanning in patients undergoing vascular surgery: Optimizing preoperative evaluation of cardiac risk. JAMA 1987;257:2185.

Geltman EM et al: Characterization of nontransmural myocardial infarction by positron-emission tomography. Circulation 1982;65:747.

Huber KC et al: Measurement of myocardium at risk by technetium-99m sestamibi: Correlation with coronary angiography. J Am Coll Cardiol 1992;19:67.

Lam JY et al: Safety and diagnostic accuracy of dipyridamole-thallium imaging in the elderly. J Am Coll Cardiol 1988;11:585.

Marshall RC et al: Identification and differentiation of resting myocardial ischemia and infarction in man with positron computed tomography, F-labeled fluorodeoxyglucose and N-13 ammonia. Circulation 1983;67:766.

Phelps ME, Mazziotta JC, Schelbert HR: *Positron Emission Tomography and Autoradiography: Principles and Applications for the Brain and Heart.* Raven, 1986.

Schwaiger M et al: Regional myocardial metabolism in patients with acute myocardial infarction assessed by positron emission tomography. J Am Coll Cardiol 1986;8:800.

Walton S et al: Phase analysis of the first pass radionuclide angiogram. Br Heart J 1982;48:441.

Wolfe CL et al: Determination of left ventricular mass using single-photon emission computed tomography. Am J Cardiol 1985;56:761.

Magnetic Resonance Imaging

Barrett EJ, Alger JR, Zaret BL: Nuclear magnetic resonance spectroscopy: Its evolving role in the study of myocardial metabolism. J Am Coll Cardiol 1985;6:497.

Bouchard A et al: Magnetic resonance imaging in pulmonary arterial hypertension. Am J Cardiol 1985;56:938.

Chan L: The current status of magnetic resonance spectroscopy: Basic and clinical aspects. West J Med 1985;143:773.

Friedman BJ et al: Comparison of magnetic resonance imaging and echocardiography in determination of cardiac dimensions in normal subjects. J Am Coll Cardiol 1985;5:1369.

Herkens RJ et al: Nuclear magnetic resonance imaging of the cardiovascular system: Normal and pathologic findings. Radiology 1983;147:749.

Higgins CB, Kaufman L, Crooks LE: Magnetic resonance imaging of the cardiovascular system. Am Heart J 1985;109:136.

McNamara MT et al: Detection and characterization of acute myocardial infarction in man with the use of gated magnetic resonance imaging. Circulation 1985;71:717.

Nienaber CA et al: Diagnosis of thoracic aortic dissection: Magnetic resonance imaging versus transesophageal echocardiography. Circulation 1992;85:434.

Omoto R et al: Evaluation of biplane color Doppler transesophageal echocardiography in 200 consecutive patients. Circulation 1992;85:1237.

Pohost GM, Canby RC: Nuclear magnetic resonance imaging: Current applications and future prospects. Circulation 1987;75:88.

Radda GK: Potential and limitations of nuclear magnetic resonance for the cardiologist. Br Heart J 1983;50:197.

Scherzinger AL, Hendee WR: Basic principles of magnetic resonance imaging: An update. West J Med 1985;143:782.

Steiner RE et al: Nuclear magnetic resonance imaging of the heart: Current status and future prospects. Br Heart J 1983;50:202.

Young SW: *Nuclear Magnetic Resonance Imaging: Basic Principles*. Raven, 1983.

Other Types of Noninvasive Investigations

Abendschein D et al: Prompt detection of myocardial injury by assay of creatine kinase isoforms in initial plasma samples. Clin Cardiol 1988;11:661.

Bates DV, Christie RV, Macklem PT: *Respiratory Function in Disease*. Saunders, 1971.

Bruce RA: Exercise testing of patients with coronary heart disease: Principles and normal standards for evaluation. Ann Clin Res 1971;3:323.

Ellis AK et al: Early noninvasive detection of successful reperfusion in patients with acute myocardial infarction. Circulation 1988;78:1352.

Epstein SE: Implications of probability analysis on the strategy used for noninvasive detection of coronary artery disease. Am J Cardiol 1980;46:491.

Jones NL: *Clinical Exercise Testing,* 3rd ed. Saunders, 1987.

Morganroth J, Parisi AF, Pohost GM: *Noninvasive Cardiac Imaging*. Year Book, 1983.

Murray JF: *The Normal Lung: The Basis for Diagnosis and Treatment of Pulmonary Disease,* 2nd ed. Saunders, 1986.

Naughton J: *Exercise Testing: Physiological, Biomechanical and Clinical Principles*. Futura, 1988.

Sobel BE, Shell WE: Serum enzyme determinations in the diagnosis and assessment of myocardial infarction. Circulation 1972;45:471.

Special Investigations: Invasive

6

The descriptions of invasive investigations in this chapter are general, including the variety of investigations available, techniques involved, indications, precautions, complications, and some broad observations about interpretation. Findings in different cardiac diseases are discussed in the chapters dealing with specific disorders. This chapter attempts to show that a range of approaches is available. Personal preference of the investigator, based upon a familiarity with a particular technique, plays a logical part in determining which procedure will be used.

It should be apparent from the term invasive that such investigations are carried out in hospitalized patients for valid indications and only after adequate preliminary appraisal. In many instances, however, invasive diagnostic methods provide important information that cannot be obtained by simpler methods of cardiac diagnosis. The patient should be advised about the nature, risks, and benefits of such procedures. It is necessary to obtain the patient's written informed consent before all studies.

BEDSIDE VERSUS LABORATORY PROCEDURES

Invasive investigations fall into two main categories: those carried out at the bedside in severely ill patients and those performed in a cardiac catheterization laboratory. There is some overlap between the two, but, in general, arterial and venous pressure monitoring and pulmonary arterial and wedge pressure recording with a Swan-Ganz catheter are done at the bedside. Formal diagnostic catheterization studies and angiography are performed in specially equipped laboratories.

BEDSIDE CATHETERIZATION

Whereas arterial blood sampling has become a routine procedure in most hospitals, arterial catheterization, together with central venous or pulmonary arterial pressure monitoring, is mainly confined to intensive care areas where specially trained personnel are constantly available to keep the catheters patent and make certain that they are appropriately positioned. This form of monitoring of the patient's hemodynamic status is indicated only in severe illnesses such as myocardial infarction with shock or heart failure and in acute pulmonary edema or in the postoperative period after cardiac surgery. The disturbance, loss of sleep, and psychologic effect on the patient must be weighed against the therapeutic benefit, ie, early recognition of complications and assessment of the effects of therapy.

ARTERIAL CATHETERIZATION

Arterial puncture is a standard and routine procedure used to obtain samples for blood gas analysis and for direct recording of arterial pressure. Arterial blood can be obtained from a number of different sites, and the principles involved are generally similar. Arterial puncture is more painful than venipuncture, and local anesthesia is advocated in all conscious patients. The risks of hemorrhage and hematoma formation are much greater than with venipuncture, especially in patients receiving anticoagulant therapy, but infection of the puncture site and the development of blood-borne infections are much less apt to occur. Local thrombosis with consequent interruption of blood supply to the distal tissues is perhaps the greatest danger.

Repeated blood sampling and arterial pressure recording are greatly facilitated by the use of an indwelling arterial catheter. This is usually a short (25 cm) plastic tube whose proximal end holds a female adapter plus stopcock. After cannulation of the artery, a plastic or plastic-coated guide wire is inserted, and after removal of the arterial needle, the catheter is passed over the guide wire into the artery. The system is flushed with heparinized saline, or a slow (0.1 mL/min) infusion of heparinized saline (1000 units in 200 mL) is maintained.

PERCUTANEOUS VENOUS & RIGHT HEART CATHETERIZATION

Venous puncture and venous catheterization present few problems in patients with large veins that have not previously been the site of multiple punctures. More peripheral, smaller veins should be used for infusions and for taking single blood samples. The larger veins in the antecubital fossa should be preserved for the introduction of catheters into the central circulation. Most difficulty is encountered in dealing with the veins of persons who habitually use intravenous drugs, especially heroin; in such patients it is sometimes necessary to make a cutdown to expose the venae comitantes of the brachial artery. Superficial veins can be made to relax by flicking the skin with a finger, by warming the arm, and, if necessary, by exercising the limb. The vein should be palpated rather than inspected to find a good puncture site, and the skin and the vein should be punctured sequentially. If a catheter is to be inserted, either a plastic fishing line or a catheter can be introduced through the needle. Successively larger catheters can be used to dilate the puncture site until a catheter with a large enough bore is introduced. For central venous pressure measurements, a plastic catheter equivalent to No. 5F is sufficient, and a percutaneous approach is often successful.

Swan-Ganz Catheter

If a balloon-tipped catheter is to be placed in the pulmonary artery (Swan-Ganz catheter), a percutaneous technique with insertion in the arm is only feasible if the patient has large veins, and a cutdown over the vein is usually needed. Catheter insertion in the subclavian or internal jugular vein provides a short, direct route to the heart and makes it easier to immobilize the catheter, but complications such as hemorrhage, air embolism, and pneumothorax are more frequent. The standard balloon-tipped catheter used to monitor pulmonary and indirect left atrial (wedge) pressure can be introduced without fluoroscopic control in most cases. The length of catheter that has been introduced should be carefully measured. When it is felt that the tip is in the right atrium, the balloon is partially inflated with air and the catheter allowed to float forward through the right ventricle with the bloodstream. *Electrocardiographic monitoring is mandatory,* and if fluoroscopic control is not available, a record of pressure at the tip is essential in order to check the position of the catheter.

Inflation of the balloon to measure indirect left atrial (wedge) pressure should be kept to a minimum to avoid pulmonary infarction. The catheter tends to move forward with blood flow, and care must be taken to ensure that it does not become accidentally wedged for long periods of time. Catheters must be kept filled with heparinized saline, as leaks in the pressure recording system that permit blood to enter the catheter readily cause blockage of the lumen.

Pressure Recording

Arterial and venous pressures are usually recorded at the bedside with strain-gauge pressure transducers. The operator should be familiar with the steps required to balance the gauge and set the operating pressure range appropriately. Provision must be made for calibrating the manometer against a column of water or mercury, setting the zero level at the middle of the thorax, and providing a drip of heparinized normal saline to flush the catheter. The physician should be familiar with the characteristics of the pressure tracings in each of the right heart chambers. The recording of indirect left atrial (wedge) pressure is checked by observing the appropriate change in the tracing when the balloon is inflated. If there is any doubt, a blood sample can be obtained. It should show a high Po_2 (about 100 mm Hg) and a low Pco_2 ($<$ 30 mm Hg).

Thermodilution Catheters

Special catheters are available for the recording of cardiac output by thermodilution. Cold saline is injected through a proximal lumen that lies in the right atrium. The resulting temperature change is recorded at the tip of the catheter in the pulmonary artery by means of a thermistor bead embedded in the wall of the catheter.

Pacemaker Catheters

Pacemaker catheters are available that incorporate electrodes appropriately placed to lie in the right ventricle when the tip is in the pulmonary artery. In emergency situations, these catheters can be inserted to pace the heart without fluoroscopic control.

Indications for Bedside Catheterization

Catheterization is most clearly indicated in patients with myocardial infarction in whom heart failure with hypotension, pulmonary edema, or shock develops. Complications such as rupture of the ventricular septum, right ventricular infarction, or papillary muscle dysfunction are best managed when hemodynamic information about cardiac output and left atrial pressure is available. Vasodilator therapy can be more closely controlled, and the course of postoperative recovery in cardiac surgical patients can be monitored efficiently. Patients with virtually any condition resulting in hemodynamic instability warranting admission to a general medical or surgical intensive care unit are also candidates for invasive monitoring (eg, patients with extensive trauma, burns, massive pulmonary embolism, cardiac tamponade, respiratory failure, or drug overdose).

Complications of Bedside Catheterization

The complications of bedside arterial and venous catheterization increase with the length of time the catheter is left in place. It is difficult to maintain sterility, especially when an incision is made in the skin. Infection is much more readily introduced through a venous than an arterial catheter, and infection of arterial puncture sites virtually never occurs. Thrombophlebitis, pulmonary embolism, and endocarditis can all occur following venous catheterization, and if phlebitis occurs, removal of the catheter and reinsertion in another site should be undertaken without delay. Even without complications, the catheter site should be changed after 72 hours. The catheter itself may be accidentally severed and may enter the right heart if care is not taken to secure it properly. Air embolism is a possible hazard, especially when the jugular vein is the site used and when the slow drip of heparinized saline used to maintain patency is exhausted and the bottle is empty.

Complications following use of a Swan-Ganz catheter include arrhythmias, pulmonary artery perforation, pneumothorax, damage to heart valves, and intravascular knot formation. Deaths have been reported, but severe complications are few considering the widespread use of such catheters.

ELECTIVE DIAGNOSTIC CARDIAC CATHETERIZATION

Cardiac catheterization has become a standard procedure for the diagnosis and assessment of severity of cardiovascular disease. It is now almost always combined with some sort of angiographic procedure. The range of possible investigations is wide, and the morbidity and mortality rates of the different procedures vary widely with the age of the patient, the severity of the disease, and the skill and experience of the operator. *Cardiac catheterization should only be undertaken by a physician who has personally seen and evaluated the patient's problem clinically before the study.* The techniques require constant practice, and the procedure should not be done occasionally in laboratories that are only used once or twice a week. The study combines anatomic diagnosis with functional assessment, and—especially in congenital heart disease—it cannot always be known what information should be obtained until the procedure is actually under way. Thus, it is not always a routine procedure in which a previously decided list of data must be obtained but rather an investigation in which the operator should be continuously aware of what has been established and what remains to be done. The study optimally requires the cooperation of a cardiologist, a radiologist, a nurse, and a technician. With the development of two-dimensional echocardiography, especially with Doppler, much of the information obtainable previously only by cardiac catheterization can be obtained by these newer noninvasive techniques. Many patients can be evaluated now prior to surgery without catheterization, especially when

the patient is young and coronary arteriography is not necessary.

Indications for Diagnostic Cardiac Catheterization

In the past, cardiac catheterization was indicated prior to cardiac surgical procedures in order to make the diagnosis as certain and complete as possible, thus providing the maximum help to the surgeon. At present, with the development of Doppler two-dimensional echocardiography, computer-automated tomography, and magnetic resonance imaging, an accurate diagnosis can be made prior to catheterization in most cases. Catheterization *must* be done prior to surgery only when it is important to assemble data about left ventricular filling pressures, left atrial pressure, the status of pulmonary vascular resistance, the presence of extracardiac abnormalities such as anomalous veins or pulmonary arteriovenous fistulas, or the anatomy of the coronary arteries. Accordingly, in most cases, catheterization is done in patients over age 40 or in younger patients with multiple risk factors to examine the coronary arteries.

However, although estimation of the severity of valvular stenosis by Doppler two-dimensional echocardiography is accurate when small or large gradients are found, with moderate gradients the severity of the stenosis depends on the flow, and in this situation the patient should be catheterized to obtain the most reliable assurance that the stenosis is severe and requires surgery. Furthermore, there are some patients in whom a reliable gradient cannot be obtained by Doppler.

In patients with moderate valvular insufficiency or calculation of shunt size, echo-Doppler can be misleading in estimation of severity, and in this case catheterization is required. Because the decision to perform cardiac surgery is so important, whenever there is doubt about the diagnosis or the severity of the lesion—or whenever clinical data are not consistent with the findings of the noninvasive techniques—catheterization should be done prior to cardiac surgery. It is not that catheterization is without possibility of error—for example, there is really no good way to measure the severity of moderate valvular regurgitation. However, the decision to proceed with cardiac surgery is an important one for the patient, and the cardiologist must be as certain as possible that the right decision is being made.

Selection of Studies

It is often more difficult to decide what studies should be undertaken in a given patient than to decide which patient should be studied. The operator must consider how much the patient can tolerate, especially the time involved in any given procedure. High-risk patients—eg, those with severe mitral stenosis, pulmonary hypertension, recent myocardial infarction, or severe aortic stenosis—are much more likely to suffer complications from prolonged procedures. It is often better to postpone part of the study to a later date than to add a procedure such as coronary arteriography to the end of a 3-hour session. The operator must always bear in mind the primary aim of the study, which may be to establish a diagnosis in a patient with congenital heart disease, measure the pressure difference and flow across an aortic valve, or measure the pulmonary vascular resistance in a patient with pulmonary hypertension.

RIGHT HEART CATHETERIZATION

Technique

The traditional approach via the right medial basilic vein at the bend of the elbow has largely been superseded by the Seldinger percutaneous approach via the femoral vein. The cephalic vein often makes an awkward bend at the shoulder, and it is impossible to enter the thorax by this route in about one-third of patients. With the Seldinger technique, a needle is placed in the femoral vein percutaneously. A guidewire is passed through the needle into the vein, and the needle is removed. A sheath over a short dilating catheter is then introduced into the vessel over the guidewire and the catheter and guidewire are removed, leaving the short plastic sheath with stopcock in the vessel. Other catheters can be placed into the vessel through the sheath.

Wedging the Catheter in a Branch of the Pulmonary Artery

When the catheter enters the pulmonary artery, a wedge pressure is obtained by advancing the catheter firmly until its tip becomes wedged in the tapering vessel. A tracing is obtained, and a and v waves are sought if the patient is in sinus rhythm or a v wave if the patient is in atrial fibrillation. The right lower lobe

of the lung is the usual site for wedging the catheter. The tracing obtained is called a pulmonary capillary (PC), or wedge, pressure tracing. At the present time, a Swan-Ganz balloon-tipped flotation catheter is almost always used to obtain the pulmonary capillary wedge pressure.

Validity of Wedge (Pulmonary Capillary) Pressure

In the 40 years since wedge pressure was first introduced, it has been repeatedly shown to give an accurate measure of left atrial pressure, delayed by about 0.1 s. An example of simultaneous left atrial and pulmonary capillary tracings is shown in Figure 6–1. Experience and judgment are needed to determine whether a satisfactory measurement of wedge pressure has been obtained, especially in patients with pulmonary hypertension, mitral stenosis, or acute mitral incompetence. The best way to determine that the catheter is wedged is by recording the pressure change as it is withdrawn. It "pops out" of the wedge position, and pressure rises at that instant, with the tracing changing from a wedge to a pulmonary arterial configuration, as shown in Figure 6–2. A catheter in the wedge position can be flushed easily, but withdrawal of blood samples may be difficult. In any case, the sample obtained is physiologically irrelevant, since the blood obtained equilibrates with an overventilated and underperfused area of lung on the way to the sampling catheter. However, the characteristic high Po_2, low Pco_2, and high pH found in wedge samples are a good means of confirming that the catheter has been properly placed to obtain a satisfactory wedge pressure tracing. Occasionally the wedge pressure may overestimate the true left atrial pressure, resulting in a falsely high gradient across the mitral valve. This is especially important in patients with tachycardia or pulmonary vascular disease and in those with mechanical valves in the mitral

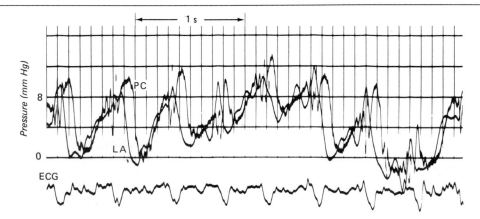

Figure 6–1. Simultaneous left atrial (LA) and wedge (PC) pressure tracings in a patient with aortic stenosis obtained during simultaneous transseptal and right heart catheterization. The patient is in atrial fibrillation,and the PC pressure can be seen to lag about 0.1 s behind the LA pressure. The waveforms are similar.

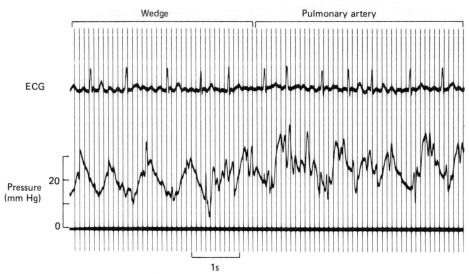

Figure 6–2. Pressure tracing and ECG showing withdrawal of a catheter from the wedge to the pulmonary artery in a patient with mitral valve disease in atrial fibrillation.

area. In these cases, direct left atrial pressures should be measured through a transseptal needle. It is also possible in a patient with an atrial septal defect to pass a catheter through the defect and to wedge the catheter in the reverse direction by pushing the catheter far out from the left atrium into a pulmonary vein. The pressure obtained resembles that of the pulmonary artery, but the measurement is liable to be incorrect in the presence of pulmonary hypertension.

PRESSURE RECORDINGS

Pulmonary Artery

Phasic and mean pulmonary arterial tracings should always be recorded in the main pulmonary artery. The right pulmonary artery is more readily entered than the left, and the lower lobes of the lungs are more easily catheterized than the upper lobes.

Right Ventricle

Right ventricular pressure tracings are conventionally recorded on withdrawal of the catheter from the pulmonary artery. Mean ventricular pressures are not obtained. Right ventricular tracings are particularly liable to be interrupted by ectopic beats, and it is difficult to place a catheter in the right ventricle in a stable position.

Blood Sampling

At the time that withdrawal tracings from the pulmonary artery are obtained, blood samples are taken from each chamber, especially if there is any question of a left-to-right shunt. A sample from the superior vena cava should be followed by a high caval or innominate vein sample if an atrial defect is suspected, because anomalous venous return into the superior vena cava must be excluded. Opinions differ about the importance of obtaining a sample from the inferior vena cava. We believe that a sample should be taken after positioning the catheter approximately 2.5 cm below the diaphragm and pointing to the left, away from the hepatic vein. This may be difficult, and streams of blood from the renal vein tend to give falsely high saturations if the catheter is placed too low.

Measurement of Cardiac Output

Cardiac output is ordinarily measured during right heart catheterization when the right heart catheter is in the main pulmonary artery (mixed venous blood) and an arterial sample is available from a systemic artery. A 3-minute expired gas collection is made, and simultaneous pulmonary arterial and systemic arterial samples are drawn during the gas collection and analyzed for oxygen content and capacity. An ECG is obtained during the gas collection to record the heart rate and to make sure that the patient is in a steady state. Alternatively, the cardiac output may be measured by the indicator dilution method, using Cardio-Green dye or thermodilution.

LEFT HEART CATHETERIZATION

Left heart catheterization is usually carried out in combination with right heart studies. The right heart data are generally obtained first.

Indications for Left Heart Catheterization

Left heart catheterization has come to be widely used in all forms of heart disease affecting the left heart, eg, mitral and aortic valve disease, coronary artery disease, and cardiomyopathy. It is not necessarily indicated in most forms of congenital heart disease, especially when the catheter can be passed from the right heart through a defect into the left heart. In some centers, an attempt is routinely made to enter all cardiac chambers in all patients. We feel that the operator should exercise judgment in choosing procedures and should tailor the study to the needs of each patient.

Different Approaches to Left Heart Catheterization

Four methods are in common use to approach the left side of the heart in adults: (1) retrograde percutaneous femoral artery catheterization, (2) retrograde brachial arterial catheterization via arterial cutdown, (3) transseptal left heart catheterization via the femoral vein, and (4) direct percutaneous left ventricular puncture.

Almost all laboratories use more than one approach to the left heart, since no one approach is always appropriate, feasible, or successful. The choice depends partly on personal preference and partly on the method used for coronary angiography in that particular laboratory.

Selection of Method

The nature of the patient's disease plays an important part in the choice of method. Most problems are encountered in patients with aortic stenosis in whom it is difficult to pass a catheter in a retrograde fashion across the aortic valve. If at all possible, the entire left heart study is performed by a single route in an attempt to minimize complications. Thus, the fact that a brachial arteriotomy will be needed to perform coronary arteriography by the Sones technique leads to the selection of the retrograde brachial arterial approach, whereas the need for a study by the Judkins technique for coronary angiography would lead to the selection of a retrograde femoral approach. Transseptal catheterization requires more skill and constant practice than any other form of left heart catheterization but is needed if balloon valvuloplasty of the mitral valve is to be undertaken or if catheterization of the left ventricle is necessary in a patient with a prosthetic mechanical valve in the aortic area.

Retrograde Percutaneous Femoral Artery Catheterization Technique

The method used to introduce the catheter is similar to that used in coronary arteriography by the Judkins technique. The femoral artery is punctured with a Cournand needle about 2.5 cm below the inguinal ligament in the groin. A guide wire is threaded via the needle to the abdominal aorta, and the needle is removed. A short (25 cm) dilator inside a plastic sheath is advanced over the wire into the artery and pushed in and pulled out of the artery two or three times. The dilator is removed, leaving the short sheath through which a catheter can be introduced. The catheter and the wire are advanced under fluoroscopic control to the ascending aorta. Several varieties of catheter are available for entering the left ventricle. If the aortic valve is normal, a pigtail catheter can usually be advanced into the left ventricle without a guide wire. Any end-hole catheter should always be used with a soft guide wire projecting 3–10 cm from its tip, because the unoccluded tip may damage the aortic valve when pushed firmly against it. The guide wire rather than the catheter is manipulated to enter the ventricle, the catheter is then advanced over the wire, and the wire is withdrawn. Because it has a curve near the tip, a right coronary artery Judkins catheter is a useful alternative to the standard Gensini Teflon catheter for entering the left ventricle. Once a catheter is in the artery, the patient should be given 2000–3000 units of heparin intravenously to prevent thrombus formation.

This approach is not advocated when the patient has iliofemoral atherosclerosis or has had peripheral vascular surgery, with or without prosthetic replacement.

Retrograde Arterial Catheterization via a Brachial Arterial Cutdown Technique

Cutting down on the brachial artery and exposing it for 1.5–2.5 cm is the method of choice for left heart catheterization from the arm. Others have successfully catheterized the brachial and axillary artery percutaneously by the Seldinger technique. Brachial artery cutdown is also used for coronary arteriography by the Sones technique. The dissection usually takes 15–20 minutes. Generous use of local anesthesia, complete familiarity with the anatomy, and an ability to distinguish between the brachial artery and the median nerve are important factors in the success of this approach. Adequate exposure through a 5-cm incision, checking for position of the vessel by palpating its pulse, and identification of the tendinous bicipital aponeurosis and its retraction laterally are helpful in the dissection. Two plastic tapes are placed around the vessel for control of hemorrhage, and the catheter is inserted either through an arteriotomy or via a puncture site that has been dilated with a tapering plastic cannula. It is helpful to put a loose pursestring suture around the site of entry into the vessel before opening it, using 5-0 silk. The hole in the vessel can then be quickly closed by tightening this suture at the end of the procedure. Alternatively, the arteriotomy can be repaired by two or three interrupted sutures.

A straight, closed-tip catheter with multiple side holes is usually used from the arm. Negotiating the bend in the subclavicular area is sometimes a problem in elderly atherosclerotic patients, but the degree of control of the catheter is much greater with this brachial approach than with the femoral approach, and crossing the aortic valve is more readily accomplished. Patients with aortic stenosis present the main problem.

Transseptal Catheterization

Transseptal left heart catheterization provides an alternative approach that is preferred in some centers. The procedure is carried out under fluoroscopic control and with a continuously visible pressure record. A special (Brockenbrough) catheter is used with a curved, tapered tip. It is adapted to a long (35-cm) needle, also curved at the tip. It is important to ensure that when the needle is fully engaged with the catheter, the two fit together to give a smooth transition, with no shoulder from catheter to needle. The catheter is first passed via the femoral vein into the superior vena cava. The needle is passed until it lies close to the tip of the catheter. The catheter and needle are rotated 45 degrees posteriorly and withdrawn into the right atrium until the catheter crosses the limbus of the fossa ovalis and impinges on the surface of the fossa. A pigtail catheter, previously passed via the femoral artery to the aortic valve, provides an important landmark indicating the point 1–3 cm below which atrial puncture is to be made. With the patient in a 45-degree right anterior oblique position, allowing a perpendicular view of the atrial septum, the needle is advanced to puncture the septum. Once the tip has entered the left atrium, the catheter is advanced over the needle to lie in the left atrium. The catheter itself, or a specially shaped guide wire passed through it, is then advanced into the left ventricle in the position shown in Figure 6–3.

The principal indication for the use of transseptal catheterization is in patients with aortic stenosis in whom a retrograde aortic catheter fails to enter the left ventricle. The development of balloon valvuloplasty (see Chapter 12) for the treatment of patients with mitral stenosis has led to more frequent performance of transseptal catheterization.

The procedure is likely to cause problems in patients with kyphoscoliosis, left atrial thrombus, left atrial myxoma, or giant left atrium. The success rate in entering the left ventricle from the atrium is not 100%, and the fact that aortography and coronary arteriography are now so commonly performed has tended to reduce the number of transseptal studies being done.

Left Ventricular Puncture

Percutaneous transthoracic left ventricular puncture is indicated when a catheter cannot be passed into the left ventricle, as in a patient with calcific aortic stenosis or after mitral and aortic mechanical valve replacement. This procedure is easier to perform and less dangerous than might be expected and is described in Chapter 13.

Measurements During Left Heart Catheterization

Left ventricular and aortic pressures constitute the principal measurements to be obtained during left heart catheterization. In investigating patients with mitral disease, the left ventricular pressure is measured together with the wedge pressure (via right heart catheterization) in order to assess the pressure difference across the mitral valve. The wedge pressure is inevitably delayed by about 0.1 s and so lags behind the left ventricular pressure. This fact, illustrated in Figure 6–4, must be taken into account in analyzing the tracings and calculating valve area. During transseptal catheterization, the gradient across the mitral valve is recorded on pulling the catheter back across the valve.

Simultaneous arterial or aortic and left ventricular pressures are recorded during transseptal catheterization to assess aortic valve hemodynamics. In retrograde catheterization, the pressures are recorded on pullback. Pressure differences within the ventricle are best sought in retrograde studies on withdrawal of the catheter from the body of the ventricle to the outflow tract. In transseptal catheterization, the operator should be careful to avoid confusing valvular and subvalvular obstructions, which tend to give superficially similar tracings.

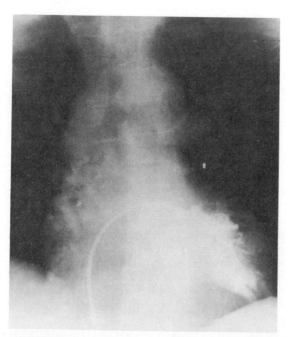

Figure 6–3. Single frame from left ventricular angiography carried out via a catheter passed transseptally into the left atrium and left ventricle.

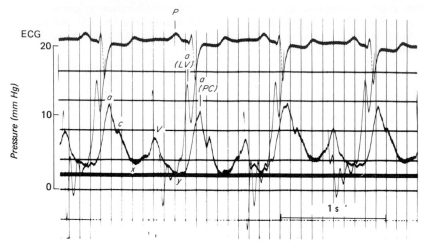

Figure 6-4. Simultaneous wedge (PC) pressure measured by the right heart route and left ventricular (LV) pressure measured by retrograde left heart catheterization. The delay in the PC tracing can be seen at the time of the a wave. The systolic LV pressure is "off scale," and the tracings show the diastolic events only.

ANGIOCARDIOGRAPHY

Angiocardiography has come to play a major role in the clinical assessment of cardiac lesions in the last 35 years. The advent of image intensifiers and cineangiography greatly improved the quality of the pictures obtained and made angiography a valuable way of visualizing the cardiovascular anatomy. Left ventricular angiography is an important means of assessing left ventricular function. The performance of the left ventricle can be assessed either by observing the speed and extent of contraction or by measuring the ventricular ejection fraction.

Technique

Pressurized injectors are conventionally used, and the dosage of contrast material and the rate of injection vary with the size of the catheter used and the size of the patient. Angiography (other than coronary angiography) requires the use of a multiple-hole catheter, usually a pig-tail catheter or—now more infrequently—a closed-tip catheter (Lehman or NIH). A small preliminary injection is always given to ensure that the catheter is appropriately positioned. This prevents the injection of large amounts of contrast material into the myocardial tissue. This complication can be serious if it occurs in either the right or the left ventricle when the catheter tip is embedded in trabeculae.

Effects of Contrast Material

A total dose of up to 2 mL/kg can be given without fear of complications. The contrast material always

affects ventricular function, so that an increase in ventricular diastolic pressure is often seen after an injection. This finding is particularly likely to occur in patients in whom ventricular function is impaired. It may last for half an hour or more and occasionally interferes with assessment of the severity of a lesion. Nonionic contrast agents are available that have less effect on hemodynamics and fewer arrhythmogenic effects.

Quality of Angiograms

Angiocardiography provides the best pictures when the dose of contrast material is large and the dye remains highly concentrated in the heart. Thus, sequential pictures of the chambers of the right and left heart are best taken when cardiac function is good. Conversely, if the contrast material is injected directly into a chamber whose function is poor (eg, the left ventricle in cardiomyopathy), the chamber tends to be well outlined because the dye stays in it so long.

CORONARY ANGIOGRAPHY

Coronary angiography has come to be an extremely important investigation that is indicated in all patients with coronary artery disease in whom surgical treatment is contemplated. It is also indicated in older patients with other lesions in whom the presence of associated coronary disease is suspected. *Coronary arteriography is less useful in the diagnosis of angina pectoris, which is based principally on the history and the electrocardiographic changes that occur with the onset of the pain.* Abnormalities in the coronary arteriogram can be present without symptoms, and the presence of lesions in an arteriogram cannot be used to show that a given patient's pain is due to ischemia.

Techniques

Two methods are in common use for coronary angiography. The Sones method involves a brachial arterial cutdown using a catheter with a tapered tip. This catheter is manipulated into the aortic root by techniques that require considerable skill in order to enter the right and left coronary arteries. Small (5–10 mL) injections of contrast material are made by hand, and cineangiographic films are taken of the coronary circulation. Multiple views are obtained, and the procedure is made easier if both the patient and the x-ray equipment can be turned at different angles.

The other technique, introduced by Judkins, uses a percutaneous femoral arterial approach. Specially shaped catheters are used for the right and left coronary arteries. The left coronary catheter enters the left coronary ostium quite readily, and little skill is needed for its placement. The right coronary catheter is slightly more difficult to place, but less skill is needed than for the Sones method. Injections of contrast material are again made by hand, and since the arms are free to be placed above the head, biplane angiography can be readily performed. The number of injections of contrast medium, the duration of the procedure, and the severity of the coronary disease

determine the morbidity and mortality rates of the Judkins technique. A coronary arteriogram obtained by means of the Judkins technique and showing a normal left coronary pattern is seen in Figure 6–5.

Left ventricular angiography should always be performed as an adjunct to coronary arteriography. Left ventricular volume and ejection fraction are measured, and localized areas of abnormal ventricular motion are sought.

No specific coronary angiographic technique is appropriate for use in every case. In some elderly atherosclerotic patients, access to the aorta via tortuous subclavian and innominate vessels may be impossible, or a previous arteriotomy may have obliterated the brachial artery, making the standard Sones technique impossible. Similarly, previous surgery for peripheral vascular disease may have obliterated the femoral vessels, or iliofemoral grafts may have been inserted at surgery, contraindicating the Judkins technique. In such cases, the axillary arteries may provide an alternative approach.

The possibility of cardiac standstill or complete atrioventricular block developing during coronary angiography has led many physicians to insert a pacing catheter into the right heart as a routine precautionary measure. These problems are less common with the use of nonionic contrast agents.

Videotape Recorders

It is important to make certain that adequate coronary arteriographic films have been obtained and that it will not be necessary to repeat the studies. Videotape recorders are used to view the results immediately and decide whether the pictures are adequate. The underlying anatomy and the distribution of atherosclerotic disease are so variable that it is difficult to be sure all aspects of the lesion have been demonstrated if only a single pass of the study on a television screen is seen.

Interpretation of Coronary Angiograms

The interpretation of coronary angiograms is of necessity subjective. While complete occlusion of a major vessel can be unequivocally recognized, the percentage of reduction in the size of the lumen may be more difficult to estimate. Multiple views outlining the vessel from different angles help in assessing the degree of obstruction. Most cardiologists using calipers estimate the percentage reduction in diameter that lesions cause. The arbitrary assignment of numerical ratings (eg, 50% or 70% obstruction) may be misleading. It is customary to assume that the narrowing is concentric, but in fact eccentric lesions are commonly seen at autopsy. With eccentric lesions, the degree of obstruction may vary in different views. The severity of the obstruction in these situations is taken from the view in which the obstruction appears to be the most severe. Unfortunately, the visually esti-

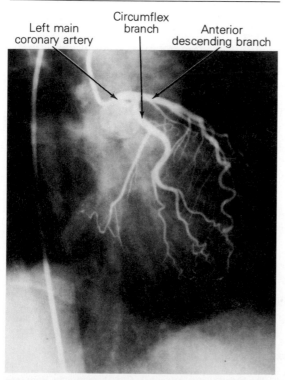

Figure 6–5. Normal left coronary arteriogram using Judkins technique. Right anterior oblique view. (Courtesy of Philips Medical Systems, Inc.)

mated degree of obstruction correlates only weakly with the degree of obstruction of the blood flow. In addition, the effects of long segments of narrowing and multiple obstructions in series cannot be adequately assessed.

Coronary Blood Velocity Measurements

Ultrasonic, transducer-tipped catheters have been developed that are small enough (No. 3F) to lie in major extracardiac coronary arteries without seriously altering the pattern of flow. The transducer is pulsed and range-gated, transmitting ultrasound at a frequency of 20 MHz. The range gate is set at about 1 cm from the transducer to sample from a relatively undisturbed area, and the Doppler shift of reflected ultrasound is measured (see Chapter 5). Spectral analysis of the signals in the audio range provides the best information about the velocity of blood flow. A simpler form of analysis using a frequency-to-voltage convertor is less accurate. The best established means of assessing the functional status of the coronary circulation is to measure the increase in blood velocity that occurs when maximal vasodilation is produced by injection of papaverine (12 mg) into the coronary artery. A four- to fivefold increase in velocity occurs in patients with normal coronary arteries.

The Doppler tracings from the left anterior descending coronary artery in a human subject with coronary disease (Figure 6–6) show that, as is always the case, flow is mainly diastolic and that the velocity profile is close to parabolic. The effects of angioplasty and of vasodilation with papaverine are shown.

OTHER DIAGNOSTIC STUDIES

Exercise During Cardiac Catheterization

Exercise is sometimes used during cardiac catheterization to evaluate the effect of stress on the hemodynamic state. However, it is difficult to do physiologic studies in supine patients lying under a fluoroscopic screen with catheters in several vessels. Although supine bicycle exercise can be done with catheters in the femoral artery and vein, it is difficult and exposes the patient to the danger of infection. If the brachial approach is used, the patient can pedal a cycle ergometer attached to the foot of the table, but even this form of exercise is less satisfactory than

A Before angioplasty

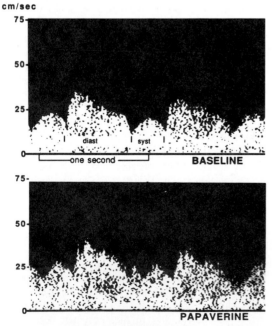

B After angioplasty

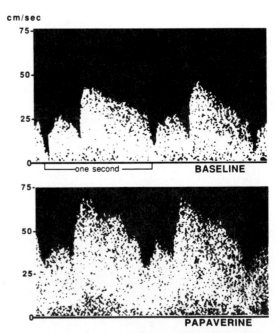

Figure 6–6. Doppler blood velocity signals from a catheter-tip ultrasonic transducer in a patient with coronary disease. The catheter was in the left coronary artery. Signals were obtained before and after an intracoronary injection of papaverine, before and after angioplasty. **A:** Before angioplasty, the blood velocity was low and showed little increase with papaverine. **B:** After angioplasty, the blood velocity was higher and showed a greater increase with papaverine. (Courtesy of P Yock.)

upright exercise on a cycle ergometer or treadmill. Exercise is most commonly used in patients with mitral valve disease and usually consists of a short, nonsteady state period of leg raising or lifting weights with both arms.

Coronary Sinus Catheterization & Atrial Pacing

Functional information about the adequacy of coronary perfusion can be obtained by coronary sinus catheterization and by right atrial pacing. It is difficult to use exercise to induce angina in the cardiac catheterization laboratory, and the less "physiologic" stress of progressive levels of tachycardia produced by atrial pacing is more frequently employed. Unfortunately, the electrocardiographic tracing and the level of left ventricular pressure provide unreliable indications of the effects of myocardial ischemia during pacing. The onset of pain and the level of lactate in the coronary sinus blood are the most valuable indicators of ischemia. Selective catheterization of different cardiac venous segments via the coronary sinus and its branches provides some degree of localization of the area of ischemia.

Electrophysiologic Studies

Intracardiac electrocardiography is used in the elucidation of difficult cardiac arrhythmias, eg, in distinguishing supraventricular and ventricular arrhythmias. Intracardiac electrograms are obtained from the conduction system as it runs in the interventricular septum near the tricuspid valve. A special catheter with four or more separate electrodes at different distances from the tip is positioned in the right heart after introduction through a right femoral vein approach. A second catheter is inserted from the arm to pace the heart by right atrial or ventricular stimulation. The timing of the electrical signals from the different electrodes against a conventional ECG is used to identify the recording site, and recordings can be obtained from the bundle of His and the right bundle. (See Chapters 14 and 15.)

Programmed stimulation of the right atrium or right or left ventricle using two to four premature stimulations is being used with increasing frequency to induce arrhythmias in the laboratory. The induced forms of arrhythmia have been shown to resemble those that occur spontaneously. The increasing use of surgical ablation of parts of the conduction system and accessory bundles of Kent has called forth these electrophysiologic studies to define the nature and likely site of origin and pathway of the arrhythmia. The effects of different drugs in the prevention and termination of different arrhythmias can also be tested. It is safer to find out the most effective regimen for suppressing the arrhythmia by having the patient experience an episode of arrhythmia in controlled circumstances in the laboratory than to give conventional treatment using trial and error. Almost any arrhythmia that is induced and persists for any length of time can be eliminated by overdrive suppression (see Chapter 15) or, as a last resort, by DC countershock (see Chapter 7).

Patients with aborted sudden death or unexplained syncope can benefit from electrophysiologic studies to determine whether ventricular arrhythmia can be induced by programmed electrical stimulation of the right or left ventricle. The efficacy of drug therapy in suppressing the arrhythmia can be investigated during the study and optimal drug therapy determined. Electrophysiologic studies to establish the optimal form of therapy are also indicated in any patient with documented ventricular tachycardia.

Provocation & Relief of Coronary Spasm

Coronary spasm has come to be recognized as a possible cause of cardiac pain; therefore, many cardiologists are using drugs to provoke and relieve vessel spasm. Some feel it is important to try to eliminate spasm as a factor in routine studies and give nitroglycerin or a calcium-blocking drug as premedication. Others reserve medication for relief of spasm when it occurs, either spontaneously during catheterization or in response to ergonovine maleate injection. The use of ergonovine to provoke coronary spasm is effective but is contrary to the principle of avoiding procedures that aggravate disease. The drug can be injected either intravenously or into the aorta in an initial dose of 0.0125 mg, which is increased every 5–10 minutes until chest pain occurs or ST-T wave changes appear on the ECG. The maximum total dose used is approximately 0.5 mg. It is generally considered dangerous to try to provoke coronary spasm outside the cardiac catheterization laboratory. The test should be confined to patients with normal coronary vessels or single-vessel disease and should be used only when the cause of chest pain is seriously in doubt. An ergonovine test may help in management of patients who are repeatedly admitted to the hospital because of pain and in whom spasm cannot be ruled out, coronary angiography shows minimal disease, and ancillary studies are negative. Previous myocardial infarction and significant hypertension are considered contraindications to the test. Hemodynamic and electrocardiographic changes should be sought after each dose of ergonovine; increases in systolic and diastolic left heart pressures are an indication to stop the test. Nitroglycerin and calcium-blocking drugs should be immediately available to reverse spasm.

In spite of all precautions, serious complications of arrhythmia, heart block, and myocardial infarction and death have been reported. The effects of systemic injections of ergonovine are not confined to the coronary circulation. It causes generalized vasoconstriction, and its effect in increasing peripheral resistance may sometimes cause cardiac pain. Ergonovine can cause chest pain from esophageal spasm. Ergonovine testing is thus a "nonstandard" procedure that should not be undertaken for the first time unless a physician experienced in using the technique is present.

Endomyocardial Biopsy

Biopsy of myocardial tissue can be carried out through a cardiac catheter. The usual site is the right ventricle in the region of the interventricular septum. A special catheter is used, and a piece of cardiac muscle is pinched off by miniature jaws activated from the hub of the catheter. The yield of diagnostic information using this method has not been great, and the principal use of the technique has been to follow the histologic changes that occur in rejection after cardiac transplantation and to adjust the dosage of immunosuppressive drugs according to what is revealed by the biopsy findings. The technique can also be used to establish the benefit of therapeutic regimens (eg, in acute myocarditis) (see Chapter 17). The procedure is painless, and complications are rare but can involve arrhythmias and even ventricular perforation and tamponade.

THERAPEUTIC PROCEDURES INVOLVING CATHETERIZATION

PERCUTANEOUS TRANSLUMINAL CORONARY ANGIOPLASTY (PTCA) (See also Chapter 8.)

The use of special balloon catheters to dilate narrowed vessels anywhere in the arterial bed, but especially in the coronary circulation, is now an accepted procedure for the palliative treatment of atherosclerosis. The design of the catheters has improved since the technique was introduced by Gruentzig in the late 1970s. Inflation of the balloon in the area of stenosis relieves the obstruction. Improvement is not necessarily only immediate. According to the Bernoulli principle, localized narrowings in blood vessels tend to become progressively more severe because the pressure in the narrowed part of the vessel tends to fall, further narrowing the vessel. Conversely, acute localized dilation tends to expand the vessel in the long run because the pressure in the previously narrowed area is increased.

The technique demands skill and judgment, and the results are related to the experience of the operator. It should only be performed in hospitals in which open heart surgery is immediately available to deal with untoward events requiring coronary bypass surgery.

Indications & Contraindications

Angioplasty is most clearly indicated in patients with single-vessel disease with medically uncontrolled angina pectoris. Short, proximal, noncalcified single lesions are the most satisfactory. The technique is least successful in lesions of the coronary ostia, and calcification in the neighborhood of the lesion is no longer a contraindication but can decrease the success of the dilation. Age is no bar, and patients with multivessel disease can also be treated by this method. Patients with unstable angina can also benefit, but restenosis at the site of dilation is more frequent in this condition. A second dilation can produce a satisfactory result.

There are now many indications for the procedure and few contraindications. Even totally occluded vessels can be reopened with a success rate of about 50%—higher if the occlusion is less than 2 months old. A recent myocardial infarct (< 20 weeks old) and a short (< 1.5 cm) narrowing increase the chances of success. If thrombus is detected at angiography, the procedure is less successful because of reocclusion with fresh thrombus.

Technique

Preliminary medication with aspirin is started before the procedure. After the lesion has been identified by coronary angiography, spasm is excluded by medication with a calcium-blocking drug and intracoronary nitroglycerin. The special catheters needed for the procedure are inserted via the femoral artery. Full anticoagulation is established with heparin, and a guiding catheter is passed to the orifice of the coronary artery in question. The balloon catheter, inserted through the guiding catheter, is passed across the obstruction using a flexible, steerable guide wire, while proximal and distal pressures are being monitored. When the position is optimal, as judged by fluoroscopy and contrast injection, the balloon is distended with weak contrast material, initially to a pressure of 3–6 atm for 15–30 seconds. Several inflations at progressively higher pressures up to 10 atm are sometimes needed, and further angiography is performed to assess the results. Special catheters with balloons that will inflate under pressures up to 20 atm and catheters that will maintain their bend with full inflation have made possible dilation of calcified lesions and lesions at bends of the artery. An example of two successful dilations is shown in Figure 6–7. The obstruction in the circumflex branch was dilated first, followed by the lesion in the anterior descending coronary artery. The balloon catheter is shown positioned within each artery in Figure 6–8.

Results

At present, 30–40% of patients with coronary disease are suitable candidates for dilation. Dilation is feasible in about 80% of such suitable candidates, and

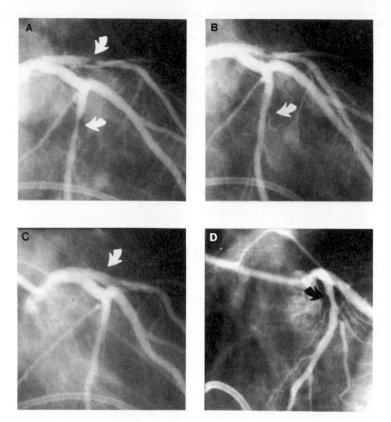

Figure 6–7. Coronary arteriograms showing effects of percutaneous transluminal coronary angioplasty in a patient with obstructions in the circumflex and anterior descending branches of the left coronary artery. In **A,** both lesions are seen. In **B,** the circumflex lesion has been dilated and the anterior descending lesion is still present. In **C,** the anterior descending lesion has been dilated. A different view is shown in **D.** (Courtesy of TA Ports.)

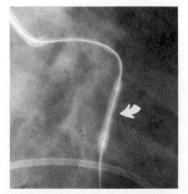 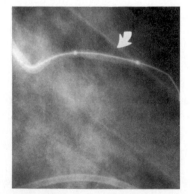

Figure 6–8. Radiographs showing a balloon catheter positioned within each of the coronary arterial lesions shown in Figure 6–7. At left, the balloon is in the circumflex lesion. At right, the balloon is in the left anterior descending lesion. (Courtesy of TA Ports.)

70–80% show objective evidence of benefit as measured by exercise testing, including electrocardiographic or radionuclear investigations. Restenosis is a serious problem and is commoner in patients in whom more than one vessel has been dilated. The rate of restenosis is about 20%, and in about 30–40% of cases a second dilation produces benefit. Lesions involving the proximal anterior descending coronary artery may have a restenosis rate of 40%. Lesions of coronary grafts are also amenable to dilation, but lesions involving branches are less suitable. The best results in vein grafts are at the anastomosis with the coronary artery. Stenoses at the aortic orifice do not dilate with balloon catheters. Old vein grafts should not be dilated, because the atheromatous material in them will embolize.

Complications

Cardiac pain or arrhythmia may develop when the catheter passes through the obstruction or the balloon is inflated. Spasm, dissection, rupture, or occlusion of the vessel by a displaced plaque may occur when the balloon is inflated. In addition, the multiple manipulations of catheters in the iliofemoral vessels of fully heparinized patients can cause vascular complications. About 2.5–5% of patients suffer myocardial infarction after angioplasty. About 2.5–5% of patients require immediate coronary bypass surgery for complications. The overall mortality rate is about 0.5–1%.

Long-Term Results

The long-term (5- to 10-year) results of angioplasty are not yet available. Restenosis is the major problem with angioplasty and appears to be the result of the intimal hyperplasia caused by stimulating the smooth-muscle cells of the media to proliferate and migrate into the intima. This is believed to be a manifestation of the "healing" process. Like coronary artery bypass surgery, the procedure is palliative, and coronary atherosclerosis is a progressive disease. Angioplasty is clearly less traumatic and less expensive than surgical treatment, but its ultimate role in the treatment of ischemic heart disease is not yet established. Numerous ongoing studies are comparing angioplasty with coronary bypass surgery. One study has shown that patients with single-vessel disease have better exercise performance on the treadmill and less exercise-induced angina if treated with angioplasty versus medical management.

OTHER TECHNIQUES

New techniques for the treatment of atherosclerotic lesions are under development. Lasers have been tried over the past few years to vaporize coronary arterial lesions. The incidence of perforation of the coronary vessel has been high enough to slow the development of this approach significantly.

An atherectomy catheter designed to bore a tunnel through a lesion is still in the experimental stage. It has been used with success in the treatment of peripheral arterial lesions. A parallel development involves the use of a catheter with a rotating piezoelectric crystal at its tip. This can produce an ultrasonic image of the interior of the vessel similar to that obtained with transesophageal echocardiography. This image should be useful as a guide to the positioning of an atherectomy catheter. The small size of the coronary vessels and the technical problems of miniaturization of the equipment make it likely that only proximal coronary lesions will be amenable to investigation and treatment with such devices.

BALLOON VALVULOPLASTY

Balloon valvuloplasty, based on the same principles as percutaneous transluminal coronary angioplasty, has come to be used extensively over the past 5 years in the treatment of valvular stenosis. The technique involves passing a catheter with a sausage-shaped balloon near its tip across the stenotic valve over a guidewire and inflating the balloon to a pressure of up to 10 atm to dilate the valve. Aortic, mitral, and pulmonary valves are also amenable to dilation, and pulmonary arterial stenoses and coarctation of the aorta are being treated similarly.

The indications for the procedure and the technical aspects are dealt with under the headings of the individual lesions. The efficacy of the treatment is roughly comparable to that of finger fracture of stenotic lesions that was the standard operative procedure 30 or more years ago. Progressive dilation, starting with a single, small-diameter (18 mm) balloon and progressing to a large balloon and a double balloon, has become the standard approach.

Dangerous tears of valve leaflets and embolization have not proved to be important complications, but problems have arisen from the placement of one or two large balloons, which are introduced via the femoral artery across the aortic valve or via two separate transseptal puncture holes into the left atrium and across the mitral valve. Frequently with valvuloplasty, mild valvular insufficiency develops or a preexisting insufficiency worsens. This technique is least successful with aortic stenosis due to calcification of the valve.

COMPLICATIONS OF CARDIAC CATHETERIZATION

COMPLICATIONS COMMON TO ALL FORMS OF CATHETERIZATION

Vessel Spasm

Spasm of the vessel into which a catheter is inserted—either an artery or a vein—almost invariably results from excessive trauma, often due to the use of too large a catheter for the size of the vessel. It is more common in young, nervous persons, and prior sedation, which is not needed routinely, may help to minimize it. Vessel spasm is now rarely seen with catheterization through the femoral artery and vein.

Vasovagal Attacks

Vasovagal attacks with bradycardia, hypotension, and ultimately loss of consciousness can occur in any study even before a catheter is introduced but are sufficiently common in coronary arteriography (especially when the catheter is near the orifice of the right coronary artery) so that atropine, 0.4–0.8 mg intravenously, is sometimes administered prophylactically. In other studies, it is sufficient to watch for the early signs—bradycardia, often associated with yawning—and to raise the patient's legs, give fluid boluses, and give atropine via the catheter.

Pulmonary Edema

Cardiac catheterization involves keeping the patient lying flat for several hours. If the patient has pulmonary congestion, this may provoke pulmonary edema. Contrast agents are high-osmolar fluids and can transiently increase blood volume. The first hint of development of edema is often restlessness, with a dry cough.

Arrhythmia

Atrial or ventricular arrhythmias are commonly provoked during cardiac catheterization. Fortunately, they usually subside upon removal of the catheter, which is thought to be responsible for their provocation by direct mechanical stimulation. Atrial arrhythmias are common when the catheter is in the right atrium in patients with atrial septal defect or mitral valve disease. Runs of ventricular ectopic beats are particularly frequent when the catheter is in the right ventricle. If the patient has left bundle branch block and electrical activation of the heart depends solely on the right bundle branch, cardiac standstill may take the place of the run of ectopic beats. With contrast injection, sinus bradycardia and even sinus arrest may occur briefly. A pacemaker should always

be available in the laboratory but is seldom needed. Ventricular tachycardia and ventricular fibrillation are rarely seen in right heart catheterization. They are most likely to occur during coronary arteriography (incidence about 0.5–1%). A sharp blow on the chest—or, if that is not successful, DC countershock—should restore sinus rhythm. A defibrillator should be available and charged in the room where cardiac catheterization is being done for use in an emergency situation.

Arteriovenous Fistula

Since cardiac catheterization involves the puncture or dissection of arteries and veins as they lie in close proximity in the groin or at the elbow, the possibility of creating an arteriovenous fistula always exists.

Dissection

Dissection of an artery by a guide wire passed up between the media and the intima is a potentially dangerous complication. The actual process of dissection is painful, and advancing guide wires while a patient is experiencing pain is ill advised. It is possible for a dissection begun in the femoral or external iliac artery to spread up into the abdominal aorta, thereby compromising blood flow to the viscera.

Broken Catheters

There is always a risk of breaking a catheter or forming a knot that cannot be extracted by manipulation. When the catheter fragment is radiopaque, it is possible to insert a long looped guide wire in the form of a snare and to extract the fragment as it is carried through the circulation. In other cases, thoracotomy may be necessary, with or without cardiotomy.

Prevention of Complications

In general, the sooner the onset of a complication is recognized, the easier it is to restore the patient's status to normal and complete the study. Most complications are due to the study, and stopping the procedure is usually an effective but unsatisfactory method of treatment.

SPECIAL COMPLICATIONS OF PARTICULAR PROCEDURES

Right Heart Catheterization

Right heart catheterization should result in minimal morbidity and a zero mortality rate in adults. Adequate data should be obtainable in 99% of cases. With the use of peripheral veins, spasm is probably the most common problem, and anatomic variations in venous anatomy may interfere with the passage of the catheter to the right atrium. With the use of the femoral, internal jugular, and subclavian veins, neither spasm nor difficulty in passage is a problem.

Left Heart Catheterization

Rarely, percutaneous femoral catheterization leads to arterial occlusion or laceration of the femoral artery. Thrombus forms on the outside of the catheter, and as the catheter is withdrawn from the vessel, a sheath of thrombus is pulled off that coils up and blocks the artery. This complication is likely to occur when the catheter is left for a long time in the arterial tree. A low cardiac output and a small femoral artery, as seen in thin female patients with mitral stenosis and raised pulmonary vascular resistance, favor the occurrence of the complication.

Following brachial arterial arteriotomy, control of hemorrhage is sometimes a problem. Hemorrhage usually stops with prolonged pressure over the vessel. On removal of the catheter at the end of the study, a jet of blood should spurt from both the proximal and distal ends of the artery. When this does not happen, the presence of a blood clot should be suspected. Gently probing the vessel with a soft plastic catheter often dislodges soft thrombus. Passage of a Fogarty balloon catheter is the next step, and a vascular surgeon should be summoned when these measures do not meet with success. Since the brachial artery can usually be tied off without compromising the circulation to the hand and arm, the complications of the brachial approach are seldom serious, but the median nerve may be damaged.

In transseptal catheterization, it is possible to puncture the free wall of the right atrium, the aortic wall, or the tricuspid valve inadvertently, and complications can be serious. Hemorrhage and tamponade are the most common causes of death from the procedure.

In direct left ventricular puncture, the principal complication is pneumothorax. If the procedure is done only in patients with severe left ventricular hypertrophy due to aortic stenosis, the danger of intrapericardial hemorrhage and tamponade is minimized.

The dangers associated with all forms of left heart catheterization are about ten times greater than those of right heart studies. Systemic embolism from thrombus forming on catheters in the left heart is much more dangerous than in the lesser circulation. With catheters on the left side of the circulation, the patient should be heparinized with 2000–3000 units, repeated in 1 hour. In addition, a slow drip of heparinized saline is maintained between flushings. Before flushing, the catheter should always be reverse-flushed by withdrawing 1–2 mL back into the syringe.

Coronary Angiography

Ventricular fibrillation or ventricular tachycardia occurs during coronary angiography in about 0.5–1% of patients with coronary disease. A sharp blow on the chest, a cough, or DC countershock should restore sinus rhythm, and in many laboratories coronary angiography is continued after this treatment has been successful. Coronary angiography is now the commonest precipitating cause of death in the cardiac catheterization laboratory in adults. The procedure is most dangerous in patients with left main coronary disease and patients with severe aortic stenosis and coronary artery disease. Progressive hypotension during and after the procedure—rather than arrhythmia—is the usual problem. Precipitation of myocardial infarction is another complication of the procedure. This may be due to embolism, trauma to the coronary ostium, or impaction of the catheter, which occludes the ostium completely.

It is important to monitor the pressure at the catheter tip at all times when the catheter is in a coronary vessel. This obviously is not possible during injection, but the operator should switch off the pressure tracings for the minimal time. Progressive damping of the pressure tracing is an important indication of the need to reposition the catheter. Spasm of the proximal part of a coronary artery can occur during coronary angiography and is usually attributed to mechanical effects of the catheter. Sublingual or intracoronary nitroglycerin is used for prevention and treatment.

The contrast material used in angiography tends to act as an osmotic load and increase the blood volume. This can lead to complications, especially in patients on the verge of pulmonary edema. It is unwise to inject large amounts of contrast material into the pulmonary arteries of patients with mitral stenosis, especially if the pulmonary vascular resistance is raised. After catheterization, the contrast agent is excreted by the kidneys, carrying fluid with it. If fluid intake is not maintained, hypovolemia and hypotension may occur.

Hypersensitivity responses to the iodine in the contrast material are rare. It seems that injections into the left side of the heart, bypassing the lungs, cause less trouble than intravenous injections, as in intravenous urography.

REFERENCES

Bedside Catheterization

Connors AF et al: Evaluation of right-heart catheterization in the critically ill patient without acute myocardial infarction. N Engl J Med 1983;308:263.

Russell RO, Rackley CE: *Hemodynamic Monitoring in a Coronary Intensive Care Unit,* 2nd ed. Futura, 1981.

Silver GM et al: Arterial complications of attempted Swan-Ganz insertion. Am J Cardiol 1984;53:340.

Swan HJC et al: Catheterization of the heart in man with use of a flow-directed balloon-tipped catheter. N Engl J Med 1970;283:447.

Cardiac Catheterization

Bloomfield DA: The nonsurgical retrieval of intracardiac foreign bodies: An international survey. Cathet Cardiovasc Diagn 1978;4:1.

Brockenbrough EC, Braunwald E, Ross J: Transseptal left heart catheterization: A review of 450 studies and description of an improved technic. Circulation 1962;25:15.

Cheitlin MD: Valvular heart disease: Management and intervention: Clinical overview and discussion. Circulation 1991;84(Suppl I):I–259.

Croft CH, Lipscomb K: Modified technique of transseptal left heart catheterization. J Am Coll Cardiol 1985;5:904.

Fogarty TJ et al: A method for extraction of arterial emboli and thrombi. Surg Gynecol Obstet 1963;116:241.

Forssmann W: Die Sondierung des rechten Herzens. Klin Wochenschr 1929;8:2085.

Grossman W (editor): *Cardiac Catheterization and Angiography,* 3rd ed. Lea & Febiger, 1986.

Haskell RJ, French WJ: Accuracy of left atrial and pulmonary wedge pressure in pure mitral regurgitation in predicting left ventricular end-diastolic pressure. Am J Cardiol 1988;61:136.

Kennedy JW et al: Complications associated with cardiac catheterization and angiography. Cath Cardiovasc Diagn 1982;8:5.

Mason JW: Endomyocardial biopsy: The balance of success and failure. Circulation 1985;71:185.

Primm RK et al: Incidence of new pulmonary perfusion defects after routine cardiac catheterization. Am J Cardiol 1979;43:529.

St. John Sutton MG et al: Valve replacement without preoperative cardiac catheterization. N Engl J Med 1981;305:1233.

Sibley DH et al: Subselective measurement of coronary blood flow velocity using a steerable Doppler catheter. J Am Coll Cardiol 1986;8:1332.

Wilson RF, White CW: Intracoronary papaverine: An ideal coronary vasodilator for studies of the coronary circulation in conscious humans. Circulation 1986;73:444.

Wilson RF et al: Transluminal, subselective measurement of coronary artery blood flow velocity and vasodilator reserve in man. Circulation 1985;72:82.

Angiography

Abrams HL (editor): *Angiography,* 2nd ed. (2 vols.) Little, Brown, 1971.

Complications and mortality of percutaneous balloon mitral commissurotomy: A report from the NHLDI Balloon Valvuloplasty Registry. Circulation 1992;85:2014.

Dodek A, Hooper RO: Coronary spasm provoked by ergonovine. Am Heart J 1984;107:781.

Gensini GG: *Coronary Arteriography.* Futura, 1975.

Hardy MB et al: Ergonovine maleate testing during cardiac catheterization: A 10-year perspective in 3,447 patients without significant coronary artery disease or Prinzmetal's variant angina. J Am Coll Cardiol 1992;20:107.

Hastey CE, Erwin SW, Ramanathan KB: Ergonovine induced coronary spasm refractory to intracoronary nitroglycerin but responsive to nitroprusside. Am Heart J 1984;107:778.

Judkins MP: Selective coronary arteriography. 1. A percutaneous transfemoral technic. Radiology 1967;89:815.

Klocke FJ: Measurement of coronary blood flow and degree of stenosis: Current clinical implications and continuing uncertainties. J Am Coll Cardiol 1983;1:31.

The NHLBI Balloon Valvuloplasty Registry: Multicenter experience with balloon mitral commissurotomy: NHLKBI Balloon Valvuloplasty Registry on immediate and 30-day follow-up results. Circulation 1992;85:448.

Sones FM, Shirey EK: Cine coronary arteriography. Mod Concepts Cardiovasc Dis 1962;31:735.

Therapeutic Interventions

Al Zaibag M et al: Percutaneous double-balloon mitral valvotomy for rheumatic mitral-valve stenosis. Lancet 1986;1:757.

Angelini P: *Balloon Catheter Coronary Angioplasty.* Futura, 1987.

Balin DS: Coronary interventions in ischemic heart disease. Curr Opin Cardiol 1991;6:524.

Bentvoglio LG et al: Percutaneous transluminal coronary angioplasty (PCTA) in patients with relative contraindications: Results of the National Heart, Lung, and Blood Institute PCTA registry. Am J Cardiol 1984;53(Suppl C):82C.

Block PC et al: Percutaneous angioplasty of stenoses of bypass grafts or of bypass graft anastomotic sites. Am J Cardiol 1984;53:666.

Clark DA: *Coronary Angioplasty.* Liss, 1987.

Dorros G et al: Percutaneous transluminal coronary angioplasty in patients with prior coronary artery bypass grafting. J Thorac Cardiovasc Surg 1984;87:17.

Gruntzig A, Kumpe DA: Technique of percutaneous transluminal angioplasty with the Gruntzig balloon catheter. AJR 1979;132:547.

Hartz AJ et al: Mortality after coronary angioplasty and coronary artery bypass surgery. (The National Medicare Experience.) Am J Cardiol 1992;70:179.

Kereiakes DJ et al: Angioplasty in total coronary artery occlusion: Experience in 76 consecutive patients. J Am Coll Cardiol 1985;6:526.

Kulick DL et al: Catheter ballon commissurotomy in adults. Part II: Mitral and other stenoses. Curr Probl Cardiol 1990;15:403.

Kulick DL et al: Catheter balloon valvuloplasty in adults. Part I: Aortic stenosis. Curr Probl Cardiol 1990;15:359.

Mabin TA et al: Intracoronary thrombus: Role in coronary occlusion complicating percutaneous transluminal coronary angioplasty. J Am Coll Cardiol 1985;5:198.

McKay RG et al: Balloon dilation of calcific aortic stenosis in elderly patients. Postmortem, intraoperative, and percutaneous valvuloplasty studies. Circulation 1986;74:119.

McKay RG et al: Balloon dilation of mitral stenosis in adult patients: Postmortem and percutaneous mitral valvuloplasty studies. J Am Coll Cardiol 1987;9:723.

O'Keefe JH Jr et al: Multivessel coronary angioplasty from 1980 to 1989: Procedural results and long-term outcome. J Am Coll Cardiol 1990;16:1097.

Rahimtoola SH: Catheter balloon valvuloplasty of aortic and mitral stenosis in adults: 1987. Circulation. 1987;75:895.

Stertzer SH et al: Lesion morphology and coronary angioplasty: Current experience and analysis. J Am Coll Cardiol 1992;19:1641.

Topol EJ (editor): *Acute Coronary Intervention*. Liss, 1987.

Vogel RA (editor): A symposium: Beyond the balloon: Complex angioplasty for the practitioner. Am J Cardiol 1992;62:3F.

Weintraub WS et al: Changing use of coronary angioplasty and coronary bypass surgery in the treatment of chronic coronary artery disease. Am J Cardiol 1990;65:183.

Electrophysiology

Eldar M, Sauve MJ, Scheinman MM: Electrophysiologic testing and follow-up of patients with aborted sudden death. J Am Coll Cardiol 1987;10:291.

Fogoros RN et al: Long-term outcome of survivors of cardiac arrest whose therapy is guided by electrophysiologic testing. J Am Coll Cardiol 1992;19:780.

Krol RB et al: Electrophysiologic testing in patients with unexplained syncope: Clinical and noninvasive predictors of outcome. J Am Coll Cardiol 1987;10:358.

Simonson JS et al: Selection of patients for programmed ventricular stimulation: A clinical decision-making model based on multivariate analysis of clinical variables. J Am Coll Cardiol 1992;20:317.

Vandepol CJ et al: Incidence and clinical significance of induced ventricular tachycardia. Am J Cardiol 1980;45:725.

Waldo AL et al: The minimally appropriate electrophysiologic study for the initial assessment of patients with documented sustained monomorphic ventricular tachycardia. J Am Coll Cardiol 1985;6:1174.

Therapeutic Procedures

7

This chapter deals with the techniques of therapeutic procedures used in the management of cardiac disorders. Whenever possible, the patient's status should be monitored by the methods described in Chapters 5 and 6 to observe the response to therapy. However, since therapeutic procedures are often needed in emergency situations, the techniques described must on occasion be used in circumstances that are less than ideal.

CARDIOPULMONARY RESUSCITATION (CPR)

All physicians must be familiar with the emergency procedures involved in cardiopulmonary resuscitation. Basic life support has now become standardized and covers the procedures used when someone collapses or is found collapsed. The more sophisticated modes of treatment undertaken by a skilled resuscitation team are covered under Advanced Cardiac Life Support, below.

Basic Life Support

Speed in providing support is essential in order to maintain oxygenation and blood flow to the brain. A delay of more than 4 minutes after the onset of respiratory or circulatory arrest is likely to compromise the chance of complete recovery.

The sequence of steps to be taken starts with the establishment of the need for resuscitation. Verbal contact and gently shaking the subject determine the level of consciousness. The rescuer calls for assistance and tells any bystander to call for help from the emergency medical services. The subject is placed supine on the nearest convenient level surface.

The sequence of treatment follows the "ABC" of CPR (Airway, Breathing, Circulation).

A. Airway:

1. Establish whether breathing is absent. Open the airway by extending the neck, lifting the chin, and pressing down on the forehead (Figure 7–1A). Do not lift up the neck in accident cases, as displacement might damage the spinal cord. Determine whether breathing is absent by looking to see if the chest is moving, listening for sounds of breathing, and holding a hand or the face close to the patient's nose and mouth.

2. If breathing is absent, make sure that the airway is patent.

3. Clear the mouth and pharynx of foreign material with a finger in the throat.

B. Breathing:

1. If steps A2 and A3 do not establish a patent airway, inflate the lungs with two breaths through the mouth (occluding the nose) or through the nose (occluding the mouth) (Figure 7–1B). The breaths should last 1–1.5 seconds. If the airway does not clear immediately, a foreign body may be obstructing the airway. Roll the person on the side, and deliver a sharp blow on the back. If this fails, apply the Heimlich maneuver (see below).

2. Feel for a carotid pulse. If a strong pulse is felt, continue mouth-to-mouth or mouth-to-nose breathing 12–15 times per minute until spontaneous breathing returns. If carotid pulsation is absent or ceases, proceed to C.

C. Circulation:

1. Deliver a short, sharp blow to the lower sternum. This is equivalent to an electric shock of about 1 J and sometimes stops ventricular arrhythmia.

2. If carotid pulsation does not return, start closed chest cardiac compression without delay, alternating chest compression and ventilation. Standing or kneeling beside the subject as shown in Figure 7–2, place the heel of one hand on the lower sternum above the level of the xiphoid. Place the other hand on top, and, with the arms extended, press down rhythmically at a rate of 80–100 strokes per minute. Aim to move the sternum 4–5 cm per stroke. After 15 strokes, stop and inflate the lungs twice as indicated in ¶B1, above. After four cycles of compression and ventilation, check the carotid pulse and reassess the situation, stopping for no more than 7 seconds. If help is available, the second person should be at the head of the subject and take over the ventilation. The rhythm should be one inflation to every five compressions.

Advanced Cardiac Life Support

Chest compression and artificial ventilation are continued while attempts to restart vital functions or stabilize the circulation are made by medical or paramedical staff who have arrived on the scene in response to calls for help. Oxygen is given by mask, electrocardiographic leads are attached, and an ECG is recorded. An intravenous infusion of normal saline

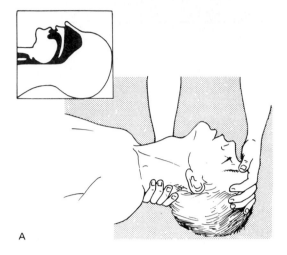

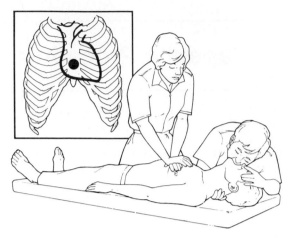

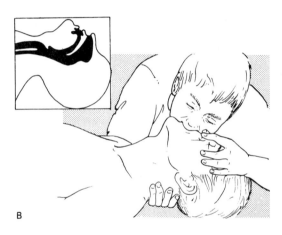

Figure 7–2. Technique of alternating external chest compression and ventilation. Heavy circle in heart drawing shows area of application of force. (Modified and reproduced, with permission, from Krupp MA, Chatton MJ, Tierney LM Jr [editors]: *Current Medical Diagnosis & Treatment 1986.* Lange, 1986.)

is started, a DC defibrillator is prepared, and an arterial sample is taken for analysis of Po_2, Pco_2, and pH. An endotracheal tube is usually inserted to facilitate lung inflation.

A team leader must try to determine the following: (1) What is the nature of the problem? (Arrhythmia? Asystole? Respiratory failure?) (2) What is the underlying cause of the problem, and is it correctable? (Myocardial infarction? Pulmonary embolism? Hemorrhage? Trauma?) (3) What further measures are needed?

Mechanism of Action of External Chest Compression

Until recently, it was assumed that the mechanism of "closed chest cardiac massage" was to squeeze the heart between the sternum and spine and thus to expel blood from the thorax. Studies have now indicated that it is the rise in intrathoracic pressure associated with chest compression that expels blood from the thorax into the extrathoracic arteries. The effect is not transmitted to the great veins, since they collapse in response to raised intrathoracic pressure. Corollaries to these findings are that "cardiac massage" should be more effective if the chest is compressed at high rather than low lung volumes and that compression during inflation is more effective than compression during deflation.

Choking on Food

Choking on food is commonly seen in restaurants in persons who have overindulged in alcohol. It is also a risk in nursing homes among elderly, debilitated, edentulous patients who may be oversedated. Acute respiratory distress associated with airway ob-

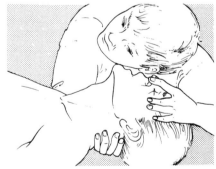

Figure 7–1. Proper performance of mouth-to-mouth resuscitation. *A:* Open airway by positioning neck anteriorly in extension. Inserts show airway obstructed when the neck is in resting flexed position and opening when neck is extended. *B:* Rescuer should close victim's nose with fingers, seal mouth around victim's mouth, and deliver breath by vigorous expiration. *C:* Victim is allowed to exhale passively by unsealing mouth and nose. Rescuer should listen and feel for expiratory air flow. (Reproduced, with permission, from Schroeder SA et al [editors]: *Current Medical Diagnosis & Treatment 1989.* Appleton & Lange, 1989.)

struction resulting from blockage by food is often apparent because the patient jumps up, coughs and splutters, and shows clear signs of respiratory distress. If airway obstruction is only partial, as evidenced by wheezing, forceful coughing, and adequate airway exchange, *do not* interfere with the patient's attempt to expel the foreign body. *If the patient is able to speak, even in a whisper, do not go on to the following steps in treatment.* If the patient cannot speak, the rescuer should take up a position behind the victim, who should stand still in the upright position. The rescuer's arms are then placed around the victim's waist, the hands formed into fists against the victim's epigastrium, and pulled in forcibly on the victim's abdomen several times **(Heimlich maneuver).** The forced expiratory air flow will usually dislodge the obstruction, at least partially, and it may then be possible to grasp it with the fingers down the throat and remove it if the patient cannot spit it out. If the victim is lying on the floor, the rescuer should kneel beside or astride the victim's body and attempt to expel the obstruction by blows with the fist to the epigastrium. If these maneuvers fail, emergency tracheostomy may have to be performed using the sharpest knife available.

Resuscitation in a Hospital Setting

All hospitals should have an emergency resuscitation team available at all times capable of responding to a telephone call for assistance anywhere in the hospital. The emergency is usually announced over a public address system or a signal flashed to the code team's beepers, and the appropriate persons— usually a cardiologist, an anesthetist, a nurse, and a surgeon—should go as quickly as possible to the scene. Basic life support procedures are instituted by persons already at the scene as described above. In a hospital setting, it is usually easier to make a rapid diagnosis because the reasons for the patient's hospitalization will be known. The same principles apply in deciding whether chest compression or mouth-to-mouth resuscitation (or both) is required, and since more than one person is usually present, one must take charge and direct operations, maintaining resuscitative measures until further assistance arrives. Note should be made of the time the resuscitation team arrives on the scene, since this will be important in deciding when to abandon resuscitation efforts if they are unsuccessful.

Emergency Defibrillation

If ventricular fibrillation or tachycardia is the cause of the emergency, defibrillation should be carried out with a minimum of delay. In emergency situations, a DC shock of 400 J is routinely given and repeated as necessary. The paddles, which should already have been smeared liberally with ECG electrode paste, are applied, one over the cardiac apex and the other over the base of the heart . Everyone except the holder of the paddles breaks physical contact with the patient, and the shock is administered by pressing the button to complete the circuit and discharge the electric impulse through the patient. Since the patient is already unconscious, no anesthetic is required. The instant of the shock is clearly visible as the patient's body jerks because of electrical stimulation of the thoracic muscles. When the response to the shock has been determined, a decision is made whether to restart chest compression and ventilation, whether to try to improve the state of perfusion and oxygenation by some other means, or whether to try another shock.

Defibrillation by Paramedical Personnel

Early treatment of patients with myocardial infarction by specially trained ambulance and fire department personnel is becoming more widespread. Administration of drugs (atropine or lidocaine) and especially electrical defibrillation are the principal forms of treatment available. The most important determinant of successful resuscitation is the promptness of initiation. The incidence of successful resuscitation is inversely proportionate to the time between the onset of collapse and defibrillation. Advances in the design and portability of equipment, use of the tongue-abdominal pathway for electrocardiographic recording, pacing, and defibrillation, and the introduction of special "foolproof" logic-based instruments may lead to improved results.

Further Measures

If defibrillation is unsuccessful, one should consider the possibility of giving lidocaine, 50 mg, as an intravenous bolus, and repeating the DC shock. The drug can be repeated up to a total dose of 500 mg. If asystole is present and a pacemaker is not immediately available, intravenous or intracardiac epinephrine (0.5 mg, or 5 mL of a 1:10,000 aqueous solution) should be tried. The drug may start cardiac contractions and produce ventricular fibrillation that can then be treated by DC countershock. Acidosis develops rapidly with cardiac arrest and inhibits cardiac contractility. Since chest compression provides only 15–20% of a normal output, acidosis must be treated in all cases that do not respond within 3–5 minutes. Since myocardial function is depressed by increases in Pco_2, the arterial pH should be maintained as close as possible to normal (pH 7.36), primarily by controlling arterial Pco_2 by effective ventilation. If the patient becomes acidotic in spite of this, sodium bicarbonate may be useful. Recently, the beneficial effects of sodium bicarbonate have been questioned, and numerous harmful consequences of its use have been documented. It should not be used until effective ventilation has been established, because it results in increased carbon dioxide production. If the patient remains in cardiac arrest for a prolonged period despite adequate ventilation, sodium bicarbonate solution, 3.75 g (44.6 meq), should be given intravenously and the dose repeated every 5 minutes until the circulation is restored. A slow infusion of 5% sodium bicarbonate at 100–150 drops/min is often more convenient. The effect of the infusion should be monitored by arterial blood gas measurements whenever possible.

If asystole is present, calcium chloride, 10 mL of a 10% solution, should be tried as a cardiac stimulant. If this fails, an external, noninvasive temporary pacemaker should be used in an attempt to restore the heartbeat. Improvements in electrode design have largely eliminated the stinging, burning pain that made external pacing intolerable in conscious patients in the past. Modifications of the stimulus duration and shape have reduced the threshold current to about 40–70 mA and greatly reduced the intensity of induced muscle contractions. External pacing can be tolerated by more than 95% of patients. Temporary external pacing can also be used to cover the insertion of an intravenous pacemaker. It can be left in a standby mode and set to pace when the heart rate falls below a specific level. It is sometimes possible to stimulate the heart to contract by tapping the precordium rhythmically about 60 times per minute with the ulnar edge of the hand, using a modified "karate chop"; if this is successful, it is much preferred to external pacing.

External pacing is only used as an emergency procedure to bridge the gap until a temporary transvenous pacemaker can be inserted. If bradycardia is present after DC countershock, atropine (0.4–0.8 mg intravenously) should be tried.

Isoproterenol is often used as a general supportive measure when the heart rate is slow. It is given as an intravenous drip with 1 mg of the drug in 500 mL of 5% dextrose in water at a rate of 0.03 mg per 5 minutes (3 mL/min). A patient who recovers should be carefully examined, transferred to an intensive care area, and observed for the development of shock and for complications arising from the precipitating cause of the original circulatory collapse.

Follow-Up Measures

After the patient has responded to resuscitative measures, evaluation of central nervous system function deserves careful consideration. Each case must be treated on its merits, and it must be decided whether the physician is prolonging life or simply prolonging dying in patients with serious brain damage. Apparently complete central nervous system recovery has been reported in a few patients who have remained unconscious for as long as a week after resuscitation. No decision concerning the irreversibility of damage due to cerebral anoxia can be made before 24 hours have elapsed after arrest. After that time, the absence of cerebral and midbrain function is highly predictive of irreversible brain damage.

Hypothermia at 30 °C for 2–3 days may lessen the degree of brain damage. It is also important to look for complications associated with resuscitation, such as broken ribs, ruptured abdominal viscera, or pneumothorax.

OXYGEN THERAPY

Oxygen therapy should be considered in all patients in whom hypoxia is present and in those who are dyspneic at rest. The objective is to maintain an arterial Po_2 greater than 60 mm Hg. Oxygen is ordinarily available as the pure 100% gas either from a cylinder or via a wall outlet in intensive care areas. How well the patient tolerates oxygen therapy depends on the benefit derived from its use. When dyspnea and hypoxia are severe at rest, as in acute pulmonary edema or in lung disease, and the oxygen both raises the arterial Po_2 and relieves the dyspnea, the patient tolerates the therapy well. If the dyspnea is not relieved by oxygen, as in right-to-left shunts, severe low cardiac output states, and shock, the patient often tolerates the mask or catheter poorly.

If oxygen therapy is well tolerated, it can increase the oxygenation of marginally perfused tissues. If the patient is disturbed by the mask or catheter used for its administration, the resulting increase in cardiac output may offset the benefits obtained.

It is difficult to achieve an alveolar oxygen level of more than 40% by the use of masks or nasal catheters, especially in dyspneic patients, and thus it is mainly in those patients in whom a small increase in alveolar Po_2 produces a large increase in arterial Po_2 that oxygen therapy is effective.

It is possible to achieve higher alveolar oxygen levels by careful administration of oxygen with a trained person in constant attendance and constant monitoring available; 100% oxygen increases the oxygen content of blood leaving the lungs in patients with normal lung function by increasing the amount of oxygen carried in solution in the blood. This effect is small in patients with normal levels of hemoglobin, amounting to 17 mL/L, or equivalent to an increase in saturation of about 8.5% in a person with an oxygen capacity of 200 mL/L. This extra oxygen does not generally produce a significant clinical effect in patients in heart failure with a low cardiac output and normal lungs. In anemic patients, however, the effects are greater, amounting to the equivalent of an increase in oxygen saturation of 34% in a patient with an oxygen capacity of 50 mL/L (hemoglobin level 3.7 g/dL).

Oxygen Therapy in Specific Conditions

Oxygen therapy is indicated in the treatment of high-altitude pulmonary edema, especially when the patient cannot return to a lower altitude, and is indicated in any other patient with pulmonary edema irrespective of the underlying cause. Oxygenation of the blood leaving the lungs is incomplete in pulmonary edema, and oxygen is usually effective and well tolerated in all but the most restless patients.

It is in patients with lung disease, especially those with cor pulmonale, that oxygen is most clearly indicated. Oxygen often reduces the pulmonary artery pressure by reversing hypoxic pulmonary arterial vasoconstriction. This may break the vicious circle responsible for right heart failure and thus play a major part in the patient's recovery. Care must be taken to avoid depressing respiration by increasing Po_2 in patients with high Pco_2, in which case the major stimulus for respiration is the hypoxia. These patients must be monitored closely and the percentage of administered inspiratory oxygen (Fio_2) lowered, so that respiration is not depressed.

Oxygen should be tried in all patients with myocardial infarction in whom severe myocardial damage has occurred. Ventilation-perfusion mismatching may be present, and hypoxia is not infrequently seen.

Positive Airway Pressure

Maintenance of a continuous positive airway pressure and the use of positive pressure to inflate the lungs have a place in the treatment of pulmonary edema. Positive end-expiratory pressure (PEEP) can be achieved by having the patient breathe from a mask fitted with a demand valve, breathing out into a tube the end of which is submerged in water to a level of several centimeters. The extra end-expiratory pressure serves to increase the lung volume and, by increasing the intra-alveolar pressure, prevents the transudation of fluid into the alveoli. A similar effect can be obtained by the use of patient-cycled respirators. The aim of their use in pulmonary edema is not to assist in lung inflation but to provide a constant positive pressure airway throughout the respiratory cycle and maintain a normal alveolar volume. They can be used with either air or oxygen, and a considerable amount of cooperation is required from the patient. This form of therapy is preferable to continuous positive pressure breathing, in which an artificial respirator actively inflates the lungs. The patient is much more likely to struggle and fight the latter type.

Ventilatory assistance is seldom needed in patients who have heart disease alone, but it may become necessary if respiratory failure also develops. Artificial ventilation via a cuffed endotracheal tube with pressure-cycled or volume-controlled respirators tends to reduce venous return and decrease cardiac output. The possibility of compromising cardiac function must be borne in mind when ventilatory assistance is used, especially in the case of older patients with coronary artery disease.

VENESECTION

Venesection is a traditional means of treating cardiac failure that is seldom used today. Venous blood is ordinarily removed from an antecubital vein with the patient semirecumbent. Blood should not be removed rapidly, and a total of 500 mL is removed in about 15 minutes through a large (16-gauge) needle. If the patient shows any evidence of distress, the foot of the bed can be raised and venous return improved. The great increase in the effectiveness of diuretic drugs has markedly reduced the need for this procedure. It is now almost confined to the treatment of hemochromatosis and of polycythemia in adult patients with cyanotic congenital heart lesions in whom cardiac surgery is not indicated (eg, Eisenmenger's syndrome).

Bloodless Venesection

The use of tourniquets applied to the limbs in rotation to reduce venous return has been advocated in the treatment of acute pulmonary edema. Blood pressure cuffs are inflated on three limbs to a level of about 40 mm Hg (between venous and arterial pressure) in order to trap blood in the periphery. The cuff is removed and reapplied on another limb in rotation every 15 minutes. Up to 700 mL of blood can be trapped in the limbs by this means.

BLOOD TRANSFUSION IN CARDIAC PATIENTS

Blood transfusion is seldom indicated in the treatment of heart disease but is not infrequently needed when anemia occurs for other reasons. The patient should always receive the transfusion in the supine position so that the earliest manifestations of pulmonary congestion can be readily recognized. The patient can then sit up to relieve pulmonary congestion while the transfusion is slowed or stopped. Packed cells should be routinely used, and transfusion should be given as slowly as possible after taking into account the underlying reason for the transfusion. The use of sodium citrate as the anticoagulant imposes a severe load on the circulation, and the use of heparinized blood is preferable.

AFTERLOAD REDUCTION
(See also Chapters 8 and 10.)

Vasodilator drugs can combat the peripheral vasoconstriction seen in acute forms of heart failure and thereby provide a useful emergency means of relieving the load on the left ventricle. Afterload reduction is particularly helpful in patients with acute aortic or mitral valve incompetence (which often causes acute pulmonary edema), because it decreases backflow across the incompetent valve. Valvular incompetence is, therefore, another indication for the use of afterload reduction as an emergency measure to tide the patient over until surgery can be performed. Afterload reduction has been demonstrated to be beneficial in chronic left heart failure, even prolonging survival in patients with severe left ventricular systolic dysfunction. It is also useful in some cases of acute myocardial infarction with heart failure.

The dose of the vasodilator drug must be carefully titrated against its effects on the systemic arterial pressure, heart rate, and cardiac output; direct monitoring of hemodynamic events is mandatory. The benefits of reducing the load against which the left ventricle must eject blood must be weighed against any increase in cardiac oxygen consumption that may result from increase in heart rate.

There is no entirely satisfactory drug with which to produce systemic vasodilation. Sodium nitroprusside is relatively short-acting and is given intravenously, and hydralazine can be given by mouth. The most frequently used afterload-reducing drugs now are the long-acting angiotensin-converting enzyme inhibitors captopril and enalapril. Both these drugs have been shown to prolong survival, perhaps because of antagonism to the increased renin-angiotensin activity seen in congestive heart failure. Lisinopril and other angiotensin-converting enzyme inhibitor drugs are rapidly becoming available. Their actions are more long-lasting, but as a result their dosage for afterload reduction may be more difficult to titrate in acute cases. Long-term therapy, however, is easier with these drugs than with the above-mentioned ones.

The optimal dosage of all of these drugs must be determined by trial and error in each individual patient. The most satisfactory regimen is to start with a small dose (15 μg/min of nitroprusside intravenously, 25 mg of hydralazine, or 6.25 mg of captopril or 5 mg of enalapril) while monitoring the hemodynamic status closely and to gradually increase the medication until a full hemodynamic response is obtained. The dose is then reduced by 15–20% to a maintenance level.

Several other drugs have been tried in an attempt to obtain longer-lasting effects. Sublingual, intravenous, or topical nitroglycerin and sublingual or oral isosorbide dinitrate have been shown to be effective, but their effects on capacitative vessels (veins) are greater, and a fall in output may occur. Their therapeutic effects are less predictable than those of intravenous drugs. Drugs such as prazosin have been used but rapidly induce tachyphylaxis, which limits their usefulness.

PERICARDIOCENTESIS
(See also Chapter 18.)

This procedure is more commonly required in chronic than in acute pericardial effusion. It is best carried out in a cardiac catheterization laboratory under fluoroscopic control, but in an emergency can be done in the patient's bed. In traumatic cases and after thoracic surgical procedures when tamponade is suspected, it is frequently combined with surgical exploration, which is needed to check for bleeding points.

The puncture site of choice is in the subxiphoid region, with the subject semirecumbent, but any precordial site can be used. The needle is directed toward the left shoulder about 30 degrees posteriorly. Once the pericardium is perforated, the stylus should be removed and the needle aspirated with a syringe. The needle used should not be too small (18-gauge or larger), especially if purulent effusion is suspected, and should have a short bevel. The procedure is more safely carried out if the exploring (chest) electrode of an electrocardiograph is connected to the needle by means of a sterile wire with alligator clips at each end. By this means, any contact between the needle tip and the myocardium can be detected as a sudden elevation of the ST segment, and inadvertent cardiac puncture can be avoided. Examples of electrocardiographic recordings obtained with the needle tip in different sites are shown in Figure 7–3. Others have recommended guiding the pericardiocentesis needle by echocardiography. The procedure is done under local anesthesia similar to that used in thoracentesis, and precautions should be taken to avoid the intercostal blood vessels that run behind the lower edges of the ribs.

It is advantageous to have a central venous pressure recording available at the time of removal of pericardial fluid. A significant fall in central venous pressure indicates that relief of tamponade has occurred, and the final pressure gives an indication of the state of right ventricular function and the level of blood volume.

All pericardial taps should be regarded as diagnostic as well as therapeutic procedures, and fluid should always be sent for appropriate laboratory examination, including culture. If a large volume of fluid is to be removed, it is helpful to insert a soft plastic catheter through the needle to avoid myocardial and coronary artery injury. We place a guide-wire into the pericardial sac, remove the needle, and thread a 6F short pigtail catheter over the wire, which is then removed. This catheter is likely to remain patent, permitting prolonged pericardial drainage. Its patency can be maintained by flushing with heparinized saline. A plastic catheter may be left in situ if effusion is deemed likely to recur rapidly. In recurrent effusions due to cancer or uremia, drugs such as antineoplastic agents, corticosteroids, or those causing inflammation and adhesions such as tetracycline can be instilled in a properly sedated patient in an attempt to prevent further effusion.*

---

*Tetracyline for this purpose is no longer available from its only manufacturer (Lederle Laboratories), though stocks on hand are

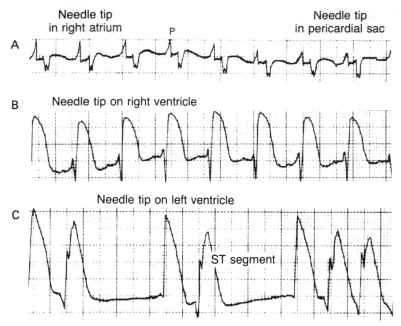

Figure 7–3. Electrocardiograms obtained from the needle tip during pericardiocentesis. In **A,** the amplitude of the P wave decreases when the needle is removed from the right atrium. In **B** and **C,** large-amplitude deflections are seen when the needle touches a ventricle, and in **C,** ectopic beats occur. (Courtesy of A Hollman.)

ELECTIVE CARDIOVERSION

Restoration of sinus rhythm by DC countershock applied to the chest, when carried out electively, is always performed with the patient under anesthesia. The procedure is painful, and analgesia with morphine or meperidine is not sufficient. Except when the atrial fibrillation has been present for less than 48 hours, anticoagulation for 2 weeks before cardioversion is recommended. The indications for the use of this treatment are similar to those for restoration of sinus rhythm by means of drugs and are dealt with elsewhere (see Chapter 15).

An antiarrhythmic agent, either quinidine by mouth (0.2 g four times daily) for 2 days before, or intravenous procainamide (0.5 g given over 5 minutes) immediately, is given before the procedure. This premedication is intended to reduce the tendency for the rhythm to revert to the precardioversion state. The premedication may on occasion restore sinus rhythm and make countershock unnecessary. An adequate 12-lead ECG should be taken at the start of the procedure. The rhythm should be identified and a lead chosen in which the characteristics of the arrhythmia are clearly seen. Lead V_1 or V_2 is usually best for patients with atrial fibrillation. The patient's recent medication must be accurately known, especially the level of digitalis dosage and, if possible, the digitalis blood level. Therapeutic levels of serum digoxin (0.8–2 ng/mL) are no bar to cardioversion, but if there is any possibility of an element of digitalis toxicity, elective cardioversion should be postponed until digitalis toxicity is resolved, or the first shock after the patient has been anesthetized should be small (about 5 J). If this small shock elicits bursts of ventricular tachycardia, cardioversion is postponed.

At least three persons should be in attendance: a nurse, an anesthesiologist, and a cardiologist. The anesthesiologist chooses the method of anesthesia; the nurse runs the electrocardiographic recording, which should also be displayed on a monitor oscilloscope if possible; and the cardiologist applies the paddles to the chest and administers the shock. The large current passing through the body must not be allowed to feed back through the electrocardiographic leads and damage the electrocardiograph. Everyone except the holder of the paddles breaks physical contact with the patient in order to avoid an electric shock. The paddles are insulated.

The minimum shock necessary to restore sinus rhythm varies. In most cases, an initial dose of 80–150 J is used in atrial fibrillation except when digitalis has been given. In that case, a trial dose of 5 J is given and the shock is gradually increased. Atrial flutter usually responds to lower doses. Electrical countershock almost always restores sinus rhythm for at least a few beats, but in many instances the abnormal rhythm recurs. If the first shock is ineffective, a

---

still being used. Possible substitutes such as doxycycline are being investigated.

second shock with a larger dose should be given. If multiple shocks (six or more) are not effective, the physician should consider leaving the patient in the abnormal rhythm, especially if it is atrial fibrillation. The dosage of antiarrhythmic drug, usually quinidine, is continued after the procedure if sinus rhythm is restored.

PACEMAKERS
(See also Chapter 14.)

Significant advances in pacemaker technology have occurred in the past decade. Simple, fixed-rate devices, used for demand pacing of the ventricle, have been superseded by externally programmable instruments that can be used to pace both atrium and ventricle and also to trigger pacing from the intracardiac electrogram. Devices that alter rate in response to parameters reflecting increases in physical activity, such as muscle activity, blood temperature, or venous oxygen saturation, now make it possible to increase the heart rate appropriately as exercise increases. Advances in the design of integrated circuits and microcomputer technology have played an important role. In addition, the design of pacing wires and electrodes has been improved, and the methods for their introduction and stabilization are now more reliable.

The four components of any pacemaking system are (1) the battery, (2) the hermetically sealed housing, (3) the lead system, and (4) the signal generator. Failure of any of these components will lead to failure of the whole system, and it was not until advances had been made in the first three that sophisticated developments in the signal generator began to be applied. The modern pacemaker is a complex instrument whose function can be changed by setting multiple switches. The pacemaker's program, which is set

at the time it is implanted, can be changed noninvasively by means of a magnet or a radio-frequency signal from a coil placed over the implanted unit. A receiver coil in the pacemaker changes the switches appropriately. The implanted unit weighs 50–100 g and is powered by a lithium battery that can last 5–15 years. The variables that can be programmed include the mode of operation (unipolar or bipolar), rate, output (in terms of voltage and duration), sensitivity, atrioventricular delay, and refractory period.

The mode of operation of the modern pacemaker is now conventionally described by a five-letter code (Table 7–1): The first letter identifies the chamber paced. The second letter denotes the chamber whose electrical activity is sensed by the pacemaker. The third letter designates the mode of response. The fourth letter describes programmable functions such as rate modulation or communicating function. The fifth letter describes antitachyarrhythmic functions such as shock. If the fourth and fifth codes are not applicable, as with an implanted defibrillator, a three-letter code is used.

The simplest, oldest form of ventricular pacemaker is thus designated "VOO," indicating that it paces the ventricle with no sensing of the patient's heartbeat. A common form of demand pacemaker is designated "VVI," indicating that it paces the ventricle, sensing the ventricular electrogram and inhibiting the pacing function for a time after sensing an appropriate R wave in the patient's electrogram.

If the standard VVI, R wave-inhibited pacemaker is inserted for sinoatrial disease, the "pacemaker syndrome" (Erbel, 1979) may develop. In such a case, when ventricular pacing starts in response to sinus bradycardia, the lack of atrioventricular coordination causes the cardiac output and blood pressure to drop to levels that cause symptoms. This drop can be aggravated by retrograde stimulation of the atrium so

Table 7–1. Code positions of international pacemaker code.[1]

I[2,3] Chamber Paced	II[3] Chamber Sensed	III Response to Sensing	IV Programmable Functions; Rate Modulation	V Antitachyarrhythmia Functions
V—ventricle A—atrium D—double O—none	V—ventricle A—atrium D—double O—none	T—triggers pacing I—inhibits pacing D—triggers and inhibits pacing O—None	P—programmable rate and/or output M—multiprogrammability of rate, output, sensitivity, etc C—communicating functions (telemetry) R—rate of modulation O—None	P—programmable rate and output for antitachyarrhythmia S—shock D—dual (P + S) O—none

[1] Modified and reproduced, with permission, from *Medtronic News*, Winter 1987/1988. © Medtronic, Inc. 1987.
[2] Positions I–III are used exclusively for antibradyarrhythmia pacing.
[3] Manufacturers often use "S" for single-chamber (A or V).

that atrial contraction occurs during ventricular systole, resulting in increased right atrial and systemic venous pulsations. With sequential pacing of the atrium and ventricle ("physiologic pacing"), blood pressure and cardiac output are maintained. Sequential pacing is, however, contraindicated if atrial flutter or fibrillation is suspected.

The standard demand pacemaker is designated as VVIPO, indicating that with this form of pacemaker (cost about $2500), the rate and output of the pacemaker can be changed noninvasively. More complex dual units with outputs to atrial and ventricular electrodes are capable of operating in several different modes and of transmitting information back to the external programming coil. This may be an intracardiac electrogram or information about the state of the switches in the unit. The ultimate level of sophistication in this system of classification of pacemakers is "DDDMO," which denotes a pacemaker that can be programmed in all the possible modes. Because of its versatility, the use of this pacemaker is rapidly increasing.

These capabilities are not achieved without raising problems. More complex pacemakers are more expensive (about $5000) and require technical expertise in programming. It is possible for a pacemaker to initiate arrhythmias or to be oversensitive and triggered either by the T wave of the ECG or by muscle action potentials from the diaphragm or chest wall muscles. If the sensitivity is set too low, the pacemaker may not fire. The program of each pacemaker must be readily available at follow-up visits and be capable of transmission over the telephone in case of emergency. Different manufacturers use different techniques and detailed information, and records must be available on a 24-hour basis. The design details of the various commercially available pacemakers are beyond the scope and intention of this book.

Pacemakers are also used to treat arrhythmias. Thus, automatic antitachycardia pacemakers (AATOP) can be used to detect supraventricular tachycardia and to initiate atrial pacing either with short bursts of depolarizations at high electrical frequency or at a rate predetermined at electrophysiologic study to interrupt the arrhythmia. Higher levels of energy are needed to treat ventricular tachycardia or fibrillation with an automatic internal defibrillator. Furthermore, at present, a thoracotomy is necessary to apply the electrode patches to the heart. Electrodes will soon be available that can be placed into the heart by a venous approach similar to the method used in placing electrodes for permanent pacemakers. These more complex varieties of pacemaker should not be used unless an electrophysiologic study has been done.

The ability to vary the modes of operation of pacemakers has made it possible to minimize the expenditure of electrical energy and thus prolong the life of the battery. In addition, it has improved the efficiency

of troubleshooting and reduced the number of pacemakers that need to be replaced.

Newer "physiologically sensing pacemakers" can sense temperature change, skeletal muscle activity, change in venous oxygen saturation, or other parameters that change with exercise and can increase the ventricular rate appropriately. Since these pacemakers have the advantage of not depending on consistent atrial depolarization, they can be used in patients with atrial fibrillation.

The increased complexity of pacemakers makes it likely that management of patients with pacemakers will require even more expertise in the future, and skill in the programming of microcomputers will be required of physicians involved in this activity. Thus, the control of pacemakers is coming to be more and more concentrated in specialized units.

Electrodes & Leads

Improvements in the design of electrodes and leads have come close to eliminating lead failure as a problem. Maintenance of a stable position for atrial electrodes has been made easier by use of J-shaped, tined, and "screw-in" electrodes. The new polyurethane lead casings are sufficiently slippery to permit simultaneous manipulation of two leads in the same vein, and reduction in the stimulation thresholds of new atrial electrodes has increased the life of the whole system.

Method of Introduction: Temporary

The transvenous approach is used unless a pacemaker is inserted at open heart surgery. The site of choice is the subclavian vein (Figure 7–4), with the external or internal jugular, femoral, or antecubital veins as alternatives. Pneumothorax, air embolism, hemorrhage, thrombosis, and phlebitis are the principal complications of the procedure. The pacemaker is almost always inserted under fluoroscopic control. The position of the leads is checked by fluoroscopy at the time of insertion, and the leads are sutured to the skin at the entry site. Use of the subclavian route of entry leaves the patient's arms free during temporary pacing. A balloon pacing catheter has been developed recently that can be inserted without fluoroscopy. Its position can be guided by recordings of the intracardiac electrogram and tests of the ability to achieve adequate capture of the ventricular impulse. In extreme emergencies, percutaneous transthoracic insertion may be required.

Permanent Pacemaker

Permanent pacemakers are now frequently placed by cardiologists rather than by surgeons. Since thoracotomy is no longer used, the creation of a subclavicular pocket to hold the pulse generator is a relatively simple procedure, compared to the positioning of the intracardiac leads. A cephalic branch of the

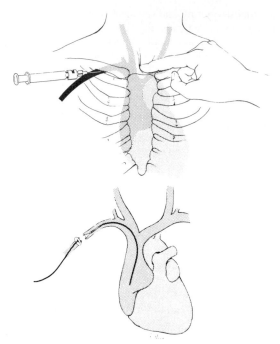

Figure 7–4. Percutaneous subclavian catheterization. (Reproduced, with permission, from Dunphy JE, Way LW [editors]: *Current Surgical Diagnosis & Treatment,* 5th ed. Lange, 1981.)

axillary vein is often used, with the subclavian or external jugular vein as an alternative. A temporary pacemaker is usually left in situ until the permanent device is functioning properly. A temporary pacemaker may sometimes be introduced to provide adequate maintenance of heart rate during insertion of the permanent device. The permanent pacemaker wires may be introduced into the vein after the skin incision has been made. When the wires have been passed into the right atrium, they are positioned under fluoroscopic control. Stylets are now available whose shape can be altered to provide appropriate curves. Placing ventricular leads is generally easier than placing atrial leads.

Checking Operation of the Pacemaker

The threshold of operation of the pacemaker must be checked by determining the minimal voltage needed to capture the rhythm. The voltage is then turned up to determine whether the diaphragm or chest wall muscles contract with each stimulus. Unipolar devices are more likely to respond to external potentials, and changing to a bipolar mode of operation may be helpful. The operation of other aspects of the pacemaker's function (eg, sensing the intracardiac electrogram) is tested and optimized. The patient's ECG is continuously monitored for the first 2 postoperative days, and a follow-up schedule, which must

be strictly adhered to, is started. An overpenetrated posteroanterior and lateral chest x-ray should always be taken before discharge. Comparison with subsequent x-rays will be important in determining whether the position of the electrodes has changed. The threshold for pacing often rises in the first few weeks after operation, and the output may well have to be adjusted at this time. A temporary pacemaker is removed when the permanent unit is working satisfactorily. Removal is always done under fluoroscopic control.

Modern pacemaking systems provide for two-way telemetry between the pacemaker and the programming system. Thus, it is possible to interrogate the implanted instrument and obtain a printout of the programmed settings (eg, set rate, refractory period, stimulus characteristics, and sensitivity). In addition, the instrument can measure and report the actual rate, amplitude, current, and energy of the stimulus and the impedance of the lead or battery. Battery impedance gives an indication of the reserve capacity of the battery. Availability of such information has greatly improved the evaluation and optimization of pacemaker function.

Indications for Pacemaker Insertion

Details of the indications for the use of pacemakers are given in chapters dealing with different diseases (Chapters 8, 14, and 15). Complete heart block with episodes of syncope is the longest-established indication, but many pacemakers are now inserted for control of bradycardia and prevention or control of arrhythmia. The principal advantage of the newer pacemakers is their ability to provide sequential atrioventricular ("physiologic") pacing. The hemodynamic benefits of this form of pacing have been shown to be significant, but the clinical benefits and the effect on prognosis are not clear. It is certainly useful in avoiding the "pacemaker syndrome" seen in some patients with VVI pacemakers, and it is capable of tracking the atrial rate so that greater increases in cardiac output can be achieved during exercise.

It has been suggested that some physicians may have been overenthusiastic in their use of pacemakers in recent years. There is still some difference of opinion about the indications for pacemaker insertion, and assessment of the benefit is mainly clinical. The huge increase in the use of this expensive form of therapy, which is usually employed in older patients, has raised problems related to the cost of health care.

Complications of Pacemakers

Migration of the pacing electrodes, with erratic pacing or sensing, is a common problem. The electrode may work its way through the myocardium into the pericardial space. This may cause chest pain, pericardial effusion, or stimulation of the diaphragm. Displacement or fibrosis around the electrode tip may necessitate an increase in the stimulating voltage or may decrease the voltage of the electrogram to a level that interferes with proper sensing. Temporary pacemakers and unipolar pacemakers are more likely to be affected by external radio-frequency emissions—eg, electric shavers, electrocautery, or magnetic resonance scanners—and some of the more modern devices are sensitive to levels of ionizing radiation used in treatment.

Surgical complications such as hemorrhage, venous thrombosis, and sepsis may occur after permanent pacemaker insertion. Problems can occur with the wires attaching the signal generator to the leads, and displacement of the intracardiac electrodes is commonest in the first 2 months after operation. Battery depletion and ultimately failure are inevitable complications that require operation for their correction.

Regular follow-up with clinic visits is often supplemented by checks on pacemaker function over telephone lines. It is important to try to prevent or alleviate the patient's natural worry over dependence on an electronic instrument.

INTRA-AORTIC BALLOON PUMPING (Counterpulsation)

This specialized circulatory support technique is used only in intensive care areas. The principle is to reduce the afterload and increase coronary perfusion by lowering the systolic and raising the diastolic pressure. A plastic balloon is placed in the thoracic aorta and alternately inflated and deflated in time with the heartbeat. Inflation takes place in diastole and deflation during systole. Improvements in design have made it possible to introduce a catheter, around which the deflated balloon is furled, percutaneously via a No. 12F sheath in the femoral artery. This technique is preferable to insertion through an arteriotomy.

This procedure is effective as a short-term measure but is not widely used outside specialized centers. Its medical use has been confined mainly to patients with cardiogenic shock following myocardial infarction and in patients with unstable angina have been treated by counterpulsation before coronary arteriography. Balloon counterpulsation has also been used preoperatively in patients going to surgery with high-risk coronary artery disease and poor left ventricular function. It has also been used in patients with acute mitral regurgitation and rupture of the ventricular septum with myocardial infarction or trauma.

It has been used in conjunction with cardiac surgery, both for the temporary support of patients with cardiogenic shock in the immediate preoperative period and for patients in the postoperative period who cannot be weaned from cardiopulmonary bypass equipment following open heart surgery. The length of time for which intra-aortic balloon pumping can be safely maintained is measured in hours rather than days. Complications include dissection of the aortoiliac arteries, ischemic changes in the legs, and migration of the balloon up the aorta. Timing of the counterpulsation may cause problems in patients with atrial fibrillation or frequent premature beats.

REFERENCES

Bernstein AD et al: The NASPE/BPEG generic pacemaker code for antibradyarrhythmia and adaptive-rate pacing and antitachyarrhythmia devices. PACE 1987;10:794.

Bregman D et al: Percutaneous intraaortic balloon insertion. Am J Cardiol 1980;48:261.

Brown CG, Werman HA: Adrenergic agents during cardiopulmonary resuscitation. Resuscitation 1990; 19:1.

Brundage BH et al: The role of balloon pumping in postinfarction angina: A different perspective. Circulation 1980;62(Suppl 2):119.

Cobb LA et al: Report of the American Heart Association Task Force on the Future of Cardiopulmonary Resuscitation. Circulation 1992;85:2346.

Dreifus LS et al: Guidelines for implantation of cardiac pacemakers and antiarrhythmic devices. J Am Coll Cardiol 1991;18:1.

Erbel R: Pacemaker syndrome. Am J Cardiol 1979;44: 771.

Furman S: The inflatable cardioverter defibrillator. PACE 1991;14:249.

Furman S, Gross J: Dual-chamber pacing and pacemakers. Curr Probl Cardiol 1990;15:123.

Emergency Cardiac Care Committee and Subcommittees, American Heart Association: Guidelines for cardiopulmonary resuscitation and emergency cardiac care. JAMA 1992;268:2171

Hargarten KM et al: Prehospital experience with defibrillation of coarse ventricular fibrillation: A ten-year review. Ann Emerg Med 190;19:157.

Hayes DL: The next 5 years in cardiac pacemakers: A preview. Mayo Clin Proc 1992;67:379.

Heimlich HJ: A life-saving maneuver to prevent food-choking. JAMA 1975;234:398.

Iseri LT et al: Fist pacing: A forgotten procedure in bradyasystolic cardiac arrest. Am Heart J 1987;113: 1545.

Isner JM et al: Complications of the intraaortic balloon counterpulsation device: Clinical and morphologic observations in 45 necropsy patients. Am J Cardiol 1980;45:260.

Mann DL et al: Absence of cardioversion-induced ventricular arrhythmias in patients with therapeutic digoxin levels. J Am Coll Cardiol 1985;5:882.

Manning JE et al: Closed-chest cardiopulmonary resuscitation: Physiology and hemodynamics. Top Emerg Med 1989;11:1.

Mirowski M et al: Implanted automatic defibrillator to convert malignant arrhythmias. N Engl J Med 1980;303:322.

Paradis NA et al: Simultaneous aortic, jugular bulb, and right atrial pressures during cardiopulmonary resuscitation in humans: Insights into mechanisms. Circulation 1989;80:361.

Parsonnet V et al: Optimal resources for implantable cardiac pacemakers. Circulation 1983;68:227A.

Rosenthal ME, Josephson ME: Current status of antitachycardia devices. Circulation 1990;82:1889.

Rudikoff MT et al: Mechanisms of blood flow during cardiopulmonary resuscitation. Circulation 1980;61:345.

Safar P, Bircher N: Cardiopulmonary Cerebral Resuscitation, 3rd ed. Saunders, 1987.

Weaver WD et al: Automatic external defibrillators: Importance of field testing to evaluate performance. J Am Coll Cardiol 1987;10:1259.

Zoll PM et al: External noninvasive temporary cardiac pacing: Clinical trials. Circulation. 1985;71:937.

Coronary Heart Disease

8

OVERVIEW OF CORONARY HEART DISEASE

Coronary heart disease is one of the most common fatal diseases in the industrialized countries. In the USA, it is the cause of one-third to one-half of all deaths and 50–75% of all cardiac deaths; approximately 500,000 people a year die from the disease. The disease affects men in the prime of life; the average age at the time of the first myocardial infarction is the mid fifties. Women are spared for about 10 years relative to men.

The importance of coronary heart disease extends beyond the high morbidity and mortality rates. Clinical manifestations are unpredictable or absent; the course is variable; and in one-third to one-half of patients, death is sudden and unexpected ("sword of Damocles"). The recognition of coronary heart disease in any of its clinical forms raises the possibility of sudden death, and even minimal symptoms may portend more serious disease.

In about 99% of cases, coronary artery disease is due to atherosclerotic changes. Other causes include syphilis, various forms of arteritis, coronary embolism, and connective tissue disorders (eg, systemic lupus erythematosus). Myocardial ischemia, the clinically relevant manifestation, is usually due to coronary atherosclerosis, but in some instances coronary artery spasm alone may be the cause. More frequently, coronary spasm complicates coronary atherosclerosis. Other causes of myocardial ischemia are unusual conditions such as coronary artery anomalies and coronary arteriovenous fistulas. Relative myocardial ischemia can occur in the absence of coronary artery disease when the demand for myocardial oxygen exceeds the ability of the normal coronary arterial tree to meet the demand. This occurs in such diseases as aortic stenosis and hypertrophic cardiomyopathy. The discussion here will be limited to atherosclerotic coronary heart disease.

GENERAL CLASSIFICATION OF CORONARY HEART DISEASE

The classification of coronary heart disease by type and degree is arbitrary and unsatisfactory, because the clinical manifestations merge into one another and represent a diverse spectrum of progressive ischemia, necrosis, spasm, fibrosis, and left ventricular dysfunction. Any of the manifestations may be the first one to appear, and the patient may present with one, develop another, and then stabilize at any manifestation. Figure 8–1 illustrates the presenting clinical manifestations in the Framingham study. The disease can have acute and chronic phases, and the patient may be critically ill during one phase and capable of full activity a few months later with or without another manifestation. The correlation between symptoms, clinical manifestations, and pathologic findings is so imprecise that one cannot be predicted on the basis of the other. The clinical expression of the various phases of coronary heart disease is not self-limited or specific. In coronary heart disease, therefore, the patient may present with—or may develop—any of the following:

(1) Asymptomatic coronary heart disease, manifested by induced myocardial ischemia.
(2) Sudden death.
(3) Stable angina pectoris; variant (Prinzmetal's) angina; coronary spasm; "silent ischemia."
(4) Unstable angina pectoris.
(5) Acute myocardial infarction.
(6) Cardiac failure.
(7) Cardiac arrhythmias or atrioventricular conduction defects.

We now believe that the transition from stable angina pectoris to an unstable phase probably represents a change in the surface of the atherosclerotic plaque—often a fracturing of the fibrous cap—with subsequent platelet aggregation, fibrin deposition, and thrombus formation; or a sudden increase in smooth muscle contraction, resulting in spasm of the coronary artery. These changes all result in abrupt critical narrowing of the coronary lumen and marked obstruction to flow, precipitating the acute clinical picture.

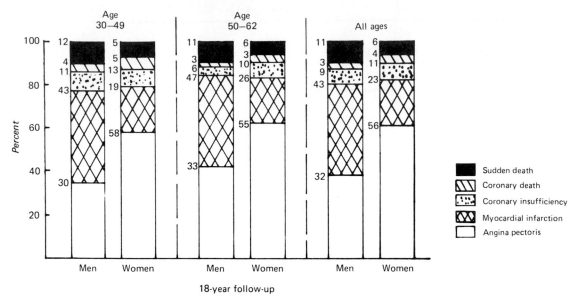

Figure 8–1. Presenting clinical manifestations of coronary heart disease: Framingham study, men and women aged 30–62 years at entry. (Reproduced, with permission, from Kannel WB: Some lessons in cardiovascular epidemiology from Framingham. Am J Cardiol 1976;37:269.)

PATHOGENESIS OF ATHEROSCLEROTIC CORONARY HEART DISEASE

The clinical entity of coronary heart disease (ischemic heart disease) must be differentiated from its underlying pathologic process, coronary atherosclerosis.

The clinical manifestations have become more common, but the pathologic process has not changed. Atherosclerosis is an age-related degenerative process, occurring with increasing frequency with advancing age. It is not inevitable, because some octogenarians have minimal or no evidence of coronary atherosclerosis at postmortem examination, but the reason for its absence in these people is unknown.

Atherosclerosis may begin early in life. During the Korean War, evidence of atherosclerosis was found in about three-fourths of young soldiers killed in battle, and about one-fourth had stenosis of at least 50% of one coronary artery.

Lesion of Atherosclerosis

Atherosclerosis occurs in the muscular and elastic arteries, including the aorta and the coronary, femoral, iliac, internal carotid, and cerebral arteries. The typical lesion is the fibrous plaque, which grossly is dull white and slightly elevated and impinges on the arterial lumen but, when uncomplicated, rarely occludes it. Histologically, it is characterized by a protrusion of smooth muscle cells containing lipids surrounded by a matrix of connective tissue cells,

collagen, elastic fibers, and mucopolysaccharides. As the fibrous plaque enlarges, it may become calcified, may undergo necrosis, may bleed internally, and may fissure and develop a superimposed mural thrombus—and in these ways may ultimately partially or completely occlude the artery. Hemorrhage into old atherosclerotic plaques in the coronary arteries may occur. The lesions are focal, tend to occur at points where the arteries branch, and do not impair flow through the artery until stenosis exceeds 70% of the lumen of the artery.

The structure of a normal muscular artery is illustrated in Figure 8–2A.

Pathogenesis of Atherosclerosis

The most accepted theory of the pathogenesis of atherosclerosis is that intimal injury caused by elevated pressure, deposition of lipid, and infiltration of hypertrophied smooth muscle cells from the media leads to obstruction of the coronary artery, fibrosis, lipid deposition, and atheroma formation, which may then undergo calcification, hemorrhage, and thrombosis (Ross, 1976). Figures 8–2B and 8–2C illustrate the effect of endothelial injury and the subsequent deposition of platelet aggregates (microthrombi) and infiltration of smooth muscle cells into the damaged intima from the media. The lipid particles that accumulate in the fibrous plaque arise from the plasma lipid flowing through the artery, as shown by the similarity of the lipid composition of the plasma and of the atherosclerotic plaque.

Arterial endothelial cells have been cultured in the

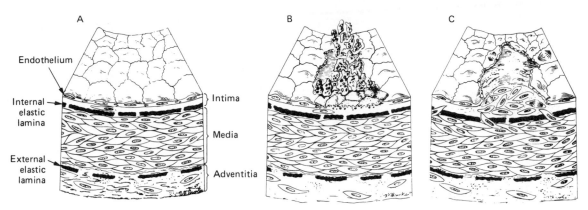

Figure 8–2. Mechanisms of production of atheroma. **A:** Structure of normal muscular artery. The adventitia, or outermost layer of the artery, consists principally of recognizable fibroblasts intermixed with smooth muscle cells loosely arranged between bundles of collagen and surrounded by proteoglycans. It is usually separated from the media by a discontinuous sheet of elastic tissue, the external elastic lamina. **B:** Platelet aggregates, or microthrombi, which may form as a result of adherence of the platelets to the exposed subendothelial connective tissue. Platelets that adhere to the connective tissue release granules whose constituents may gain entry into the arterial wall. Platelet factors thus interact with plasma constituents in the artery wall and may stimulate events shown in the next illustration. **C:** Smooth muscle cells migrating from the media into the intima through fenestrae in the internal elastic lamina and actively multiplying within the intima. Endothelial cells regenerate in an attempt to re-cover the exposed intima, which thickens rapidly owing to smooth muscle proliferation and formation of new connective tissue. (Reproduced, with permission, from Ross R, Glomset JA: The pathogenesis of atherosclerosis. [Part 1.] N Engl J Med 1976;295:369.)

laboratory, allowing direct study of the role of injury, risk factors, and low-density lipoprotein receptor defects in endothelial damage.

Coronary artery embolism is the cause of 10% of myocardial infarctions. (See also Chapter 20.) Mural thrombi occur in the left atrium or left ventricle in patients with valvular (usually mitral) heart disease, previous myocardial infarction, cardiomyopathy, and chronic atrial fibrillation due to any cause. Bits of the thrombi break off and occlude any of the branches of the left coronary artery, usually the more distal ones.

Diagnosis of Stenosis by Coronary Arteriography

Coronary arteriography, which is used to delineate the luminal anatomy of the coronary arteries, often underestimates the extent of coronary stenosis shown at autopsy. There is usually good agreement between the radiologic interpretation of the coronary arteriogram and the findings of the pathologist if the stenosis exceeds 85%; if the stenosis is less than 85%, or if the lesions are peripheral, there is great disagreement about the degree of stenosis. Furthermore, the lesions may be obscured in one radiologic plane, and multiple views in different projections are required to avoid missing or underestimating the lesions. Proximal lesions are more prevalent and more severe than distal ones—a fact of considerable operative significance. Not only do proximal lesions more adversely affect blood flow to the myocardium, but the beneficial ef-

fect of bypassing a proximal stenosis is correspondingly greater. Collateral vessels between a relatively normal coronary artery and a companion coronary artery distal to a stenosis are found in practically all cases of severe stenoses—compensating, in part, for the decreased flow through the stenotic channel.

Risk Factors in the Development of Atherosclerosis

The major risk factors are age, a family history of atherosclerosis, hyperlipidemia, male gender, hypertension, diabetes, and cigarette smoking. Less important factors are the use of oral contraceptives and the imbalance between the vasodilating and vasoconstrictive prostaglandin products prostacyclin and thromboxane. Controversial factors are physical inactivity, personality and sociocultural factors, and prostacyclin deficiency. Combinations of risk factors greatly enhance the probability of a cardiovascular event.

The mechanisms by which these risk factors operate to enhance the likelihood of atherosclerosis are not precisely known. A comprehensive analysis of risk factors and the response to interventions has been published by Stamler (1984).

A. Hyperlipidemia: Hyperlipidemia is thought to foster atherogenesis by increasing the deposition of lipid in the intima because of its increased concentration in plasma. The importance of lipid disorders is strikingly emphasized by the course of coronary disease in hypercholesterolemia. By age 60, myocardial infarction has been shown to occur in 85% of hyper-

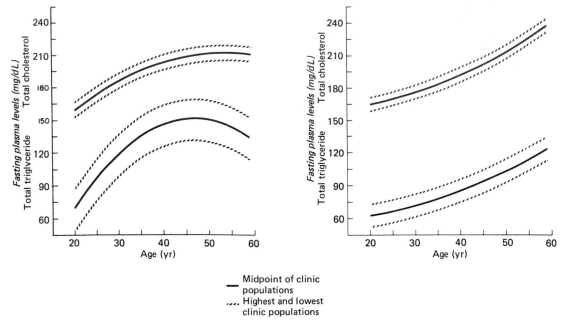

Figure 8–3. Regression estimates of mean plasma lipid values by age and clinic. **Left:** White males, aged 20–59 years. **Right:** White females not taking sex hormones, aged 20–59 years. (Reproduced, with permission of the American Heart Association, Inc., from Heiss G et al: Lipoprotein-cholesterol distributions in selected North American populations: The Lipid Research Clinics Program Prevalence Study. Circulation 1980;61:302.)

cholesterolemic subjects in contrast to 20% of the population at large (Slack, 1969).

Patients with type II hypercholesterolemia on a low-fat, low-cholesterol diet given cholestyramine had a reduction of plasma cholesterol and decrease in the incidence of coronary heart disease, nonfatal myocardial infarction, progression of coronary disease by angiography, and death (Brensike, 1984; Lipid Research Clinics Program, 1984; Levy, 1984). Patients taking gemfibrozil had a considerable decrease in triglycerides and a modest increase in HDL cholesterol (Manninen, 1988). In a meta-analysis of 22 randomized clinical trials of cholesterol-lowering regimens to prevent coronary heart disease, there was a significant reduction in the risk of nonfatal myocardial infarction and cardiac deaths in the treated group as compared with the control group. These involved 40,000 persons, and the reduction in incidence of coronary disease was related to both the degree and the duration of cholesterol reduction. In trials with less than 4 years of treatment, a 10% reduction in cholesterol led to a 10% reduction in the incidence of coronary artery disease. In trials of longer duration, a similar reduction in cholesterol led to an approximately 20% reduction in the incidence of coronary disease. These data, together with the latest controlled trials of lipid-lowering drugs showing a halt in the progression and even regression of coronary artery obstruction discussed below, strongly support the use of diet and cholesterol-lowering drugs in the treat-

ment of hypercholesterolemia. However, there are several subgroups of HDL, not all of which may be equally important in pathogenesis. Data on the fasting plasma triglyceride and total cholesterol levels in both men and women in a large series of subjects are presented in Figure 8–3.

The estimated sex- and age-adjusted plasma cholesterol and triglyceride levels in control subjects were found by Goldstein (1973) to be, respectively, 270 and 147 mg/dL at the 90th percentile; 285 and 165 mg/dL at the 95th percentile; and 314 and 200 mg/dL at the 99th percentile. More recent data indicate that a plasma cholesterol level of 240 mg/dL (6.21 mmol/L) falls at the 75th percentile in the population of middle-aged adults. This is considered a moderate risk; a high risk is 265 mg/dL (6.85 mmol/L) (Bernstein, 1985). Cholesterol and triglyceride values in survivors of myocardial infarction are often in the top 20% of the levels found in control subjects.

B. High-Density Lipoproteins (HDL): A decrease in HDL may be more important than an increase in low-density lipoprotein (LDL) or total cholesterol in the pathogenesis of atherosclerosis (Figure 8–4). The ratio of HDL cholesterol to total cholesterol (< 0.15) may be a better predictor of coronary disease than either level alone, or levels of apoprotein (Apo) A, B, or E (Schmidt, 1985). HDL increases the absorption of cholesterol from peripheral tissues, including the arterial wall ("scavenger" effect), and

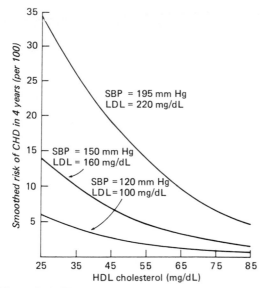

Figure 8–4. Risk of coronary heart disease according to levels of high-density lipoprotein cholesterol in 55-year-old men. Framingham study 24-year follow-up. (CHD, coronary heart disease; SBP, systolic blood pressure; LDL, low-density lipoprotein; HDL, high-density lipoprotein.) (Reproduced, with permission, from Kannel WB, Castelli WP, Gordon T: Cholesterol in the prediction of atherosclerotic disease. Ann Intern Med 1979;90:85.)

transports it to the liver, where metabolic breakdown and excretion occur. The cholesterol in atheroma is derived from that in the plasma, whereas that in the arterial wall is normally synthesized in situ. Decreased HDL may impair the clearance of cholesterol from the arterial wall, leading to an imbalance between filtration of cholesterol from plasma and its clearance, thereby causing increased deposition of cholesterol.

The mechanism of familial hypercholesterolemia is thought to be a primary genetic defect in the cell membrane surface receptors that bind LDL, the major cholesterol-containing lipoprotein in plasma. In the homozygous form, functional LDL receptors are greatly decreased or completely absent in cultured fibroblasts, amniotic fluid cells, smooth muscle cells, or lymphocytes; in the heterozygous form, more LDL receptors are present, but there are fewer than normally is the case. When this occurs, lipoprotein cannot bind to receptors and enter cells to be used for intracellular metabolism and membrane synthesis. Premature atherosclerosis may occur (most markedly in the homozygous form), and there may be other signs such as tendon and plantar xanthomatosis. The system that regulates the rate of cellular uptake of LDL is complex because of the number of alternative pathways for dealing with excessive serum cholesterol when there are few or no LDL receptors.

The pathogenetic role of Apo B-100 located on the LDL receptor, as well as other species, such as Lp(a) lipoproteins, which contain a protein analogue of plasminogen, is being actively investigated; their genetic features have suggested that they may be independent risk factors.

Several studies have supported this hypothesis. Normalization of the serum cholesterol occurred in a child with homozygous familial hypercholesterolemia, severe coronary disease, and multiple myocardial infarctions following cardiac and liver transplantation (East, 1986). In another report, cultured amniotic fluid cells were studied from a 20-week-old aborted fetus whose brother had died at age 8 years of homozygous hypercholesterolemia. The cells showed an almost complete absence of LDL cell surface receptors. The serum cholesterol of the fetus was nine times the average of control fetuses of the same age (Brown, 1978). More recently, studies of Watanabe-heritable hyperlipidemic rabbits have also supported this theory (Goldstein, 1983). This strain of rabbits has a genetic defect and disease similar to those found in humans. Striking hypercholesterolemia and atherosclerosis develop even when the rabbits are fed a cholesterol-free diet.

The evidence of the importance of hypercholesterolemia as a risk factor is sufficiently convincing that the American Heart Association has published dietary guidelines (AHA Nutrition Committee, 1988) to prevent cardiovascular disease in healthy adults. For those with serum cholesterol above 240 mg/dL (6.21 mmol/L) total fat intake should be less than 30% of calories—reduced to obtain ideal weight for the individual—with approximately equal amounts of saturated and unsaturated fat; cholesterol intake should not exceed 300 mg/d; of total calories, carbohydrate intake (especially complex varieties) should be about 50% and protein intake about 15–20%. Sodium and alcohol intake should be moderate. When the patient has coronary disease or two or more risk factors—including male sex, cigarette smoking, hypertension, a family history of premature coronary disease, HDL cholesterol less than 35 mg/dL, diabetes mellitus, a history of cerebrovascular or peripheral arterial disease, or severe obesity ($\geq$ 30% overweight)—the goal should be to reduce total cholesterol to under 200 mg/dL and LDL cholesterol to under 130 mg/dL (Working Group on Management of Patients With Hypertension and High Blood Cholesterol, 1991).

C. Hypertension: Hypertension increases the filtration of lipid from plasma to the intimal cells by virtue of increased arterial pressure, especially in the presence of elevated plasma lipids. Hypertension as well as hyperlipidemia may injure the intima, leading to platelet aggregation and proliferation of smooth muscle cells in the media. Increased susceptibility to injury from shear forces, torsion, and lateral wall pressure changes may also be important. Hypertension is a common risk factor in the pathogenesis of atherosclerosis; atherosclerotic complications constitute the most common causes of death in hypertensive patients.

The average degree of coronary artery sclerosis in a large group of routine autopsies was grade 9 (on a scale of 1–10) in hypertensives in the 40- to 49-year age group, whereas this degree of coronary sclerosis was not reached in nonhypertensives until age 60–70 years (Lober, 1953). Purely hypertensive complications (cardiac failure, accelerated or malignant hypertension, hemorrhagic stroke, and renal failure) have been sharply reduced by present-day antihypertensive treatment. The evidence for reduction of atherosclerotic complications (myocardial infarction or cerebral infarction) is less convincing. In the Hypertension Detection and Follow-Up Program Study, patients who received stepped-care treatment had significantly decreased mortality rates following acute myocardial infarction as compared with patients who received referred care. In other clinical trials, patients with diastolic pressures of 90–104 mm Hg and no major target organ damage or electrocardiographic abnormalities at baseline did not have a significantly decreased incidence of coronary disease following antihypertensive treatment. However, in these cases, mortality rates associated with coronary heart disease were 40% lower in the group receiving stepped care (Stamler, 1984).

D. Diabetes: The asymptomatic hyperglycemia of adults with diabetes mellitus may be a risk factor independent of and additive to the effect of blood pressure and serum lipids. Diabetes affects the capillary basement membrane (microangiopathy) of all tissues. It produces abnormalities in the myocardium, in small coronary vessels, and in the major arteries. Pathologically, atherosclerosis occurs more frequently and at an earlier age in diabetic patients (Waller, 1980). The adverse effect of diabetes on cardiovascular disease cannot be explained by known risk factors. The roles of serum glucose and serum insulin are unknown, and the conclusions are conflicting. Even when coronary disease is excluded, rates of cardiac failure in diabetes are increased; this may be due to diabetic cardiomyopathy unrelated to small-vessel disease causing diastolic left ventricular dysfunction and decreased ventricular compliance. It is not rare to see angina and myocardial infarction in young people with type I (insulin-dependent) diabetes mellitus. In subjects with impaired glucose tolerance, the mortality rate from coronary heart disease was approximately doubled as compared with that in patients with normal glucose tolerance after a 7 1/2-year period of observation (Fuller, 1980). Control of hyperglycemia in type II (non-insulin-dependent) diabetes mellitus has not been shown to influence subsequent coronary disease. Rigid control of type I diabetes has been claimed by some to be preventive, though this opinion has been challenged.

E. Family History: A positive family history may reflect (1) genetic predisposition to the development of hypertension, hyperlipidemia, or diabetes; or (2) environmental influences such as diet, stress, and life-style; or (3) protective genetic influences such as HDL cholesterol levels. After all known risk factors for coronary disease are eliminated, there is still a twofold risk of myocardial infarction among first-degree relatives of survivors of myocardial infarction as compared with first-degree relatives of those who have not had myocardial infarction (ten Kate, 1982). Sons of fathers with coronary disease were found both to develop the disease earlier and to die at an earlier age than their fathers (Hamby, 1981).

For men under age 55, a coronary death in a first-degree male relative under age 55 increases the risk of coronary death to three times that of the general population. For women under age 65, a coronary death in a first-degree male relative under age 55 increases the risk of coronary death to five times that of the general population (Slack, 1968). The risk of coronary death in these cases is greater than it is in middle-aged men with elevated serum cholesterol or blood pressure. Men with a risk of dominantly inherited familial hypercholesterolemia have a 15-fold increase in risk, and 50% die of coronary heart disease before age 60 (Slack, 1969). The British Regional Heart Study, which in the past has minimized the effect of unknown versus known risk factors, has shown that most of the risk associated with parental history is unexplained by the ordinary risk factors, suggesting an independent genetic risk (Phillips, 1988).

F. Cigarette Smoking: The principal importance of cigarette smoking is that it precipitates arrhythmias and is a factor in sudden death in patients with coronary artery disease. In addition, *smoking is a definite risk factor in promoting atherosclerosis*. Cigarette smoking is strongly associated with reduced serum HDL cholesterol, and this may be one of the mechanisms for its adverse effect. Cigarette smoking is the most prominent risk factor for myocardial infarction in women under age 50 years. The incidence of sudden death is significantly greater in smokers (Figure 8–5). The risk of cigarette smoking is independent of other major risk factors but aggravates them. The risk is reduced when smoking is stopped. The mechanism of atherogenesis due to cigarette smoking is not clear. Chewing tobacco is also thought to be a risk factor.

The frequency of cigarette smoking is high in patients with atherosclerosis; at the outset of the Framingham study, in 1949, 60% of the men and 40% of the women were smokers. Cigar and pipe smoking are less important as risk factors.

G. Prostaglandins: The pathway of prostaglandin synthesis from arachidonic acid is illustrated in Figure 8–6. Blood platelets synthesize thromboxane (TXA_2), which both aggregates platelets and constricts arteries. Endothelial cells synthesize prostacyclin (PGI_2), which inhibits platelet aggregation and dilates arteries. Both TXA_2 and PGI_2 are local

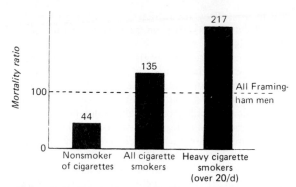

Figure 8–5. Framingham study 12-year follow-up mortality ratios for sudden death in nonsmokers, all smokers, and heavy smokers among men originally aged 30–62. (Modified and reproduced, with permission, from Kannel WB: *Habits and Coronary Heart Disease. The Framingham Heart Study.* Public Health Service Publication No. 1515, National Heart Institute, 1966.)

hormones, which by their balance affect coronary blood flow. It has been speculated that imbalance, especially if TXA_2 is predominant, may foster atherosclerosis (Vane, 1983), and a number of researchers are testing this hypothesis.

H. Estrogens and the Menopause: Women taking estrogens have an average HDL cholesterol ap-

proximately 20% higher than those not taking the compounds.

Coronary disease in young menstruating women is rare—much rarer than in men of the same age—and it usually occurs in association with one of the other major risk factors noted above. However, there is an unexplained substantial increase in cardiovascular disease with menopause—especially surgically induced menopause—most evident in the age group from 40 to 44 years. The mechanisms by which the menopause influences coronary disease have not been established.

Premenopausal women with severe hypertension (diastolic pressure > 120 mm Hg) are not protected from coronary disease.

I. Oral Contraceptives: There is increasing evidence that women taking oral contraceptives, especially agents with high estrogen content, have an increased risk of myocardial infarction, particularly if they are cigarette smokers, are older than 35, and have been taking the drugs for longer than 5 years. The mechanism is unclear. The rate of infarction is increased three- to fourfold in women under age 50, as compared with women who have never used the agents (Slone, 1981). It remains to be determined whether the agents with lower estrogen content will lessen or nullify the increased risk.

J. Physical Inactivity: A sedentary habit of life may produce its effects through associated obesity,

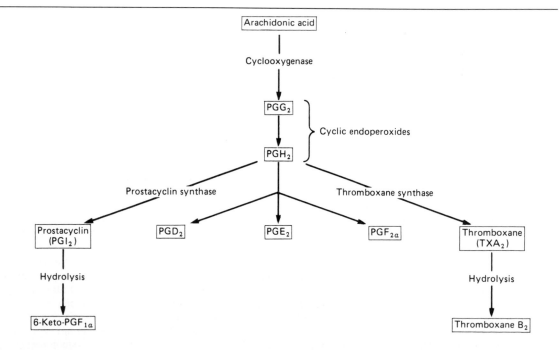

Figure 8–6. Pathway of prostaglandin biosynthesis. (Redrawn, modified, and reproduced, with permission, from Kuo PT: Lipoproteins, platelets, and prostaglandins in atherosclerosis. Am Heart J 1981;102:949.)

which may predispose to diabetes and possibly hypertension. Obesity per se is a marginal risk factor. Preliminary data suggest that because inactive people have fewer collateral coronary vessels, physical inactivity may merely decrease the chance for survival when myocardial infarction occurs; it does not influence the atherosclerotic process itself. The high incidence of myocardial infarction in vigorous northeastern Finns who consume a diet high in saturated fats and cholesterol suggests that exercise affords only minimal protection against coronary disease. Although exercise improves morale and fitness, lessens the occurrence of evidence of left ventricular function, and provides a sense of well-being, cardiovascular morbidity and mortality rates are not convincingly decreased (as independent risk factors) by exercise programs. The National Exercise and Heart Disease Project (Shaw, 1981) found that mortality rates did not differ significantly between men who engaged in high-intensity exercise for approximately 3 years after a myocardial infarction and those who did not. The Ontario Exercise Heart Collaborative Study (Rechnitzer, 1983) found that the recurrence rate of myocardial infarction over a 4-year period did not differ significantly in men who participated in a program of high-intensity exercise compared with those who participated in light exercise. The number of fatal and nonfatal reinfarctions did not differ between the two groups.

In the Framingham Heart Study cohort, overall mortality, cardiovascular disease mortality, and coronary heart disease mortality were all inversely related to the level of physical activity reported. The benefits of physical activity compared with the other risk factors were less impressive, though independent of the other risk factors (Kannel, 1979). Salonen et al (1988) reported that when corrected for other risk factors, much of the effect of leisure-time inactivity was shown to be unrelated to mortality risk. Activity at work still seemed to be protective.

Opinions about the benefits of physical exercise in preventing coronary disease or its complications are conflicting. Confounding factors such as family history, the association of other risk factors, preselection of individuals, the large number of dropouts from the studies, and the difficulty in quantifying the amount of exercise make interpretation difficult. The independent preventive benefits of vigorous exercise programs appear to be slight and not as clear-cut as the primary risk factors of high serum cholesterol, hypertension, positive family history, smoking, or diabetes. In general, physiologic benefits and better fitness may accrue from exercise programs, but lack of exercise is not a proved specific risk factor.

K. Personality, Sociocultural, and Psychosocial Factors: Rosenman (1976) has postulated that personality and behavior characteristics such as pressure of time and work, competitiveness, and aggressiveness (type A) are variables independent of other risk factors. They found that the incidence of coronary disease was lower in type B (more relaxed) individuals.

However, multicenter trials found no relation between type A behavior and subsequent coronary disease in subjects previously free of it (Multiple Risk Factor Intervention Trial Research Group, 1982) or in late cardiac morbidity or mortality rates in survivors of acute myocardial infarction (Case, 1985). These studies throw doubt on the independent specificity of type A characteristics but not necessarily of other personality traits that may be risk factors. Hostility, anger, and depression are possible components of the type A personality that may be important (Ragland, 1988).

L. Endothelial Factors: Endothelium-derived relaxing factor, released from endothelial cells, is undergoing investigation as a possible cause of increased endothelial permeability and endothelial damage, influencing stimulation of smooth muscle cells of arterial walls. In addition, the endothelium is now known to display a large number of synthetic, secretory, and metabolic functions involving a variety of vasoactive substances that influence coronary arterial tone, platelet adhesion, and antithrombotic activity. These substances modulate coronary arterial tone, inhibit platelet adhesion and thrombus formation, and may affect permeability of the intima to circulating substances such as lipoproteins. This developing field of vascular biology may yield a great deal of information about the pathogenesis of atherosclerosis and coronary heart disease (Bassenge, 1988).

Each risk factor discussed above is not only significant in itself but is also additive and perhaps synergistic when combined with one or more other risk factors. Hypertension and atherosclerosis, for example, are independent disease processes, yet hypertension accelerates atherosclerosis. The same is true when cigarette smoking is combined with one of the other risk factors.

Pathogenesis of Coronary Heart Disease

The Framingham study was designed to determine the factors influencing the development of coronary heart disease in 2282 men and 2845 women aged 30–62 in Framingham, Massachusetts, who were found to be clinically free of coronary heart disease when entering the study. Through clinical examinations at 2-year intervals and other methods of follow-up over more than 20 years, the study has traced the natural history of the various manifestations of coronary disease, as well as stroke and peripheral artery disease, and has meticulously related their development to host and environmental factors. The study has provided an elaborate epidemiologic survey of coronary disease and has determined risk factors that increase the likelihood of developing coronary disease. These have been discussed above with respect to atherosclerosis. When atherosclerosis significantly occludes the coronary artery, impairing flow, coronary heart disease ensues.

In patients with unstable angina, intracoronary angioscopy at the time of coronary surgery reveals rupture of the intimal atherosclerotic plaque with hemorrhage and platelet and fibrin aggregation. This partial obstruction causes prolonged myocardial ischemia or early myocardial infarction. In contrast, patients with stable angina rarely have such rupture. The mechanisms for the sudden change in plaque morphology are unknown (Forrester, 1987). Arteries with advanced atherosclerotic plaques show alteration and fragmentation of the elastic fibers of the media as well as softening due to increased growth substances and lipid content. This is particularly true at the margin of the plaque. With narrowing of the lumen, there is increased velocity of flow and increased wall shear stress. This, in combination with fluctuations in blood pressure, vascular tone, and even torque stress due to twisting and bending of the artery as the heart beats, may lead to plaque rupture (Fuster, 1992).

Thrombosis usually superimposed on a stenotic atherosclerotic lesion is the most frequent cause of myocardial infarction. Such lesions were found in more than 80% of patients with acute infarction studied by coronary arteriography in the first few hours (DeWood, 1980). Ruptured plaques with intimal hemorrhage and occlusive thrombosis were identified in 82% of patients with fatal ischemic disease (Falk, 1983).

The exact reasons for the apparently haphazard onset of angina, myocardial infarction, ventricular arrhythmias, or sudden death are often unknown.

A. Pathophysiology of Coronary Blood Flow: Myocardial oxygen extraction is almost complete even when coronary blood flow is normal. There is thus little reserve capacity to increase oxygen delivery. When delivery is insufficient, anaerobic metabolism is initiated with the production of lactate from glycogen. The presence of increased lactate production can be determined by comparing the lactate content in the coronary sinus with that in arterial blood.

Coronary blood flow is increased further by vasoactive substances that, as a result of hypoxia, increase flow by causing coronary vasodilation. Vasoactive substances include potassium, lactate, adenosine, and prostaglandins. When myocardial ischemia occurs from decreased coronary perfusion or increased myocardial oxygen demand, the rate of diastolic relaxation of the ischemic muscle decreases, resulting in stiffening of the left ventricle; decreased systolic contraction; anaerobic metabolism with lactate production; a change in transmembrane potentials, resulting in ST–T wave changes; arrhythmias; and angina pectoris.

Another important factor in regulating coronary blood flow is autoregulation, which relates intra-arterial pressure to vascular tone. For example, in hypertension, blood vessels may stretch, causing contraction of arteriolar muscle. In myocardial ischemia, local vascular pressure levels may fall, causing vasodilation, probably through an endothelial mechanism such as the production of adenosine, endothelium-relaxing factor, or other substances. Brief coronary occlusion results in a fall in intracoronary pressure and induces vasodilation.

Pathologic studies have shown that the subendocardium is more vulnerable to myocardial ischemia or transmural infarction than the subepicardium. During systole, the subendocardial coronary flow is opposed by pressure in the left ventricular cavity, whereas subepicardial flow is not. The extravascular forces acting on the intramural coronary arteries therefore reduce flow to the subendocardium, especially during exercise (Dole, 1987).

Myocardial ischemia, which results when coronary blood flow is inadequate to meet the demands of the muscle at any moment, may be due to decreased oxygen supply (vasoconstriction, spasm, or obstruction) or increased demand. The latter occurs when factors such as heart rate, left ventricular wall stress, inotropic state of the myocardium, or preload cause increased myocardial oxygen consumption. Myocardial ischemia is regional, not global, and results from decreased perfusion in the area of a particular stenosed coronary artery. Myocardial ischemia can be documented by regional myocardial perfusion defects, decreased regional wall motion abnormalities, and ST elevation or depression on the ECG. Coronary spasm due to alpha-adrenergic receptor-mediated coronary constriction has been shown to be responsible for (1) variant (Prinzmetal's) angina; (2) worsening of some cases of stable angina of effort; and (3) infrequently, induction of myocardial infarction, presumably because of platelet adhesion and aggregation resulting from endothelial injury consequent to the spasm (Maseri, 1980).

B. Pathologic Lesions and Serum Lipoprotein Studies: Patients with abnormal serum lipoprotein values who died of coronary heart disease showed at autopsy 75% stenosis of at least one, and often of three, coronary arteries. A similar degree of stenosis is sometimes found in persons who had normal serum lipoproteins. Thus, lipoprotein abnormalities are not essential to the development of atherosclerosis.

Arteriograms of patients studied within 1 year after onset of ischemic symptoms reveal stenosis of one to three coronary arteries. These changes may be seen very soon after onset of symptoms; this suggests that extensive atherosclerosis and even complete occlusion can precede the onset of symptoms.

C. Onset of Myocardial Infarction: Three mechanisms have been postulated to explain the onset of myocardial infarction: coronary thrombosis, subintimal hemorrhage, and coronary artery spasm (see above). Maseri (1983) believes that coronary spasm leads to platelet adhesion and aggregation, which in turn lead to a sequence of events ending in thrombosis that may cause myocardial infarction. (See also Angina Pectoris.)

Current prevailing opinion is that the vast majority of acute myocardial infarctions begin with fissuring of an atherosclerotic plaque, leading to platelet adhesion, platelet aggregation, and activation of thrombus formation. There is a variable contribution of increased local vascular tone, and all of these events lead to sudden, severe obstruction of the coronary arterial lumen and a marked decrease in coronary blood flow to the involved myocardium (Davies, 1985; Fuster, 1985).

D. Ventricular Arrhythmias: Fibrosis and chronic ischemia of subendocardial fibers ("blighted zone") containing Purkinje cells induce variable excitability, automaticity, velocity of conduction, refractory periods, and repolarization in neighboring fibers, leading to electrical instability with ventricular fibrillation and sudden death. Ventricular fibrillation is the chief mechanism of cardiac arrest in apparently healthy individuals and in those with known coronary disease who have been resuscitated after apparent death in cardiac arrest. Sudden death is rarely due to conduction defects or Stokes-Adams attacks in the absence of acute anterior myocardial infarction. Emotional factors, with intense sympathetic discharge from the central nervous system, have been incriminated in some patients who have developed ventricular tachycardia or fibrillation or acute myocardial infarction. Vagal stimulation may decrease the heart rate and lead to an increased incidence of arrhythmia, aggravated by sympathetic stimulation.

E. Unusual Demands and Myocardial Ischemia: Unusual demands (unaccustomed severe exertion, rapid ventricular rates, intense emotion, acute hypoxemia, severe anemia, or blood loss) on a myocardium already compromised by decreased flow from coronary artery stenoses may precipitate local chemical and pathophysiologic events in patients with coronary atherosclerosis and may explain unexpected myocardial infarction.

F. Mural Obstruction of Left Anterior Descending Coronary Artery: Muscular bridges may obstruct the left anterior coronary artery in its intramyocardial portion and may rarely lead to myocardial ischemia and sudden death in the absence of coronary atherosclerosis (Morales, 1980).

Basis for Diagnosis

Coronary heart disease is characterized by a wide variety of clinical manifestations ranging from asymptomatic to stable angina pectoris, silent myocardial ischemia (with or without angina pectoris), coronary artery spasm, unstable angina, acute myocardial infarction, and sudden death. The basic disease is almost always coronary atherosclerosis. Its course is

variable, and symptoms and signs may occur singly or in combination, often with asymptomatic intervals.

The basis for clinical diagnosis is a history of angina pectoris, myocardial infarction, cardiac failure, or arrhythmias. Risk factors must be noted and evaluated. Various exercise and noninvasive tests can be used to evaluate possible abnormalities in coronary circulation and degrees of myocardial ischemia and dysfunction. Ultimately, however, coronary angiograms must be used to outline the coronary arteries. Localized impaired contractility or aneurysmal dilation can be determined by contrast ventricular arteriography, radionuclide angiography, or two-dimensional echocardiography. The evaluation of patients with coronary disease may be complex and is best performed by cooperating specialists in related disciplines.

CLINICAL VARIETIES OF CORONARY HEART DISEASE

LATENT CORONARY HEART DISEASE

Initial Manifestations in Latent Coronary Heart Disease

Sudden death may be the first and only clinical manifestation of coronary heart disease; this means that asymptomatic coronary heart disease must have existed in the time immediately preceding this event.

Middle-aged individuals may present not with angina but with ventricular arrhythmias or atrioventricular or bundle branch conduction defects that may be the first manifestation of coronary heart disease. Asymptomatic atrial fibrillation is rarely such a manifestation, because it is uncommon even in patients with stable angina pectoris. Stokes-Adams attacks in patients with complete atrioventricular block usually occur during the initial phase of acute myocardial infarction or in the months following an acute anterior myocardial infarction, but Stokes-Adams attacks occur infrequently as an isolated manifestation of coronary disease in otherwise asymptomatic patients. Short bursts of ventricular premature beats or nonsustained ventricular tachycardia are a more important manifestation and may be the precursors of ventricular fibrillation and sudden death, especially in the setting of impaired left ventricular function. Ventricular premature beats, however, are so common and variable in the older population at large that it is difficult to classify them as manifestations of asymptomatic coronary disease. Furthermore, various studies have shown that premature beats in the absence of clinical coronary disease do not presage sudden death.

Noninvasive Investigation of Possible Myocardial Ischemia in Asymptomatic Individuals (Silent Ischemia)

Increasingly, efforts are being made by use of noninvasive tests to recognize the presence of ischemic coronary disease in asymptomatic individuals who want to be reassured about the absence of coronary disease. These include persons whose occupations have public safety implications (airline pilots, bus drivers, railroad engineers); executives being considered for promotion or transfer to a new position; persons at high risk of coronary disease by virtue of a history of early coronary disease in first-degree relatives; persons who have multiple risk factors for coronary disease (familial hypercholesterolemia, hypertension, diabetes); and middle-aged persons who simply want the evaluation.

Although ST segment depression in response to exercise cannot be used to make a diagnosis of coronary heart disease, it is useful in identifying a subgroup of asymptomatic subjects among whom the risk of developing a clinical manifestation of coronary heart disease in the future is increased. Gibson (1989) evaluated ten studies in the literature reporting a total of 7692 asymptomatic patients followed for 6.2 years after an exercise test. Clinical development of coronary artery disease occurred in 21.7% of those with ST segment depression and in 4.5% of those without, for a risk ratio of 4.9.

In these studies, the development of angina pectoris was the most frequent clinical manifestation of coronary artery disease. The studies of McHenry (1984), Fleg (1990), and Josephson (1990) all indicate that while an abnormal exercise test is predictive of the future development of angina, it is not significantly associated with an increased risk of sudden death or nonfatal myocardial infarction.

In patients with coronary risk factors, the stress test can predict a subgroup who are at higher risk of death on follow-up. The Multiple Risk Factor Intervention Trial Research Group (1985) evaluated exercise-induced ST segment depression in 12,016 patients with a follow-up of 7 years. The mortality rate in those with ST segment depression was 3.7% compared with 1.5% in those without, for a risk ratio of 2.5. Gordon (1986) reported the Lipid Research Clinic Study, in which 3718 patients were exercised and followed for 8.6 years. On follow-up, the mortality rate with ST segment depression on exercise was 8.6%, and in those without ST segment depression it was 0.9%, for a risk ratio of 9.6.

Controversy exists over the desirability of performing such noninvasive procedures as electrocardiography or radionuclide studies at rest or after exercise, because of the likelihood of both false-positive and false-negative tests. The sensitivity, specificity, and predictive value of such tests (see below and Figure 8–9) depend upon the selection of subjects, the criteria for a positive test, the degree of stenosis of the coronary artery, the presence of noncoronary cardiac disease, and the skill of the cardiologist. The procedure to be followed in the event of a positive test is also controversial. Should one proceed to coronary arteriography if the exercise ECG shows significant ST depression in an asymptomatic middle-aged man? (See Noninvasive Tests.)

Ambulatory electrocardiography and continuous electrocardiography at rest have shown that patients with known coronary heart disease may have "silent ischemia"—prolonged episodes of asymptomatic ST segment depression consistent with ischemia. Most episodes of ischemia have been shown by monitoring to occur without anginal pain (Figure 8–7). Patients with frequent, prolonged episodes of severe silent ischemia may develop myocardial infarction; the associated ventricular arrhythmias may cause sudden death. Silent ischemia is important because the patient is unaware of it and may initiate or continue

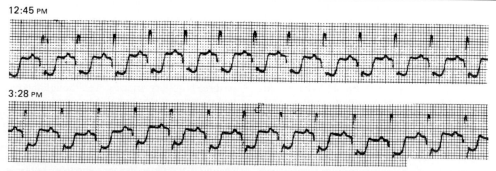

12:45 PM

3:28 PM

Figure 8–7. Holter monitor ECG of a 65-year-old man showing marked ST depression of myocardial ischemia when the patient carried out his ordinary work routine as a salesperson. There were no symptoms during the time of the ischemic changes on the ECGs, but angina pectoris of effort occurred at other times. (Courtesy of W Atchley.)

activities that aggravate it. Most patients with numerous episodes of silent ischemia also have ST segment depression on exercise testing. The 7-year prognosis in coronary patients with silent ischemia is similar to that for patients with chest pain (Weiner, 1987). Patients with documented coronary heart disease with silent ischemia in response to exercise had the same prognosis at 5 years as those with no ST segment depression, whereas those with symptoms and ST segment depression had a much worse 5-year prognosis (Mark, 1989). Treatment with calcium entry blockers or beta-blockers, alone or in combination, decreases the incidence of transient silent myocardial ischemia. Whether this decreases morbidity and mortality is as yet unknown.

SUDDEN DEATH

Sudden death is the first and only clinical manifestation of coronary heart disease in about one-fourth of patients. Most sudden deaths are not totally unexplained or unexpected; often, the patient has had coronary or hypertensive heart disease or has recently sought medical care for symptoms that were disregarded or misinterpreted. One study showed that about a third of the patients had seen a physician within 2 weeks before death complaining of various prodromal symptoms. The recurrence rate of ventricular tachycardia becoming ventricular fibrillation—the mechanism of "sudden death syndrome"—is high: about 30% in the first year and 50% by 3 years (Cobb, 1975; Cobb, 1980).

Survivors of out-of-hospital ventricular fibrillation subsequently studied by cardiac catheterization and coronary arteriography demonstrated a high prevalence of advanced coronary atherosclerosis (in one or more major coronary arteries), and three-fourths had abnormalities of left ventricular wall motion, indicating the likelihood of previous myocardial infarction. Of the patients who were resuscitated but died in subsequent months, at least two-thirds had "recurrent sudden death," indicating that the final event was similar to the initial event, usually ventricular fibrillation.

Electrophysiologic studies in survivors of cardiac arrest have revealed inducible sustained or unsustained ventricular tachycardia in about three-fourths of patients. Treatment of these patients with conventional drugs or newer drugs such as amiodarone decreases the likelihood of recurrence of cardiac arrest, especially if these drugs prevent induction of ventricular tachycardia at electrophysiologic study. The Cardiac Arrhythmia Suppression Trial (CAST) study (1988), which used type Ic antiarrhythmic drugs that were effective in suppressing ventricular ectopy, was stopped prematurely because of a higher death rate in the patients given drugs. There is, therefore, no place for empirical drug therapy in patients with sustained ventricular tachycardia—with the possible exception of amiodarone (Moosvi, 1990) (see Chapter 15).

Electrophysiologic study of survivors of out-of-hospital cardiac arrest revealed that 79% had inducible ventricular arrhythmias, suppressed by drugs or surgery in 72%. The high-risk patients for recurrent cardiac arrest were those with a left ventricular ejection fraction under 30%, persistence of inducible ventricular arrhythmias, and absence of cardiac surgery (Wilber, 1988).

Use of the signal-averaged ECG (SA-ECG), a high-sensitivity ECG analyzing the high-frequency components of the terminal portion of the QRS, is being evaluated as a means of identifying patients among whom electrophysiologic study might induce sustained monomorphic ventricular tachycardia. In those without abnormal late high-frequency potentials (negative SA-ECG), inducibility of sudden arrhythmias is low. This technique has been applied to patients after acute myocardial infarction. Serial SA-ECGs on 220 survivors of acute myocardial infarction showed abnormal late potentials in 23% and no such potentials in 77% (Verzoni, 1989). Spontaneous normalization of the SA-ECG occurred in 70% of those with abnormal SA-ECGs. Only three patients died suddenly, and three had late, sustained ventricular tachycardia. In those with abnormal SA-ECGs, 8% had an arrhythmic event compared with 0.6% of those with negative SA-ECGs. The problem with the SA-ECG after acute myocardial infarction is that a significant number change from normal to abnormal and vice versa. The appropriate time to do the SA-ECG is not clear. The technology is being evaluated (el-Sherif, 1989).

Patients with recurrent ventricular arrhythmias associated with cardiac arrest should undergo two-dimensional echocardiography or left ventricular angiography to identify ventricular aneurysm, which occurs in a substantial percentage of these patients. If an aneurysm is found, aneurysmectomy and endocardial resection should be considered (see Prevention of Sudden Death, below). In patients who are noninducible upon electrophysiologic study, consideration should be given to low-dose amiodarone or implantation of an automatic internal defibrillator (DiMarco, 1990).

One-fourth of deaths due to coronary disease in the USA and UK are investigated by a coroner. Autopsy usually discloses severe atherosclerosis involving two or three coronary arteries even though the patient had had no prior symptoms. Of patients who died within an hour after onset of the acute episode, more than 90% had coronary artery disease. Recent coronary thrombosis, intramural or subintimal hemorrhage, and recent myocardial infarction are also found, suggesting that sudden death is due to arrhythmia, probably ventricular fibrillation. This hypothesis is reinforced by the ECGs obtained by mobile coronary ambulance crews, which demonstrated ventricular fibrillation in most patients who have collapsed and were apparently "dead." If and when these patients are resuscitated and subsequently studied, myocardial infarction can be demonstrated in half of them, but a history of cardiovascular disease can be elicited in about three-fourths of patients. Interviews with relatives of people who died indicate that the most significant relationship between sudden death and other identifiable factors was that with acute psychologic stress (Myers, 1975). The age-adjusted incidence of sudden death increased with increasing blood pressure, serum cholesterol, relative weight, and cigarettes smoked per day at the time of the initial examination in the Framingham study (Kannel, 1982).

Differential Diagnosis

In deaths investigated by the coroner's office, sudden unexpected, unexplained deaths that occur within 1 hour after onset of symptoms are almost always due to coronary heart disease. When death is delayed more than 2 hours, coronary disease is less commonly the cause but is still the cause in at least half of cases. Other causes are overwhelming sepsis; other cardiac disorders such as myocarditis, cardiomyopathy, aortic stenosis or aortic dissection; cerebral hemorrhage; shock due to any cause; or bowel obstruction. The so-called cafe coronary, which is due to tracheal obstruction by food while eating, may be confused with sudden death from coronary disease.

Prevention of Sudden Death

Sudden death can be prevented both by management of cardiac arrest or acute myocardial ischemia and by longer-term approaches designed to prevent cardiac arrest. Since most deaths due to coronary heart disease occur suddenly, usually owing to ventricular fibrillation, successful resuscitation depends upon how quickly trained persons can institute appropriate measures to sustain the patient until defibrillation can be accomplished. There is no doubt that lives have been saved in communities where specially equipped, trained paramedics are available and can reach the patient within 2–3 minutes, recognize arrhythmias, administer atropine or lidocaine, and accomplish defibrillation (Cobb, 1992).

About two-thirds of patients who are resuscitated subsequently testify to having had premonitory symptoms such as chest discomfort, excessive fatigue, or just a sense of "not feeling well" in the preceding 1–2 weeks, and one-fourth of them saw a physician in the preceding 1–2 days, not necessarily for a recognizable cardiac complaint. However, because so many sudden deaths are unwitnessed or occur so soon after the development of acute symptoms that the mobile coronary care team cannot arrive in time, it can be fairly stated that most patients with ventricular fibrillation do not survive—even those resuscitated during the acute phase. Of the 40–60% who were initially resuscitated, only about 30% of 1106 patients

found to be in ventricular fibrillation by the mobile team were eventually discharged from the hospital (Cobb, 1980). The ultimate survival rate is much lower in those found to be without electrical activity on ECG, in those still in ventricular fibrillation when brought to the emergency department, and in those over age 70.

A. Coronary Care Unit: Prompt diagnosis of acute myocardial ischemia, preferably in coronary care units, and immediate recognition and treatment of ventricular arrhythmias, ventricular fibrillation, cardiac failure, and cardiogenic shock may prevent secondary ventricular fibrillation. (See Acute Myocardial Infarction, below, for discussion of the early recognition and treatment of the sequelae of acute myocardial ischemia or infarction—eg, conduction defects, arrhythmias, extension of infarction, ventricular septal defect, papillary muscle dysfunction, subacute rupture with pseudoaneurysm, and left ventricular aneurysm.)

B. Automatic Implantable Defibrillator: (See Chapter 15.) This device monitors cardiac rhythm continuously and is designed to detect ventricular fibrillation or ventricular tachycardia and deliver automatically a discharge of 25 J within 20 seconds. It has now been used successfully in patients who have had a number of cardiac arrests and have not responded to multiple antiarrhythmic drugs. Problems are discussed by Scheinman (1988); modifications are being devised, with a transvenous electrode system being developed as well as more extensive programmable functions such as antitachycardia pacing capability and telemetry (Troup, 1989). Automatic external defibrillators are receiving renewed attention, and further experience is awaited.

C. Cigarette Smoking: The relationship between cigarette smoking and sudden death has been conclusively documented. In cases studied by the coroner's office, for example, sudden deaths from coronary heart disease are two to three times as common in smokers as in nonsmokers, which suggests that cigarette smoking may predispose to ventricular fibrillation in susceptible individuals. Smoking results in an increase in serum catecholamines that may be arrhythmogenic. Although sudden death occurs at an older age in women than in men, it occurs in younger women who are heavy smokers. The electrophysiologic mechanism by which smoking causes ventricular fibrillation in patients with coronary artery disease is not fully understood, but it is probably related to the arrhythmogenic properties of increased sympathetic and catecholamine stimulation.

D. Drug Therapy: Preventive measures may include long-term use of beta-adrenergic-blocking agents, possible long-term use of calcium entry-blocking agents, use of antiplatelet drugs, and vigorous use of antiarrhythmic agents selected by electrophysiologic studies in high-risk patients, especially those with previous episodes of ventricular tachycardia or fibrillation or with known coronary disease and complex ventricular arrhythmias. The results of the CAST study have made empirical treatment of ventricular arrhythmias, even guided by proved suppression on 24-hour electrocardiographic monitoring, contraindicated with the possible exception of amiodarone (CAST, 1989). A sustained effort should also be made to treat risk factors for coronary disease.

E. Physical Activity: The high incidence of both coronary disease and coronary deaths in the lumberjacks of northeastern Finland indicates that strenuous physical activity does not protect against coronary disease. Increased physical activity may lead to increased food intake, and there is some evidence that serum cholesterol is slightly higher in eastern than in western Finland, where the coronary mortality rate in men is half that in eastern Finland.

F. Surgical Measures: Coronary bypass surgery has been shown to decrease the incidence of sudden death in patients with left main coronary stenosis exceeding 70% and probably in patients with three-vessel coronary disease associated with easily induced ischemia and only moderately impaired left ventricular function.

Emergency Measures

A. Resuscitation: (See also Chapter 7.) Emergency rooms should be equipped for immediate monitoring and resuscitation. The value of resuscitation efforts on behalf of patients with ventricular fibrillation has been demonstrated in a number of community studies in which the 1-year survival rate of those who were resuscitated was about 70%. Resuscitated patients with primary ventricular fibrillation are often able to return to work with adequate left ventricular function. However, the likelihood of recurrence of ventricular fibrillation increases within the next year, and the long-term prognosis is guarded unless effective antiarrhythmic agents or other treatment methods such as automatic internal defibrillators are used and attention is paid to social, psychologic, and environmental factors in order to reduce adrenergic impulses operating through the central nervous system that may produce coronary vasoconstriction.

B. Patient Education: The high mortality rate of ventricular fibrillation in acute myocardial infarction and the high incidence of sudden death within 1–3 hours after the acute ischemic episode have highlighted the need for shortening the interval between onset of symptoms and admission to a coronary care unit. There should be no delay in getting the patient to the hospital, and this means within 1 hour at most after onset of symptoms. The best advice is to get to the hospital and *then* call the personal physician.

In spite of public education efforts, even patients with previous coronary heart disease and those who have been told to seek immediate care should new symptoms or a change of symptoms appear sometimes delay seeking medical care, perhaps because patients fail to realize the significance of the symptoms or try to combat the fear of death with the psychologic mechanism of denial.

Although excessive physical activity or intense emotion may be responsible in some instances, especially when death is instantaneous (within seconds), most sudden deaths occur during the patient's usual activities and not as a result of some determinable unusual event.

Delays in treatment in the emergency room must be minimized. Patients who are not accustomed to strenuous physical exertion should be warned of its risks, especially in a setting of emotional stress or on unusually cold and windy or hot and humid days. Shoveling snow after dinner and pushing stalled automobiles in cold weather are particularly dangerous activities. Hot, humid weather increases the blood flow to the skin and increases the work of the heart.

C. Reversibility of Sudden Death: Sudden death due to primary ventricular fibrillation is reversible in many cases. Many survivors have had no episode of acute myocardial infarction after resuscitation, as shown by serial enzyme determinations and electrocardiographic examinations. Most have the same left ventricular function 1 year later as they had before the episode of fibrillation. Furthermore, when cardiac arrest occurs during electrocardiographic monitoring of these patients, the arrhythmia is ventricular fibrillation rather than ventricular standstill.

D. Defibrillation: When ventricular fibrillation occurs in coronary care units, it often is preceded by ventricular tachycardia or multifocal ventricular premature beats. A small electric shock during this period may depolarize the reentry circuit, terminating the ventricular tachycardia. A sharp thump on the chest is not quite as effective but may do the same. Electrophysiologic studies have demonstrated that myocardium which has been damaged by fibrosis or by ischemic episodes has a variable recovery of excitability and duration of refractoriness in neighboring cells; this can lead to multiple reentry circuits, which in turn may initiate ventricular fibrillation. Prompt treatment of ventricular tachycardia in susceptible patients may prevent ventricular fibrillation. Use of the automatic implanted defibrillator is increasing (Scheinman, 1988; Troup, 1990). (See Chapter 15.)

E. Café Coronary: See Cardiopulmonary Resuscitation, p 132.

ANGINA PECTORIS; VARIANT (PRINZMETAL'S) ANGINA (CORONARY SPASM); SYNDROME X

Angina pectoris is usually due to atherosclerotic coronary heart disease, but it can occur as a result of severe aortic stenosis or insufficiency or hypertrophic obstructive cardiomyopathy; syphilitic aortitis; increased metabolic demands (eg, in hyperthyroidism

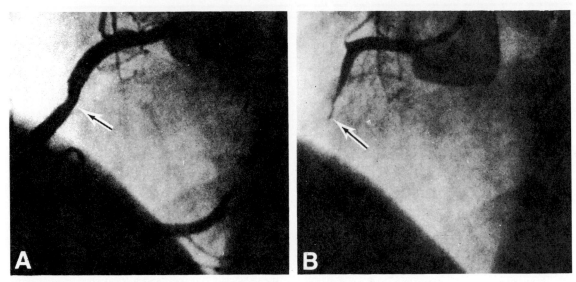

Figure 8–8. Arteriograms of the right coronary artery in left anterior oblique projection demonstrate localized 40% narrowing in the proximal right coronary artery **(arrow)** after nitroglycerin **(A)** and total obstruction in the same area **(arrow)** after ergonovine maleate **(B).** Angina and ST segment elevation in the inferior electrocardiographic leads developed during spasm. (Reproduced, with permission, from Heupler FA Jr, Proudfit WL: Nifedipine therapy for refractory coronary arterial spasm. Am J Cardiol 1979;44:798.)

or after thyroid therapy); marked anemia; paroxysmal tachycardias with rapid ventricular rates; emboli, arteritis, or, as has recently been reemphasized, coronary spasm. The underlying mechanism is a discrepancy between myocardial demands for oxygen and substrate and the amount delivered through the coronary arteries. Four groups of variables determine the production of relative or absolute myocardial ischemia

(1) Limitation of oxygen delivered by the coronary arteries:

(a) Vessel factors: Atherosclerotic narrowing; inadequate collateral circulation; reflex narrowing in response to emotion, cold, upper gastrointestinal disease, or smoking.

(b) Blood factors: Anemia, hypoxemia, polycythemia (increased viscosity).

(c) Circulatory factors: Fall in blood pressure due to arrhythmias, bleeding, and Valsalva's maneuver; decreased filling pressure of or decreased flow to the coronary arteries due to aortic stenosis or insufficiency.

(2) Increased cardiac output:

(a) Physiologic factors: Exertion, excitement, digestive and metabolic processes following a heavy meal.

(b) Pathologic factors (high output states): Anemia, thyrotoxicosis, arteriovenous fistula, pheochromocytoma.

(3) Increased myocardial demands for oxygen: Increased work of the heart, as in aortic stenosis, aortic insufficiency, hypertension; increased oxygen consumption due to thyrotoxicosis or to any state characterized by increased catecholamine secretion (pheochromocytoma, strong emotion, hypoglycemia).

Patients who develop exercise-induced angina during cardiac catheterization show a rise in arterial pressure and left ventricular end-diastolic pressure just before the appearance of angina and the ischemic changes in the ECG. Myocardial oxygen consumption increases similarly. The changes indicate that left ventricular failure or decreased compliance often coincides with or even precedes the appearance of angina.

(4) Decreased myocardial supply secondary to coronary artery spasm (coronary spasm): Coronary artery spasm contributes to manifestations of ischemic cardiac disease (Figure 8–8). **Variant angina,** first described by Prinzmetal (1959) as occurring at rest and sometimes relieved by exercise, has been attributed to spasm of the large coronary arteries, because coronary arteriograms are frequently normal or show minimal coronary artery disease. In patients with variant angina, ergonovine, a powerful coronary vasoconstrictor, can provoke localized coronary artery spasm. The ECG may show elevation and not depression of the ST segment during pain. Variant angina occasionally occurs in patients with minimal coronary stenosis, but it more usually occurs in patients with substantial coronary artery lesions.

Decreased coronary blood flow results from coronary spasm in the absence of increased myocardial demands. Furthermore, it has been shown that angina pectoris and even myocardial infarction may occur in the absence of visible obstructive coronary artery disease (normal coronary arteriogram). It has therefore been postulated that coronary artery spasm alone in the absence of arteriosclerotic coronary artery disease may be sufficient to produce myocardial ischemia and infarction, though most instances of coronary spasm occur in the presence of coronary stenoses.

Transient localized spasm relieved by nitrates has been noted in about 5% of cases during coronary angiography. Spasm may be confined to an area near the tip of the catheter and therefore is presumably due to mechanical irritation, or it may occur some distance away from the catheter, in which case it is thought to indicate neural or neurohumoral activation. It is therefore necessary to exclude spasm before diagnosing organic stenosis of a coronary artery during coronary arteriography, and it is routine to obtain the arteriogram in multiple views and to give sublingual nitroglycerin or isosorbide dinitrate in an attempt to reverse possible catheter-induced spasm.

Myocardial infarction has been seen in the absence of either obstructive coronary artery disease, coronary spasm, or diseases such as aortic stenosis that are associated with an increased myocardial oxygen demand. In these cases, either a hidden, missed lesion on angiography or coronary embolism with subsequent fibrinolysis has been invoked.

Angina pectoris in patients with normal coronary arteriograms—so-called syndrome X—has also been described. In these patients, abnormal ST segment depression on exercise testing and even myocardial lactate production has indicated that this discomfort is probably angina due to myocardial ischemia. The present explanation is that these patients have an abnormal coronary vascular reserve. There is an abnormal increase in coronary vascular resistance in response to vasoconstrictive influences and an inability to vasodilate to meet increases in myocardial oxygen demands.

The exact nature of this disease is unknown, but it is probably related to some local factors that autoregulate coronary vascular resistance. These are paracrine hormones, endothelium-derived relaxing factor (EDRF), and endothelin, a vasoconstrictor that functions as a calcium channel agonist. Abnormalities of release of these hormones or of their effects on smooth muscle may be the problem in syndrome X (Bertolet, 1991). The long-term outcome of patients with syndrome X is markedly different from that of patients with angina due to epicardial coronary artery disease (Bemiller, 1973). A recent study of 88 syndrome X patients revealed a 97% survival rate after a follow-up of 9.2 years. Only one patient died of documented myocardial infarction. Angina decreased in about half, remained unchanged in 20%, and worsened in about 25% (Voelker, 1991). These patients

should be treated with antianginal medications and reassured as to the excellent prognosis.

Clinical Findings

The term "angina" denotes a specific type of chest discomfort associated with myocardial ischemia and is now used only in that sense when describing chest discomfort. Pain in the chest is one of the most common complaints the physician is called upon to assess.

A. Symptoms:

1. Characteristics of anginal pain– (See also Chapter 2.) The discomfort is described by most patients as a sensation of tightness or pressure that starts in the center of the chest and subsequently radiates to the lower jaw, to the inner surface of the left arm, and to the ulnar surface of the fourth and fifth fingers.

a. Precipitating factors– The pain is induced by anything that increases the oxygen requirements of the myocardium; examples are exercise, sexual activity, emotional stress, cold weather, wind, a large meal, anemia, an increase in blood pressure, tachycardia, high altitude, and decreased oxygen content of the inspired air. The essential features of the history include the circumstances that precipitate or relieve the discomfort and the characteristics of the discomfort itself, including its location, radiation, and duration. The essential feature is that the discomfort is precipitated in circumstances that increase the oxygen demands of the myocardium; the most common occasion is during walking, especially when the patient is hurrying or walking up an incline or a flight of stairs.

Usually the discomfort subsides promptly if the patient stands or sits quietly. If other factors upset the balance between myocardial oxygen supply and demand, less activity is required to produce angina, especially after meals, during times of emotional excitement, or on exposure to a cold wind. Heavy meals and strong emotion can provoke an attack even with trivial exertion.

The discomfort of angina of effort lasts but a short time if the effort is discontinued—almost always less than 10–15 minutes and usually much less. The discomfort develops and subsides fairly quickly but not abruptly. If the effort is continued unabated, the discomfort increases until the patient must stop. Occasionally, a patient learns to decrease activity until discomfort subsides and thus "walks through" the angina. Alternatively, the heart rate and blood pressure may have inappropriately increased at the beginning of exercise and then, while exercise continues, decreased to levels appropriate to the activity, thus reducing myocardial oxygen demand, whereupon the angina abates.

b. Quality of anginal pain– Patients describe anginal pain as pressing, squeezing, a tightness, a weight on the chest—rarely as though the chest is in a vise. They may describe it as burning and may have difficulty finding the right word but will convey the type of discomfort by pressing on the chest with both hands. Many patients use the term discomfort or distress rather than pain and will answer "No" to the question, "Do you have or have you had chest pain?" The pain is rarely stabbing, lancinating, pointed, or piercing. Anginal pain is rarely influenced by respiratory movements or exactly reproduced by direct chest pressure.

c. Location of anginal pain– The pain usually covers a fairly broad area in the central chest and has diffuse, ill-defined edges. Although it may be dominantly left precordial, it almost always involves the central chest and is rarely solely left precordial, lateral, or epigastric. Anginal pain may involve the lower area of the sternum and extend into the epigastrium. Rarely is there localized tenderness during or between attacks—in contrast to patients with musculoskeletal or radicular disease, in whom this is common.

d. Radiation of anginal pain– The pain radiates to the lower jaw (never to the upper jaw), upper neck, left shoulder, and the inner surface of the arm to the ulnar surface of the hand in the fourth and fifth fingers. It may be felt only as a sensation of pressure across the volar surface of the wrist. Rarely, a patient with angina may go to the dentist with a "toothache" or to an orthopedist complaining of upper back pain. Chest discomfort is often the only symptom, but there may be associated dyspnea if there is some element of left ventricular failure during episodes of pain.

The pain or discomfort of angina pectoris is a visceral pain from the heart referred from C8–T4 segmental dermatomes. Small pain fibers run with the autonomic nerves and enter the spinal cord in the C8–T4 segments. As with all visceral pain, it is poorly localized. The diaphragm is innervated by T4, and neck pain may be related to the cutaneous pattern of this segment. The thumb is innervated by C5 and C6 and is rarely involved in anginal pain.

e. Ease of production of pain– The ease of production of the pain during effort varies on different days, often depending upon how the patient feels emotionally, whether the patient is out of doors or not, how cold and windy it is, and how much time has elapsed since eating. All of these factors increase the determinants of myocardial oxygen demand, including heart rate and blood pressure. When patients with stable chronic angina are exercised in a comfortable laboratory on an empty stomach in a relaxed state of mind, the amount of exercise required to induce pain is fairly constant (within 10%).

f. Patient response to pain– Patients learn to avoid pain by recognizing the earliest manifestations of pressure or tightness in the chest when they are walking or start to get excited. Most patients must slow down or stop walking and stand still, since otherwise the pain worsens until they are forced to stop. A patient may have discomfort hurrying to the bus in the morning but may find that a similar amount of effort later in the morning or in the afternoon causes no discomfort. Similarly, an individual may have discomfort during the first one or two holes of golf and then play the rest of the game in comfort. This uncommon "second wind" phenomenon is presumably explained by local vasodilation caused by metabolites accumulated during the ischemic pain period.

g. Coronary artery spasm (Prinzmetal's variant angina)– Prinzmetal's variant angina differs from ordinary angina of effort in that it is more apt to occur at rest than with effort, may occasionally be relieved with exercise, may occur at odd times during the day or night (even awakening patients from sleep), and is more likely to be associated with various types of arrhythmias or conduction defects; the ST segment is more commonly elevated rather than depressed, as occurs during angina of effort. If the angina is provoked by exercise, that is more likely to happen in the morning than in the afternoon. Angina can also be precipitated in some patients by hyperventilation.

There are hemodynamic differences as well. Patients with variant angina usually have no history of previous myocardial infarction, whereas those with the usual angina of effort often have such a history. Variant angina is more common in women under age 50, whereas angina of effort is uncommon in women of this age in the absence of severe hypercholesterolemia, hypertension, or diabetes mellitus. Both variant angina and angina of effort respond rapidly to sublingual nitrates as well as to nifedipine.

The pathogenesis of coronary artery spasm is not yet understood but seems to be an abnormal localized response of a segment of the epicardial coronary artery to vasoconstrictive influences. Since there is frequently some underlying abnormality in the area of the spasm—usually a nonobstructive atherosclerotic plaque—it is possible that the endothelium is abnormal and may not be producing EDRF appropriately or may be overproducing other vasoconstrictive substances such as endothelin. The vasoconstrictor endothelin is produced by the endothelial cell converting a circulating prohormone "big" endothelin, which is produced in the liver. Other vasoconstrictors such as angiotensin II and vasopressin as well as thrombin all stimulate the production of endothelin.

Toyo-oka et al (1991), in studying patients with Prinzmetal's angina, demonstrated that endothelin serum levels are higher both in peripheral and coronary venous blood in patients with coronary spasm than in those without spasm. It is postulated that endothelin may not itself cause the spasm but that it may sensitize the vascular smooth muscle to other vasoconstrictive stimuli and potentiate their action. There is also activation of both coagulation and platelet aggregation that predispose to thrombus formation.

Angina has been provoked by ergotamine used for the treatment of migraine and has been specifically induced by ergonovine for diagnosis during coronary arteriography. Because the resulting spasm may be intense and may induce severe ischemia, arrhythmias, or myocardial infarction, ergonovine should be used in small doses, under close clinical observation, and with resuscitation equipment at hand. Because the induced coronary spasm may be resistant to sublingual nitroglycerin and may respond only to intracoronary nitroglycerin or nifedipine, ergonovine stimulation should be done only at the time of coronary arteriography.

Coronary artery spasm due to neurohumoral influences may occur in patients with or without coronary artery stenoses and may play a role in the frequent association of emotional events and angina pectoris. Spontaneous coronary artery spasm has been associated with ventricular arrhythmias in many patients during ambulatory monitoring. These arrhythmias can be seen to follow significant ST elevation or depression; they may be life-threatening and have caused cardiac arrest (Fellows, 1987). Drugs to combat myocardial ischemia may prevent the cardiac arrhythmias associated with coronary spasm.

2. Interpretation of pain of angina pectoris– In about one-fourth of patients, there are no objective clinical findings of coronary atherosclerosis, and interpretation of the symptom must be based on the history alone. The diagnosis may be simple or extremely difficult. The diagnosis of angina is more probable if there is electrocardiographic evidence of myocardial ischemia or a history of myocardial infarction. The likelihood that an uncertain history represents angina is increased by the presence of resting or induced myocardial ischemia or of other atherosclerotic manifestations such as intermittent claudication, cerebral ischemic attacks, or bruits over the major arteries. Significant epicardial coronary stenoses are revealed by coronary arteriography in about 90% of patients with typical angina pectoris, in 50% with atypical angina, and in only 5% with nonanginal chest pain (Alison, 1978).

3. Induction of pain as support for the diagnosis of angina– The diagnosis is strongly supported (1) if the patient's chest discomfort is induced by procedures that increase myocardial oxygen demand (such as exercise, rapid atrial pacing, or isoproterenol infusion) and if production of chest discomfort is associated with electrocardiographic evidence of myocardial ischemia; (2) if wall motion contraction abnormalities can be demonstrated with exercise by radionuclide angiography or echocardiography; (3) if thallium perfusion defects are seen during exercise, with redistribution at rest; or (4) if transiently raised left ventricular end-diastolic pressure occurs with evidence of left ventricular dysfunction. Continuous electrocardiographic tape recordings (Holter) for 12–24 hours can be used to look for the presence of ischemic ST segments during episodes of pain or in the absence of pain (Figure 8–7).

Coronary arteriography is rarely justified for diagnosis alone except in unusual circumstances.

B. Signs: Examination is often completely negative in patients with angina pectoris who have not had a previous myocardial infarction and who show no evidence of hypertensive or aortic valve disease. During an attack, the systolic and diastolic blood pressures are usually significantly elevated, and there may be a third or fourth heart sound, pulsus alternans, transient pulmonary rales, or the apical murmur of mitral regurgitation.

C. Hemodynamic Observations: The clinical signs mentioned in ±B, above, have been shown in some patients during cardiac catheterization. The pulse rate may be increased, and carotid sinus massage to slow the ventricular rate may abruptly reverse the increase. This maneuver (carotid sinus massage) with relief of chest discomfort can be used as a diagnostic test.

D. Laboratory Findings: Routine laboratory findings in stable angina pectoris are usually normal. Possible contributing factors that should be investigated include anemia, hypercholesterolemia, hypertriglyceridemia, low HDL, diabetes mellitus, hypoglycemia, hypo- or hyperthyroidism, and upper gastrointestinal tract diseases.

E. Imaging Studies: A chest x-ray is valuable to exclude pulmonary or skeletal abnormalities that might be the cause of pain. Occasionally, calcified coronary arteries can be seen on the chest film. These appear as parallel calcified lines in the place where the left anterior descending or right coronary artery runs. Calcification in the area of the aortic valve occasionally gives evidence of aortic stenosis.

Figure 8–9 indicates the specificity and sensitivity of noninvasive tests in the diagnosis of angina pectoris and defines the terms used. Noninvasive tests are described in the next section, followed by a section on invasive special procedures.

F. Electrocardiographic Findings: The resting ECG is normal in about one-fourth of patients with stable angina. In the remainder, abnormalities include patterns of left ventricular hypertrophy, old myocardial infarction, nonspecific ST–T abnormalities, and atrioventricular or conduction defects.

Noninvasive Tests

Noninvasive tests may be important because a clear history of angina pectoris is sometimes difficult to obtain.

A. Routine ECG: An electrocardiographic abnormality on routine examination may reveal unexpected characteristic features of previous myocardial infarction such as typical abnormal Q waves or unequivocal ST–T abnormalities. Acute myocardial infarction may occur without symptoms, or the symptoms may be so atypical that the diagnosis of old infarction can

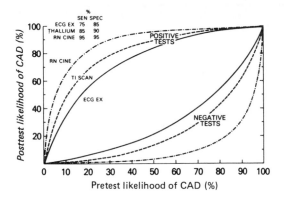

Definitions

Predictive value of a positive test
= The probability that a patient has disease, given a positive test outcome

$$= \frac{\text{Number of patients with disease}}{\text{Total number of patients with a positive test}}$$

Predictive value of a negative test
= The probability that a patient does not have disease, given a negative test outcome

$$= \frac{\text{Number of subjects without disease}}{\text{Total number of subjects with a negative test}}$$

Sensitivity
= The probability a patient with disease will have a given test result

$$= \frac{\text{Number of patients with disease with a given test result}}{\text{Total number of tested patients with disease}}$$

Specificity
= The probability a patient without disease will not have the given test result

$$= \frac{\text{Number of disease-free subjects not showing the test result}}{\text{Total number of disease-free subjects tested}}$$

Pretest likelihood (= prior probability)
= The probability of disease in a subject to be tested

$$= \frac{\text{Number of patients with disease in the test population}}{\text{Total number of patients in the test population}}$$

Posttest likelihood (= posterior probability)
= The probability of disease in a subject showing a given test result

$$= \frac{\text{Number of patients with disease showing a given test result}}{\text{Total number of subjects showing the test result}}$$

Figure 8–9. Probability of coronary artery disease (CAD). Comparison of electrocardiographic exercise testing (ECG EX), thallium perfusion scanning (TI SCAN), and radionuclide cineangiography (RN CINE). (Sensitivity [SEN] and specificity [SPEC] values are approximations derived from published series.) (Reproduced, with permission, from Epstein SE: Implications of probability analysis on the strategy used for noninvasive detection of coronary artery disease: Role of single or combined use of exercise electrocardiographic testing, radionuclide cineangiography and myocardial perfusion imaging. Am J Cardiol 1980;40:491.)

Table 8–1. Criteria for diagnosis of coronary disease with exercise stress test (assuming normal baseline ECG and no digitalis).

- Horizontal downsloping ST depression $\geq$ 1 mm (2 mm in some studies).
- Duration of ST depression > 3 minutes.
- Angina pectoris during or immediately after the test.
- Exercise associated with hypotension or blood pressure < 130 mm Hg.

only be made on the basis of electrocardiographic abnormalities.

B. Stress Electrocardiographic Tests: (See also Chapter 5.) Induction of chest discomfort or flat or downsloping ST segments by exercise has for many years been the commonest noninvasive technique used to provide objective evidence of myocardial ischemia. The current method uses a cycle ergometer or treadmill and the Bruce protocol, with progressive, graded exercise (stages I–VI). The physician may terminate the exercise at any stage (see Precautions, below).

1. Criteria for a positive electrocardiographic stress test– Table 8–1 sets forth the criteria for the diagnosis of coronary disease.

The original criteria for a positive test were the same for all studies, consisting of a horizontal downsloping ST segment depression of a degree that varied from 1 mm to 1.5–2 mm. Refinements of the electrocardiographic stress tests attempt to measure the degree of positivity and not merely to classify results as positive or negative. Factors considered in these refinements include the contour, depth, and area of the ST segment change (depression or elevation); the time of appearance (which stage of the Bruce protocol); the duration of the ST segment changes; the pulse rate achieved in relation to the maximum predicted for the age and sex of the patient; the coexistent development of anginal pain; and the appearance of hypotension or complex ventricular beats during exercise. These have led to attempts at quantitative grading of symptoms in order to permit gradations of positivity by combining the ECG and clinical responses. A strongly positive test consists of marked ST changes (> 2 mm) that (1) appear early and at a heart rate less than 85% of predicted maximum and (2) are associated with angina, hypotension, or complex arrhythmias. Additional refinements include having the patient perform the exercise test following use of beta-adrenergic-blocking agents or with a hand placed in ice water, so that the effects of a cold pressor and an exercise ECG are combined. It is difficult to interpret many of the published reports, because different criteria are used by different authors (Detrano: The diagnostic accuracy, 1989).

It seems clear, however, that the greater the abnormality, the more marked the positivity and the more likely the presence of multivessel disease, including left main coronary disease. Care must be taken not to

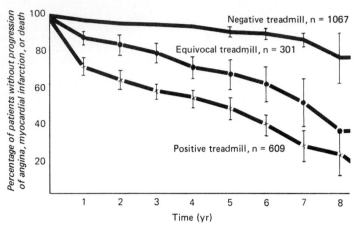

Figure 8–10. Life table display of an 8-year experience of absence of complications in approximately 2000 ambulatory individuals who had a negative, equivocal, or positive (ST depression of 1.5 mm or more) treadmill response. (n, number of patients.) (Reproduced, with permission of the American Heart Association, Inc., from Ellestad MH, Wan KC: Predictive implications of stress testing: Follow-up of 2700 subjects after maximum treadmill stress testing. Circulation 1975;51:363.)

interpret a J junction depression as a positive test, because this occurs often in normal individuals, is of short duration, and immediately precedes the ST segment. Upsloping ST depression likewise is less significant than downsloping depression, and it may occur when a deep J junction ascends to the T wave. Elevated ST segment changes may also occur, perhaps because of the association of coronary spasm with the effort. ST segment elevation with exercise in leads with Q waves does not correlate with ischemia but may be associated with a severe wall motion abnormality.

2. Precautions during exercise stress test– Exercise should not be performed if an acute myocardial infarction or unstable angina is diagnosed or suspected or if the patient is in a condition in which exercise would be unwise. Acute myocardial infarction may be precipitated if exercise testing is done in patients with acute or subacute myocardial ischemia and with pain of recent origin. The test must be done under the supervision of a physician, who should observe and examine the patient during the exercise and be able to perform resuscitative measures in the event of ventricular tachycardia or fibrillation. Electrocardiographic recording should be obtained continuously during exercise so the test can be stopped if necessary. Rate-limited (not symptom-limited) stress exercise tests 7–14 days following infarction can stratify patients into high- and low-risk groups.

3. Prognostic significance of a positive exercise stress test– Ellestad (1975) and Bruce (1977) both have shown that patients who have had positive exercise studies have increased rates of subsequent clinical coronary disease or death due to coronary disease (Figures 8–10 and 8–11).

4. General significance of a positive exercise stress test– There is controversy about the desirability of performing exercise tests in asymptomatic middle-aged persons. Some of the same considerations pertain to patients with probable or definite angina pectoris. The specificity and predictive accuracy of an abnormal exercise ECG test is high in symptomatic individuals but generally less than 50% in asymptomatic individuals. The prevalence of the disease in the population being studied influences the reliability of any test. Even marked ST depression may represent a false-positive test, and a negative test is unreliable in excluding coronary disease. In a recent meta-analysis of 150 studies, the mean weighted sensitivity of 0.1 mV ST segment depression for significant coronary artery disease by arteriography was 68% (range, 23–100%), which means that 32% of patients with angiographic coronary disease had a negative exercise ECG (Gianrossi, 1989). All clinical data must be taken into account in the interpretation of a positive test. (See Figure 8–9.) False-positive exercise ST segment depression occurs in about 11% of tests. Sensitivity varies from 35% in one-vessel disease to 86% in three-vessel disease (Martin, 1972).

Patients with known coronary disease can be divided into low- and high-risk subgroups on the basis of ease of production of pain and duration of exercise or electrocardiographic changes. Figure 8–12 shows a greatly increased survival rate in the low-risk group. Because patients with multivessel disease are at higher risk, stress ECG has been used to identify them. In a meta-analysis of 62 studies reported, Detrano (Exercise-induced, 1989) found a weighted mean sensitivity of 0.1 mV ST segment depression for identifying patients with multivessel disease of

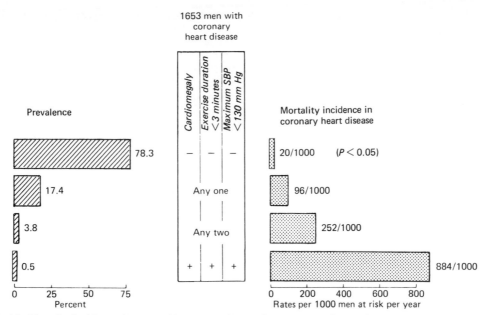

Figure 8–11. Mortality incidence in men with coronary heart disease, according to the presence or absence of three predictors: cardiomegaly, peak systolic pressure less than 130 mm Hg, and exercise duration not exceeding 3 minutes. P for the first row applies in combination with the second, third, and fourth rows and is based on Poisson confidence intervals. (SBP, systolic blood pressure.) (Reproduced, with permission, from Bruce RA: Exercise for evaluation of ventricular function. N Engl J Med 1977;296:671.)

81% (range, 40–100%) and specificity of 66% (range, 17–100%).

Exercise testing is also useful in the assessment of left ventricular function, especially if the symptoms seem out of proportion to other clinical findings. Comparison of the exercise capacity of the patient during exercise and at rest may reveal the onset of angina, dyspnea, or hypotension on slight effort of short duration and is therefore an important index of cardiac function. Noting changes on the ECG in association with maximal oxygen uptake during exercise also gives useful information about cardiovascular function.

C. Radioisotope Studies: If patients with atypical chest pain thought possibly to be anginal have negative or equivocal exercise stress studies or if the presence of abnormalities at rest (such as conduction defects, ST–T changes, or changes due to medication) makes interpretation of stress ECG unreliable, radioisotope evaluation with thallium-201 or the newer technetium-99m-sestamibi during exercise and after redistribution should be obtained. Hypoperfusion (myocardial ischemia) with a discrete defect or "cold spot" that disappears after redistribution of the isotope a few hours later is a more reliable indication of ischemia than electrocardiographic exercise studies. False-negative results occur in a small percentage of patients. If the patient cannot exercise because of musculoskeletal problems, claudication, or

generalized instability, coronary vasodilation with intravenous dipyridamole or with adenosine with thallium imaging has been successful in identifying areas of decreased perfusion. These vasodilators decrease coronary vascular resistance and can increase coronary blood flow to four or five times the normal value. Those areas of myocardium supplied by obstructed vessels have lesser increases in myocardial blood flow and for that reason, upon injection of a radioisotopic perfusion agent, will be relative "cold spots" compared with myocardium supplied by the normal coronary vessels (Ranhosky, 1990).

Radionuclide angiography, at rest and with exercise, has been used in patients with angina pectoris. It may be more sensitive than thallium-201 perfusion during exercise but is less specific for coronary disease. Whereas the appearance and disappearance of hypoperfusion defects with thallium indicate the presence of myocardial ischemia, radionuclide angiography assesses overall and regional left ventricular function by determining ejection fraction and the location and degree of wall motion (contraction) abnormalities. Ejection fraction can be determined from the difference between the systolic and diastolic isotope images of left ventricular volume. Outlines of these images in both phases of the cardiac cycle also allow various segments of the left ventricle to be analyzed for localized areas of hypokinesia, akinesia, or dyskinesia. These areas correlate positively with

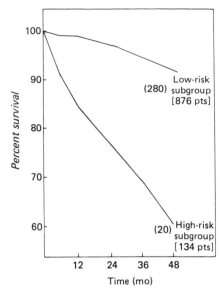

Figure 8–12. Cumulative life table survival rates in low and high-risk subgroups. Numbers in parentheses represent the number of patients followed for 48 months. Numbers in brackets represent the number of patients in each subgroup. The low-risk subgroup includes those patients with a negative test or exercise duration ≥ stage IV or a maximum heart rate ≥ 160. The high-risk subgroup includes those patients with a positive test and exercise duration < stage III. (Reproduced, with permission of the American Heart Association, Inc., from McNeer JF et al: The role of the exercise test in the evaluation of patients for ischemic heart disease. Circulation 1978;57:64.)

myocardial fibrosis found at autopsy. Many patients with angina pectoris have had previous myocardial infarction. A low ejection fraction (< 0.4) alone—or especially with clinical risk factors—is an adverse prognostic sign following myocardial infarction (Moss, 1983).

If a thallium defect is present at rest but does not increase and then resolve during and after exercise, one cannot infer the induction of myocardial ischemia or even the presence of an old myocardial infarct. The defect at rest may represent scar from any cause or chronic myocardial ischemia. The appearance and disappearance of a thallium defect is necessary to document that myocardial ischemia has been induced.

Two new radioisotope perfusion imaging agents have recently been introduced, both tagged with technetium-99m: teboroxime and sestamibi (technetium-99m hexakis-2-methoxy isobutyl isonitrile). They were developed because of the suboptimal quality of thallium-201 for gamma camera imaging. Teboroxime labeled with technetium-99m accumulates rapidly in the myocardium to an extent proportionate to the myocardial blood flow, but it stays in the heart muscle only a short time, and imaging must be done within 5 minutes after administration. For this reason, experience with this substance is limited.

Technetium TC 99m sestamibi has a peak myocardial extraction rate lower than that of thallium-201, but because of its higher retention efficacy the net myocardial accumulation of sestamibi is similar to that of thallium. The energy of technetium is better for imaging, especially for SPECT (single-photon emission computed tomography).

Sestamibi is accumulated to an extent proportionate to coronary blood flow and is dependent on uptake by viable myocardial cells. Unlike thallium-201, there is negligible redistribution, so the myocardial flow conditions at the time of injection remain the same for a relatively long time, allowing for less time-dependent imaging after exercise. Later, a single injection may be done at rest to see whether at lower demands for coronary blood flow previous "decreased" areas of perfusion are now similar to areas perfused by normal coronary arteries. Another advantage was reported by Villanueva-Meyer et al (1990), who demonstrated that simultaneous measurement of myocardial perfusion and left ventricular ejection fraction by first-pass imaging from a single injection of technetium-99m sestamibi is feasible. Experience with this imaging agent is continuing to accumulate (Berman, 1990).

D. Two-Dimensional Echocardiography: Two-dimensional echocardiography is valuable for qualitative but only for approximate quantitative evaluation of left ventricular function in patients with angina pectoris. It is difficult to perform and evaluate during exercise. However, there is increasing experience with postexercise two-dimensional echocardiography with and without dipyridamole infusion. Dipyridamole increases the sensitivity of the postexercise two-dimensional echocardiogram without decreasing the specificity compared with conventional exercise electrocardiography or even postexercise two-dimensional echocardiography without dipyridamole (Armstrong, 1988; Picano, 1991).

Echocardiography after infusion of dobutamine has been used to precipitate myocardial ischemia, which causes wall motion abnormalities in patients with coronary artery disease. With ischemia there is a failure of that segment of myocardium to develop hyperkinesis. In one study, the sensitivity for detecting coronary disease with luminal narrowing of 50% or more was 95% with a specificity of 82% and sensitivity of 92%. There were no differences in sensitivity of detecting disease among the three major coronary artery systems (Segar, 1992).

Two-dimensional echocardiography is valuable in identifying left ventricular aneurysm and associated pericardial effusion and for estimating ejection fraction. Left ventricular angiography and coronary angiography are the reference standards against which the noninvasive radioisotope studies must be judged.

E. Comparison of Exercise Electrocardiographic Testing, Radionuclide Studies at Rest and Exercise, and Coronary Arteriography: (See

Figure 8–9.) There is significant correspondence of results in these three methods of evaluation. Generally, hypoperfusion (transient or permanent) with thallium-201 or sestamibi is more specific than stress electrocardiographic tests. With exercise electrocardiography, localization of the ischemia is not possible; with radioisotope perfusion studies, areas of ischemic myocardium can usually be localized.

The greatest sensitivity (the proportion of patients with established coronary disease who have a positive test) and specificity (the proportion of negative tests in patients proved not to have coronary disease) will be obtained when all three tests (electrocardiography, radioisotope perfusion, and radionuclide angiography) are combined. The ultimate diagnostic procedure to establish coronary stenoses is invasive coronary arteriography combined with contrast ventriculography.

F. Newer Investigational Noninvasive Procedures: A number of experimental approaches are under development to image the coronary arteries noninvasively and detect ischemic myocardium and differentiate it from infarcted or fibrotic myocardium. **Digital subtraction angiography** is performed with injection of small amounts of a contrast agent at the aortic root or directly into the coronary arteries. The video image is computer-digitized on-line. These images can be enhanced in definition by computer subtraction of a mask of a digitized image frame acquired before contrast injection. Because the coronary arteries are small-diameter vessels moving with cardiac contraction, movement artifacts have kept this technique from being practical for imaging the coronary arteries. However, it is an excellent technique for doing ventriculography with minimal contrast or even from an intravenous injection. Furthermore, by measurement of myocardial time-density curves and of the time required for appearance of contrast in the myocardium after rapid intracoronary artery injection, valuable information about myocardial blood flow can be obtained as well. These techniques are for the most part under development but offer promise of clinical utility in the future (Zijlstra, 1988; Kussmaul, 1990).

Positron emission tomography (PET scanning) is most useful in identifying viable myocardium where both perfusion and metabolic activity are seen to be present. This is accomplished by injecting generator-produced rubidium-82 or cyclotron-produced N-13 ammonia for perfusion data and cyclotron-produced fluoro-18-deoxyglucose for metabolic data. These techniques can identify nonperfusible defects seen on thallium-201 scintigraphy as being still viable (Camici, 1989). This technique is also more specific than thallium scanning or exercise electrocardiography (Demer, 1989).

Magnetic resonance spectroscopy is still experimental at present but may in the future, with the development of larger magnets, yield important information about myocardial metabolism noninvasively.

Computerized tomography (CT scanning) has proved valuable in detecting calcification in coronary arteries, and this has been highly correlated with the presence of coronary atherosclerosis. In patients under age 65, it may also correlate with the presence of significant coronary artery obstruction (Tannenbaum, 1989). After contrast injection, CT scanning has proved highly accurate in determining the patency of saphenous vein bypass grafts (Stanford, 1988). Obviously, both CT scanning and MRI are highly accurate in identifying and quantifying scarred areas of the myocardium. With rapid-acquisition cine mode MRI or CT scanning, wall motion abnormalities can also be detected and quantified. However, at present these techniques add little to radioisotope or two-dimensional echocardiographic techniques. Attempts are under way to characterize tissue differences by MRI with and without contrast agents in order to identify infarcted myocardium.

Invasive Special Procedures

A. Coronary Arteriography: Because of its risk potential, coronary arteriography should not be used solely for diagnosis and prognosis. The procedure involves only a slight risk in experienced hands. The anatomy of the coronary arteries cannot be predicted from the history of angina and the patient's responses to exercise testing. Patients with stable angina may have one-, two-, or three-vessel disease. Even in mild angina there may be major stenoses of two or three coronary arteries; thus, coronary angiograms are required if the physician wishes to know the anatomy of the coronary arteries in any particular case.

The anatomy and distribution of the coronary arteries and the topography of infarction are illustrated in Figure 8–13. Multiple views and projections are usually necessary to evaluate the coronary angiogram. Figure 8–14 shows examples of branches of the right and left coronary arteries seen in left anterior oblique and right anterior oblique coronary angiograms.

1. Complications– Nationwide surveys have shown that the morbidity and mortality rates associated with coronary arteriography are directly related to the experience of the operator and the frequency with which the procedure is done in the particular hospital. Ventricular fibrillation, acute myocardial infarction, hemorrhage, and thrombosis of the artery are the major problems encountered. Embolism is the least common complication. The mortality rate in various series is about 0.1–0.5%. The risk rises with the degree of severity of left main coronary artery disease. The use of contrast media in patients with renal insufficiency can increase renal failure caused by diabetes, at times requiring temporary hemodialysis. The development of water-soluble contrast media that are either isosmotic or of low osmolality and which are either nonionic or contain physiologic concentrations of calcium ions provides contrast with fewer hemodynamic and electrocardiographic

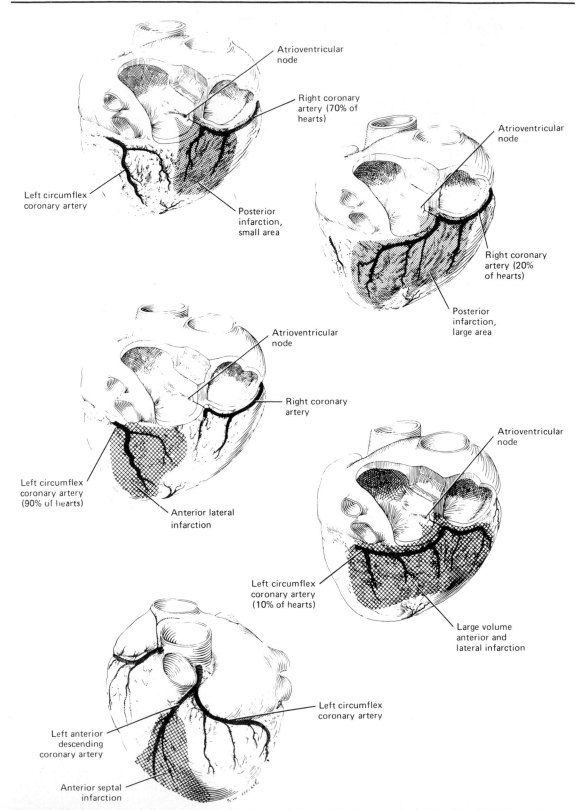

Figure 8–13. Anatomy and distribution of the coronary arteries and the topography of infarction. (Modified and reproduced, with permission, from James TN: Arrhythmias and conduction disturbances in acute myocardial infarction. Am Heart J 1962;64:416.)

RIGHT CORONARY SYSTEM

LEFT CORONARY SYSTEM

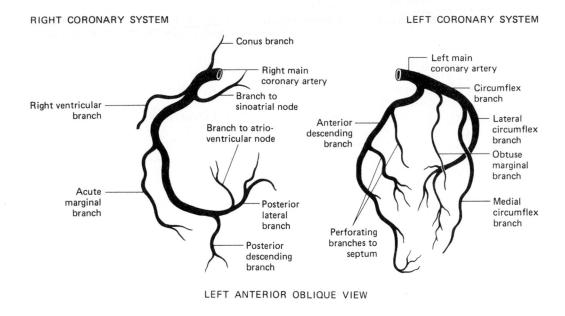

LEFT ANTERIOR OBLIQUE VIEW

RIGHT CORONARY SYSTEM

LEFT CORONARY SYSTEM

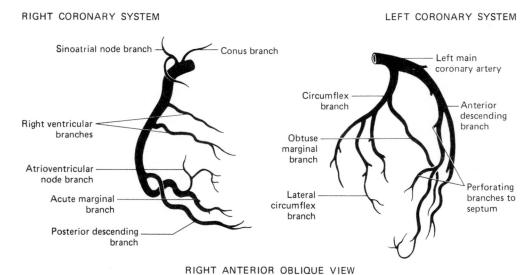

RIGHT ANTERIOR OBLIQUE VIEW

Figure 8–14. Example of branches of the left and right coronary arteries as seen in the usual coronary angiograms, left and right oblique views. (Modified and reproduced, with permission, from Cosby RS et al: Clinicoarteriographic correlations in angina pectoris with and without myocardial infarction. Am J Cardiol 1972;30:472.)

changes than the hyperosmotic ionic agents. These agents may also be safer, causing fewer episodes of ventricular arrhythmia and hypotension, and may have less tendency to precipitate renal insufficiency (Reagan, 1988), though this has yet to be proved. A recent study by Hirshfeld (1990) of over 4500 angiograms using conventional contrast agents found a very low incidence of major complications (1.3%) and suggested—because the cost is so much greater—that the newer agents be used only for pa-

tients at high risk for complications, those with severe hemodynamic instability, or those with ventricular arrhythmias (Brinker, 1990).

The interpretation of coronary angiograms is hampered by the difficulty of quantitating partial stenosis, of determining the significance of collaterals, and of deciding whether arterial spasm or technical artifacts are present. The tendency in qualitatively interpreting the coronary arteriogram is to underestimate the severity of lesions. Quantitative coronary arteriography, where all dimensions of the lesion are taken into consideration, can better estimate the functional severity of the lesion (Brown, 1986).

2. Indications for coronary arteriography– A number of studies have shown that survival in patients with angina pectoris depends upon (1) the dominance (whether posterior descending coronary arteries come from right or left systems) of the stenotic artery; (2) the location, severity, and number of coronary stenoses (whether there is a single severe proximal stenosis or more moderate multiple distal stenoses); (3) the proximity of the stenosis to the first perforator (left anterior descending); (4) left ventricular function as estimated by the ejection fraction, left ventricular volumes, and the presence and degree of wall motion abnormalities; and (5) the presence and adequacy of collateral circulation.

Coronary arteriography is indicated for the following classes of patients:

(1) Patients being considered for revascularization procedures (coronary bypass surgery or percutaneous transluminal coronary angioplasty [PTCA]) because of disabling stable angina and failure to improve on an adequate medical regimen.

(2) Patients with angina controlled by medical management where noninvasive evaluation reveals large amounts of myocardium at risk.

(3) Patients being considered for coronary bypass surgery or PTCA because of myocardial infarctions in rapid succession, if residual ischemia can be demonstrated, or because of repeated unstable angina causing hospital admissions, or with a single episode of unstable angina where noninvasive evaluation reveals large amounts of myocardium at risk.

(4) Patients with aortic stenosis or mitral valve disease with angina pectoris, to determine whether the angina is due to coronary disease. Severe angina in the presence of aortic stenosis is associated with coronary artery stenosis in about half the cases.

(5) Patients who have had coronary bypass surgery or PTCA with initial improvement and subsequent relapse of symptoms, to determine whether the bypass graft is patent or occluded.

(6) Patients with coronary disease, ischemic cardiomyopathy, and cardiac failure where a mechanical lesion, such as mitral regurgitation, ventricular septal defect, or ventricular aneurysm, is suspected.

(7) For diagnostic purposes in patients who have chest pain of uncertain cause believed not to be anginal, if the patient will be benefited in knowing for certain that the pain is not due to coronary disease.

B. Contrast Left Ventricular Angiography: (See also Chapter 6.) Left ventricular cineangiograms should be performed in conjunction with coronary arteriograms because of the information the former give on left ventricular function; size of the heart during systole and diastole; wall motion abnormalities; the presence of ventricular aneurysm; and the absence of other conditions such as valvular disease,

hypertrophic cardiomyopathy, mitral valve prolapse, and other unsuspected abnormalities. It is unwise to perform coronary arteriography without contrast left ventricular angiography where there are no contraindications. If renal failure is present, radioisotope angiography can replace ventricular angiography.

Differential Diagnosis of Anginal Pain

The differential diagnosis of chest pain requires great skill in history taking. The physician can usually decide that the pain is or is not angina, but in some cases even the most careful and thoughtful inquiry may leave the issue in doubt. Chest pain in someone with coronary disease is not necessarily angina.

A. Psychophysiologic Reactions: Psychophysiologic cardiovascular reactions are a loosely defined group of disorders having in common dull aching chest pains often described as "heart pain," lasting hours or days, often aggravated by exertion but not promptly relieved by rest. Darting, knifelike pains of momentary duration at the apex or over the precordium are often present also. Emotional tension and fatigue make the pain worse. Hyperventilation, palpitations, fatigue, and headache are also usually present. Constant exhaustion is a frequent complaint.

B. Anterior Chest Wall Syndrome: This disorder is characterized by sharply localized tenderness of intercostal muscles, and pressure at these sites reproduces the chest pain. Sprain or inflammation of the chondrocostal junctions, which may be warm, swollen, and red (so-called Tietze's syndrome), may result in diffuse chest pain that is also reproduced by local pressure; this is an extremely unusual entity. Intercostal neuritis (herpes zoster, diabetes mellitus) may confuse the diagnosis.

Xiphoid tenderness and lower sternal pain may arise from and be reproduced by pressure on the xiphoid process.

Any of the above may also occur in a patient with angina.

C. Degenerative Thoracic or Cervical Spine Disease: Thoracic or cervical spine disease (degenerative disk disease, postural strain, "arthritis") involving the dorsal roots produces sudden sharp, severe chest pain similar to angina in location and "radiation" but related to specific movements of the neck or spine, recumbency, straining, or lifting, and there are usually sensory changes in the skin. Pain due to cervical thoracic disk disease involves the outer or dorsal aspect of the arm, thumb, and index fingers rather than the ring and little fingers, as in angina pectoris.

D. Gastrointestinal and Esophageal Disorders: Peptic ulcer, chronic cholecystitis, cardiospasm, and functional gastrointestinal disease are often suspected because some patients indisputably obtain relief from angina by belching. In these disorders, symptoms are related to food or alcohol intake rather than physical exertion. X-ray and fluoroscopic study are helpful in diagnosis. The pain is relieved by appropriate diet and drug therapy.

Esophageal disorders, either reflux esophagitis or esophageal motility disorders—including diffuse esophageal spasm, hypertensive lower esophageal sphincter, and high-amplitude peristaltic contractions ("nutcracker esophagus")—can all mimic angina pectoris (Richter, 1989). Not only the quality of the discomfort but the length of time it lasts, its radiation to the left arm and neck, and even its precipitation by exercise can all be similar to the discomfort of myocardial ischemia. Esophageal discomfort is often longer-lasting and is more likely to occur on recumbency or at night—or after bending over—or to be accompanied by "sour belching," or waterbrash, and is likely to be relieved by antacids. Esophageal motility disorders can be diagnosed by esophageal manometry and placebo-controlled provocative testing with acid perfusion or edrophonium chloride in 25–50% of patients with known coronary artery disease (Hewson, 1990). Although not all chest pain in patients with coronary disease is angina pectoris, an important dictum is that esophageal disorders are not diagnosed until discomfort from coronary artery disease is excluded.

E. Shoulder Origin of Pain: Degenerative and inflammatory lesions of the left shoulder or cervical rib and the scalenus anticus syndrome differ from angina in that the pain is precipitated by movement of the arm and shoulder, paresthesias are present in the left arm, and postural exercises and pillow support to the shoulders in bed give relief.

F. Pain of Pulmonary Hypertension: "Tight" mitral stenosis or pulmonary hypertension resulting from chronic pulmonary disease can on occasion produce chest pain which is indistinguishable from that of angina pectoris, including ST segment depression possibly from right ventricular myocardial ischemia. The clinical findings of mitral stenosis or of lung disease are evident, and the ECG invariably discloses right axis deviation or right ventricular hypertrophy. Pulmonary embolism must also be considered.

G. Spontaneous Pneumothorax: Spontaneous pneumomediastinum or pneumothorax may cause chest pain as well as dyspnea and create confusion with angina pectoris as well as myocardial infarction.

H. Pericarditis: See Chapter 18.

Complications

The major complications of stable angina are unstable angina, myocardial infarction, arrhythmias, and sudden death.

Treatment

Treatment will be discussed in three main categories: (1) overall considerations, (2) treatment of the acute attack of angina pectoris, and (3) management

of chronic angina pectoris. One must exclude acute myocardial infarction, evaluate the presence of an old infarction or segmental wall motion abnormalities, and evaluate left ventricular function.

A. Overall Considerations:

1. Approach to atherosclerosis in general– One must distinguish between efforts to prevent or relieve anginal pain; efforts to prevent myocardial infarction or arrhythmias; and efforts to avert the fundamental process of atherosclerosis.

2. Treatment of hypercholesterolemia– The evidence is now convincing that hypercholesterolemia is a major cause of coronary artery disease. The critical element in cholesterol control is the hepatic LDL receptor. A high cholesterol and saturated fat intake suppresses this receptor, which leads to an increase in LDL cholesterol. High carbohydrate intake stimulates the hepatic synthesis of triglycerides and raises the very low density lipoprotein (VLDL) (Grundy, 1990).

In the average case of hypercholesterolemia, treatment should be begun when cholesterol levels are equal to or exceed 240 mg/dL (LDL cholesterol 160 mg/dL)—a level that includes 25% of the adult population. If the patient has other risk factors, treatment can be started at a lower level (serum cholesterol > 200 mg/dL or LDL cholesterol > 130 mg/dL). The initial step in treatment is dietary and may be sufficient for many people. The diet should be sufficiently low in calories to reduce weight to that ideal for the individual. Fat should be less than 30% of total calories (divided equally between saturated and unsaturated fat). Cholesterol intake should be 250–300 mg/d. Protein should be 15%, and carbohydrates including alcohol should be about 55% of calories (AHA Nutrition Committee, 1988). High alcohol intake causes considerable increase in serum triglycerides. The diet should be employed for 1–3 months and the serum cholesterol, low-density lipoprotein cholesterol (LDL), and high-density lipoprotein cholesterol (HDL) determined before and after the dietary phase of treatment.

If dietary treatment does not lower the serum cholesterol to approximately 200 mg/dL, the next step in the past was the use of bile acid-binding resins (cholestyramine, 20–30 g/d, or colestipol, 20 g/d), combined with nicotinic acid, in divided doses, starting with 100 mg three times daily and increasing slowly to 3–7.5 g/d. Nicotinic acid inhibits secretion of VLDL, the LDL precursor, thus decreasing LDL and VLDL. It also inhibits the catabolism of HDL, thereby raising its serum level. The resins are often unpleasant to take and produce gastrointestinal symptoms. They bind the bile acids in the bowel and increase the removal of LDL from the plasma. Nicotinic acid causes flushing of the skin, especially in the early phase of treatment (Kane, 1990), which can be prevented by taking an aspirin tablet 20–30 minutes before the nicotinic acid, thus blunting the prostaglandin-mediated effect. Hepatic transaminase levels can rise with this drug up to three times normal. Serious hepatic toxicity is rare. Since uric acid and fasting blood glucose also may rise, nicotinic acid should be avoided in diabetics and in patients with gout.

Alternatively, and probably increasingly in the future as a primary drug, patients can be given lovastatin, pravastatin, or simvastatin, all of which inhibit HMG-CoA reductase and reduce the synthesis of cholesterol. Other HMG-CoA reductase inhibitors will soon be available. However, another mechanism—perhaps the main one—is through an increase in LDL receptor activity rather than a decrease in cholesterol synthesis (Grundy, 1988). The beginning dose of lovastatin, the first HMG-CoA reductase inhibitor available, is 10–20 mg twice daily, titrated to 20–40 mg twice daily. Serum cholesterol, LDL, and apolipoprotein B (Apo B) are reduced about 20–40%, depending upon the initial cholesterol level. The other drugs probably have a similar effect. There is about a 10–30% decrease in plasma triglycerides and a tendency for HDL cholesterol to increase by 2–15%. Lovastatin has few side effects. Serum transaminases may increase. Lovastatin should be stopped if the increase is threefold, but this is rare. Opacities of the lens without visual disturbances, although early thought to be a problem, have not been seen in large studies, and yearly ophthalmologic examination is no longer deemed necessary. If myositis occurs, the drug should be stopped. Lovastatin increases HDL only slightly; if further experience indicates that a rise in HDL is essential, gemfibrozil, 0.6–1.2 g/d, may be substituted because it raises the HDL while decreasing total cholesterol. Side effects include gastrointestinal symptoms and myopathy (Frick, 1987). Elevations of creatine kinase up to twice normal are not unusual and do not require withdrawal of the drug. Lovastatin and gemfibrozil or cyclosporine should not be given together because of the risk of severe myositis. Myopathy has also been seen when erythromycin and niacin are combined.

All of the above drugs except gemfibrozil are complementary; if the plasma cholesterol is not reduced to around 200 mg/dL and if the LDL cholesterol is not reduced to 160 mg/dL or less, "triple therapy" (resin, nicotinic acid, and lovastatin) can be instituted, resulting in a greater effect (Malloy, 1987; Prihoda, 1992).

The place of vigorous cholesterol-lowering measures in people without clinically manifest coronary artery disease—primary prevention—is not as clearly defined as in the population with already manifest coronary disease—secondary prevention. A number of primary prevention trials involving more than 40,000 subjects where serum cholesterol has been lowered moderately ($\approx$ 15%) have been subjected to meta-analysis (Yusuf, 1988). The overall results suggest that a 10% reduction in serum cholesterol leads to a 20% reduction in the development of coronary artery disease.

Using the published data concerning the benefits of reduction of cholesterol in the population, a computer model has been created predicting the benefits of treating hyperlipidemia in the general population to prevent coronary heart disease (Grover, 1992). The model was validated by comparing the computer estimates with the observed results in three primary coronary heart disease prevention trials (LRC Trial, the Helsinki Heart Study, and MRFIT). The forecast is that in the population with serum cholesterol levels between 200 and 300 mg/dL (5.2–7.8 mmol/L), if serum cholesterol is lowered 5–33%, the average life expectancy would be increased by 0.03–3.16 years and that the average onset of symptoms of coronary heart disease would be delayed by 0.06–4.98 years.

An argument against vigorous reduction of serum cholesterol in the general population is the observation in many of the lipid-lowering trials that there has been an increase in deaths from cancer and from suicides and accidents. It is not clear whether this is related to the lipid-lowering diet or drugs, but the observation does suggest that cautious appraisal of the possible risks should precede vigorous cholesterol reduction in asymptomatic patients with cholesterol levels between 220 and 240 mg/dL.

Several reports are now available of angiographically evaluated trials of lipid-lowering strategies and drugs in patients with hypercholesterolemia and known coronary artery disease. These studies have conclusively documented a marked decrease in the progression of coronary atherosclerotic lesions, modest regression of lesions, decreased formation of new lesions, and a moderate reduction in coronary events. These trials included the Lifestyle Heart Trial, in which changes in life-style—including a vegetarian diet, cessation of smoking, and stress management—showed a decrease in progression and minimal regression when cholesterol was lowered in men with previously known coronary heart disease (Ornish, 1990).

The Program on Surgical Control of the Hyperlipidemias (POSCH) trial involved 838 patients who had survived a first myocardial infarction in which partial ileal bypass markedly lowered cholesterol; the mean follow-up was 9.7 years. Overall mortality and morbidity due to heart disease was not reduced in comparison with a control group, but death due to coronary heart disease and confirmed nonfatal myocardial infarction combined were 35% lower in the operated group ($P < .001$) (Buchwald, 1990).

The Familial Atherosclerosis Treatment Study (FATS) tested colestipol-niacin and colestipol-lovastatin combinations and reported in a 2.5-year follow-up that 46% of the patients in the conventionally treated group progressed by coronary arteriography compared with 21–25% in the drug treatment group. There was no regression in the conventionally treated group, in comparison with 32–39% regression of the drug treatment group. There was also a significant decrease in clinical coronary events in the drug treatment group compared with the control group (Brown, 1990).

The UCSF Specialized Center of Research (UCSF-SCCR) interventional trial after coronary angiography randomized 72 patients with heterogeneous familial hypercholesterolemia to a conventional treatment and an aggressive drug therapy group. After 2 years, there was minimal progression in the percentage of obstructed area in the control group and regression in the treated group (Kane, 1990).

The Cholesterol-Lowering Atherosclerosis Study (CLAS) tested combined drug therapy with colestipol and niacin against conventional therapy and repeated coronary arteriography after 2 and 4 years. This study also showed marked decrease in progression (52% nonprogression in the drug group versus 15% in the placebo group and new lesion formation in 18% of the drug group compared with 69% of the conventionally treated group (Cashin-Hemphill, 1990). It therefore appears that lowering cholesterol—at least in patients with an elevated cholesterol and known coronary artery disease—is essential treatment.

Prevention of coronary disease should be started in childhood or adolescence, because hypertension and genetic disorders of lipid and carbohydrate metabolism are manifest early in life.

3. Prevention of myocardial infarction–
Prevention of myocardial infarction is one of the aims of treatment of angina. While most infarctions come "out of the blue" and cannot be predicted by patient or physician, an effort should be made to avoid factors that sometimes precipitate the event. The list includes physical stresses (eg, bursts of unaccustomed strenuous activity, shoveling snow in the cold after a heavy meal, running with heavy luggage to a departure gate) and emotional stresses associated with a rise in blood pressure or coronary vasoconstriction (eg, arguments at home or on the job). The physician should help patients to develop insight into the effects of stress and to learn healthy ways of responding to it. In spite of such efforts, however, acute myocardial infarction may develop without apparent reason at any time.

4. Risk factors–
It is desirable to eliminate or control known risk factors (hyperlipidemia, hypertension, diabetes, cigarette smoking, emotional stress, obesity) that aggravate atherosclerosis. Cigarette smoking, which may precipitate ventricular arrhythmias and sudden death in patients with coronary disease, should be stopped permanently. There is no statistically convincing evidence that physical fitness achieved by exercise programs prolongs life. Weight reduction decreases the work of the heart, and a reducing diet low in calories and animal fats is desirable. Sedatives or tranquilizers may reduce the frequency of attacks but are of only marginal benefit

Table 8–2. General principles of medical treatment of stable angina pectoris.

---

1. Use sublingual nitroglycerin or nifedipine for acute relief when discomfort starts or sublingual or oral isosorbide dinitrate for prevention of attacks or more prolonged effect.
2. Use transdermal nitroglycerin for long-term effect, including nocturnal discomfort.
3. Use beta-blockers to prevent attacks, lower blood pressure, and prevent or treat ventricular arrhythmia; if coronary spasm is present, use calcium entry-blocking agents.
4. Avoid physical and emotional factors that precipitate the pain.
5. Avoid exercise in the presence of other precipitating factors that increase work of the heart (cold weather, heavy meals, emotional upset).
6. Exercise caution in the face of unusual and unaccustomed effort.
7. Reduce work activity (speed of effort, regulation of time, intermittent rest periods).
8. Treat hypertension if present.
9. Treat arrhythmias if present.
10. Treat cardiac failure if present.
11. Stop cigarette smoking.
12. Reduce weight if overweight.
13. Manage adverse emotional responses.
14. Institute supervised physical fitness program (perhaps beneficial).

---

except in hyperactive or emotionally stressed individuals.

B. Treatment of Acute Attack of Angina Pectoris:
(Table 8–2.) (See also Abrams, 1992.) Nitrates and amyl nitrite are the drugs of choice to terminate an acute anginal attack. Nitrates enter the smooth muscle cell and are cleaved to inorganic nitrite, requiring sulfhydryl groups, and then to nitric oxide, which has been identified as endothelium-derived relaxing factor (EDRF). This induces an increase in cyclic guanosine monophosphate (cGMP), which accelerates calcium release from vascular smooth muscle cells and therefore relaxation. Nitrate-induced vasodilation is not endothelium-dependent (Thadani, 1988). Nitrates are available in sublingual tablets, spray, buccal, standard, and slow-release forms; as transcutaneous ointment and as transdermal patch formulations; and for intravenous administration. The choice of drug and dosage depends on the patient's experience. Nitroglycerin must be fresh (replenish supplies every 6 months), kept in a tightly closed glass container, and stored in a refrigerator. A 0.3 mg tablet dissolved sublingually is usually sufficient, but the dose may be increased to 0.4–0.6 mg if needed. A burning sensation on the tongue, flushing, or a headache are to be expected if the drug is active. Transcutaneous nitroglycerin is effective for 8–12 hours and may be valuable in nocturnal angina.

Crushing an amyl nitrite ampule and inhaling the vapor gives relief in 10–45 seconds. Some patients dislike the odor and the attention drawn to them by the procedure. Isosorbide dinitrate, 2.5–10 mg dissolved sublingually, acts somewhat more slowly. (The chewable preparation is irregularly absorbed.) Pentaerythritol tetranitrate has not been much used recently. If these preparations are ineffective even in larger doses or are poorly tolerated, nifedipine, 10 mg sublingually, may be of benefit.

All preparations mentioned (except for nifedipine) have a half-life of less than 10 minutes, and all cause relaxation of vascular smooth muscle. This results in peripheral pooling of blood and decreased venous return, thereby lowering ventricular volume, intraventricular pressure, and cardiac output, causing reduced oxygen demand of the myocardium. Cineangiography can demonstrate decreasing venous return, with relaxation of large veins, decreased cardiac volume, and left ventricular filling pressure and increasing ejection fraction of the left ventricle. Total coronary blood flow does not appear to be increased, but there may be some redistribution of blood flow, eg, vasodilation of epicardial coronary arteries. Coronary artery vasodilation does occur with nitrates, and if there is an intact media with smooth muscle, even high-grade eccentric obstructive lesions may have their lumen size significantly increased, thereby markedly increasing blood flow to ischemic myocardium. This is especially true in response to exercise (Gage, 1986). An additional benefit of nitroglycerin and its production of nitric oxide is that nitric oxide has been shown to be an inhibitor of platelet adhesion under all flow conditions. This could be of particular benefit in preventing platelet adhesion beyond high-grade coronary lesions (de Graaf, 1992).

If patients with angina due to coronary spasm do not respond rapidly to nitrates, coronary vasodilators such as verapamil, diltiazem, or nifedipine may be given not only in Prinzmetal's variant angina but also in the usual angina of effort in which spasm may be superimposed.

The major untoward effects accompanying relief of angina are the result of vasodilation (flushing, dizziness, throbbing headache, tachycardia, faintness [orthostatic hypotension]), and the patient should therefore sit or lie down when using nitrates or amyl nitrite. Obviously, the patient should cease whatever activity brought on the acute attack until the pain is gone. In a few patients, carotid sinus massage or Valsalva's maneuver may provide relief.

C. Management of Chronic Angina Pectoris:

1. Avoidance of precipitating factors– Patient and physician should review carefully the situations causing physical or emotional stress that result in anginal attacks and should make specific plans to avoid or diminish these situations. If this proves unfeasible, drug prophylaxis should be considered. Less obvious precipitating factors are paroxysmal arrhythmias, hypotension, hyperthyroidism, left ventricular outflow obstruction, left ventricular failure, anemia, and obesity. Left ventricular failure may be obvious or incipient, and treatment with digitalis or diuretics (or both) may be helpful.

2. Drug prophylaxis– (Table 8–3.)

a. Nitrates– When undertaking an activity that usually causes acute angina, the patient can prevent angina by use of sublingual nitroglycerin in a dosage known to be effective; prevention, however, is brief. For longer-lasting prevention, nitroglycerin ointment, 1/2–2 inches of 2% ointment placed on a hairless area of skin, can be effective for 3–6 hours. Topical slow-release preparations (5–30 mg), which provide prophylaxis for 6–12 hours and are particularly suitable for nighttime use, are used in the form of transdermal patches of ointment placed on a hairless area of skin and covered by plastic. When this form of medication is discontinued, the dosage must be tapered over a 2-week period. These preparations can increase exercise tolerance and can prevent coronary spasm of variant angina. Side effects include headache and hypotension.

Another longer-lasting nitrate medication is isosorbide dinitrate, 10–30 mg orally every 4–6 hours. When taken at bedtime, this agent tends to prevent nocturnal pain. Tachyphylaxis may result from con-

Table 8–3. Effects of antianginal drugs on myocardial supply and demand.[1]

Index	Nitrates	β-Adrenergic Blockers	Calcium Entry Blockers
Maximum venous oxygen supply			
Coronary resistance	↓↓	→↑	↓↓↓
Left ventricular diastolic pressure on small vessels	↓↓↓	↑	→↓
Coronary collateral circulation	→↑	→	→↑
Diastolic filling period	→↓	↑↑↑	↑↑↑→↓ [2]
Maximum venous oxygen demand			
Left ventricular systolic blood pressure	↓	↓	↓↓
Left ventricular diastolic volume	↓↓↓	↑	↓→
Heart rate	↑→	↓↓↓	↓→↑ [3]
Contractility	↑→	↓↓	↓→↑ [4]

[1] Modified and reproduced, with permission, from McCall D et al: Calcium entry blocking drugs: Mechanisms of action, experimental studies, and clinical uses. Curr Probl Cardiol (O'Rourke RA, editor) 1985; 110 [No. 8]:56.
[2] Depends on drug: verapamil and diltiazem decrease heart rate; nifedipine can reflexly increase heart rate.
[3] Depends on drug: diltiazem and verapamil decrease; nifedipine may increase reflexly.
[4] If decrease in blood pressure leads reflexly to increased adrenergic stimulus, contractility can also increase.

Table 8–4. Oral beta-adrenergic blocking drugs.

Agent	Cardio-selectivity	Intrinsic Sympathetic Activity	Half-Life	Lipid Solubility	Average Daily Dose
Acebutolol	Yes	Yes	3–4 hours	Slight	200–600 mg once or twice daily
Atenolol	Yes	No	6–9 hours	Yes	50–100 mg once daily
Labetalol	No	No	5.5–8 hours	Yes	200–800 mg in two divided doses
Metoprolol	Yes	No	3–6 hours	Yes	50–150 mg in two divided doses
Nadolol	No	No	12–14 hours	No	20–120 mg once daily
Pindolol	No	Yes	3–5 hours	Slight	5–20 mg in two divided doses
Timolol	No	No	4–6 hours	Slight	5–20 mg in two divided doses
Propranolol	No	No	4–6 hours	Moderate	180–240 mg in two or three divided doses

stant nitrate administration, perhaps as a result of diminished availability of sulfhydryl groups, leading to reduced formation of cGMP; rest periods of 12–18 hours may restore effectiveness; to prevent tachyphylaxis, the best dosing regimen for isosorbide is three times daily (Thadani, 1988).

b. Beta-adrenergic-blocking agents– Propranolol, timolol, atenolol, nadolol, metoprolol, and other similar agents are beneficial because of their hemodynamic effects (decreased heart rate, blood pressure, and contractility), all of which decrease myocardial oxygen requirements. They also may prevent cardiac arrhythmias and decrease the likelihood of myocardial infarction or sudden death. Beta-blockers may have antiatherogenic effects with decrease in stress-induced endothelial injury and perhaps stimulation of prostacyclin synthesis. They also have an antithrombotic effect resulting from decreased endothelial injury, reduced platelet deposition, increased prostacyclin synthesis, and perhaps even an increase in fibrinolysis (Olsson, 1990). An adverse effect of beta-blockers on atherogenesis is a tendency to increase low-density lipoproteins.

Beta-blockers have been used for prophylaxis (see Table 8–4). These drugs should not be given to patients with a history of ventricular failure, bronchospasm, or atrioventricular conduction defects. Decreased ejection fraction is no contraindication to the use of beta-blocking drugs. If the patient has had clinical heart failure, beta-blockers should be avoided but still may be useful if started in very small doses (5 mg metoprolol per day) with gradual increase in dose (Lichstein, 1990). (See Chapter 10.) Undesirable effects of beta-blocking agents include slowing of the heart rate, with an increase in end-diastolic volume and an increase in ejection time. These deleterious effects are commonly counteracted by the concomitant use of nitrates.

Among the growing number of beta-blockers, cardioselective drugs may be of wider use because they are less likely to cause bronchospasm. Beta-blockers must not be withdrawn abruptly, because myocardial ischemia or infarction may be precipitated.

c. Calcium entry-blocking agents– Agents of this class (eg, nifedipine, verapamil, diltiazem) inhibit calcium influx and decrease the myocardial contractile force, which in turn reduces myocardial oxygen requirements (see Table 8–5). These agents also decrease arteriolar tone and systemic vascular resistance, resulting in decreased arterial and intraventricular pressure—again reducing myocardial oxygen requirements. They tend to relieve and prevent focal coronary artery spasm; this is important in variant angina, for which they are effective treatment. Calcium blockers are effective in the long-term management of chronic stable angina, with an increase in exercise duration and a significant delay in the onset of effort angina. They are likewise helpful in unstable angina, cardiac arrhythmias, hypertrophic cardiomyopathy, and hypertension. In unstable angina with

Table 8–5. Oral calcium entry-blocking drugs.

	Inhibition of Atrioventricular Conduction	Coronary Vasodilatation	Decreased Inotropic Action	Hypotension, Edema	Dose (Initial; Daily)[1]
Verapamil	+++	++	++	++	40–80 mg; 240–360 mg
Diltiazem	+ to ++	++	+	+	30–60 mg; 180–240 mg
Nifedipine	0 to +	+++	0	+++	20 mg; 40–120 mg

[1] Given in divided doses.

coronary spasm, patients who fail to respond favorably to rest, sedation, nitrates, and beta-blockers may respond to nifedipine (10–20 mg two or three times daily), verapamil (80–120 mg two or three times daily), or diltiazem (30–90 mg two or three times daily). This may permit deferral of invasive diagnostic studies and coronary surgery until conditions have stabilized. However, the three drugs have different hemodynamic and electrophysiologic actions: nifedipine has the greatest vasodilator effect; verapamil has the greatest inhibiting effect on the atrioventricular node; and diltiazem has effects intermediate between these two agents. Vasodilation induced by nifedipine may cause reflex tachycardia that may precipitate angina pectoris; this effect can be prevented, if the patient does not have cardiac failure, by concomitant use of a beta-blocker. The combination must be used with caution because both nifedipine and beta-blockers have negative inotropic effects.

Recently, the anti-ischemic effect of diltiazem and nifedipine has been questioned (Stone, 1990). This study compared propranolol, diltiazem, and nifedipine in the treatment of ambulatory ischemia in patients with stable angina pectoris. The investigators found that the number of anginal attacks was significantly reduced by both diltiazem and propranolol, but the number of ischemic episodes on ambulatory electrocardiography was decreased only with propranolol. Nifedipine had no anti-ischemic effect. Because diltiazem decreased the heart rate less than propranolol and because nifedipine even increased the heart rate, the conclusion was reached that the most important anti-ischemic mechanism of these drugs is reduction of myocardial oxygen consumption (Böhm, 1990; Mitrovic, 1990).

d. Aminophylline– In some patients with incipient left ventricular failure and bronchospasm, aminophylline, 250–500 mg in rectal suppositories, may provide relief of angina and dyspnea.

3. Control of ventricular premature beats and ventricular arrhythmias– Ventricular arrhythmias are common in patients with coronary heart disease. They may occur in one-third to one-half of patients following the ST depression, representing silent ischemia during ambulatory monitoring (Stern, 1992). Arrhythmias may precipitate myocardial ischemia, angina pectoris, and sudden death by decreasing cardiac output and coronary perfusion and inducing ven-

tricular fibrillation. Both ventricular premature beats and the more complex ventricular arrhythmias are more apt to be noted by 24-hour ambulatory electrocardiographic monitoring than by graded exercise. One-third to one-half of patients with no premature ventricular beats (or only one) on a routine ECG show a variety of ventricular premature beats that are frequent, multiform, or early or occur in runs when monitoring is employed. The frequency and complexity of ventricular premature beats is similar in coronary patients with and without a history of myocardial infarction (Table 8–6).

Because most cases of sudden death syndrome are due to ventricular fibrillation often preceded by ventricular premature beats, conventional wisdom has assumed that control of the premature beats may prevent ventricular fibrillation and sudden death. Patients with poor left ventricular function are more likely to have "malignant" ventricular arrhythmias and therefore a significant risk of sudden death. Anti-

Table 8–6. Comparison of the nature of complex ventricular premature complexes (VPCs) during 1 hour of baseline monitoring in coronary heart disease patients with and without prior myocardial infarction (MI).[1]

	Angina Only		Prior MI	
	(n)	(%)	(n)	(%)
Men with any complex form in 1 hour	65	100.0	462	100.0
Qualitative features				
Early VPC (R on T)	12	18.5	83	18.0
Runs of 2 or more VPCs	19	29.2	172	37.2
Early and/or runs	27	41.5	202	43.7
Bigeminy	26	40.0	208	45.0
Multiform VPCs	53	81.5	362	78.4
Multiformity is sole complex feature	28	43.1	158	34.2
Total number of VPCs in 1 hour				
1–9	12	18.5	109	23.6
10 or more	53	81.5	35.3	76.4

[1] Reproduced, with permission, from the American Heart Association, Inc., Ruberman W et al: Ventricular premature complexes in prognosis of angina. Circulation 1980:61:1172.

arrhythmic drugs may decrease ventricular premature beats, but with the exception of beta blockers (see above), it has not been established that they prevent sudden death. The CAST trial, using encainide and flecainide—drugs that were shown to markedly suppress ventricular premature complexes—was terminated when the treatment group was shown to have a significantly higher mortality rate than the placebo group. Moricizine was continued, but even this arm was stopped because of a tendency to increased mortality in the moricizine group compared with the placebo group. The proarrhythmic effect of the drugs presumably negated the antiarrhythmic effect (CAST, 1989).

4. Treatment of hypertension– Episodes of angina are often preceded by rises in blood pressure, and treatment of hypertension may be valuable in these patients (see Chapter 9). Beta-adrenergic and calcium entry blockers may be particularly effective, because they may relieve the symptoms of angina pectoris, lower the blood pressure, and prevent ventricular arrhythmias. Beta-blockers can also be combined with hydralazine in the treatment of hypertension in patients with angina pectoris, in order to prevent the reflex tachycardia that results from the vasodilator.

5. Treatment of cardiac failure if present– (See Chapter 10.)

6. Social and psychologic factors– Knowing that one has "a bad heart" is a heavy psychologic burden, and some patients respond by denial, anger, depression, or regression. Sympathetic listening and discussion are an essential part of good management. The high percentage of patients (50–60%) who report decreased frequency of attacks and decreased need for nitroglycerin when given a placebo attest to the role of emotional factors in increasing the frequency of anginal attacks. An attempt should be made to improve the patient's general emotional health and state of mind. Factors that cause unhappiness, resentment, or hostility should be eliminated if possible. Everyone associated with the patient must be considered as a possible source of emotional stress, including the employer, colleagues at work, spouse, and children. The physician who has a good personal relationship with the patient is in the best position to suggest creative solutions to problems of this sort.

Patients with driving personalities who lead hectic lives must learn to moderate their activities, quit smoking, use alcohol only in moderation, take rest periods in the afternoon and frequent short holidays, and avoid all activities shown by experience to bring on attacks. Rest and relaxation in a totally different environment often produce dramatic results when drugs do not.

7. Anticoagulant therapy– Anticoagulants have been tried, both in patients with angina of effort and in patients who have survived an acute infarction, in order to prevent subsequent infarction and death, but until recently the results have shown only minimal benefit if any. There have been two studies using warfarin—both after acute myocardial infarction—which have shown significant decreases in mortality and reinfarction rates compared with placebo (Sixty Plus Reinfarction Study Research Group, 1980; Smith, 1990). These studies will be discussed in the section on myocardial infarction. There is no indication that anticoagulation is beneficial to patients with angina pectoris if there has been no recent acute myocardial infarction (Jafri, 1991).

8. Antiplatelet therapy– There is excellent evidence that aspirin will reduce the incidence of acute myocardial infarction and death in patients with unstable angina (see Unstable Angina). The ISIS-2 study—in patients admitted with a suspected acute myocardial infarction—showed a decrease in mortality rate equal to the effect of intravenous streptokinase and additive to it (see Acute Myocardial Infarction).

In patients with angina pectoris or after recovery from myocardial infarction—or in primary prevention of coronary events—the evidence of benefit has been less impressive. Only the PARIS-II study of 3128 patients after acute myocardial infarction—starting aspirin and dipyridamole 1–6 months after the infarction—showed a significant reduction (24%) in combined cardiac deaths or nonfatal myocardial infarction (11.8% placebo to 9.0% drug). There was no significant difference in all-cause mortality (Klimt, 1986).

The Physicians Health Study and a study by Peto in the United Kingdom tested aspirin versus placebo in a primary prevention trial in men. Both trials showed no differences in overall mortality, but in the Physicians Health study there was a 44% decrease in myocardial infarction in men over 55 years of age (Steering Committee of the Physicians Health Study Research Group, 1989; Peto, 1988). A subgroup of 333 men in the Physicians Health Study had stable angina pectoris but no previous myocardial infarction. After controlling for other risk factors, it was concluded that the patients taking aspirin every other day had an overall 87% reduction in risk for developing a myocardial infarction compared with the group taking placebo ($P < .001$) (Ridker, 1991).

A meta-analysis of 31 randomized trials of a variety of antiplatelet therapies of about 29,000 patients with ischemic vascular disease showed an overall decrease in vascular mortality of 15% and in nonfatal vascular events, including stroke and myocardial infarction, of 30% (Antiplatelet Trialists' Collaboration, 1988). There is no evidence favoring a particular dose of aspirin or any other antiplatelet drug such as sulfinpyrazone or dipyridamole. For this reason, it is recommended that patients with known coronary artery disease take 325 mg of aspirin per day or every other day.

9. Increased physical activity– Because of the beneficial physiologic and psychologic effects associated with greater fitness, patients often feel better while in an exercise program, but there is no convincing evidence that it prevents coronary disease. A planned program of daily exercise may not prevent myocardial infarction and death. The same degree of exercise that is well within the bounds of tolerance in the laboratory or on a pleasant day may not be tolerated under less favorable circumstances.

10. Referral for coronary angiography and possible surgery– See Coronary Heart Surgery, below, for indications for coronary bypass surgery or percutaneous transluminal coronary angioplasty (PTCA) in patients who have unacceptable angina pectoris.

11. Preparation for survival–

a. Education of family– When an attack occurs, the patient should be taken promptly to a nearby hospital with good coronary care facilities unless mobile ambulance crews trained in resuscitation are readily available.

b. Education of lay people and ambulance crews– Various communities provide physician and lay educational programs in order to minimize the time between onset of symptoms of a coronary event and hospitalization. Emergency paramedics and medical technicians in specially equipped ambulances and fire department personnel with rescue vehicles have been taught to recognize arrhythmias, to accomplish defibrillation, and to inject drugs such as atropine and lidocaine. Good prehospital care of this kind in patients with angina can be lifesaving.

Prognosis

A. Overall Mortality Rate: The overall mortality rate of patients with stable angina varies from 0.3% to 8% per year, averaging 4% (Frank, 1973). The influence of congestive heart failure and hypertension is shown in Figure 8–15. Factors adversely influencing survival include complex arrhythmias, easily induced myocardial ischemia, large perfusion or contraction abnormalities, low ejection fraction, and left main coronary artery disease. Sudden death is usually seen in patients with multivessel coronary disease. When sudden death occurs in patients with single-vessel disease, it most frequently involves the left anterior descending coronary artery. In general, mortality is related to the amount of left ventricular myocardium that either is nonfunctioning or may become nonfunctioning because of continued ischemia.

The causes of death are listed in Table 8–7. Note that one-third of the deaths are sudden deaths.

B. Role of Coronary Artery Anatomy: Angina is often the initial manifestation of coronary disease, and the prognosis depends chiefly on the extent of disease of the coronary arteries (Figure 8–16) and the left ventricular function. The mortality rate is higher when left ventricular function is impaired. Three-vessel disease with diffuse left ventricular functional abnormalities with a low ejection fraction was found

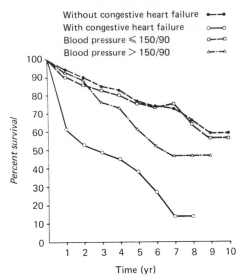

Figure 8–15. Survival with coronary artery disease related to heart failure and blood pressure. (Reproduced, with permission of the American Heart Association, Inc., from Burggraf GW, Parker JO: Prognosis in coronary artery disease: Angiographic, hemodynamic, and clinical factors. Circulation 1975;51:146.)

by Sheldon (1975) to have an almost 100% 5-year mortality rate, whereas 3-vessel disease with normal left ventricular function had a 35% 5-year mortality rate. Most deaths occur in the year following the onset of myocardial infarction.

Another means of estimating the severity of coronary disease involves recognition of the extent of coronary calcification by fluoroscopy in one, two, or three vessels (Margolis, 1980) and now by ultrafast CT (Agatston, 1990).

C. Importance of Previous Myocardial Infarction: Patients presenting with angina pectoris may have had a previous myocardial infarction that either was silent or coincided with the onset of angina. The mortality rate of such patients is higher than that of

Table 8–7. Causes of death in patients with stable angina pectoris.[1]

Cause	Number	Percent of Deaths
Noncardiac	8	11
Sudden (outside hospital)	24	34
Chronic congestive heart failure	10	14
Acute myocardial infarction		
Arrhythmia	16	23
Pump failure	13	18
TOTAL	71	100

[1] Reproduced, with permission, from the American Heart Association, Inc., Burggraf GW, Parker JO: Prognosis in coronary artery disease: Angiographic, hemodynamic, and clinical factors. Circulation 1975;51:146.

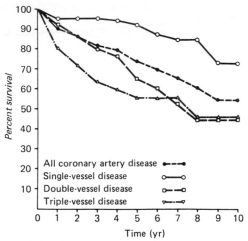

Figure 8–16. Survival related to extent of coronary artery involvement. (Reproduced, with permission of the American Heart Association, Inc., from Burggraf GW, Parker JO: Prognosis in coronary artery disease: Angiographic, hemodynamic, and clinical factors. Circulation 1975 51:146.)

patients who have not had a previous myocardial infarction. Patients who have had a previous myocardial infarction with diffuse fibrosis from healed ischemic areas often have evidence of left ventricular failure; in these patients, the 2-year mortality rate is 40–50% regardless of the number of vessels involved. Patients with orthopnea and paroxysmal nocturnal dyspnea have enlarged hearts and an unfavorable prognosis.

The anatomic changes revealed by coronary arteriography show that the most hazardous lesion is stenosis of the left main coronary artery and then (in decreasing order of risk) the left anterior descending, the left circumflex, and the right coronary artery. Patients with stenosis of the left main coronary artery have at least twice the mortality rate over a period of 1–3 years of those with equivalent stenoses in the other two vessels.

D. Need for Better Definition of Stenosis: Better methods are needed to define precisely the location and degree of stenosis and the amount of blood flow across stenotic coronary vessels. There appears to be little practical advantage to using digital-based densitometry rather than hand-held calipers in evaluating the degree of coronary stenosis (Theron, 1990). Intravascular ultrasound, using a wire with an echo-Doppler chip through a coronary catheter, can image in great detail the lumen and wall of the coronary artery; the intima and the media can be differentiated. Atheromatous plaques can be visualized in detail, including surface characteristics, the depth into the wall that they extend, and the presence of thrombus or platelet aggregations on their surface.

The clinical use intravascular ultrasound is still evolving (Tobis, 1991). Using this technique, local coronary blood flow can also be estimated, and by injecting a vasodilator and observing the increase in flow as measured by velocity, an index of coronary vascular resistance reserve is possible.

Angioscopy is another exciting new technique now being developed (Mizuno, 1992). By directly visualizing the lumen after flushes of saline, atherosclerotic plaques can be observed directly. Ramee (1991) described coronary angioscopy before and after angioplasty. They found a high prevalence of thrombus and plaque dissection in patients with unstable angina, infrequently detected by angiography.

E. Assumption of Coronary Disease With Normal Angiograms: Possible explanations of normal coronary arteriograms in the presence of what is considered to be definite angina pectoris or a clear history of myocardial infarction include improper technique, errors of interpretation, small-vessel coronary disease, recanalization of a previously thrombosed single coronary artery, previous prolonged coronary spasm, or lysis of a previous embolus or thrombus (Michaelson, 1977).

About 5–10% of patients with recurrent myocardial infarction are believed to have had angina pectoris in spite of normal coronary angiograms. One must always exclude vasculitis and arteritis as the cause of angina in patients with normal coronary angiograms. Rheumatic disease, connective tissue disorders, and syphilis involving coronary arteries must be excluded as causes of vasculitis.

UNSTABLE ANGINA PECTORIS

The foregoing discussion pertained to stable angina of effort, in which condition patients can relate frequency of angina to effort expended, emotional state, weather, and meals, and the occurrence of attacks is relatively predictable within a broad range of activities. Intermediate between this stable angina and acute myocardial infarction is a clinical state variously referred to as unstable angina, acute coronary insufficiency, and preinfarction angina.

Definition of Unstable Angina

Patients with unstable angina are not a homogeneous group but can be divided into several subgroups. This may explain the widely differing estimates of prognosis in these patients.

The usual condition is **crescendo** or **progressive angina,** in which a patient known to have had stable angina of effort (1) develops angina on less exertion, (2) develops angina at rest or during sleep, (3) has pain with a somewhat different duration or radiation, (4) has pain that is not relieved as promptly with nitroglycerin as before, or (5) has angina that gradually worsens over a period of days and in many instances develops into acute myocardial infarction. However, infarction often does not follow. Some patients with unstable angina have already had a small myocardial infarction. Its divergent features in patient subgroups may explain the different mortality rates in unstable angina. Angina that occurs for the first time in a patient is also considered unstable because it may result in acute myocardial infarction. However, the patient with first-time angina is more likely to have one-vessel disease than is the patient with chronic stable angina. Unless it occurs at rest and requires hospitalization, first-time angina has a better prognosis than does angina that progresses to pain at rest or is of the crescendo type and recurs at increasingly shorter intervals or lesser degree of effort or lasts longer. Angina at rest without provocation has the worst prognosis, especially if associated with ST segment changes. Rest angina, especially with ST depression, is the most predictive of the various clinical presentations to have a poor prognosis (Gazes, 1973).

Pathophysiology of Unstable Angina

The pathophysiology of unstable angina is uncertain when aggravating factors such as arrhythmias, cardiac failure, and anemia are excluded. Coronary occlusion or near occlusion due to subintimal hemorrhage or rupture of an atherosclerotic plaque, clumping of platelets or fibrin, or coronary spasm may be involved. Angioscopy by direct vision at the time of surgery has revealed ruptured plaques with hemorrhage and incomplete thrombosis in unstable but not in stable angina (Sherman, 1986). Reduced regional coronary blood flow is the mechanism for rest angina; this can be due to increased metabolic demands or to decreased flow caused by coronary obstruction or spasm but in most cases is probably due to a fracture in the fibrous atheromatous cap with platelet aggregation and thrombus formation.

Most patients with unstable angina and chest pain at rest have coronary obstruction, but about one-third have decreased coronary blood flow due at least in part to coronary vasoconstriction. With platelet aggregation and activation, vasoactive substances such as serotonin and thromboxane A_2 are released that are vasoconstrictors in the absence of normal endothelium (Golino, 1991). Many episodes of such pain are associated with ST elevation and decreased left ventricular wall motion. In these episodes, Chierchia (1983) found no changes in pulse or blood pressure prior to the pain and the heart rate-blood pressure product was not altered, indicating that myocardial oxygen demand was not increased. The National Cooperative Study Group to Compare Surgical and Medical Therapy (Russell, 1980) in unstable angina found that two-thirds of patients with unstable angina had ST depression during chest pain and about one-third had ST elevation.

Coronary arteriography in patients with unstable angina reveals that 40–60% have multivessel disease, 10–15% have a left main coronary lesion, 20–30% have single-vessel disease (frequently the left anterior descending coronary), and 10% have no significant obstruction (Conti, 1973; Weiner, 1987). The coronary angiographic findings vary with the population studied. In a study comparing the angiographic findings in patients with unstable angina, some of whom had no previous history of angina or myocardial infarction versus those with such a history, the group with new-onset unstable angina without a preceding history of angina or myocardial infarction had more subjects with single-vessel disease (43% versus 27%) and fewer with three-vessel disease (23% versus 35%) (Roberts, 1983). Ambrose (1986) described the angiographic morphology of coronary lesions in patients with unstable angina as eccentric lesions with overhanging edges, jagged borders, or both as common configurations. Williams (1988), performing coronary arteriography within 5 days after onset of the discomfort in 101 consecutive patients with unstable angina, described complex morphology in 61% and thrombus alone in 27% of patients. The presence of complex morphology and thrombus was associated with an increased number of coronary events such as myocardial infarction, death, or need for revascularization. This is supported by other studies (Bugiardini, 1991). The morphology of the lesion, which can be determined only by coronary arteriography, may have prognostic importance, and this is one argument for early coronary arteriography in unstable angina.

Classification & Symptoms of Unstable Angina

It is logical to subdivide unstable angina as follows: (1) initial angina that promptly subsides with bed rest, which has a relatively good prognosis; (2) initial angina that continues despite bed rest and medical treatment; (3) crescendo angina in patients with previous stable angina; (4) angina at rest or during sleep; and (5) angina that changes in character and duration.

A. Puzzling Diagnosis of Unstable Angina: When unstable angina is the first manifestation of coronary disease, the diagnosis can be very puzzling because there is no history of angina of effort. Often the patient states that effort does not induce pain but that pain occurs at unpredictable times during periods of rest. But the quality of the discomfort is typical of ischemic pain.

B. Possible Presence of Unproved Myocardial Infarction: Radioisotope imaging may help identify areas of myocardial necrosis in this group of patients (see Chapter 5). *Discrete* resting hypoperfusion defects with thallium-201 or sestamibi indicate a myocardial infarction. *Diffuse* hypoperfusion occurs with unstable angina and should not be used to diagnose infarction.

C. Hazards of Unstable Angina: The develop-

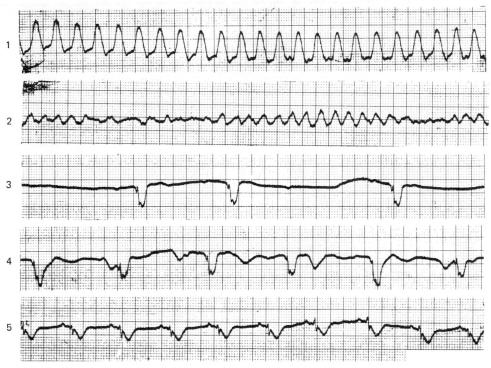

Figure 8–17. Sequential changes after cardiac arrest in a 55-year-old woman with unstable angina: Strip 1 shows ventricular tachycardia. Strip 2 shows ventricular fibrillation. Strip 3 shows idioventricular rhythm after defibrillation. Strip 4 shows ventricular premature beats. Strip 5 shows sinus rhythm. (Courtesy of K Gershengorn.)

ment of unstable angina should be thought of as a sign of an increase in coronary artery obstruction due to a change in an atherosclerotic plaque, which for a period of time will have an increased risk of sudden occlusion by spasm or thrombus. The possibility of development of an acute myocardial infarction within the next few hours, days, or weeks after the development of unstable angina makes it a hazardous manifestation of ischemic heart disease. Acute myocardial infarction or sudden cardiac death occurs in 10–15% of unstable angina patients on follow-up (Mulcahy, 1985). The mortality rate of acute myocardial infarction is greatest in the first few hours (see Acute Myocardial Infarction); therefore, it is prudent to monitor all patients with unstable angina in a coronary care unit for at least 2 days both because they might be developing a myocardial infarction that can become obvious at any time and because unstable angina may be associated with serious ventricular arrhythmias requiring immediate care (Figure 8–17). Restriction of all activity and appropriate medication (see below) may turn the tide, and infarction may be prevented.

Treatment

A. Medical Therapy: The goals of treatment are to increase blood flow to the myocardium, relieve pain, prevent myocardial infarction, and enhance survival. With unstable angina, the goals of therapy are to control the major determinants of oxygen demand, decreased platelet and fibrin aggregation, and coronary spasm. If the coronary arteries are severely stenotic, an ordinary stimulus causing a small degree of vasoconstriction or minor changes in cardiac work can cause intermittent ischemia. If transdermal or sublingual nitrates do not relieve pain, give nitroglycerin intravenously in an initial dose of 5 μg/min, increased by 5 μg increments at 2- to 5-minute intervals until pain is relieved or systolic pressure decreases by 20 mm Hg. The average maximal rate of infusion is about 50 μg/min.

Vigorous medical therapy with bed rest, nitrates, beta-adrenergic and calcium entry-blocking agents as well as other vasodilator therapy should be used, because in many patients with unstable angina but without infarction the acute process subsides. This probably occurs as a result of stabilization of the disrupted atherosclerotic plaque.

Beta-blockers reduce myocardial oxygen consumption and metabolic demands. They do not cause dilation of the large coronary arteries and do not prevent ergonovine-induced spasm. Begin with 20 mg of propranolol or its equivalent with atenolol or metoprolol and increase the total daily dosage to 300 mg/d in divided doses every 4 hours until bradycardia (< 50 beats/min) or hypotension (< 90–100 mm Hg systolic) occurs. An ultra-short-acting beta-blocker such as esmolol, a rapidly metabolized cardioselective beta-adrenergic blocker administered by continuous intravenous infusion has been used. This is especially useful if there is a relative contraindication to the use of beta-blockers such as a past history of congestive heart failure, since the hemodynamic effects of the esmolol are reversed within 30 minutes after cessation of infusion (Wallis, 1988).

Calcium entry blockers do cause dilation of the large coronary and other large arteries and prevent ergonovine-induced spasm. (Maseri, 1983) For angina at rest, calcium entry-blocking agents are superior to beta-blockers; nifedipine can be given, 10 mg three times a day. Side effects of calcium entry blockers are headache, peripheral edema, constipation, hypotension, and dizziness. Verapamil should be used with caution if the ejection fraction is less than 30%. The combination of a beta-blocker and a calcium entry blocker may be more effective than either alone. Unfortunately, neither beta-adrenergic blockers nor calcium entry blockers, although they are effective in reducing or abolishing episodes of angina, have been shown to significantly reduce mortality or progression to myocardial infarction (Cohen, 1989).

Activity should be restricted. Recurrent pain at rest lasting 10–15 minutes and requiring opiates occurs in about 20% of patients despite full medical treatment. Aspirin and heparin have been shown to be effective in reducing nonfatal myocardial infarction and death in unstable angina patients. Aspirin was reported to decrease the incidence of acute myocardial infarction and the mortality rate by 50% in a 12-week trial in patients with unstable angina. There was no increase in bleeding complications in aspirin-treated patients (Lewis, 1983). Cairns (1985) randomized patients to aspirin 1300 mg/d, sulfinpyrazone 800 mg/d, a combination of the two, and placebo. After a mean follow-up time of 1 1/2 years, they found about a 50% reduction in deaths due to myocardial infarction and nonfatal myocardial infarctions in the patients taking aspirin.

In the PARIS-II study (Klimt, 1986), in non-Q wave myocardial infarction—a syndrome closely related to unstable angina—aspirin plus dipyridamole were used in secondary prevention; there was a 53% reduction in deaths and coronary events compared with placebo.

Theroux (1988), in a placebo-controlled trial, compared aspirin, heparin, and, for the first time, the combination of the two with either alone. There was a 50% reduction in cardiac events in the patients taking aspirin or heparin. The study was too small to identify one antithrombotic regimen as better than another (Theroux, 1988).

These studies all have limitations. The Lewis study had difficulties with precise diagnosis of unstable angina, and 81.7% of patients meeting the original diagnostic criteria were excluded. In the high-dose aspirin trial, there was a high percentage of withdrawal for side-effects, and in the heparin trial almost half of the patients had to have PTCA within 6 months. Despite these objections, the data are strong enough to recommend immediate institution of aspirin, 325 mg/d, the first one chewed, or heparin (or both) in all patients with unstable angina.

A Veterans Administration multicenter, randomized, prospective study compared intensive medical therapy with coronary bypass surgery (followed by medical therapy) in men with unstable angina. The 2-year survival rate did not differ between the two groups, though a subgroup with significantly reduced ejection fraction prior to surgery had a reduced mortality rate with surgery. The operative mortality rate was 4.1%. The rate of crossover from medical to surgical therapy after 2 years was 34% (Luchi, 1987). It thus does not appear to be necessary to consider revascularization as the first approach in patients with unstable angina without first employing medical management.

B. More Aggressive Therapy: If it becomes clear that medical treatment is ineffective after 24–48 hours, an aggressive approach can be initiated. Intra-aortic balloon pumping controlled by hemodynamic monitoring may decrease myocardial ischemia and relieve angina, but technical difficulties and later problems from the leg in which the balloon was introduced must be considered. Intravenous nitroglycerin often controls the symptoms, but they may recur when the drug is stopped. When stabilization occurs, one can proceed to coronary arteriography, and if the stenotic lesions are anatomically suitable, coronary bypass surgery or percutaneous transluminal angioplasty can be performed. Early surgical treatment is confined to the 10–20% of cases that fail to respond to maximum medical treatment; nifedipine or other calcium entry-blocking agents relieve rest angina in 75% of those patients who fail to get relief with nitrates and beta-blockers.

Because of the frequency with which angina recurs in patients with crescendo or unstable angina after discharge from the hospital, exercise electrocardiography and possibly radionuclide studies are usually performed just before discharge at 7–14 days. If early, markedly positive ischemic ST changes or complex ventricular arrhythmias are found, coronary arteriography is recommended with a view to performing revascularization. Patients with multivessel disease and evidence of ischemia are usually referred for coronary bypass surgery.

Coronary angioplasty (PTCA) has been used but confined to the vessel responsible for the severe ischemia; any other lesions have been left alone. Since there is a higher risk of complications if PTCA is done early after onset of unstable angina, an attempt is made to treat medically and to delay PTCA for 48–

72 hours. Most patients have had relief of angina, increase in functional capacity, and objective improvement in previously ischemic myocardium, as seen with exercise electrocardiographic testing and thallium-201 images.

Employing this strategy, de Feyter et al (1988) reported revascularization in 422 patients with unstable angina. PTCA was done in 200 patients with success—as defined by improvement in clinical signs of ischemia—and successful dilation of the lesion was obtained in 89.5% of cases. Complications occurred in 10.5%, with death in 0.5%, myocardial infarction in 8%, and need for urgent coronary bypass surgery in 9%. After 1 year there was angiographic evidence of restenosis in one-third of the patients.

Since thrombus is not infrequently seen in patients with unstable angina, the question of thrombolysis has been raised. No conclusive evidence is available that thrombolysis benefits these patients. If thrombus is seen on coronary arteriography, treatment with thrombolysis might be beneficial (Ambrose, 1989).

Prognosis

The prognosis of unstable angina is controversial because of the difficulties of definition discussed above. The outcome is influenced by (1) the extent and nature of the anatomic disease in the coronary arteries, (2) the presence or absence of a previous myocardial infarction or multiple areas of wall motion abnormalities, including fibrosis; (3) the existence of acute myocardial infarction, which may be suggested by ST segment abnormalities, new Q waves, or an increase in serum enzymes by serial determination; and (4) other factors such as cardiac failure, ventricular arrhythmias, and hypertension or hypotension.

The imbalance between supply and demand of oxygen, even at rest, is precarious, and myocardial ischemia and myocardial necrosis can be imminent if demands are even slightly raised, as after meals or during bathing or defecating.

The natural history of unstable angina has been changed by both medical management and revascularization. Before beta-blockers were introduced, the 1-year mortality rate in patients with severe rest angina and electrocardiographic changes was estimated to be 40%. With progressive angina, the annual mortality rate was much lower, between 2% and 5% (Gazes, 1973; Patterson, 1988).

A. Differentiation of Unstable Angina and Myocardial Infarction: It may be very difficult to differentiate unstable angina from myocardial infarction that is already present. In a patient with prolonged or rest pain, infarction must be ruled out by the absence of ischemic changes in the ST–T segment, the absence of serum enzyme elevations, and the absence of discrete increased uptake on radioisotopic imaging with technetium ^{99m}Tc pyrophosphate. Serum enzyme measurements and myocardial imaging may demonstrate that infarction has already occurred in some patients in whom the ECG failed to show infarction.

B. Prospective Studies to Establish Prognosis: Accurate prognosis is particularly important because it influences the choice of therapy. There is a need to establish the prognosis for sharply defined subgroups. At present, the mixing of different subgroups in reported series results in widely differing estimates.

C. Effect of Treatment on Prognosis: The prognosis of unstable angina is influenced by the treatment given. It is not reasonable to compare the outcome in patients who are ambulatory and at work with others who are at strict bed rest.

The evidence is not convincing that survival rates are improved by treating unstable angina as an acute surgical emergency. In most cases, symptoms are relieved by medical treatment. Immediate revascularization should be performed if angina at rest continues despite vigorous medical management.

If medical management eliminates angina, the patient should be risk-stratified at 7–14 days by stress testing with or without thallium-201 or sestamibi and a decision made for revascularization on the basis of ventricular function and the magnitude of areas of residual ischemia.

ACUTE MYOCARDIAL INFARCTION

In myocardial infarction, there is ischemic necrosis of a variable amount of myocardial tissue as a result of an abrupt acute decrease in coronary flow or an equivalent abrupt increase in myocardial demand for oxygen that cannot be supplied by an obstructed coronary artery. Coronary flow may be impaired by a thrombus in one of the coronary arteries, by hemorrhage within or beneath an atherosclerotic plaque, or by coronary vasoconstriction or spasm. Decreased coronary flow may be due to shock, dehydration, or hemorrhage, leading to poor perfusion of all tissues, including the myocardium. Rapid ventricular rates due to ventricular tachycardia or uncontrolled atrial fibrillation may also contribute to myocardial ischemia because of the decreased diastolic filling time. Transient temporary ischemia is reversible, but persistent ischemia (approximately 1 hour) results in gradual necrosis spreading from the subendocardial area toward the epicardium.

The site and extent of necrosis depend upon the degree of occlusion of the coronary artery, the disproportion between flow and demand resulting from the anatomic distribution of stenoses within the coronary vessels, the adequacy of the collateral circulation between neighboring coronary arteries, and the presence and extent of previous infarctions. The infarct may involve the full thickness of the myocardium from endocardium to epicardium (transmural infarction) or may be confined to the subendocardium (nontransmural, non-Q wave, subendocardial infarction). An infarct is usually caused by a thrombus in the coronary artery overlying a fractured or ulcerated atherosclerotic plaque in the distribution of acute myocardial infarction (DeWood, 1980). Acute myocardial infarction may occur from other causes such as acute hypotension or coronary spasm with or without thrombosis. Coronary occlusion and acute myocardial infarction are independent entities. A thrombus may occlude a branch of the coronary artery without producing myocardial infarction. Conversely, infarction may occur in the absence of coronary thrombosis. One must keep in mind the three distinct entities: (1) coronary atherosclerosis (a pathologic finding that may or may not be associated with coronary heart disease), (2) coronary thrombosis, and (3) myocardial infarction.

Although infarction of the left ventricle is usually assumed when one refers to myocardial infarction, right ventricular infarction is not rare and is usually associated with the inferior myocardial infarction resulting from occlusion of the right coronary artery.

The left anterior descending artery is most commonly occluded; this results in infarction of the anteroseptal portion of the left ventricle. Less commonly, occlusion of the right coronary artery leads to infarction of the inferior and posterior left ventricle. Least common is occlusion of the left circumflex artery, producing anterolateral myocardial infarction. When complete occlusion of the left main coronary artery occurs, massive infarction of the left ventricle often results. Decrease in coronary flow in occlusive disease of the coronary artery usually implies occlusion of at least 80% of the diameter of the artery. A lesser degree of coronary stenosis may increase coronary resistance, preventing the required coronary flow increases during exercise (Klocke, 1983).

Premonitory Manifestations

Reports of premonitory symptoms such as weakness, shortness of breath, and vague chest discomfort days or weeks before the event in 50–75% of patients with acute myocardial infarction indicate the presence of progressive myocardial ischemia, suggesting that the onset is not as "unexpected" as was once thought.

Clinical Findings

A. Symptoms:

1. Pain– Pain is the classic dominant feature of acute myocardial infarction that compels the patient to seek help. It is similar in quality to angina pectoris and may be described as a heaviness or tightness or a great weight sitting on the chest rather than as pain. The pain is similar to angina of effort in location and radiation, but it may radiate more widely. Not only may it radiate more widely to the lower jaw and teeth,

neck, left shoulder, upper back, or down the left arm to the two fingers innervated by the ulnar nerve (as with angina of effort), but it may also involve the upper posterior thoracic area, and the patient may think there is an orthopedic problem. The pain is more severe than that of angina of effort, does not subside with rest, builds up rapidly, may wax and wane, and may reach maximum severity in a few minutes. Nitroglycerin has little or no effect. The pain may last for hours if unrelieved by narcotics and may be unbearable. The severity of chest pain is not related to the severity or size of the infarct, and the physician must not be misled into considering the event a minor one because the symptoms are not devastating. Myocardial infarction can occur without any pain or discomfort (Maseri, 1992). The incidence of "silent" or unrecognized nonfatal myocardial infarctions found on subsequent routine ECGs was 25% in the Framingham study.

2. Systemic manifestations– An indirect measure of the amount of necrotic tissue is the magnitude of the systemic response to acute infarction as evidenced by fever, tachycardia, leukocytosis, and increase in the sedimentation rate. These systemic signs of tissue necrosis usually appear 24–48 hours after the onset of the initial pain and are related to the amount of tissue that has undergone necrosis.

Because necrosis appears 24–48 hours after the initial onset of pain, the temperature course follows this time interval. Substantial fever that is present at onset of pain or occurs after the fifth or sixth day should raise the question of some independent cause of fever. Patients with pulmonary infarction, for example, may have fever on the day of onset of chest pain, whereas in acute myocardial infarction the fever is delayed.

3. Sweating, weakness, and apprehension– The patient often breaks out into a cold sweat, feels weak and apprehensive, and moves about, seeking a position of comfort—in contrast to the discomfort of angina of effort, in which the patient's instinct is to stand still or to sit or lie down.

4. Light-headedness, dyspnea, and hypotension– In association with the pain and sweating, the patient may feel weak, faint, and light-headed. Syncope may occur if there is a rapid onset of ventricular tachycardia or fibrillation or an atrioventricular conduction defect with a Stokes-Adams attack. Syncope and manifestation of cerebral infarction are presumably the effects of decreased cardiac output on a compromised carotid or cerebral arterial supply to the brain.

The presence or absence of pain is important in evaluating the significance of hypotension, especially at the onset of acute myocardial infarction. The vasomotor response to acute pain is hypertension in some individuals but abrupt decrease in cardiac output and vasodilation in muscles and skin in others, resulting in hypotension with poor tissue perfusion manifested by cold, clammy skin; a gray appearance; sighing respirations; tachycardia; and low blood pressure. These signs must not be taken as evidence of cardiogenic shock until pain is relieved by appropriate medication (see below).

Ventricular arrhythmias in the first few hours after an acute infarction may cause hypotension aggravated by the pain and fear engendered by the infarct. There is marked activation of the sympathetic nervous system with the onset of acute myocardial infarction; sharp increases in serum levels of catecholamines are arrhythmogenic. The myocardium often responds to acute ischemia with variable electrophysiologic changes of excitability and refractoriness, increased vulnerability to ventricular ectopia, and ventricular fibrillation.

5. Nausea, vomiting, and "indigestion"– Nausea and vomiting are not rare. The discomfort may extend into the epigastrium and be associated with sensations of indigestion and bloating, so that the patient takes antacids for supposed acute indigestion, but without benefit.

6. Pulmonary edema and left ventricular failure– In 10–20% of cases, the pain is minor or entirely absent and may be misinterpreted or overshadowed—especially in elderly or diabetic patients — by the presence of acute pulmonary edema, rapidly developing left ventricular failure, profound weakness, shock, dyspnea, or cough or wheezing of acute left ventricular failure.

7. Retrospective diagnosis– In perhaps 10% of cases, the initial symptoms are mild enough so that the diagnosis is only recognized in retrospect, when an ECG is taken months later. This is particularly true in patients with autonomic nervous system dysfunction due to diabetes mellitus and in the elderly. The patient may fail to realize that myocardial infarction has occurred, because the pain lasts only 30 minutes and is unrelated to effort, with onset at rest or even during sleep. A patient with previous angina of effort will recognize the unusual features, particularly the severity, radiation, and duration of the discomfort and its failure to respond to nitroglycerin; however, a patient who has not had angina of effort may interpret the discomfort as indigestion or musculoskeletal disease or may merely complain of feeling unwell.

B. Signs: The signs of acute myocardial infarction may be trivial, or the patient may be at the point of death when first seen. The clinical picture is related to the size and extent of the infarction, the presence of previous infarction with left ventricular dysfunction, and the adequacy of the collateral circulation.

1. Initial signs– The initial signs may be more severe than those found 1–2 hours later, especially if the patient has had a ventricular arrhythmia, marked bradycardia with poor output, or abrupt left ventricular failure that subsided as compensatory reflex mechanisms came into play.

2. Signs in mild cases– In mild cases the patient may appear well, with dry skin, normal pulse and blood pressure, and complaining only of prolonged substernal discomfort.

3. Signs in more severe cases– In more severe cases the patient appears acutely ill and may have marked hypotension with low cardiac output; tachycardia; cold, clammy, sweaty skin; and a gray (ashen) appearance due to peripheral cyanosis. If cerebral perfusion is impaired, the patient may be mentally dull and confused and may have either tachycardia or bradycardia. The cardiac findings may be only an S_4 gallop or may include an S_3 gallop, a paradoxically split S_2, or the murmur of mitral regurgitation. At the onset of acute myocardial infarction, the temperature is usually normal. Fever is delayed for 24-72 hours and is due to myocardial necrosis, which takes time to develop.

4. Combination of shock and cardiac failure– A patient with clinically apparent shock with a systolic pressure less than 80 mm Hg and a urine output less than 20 mL/h may show signs of left ventricular failure with an S_3 gallop rhythm, pulsus alternans, and bilateral rales. The gallop and rales may remain the same or rapidly progress to acute pulmonary edema or right-sided congestive heart failure. The chest x-ray confirms left ventricular failure by haziness in the central lung fields (caused by transudation into the alveoli) or redistribution of flow to the upper lobe (if there is interstitial edema). Kerley B lines may also occur after some days but may be out of phase with the clinical signs, and there may be hemodynamic evidence of raised pulmonary artery diastolic pressure. Although the radiologic signs lag behind the hemodynamic ones, x-ray offers valuable evidence of cardiac failure, especially when raised wedge pressure is present.

The systemic venous pressure may be raised as shown by examination of the neck veins; and when hemodynamic studies are done, the right atrial pressure is elevated. With fever, perspiration, decreased fluid intake, and even vomiting. hypovolemia may result, in which instance the right atrial pressure is low and volume repletion is indicated.

Right ventricular infarction must be considered in patients with inferior myocardial infarction who have right ventricular failure with raised systemic venous pressure, low cardiac output and hypotension, but little evidence of left ventricular failure. The right atrial pressure is often higher than the wedge pressure. There is frequently right-sided S_4 or S_3 gallop along the left sternal border, and on electrocardiography the ST segment elevation occurs in right-sided V leads as well as V_1 and V_2. Hypokinesis or akinesis localized to the right ventricle (on two-dimensional echocardiography or gated blood pool angiography) and abnormal radionuclide uptake localized to the right ventricle aid in the diagnosis. Recognition is important because diuretic therapy is inadvisable and prognosis is better than when right ventricular failure complicates left ventricular failure from anterior infarction.

C. Laboratory Findings:

1. White count and erythrocyte sedimentation rate– The white blood count and sedimentation rate are normal at onset and rise with the fever as myocardial necrosis occurs. As the necrotic area of myocardium extends toward the epicardium, pericarditis may be recognized by pericardial friction rub, but this is often delayed until at least the second day and is transient, usually lasting not more than 2–4 days, and may be intermittent. If the pericardial friction rub occurs within 24 hours after the onset of pain, the diagnosis is more likely to be pericarditis than acute myocardial infarction. High fever and leukocytosis indicate extensive infarction in the absence of pneumonia or other diseases. The sedimentation rate often remains elevated for 2–3 weeks after the white blood count and temperature have returned to normal.

2. Myocardial enzymes– With necrosis of cells, myocardial enzymes appear in the serum. The myocardial band (MB) isoenzymes of creatine kinase (CK) are found within 6 hours. These isoenzymes are derived exclusively from myocardial cells, as compared with the total CK, which may enter the serum from muscle, brain, liver, small bowel, or uterus (Figure 8–18). Small amounts of the MB isoenzymes may be found in these tissues. Serum glutamic-oxaloacetic transaminase (SGOT; also knows as aspartate transaminase [AST]) may not rise for 6–12 hours and returns to normal in 5–7 days; CK reaches its peak concentration in the serum in 18–24 hours and is usually normal in 3–4 days. Serum lactate dehydrogenase (LDH) takes longer to rise—about 24 hours—peaks at 3 days, and may remain elevated for 7–9 days; for this reason, measurement of LDH, especially the fastest electrophoretic isoenzyme of LDH, may be valuable when the patient is not seen until a few days have elapsed after an acute episode of pain, because these enzymes may remain positive after the MB CK isoenzymes have returned to normal. Serial determinations of enzymes every 2 hours make it possible to determine the area under the time curve of the increase and decrease in the enzyme and thus permit an estimate of the magnitude of the infarction. An early peaking of CK in the serum at 8–12 hours is consistent with the occurrence of reperfusion.

Recently, the MM and MB isoenzymes of CK have been further subdivided—MM into three and MB into two subforms. They are released from the infarcted myocardium rapidly and appear in the blood early, because these are small molecules. With myocardial injury, MM_3 and MB_2 are released and enzymatically converted in the plasma to different subforms. Therefore, with myocardial necrosis, there is a shift in the ratio of these two subforms relative to their plasma-derived counterparts, and this occurs early, before there is a rise in total CK. In a recent study, analysis

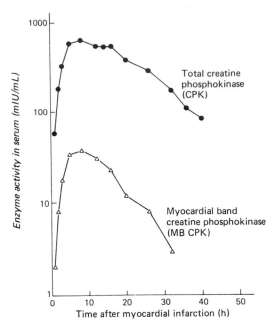

Figure 8–18. Serial changes in total serum CPK activity and serum MB CPK activity in a patient with hemodynamically uncomplicated acute myocardial infarction. The disappearance rate of MB CK activity exceeded the corresponding rate for total CPK. MB denotes myocardial band of CPK. (Reproduced, with permission, from Sobel BE, Roberts R, Larson KB: Estimation of infarct size from serum MB creatine phosphokinase activity: Application and limitations. Am J Cardiol 1976;37:474.)

of MB subforms reliably detected myocardial lesions in 59% of patients within 2–4 hours after onset and in 92% of patients by 4–6 hours (Puleo, 1990). This development gives promise for rapid, early diagnosis of myocardial infarction.

D. Electrocardiographic Findings: A myocardial infarction of significant size, especially if transmural and anterior, produces characteristic electrocardiographic changes in about 95% of patients. Five examples of the electrocardiographic changes in myocardial infarction are seen in Figures 8–19 to 8–23.

1. Early unchanged ECG– At the onset of infarction, the ECG occasionally may be within normal limits. A normal ECG at this stage should not rule out the diagnosis. If the initial ECG is within normal limits and if infarction subsequently evolves, it is usually small and uncomplicated (Slater, 1987).

2. Early electrocardiographic changes– The characteristic pattern may be delayed for hours or days, and the initial slightly convex ST elevation seen over septal leads V_{2-4} in anteroseptal myocardial infarction, over lateral leads V_{5-6} anterolateral infarction, and in inferior leads II, III, and aVF in inferior infarction may be subtle and difficult to distinguish from the normal variant of early repolarization. Over

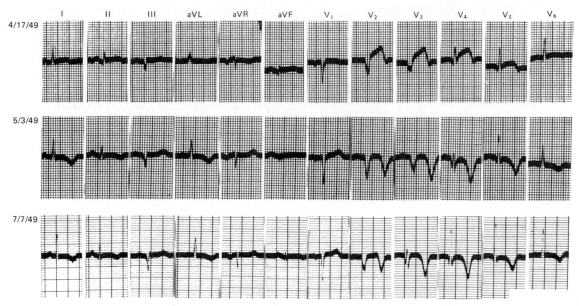

Figure 8–19. ECG of a 65-year-old man with anteroseptal myocardial infarction. Electrocardiographic findings of acute anteroseptal infarction with serial changes were noted on 4/17/49—1 month after the patient developed pain in the posterior aspect of the upper chest that awakened him from sleep and required injection of an analgesic. The pain had recurred the next day, spread to the anterior chest, and was recurrent at rest for the month prior to 4/17/49. The ECG shows a QS complex with elevated ST and late inversion of the T wave, which progressively developed in the 3 months indicated by the dates. Sequential changes resulted in a significant Q wave in V_3 followed by deep inversion of the T wave in V_2–6.

a period of hours or days, however, the characteristic evolution occurs, with subsequent symmetric inversion of T waves in the leads that initially showed convex elevated ST segments.

3. Evolving ECG– An unequivocal diagnosis can be made if characteristic broad Q waves (≥ 0.04 S) are present in leads with convex elevated ST segments that subsequently evolve to symmetrically inverted T waves. Q waves are more significant than QS complexes, particularly in the right precordial (V_1–$_3$) or septal leads (V_2–$_4$) or in the inferior leads (II, III, aVF) in horizontal heart position with left axis deviation. The diagnosis is strongly supported if there is a broad (≥ 0.04 s) slurred, wide Q wave with an amplitude exceeding 30% of that of the succeeding R wave, which is slightly slurred in its upstroke—and especially if a previous ECG did not show the Q waves.

4. Serial changes– The diagnosis is less certain if there are no diagnostic Q waves, as is the case with nontransmural (non-Q wave) infarctions. In these instances, serial changes with waxing and then waning of the ST–T abnormalities are more reliable than static changes. If the patient is seen after the infarction has been present for some days and there is no previous ECG for comparison, the initial ST–T changes may appear nonspecific, and further serial records over days to weeks may be necessary before

one can interpret the electrocardiographic changes as diagnostic.

5. ECG in presence of old infarct– The interpretation is more difficult if the patient has had previous myocardial infarction, if there is left bundle branch block or significant conduction defects in the peripheral Purkinje system, or if there is underlying left ventricular hypertrophy or digitalis effect. In these cases, the presence of diagnostic Q waves or characteristic serial evolution of the ST–T abnormalities is required to establish the electrocardiographic diagnosis of myocardial infarction; radioisotopic methods may be especially useful. In the presence of Wolff-Parkinson syndrome, the ECG cannot be used in making the diagnosis of myocardial infarction.

6. Return to normal ECG– The usual evolution of the ST–T changes takes several weeks, but in minor infarction this may occur within 10 days. When the acute infarction is characterized only by ST–T changes (non-Q wave infarction and inferior myocardial infarction), the ECG may return completely to normal in about 20–30% of patients; a normal ECG therefore does not exclude a previous infarction.

7. Abnormal Q waves– Abnormal Q waves, defined as initial negative deflections followed by positive deflections—in contrast to QS complexes, which

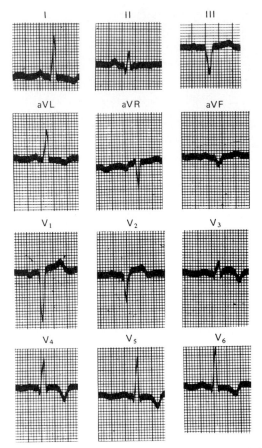

Figure 8–20. ECG of a 59-year-old man showing old inferior myocardial infarction (slurred QS in aVF and slurred Q in lead II) and more recent anteroseptal myocardial infarction with associated left ventricular conduction defects (inverted T waves in V_{3-6}, I, and aVL with a slurred Q in V_3 and a slurred QRS complex in V_4).

are negative deflections not followed by positive ones—have greater diagnostic value than ST–T abnormalities. An abnormal Q wave of 0.04 s, especially if slightly slurred and followed by a slurred upstroke of the R wave, is considered diagnostic of anterior infarction when it occurs in the precordial leads and of inferior infarction when it occurs in lead aVF. One-half to two-thirds of patients with abnormal Q waves have localized segmental wall motion abnormalities demonstrable by left ventricular angiography in the area of the myocardium in which infarction is inferred from the abnormal Q wave. The total long-term mortality rate over time is similar in both Q wave and non-Q wave infarctions. The Q wave variety has a higher in-hospital mortality, but the non-Q wave infarction has a higher later mortality, probably because the original infarct was incomplete, leaving viable but ischemic, jeopardized myocardium.

Initial force abnormalities (abnormal Q waves) may be transient and due to functional impairment

resulting from hypoxia or ischemia or the development of collateral blood flow and may disappear as the infarct heals. The presence of an abnormal Q wave, therefore, does not mean myocardial scar, death of cells, or permanent damage. During left ventricular angiography the abnormal Q waves may disappear, and segmental areas of hypokinesia or asynergy may contract more normally when the load on the myocardium is decreased following administration of nitroglycerin or hydralazine.

Conduction defects that alter pathways of activation may influence the appearance and course of abnormal Q waves. The waves may disappear when left bundle branch block develops, only to reappear when the conduction delay disappears in intermittent block, as sometimes occurs during the course of an acute infarction.

Persistent abnormal Q waves are not a reliable sign of ventricular aneurysm. Many patients with abnormal Q waves do not have aneurysms, although they may have segmental localized contraction abnormalities.

In aVF, the most reliable sign of inferior infarction is an abnormal Q wave 0.04 s wide with a depth of at least 30% that of the succeeding R wave, with an associated significant abnormal Q wave in lead II. Small abnormal Q waves may appear in aVF in a vertically placed heart in normal individuals. An abnormal Q wave in aVF is more significant if the patient has a leftward QRS axis than if the QRS axis is vertical. The diagnosis is considered to be firmly established when typical evolutionary serial electrocardiographic changes occur in the presence of progressive increases in serum enzymes (particularly the MB isoenzymes of CK) and a compatible clinical history.

E. Radioisotope Studies of Myocardial Infarction: (See Figures 8–24 to 8–27.) Coronary perfusion studies using thallium-201 in patients with previous myocardial infarction have shown decreased *resting* perfusion in the area of myocardial infarction. By contrast, in patients with angina pectoris they have shown decreased perfusion under the stress of *exercise,* which some hours later redistributes to normal (see also Chapter 5). Quantitative thallium-201 scans have been used to determine the location, extent, and persistence of myocardial ischemia at the time of the acute infarction and later before hospital discharge. Perfusion defects in areas distant from that of the acute infarction indicate additional areas of ischemia. Multiple thallium-201 defects usually predict multivessel and more extensive disease with a greater likelihood of left ventricular dysfunction (Beller, 1991). When the patient has not been able to exercise, thallium-201 has been injected after atrial pacing or coronary vasodilation (using intravenous dipyridamole or adenosine) to identify areas of decreased perfusion and thus ischemic myocardium.

Right ventricular infarction can be diagnosed by radioisotope studies as well as clinical findings. Ab-

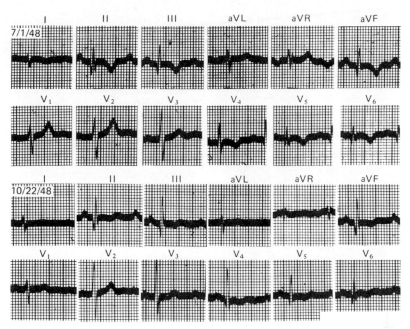

Figure 8–21. ECG of a 59-year-old man with inferolateral myocardial infarction who had dyspnea on exertion for 6 months as well as angina of effort and anginal pain on awakening that lasted about 2 weeks (up until 2 months before the time of the first tracing). Blood pressure was 140/90 mm Hg. Note the prominent Q and inverted T waves in leads II, III, aVF, and V_{4-6} in the record of 7/1/48. The abnormalities have improved in the record of 10/22/48.

normal intravenous technetium ^{99m}Tc pyrophosphate uptake can be localized to the right ventricle, or localized hypokinesis of the right ventricle may be evident on gated blood pool angiography. Infarction of the right ventricle may explain predominant right ventricular failure in patients with acute inferior myocardial infarction.

Thallium isotopic perfusion scans do not show small perfusion defects, and reproducibility is variable unless maximum exercise is performed. Resolution of isotopic scans is imperfect, but the reliability of scanning is improved by the use of computer techniques. Presently, most laboratories are using SPECT techniques for performing tomographic "slices" of the radioisotopic myocardial image in frontal, horizontal, and cross-sectional planes. This technique has permitted improved detection, localization, and determination of magnitude of perfusion defects corresponding with areas of ischemia or infarction.

In contrast to thallium-201, which reveals defects in perfusion ("cold spots"), infarct-avid scintigraphy employs intravenous technetium-99m pyrophosphate, which has the advantage of being actively taken up by acutely infarcted myocardial cells (but not old scar), producing discrete, well-localized "hot spots" in transmural acute infarction. Technetium pyrophosphate has limitations in non-Q wave infarction, because diffuse uptake can be seen. Such uptake may also occur in patients with ventricular aneurysms in the absence of infarction and will cause false-positive interpretations.

A new infarct-avid imaging technique involves the intravenous injection of radiolabeled myosin-specific antibody and its scintigraphic detection in necrotic myocardium. This antibody will bind to the intracellular myosin when the cell membranes are disrupted by necrosis. As with ^{99m}Tc pyrophosphate, one must wait 24 hours for the agent to be cleared from the blood pool before myocardial imaging can be done. Discrete uptake in an area of myocardium is specific for necrosis. In one multicenter study, antimyosin antibody imaging has yielded a 92% sensitivity for identifying acute Q wave infarction (Johnson, 1989).

As imaging techniques improve, especially with three-dimensional computer processing, it is becoming possible to more accurately determine the size of an infarct, especially if it is anterior. The quantitative estimate of the size of the infarct by radionuclide technique correlates significantly with serial serum enzyme determinations and hemodynamic measurements. The methods are complementary. In patients with old myocardial infarction or myocardial scars, image perfusion defects may be diagnostic of an old infarction or scar at a time when only nonspecific ST segment abnormalities without Q waves are present in the resting ECG. Defects that are present both at rest and following exercise are usually due to fibrous scar rather than to ischemic but viable myocardium.

F. Size of Myocardial Infarct: As a result of the factors mentioned earlier that influence myocardial ischemia, the artery occluded in an extensive myocar-

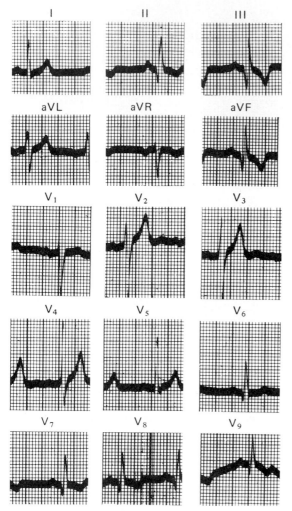

Figure 8–22. Inferior myocardial infarction with typical findings of prominent Q in leads II, III, and aVF, with inverted T waves in these leads and in the posterolateral leads (V$_{7-9}$) in the seventh interspace but no diagnostic findings in the routine lateral leads (V$_{4-6}$).

dial infarction cannot always be predicted accurately. Although we describe myocardial infarction as a disease entity, it is more useful to consider it as a continuum of increasing necrosis from a few cells to massive infarction. The former results in a mild illness mainly with cardiac pain (see below), without disturbance in left ventricular function, and with minimal serum enzyme elevations, although the pattern on the ECG may be diagnostic. When necrosis involves many cells and a large area, especially if there has been previous infarction with segmental scars, the clinical picture is complicated by the presence of ventricular arrhythmias, cardiogenic shock, left ventricular dysfunction with cardiac failure, conduction defects, cardiac arrest, and death. The physician therefore must attempt to estimate the extent of the infarction in terms of its impact on the circulation as well as its site and size. The former is a function of the extent of the previous as well as the current myocardial infarction, which limits left ventricular function. If the amount of previous myocardial scarring is extensive, even a small additional myocardial infarction may produce severe clinical manifestations of cardiogenic shock and failure.

Methods for measuring the size of the myocardial infarction include the following: (1) determination of the extent of abnormalities on the ECG and location of the Q, ST, and T wave changes, whether they occur in just a few leads over the lateral chest or extend across the entire anterior precordium and perhaps the inferior wall as well; (2) ST mapping, in which the magnitude and persistence of ST segment elevation using multiple precordial leads are added up and averaged over a period of days; (3) serial determinations of MB isoenzymes of CK released into the serum by necrosing myocardial cells; (4) pyrophosphate ^{111}In-labeled antimyosin and thallium radioisotope uptake studies; (5) hemodynamic studies; and (6) cineangiography.

The greater the isoenzyme rise or the larger the portion of the myocardial image with uptake of

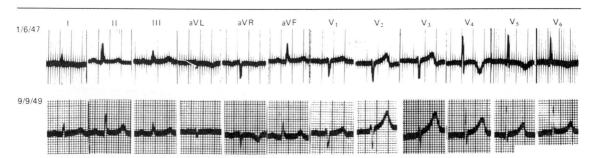

Figure 8–23. ECG of a 63-year-old man with myocardial infarction. The electrocardiographic abnormalities characteristic of myocardial infarction on the first tracing have completely disappeared in the second tracing obtained 2 years later. (Inverted T waves in V$_{4-6}$.)

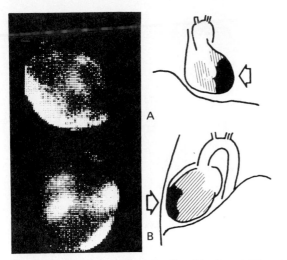

Figure 8–24. Anterolateral infarction. The frontal **(A)** and left lateral **(B)** scintiscans show an area of diminished activity **(arrows)** at the site of infarction. (Reproduced, with permission, from Wackes FJT et al: Noninvasive visualization of acute myocardial infarction in man with thallium-201. Br Heart J 1975;37:741.)

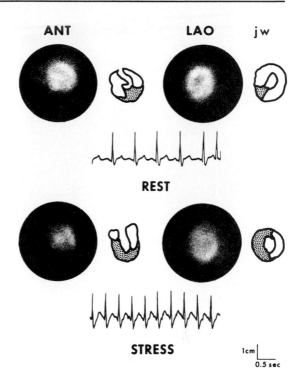

SCA : 80% LAD, 90% RCA

Figure 8–25. Isotopes in myocardial infarction. Man, age 58, with a negative treadmill test but showing, at rest, a residual old infarct abnormality, worse with exercise after administration of thallium. Selective angiogram shows left anterior oblique artery 80% stenotic and right coronary artery 90% stenotic. (ANT, anterior; LAO, left anterior oblique; SCA, selective coronary angiogram; LAD, left anterior descending artery; RCA, right coronary artery.) (Reproduced, with permission, from Botvinick EH et al: Myocardial stress perfusion scintigraphy with rubidium 81 versus stress electrocardiography. Am J Cardiol 1977;39:364.)

pyrophosphate—the larger the perfusion defect with thallium or sestamibi—the greater the volume of myocardial necrosis. Radioisotope perfusion studies cannot always distinguish between infarction and severe ischemia with viable myocardium. Using computer-assisted methods, a thallium defect score can be determined that correlates with infarct size and subsequent mortality rate (Silverman, 1980). Positive scans are usually negative within the first few hours but become positive, showing perfusion defects, in about 12 hours after intravenous injection of the radioisotope. Serial studies can then be done to follow the course, which may demonstrate an increase or decrease in the size of the infarct or allow a small infarction to become visible.

G. Determination of Wall Motion Abnormalities and Left Ventricular Function by Radioisotope and Two-Dimensional Echocardiographic Studies: Two-dimensional echocardiograms can determine left ventricular function and the presence of complications such as ventricular aneurysm, pseudoaneurysm, ventricular septal defect of papillary muscle dysfunction, or ventricular thrombi. Localized and global ejection fraction and impaired regional wall motion by two-dimensional echocardiograms may be the earliest finding in acute coronary occlusion (Gibson, 1982). The presence of extensive wall motion abnormalities outside the immediate acute infarcted area is associated with more severe disease and a worse prognosis for survival (Gibson, 1983).

Peels et al (1990) performed two-dimensional echocardiography in the emergency department before any therapy in 43 patients with suspected acute myocardial infarction. They found a sensitivity of 92%, a specificity of 53%, and a negative predictive accuracy of 94% for diagnosing myocardial infarction. Because a positive finding can represent either severe ischemia without infarction or old infarction, the most valuable use of this technique is when it is normal in a patient with chest pain, thus giving powerful evidence against infarction.

There are also at least two noninvasive radioisotope techniques by which wall motion abnormalities and left ventricular function can be estimated. The first is by the recording of images during both systole and diastole after a bolus injection of technetium-labeled albumin, "gated" (synchronized) to the ECG. Disturbances in wall motion can be recognized, and localized areas of hypokinesia or dyskinesia can be

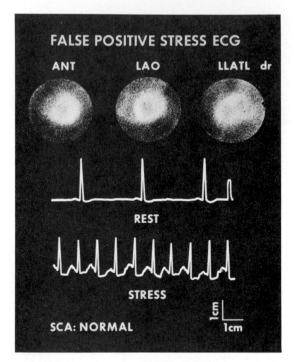

Figure 8–26. Isotopes in myocardial infarction. Positive stress test (?false-positive) with normal image and normal coronary angiogram—not on digitalis. (ANT, anterior; LAO, left anterior oblique; LLATL, left lateral; SCA, selective coronary angiogram.) (Modified and reproduced, with permission, from Botvinick EH et al: Thallium 201 myocardial perfusion scintigraphy for the clinical clarification of normal, abnormal, and equivocal electrocardiographic stress tests. Am J Cardiol 1978;41:43.)

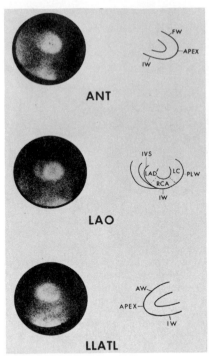

Figure 8–27. Isotopes in myocardial infarction. Normal thallium 201 perfusion image. (ANT, anterior; LAO, left anterior oblique; LLATL, left lateral; FW, free wall; IW, inferior wall; IVS, interventricular septum; LAD, left anterior descending artery; RCA, right coronary artery; LC, left circumflex artery; PLW, posterior lateral wall; AW, anterior wall.) (Modified and reproduced, with permission, from Botvinick EH et al: Thallium 201 myocardial perfusion scintigraphy for the clinical clarification of normal, abnormal, and equivocal electrocardiographic stress tests. Am J Cardiol 1978;41:43.)

noted. Ejection fraction can be determined from the difference between the systolic and diastolic isotope image. Similar images can be obtained on first-pass imaging of technetium-99m sestamibi. The second method is by the so-called single-pass nucleotide angiogram, in which technetium ^{99m} pertechnetate is given intravenously and a computerized, summated series of cardiac cycles is obtained. These cycles resemble a dye-dilution curve. Localized abnormalities of wall motion and ejection fraction can be noted. Both methods correlate reasonably well. Radioisotope special techniques such as radionuclide angiography to determine wall motion abnormalities require expensive equipment and highly technically trained physicians and are not essential in most patients with acute myocardial infarction.

MRI and fast CT scanning can also reveal wall motion abnormalities and their extent. In addition, there is some evidence that there is a difference in signal intensity between necrotic myocardium and normal or scarred myocardium (Johns, 1990). This is still in the experimental stage and at present is of little use in the clinical setting.

H. Minor Myocardial Infarction: The diagnosis of minor myocardial infarction is often obvious only in retrospect when one reviews the entire sequence of events of the illness. Slight increases in serum enzymes, relatively minor ST–T abnormalities, slight fever, the presence of transient gallop rhythm, and serial radioisotopic scans may permit diagnosis. However, myocardial infarction may extend and hemodynamic manifestations may worsen, and a patient who originally presented with what appeared to be minor myocardial infarction may develop a more severe variety. Furthermore, even a small area of myocardial necrosis may induce ventricular arrhythmias or conduction defects, which occasionally may cause death.

In general, mild and nontransmural infarction has a lower mortality rate than transmural infarction. Patients with transmural infarction may have a higher prevalence of previous myocardial infarction and therefore a greater area of total myocardial infarction, new and old, than those with nontransmural infarction.

Table 8–8. Incidence of dysrhythmias among 284 patients seen within the first hour, 1966–1969.[1]

Dysrhythmia	Number of Patients				Total Number of Patients
	Within 1 Hour	Within 2 Hours	Within 3–4 Hours	After 4 Hours	
Bradyarrhythmia	88 (31%)	10 (3.5%)	6 (2%)	21 (7%)	125 (44%)
Ventricular ectopic beats	70 (25%)	35 (13%)	16 (6%)	41 (14%)	163 (57%)
Ventricular fibrillation	28 (10%)	12 (4%)	2 (0.7%)	12 (4%)	54 (19%)
Ventricular tachycardia	10 (3.5%)	16 (6%)	6 (2%)	55 (19%)	87 (31%)
Atrial fibrillation/flutter	11 (4%)	0	0	15 (5%)	26 (9%)
Supraventricular tachycardia	1 (0.4%)	0	0	10 (3.5%)	11 (4%)

[1] Reproduced, with permission, from Adgey AA et al: Acute phase of myocardial infarction. Lancet 1971;2:501.

Course & Complications

In mild cases, after chest pain is relieved by morphine or one of its analogues, the course is uneventful, with no evidence of arrhythmia, cardiac failure, or cardiogenic shock. In more severe infarction, and even in some milder cases, the most common finding is the development of arrhythmias. The most lethal development is cardiogenic shock. Extension of the infarcted area to the epicardium causes pericarditis in about 10% of cases, usually pericardial pain combined with a transient pericardial friction rub.

A. Arrhythmias:

1. Tachyarrhythmias– (See also Chapter 15.) Within hours after an episode of acute myocardial infarction, ventricular arrhythmias are common (ventricular premature beats in 10–15% and ventricular fibrillation in 5–10% of cases). The incidence is higher in patients seen within the first hour (Table 8–8). The ventricular premature beats may be single or may occur in salvos; may occur frequently or only occasionally; or may be repetitive and lead to ventricular tachycardia or fibrillation. There is an increase in automaticity, a slowing of conduction and repolarization, and at the same time increased sympathetic and catecholamine stimulation. All of these changes are potentially arrhythmogenic. The ischemic cells are usually the site of onset of abnormal activation leading to arrhythmia. Severe ventricular arrhythmias are 10–20 times more common in the first 4 hours than they are on the second day; for this reason, patients are ideally admitted as soon as possible to a coronary unit with specially trained personnel and equipment permitting continuous electrocardiographic monitoring. The great frequency of early ventricular arrhythmias explains the high mortality rate before the patient receives treatment. The abrupt development of ventricular tachycardia or ventricular fibrillation may result in cardiac arrest.

a. Ventricular fibrillation– Patients who develop primary ventricular fibrillation (ie, fibrillation occurring early in acute myocardial infarction in the absence of cardiac failure or shock have a higher in-hospital mortality rate than those in whom the arrhythmia occurs late (Volpi, 1987). When ventricular fibrillation or cardiac arrest follows the development of shock or heart failure, it is considered secondary to the poor left ventricular function and not to primary electrical instability of the ischemic myocardium. Prompt recognition and treatment of ventricular arrhythmias in the coronary care unit (see Treatment, below) has been a major factor in reducing the mortality rate of acute infarction in the hospital and in mobile ambulance units. Continuous monitoring of the patient, with a monitor both at the bedside and at the nursing station, permits immediate recognition of the abnormal rhythm, which must be treated promptly (within 30 seconds in the coronary care unit but within 3 minutes elsewhere) in order to prevent irreversible cardiac or cerebral damage. Sudden cardiac death in acute ischemia is usually due to ventricular fibrillation, and at autopsy most patients have severe coronary disease with two- or three-vessel involvement; occasionally, only a single vessel is diseased. Although most episodes of ventricular fibrillation occur very early in the course of acute myocardial infarction, a small percentage develop late in the hospital course, especially in those patients with anteroseptal myocardial infarction complicated by right or left bundle branch block. Late arrhythmias are usually reentrant tachyarrhythmias, and their significance is related to the degree of left ventricular dysfunction.

b. Other tachyarrhythmias– (See also Chapter 15.) Accelerated idioventricular rhythm occurs in about 15–25% of patients. It is often heralded by ventricular premature beats with varying coupling intervals combined with sinus bradycardia. It is usually due to enhanced automaticity but may be expressed as an "escape" rhythm, when the sinus rate slows down. Idioventricular rhythms are "benign," because the heart rate is usually relatively slow (60–100/min) and because they infrequently lead to ventricular tachycardia with more rapid rates (150–180/min) or ventricular fibrillation. This is not always true, however; close observation is required, and the possibility of ventricular tachycardia must be considered when ventricular rates exceed 100–110/min. There are occasional cases in whom ventricular tachycardia of the same morphology occurs at double the rate of the accelerated idioventricular rhythm, suggesting that

Table 8–9. Frequency of supraventricular arrhythmias in acute myocardial
infarction (222 instances in 154 patients).[1]

Type of Arrhythmia	Alone (n)	Combined (n)	Total (n)	Incidence (%)	Mortality Rate (%)
Supraventricular premature contractions	70	58	128	36	24
Supraventricular tachycardia	20	35	55	16	25
Atrial flutter or fibrillation	5	34	39	11	41

[1] Reproduced, with permission, from Cristal N, Szwarcberg J, Gueron M: Supraventricular arrhythmias in acute myocardial infarction: Prognostic importance of clinical setting; mechanism of production. Ann Intern Med 1975:82:35.

the latter rhythm was in fact ventricular tachycardia with a 2:1 exit block.

Atrial arrhythmias, including paroxysmal atrial fibrillation or tachycardia, are less common, are usually short-lived, and do not require rigorous treatment (such as cardioversion) unless symptoms appear or hemodynamic deterioration occurs. Their frequency is illustrated in Table 8–9.

When the ventricular rate is rapid—exceeding 140–150 beats/min in atrial fibrillation or atrial tachycardia—coronary perfusion may be decreased and cardiac output may fall. If the patient has incipient left ventricular failure it may worsen, and the adverse hemodynamic effects may increase the area of infarction. In these situations, cardioversion should be used promptly. If the ventricular rate is slower and the patient is tolerating it well without symptoms or hemodynamic change, one may use antiarrhythmic agents such as digitalis, verapamil, or adenosine. Rapid atrial pacing to interrupt the reentrant cycle can be used if digitalis toxicity is probable. Atrial pacing is not useful in atrial fibrillation. The therapy of choice for supraventricular tachycardia is intravenous verapamil or adenosine (see Chapter 15 for dosage).

2. Bradyarrhythmias– (See Table 8–10 and Chapter 15.) At the onset of acute infarction, sinus bradycardia or sinus standstill may occur in 10–20%

of cases, causing junctional escape or idioventricular rhythm. Bradycardia is due to the Jarisch-von Bezold vagal reflex, a chemoreflex which is triggered by chemical stimuli (possibly histamine) from the left ventricular wall or coronary artery and which causes bradycardia or hypotension. Involvement of the sinoatrial nodal artery in right coronary artery occlusion with inferior or posterior myocardial infarction may also cause bradycardia. Most of the slow heart rates noted in the early stages following an acute infarction are due to sinus bradycardia. Sinoatrial block and atrioventricular block are infrequent. Most patients with cardiac arrest have ventricular fibrillation and not sinoatrial or atrioventricular block when first seen.

Slow heart rates (< 45/min) allow for a greater degree of nonhomogeneity of excitability and refractoriness in neighboring fibers, and arrhythmias are thus more common in these patients. Vagal hyperactivity may exert a beneficial effect on attenuating the decrease in ventricular fibrillation threshold evoked by sympathetic stimulation. If evidence of poor cardiac output is present with slow heart rates at the onset of acute myocardial infarction, atropine, 0.3–0.6 mg intravenously, is often beneficial but may produce sinus tachycardia and ventricular arrhythmias if high or repetitive doses are used.

B. Atrioventricular Conduction Defects: Atrio-

Table 8–10. Incidence of bradyarrhythmias among 284 patients related to time after onset of symptoms and site of infarction, 1966–1969.[1]

Site of Infarction	Number of Patients				Total Number of Patients
	Within 1 Hour	Within 2 Hours	Within 3–4 Hours	After 4 Hours	
Sinus or nodal bradycardia	75 (26%)	9 (3%)	5 (2%)	19 (7%)	108 (38%)
Anterior infarct	24 (18%)	5 (4%)	1 (0.7%)	2 (1.5%)	32 (24%)
Posterior infarct	48 (36%)	4 (3%)	3 (2%)	16 (12%)	71 (53%)
Atrioventricular block, second degree or complete	17 (6%)	2 (0.7%)	1 (0.4%)	8 (3%)	28 (10%)
Anterior infarct	1 (0.7%)	0	1 (0.7%)	1 (0.7%)	3 (2%)
Posterior infarct	15 (11%)	2 (1.5%)	0	7 (5%)	24 (18%)

[1] Reproduced, with permission, from Adgey AA et al: Acute phase of myocardial infarction. Lancet 1971;2:501.

ventricular conduction defects are common in acute myocardial infarction, occurring in about 10% of patients, and are associated with a mortality rate of about 50% in third-degree or Mobitz type II block. (See Chapter 14.)

1. Conduction defects in anterior infarction– Atrioventricular and intraventricular conduction defects are more hazardous in the presence of anterior myocardial infarction because they represent widespread necrosis in the ventricular septum, often involving the bundle of His and its branches and frequently resulting in impaired left ventricular function and hypokinesia. The conduction defect may be recognized early during electrocardiographic monitoring in the coronary care unit. The patient may develop a left anterior fascicular block with left axis deviation of –45 to –60 degrees; this indicates damage to the left anterior superior fascicle of the left bundle with or without right bundle branch block.

2. Stokes-Adams attacks– The patient may also develop partial atrioventricular block with prolongation of the PR interval ($>$ 0.21 s) or may have second-degree atrioventricular block with dropped beats (Mobitz type II). The change from a first-degree atrioventricular block or a left anterior fascicular block to second-degree and then complete atrioventricular block with Stokes-Adams attacks may occur within hours, and immediate prophylactic placement of a temporary artificial pacemaker is essential. When complete atrioventricular block occurs in anterior infarction, the ventricular escape pacemaker is usually below the area of destruction in the septum, in one of the branches of the left or right bundle, or even in the ventricular myocardium; as a result, the QRS complex is usually wide ($>$ 0.12 s) and the rate of discharge of the ectopic pacemaker in one of the fascicles is usually slow and unreliable. The availability of a practical external temporary pacemaker that can capture the cardiac rhythm allows time to place an intravenous wire for temporary pacing if needed.

3. Conduction defects in inferior infarction– Conduction defects occur two to four times more frequently in acute inferior myocardial infarction than in anterior infarction (Table 8–10.) In inferior myocardial infarction, the situation is more favorable when atrioventricular conduction defect occurs late, because the damage is usually to the atrioventricular node and is more ischemic than destructive. In such instances, although there are exceptions, the patient may have a partial atrioventricular block with a prolonged PR interval or may have second-degree atrioventricular block—so-called Wenckebach phenomenon or Mobitz type I—rather than 2:1 atrioventricular block with dropped beats, Mobitz type II (see Chapter 14). Although about one-sixth of patients with acute inferior infarction have a high degree of atrioventricular block, death is due chiefly to a power failure and not to Stokes-Adams attack. High-degree block is present in half of cases when the patient is first seen in the hospital; it occurs less frequently after the first few days. The mortality rate is higher when the block occurs early. The insertion of a right ventricular pacemaker has not been found to reduce the mortality rate.

4. Infrequency of Stokes-Adams attacks in inferior infarcts– When complete atrioventricular block occurs in the presence of inferior myocardial infarction, the pacemaker is in the junctional region; the QRS is usually narrow ($<$ 0.11 s), and the heart rate is faster (about 60/min) because the cardiac pacemaker is high in the conduction system. Because of the rarity of Stokes-Adams attacks in this setting, a conservative approach is usually recommended with continued monitoring rather than insertion of a temporary right ventricular pacemaker, unless the block occurs very early and is associated with hemodynamic deterioration. This decision must be individualized and must be considered tentative at present.

5. Complete infranodal block– Complete infranodal block is uncommon in patients with *preexisting* bundle branch block, but in about one-fourth of patients, right bundle branch block or left anterior hemiblock *develops* during acute myocardial infarction. Prophylactic pacing is advised in these latter instances because of the suddenness with which complete block may occur. The abrupt appearance of bundle branch block is an unfavorable sign and is associated with an increased frequency of both atrioventricular block and cardiac failure, with a higher mortality rate than in patients who do not develop bundle branch block.

6. Bilateral bundle branch block– Bilateral bundle branch block is diagnosed when block of either the right or the left bundle is associated with any degree of atrioventricular (bifascicular) block or when there are conduction defects in both branches. The mortality rate is high in these patients. The usual causes of death are ventricular arrhythmias and cardiac failure, rather than complete atrioventricular block. The use of temporary prophylactic pacemakers may be warranted but remains controversial.

The indications for *permanent* ventricular pacing in patients who have developed complete atrioventricular block during acute myocardial infarction are controversial. Some authors have asserted that patients with bifascicular block who develop complete atrioventricular block during the acute infarction are at high risk of recurrent complete atrioventricular block with sudden death if permanent pacing is not performed. Others disagree. Further prospective studies are required to determine whether death can be prevented by insertion of a permanent pacemaker in this specific subset of patients. If high-degree atrioventricular block—including complete heart block—persists after acute myocardial infarction, then a permanent pacemaker is warranted.

C. Cardiac Failure:

1. Acute left ventricular failure– Acute left ventricular dysfunction resulting from acute myocardial infarction may lead to unremitting pump failure or may be transient and associated with acute pulmonary edema, subsiding with relief of pain. The pathogenesis of cardiac failure is related to the quantity of nonfunctioning myocardium. Not only can systolic dysfunction cause failure, but diastolic dysfunction with stiffening of the myocardium can result in a rise in left ventricular filling and pulmonary capillary pressures, causing similar symptoms that are reversible if ischemia is relieved. Cardiac failure is the cause of death in two-thirds of hospital deaths occurring after 4 hours.

2. Milder cases of left ventricular failure– In less severe cases, the existence of left ventricular failure can be inferred on the basis of dyspnea, pulmonary rales, S_3 gallop rhythm, pulsus alternans, raised venous pressure, radiologic evidence of pulmonary venous congestion or redistribution of fluid to the upper lobes. If there is alveolar edema, bat's wing infiltrates near the hilar areas of the lungs may be seen. Increased heart size, sinus tachycardia, and an S_3 gallop rhythm may be the only signs.

Serial chest films parallel the hemodynamic changes (see below), and the greater the degree of pulmonary venous congestion on admission, the higher the mortality rate. The absence of pulmonary venous congestion in association with normal heart size is an excellent prognostic sign.

3. Bedside hemodynamic monitoring– Monitoring of right atrial and pulmonary artery wedge pressure during the course of acute infarction can be performed with the balloon-tipped Swan-Ganz catheter, which allows repeated measurements of pressure and oxygen saturation in the right side of the heart in the coronary care unit with little disturbance to the patient. Serial determinations of cardiac output utilizing thermodilution (see Chapters 4 and 6) and computerized techniques also make it possible for patients with left ventricular dysfunction to be monitored intermittently for the purpose of determining right atrial pressure, pulmonary arterial pressure, pulmonary arterial wedge pressure, and cardiac output (Table 8–11). Treatment can be individualized on the basis of abnormalities disclosed by these studies. Serial determinations of indices of left ventricular performance such as cardiac output, stroke output, or stroke work index can be compared with left ventricular filling pressure by inflating the balloon at the tip of the catheter wedged into the pulmonary artery. One can then determine whether left ventricular function is improving or deteriorating.

With more severe manifestations on presentation, the mean pulmonary artery wedge or diastolic pressure (left ventricular filling pressure) increases, the left ventricular end-diastolic volume increases, the ejection fraction falls, and the cardiac output decreases. Subsets of acute myocardial infarction in cardiac failure have been defined by relating the left ventricular filling pressure to stroke work or cardiac index, which describes left ventricular performance. When the end-diastolic pressure is high and the stroke work index or cardiac index is low, the prognosis is worse (Table 8–12).

Right ventricular failure secondary to right ventricular infarction can be treated with volume expansion (not diuretics) and inotropic agents such as dopamine or dobutamine to increase right ventricular output. Occasionally with atrioventricular block and right ventricular infarction, the loss of atrial "kick" can markedly depress stroke volume. In these cases, an atrioventricular dual-chamber pacemaker can be used that will increase stroke volume. Hypotension should be treated with dopamine. If the blood pres-

Table 8–11. Hemodynamic subsets in cardiac failure and shock.[1,2]

Diagnosis	Arterial Blood Pressure	Cardiac Output	Right Atrial Pressure	Pulmonary Wedge Pressure	Systemic Vascular Resistance
Normal	N	N	N	N	N
Cardiogenic shock	↓	↓	N or ↑	↑	↑
Hypovolemia	↓	↓	↓	↓	↑
Inappropriate vasodilation	↓	N or ↓	N or ↓	N or ↓	↓
Septic shock	↓	↑	N or ↓	N or ↑	↓
Right ventricular infarct	↓	↓	↑	N or ↓	N or ↑
Pulmonary embolism	↓	↓	↑	N or ↓	N or ↑
Tamponade	↓	↓	↑	↑	N or ↑
Heart failure	N or ↓	N or ↓	N or ↑	↑	N or ↑
Overtransfusion	N or ↑	↑	↑	↑	N or ↓

[1] Modified and reproduced, with permission, from Parmley WW, Chatterjee K: Cardiology. Lippincott 1987.
[2] ↓, decreases; ↑, increases; N, no significant increase or decrease.

Table 8–12. Mortality rates in clinical and hemodynamic subsets in acute myocardial infarction.[1,2]

Subset	Pulmonary Congestion (PCP >18 mm Hg)	Peripheral Hypoperfusion (CI <2.2 L/min/m²)	Mortality Rate	
			Clinical (%)	Hemo-dynamic (%)
I	−	−	1	3
II	+	−	11	8
III	−	+	18	23
IV	+	+	60	51

[1] Reproduced, with permission, from Forrester JS, Waters DD: Hospital treatment of congestive heart failure: management according to hemodynamic profile. Am J Med 1978;65:173.
[2] PCP = Pulmonary capillary pressure; CI = Cardiac index

sure is maintained but right ventricular failure persists, vasodilator therapy can be added.

4. Bedside echocardiography– Echocardiography at the bedside can complement hemodynamic studies and allow estimation of left ventricular dimensions and regional wall motion, septal and posterior myocardial wall contraction, size of the left atrium, and ejection fraction. Echocardiography can support the diagnosis of severe left ventricular failure in acute myocardial infarction by showing greatly increased left ventricular dimensions and a wide E point separation between the maximum excursion of the anterior mitral valve leaflet and the ventricular septum (see Figure 10–4).

In the two-dimensional echocardiogram, poor ventricular function is recognized as a dilated, poorly contracting, minimally thickening wall. There can be scarring and thinning of the wall resulting from an old infarction; dyskinesia of the wall, as seen in a new infarction; and complications of acute myocardial infarction, such as pericardial effusion, mitral or tricuspid valve regurgitation, ruptured septum, and severe mitral regurgitation.

5. Factors precipitating cardiac failure– Although cardiac failure may develop insidiously, it may appear abruptly, often associated with cardiogenic shock following an arrhythmia or pulmonary infarction or following complications such as perforation of the ventricular septum or dysfunction or rupture of the papillary muscle with the development of acute mitral regurgitation (see below).

6. Mechanical complications of acute myocardial infarction–

a. Infarction or rupture of a papillary muscle leading to acute mitral regurgitation– An abrupt, harsh systolic murmur and thrill are heard at the apex, and the patient may experience severe left ventricular failure or cardiogenic shock. Regurgitation of the mitral valve occurs because now the valve lacks uniform support during systole and part of the mitral leaflet prolapses during cardiac contraction. The sudden volume load on the left ventricle results in a marked increase in diastolic filling pressure and pul-

monary edema. The tip of the papillary muscle, usually the posteromedial muscle, can infarct and rupture, tearing off one or more chordae tendineae and leading to physical and clinical signs of acute mitral regurgitation and failure.

The diagnosis can be made noninvasively with Doppler echocardiography to quantify the mitral regurgitation and a Swan-Ganz catheter to demonstrate large v waves on the pulmonary capillary wedge pressure tracing (Kaul, 1990). Minor degrees of papillary muscle dysfunction due to ischemia are commonly found if careful auscultation is performed daily to search for a late or pansystolic murmur.

When mitral regurgitation is severe, treatment consists of afterload reduction with vasodilators, diuretics, and dopamine if the patient is hypotensive. If vigorous medical therapy is ineffective, intra-aortic balloon assist can be used. At this stage, mitral valve repair or replacement is required as soon as possible.

b. Perforation of the ventricular septum (acquired ventricular septal defect)– Perforation can occur anywhere in the ventricular septum but is usually distal, near the apex. It usually occurs toward the end of the first week after onset of myocardial infarction. As with papillary muscle rupture, the complication is heralded by the abrupt appearance of a harsh systolic murmur and thrill and symptoms and signs of cardiac failure or cardiogenic shock. The diagnosis can be made by two-dimensional echocardiography and Doppler, which can identify a high-velocity jet across the septum and even visualize and localize the defect itself. With injection of "contrast" consisting of agitated saline with microbubbles into the right heart, negative contrast of an "unopacified" jet of blood can be seen entering the right ventricle through the defect, thus localizing it. The diagnosis can be confirmed and quantified by finding a left-to-right shunt at the ventricular level, using a Swan-Ganz catheter.

Differentiation from ruptured papillary muscle can be difficult because of the similar presentation of abrupt systolic murmur and rapid development of cardiac failure or cardiogenic shock. Differentiation can best be made by demonstrating ventricular septal defect by two-dimensional echo-Doppler and left-to-right shunt and papillary muscle rupture by a large v wave in the wedge pressure. Cardiac catheterization can confirm the diagnosis but, unless coronary arteriography is done, is not needed to identify or quantify the magnitude of the shunt or the valvular insufficiency prior to surgical intervention (Kaul, 1990).

As in papillary muscle rupture, treatment for acquired ventricular septal defect is early vigorous medical therapy to stabilize the patient if possible. If the patient's hemodynamic status worsens, urgent surgery is necessary to close the septal defect. The patient can be temporarily markedly improved by either afterload reduction with nitroprusside or converting enzyme inhibitors. Placement of an intra-aortic balloon pump can be very helpful in temporarily improving the hemodynamic state of the patient. The timing of surgery has been debated: one hopes to delay it until "good scar tissue" has been formed; but clinical deterioration is often so rapid that surgery cannot wait. The current practice is to proceed to surgery once hemodynamically severe mitral regurgitation or a large left-to-right shunt through the ruptured septum is identified (Lemery, 1992).

c. Rupture of the heart– This is an uncommon event (5%) but may cause sudden death owing to acute hemopericardium and tamponade. Rupture may be "subacute," with slight penetration of the epicardium to the pericardium, escape of blood, and worsening of the clinical picture. Penetration of a weakened epicardial wall with hemopericardium may be recognized by a change in symptoms and by echocardiography, and immediate surgery has been successful in some patients. Cardiac rupture is more common during the first week, but it can occur later. If the cardiac rupture is contained by the pericardium, a false "aneurysm" develops. This is very unstable and can rupture abruptly at any time; therefore, surgical closure is necessary.

7. Evaluating left ventricular function– The ejection fraction, which can be estimated serially by radioisotope study or by echocardiography, can be used to estimate the size of the infarct and the effectiveness of left ventricular function and helps to determine prognosis.

D. Cardiogenic Shock: Cardiogenic shock with hypotension and poor tissue perfusion with oliguria and cerebral obtundation may be present at the onset of a massive infarction or may develop insidiously and progressively over the next few days. It is more apt to occur when there has been previous infarction or when the current infarction is so massive that at least 40% of the left ventricle is severely damaged. The patient frequently has signs of low cardiac output such as a thready pulse, low pulse pressure, and an S_3 gallop. A mitral regurgitation murmur may be present, as well as rales and other peripheral signs of congestive heart failure. Patients with cardiogenic shock frequently have three-vessel coronary artery disease, severe proximal left anterior descending artery stenosis, or left main coronary artery stenosis. Cardiogenic shock is more common than congestive failure in patients dying from "pump failure" after acute myocardial infarction. It is the most frequent cause of death in the hospital following acute infarction. The large area of damaged myocardium frustrates successful medical treatment.

Hemodynamic studies in patients with cardiogenic shock demonstrate a high left ventricular filling pressure, low cardiac output, low stroke work index, severe hypotension, and no evidence of hypovolemia. Severe cardiogenic shock is a dread event, and patients usually die within a few days. The prognosis is poor even in somewhat milder cases, and aggressive therapy is warranted. Following stabilization by temporary circulatory assist mechanisms such as aortic balloon counterpulsation, vasodilator therapy if blood pressure is high enough for the patient to benefit, and inotropic agents, coronary arteriography and left ventricular cineangiography are performed with a view to possible emergency operation. Cineangiography may also demonstrate the presence of perforation of the ventricular septum or gross mitral regurgitation as well as evidence of hypokinesia or akinesia or left ventricular aneurysm that may require surgical treatment. Even when salvage during the acute episode is possible by heroic effort, 1- or 2-year survivals are infrequent because of the severity of myocardial disease. Left ventricular asynergy with dyskinesia is more common than true aneurysm and occurs in most patients after transmural infarction. In patients who have recovered from cardiogenic shock or cardiac failure after an acute infarction and are doing well, the Swan-Ganz catheter can be removed and a search for akinetic segments or ventricular aneurysm performed by noninvasive techniques with radioisotopes (Figure 8–28) or two-dimensional echocardiography. If the patient has persistent or recurrent symptoms of cardiac failure or recurrent ventricular arrhythmias after successful initial management, left ventricular angiography is usually required. Mitral regurgitation from papillary and free wall muscle dysfunction and ventricular septal defect from perforation of the septum should always be considered with a view to possible surgical treatment in patients who have had cardiogenic shock or cardiac failure.

E. Arterial Embolism: Mural thrombi occur in some series in up to 50% of patients with acute myocardial infarction, especially in patients with anterior and apical infarction with akinetic wall motion. Thrombus is rarely seen in patients with inferior wall myocardial infarction. Thrombi are most likely to be found when the echocardiogram is done at 5–7 days postinfarction.

Although mural thrombi occur frequently, systemic emboli are less common, occurring in about 5% of patients with acute myocardial infarction—most of-

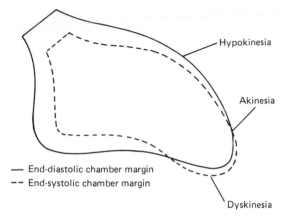

Figure 8–28. Segmental wall motion is analyzed by superimposing end-systolic chamber outline on end-diastolic chamber outline from left ventricular angiograms. Inward excursion is qualitatively estimated as mild, moderate, or severe hypokinesia, akinesia (no systolic motion), and dyskinesia (paradoxic outward systolic motion). (Reproduced, with permission, from Alderman EL: Angiographic indicators of left ventricular function. JAMA 1976;236:1055. Copyright © 1976 by the American Medical Association.)

ten at the end of the first week or into the second week—although emboli can occur at any time after infarction, even weeks or months later. In patients with mural thrombus, emboli are more likely to occur when the thrombus is pedunculated and mobile in the left ventricular cavity. Systemic emboli are less common if mural thrombi are not demonstrated (Stratton, 1987). Anticoagulation first with heparin followed by warfarin is recommended when mural thrombus is seen. Although there is controversy about how long anticoagulation should be continued, we recommend continuing warfarin for 3–6 months postinfarction.

F. Phlebothrombosis and Pulmonary Embolism: These complications are less common now than when prolonged bed rest was recommended for acute infarction. Phlebothrombosis with or without pulmonary embolism occurs in approximately 10% of patients with acute myocardial infarction. Fatalities are rare.

G. Cerebral Infarction: The fall of arterial pressure associated with acute infarction in a patient with a compromised cerebral arterial blood supply may produce cerebral infarction. One should suspect acute myocardial infarction in all patients who develop cerebral infarction and should obtain an ECG. Cerebral embolism secondary to a mural thrombus in the left ventricle may also cause cerebral infarction, but the event is usually later in the course of acute myocardial infarction and is of sudden onset.

H. Acute Renal Failure: Following prolonged hypotension and shock, patients may develop acute tubular necrosis with oliguria, anuria, and acute renal failure. Renal failure may also develop if vasodilator therapy with sodium nitroprusside is unusually vigorous, producing prolonged hypotension.

I. Pericarditis: Extension of the transmural infarct to the epicardial surface may result in inflammatory changes in the pericardium, possibly with hemopericardium, especially if anticoagulants have been used. Pericardial friction rub is rarely heard in the first 24 hours after an infarction but is common on the second to fifth days postinfarction. It is frequently asymptomatic and often very transient. The pain of pericarditis differs from that of myocardial infarction in that it is affected by inspiration, movement in bed, and swallowing and is often relieved by leaning forward. Definitive diagnosis depends upon recognition of a pericardial friction rub (in about 15% of patients), which may be triphasic if the heart rate is slow but may appear to be uniphasic if the rate is rapid. The rub is usually heard along the left sternal border, is harsh and grating in quality, may be intermittent, and may last only a few hours or days.

J. Cardiac Hypertrophy: Cardiac hypertrophy is uncommon in uncomplicated coronary heart disease but develops if myocardial infarction with cardiac failure ensues or if hypertension has been present. The average heart weight in fatal cases of acute myocardial infarction is just over 400 g, slightly heavier than normal.

Prevention

Unstable angina should be treated vigorously. If unstable angina occurs after myocardial infarction, coronary arteriography should be performed and revascularization is warranted when a region of ischemic but viable myocardium can be revascularized. Serum lipids should be reduced with a low-calorie, low-cholesterol, low-saturated-fat diet. Resins such as cholestyramine and colestipol should be combined with nicotinic acid or lovastatin.

Lovastatin is started at a dose of 10–20 mg once daily and increased monthly by 20 mg to a maximum dosage of 40 mg twice daily. Therapy should attempt to reduce the serum cholesterol to 180 mg/dL and the LDL cholesterol to no more than 160 mg/dL. Lovastatin is a 3-hydroxy-3-methylglutaryl coenzyme-A (HMG-CoA) reductase inhibitor. The mechanism by which lovastatin works is in question. There appears to be a compensatory increase in HMG-CoA reductase synthesis to overcome inhibition of the enzyme, and the major mechanism for cholesterol lowering is an increase in LDL receptor activity (Grundy, 1988).

The main side effects have been a rise in muscle and liver enzyme values in 2% of patients. Rhabdomyolysis is rare and more likely to occur if the drug is given in conjunction with gemfibrozil, niacin, or cyclosporine. Although cataracts were described in dogs, this has not been a problem in humans. Liver function tests should be performed 3–6 weeks after starting lovastatin and repeated in 6 months.

Primary prevention of coronary artery atherosclerosis by attention to other risk factors and the use of agents that prevent platelet aggregation is undergoing therapeutic trial, and the results are suggestive. Beta-blocking drugs have prevented reinfarction and death in a number of studies. Unusual physical or psychologic stress has been thought to precede the acute occurrence of myocardial infarction in some cases, but retrospective studies do not as a rule disclose any activities that might explain the cardiac event.

Treatment

Patients are ideally treated at the onset of myocardial infarction in a coronary care unit equipped for continuous monitoring of the ECG, with alarm signals, arterial and venous pressure recording, pacemaker insertion and resuscitation equipment, and specially trained nurses and physicians in attendance. Facilities for introduction of bedside Swan-Ganz balloon catheters for determination of intracardiac pressures and oxygen content in the right heart, pressure transducers for determination of direct intra-arterial pressure, and equipment to determine the cardiac output by the thermodilution method are valuable in the individualized management of severe manifestations occurring during the course of acute myocardial infarction. Equipment for taking bedside chest films, an echocardiograph, and perhaps equipment to determine the wall motion and perfusion status of the myocardium utilizing radioisotopes are also desirable, either in the unit or nearby.

Every effort must be made to recognize arrhythmias early and to recognize and treat complications of acute myocardial infarction that would otherwise be diagnosed by direct hemodynamic monitoring. The minimum requirements are constant surveillance and a trained person who can respond immediately if arrhythmias or other complications occur.

In smaller hospitals, criteria for admission to the coronary care unit must be established to select patients who will benefit most from the services available. The major benefit of the coronary care unit is that it makes possible early recognition of severe ventricular arrhythmias, which may be the prelude to ventricular fibrillation and sudden death. Patients with mild initial episodes of myocardial infarction are at less risk, though arrhythmia may develop and ventricular fibrillation can occur early. Patients with a good clinical story for prolonged myocardial ischemia with a normal ECG, even if a myocardial infarction evolves, have an excellent prognosis with few complications and can safely be followed in a monitored bed on the ward (Slater, 1987). Priorities for selection of patients for admission to a limited coronary care unit are not universally agreed upon and may vary with time and place.

A. Home Care of Acute Myocardial Infarction: Where coronary care units are not available, home care for patients with initially mild acute myocardial infarction is acceptable if the minimum requirement for constant surveillance and ready availability of effective treatment of arrhythmias can be met.

B. Hospital Care of Acute Myocardial Infarction: The goals of hospital therapy are (1) to relieve pain and anxiety; (2) to prevent and treat serious ventricular arrhythmias; (3) to recognize ventricular fibrillation immediately and give treatment to prevent sudden cardiac death; (4) to recognize the presence of cardiac failure and treat it vigorously so as to prevent extension of the myocardial infarction; (5) to attempt to decrease the extent of the infarcted and ischemic myocardium; (6) to protect the damaged myocardium by increased rest and judicious ambulation; (7) to risk-stratify the patient at the end of hospitalization; and (8) to improve survival.

1. Immediate measures– (See Emergency Measures for sudden death, p 157.) The risk of ventricular fibrillation and sudden death is greatest in the first 4 hours. Patients with acute myocardial infarction should enter the coronary care unit as soon as possible so that defibrillation can be performed if needed. The extension of coronary care capability to specially equipped ambulances and fire department vehicles manned by personnel trained in defibrillation and resuscitation (so-called pre-coronary care) may reduce the number of deaths in the first hour after the attack.

Upon arrival in the emergency department, an ECG should be performed immediately. If the ECG shows elevation of ST segments consistent with acute myocardial infarction, a nitroglycerin tablet, 0.4 mg, should be given sublingually. It can be repeated in 5 minutes. If there is no relief, no dramatic decrease in ST segment elevation, and the patient is less than 6 hours from onset of the discomfort (some authorities say 12 hours), the patient without contraindications is a candidate for thrombolysis (see below). An aspirin tablet should be chewed immediately, and aspirin should be continued thereafter at a dosage of 0.3 g/d. If the ECG shows ST–T wave changes other than ST segment elevation or if more than 6 hours have elapsed since the onset, the patient should be transported to the CCU immediately under continuous electrocardiographic monitoring.

At this point, a decision is made about whether thrombolytic therapy is indicated. This subject is considered in detail later in this chapter.

2. Relief of pain– Relief of pain is the first requirement if cardiac rhythm is satisfactory. Pain may cause nausea and vomiting, hypertension or hypotension, sinus tachycardia, sweating, and restlessness due to acute anxiety.

If the pain is severe or if the patient is in shock, give morphine sulfate, 2–5 mg slowly intravenously, repeated every 15 minutes until pain is relieved, or, less desirably, meperidine (pethidine; Demerol), 25–50 mg intravenously, repeated in 15 minutes if necessary. If the pain is not severe but bad enough to be disturbing, give morphine, 10–15 mg intramuscularly, repeated in 1 hour if necessary; or meperidine, 50–100 mg intramuscularly. Morphine or meperidine should not be repeated, however, if respirations are less than 12/min. The patient should be kept supine following injection of morphine to avoid hypotension and fainting. Monitoring of respirations is necessary.

If the pain is not relieved by opiates or oxygen (see below), aminophylline can be given, 0.5 g slowly intravenously at a rate of 1–2 mL/min. Pentazocine is not recommended as an alternative analgesic for pain of myocardial infarction, because it increases left ventricular filling pressure and cardiac work. Nitroglycerin sublingually or isosorbide dinitrate orally may relieve pain, but the drug must be stopped if tachycardia or hypotension develops. If sublingual nitroglycerin is ineffective, one should start intravenous nitroglycerin, 5–10 μg/min, rapidly titrated upward at increments of 5–10 μg/min, until relief of angina occurs or the mean blood pressure falls by 10 mm Hg. The mean blood pressure should remain above 80 mm Hg—otherwise, hypoperfusion of ischemic areas can occur (Flaherty, 1992). Beta-blocking drugs may relieve persistent pain but should be used cautiously because of their negative inotropic action.

3. Rest–

a. Sedation– Patients with acute myocardial infarction are apprehensive and anxious and often have a feeling of impending doom. Opiates, in addition to relieving pain, produce physical and mental rest by allaying anxiety; if they are ineffective, drugs such as diazepam, 2.5–5 mg orally every 4–6 hours, may be helpful. If pain is not a problem and patients are restless and unable to sleep, sedatives should be used as necessary, because adequate sleep is vital for physical and mental rest.

b. Bedside care– During the first day or two, patients with myocardial infarction should be at bed rest. Diet should be mild, low-calorie, and low-residue, with multiple small feedings. Most patients find that a bedside commode, with help getting on and off, requires less effort than use of a bedpan. Patients not in hemodynamic trouble or on a respirator can feed themselves, but modified bed rest is advisable for at least the first week. In mild, uncomplicated cases, sitting should begin after 3 days with 30 minutes in a chair, the time being progressively increased depending upon individual response.

4. Oxygen– The decreased cardiac output and pulmonary venous congestion associated with acute myocardial infarction often result in decreased arterial Po_2; levels as low as 50 mm Hg during breathing of room air are not uncommon. Hypoxemia of this degree may contribute to the development of ventricular arrhythmias, hypotension, unrelieved chest pain, and left ventricular failure. Oxygen by face mask at flow rates of 6–10 L/min is preferable to intranasal oxygen. Positive pressure breathing is often resisted by the patient, decreases venous return and cardiac output, and may aggravate myocardial ischemia. Other procedures for the management of left ventricular failure with dyspnea are preferable (see below).

5. Anticoagulant therapy– Anticoagulant therapy during the acute phase is controversial. In the past, three major trials looked at anticoagulation during acute myocardial infarction using warfarin or similar drugs. These trials showed no major impact on the outcome of acute myocardial infarction. A recent analysis of 20 trials involving 5700 patients with suspected acute myocardial infarction revealed a 20% reduction in likelihood of death as well as significantly less deep venous thrombosis, pulmonary embolism, stroke, and reinfarction in patients receiving either subcutaneous or intravenous heparin compared with placebo (MacMahon: Circulation, 1988).

Left ventricular mural thrombi can be identified in 20–40% of acute myocardial infarctions, especially in anterior wall myocardial infarction (Keren, 1990). Anticoagulants have also been shown to decrease the incidence of residual thrombi in the left ventricle and to decrease the incidence of clinical embolic events (Turpie, 1989). We are at present not routinely anticoagulating all patients with acute myocardial infarction.

Anticoagulants are not used routinely in patients with mild attacks. In older patients with cardiac failure in whom prolonged bed rest is anticipated, anticoagulation is often given to prevent venous thrombosis and possible pulmonary emboli unless there are contraindications such as a history of bleeding, peptic ulcer, or hepatic insufficiency. Such prophylactic therapy is given as subcutaneous heparin 5000 units every 12 hours. Anticoagulants can be stopped when patients are fully ambulatory. For treatment of acute attacks, randomized studies favor continuous rather than intermittent intravenous heparin therapy, because major bleeding episodes appear to be more common when boluses of heparin are given intravenously at 4-hour intervals than when heparin is given as a continuous intravenous drip of 1000–1500 units/h. An intravenous loading dose of 100 units/kg is often given in order to keep the clotting time at 15–20 minutes. If there are systemic emboli, warfarin should be used. A possible indication is echocardiographic visualization of a large thrombus. Anticoagulation is at best only marginal in the light of the low incidence of thromboembolic complications currently observed in patients with acute myocardial infarction.

6. Antiplatelet therapy– Evidence that antiplatelet therapy reduces the incidence of acute myocardial infarction and death in patients with unstable angina is compelling (Lewis, 1983; Cairns, 1985) and raises the possibility that aspirin would be beneficial in the treatment of acute myocardial infarction. This hypothesis was tested in the Second International Study of Infarct Survival (ISIS-2). In this study, over 17,000 patients suspected of having an acute myocardial infarction were randomized to 1–5 million units of intravenous streptokinase, 160 mg of aspirin, a combination of both, or placebo. Five weeks after randomization, those taking aspirin showed a 23% reduction in risk of cardiovascular death, a 50% reduction in risk of nonfatal reinfarction in hospital, and a 46% reduction in nonfatal stroke in hospital—all highly significant results (Figure 8–29). This study alone justifies the use of aspirin during and after acute myocardial infarction if there are no contraindications.

7. Beta-adrenergic-blocking agents– Beta-adrenergic-blocking agents can decrease blood pressure, heart rate, and myocardial contractility, thereby decreasing myocardial oxygen demand and myocardial ischemia. The prolongation of diastole may improve subendocardial perfusion. The marked increase in sympathetic tone and catecholamines seen early after onset of myocardial infarction results in increased arrhythmogenic potential that can be diminished with beta-blocking agents (Yusuf, 1990).

No consensus has been reached about the use of these drugs during an acute myocardial infarction. The ISIS-1 study used atenolol within 12 hours after onset of acute myocardial infarction in over 16,000 patients and showed a small but significant ($P < .02$) reduction in mortality rate from 4.3% to 3.7%. There

were also favorable trends in reinfarction rate and cardiac arrest (ISIS-1, 1986). In the TIMI-II trial, metoprolol was used in conjunction with thrombolytic agents. The frequency of reinfarction was reduced (TIMI Study Group, 1989). In the absence of clinical left ventricular failure and other contraindications to beta-blocking drugs such as obstructive pulmonary disease—and especially in patients with hypertension, tachycardia, or continued angina—beta-blocking drugs are indicated. All of the beta-blocking agents are effective except those with intrinsic sympathomimetic activity. The recommendation is to use metoprolol, 5 mg intravenously, every 2 minutes for three doses. Fifteen minutes after the last dose, 50 mg orally every 6 hours is given for 48 hours and 100 mg twice daily thereafter.

8. Nitrate therapy– Nitrates are preload-reducing agents that pool venous return and decrease the ventricular filling pressure and diastolic volume. They also decrease systemic vascular resistance and decrease arterial pressure. These two actions decrease myocardial oxygen demand and myocardial ischemia. They also dilate epicardial coronary arteries even in some areas of atherosclerotic occlusive disease, thus increasing coronary blood flow through the obstructed vessel, further decreasing myocardial ischemia.

Initially, patients are given sublingual nitroglycerin, 0.4 mg, unless the systolic pressure is under 90 mm Hg or there is tachycardia. Later, transdermal nitroglycerin can be substituted, but initially we avoid long-acting nitrates. The closest control is obtained with intravenous nitroglycerin. For many years, this was considered to be harmful in acute myocardial infarction. Since that time, experimental and clinical studies have shown a possible decrease in myocardial infarct size, a decrease in ventricular remodeling with the result of smaller end-systolic and diastolic left ventricular volumes, and even a decrease in mortality rate (Jugdutt, 1988). In meta-analysis of pooled studies of intravenous nitrates in acute myocardial infarction, the mortality rate is reduced by 10–30% (Yusuf, 1988).

When starting intravenous nitroglycerin, a 15 μg bolus is given and a pump-controlled infusion of 5–10 μg/min is started. Dosage can be increased by 5–10 μg/min every 5–10 minutes while hemodynamic responses are monitored. The end point should be the control of symptoms or a decrease in the mean arterial pressure of 10% in normotensive patients or 30% in hypertensive patients, always maintaining a systolic pressure over 90 mm Hg. Other end points are an increase in heart rate of 10 beats/min but less than 110 beats/min or a decrease in pulmonary artery end-diastolic pressure of 10–30%. If doses over 200 μg/min are needed, other vasodilators, such as nitroprusside, should be used.

9. Drugs to prevent ventricular remodeling– After acute myocardial infarction, there is a loss of

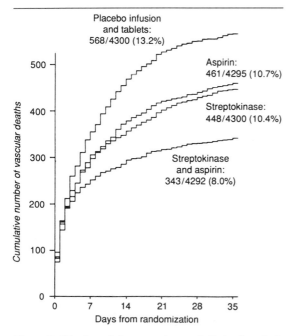

Figure 8–29. Cumulative vascular mortality in days 0–5. (Reproduced, with permission, from ISIS-2 (Second International Study of Infarct Survival) Collaborative Group: Randomised trial of intravenous streptokinase, oral aspirin, both, or neither among 17,187 cases of suspected acute myocardial infarction: ISIS-2. Lancet 1988;2:349.)

functioning myocardium, which, when of sufficient magnitude, results in a decrease of ventricular function. Subsequently, with a large myocardial infarction, the left ventricle dilates, and with decreased function there is an increase in left ventricular diastolic and systolic volumes and a decrease in ejection fraction (Rouleau, 1991). The neurohumoral system is also activated, including the sympathetic nervous system and catecholamines, as well as the renin-angiotensin system. This occurs even without clinical congestive heart failure. There is evidence that unloading the left ventricle with either angiotensin-converting enzyme inhibitors (Sharpe, 1991) or nitroglycerin (Jugdutt, 1988) favorably affects this remodeling, resulting in a smaller left ventricular end-diastolic and end-systolic volume and a higher ejection fraction. When these drugs should be started is in question. A recent study (Swedberg, 1992) has reported that enalapril, when started within 24 hours after onset of myocardial infarction, does not improve survival during the months after infarction.

Several large studies have evaluated the use of these drugs in patients after acute myocardial infarction. The Survival and Ventricular Enlargement (SAVE) Trial is a double-blind, placebo-controlled study of the use of captopril in over 2000 patients with acute myocardial infarction and a left ventricular ejection fraction of 40% or less but without overt heart failure or symptoms of myocardial ischemia. The drug was started 3–16 days postinfarction. The end points were death and the effects on left ventricular end-diastolic and end-systolic volume and ejection fraction (Moye, 1991). Follow-up was for 42 months. Mortality from all causes was significantly reduced in the captopril patients versus placebo patients (20% versus 25%) with a reduction in risk of 19%. Interestingly, the incidence of both fatal and nonfatal cardiovascular events was significantly reduced in the captopril group by 21%. Death from cardiovascular causes was reduced by 37%, the development of congestive heart failure by 22%, and recurrent myocardial infarction by 25%. All benefits were seen even in those patients taking aspirin, thrombolytic agents, and beta blockers, suggesting that treatment with captopril leads to additional improvement in outcome after acute myocardial infarction (Pfeffer, 1992). After myocardial infarction resulting in reduced ejection fraction, angiotensin-converting enzyme inhibitors should be used.

The International Studies of Infarct Survival (ISIS-4) Collaborative Group are studying the effects of 1 month of captopril versus placebo or 1 month of oral controlled-release mononitrate versus placebo in patients with acute myocardial infarction (ISIS-4 Collaborative Group, 1991). When completed, this study should establish whether converting enzyme inhibitors or nitrates (or both together) will be useful in reducing the mortality rate after acute myocardial in-

farction and, if so, when they should be started (Pfeffer, 1991).

Thrombolytic Reperfusion Agents

Angiography in the early hours after acute myocardial infarction has demonstrated complete occlusion with thrombosis in 87% of patients (DeWood, 1980). Efforts to recanalize the occluded artery and reestablish coronary arterial flow by thrombolysis have been employed to permit survival of myocardium in patients in whom irreversible necrosis had not occurred and limit the area of infarction. After occlusion, myocardial necrosis develops rapidly, starting about 20 minutes after obstruction in the subendocardium and proceeding to the subepicardium, with the majority of the myocardium at risk infarcted by 4–6 hours. If residual perfusion is present either because of incomplete obstruction or because of collaterals, the time course is prolonged.

A. Intracoronary Infusion: The first convincing evidence that fibrinolytic agents could establish patency of an occluded coronary artery when given early in the course of an acute myocardial infarction was with the infusion into the coronary artery of streptokinase (Chazov, 1976). Intracoronary infusions of streptokinase given within 3–4 hours of the onset of symptoms have been shown to restore the patency of the thrombosed artery in about 60% of cases; however, a highly skilled team with a standby catheterization laboratory is necessary, and that was a significant problem in establishing this treatment for general use. Myocardial perfusion and ejection fraction have improved in these cases. In some patients, immediate relief of angina is achieved, reversal of elevated ST segments occurs, and abnormal ECGs change toward normal. Cardiogenic shock may be reversed in some cases.

B. Intravenous Therapy: Intravenous thrombolysis has replaced intracoronary use because it can be administered in hospitals without catheterization laboratories and accomplishes patency, and therefore reperfusion, at least 1 hour earlier. Given the time course of myocardial necrosis after coronary occlusion, the earlier the fibrinolytic agent results in reperfusion, the more myocardium is salvaged (Tiefenbrunn, 1992).

Three fibrinolytic agents have at present been approved by the FDA for intravenous use in acute myocardial infarction: (1) **Streptokinase,** which complexes with plasminogen, which then converts circulating and fibrin-fixed plasminogen to plasmin, which lyses fibrin. This streptokinase-plasminogen complex results in circulating plasmin, which causes a systemic fibrinolysis with consumption of prothrombin, factors V and VIII, fibrinogen, plasminogen, and fibrin degradation products. Because it is a bacterial product, it is antigenic. (2) **Tissue plasminogen activator** (tPA), which is a product of recombinant DNA technology (sometimes abbreviated rt-PA). This drug is by itself inactive, but in the presence of fibrin it has a high affinity for plasminogen, thereby activating plasminogen in contact with fibrin on the surface of a thrombus. Unlike streptokinase, tPA is relatively thrombus-specific and produces less of a generalized lytic state. There are two forms of tPA, a single-chain form, alteplase, and a two-chain duteplase form. (3) **Anisoylated plasminogen streptokinase activator complex** (anistreplase; APSAC). This agent is a complex of streptokinase and lys-plasminogen with a *p*-anisoyl group placed in the catalytic center of the molecule (Anderson, 1988). In the intact state, APSAC is an inactive complex, but when injected into the blood, hydrolysis of the anisoyl group occurs, producing the active streptokinase-plasminogen complex. This produces fibrinolysis with a half-life of approximately 120 minutes, compared with the 15- to 20-minute half-life of streptokinase and the ultrashort half-life of 5 minutes for tPA.

Two other fibrinolytic agents are (1) **urokinase,** which acts on plasminogen, converting it to plasmin directly; and (2) **pro-urokinase** (single-chain urokinase-type plasminogen activator) (SCU-PA) (Bode, 1988). Urokinase is not antigenic, but it is not yet approved for use in acute myocardial infarction. Pro-urokinase is still in the experimental stage of development.

Although many placebo-controlled trials of streptokinase and tPA had been conducted, the huge GISSI trial was the first to show that fibrinolysis lowers the mortality rate in acute myocardial infarction (Gruppo Italiano, 1987). At 21 days, the rate was 10.7% in the treated group and 13% in the control group. Reduction in mortality was inversely related to the time after onset of symptoms that streptokinase was given. Under 1 hour after onset, there was a 50% reduction in mortality rate. When the drug was given during the first 3 hours, there was a 25% reduction; between 3 and 6 hours, there was an 18% reduction; and after 6 hours there was no benefit. In this study, only anterior wall infarctions benefited, and no benefit was shown in patients with Killip class III or class IV status or those with non-Q wave infarction.

Subsequent to the GISSI study, the ISIS-2 study involved over 17,000 patients randomized to four groups: streptokinase, aspirin, streptokinase plus aspirin, and placebo. The 5-week mortality rate revealed a 26% reduction in mortality with streptokinase alone, a 21% reduction with aspirin alone, and a 40% reduction with streptokinase and aspirin together (Figure 8–29). Admission to this study was by suspicion of acute myocardial infarction up to 24 hours after onset, and a small benefit in reduction of mortality was seen up to 24 hours after onset (ISIS-2, 1988). Numerous trials have shown similar reductions in mortality rates with tPA and APSAC compared with placebo (Wilcox, 1988; AIMS Trial Study Group, 1988).

The relative ability of tPA versus streptokinase to result in reperfusion within 90 minutes was studied in the Thrombolysis in Myocardial Infarction (TIMI-I) trial, where angiographic reperfusion occurred in 62% of tPA patients versus only 31% of streptokinase patients (Chesebro, 1987). The European Cooperative Group (ECSG-I) reported a 70% 90-minute patency rate with tPA compared with a 55% rate with streptokinase (European Cooperative Study Group, 1985). Patency rates with APSAC have been similar to those with tPA.

There is an ongoing debate about which agent is best, but several recent trials have shown no difference in mortality rate, reinfarction rate, or final left ventricular function between streptokinase and tPA; these include the GISSI-2 study, which randomized patients to tPA or streptokinase within 6 hours after onset (Gruppo Italiano, 1990); and the International tPA/Streptokinase Trial, which randomized over 20,000 patients, including 12,000 patients in the GISSI-2 study (International Study Group, 1990). In the latter study, 12,500 units of subcutaneous heparin started 12 hours after the thrombolytic agent was shown to have no benefit on mortality rate. The incidence of all strokes was greater in the tPA group compared with the streptokinase group (1.3% versus 0.9%), and major bleeding was more frequent with streptokinase than with tPA (0.9% versus 0.6%).

The ISIS-3 trial (presented in a preliminary report at the American College of Cardiology meeting at Atlanta, March 1991) randomized over 20,000 patients to streptokinase, APSAC, or tPA in the form of duteplase. All patients received aspirin and subcutaneous heparin started 4 hours after the fibrinolysis was initiated. No difference in mortality rate among the three fibrinolytic therapies was found. Reinfarction was lowest with duteplase, and hypotension and allergic reactions were more common with streptokinase and anistreplase. The lowest incidence of strokes and probable intracranial hemorrhage was seen with streptokinase. No benefit was shown with subcutaneous heparin.

There are differences among these agents that account for theoretical or actual benefits and disadvantages. Streptokinase is a foreign protein derived from the *Streptococcus* organism that elicits antibody production and allergic reactions, which makes giving it on a second occasion undesirable. Additionally, streptokinase, because of the rapid generation of plasmin and bradykinin, causes hypotension in some patients. Anistreplase (APSAC) produces these vasodilating substrates more slowly but still produces occasional episodes of hypotension.

Recombinant tissue plasminogen activator is more fibrin-specific and therefore produces less of a generalized lytic state and less chance of hemorrhage compared with streptokinase. A disadvantage is that it has a short half-life of about 5 minutes. Since fibrin and thrombolysis activate platelets, rethrombosis is prob-

Table 8–13. Indications for and contraindications to thrombolytic therapy.

INDICATIONS FOR THROMBOLYTIC THERAPY

- Patients presenting with chest pain or discomfort consistent with acute myocardial infarction and ≥ 1 mm of ST elevation in 2 contiguous ECG leads or in 1 lead reflecting the inferior wall of the heart.
- Ideally, where fibrinolytics can be administered in less than 6 hours after onset of pain. Less benefit is seen where fibrinolytics are given 6–12 hours after onset, and only questionable benefit is seen between 12 and 24 hours after onset.
- There is no definite upper age limit. Mortality benefit is seen in patients over 75 years of age.
- There are no absolute age or time from onset contraindications. The younger the patient and the shorter the time after onset, the more the benefit outweighs the risk in those with relative contraindications.

CONTRAINDICATIONS TO THROMBOLYTIC THERAPY
(The major side-effect seen with thrombolytic therapy is hemorrhage).

Absolute Contraindications
- Active or recent (< 2 weeks) internal bleeding.
- History of cerebrovascular hemorrhage.
- Blood pressure > 200/120 mm Hg.
- Prolonged or traumatic cardiopulmonary resuscitation.
- Suspected aortic dissection or pericarditis.
- Hemorrhagic ophthalmic conditions such as diabetic hemorrhagic retinopathy.
- Recent (< 2 weeks) head trauma, CNS surgery, or known intracranial neoplasm.
- Known allergy to streptokinase or anistreplase (APSAC). (Can use tPA or urokinase.)
- Pregnancy.
- Recent surgery (< 2 weeks) that could be a source of internal bleeding.

Relative Contraindications
- Head trauma or surgery (> 2 weeks).
- Recent severe hypertension with or without treatment.
- Active peptic ulcer.
- History of cerebrovascular accident.
- History of bleeding diathesis or current use of anticoagulants.
- Significant hepatic dysfunction.
- Use of streptokinase or anistreplase (APSAC) < 9 months before. (Does not apply to use of tPA or urokinase.)

[1] Adapted, with permission, from Gunnar, 1990.

ably more common with tPA than with the longer-acting streptokinase. It is possible that with proper antiplatelet drugs and anticoagulation, early reocclusion could be prevented and the ultimate benefit of tPA improved over that seen with streptokinase.

Table 8–13 lists the indications and contraindications for thrombolytic therapy as adapted from the ACC/AHA Task Force on Treatment of Acute Myocardial Infarction (Gunnar, 1990).

There is strong evidence in recent large trials that early administration of SK—with or without associated aspirin—and of tPA improve left ventricular function (especially in patients with anterior infarction) and reduce mortality rates in acute myocardial

infarction treated within 3–4 hours of the onset of infarction (Gruppo Italiano, 1987; ISIS-2 Collaborative Group, 1988). Which of the various thrombolytic agents will prove to be the most effective remains to be seen. Researchers are currently considering the possible added effectiveness of combining various thrombolytic and antiplatelet agents that act by different mechanisms.

Myocardial reperfusion is being intensively investigated in various centers; many questions still unsettled may be resolved in the near future (Topol, 1988).

C. Reocclusion and Residual Stenoses: One important problem with fibrinolytic agents is the reocclusion rate. When data from nine studies were pooled, 61 of 311 patients (17%) had angiographically documented reocclusion. In a cooperative study utilizing tPA, a late reocclusion was found in three of 60 patients (Verstraete, 1987). Some studies found a higher rate of reocclusion.

The use of heparin as an adjunct to fibrinolytic therapy is under investigation. The TAMI-III trial (Topol, 1989) randomized patients who received tPA to immediate intravenous heparin versus placebo, and at 90 minutes the patency rate for the infarct-related artery in both was an identical 79%. The more recent Heparin-Aspirin Reperfusion Trial (HART) (Hsia, 1990) compared immediate intravenous heparin with oral aspirin after tPA. After 18 hours, patency of the infarct-related artery was 82% in the heparin group and 52% in the aspirin group. The report from the European Cooperative Study Group Trial (ECSG-6) is that in 652 patients post-tPA and aspirin, patients given intravenous heparin had an 83% patency rate at 81 hours compared with 75% when no heparin was given.

The GUSTO Trial (Global Utilization of Streptokinase and tPA for Occluded Coronary Arteries) will compare alteplase given as a front-loaded dose with streptokinase and with a combination of tPA and streptokinase with and without intravenous heparin in about 40,000 patients. The primary end point will be mortality, and angiographic studies will allow patency rate to be correlated with clinical outcome.

The present recommendations for dosages of the various fibrinolytic agents are listed in Table 8–14.

After effective fibrinolysis, severe obstructive lesions may remain in the affected coronary artery in many patients. Some cardiologists have recommended performing immediate angioplasty in these patients to decrease the residual occlusion. In addition, some patients fail to reperfuse with thrombolysis, and "rescue angioplasty" has been advocated in these patients. However, three definitive studies conclude that immediate angioplasty after thrombolysis is no more effective and may be associated with a higher complication rate (occlusion, emergency surgery, and death) than elective coronary arteriography and angiography delayed 24 hours to 10 days after the fibrinolysis (Topol, 1987; Simoons,

Table 8–14. Recommended dosages of fibrinolytic agents.

Thrombolytic Agent	Dosage and Comments
Streptokinase	1.5 million units over 1 hour IV. Heparin can be started IV 4 hours after the streptokinase and maintained for 48 hours.
tPA	• 10-mg bolus IV, 50 mg in the first hour, 20 mg in the second and third hours. • Rapid or front-loading: 　15 mg IV bolus 　0.75 mg/kg over 30 minutes 　0.50 mg/kg over 60 minutes In both of these schedules, the total dose is ≤ 100 mg. Heparin can be started IV immediately after tPA is given and maintained for 48 hours.
Combined tPA and streptokinase	tPA, 1 mg/kg over 60 minutes, 10% as a bolus (total dose ≤ 90 mg); and streptokinase, 1 million units over 1 hour. Start IV heparin after thrombolysis and maintain for 48 hours.
Anistreplase (APSAC)	30 units IV over 5 minutes.

1988; TIMI Research Group, 1988). From these data it is apparent that angioplasty is generally unnecessary soon after tPA and should be undertaken only if ischemia recurs. The TIMI II B trial concludes that comparison of patients randomized to delayed catheterization and angioplasty with those randomized to predischarge, low-level exercise stress testing to determine ischemia showed equal mortality rates, reinfarction rates, and ejection fraction on hospital discharge and 1 year later (TIMI Study Group, 1989; Zaret, 1992; Williams, 1992). The patients randomized to exercise stress testing received coronary arteriography and revascularization only if important ischemia, was documented symptomatically or by the stress test. Thus, patients who do well after thrombolysis can be ambulated and the presence of residual ischemia determined by a low-level exercise stress test. Those without recurring angina or significant ischemia on the exercise test can be managed medically without coronary arteriography—a significant advantage in community hospitals (Rogers, 1991).

D. Postthrombolytic Therapy: Most recommendations for drug treatment after thrombolysis are based on hypothetical reasoning and are therefore unproved. After thrombolysis, there is usually still severe obstruction and residual thrombus. With an unstable plaque, there is danger of platelet deposition and rethrombosis as well as vasospasm (Gunnar, 1990; Roberts, 1991; Popma, 1991).

After thrombolysis, we administer drugs as follows: (1) intravenous heparin, starting immediately after thrombolysis and continuing for 48 hours; (2) aspirin, one 325 mg tablet chewed immediately, followed by one 0.3 g tablet daily; (3) intravenous or

topical nitroglycerin for 24–48 hours; and (4) in the absence of contraindications, a beta-blocking agent such as metoprolol, 5 mg every 15 minutes for three doses, followed by 50 mg twice daily.

The TIMI II study demonstrated that when beta-blockers were started within 2 hours after onset, there was a reduction in mortality rate and nonfatal reinfarction; when started within 4 hours after hospitalization, there was a reduction in nonfatal reinfarction and recurrent ischemia (TIMI Study Group, 1989).

E. Newer Antiplatelet and Antithrombotic Agents: More effective antiplatelet and antithrombotic agents are under development. These include thromboxane synthase inhibitors and thromboxane and serotonin receptor antagonists. Monoclonal antibodies against platelet membrane receptors and von Willebrand factor have been developed. Antibodies against the glycoprotein IIb–IIIa, which functions as the major platelet membrane receptor for fibrinogen, has demonstrated effectiveness in in vitro models and during thrombolysis (Mickelson, 1990; Fareed, 1992).

Antithrombotic substances are also being evaluated. Hirudin and other antithrombin III-independent substances which, unlike heparin, do not require a cofactor for thrombin inhibitory activity can inhibit free as well as clot-bound thrombin. These substances have no natural inhibitors—unlike heparin, which is inhibited by platelet factor 4 and by fibrin monomers present at the site of thrombus formation. These substrates are more effective than heparin in in vitro models of arterial thrombosis and are able to accelerate time-to-clot lysis. If they prove to be safe in humans, they will be valuable for preventing reocclusion after thrombolysis.

F. Primary Angioplasty Without Preceding Thrombolysis: Primary angioplasty of the infarct-related coronary artery without prior thrombolysis has been advocated if the vessel can be opened within 4–6 hours after onset of pain. Centers with the most experience have reported opening of the infarct-related artery in 90% of patients with a mortality rate, requirement for emergency bypass surgery, and long-term results as good as or better than those reported with thrombolysis (Kalin, 1990). This approach has the disadvantage of requiring a catheterization laboratory and an experienced team immediately available, but it is especially valuable in patients with acute myocardial infarction who have a contraindication to thrombolysis. It is also the better strategy in patients with acute myocardial infarction and profound congestive heart failure or cardiogenic shock (Lee, 1991).

G. Coronary Bypass Surgery in Acute Myocardial Infarction: In general, there is little place for coronary bypass surgery in the presence of an acute, uncomplicated Q wave myocardial infarction, though there are still advocates for this type of revascularization (ACC/AHA Task Force, 1991; DeWood, 1989).

If the patient has recurrent myocardial ischemia unresponsive to medical therapy, coronary arteriography is indicated. If there is significant myocardium at risk and if the angioplasty of the culprit vessel is contraindicated, bypass surgery is indicated. In the presence of a non-Q wave myocardial infarction, recurrent ischemia unresponsive to medical therapy is managed like unstable angina. Here bypass surgery is attended by the same excellent results as are seen in unstable angina (Ryan, 1990).

General Clinical Observation

After the patient has been relieved of pain, reassured, sedated, given oxygen, and made comfortable in bed with monitoring devices in place, further therapy depends on the presence or absence of complications.

The physician must be prepared to deal with the patient's regression, denial, anger, and hostility as well as anxiety, because emotional stress adversely affects the course of the disease and its management. The physician's manner is most important in minimizing emotional responses to the illness. Neither excessive gravity nor excessive optimism is warranted; realistic optimism is always both justified and therapeutic.

Clinical observation by the physician at hourly intervals during the first day is required to make certain that pain does not return and that hypotension, cardiogenic shock, ventricular arrhythmias, and cardiac failure do not occur. The function of constant observation by special coronary care nurses is to alert the physician to any new symptoms such as dyspnea, embolism, palpitations, mental confusion, oliguria, syncope or near-syncope from heart block, or arrhythmias.

Activity Following Uncomplicated Infarction

Increasingly, patients are being encouraged to increase their activity in bed after the first 2 days, to sit up on the third or fourth day, and to walk about the room on the fifth to seventh days, provided the course has been mild and uncomplicated and the patient tolerates the increased activity without incident. Cautious controlled ambulation allows the patient with mild myocardial infarction and a good home situation to leave the hospital between the tenth and fourteenth days. In the future, discharge after successful thrombolysis may be safe as early as the fourth hospital day, but this is still under investigation (Mark, 1991). Early hospital discharge is unwise if, during the acute phase of infarction, the patient has had multiple ventricular premature beats, ventricular tachycardia or fibrillation, second- or third-degree atrioventricular block, cardiac failure with pulmonary edema or cardiogenic shock, sinus tachycardia, systemic hypotension, atrial arrhythmias, or any evidence of extension of the infarction. These complications eliminate from early ambulation at least half of patients with infarction.

During ambulation and before discharge, the response of the patient should be monitored, so that the pulse rate and blood pressure can be observed and the presence of symptoms determined. If recovery is not smooth, the process of rehabilitation can be slowed until a stable state occurs. The object is for the patient to be partially self-sufficient before discharge.

Exercise Testing Before Hospital Discharge

Many centers recommend submaximal exercise testing approximately 7–14 days after an uncomplicated acute myocardial infarction, just before hospital discharge, in order to estimate long-term prognosis. Low-level exercise testing (with close monitoring of the patient, the ECG, and blood pressure and with resuscitation equipment immediately available) can be limited either by heart rate (up to 120–130/min) or by symptoms. Patients are exercised to the approximate metabolic equivalent of activity that they would be expected to engage in at home (about 4 METS). Patients who have a positive electrocardiographic stress test with ST depression of greater than 1 mm or who show complex ventricular arrhythmias have a greater likelihood of reinfarction, sudden death, and cardiac death in the following 1–2 years (Moss, 1987; O'Rourke, 1991). These patients usually have impairment of left ventricular function, which is an independent prognostic factor.

Results of low-level exercise testing are helpful in estimating prognosis, planning activities following discharge from the hospital, and adjusting treatment. Opinions differ as to whether ST depression or complex ventricular arrhythmias are more significant; the duration of exercise that can be performed and evidence of left ventricular dysfunction are thought by some to be more important than either of the other two findings. An important secondary result of the predischarge exercise test is reassurance of the patient and the family when exercise can be performed without significant symptoms or abnormal findings. If there is any question about the patient's ability to perform even low-level exercise, it should be postponed for 3 weeks.

The following are adverse prognostic signs: ST segment depression at a low heart rate; inability to increase the heart rate or the systolic blood pressure by 10 mm Hg; a fall in systolic pressure of 10 mm Hg or more; the inability to walk into the third stage of the Bruce protocol; the development of angina at a low heart rate; the development of rales; and an S_3 gallop.

In managing patients who have had an uncomplicated acute myocardial infarction, there are compelling arguments for postponement of exercise stress testing until 3 weeks postinfarction, when a symptom-limited exercise test can be performed. This delay is associated with a very low incidence of death or recurrent infarction in properly selected patients and can be used for evaluation of functional aerobic capacity as well as for prognostication (DeBusk, 1989; Gibson, 1991). Patients with a negative exercise electrocardiographic response to a 7 METS score or higher workload at 3 weeks have a 1-year mortality rate of less than 2% (Gunnar, 1990).

An exercise program begun early after myocardial infarction and continued for several months was found to have neither adverse nor beneficial physiologic effects. Most patients had marked spontaneous recovery after 3 months with or without the exercise program; after 3 months, no further spontaneous improvement was the rule (Sivarajan, 1982).

Treatment of Complications

A. Arrhythmias:

1. Ventricular arrhythmias– (See also Chapter 15.) The most common adverse event (approximately 90% of acute myocardial infarctions seen within the first 4 hours) (Table 8–8) is the development of an arrhythmia. Ventricular premature beats are common and must be recognized and treated promptly; they indicate either increased irritability from enhanced spontaneous depolarization of the damaged myocardial cells or reentry phenomena from currents of injury set up by impaired conduction and delayed repolarization in neighborhood fibers. Frequent (> 6/min), closely coupled, or multiform ventricular premature beats or ventricular tachycardia should be treated with lidocaine, 50–100 mg intravenously, followed by an infusion at a rate of 1–2 mg/min. In some centers, lidocaine is begun as a prophylactic measure immediately upon admission to the coronary care unit. Although lidocaine reduces the incidence of ventricular tachycardia and fibrillation, studies have not shown a reduction in overall mortality, perhaps because of an increased incidence of asystole (Gunnar, 1991; MacMahon: JAMA, 1988). Lidocaine toxicity occurs at lower dosages in the elderly and in those with congestive heart failure and renal or hepatic disease. If lidocaine is ineffective or produces central nervous system symptoms of confusion or excitement (usually when the drug is given at a higher rate of infusion), alternative drugs may be used, including procainamide, in a loading dose of 20–50 mg/min up to a total dose of 1 g, followed by maintenance infusion of 1–4 mg/min; or quinidine gluconate, in a loading dose of 0.8 g diluted in 100–200 mL of glucose and water, 1 mL/min. If necessary, a maintenance infusion of quinidine may be given, not to exceed 6 μg/mL. Quinidine can be controlled by monitoring blood levels. Do not exceed 6 μg/mL in the steady state infusion. Patients started on beta-blocking drugs have a decreased incidence of ventricular premature beats as well as of more malignant ventricular arrhythmias. If the patient has been receiving digitalis or has hypokalemia resulting from diuretic therapy, potassium salts may be given orally or intravenously depending upon the urgency of need. Prompt treatment of ventricular arrhythmias is indicated to prevent ventricular fibrillation and cardiac arrest.

2. Ventricular tachycardia and fibrillation– Ventricular tachycardia is an emergency and, if not rapidly converted with intravenous lidocaine, should be terminated by electrical cardioversion. Ventricular tachycardia will also respond to intravenous magnesium sulfate. Ventricular fibrillation should be instantly recognized by the alarm system at the nursing station, and defibrillation should be accomplished within 30 seconds. Defibrillation should be performed by specially trained personnel, because delay compromises not only cardiac function but also cerebral function. After defibrillation, lidocaine is given by constant intravenous infusion in a dosage of 1–2 mg/min in order to prevent recurrence. This may be discontinued in 24–48 hours if there is no recurrence. If this is ineffective, procainamide or bretylium can be used.

3. Other ventricular or junctional arrhythmias– Nonparoxysmal ventricular tachycardia (accelerated idioventricular rhythm) with junctional tachycardia and aberrant conduction may occur early in the course of acute myocardial infarction and may be confused with either ventricular tachycardia or complete atrioventricular block. Because the prognosis with these arrhythmias is better than that of ventricular tachycardia in general, supportive care is usually sufficient and defibrillation is rarely needed if the differential diagnosis can be made.

4. Atrial arrhythmias– Atrial arrhythmias occur less frequently (about 15% of cases) than ventricular ones. The most common atrial arrhythmia is atrial fibrillation. It is usually transient, lasting hours or 1–2 days, unless the ventricular rate is rapid and hemodynamic deterioration occurs. Treatment consists of digitalization or slowing the ventricular rate with beta-blockers or verapamil. Urgent treatment is cardioversion. Conservative therapy is usually more desirable. If frequent atrial premature beats occur—especially if they produce hemodynamic deterioration with resultant symptoms—they should be treated with quinidine sulfate, 0.3 g orally every 4–6 hours. Frequent premature beats often presage atrial fibrillation and may result in a fall in arterial pressure that decreases coronary perfusion and may increase the size of the infarct.

5. Late ventricular fibrillation– The frequency of ventricular fibrillation (10–20% overall) decreases with time and with healing of the infarction. Electrocardiographic monitoring should be continued for several days after the last episode of ventricular arrhythmia. Ideally, patients should not be transferred to general medical wards without monitoring equipment but should, if possible, be transferred to an intermediate unit where they can be monitored for another 2 days until it is clear that ventricular arrhythmias are not recurring. Late ventricular tachycardia is frequently seen in patients with left ventricular ejection fractions of 40% or less and indicates a poor prognosis (Rodriguez, 1992).

B. Cardiac Failure and Cardiogenic Shock: Left ventricular performance is impaired to some degree in all patients with acute myocardial infarction. A first myocardial infarction of minor extent in a patient with no underlying cardiac disease usually produces little or no impairment of left ventricular performance as judged by symptoms and signs and by hemodynamic monitoring of cardiac output, left ventricular filling pressure, and arterial pressure, but it may cause hypokinesia on radioisotope wall motion studies. If the infarction is large and occurs in an area of previous infarctions with large areas of scar and borderline compensation, the patient may rapidly develop severe cardiac failure. Possibilities thus range from no clinical evidence of impaired cardiac function to cardiogenic shock with a very high (80%) mortality rate. It is thus appropriate to discuss the subject as a continuum with treatment individualized according to the degree of severity (Table 8–15).

1. Mild and moderate cardiac failure– Some degree of cardiac failure, usually left ventricular failure, can be detected in 20–50% of patients with more than mild acute myocardial infarction. The patient may have dyspnea, pulmonary rales, diastolic gallop rhythm, and accentuated hilar congestion on chest x-ray. The typical central congestion with bat's wing densities does not occur unless the patient develops acute pulmonary edema. The radiologic findings may

Table 8–15. Acute myocardial infarction: Suggested therapeutic measures in relation to hemodynamic indices.[1]

Left Ventricular Stroke Work Index	Left Ventricular Filling Pressure	Therapy
Normal	Normal	Observation
Normal	Raised	Diuretics
Decreased	Decreased or normal	Volume expansion
Moderately decreased	Raised	Afterload reducing agents with or without diuretics
Markedly decreased (cardiogenic shock)	Raised	Intra-aortic balloon counterpulsation and afterload reducing agents. Use inotropic agents if other measures do not increase cardiac output, eg, dopamine or dobutamine.

[1] Modified and reproduced, with permission, from Chatterjee, K, Swan HJC: Hemodynamic profile of acute myocardial infarction. In: *Myocardial Infarction*, Corday E, Swan HJC (editors). Williams & Wilkins, 1973.

be out of phase with the clinical findings because they take longer to develop and to regress. In patients who are being monitored by means of a bedside Swan-Ganz catheter, elevated pulmonary venous wedge pressure may be noted before the radiologic changes occur.

If left ventricular failure is minimal or subclinical, treatment can be conservative, with oral diuretics (eg, hydrochlorothiazide, 50–100 mg orally), oxygen, and avoidance of sodium-containing fluids and food. Hemodynamic intracardiac monitoring is *not necessary,* because the left ventricular filling pressure is usually normal (< 12 mm Hg) and the cardiac index is also normal (> 2.5 L/min/m^2). The prognosis is good (mortality rate $\approx 6\%$).

2. More severe cardiac failure– Left ventricular failure not promptly relieved by cautious sublingual nitroglycerin beginning with 0.4 mg or by diuretic therapy requires more aggressive management (see below). Begin with hemodynamic monitoring of the arterial pressure, pulmonary venous wedge pressure (left ventricular filling pressure), and cardiac output utilizing the Swan-Ganz catheter. The stroke work index can be computed from these measurements, and rational therapy can be directed at the specific hemodynamic abnormality.

Right ventricular infarction, which rarely occurs without left ventricular inferior infarction, is often not recognized and may be responsible for right ventricular failure. The clinical diagnosis is usually suspected from the presence of high jugular and right atrial pressures, which are often higher than the left ventricular filling pressure, or from the presence of a right-sided S$_3$ or S$_4$ gallop; two-dimensional echocardiography and gated blood pool scans may establish the diagnosis. It is important to recognize right ventricular failure in right ventricular infarction, because the high jugular venous pressure helps generate right ventricular flow; venodilators and diuretics should be avoided. Fluid replacement fosters right ventricular output. Arterial vasodilators (see below) may be used to reduce the afterload.

a. Volume replacement– When monitoring reveals that left ventricular filling pressure is low (< 12 mm Hg) and cardiac output is normal despite the low arterial pressure, hypovolemia is the most probable cause. Treatment consists of volume replacement by the intravenous route in 200- to 300-mL increments with dextrose in water or half-normal saline every 5–10 minutes until the left ventricular filling pressure rises to 18 mm Hg. If cardiac output does not increase as the left ventricular filling pressure rises to 15–20 mm Hg, volume replacement should be stopped to prevent pulmonary edema.

b. Diuresis– If the only hemodynamic abnormality is a raised left ventricular filling pressure but blood pressure and cardiac output are normal, more vigorous diuresis can be obtained with large doses (80–160–320 mg) of furosemide. Excessive diuresis

Table 8–16. Vasodilators useful in cardiac failure in acute myocardial infarction.[1]

Vasodilator	Advantages	Disadvantages	Dose Range
Nitroprusside	High potency; immediate effect; half-life extremely short.	Requires hemodynamic monitoring.	15–400 μg/min intravenously.
Phentolamine	High potency; rapid action.	Requires hemodynamic monitoring.	0.25–1 mg/min intravenously.
Isosorbide dinitrate	Sublingual or oral administration.	Less potent than nitroprusside and phentolamine.	2.5–5 mg sublingually; 10–30 mg orally (ingested).
Nitroglycerin ointment	Prolonged duration of action (up to 6 hours); removable.	Topical use may not be well accepted by patients.	1.5–4 inches cutaneously.
Nitroglycerin, transdermal	Continuous well-controlled absorption for 12–24 hours; removable.	May cause headache or hypotension.	2.5–30 mg/24 h.
Nitroglycerin, intravenously	Rapid, potent action; decreases preload.	Requires hemodynamic monitoring with close observation; danger of severe hypotension.	Begin 5 μg/min (well diluted—see manufacturer's insert); increase 2.5–5 μg every 5–10 min; titrate to desired effect.
Nifedipine	Coronary spasm.		10–20 mg 3 times daily orally.
Verapamil	Coronary spasm; paroxysmal atrial tachycardia.		80–120 mg two or three times daily orally.

[1] Modified and reproduced, with permission, from Forrester JS, Waters DD: Hospital treatment of congestive heart failure: Management according to hemodynamic profile. Am J Med 1978;65:173.

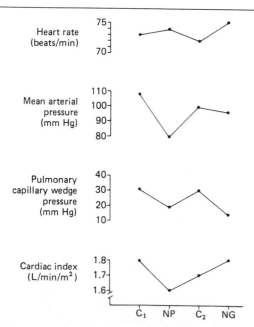

Figure 8–30. Hemodynamic changes following administration of nitroprusside (NP) and nitroglycerin (NG) in a patient with acute myocardial infarction. C_1 and C_2 refer to control periods. (Adapted and reproduced, with permission of the American Heart Association, Inc., from Armstrong PW et al: Vasodilator therapy in acute myocardial infarction: A comparison of sodium nitroprusside and nitroglycerin. Circulation 1975;52:1118.)

must be avoided because the patient may become dehydrated and hypovolemic.

c. Vasopressors– Some patients with acute myocardial infarction have hypotension with impaired tissue perfusion primarily due to failure of compensatory peripheral vasoconstriction without a substantial change in filling pressure or cardiac output; these patients often respond with a rise in arterial pressure to the inotropic action of sympathetic amines (norepinephrine, dopamine, or dobutamine) that stimulate the beta-adrenergic receptors of the heart. These drugs are a temporary measure to allow the use of vasodilators or intra-aortic balloon assist (see below). They should be infused at a slow rate to avoid tachycardia, marked increases in blood pressure, and ventricular arrhythmias.

d. Vasodilator therapy– (See Table 8–16.) When cardiac dysfunction is more severe, with reduced cardiac output, increased left ventricular filling pressure (above 20 mm Hg), and arterial blood pressure at or above 90 mm Hg, vasodilator therapy can be cautiously started while the hemodynamic result is monitored. Drugs such as nitroglycerin, sodium nitroprusside, trimethaphan, and phentolamine, given by intravenous drip, decrease the impedance to left ventricular ejection; reduce left ventricular volume and filling pressure; decrease myocardial oxygen consumption; improve perfusion to the brain (Figure 8–30), kidneys, and heart; and may improve the left ventricular stroke work index. Temporary improvement may tide the patient over a critical period (Chatterjee, 1979; Matthay, 1988). The CONSENSUS II study, where enalapril was started within 24 hours after the onset of acute myocardial infarction, did not improve survival during the 6 months after infarction (Swedberg, 1992). Dopamine or dobutamine should be tried in low-output states with hypotension. Intravenous amrinone or milrinone has been found useful at times. The combination of vasodilator therapy and inotropic therapy may be helpful if the blood pressure is low, with hypoperfusion combined with a high filling pressure documented by hemodynamic monitoring.

Nitroglycerin given sublingually in the acute phase of acute myocardial infarction may decrease the wedge pressure but may also produce arterial hypotension with or without bradycardia. The same effect may occur with intravenous nitroglycerin or intravenous sodium nitroprusside, but the dose must be titrated to avoid hypotension. In less severe cases, transdermal nitroglycerin can be used with appropriate safeguards in acute myocardial infarction; this may reduce the left ventricular filling pressure with only a slight fall in arterial pressure.

Efforts should be made to raise arterial pressure to about 100 mm Hg with vasopressors before vasodilator therapy unless vasodilators are required to relieve symptoms of pulmonary venous congestion when cardiac failure is severe. If the patient has cardiogenic shock and a low urine output, dopamine can be tried to increase the urine output and cardiac output and raise the blood pressure. Low doses of dopamine at the 3–5 μg/kg/min level increase renal blood flow and stroke volume by stimulation of β_1-adrenergic receptors and dopaminergic receptors. Peripheral vasoconstriction increases little. At higher doses, there is a dose-dependent stimulation of chronotropic, arrhythmogenic, and vasoconstrictor effects mediated by alpha-adrenergic receptors. This increases afterload and may decrease tissue and kidney perfusion. The average dose of dopamine is 15–20 μg/kg/min. Dopamine may increase the myocardial oxygen consumption. The physician must be cautious in treating severe left ventricular failure with dopamine because of the danger of worsening of myocardial function. Therefore, the dose should be titrated upward very cautiously to doses of 20 μg/kg/min. There is little to be gained by further increases.

e. Aortic balloon counterpulsation– If it is not possible to raise blood pressure with vasopressors, aortic balloon counterpulsation may, in some patients, be a dramatically effective temporary method of raising arterial pressure so that vasodilator therapy can be started; this technique is associated with morbidity and should be used only by skilled personnel. Counterpulsation decreases aortic pressure during systole and increases it in diastole. Decreasing systolic pressure decreases impedance to left ventricular ejection and reduces afterload and the work of the left ventricle. Raising the pressure during diastole increases coronary perfusion and improves left ventricular function. In refractory heart failure without shock, arterial counterpulsation decreases ischemic pain, improves cardiac failure, and increases survival (Kern, 1991). Other left heart assist devices have been developed for temporary support of the circulation. These devices are external pumps, with the intravascular lines placed percutaneously. They are rarely used with acute myocardial infarction except as a bridge to cardiac transplantation (George, 1991).

f. Combination of aortic balloon counterpulsation and vasodilator therapy– Counterpulsation followed by vasodilator therapy with sodium nitroprusside or nitroglycerin may significantly improve left ventricular "pump" function in cardiogenic shock and thus reduce the mortality rate. Treatment with hydralazine, nitroprusside, and dopamine may make counterpulsation unnecessary in some patients. The long-term prognosis in patients who have needed balloon assist for cardiogenic shock is still poor (approximately 10% survival after 1 year), because of the extensive underlying disease implied by the presence of cardiogenic shock.

g. Counterpulsation as prelude to angioplasty and cardiac surgery– Invasive balloon counterpulsation can be used as a temporary measure to tide the patient over acute "pump failure" and make it possible to perform coronary angiograms as well as to explore the feasibility of coronary angioplasty or coronary bypass surgery. Any patient with acute myocardial infarction who needs aortic balloon counterpulsation should have immediate coronary arteriography to determine if coronary revascularization is possible. The surgical mortality rate in patients recovering from cardiogenic shock is high. The feasibility and desirability of operative intervention remain uncertain. Coronary angioplasty appears to be the best hope for salvage in the patient with cardiogenic shock (Lee, 1991).

h. Hemodynamic parameters guiding treatment– The poor response to medical as well as surgical therapy in patients with cardiogenic shock can be appreciated when one considers that at least half of the left ventricle is often damaged in such patients. Left ventricular stroke work is usually less than 20 g-m/m^2 and often less than 15 g-m/m^2, and hypoxemia with P_{O_2} of less than 40–50 mm Hg is frequently found. The high wedge pressure induces dyspnea; impaired peripheral perfusion from the decreased cardiac output results in cold, clammy skin, cerebral obtundation, and poor urine output.

i. Value of hemodynamic monitoring in prognosis– Monitoring of the hemodynamic parameters is valuable in prognosis (Table 8–16). Patients with left ventricular filling pressures under 15 mm Hg and stroke work indices of more than 35–40 g-m/m^2 have a mortality rate of 6%, whereas if the filling pressure exceeds 20 mm Hg and the stroke work index is less than 15–20 g-m/m², the mortality rate is 80% (Shah, 1991). In patients with a poor prognosis, aggressive therapy is warranted before severe deterioration occurs. The response of the patient determines the drugs used and their dosages, and these are varied as treatment proceeds. If the blood pressure falls, the physician cannot continue administration of the sodium nitroprusside or nitroglycerin and must use pressor agents to raise the blood pressure.

j. Digitalis– Digitalis is infrequently used today in the treatment of cardiac failure due to acute myocardial infarction, because of its tendency to cause ventricular arrhythmias and its relatively low effectiveness against severe left ventricular pump failure. Digitalis may be tried, however, unless the failure is mild. If ventricular arrhythmias develop, it is difficult to decide whether they are due to digitalis or myocardial ischemia. Digitalis should be used if the patient has atrial fibrillation with a rapid ventricular rate.

C. Conduction Defects:

1. Stokes-Adams attack with heart block (complete atrioventricular conduction defect)– (See Chapter 14.) *This is an emergency!* Complete heart block complicates acute myocardial infarction in 6–10% of cases; it has a high mortality rate (about 60% untreated) if the block is infra-His with wide QRS ventricular escape and usually lasts less than a week. Complete block at the atrioventricular node with narrow QRS ventricular escape is less malignant and associated with a lower mortality rate. This occurs primarily with inferior wall myocardial infarction. Progression of the electrocardiographic changes of heart block may be rapid and lead to complete atrioventricular block and Stokes-Adams attacks. Complete heart block can often be treated by a ventricular pacemaker. At present, external pacemakers are available that can be used temporarily until a wire electrode can be placed in the right ventricle. Pacing at a rate of 70–80/min may greatly improve cardiac output and tissue perfusion and prevent Stokes-Adams attacks. Temporary pacemakers are usually left in place for 3 days after the atrioventricular conduction becomes normal. A permanent pacemaker may be considered in anterior infarction associated with Stokes-Adams attacks. The mortality rate is said to be reduced if a permanent pacemaker is used in patients with acute anterior myocardial infarction who have developed complete atrioventricular block in association with bifascicular block during the acute attack; the data supporting this opinion are still incomplete and contradictory. Death during a Stokes-Adams attack with syncope is rare in the presence of inferior myocardial infarction.

2. Second-degree heart block, Mobitz I and II– (See Chapter 14.) Second-degree atrioventricular block with Wenckebach pauses (see below) (Mobitz I) and *narrow* QRS complexes is not routinely paced if the patient has inferior infarction. Stokes-Adams attacks are uncommon in inferior infarction with nar-

row QRS complexes, even if complete block develops. They are common in anterior infarction with *wide* QRS complexes. The block is usually within the bundle of His or in the bundle branches, with wide QRS complexes (Mobitz II); Stokes-Adams attacks with fatalities occur if the patient is not protected by a pacemaker.

3. Prophylactic demand pacemakers in Mobitz II block– (See Chapter 14.) Because asystole may occur unpredictably, electrode catheters should be placed prophylactically in patients with anterior infarctions who have bifascicular block, complete atrioventricular block, or type II Mobitz atrioventricular block or in those who have inferior infarctions with early complete atrioventricular block, especially if there is hemodynamic deterioration from the slow ventricular response (Lavie, 1990). Infusions of lidocaine should be given to prevent ventricular fibrillation if atrioventricular block subsides and competition occurs with the patient's own pacemaker.

4. Sinus bradycardia– Sinus bradycardia, especially in inferior infarction, may precede atrioventricular block and provide a setting in which ventricular arrhythmias can occur. Furthermore, when hypotension and decreased cardiac output occur with bradycardia in acute myocardial infarction, perfusion of the vital organs may be inadequate. Atropine, 0.4–0.8 mg intravenously, is desirable in such situations, with close observation to determine its effectiveness and side effects, since ventricular arrhythmias may result. If atropine is ineffective or if the bradycardia is marked or associated with sinoatrial or atrioventricular block, a temporary prophylactic transvenous demand pacemaker should be inserted into the right ventricle.

D. Other Complications:

1. Thromboembolic phenomena– These are usually manifested by phlebothrombosis resulting from enforced bed rest. Pulmonary embolism and arterial emboli from mural thrombi in the left ventricle occur infrequently. Two-dimensional echocardiography at 5–7 days postinfarction can detect ventricular mural thrombi (Keren, 19901). Anticoagulants should be administered promptly.

2. Renal failure– Early oliguria and anuria are due to cardiogenic shock; late renal failure may be due to prolonged hypotension caused by vasodilator therapy. Early vigorous treatment of cardiogenic shock and caution in the use of vasodilator agents should decrease the incidence of renal failure. If renal failure with acute tubular necrosis develops after the patient has been stabilized with respect to cardiogenic shock and left ventricular failure, hemodialysis or peritoneal dialysis is indicated.

3. Perforation of the interventricular septum and mitral insufficiency due to papillary muscle and left ventricular wall dysfunction or rupture– These complications may occur together but are usually separate untoward events. Either may result in abrupt worsening of left ventricular failure. Two-dimensional echocardiography with Doppler can differentiate between these various complications, though when the diagnosis is made, catheterization and coronary arteriography usually precede operative repair. Two-dimensional echocardiograms are effective in diagnosing septal rupture because they provide direct visualization of the septal defect and show air bubbles entering the left ventricle via the septal rupture following intravenous saline contrast injection. Color Doppler is most valuable in detecting the site of ventricular rupture (Smyllie, 1989). Whenever possible, surgical repair of the ventricular septal defect or replacement of the mitral valve should be delayed until the lesion has been stabilized by vigorous treatment of cardiac failure (see Chapter 10). Aortic balloon counterpulsation can hemodynamically stabilize the patient. However, if the patient has developed severe hemodynamic abnormalities, surgery is advised immediately after stabilization of the patient to the best degree possible. Patients having acute mitral insufficiency with acute left ventricular failure requiring surgery have marked pulmonary venous congestion, a very high v wave, raised mean pulmonary capillary wedge pressure, and a reduced cardiac index (< 2.5 L/min/m²). In both ventricular septal defects and mitral insufficiency, vasodilator therapy may improve or correct cardiac failure, so that surgical repair can be performed with an acceptable mortality rate. Results of surgical repair of both of these lesions are gratifying and allow restoration of normal activity (Lavie, 1990).

4. Left ventricular aneurysm–

a. Spectrum of left ventricular contraction abnormalities– Acute necrosis of a portion of the left ventricle, with resulting healing by fibrosis and scar, may lead to a spectrum of disorders of contraction of the left ventricle, varying from hypokinesia or akinesia of a segment that is fully scarred to a definite left ventricular aneurysm with well-demarcated paradoxic outpocketing during systole. This can be established by two-dimensional echocardiography, radionuclide angiography, or cineangiography. Aneurysms, however, may not be disclosed on physical examination or chest x-ray; two-dimensional echocardiography may be diagnostic and differentiate pseudoaneurysm from true aneurysm—the former is really a contained rupture of the myocardium and has a narrow neck in communication with the left ventricular cavity; the latter has a wide neck (Figures 8–31 and 8–32).

b. Consequences of ventricular aneurysms– With loss of contracting myocardium, dilation of the left ventricle occurs. This in addition to the sympathetic stimulation of the contracting myocardium increases myocardial oxygen demand and the requirement for increased myocardial flow. The force of left ventricular contraction is wasted by distention of the

acute aneurysm, increasing the work of the left ventricle. Later, as the aneurysm becomes fibrotic, it is no longer distensible; insufficient contracting muscle then remains, and cardiac enlargement and failure may ensue. This may lead to persistent cardiac failure or ventricular arrhythmias, or both. When persistent left ventricular failure follows the healing of an acute myocardial infarction, the possibility of left ventricular aneurysm should be excluded by two-dimensional echocardiograms or radionuclide angiograms, and if an aneurysm is found it should be resected surgically if the remaining portion of the left ventricle has adequate function (see below). Areas of fibrous scarring together with myocardium receiving diminished perfusion, with possible ischemia on effort, may surround the area of the left ventricular aneurysm and result in frequent ventricular arrhythmias that often are disabling or fatal.

c. Surgical resection of aneurysms– Surgical resection can abolish the ventricular arrhythmias as well as slow the development of cardiac failure in many patients. In patients who have ventricular tachycardia resistant to conventional medical therapy, endocardial electrophysiologic mapping should be performed prior to resection of the aneurysm to determine the site of origin of the ectopic activity so that it will be included in the resection. Search for left ventricular aneurysm can be very gratifying; although the mortality rate is up to 15%, the results may be dramatic. In over 1000 patients from the Coronary Artery Surgery Study (CASS) Registry, the surgical mortality rate was 7.9% (Faxon, 1986). Surgery should be deferred if possible for 4–10 weeks until cardiac failure has stabilized. All obstructed coronary arteries should be bypassed. Resection of left ventricular aneurysm is often effective in relieving cardiac failure. Resection is unwise unless there is sufficient remaining contracting myocardium (at least 50% of the total left ventricle) to support left ventricular function. Surgical treatment is not indicated in patients with generalized hypokinesia with severe cardiac failure. A small left ventricular aneurysm in the absence of cardiac failure or severe ventricular arrhythmias is likewise not an indication for surgical resection, because it does not influence prognosis. Long-term follow-up after repair of left ventricular aneurysms, usually with associated bypass grafting, showed 10-year survival to be 57% with event-free (death, myocardial infarction, and reparative coronary surgery) survival of 41% (Baciewicz, 1991).

5. Cardiac rupture and false aneurysm– The rupture may be subacute with a small perforation into the pericardium and can be diagnosed on the basis of pericardial pain or effusion or by the recognition of a false aneurysm on two-dimensional echocardiogram or radionuclide angiogram. Progressive enlargement of a "false" or pseudoaneurysm of the left ventricle may result from a small cardiac rupture, with only the parietal pericardium preventing the expanding false

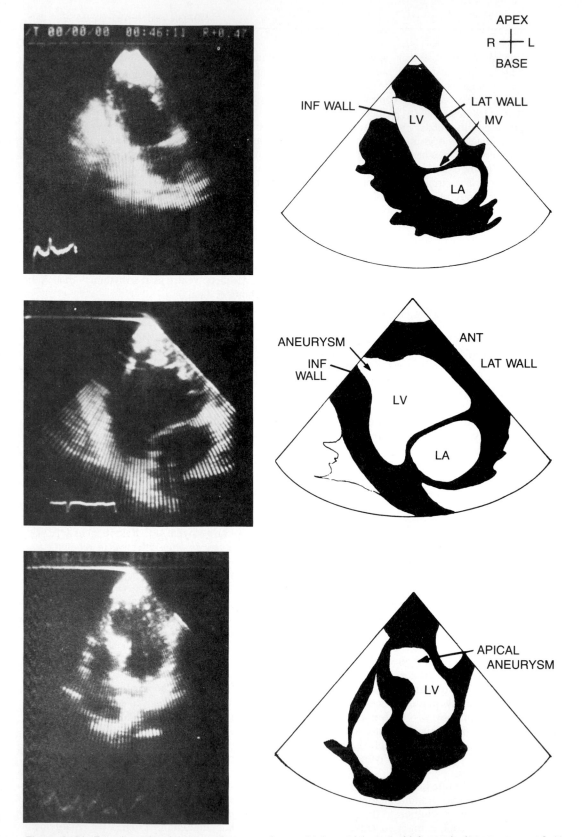

Figure 8–31. Two-dimensional echocardiograms of normal left ventricle and of left ventricular aneurysms. **A:** Normal left ventricle and mitral valve in a modified right anterior oblique position representing a hemiaxial equivalent taken through the apex. **B:** Considerably dilated left ventricle with an aneurysm on the inferior wall. **C:** Apical aneurysm with slightly enlarged left ventricular cavity. (Courtesy of NB Schiller.)

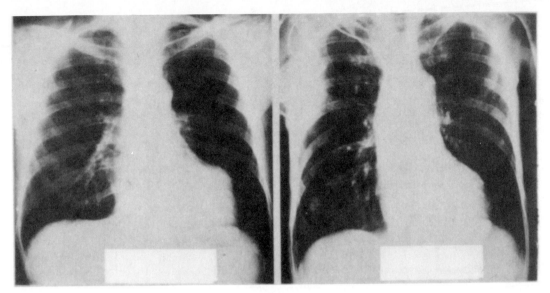

Figure 8–32. Ventricular aneurysm in two patients. **Left:** Classic x-ray findings of a discrete left ventricular aneurysm. **Right:** Film from a patient who at autopsy was found to have diffuse thinning and aneurysmal dilation of the entire apical region of the left ventricle. (Reproduced, with permission, from Davis RW, Ebert PA: Ventricular aneurysm: A clinical-pathologic correlation. Am J Cardiol 1972;29:1.)

aneurysm from rupturing. With time it may rupture, usually into the left pleural cavity. The false aneurysm is readily identified by two-dimensional echocardiography, by radionuclide angiography, and by contrast angiography. When discovered, these all require surgical repair (Bolooki, 1990).

6. Pericarditis– Although pericarditis occurs in about 15% of patients with acute myocardial infarction, pericardial tamponade is rare. The usual occurrence of pericarditis is around the third or fourth day. Involvement of the pericardium contraindicates anticoagulant therapy, because extensive bleeding in the pericardium may result in tamponade. The differential diagnosis between acute pericarditis and acute myocardial infarction may be difficult, especially if the patient is not seen until the second or third day. Most helpful is a pleuritic component to the chest pain that is common in pericarditis. Electrocardiographic abnormalities due to involvement of the epicardium and pericardium may complicate the interpretation of electrocardiographic patterns, especially if the patient has a nontransmural infarct. Two-dimensional echocardiography may show pericardial fluid.

7. Rare post-myocardial infarction syndromes–
a. Dressler's syndrome– Pericarditis, pericardial friction rub, and fever, with or without pneumonitis, may occur weeks or months after acute myocardial infarction in a small number of patients. It has been considered to be a hypersensitivity reaction similar to postcardiotomy syndrome (see Chapter 18). It must be differentiated from a new myocardial infarction, pulmonary infarction, pneumonia, or cardiac

failure. It subsides spontaneously in a few days or weeks, but improvement is more rapid if corticosteroids or indomethacin is given. Anticoagulants should not be used because of the hazards of hemorrhagic pericardial effusion.

b. Shoulder-hand syndrome– A syndrome consisting of stiffness, limitation of motion, and pain in the shoulder and arm (especially the left) following myocardial infarction is now rare. The condition probably was due to disuse of the arms and shoulders when strict limitation of activity for weeks was recommended for acute myocardial infarction. It may last for days or weeks and is benefited by symptomatic treatment, including physical therapy.

E. Convalescent Activity and Rehabilitation:
1. Initial period of rest–
a. Rest in bed– The period of rest in bed depends on the severity and size of the infarction and the presence or absence of complications.

b. Ambulation– If the infarction is mild and if the family can provide all required services, the patient who can perform 3 METS (metabolic energy equivalents) of exercise without symptoms (1 MET is the energy expenditure per kilogram per minute at rest—about 3.5–4 mL of oxygen per minute) may go home early in the second week. Walking at 2.5 mph, dressing, or taking a shower requires 3 METS.

c. Resuming full activity– As a guide, 1–2 weeks of relative rest are followed by 2 or 3 weeks of slowly increasing activity, including walking and slow stair climbing; and then several weeks of progressive activity before return to part-time work.

Even in uncomplicated cases, the patient who has previously been normally active requires 6–8 weeks of convalescence before returning to full preinfarction activity. Improvement in exercise tolerance progressively continues up to 3–6 months and depends on how rapidly the patient increases activity.

d. Usual practice of ambulation– When the patient first begins to walk slowly, the physician or the nurse should be present to note any deleterious effects that might occur. The patient should not leave the hospital until the activity status has progressed to the stage of relative self-sufficiency. Early ambulation and self-sufficiency improve morale, prevent cardiac invalidism, and restore the patient's confidence in his or her ability to resume a normal life. Progressive increases in ambulatory effort should be possible without chest pain, dyspnea, or undue tachycardia or fatigue. Severe physical exertion should be avoided for at least 2 months, in order to prevent left ventricular dilation and subsequent hypertrophy. A balance must be achieved between excessive exertion too early and prolonged inactivity and invalidism.

2. Later rehabilitation– Rehabilitation programs utilize the services of physical therapists with the object of encouraging the patient to return to normal activity without neurocirculatory asthenia or cardiac neurosis. Formal monitored exercise programs restore physical objective evidence of the level of activity that can be safely performed both recreationally and on the job (Fletcher, 1992).

a. Electrocardiographic monitoring during activity– Twelve-hour electrocardiographic monitoring (eg, with a Holter monitor) when the patient first resumes activity (usually about 3 weeks in uncomplicated cases) may alert the physician to the presence of residual myocardial ischemia or left ventricular arrhythmias, especially if asymptomatic, and may require a reduction in activity or the use of antiarrhythmic drugs (Reis, 1992).

b. Use of graded exercise and Holter electrocardiographic monitoring in early postinfarction period– Graded, limited exercise with cycle ergometers or treadmills up to a ventricular rate of about 130/min is often performed, 7–14 days after uncomplicated acute myocardial infarction; the presence and degree of flat or downsloping ST segment abnormalities or the presence of ventricular premature beats provides an estimate of recovery and has prognostic significance. Patients with ischemic ST depression or complex ventricular premature beats with low-level exercise during early postinfarction exercise have a significantly higher incidence of new infarction or ventricular fibrillation with "sudden death syndrome" in the succeeding 1–2 years (DeBusk, 1980). Before performing this early exercise test, patients should be free of complications such as cardiac failure, arrhythmia, and conduction defects, and the test should be stopped if the patient develops undue fatigue, angina, frequent or complex premature beats, or marked ST depression. The physician must be aware of drugs that the patient may be taking.

Numerous studies have shown the benefit of low-level exercise testing before leaving the hospital. In reviewing studies of exercise testing after myocardial infarction in which follow-up for cardiac end points was done, a consistent finding is that the 1-year mortality rate is higher in those patients in whom it was clinically believed that exercise testing was contraindicated compared with those who were felt capable of undergoing an exercise test. Therefore, the clinical assessment that the patient can undergo a predischarge exercise test already identifies that patient as being at low risk (Detrano, 1988). In a comprehensive review of exercise testing after myocardial infarction, five exercise test variables were linked with prognosis: (1) exercise ST segment deviation—usually depression, occasionally elevation; (2) exercise-induced angina; (3) inability to reach a heart rate of 130/min or 5 METS; (4) exercise-induced ventricular arrhythmias; and (5) inadequate blood pressure response to exercise. However, from study to study, the prognostic importance of each of these factors differed. In one study (Froelicher, 1986) of 225 men with uncomplicated myocardial infarction, the presence of ST segment depression or elevation was associated with an eightfold greater risk of dying during the year following the infarction. Exercise-induced angina was not an independent risk factor (Waters, 1985). Other studies (Mark, 1988; Krone, 1992) have shown that exercise-induced angina was associated with a threefold risk of subsequent death. Some studies have indicated that the presence of ischemia as manifested by ST segment shifts or angina was the most important indicator; in others, exercise-induced ventricular dysfunction as evidenced by poor exercise capacity or failure to increase blood pressures was most important.

Radioisotope perfusion studies with thallium-201 or sestamibi improve the sensitivity of detecting ischemia over treadmill testing alone (Gibson, 1991). The frequency of exercise-induced ischemia is almost twice as high with scintigraphy as with electrocardiographic changes alone (56% versus 29%). The patients most at risk of dying are those with a left main coronary artery lesion and those with three-vessel disease and a decreased ejection fraction after myocardial infarction. These are the high-risk patients, and treadmill exercise testing without scintigraphy has about a 90% sensitivity in identifying these patients. Therefore, the extra sensitivity provided by scintigraphy perfusion scanning is useful mostly in better identifying patients with one- or two-vessel disease, ie, those at lower risk. If parameters other than ST segment shifts are taken into account, such as inability to exercise to the third stage of the Bruce protocol or inability to raise the blood pressure with exercise, the difference between exercise testing with scintigraphy and without scintigraphy is even less striking.

Risk stratification: Initial presentation

Acute myocardial infarction

↓

Thrombolytic therapy?

— No → Risk stratify

Yes

↓

Reperfusion?
• Pain relief and
• ST resolution

— No → Risk stratify

Risk stratify

↓

High risk?
• ECG changes
  a. extensive
  b. anterolateral
  c. inferoposterior
• Previous infarction
• Hypotension
• Congestion (rales)
• Severe pain

Yes ↓

No →

Emergency coronary angiography
(transfer?)

↓ ↘

Yes ↓

Medical therapy

Coronary angioplasty   Coronary bypass surgery

Risk stratification: Days 1–5

↓

Ischemia? — Yes → Coronary angiography
• Recurrent angina
• Recurrent ST elevators

No ↓   Yes →

Coronary angioplasty   Coronary bypass surgery

Extensive jeopardized myocardium?
• "Flash" pulmonary edema
• Anterior non-Q wave infarction

↓

No

↓

Predischarge risk stratification

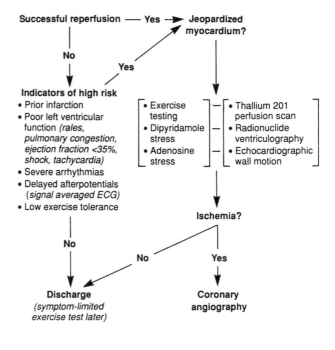

Risk stratification: Predischarge

Successful reperfusion — Yes → Jeopardized myocardium?

No ↓   Yes ↗

Indicators of high risk
• Prior infarction
• Poor left ventricular function *(rales, pulmonary congestion, ejection fraction <35%, shock, tachycardia)*
• Severe arrhythmias
• Delayed afterpotentials *(signal averaged ECG)*
• Low exercise tolerance

[• Exercise testing
• Dipyridamole stress
• Adenosine stress] — [• Thallium 201 perfusion scan
• Radionuclide ventriculography
• Echocardiographic wall motion]

↓

Ischemia?

No ↙   Yes ↓

No ↓

Discharge
(symptom-limited exercise test later)

Coronary angiography

Figure 8–33. Risk stratification. **Left:** In-hospital risk stratification strategies. **Initial presentation:** Evaluation for high risk and potential for myocardial salvage. *Days 1–5:* Evaluate for recurrent ischemia or extensive jeopardized myocardium. **Right:** Predischarge risk stratification. Evaluate for factors suggesting poor prognosis after hospital discharge. In addition to the strategy listed by the AHA/ACC Joint Task Force, noninvasive evaluation for jeopardized myocardium may indicate the need for angiography in selected patients with potential procedural morbidity (advanced age, significant renal impairment, or extensive peripheral vascular disease) who have indicators of high risk. (Reproduced, with permission, from Krone RJ: The role of risk stratification in the early management of a myocardial infarction. Ann Intern Med 1992;116:223.)

Three strategies are recommended for predischarge or early postdischarge exercise evaluation after acute myocardial infarction (Gunnar, 1990), depending on whether there are clinical indicators of high risk such as congestive heart failure or recurrent angina. The approaches depend on an early submaximal treadmill test predischarge and a symptom-limited exercise test at 3 weeks, with or without a scintigraphic perfusion study (Figure 8–33). It is still not clear whether it is better to perform a low-level predischarge stress test with or without thallium-201 scintigraphy in clinically low-risk patients than to wait 3 weeks and do a symptom-limited stress test (Kotler, 1990). In patients who are unable to exercise, dipyridamole or adenosine vasodilation with thallium scintigraphy has been advocated (Beller, 1991). The results appear to be equivalent to thallium-201 exercise scintigraphy (O'Rourke, 1991).

Performing a predischarge exercise test has other advantages. Ability to perform the exercise test is usually a source of great encouragement to the patient. At 1 month the patient has regained about 70% of preinfarction exercise tolerance, and recovery is usually complete by 3–6 months. Sexual activity in both sexes may be resumed after 1–2 months when the patient has shown the ability to tolerate a heart rate of 130/min. Properly supervised rehabilitation exercise programs have been shown to be safe and helpful in that they foster a sense of well-being, decrease anxiety, and induce a healthier emotional response to the life-threatening event; they have not been shown to prolong life or decrease the frequency of recurrence of myocardial infarction.

Special Precautions in Patients at Increased Risk

The high-risk patient likely to have recurrent acute myocardial infarction or sudden death is one who has survived a previous episode of "sudden death syndrome" or acute myocardial infarction and who has frequent or complex ventricular premature beats as well as a decrease in left ventricular function (ejection fraction ≤ 40). Monitoring such patients electrocardiographically will indicate whether the premature beats are simple or complex. In addition to ambulatory electrocardiographic monitoring, high-risk patients should have radioisotope or echocardiographic evaluation of wall motion and ejection fraction 1–2 weeks after the acute episode. Multiple areas of hypokinesis or dyskinesis indicating myocardial fibrosis correlate with frequent ventricular premature beats, and the combination of complex ventricular premature beats and poor left ventricular function considerably increases the likelihood of sudden death and is an indication for coronary angiography with a view to possible angioplasty or coronary surgery. If neither is present, the prognosis is good.

Prognosis

Patients who had a previous myocardial infarction and findings during the second infarction of severe cardiac failure, shock, high left ventricular filling pressure, sinus tachycardia, low ejection fraction, decreased cardiac index, and decreased left ventricular stroke work all had significant left ventricular impairment and a correspondingly worse outcome (Moss, 1983; Moss, 1987).

A. Overall Mortality Rate: The overall prehospital and in-hospital mortality rate during the first month after acute myocardial infarction is about 30%. Most of the deaths occur in the first 12 hours; one-fourth result from ventricular fibrillation in the first 1–2 hours. With mild attacks and no complications, the hospital mortality rate is less than 5%, but the average hospital rate is about 10–15%. It is 50% higher in recurrent than in initial infarctions, but cardiac rupture occurs more frequently with the first infarction. Early recurrence or extension of acute myocardial infarction takes place in approximately 15% of patients, is most likely to occur in non-Q wave infarctions, and can be diagnosed by the reappearance of MB isoenzymes of plasma CK. These patients are at increased risk. Overall figures are misleading in estimating prognosis. Since the average delay between onset of symptoms and arrival at the hospital is 4–6 hours, arrival of the patient alive at the hospital is itself a favorable prognostic sign with respect to electrical instability but not necessarily to pump failure.

B. Factors Influencing Survival: Over a 5-year period, 3-vessel disease with poor left ventricular function has at least 10 times the mortality rate of single-vessel disease with good left ventricular function (Table 8–17). At present, the prognosis is influenced favorably by surgical treatment for (1) repair of perforated ventricular septum; (2) replacement of the mitral valve when there is gross mitral regurgitation resulting from papillary muscle dysfunction; (3) resection of left ventricular aneurysm associated with left ventricular failure; and (4) coronary bypass or angioplasty when the artery involved is the left main coronary artery or in proximal 3-vessel disease with only moderately impaired left ventricular function. Thrombolytic agents improve prognosis, especially if given within 6 hours after onset, but long-term data are limited.

C. Life Adjustment After Myocardial Infarction: Patients who were actively employed before an acute infarction are more likely to seek work than those who were not employed before the attack. Only one-third of patients surviving an infarction actually return to their jobs. The prognosis for return to work is less good if the patient is depressed or denies the illness.

D. Variable Postinfarction Health: A long period of good health often follows an initial episode of angina or myocardial infarction. Others may pursue a

Table 8–17. Mortality rates following coronary arteriography by number of vessels diseased and by symptoms of congestive heart failure (CHF).[1] (Mean duration of follow-up = 21 months.)

Vessels Diseased (n)	No Symptoms of CHF			Symptoms of CHF		
	Dead (n)	Alive (n)	Mortality Rate (%)	Dead (n)	Alive (n)	Mortality Rate (%)
None	2	87	2.2	1	8	11.1
One	1	39	2.5	1	5	16.7
Two	4	32	11.1	9	5	64.3
Three	8	28	22.2	7	9	43.8
TOTAL	15	186	8.1	18	27	40.0

[1] Modified from Oberman (1972). Reproduced, with permission of the American Heart Association, Inc., from Kouchoukos NT, Kirklin JW, Oberman A: An appraisal of coronary bypass grafting. Circulation 1974;50:11.

downhill course following acute myocardial infarction, with progressively worsening symptoms and recurrent infarctions. In general, the prognosis worsens with increasing ventricular dysfunction and increasing areas of persistent ischemic myocardium.

Evaluation of Post-Myocardial Infarction Patients

The mortality rate in the first year after hospital discharge following uncomplicated acute myocardial infarction varies from 7% to 10%. Patients with a complicated course (cardiac failure, cardiogenic shock, low ejection fraction, complex ventricular arrhythmias, conduction defects) have a significantly higher mortality rate that may approach 30–50% in the first year (Epstein, 1982; Moss, 1987). (See also Figure 8–34.)

Because of variability in the clinical course following acute myocardial infarction, it seems prudent to evaluate patients recovering from infarction to identify high-risk subgroups for possible further diagnostic or therapeutic intervention. It is important to note evidences of continuing ischemia, left ventricular dysfunction, complex ventricular arrhythmias, unrecognized ventricular aneurysm, ventricular septal defect, or papillary muscle dysfunction with mitral regurgitation.

Low-level electrocardiographic exercise stress testing and 24-hour Holter electrocardiographic monitoring performed just before hospital discharge will demonstrate any evidence of residual ischemia or complex ventricular arrhythmias. High-risk patients include those whose continuing ischemia is demonstrated by a markedly positive ECG, those who have had congestive heart failure before leaving the hospital, and those who have recurrent postinfarction angina. Coronary and left ventricular angiography is usually advisable before such patients leave the hospital.

Unless the situation is critical, the patient is usually discharged from the hospital on medical therapy with nitrates and beta-adrenergic or calcium entry-blocking agents; on aspirin, 325 mg/d; is given advice about restricted activities; and is advised to return in 4 weeks for clinical evaluation.

If clinical and noninvasive studies reveal no angina or ischemia, a good ejection fraction (> 50%), and no complex arrhythmias, no further investigation is required, and the patient is given medical treatment as for stable angina. If at 6 weeks there is persistent ischemia, complex ventricular arrhythmias, or significant left ventricular dysfunction with an ejection fraction of 30–40% or less, coronary and left ven-

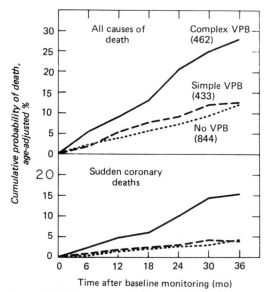

Figure 8–34. Mortality rates over 3 years after baseline monitoring in relation to ventricular premature beats (VPB) in the monitoring hour. (Reproduced, with permission, from Ruberman W et al: Ventricular premature beats and mortality after myocardial infarction. N Engl J Med 1977;297:750.)

tricular angiograms are advised to assess the coronary anatomy, to estimate the amount of myocardium at risk, and to consider angioplasty or coronary surgery. Both the number of vessels involved and the degree of left ventricular dysfunction are important in prognosis (see Table 8–16). The importance of complex ventricular arrhythmias can be seen in Figure 8–34.

In the patient with postinfarction angina, a strongly positive electrocardiographic stress test and multiple wall motion abnormalities raise the possibility of significant stenosis of the left main coronary artery or multivessel disease with a substantial area of the myocardium at jeopardy. If these are documented by angiography and left ventricular function is only moderately impaired, coronary bypass surgery is considered. If, however, severe proximal stenosis of the left anterior descending coronary artery is found, angioplasty may be considered. If considerable left ventricular failure due to coronary cardiomyopathy is found (ejection fraction $\leq$ 20–30%) without substantial areas of ischemic myocardium, medical and not surgical treatment is advised (Krone, 1992).

If investigation reveals a localized, well-demarcated ventricular aneurysm and if the patient has chronic cardiac failure, surgical resection is indicated.

An algorithm for the risk stratification of patients after acute myocardial infarction is presented in Figure 8–33.

Late Prognosis
Following Myocardial Infarction

The prognosis after infarction is worse (1) the greater the area of infarction during the acute episode; (2) the more severe the evidence of left ventricular dysfunction after myocardial infarction (Moss, 1987; Figure 8–35); (3) the greater the magnitude and number of areas of wall motion hypokinesis, akinesis, or dyskinesis; (4) the more marked the ST segment depression on exercise (especially if the ST change occurs early at a relatively low heart rate below the predicted maximum); (5) the greater the fall in ejection fraction with exercise; (6) the more prominent or persistent the complex ventricular arrhythmias during exercise or during long-term ambulatory electrocardiographic monitoring; (7) the greater the number of stenosed coronary arteries, especially if the stenoses are proximal and involve the left main coronary vessel; or (8) if the infarction is recurrent, especially with non-Q wave infarction.

A large, poorly contracting left ventricle without a well-demarcated aneurysm is usually associated with left ventricular failure and has a poor prognosis.

The mortality rate of patients who survive an acute infarction is higher during the first 3–12 months than later. Patients with anterior infarction who have had transient complete atrioventricular block are at substantial risk of sudden death within the year, and permanent pacemakers are considered more often. Patients who have had severe cardiac failure have a

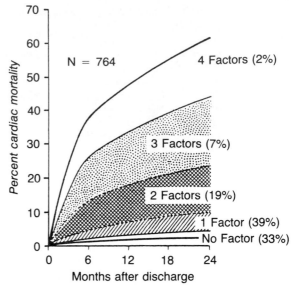

Figure 8–35. Mortality curves after discharge and zones of risk, according to number of risk factors. The risk factors were New York Heart Association functional class II–IV before admission, pulmonary rales, occurrence of ten or more ventricular ectopic depolarizations per hour, and a radionuclide ejection fraction below 0.4. (Reproduced, with permission, from Moss AJ: The Multicenter Post-Infarction Research Group: Risk stratification and survival after myocardial infarction. N Engl J Med 1983;309: 331.)

higher mortality rate in the 1–2 years following infarction.

Secondary Prevention
of Myocardial Infarction
& Sudden Death

A. Vigorous Treatment of Risk Factors: See p 147 for discussion of serum lipids.

B. Antiarrhythmic Agents: About 60% of patients with coronary heart disease are victims of sudden death. Those with complex ventricular arrhythmias following acute myocardial infarction are more likely to die suddenly or have early cardiac death, and patients have been given conventional and investigative antiarrhythmic drugs in various trials. Although the prevalence of simple and complex ventricular premature beats was reduced in most studies, there was no convincing evidence that sudden death was prevented.

Antiarrhythmic agents do not remove the anatomic substrate necessary for the generation of arrhythmias but do alter the myocardium by influencing conduction, prolonging refractoriness, or removing arrhythmic trigger mechanisms. In patients with recurrent sustained ventricular tachycardia—especially if refractory to changes and if associated with ventricular aneurysms—electrophysiologic mapping and surgical or catheter ablation of the trigger areas can be successful (Weiss, 1991).

The hypothesis that fatal ventricular arrhythmias could be prevented if drugs which eliminated ventricular ectopy were used was tested using class Ic drugs, flecainide and encainide, in the CAST study (Cardiac Arrhythmia Suppression Trial Investigators [CAST], 1989). The trial was stopped because of increased numbers of deaths in the antiarrhythmic drug group compared with the placebo group, perhaps because of the proarrhythmic effect of these powerful antiarrhythmic drugs. The only drugs so far proved to decrease the incidence of sudden death in post-myocardial infarction patients have been the class II (beta-adrenergic-blocking) drugs, which have both bradycardiac and anti-ischemic action. Calcium channel-blocking drugs—class IV agents—do not seem to affect or actively increase mortality (Yusuf, 1987).

Class III agents, amiodarone and sotalol, which prolong refractoriness and slow the rate of ventricular tachycardia—an antifibrillatory activity—show more promise (Nademanee, 1990). One randomized study showed a decreased mortality rate in survivors of acute myocardial infarction with high-grade ventricular ectopy in those on low-dose amiodarone (1000 mg/d for 5 days and then 200 mg/d) compared with placebo (Burkart, 1990).

Other approaches to selecting patients who may be at high risk are being pursued. Use of the signal-averaged ECG (SA-ECG) is being investigated (O'Rourke, 1991). It appears to have an excellent negative predictive accuracy (95%) but a low positive predictive accuracy (15%). This means that if the SA-ECG is negative, the patient has a low risk of having sustained ventricular tachycardia or sudden death on short-term follow-up. A patient with a positive SA-ECG has only a 15% chance of having such an arrhythmia (Steinberg, 1992).

The use of **electrophysiologic stimulation** (EPS) to induce sustained ventricular tachycardia in survivors of acute myocardial infarction and thus find those at risk of spontaneous sustained ventricular arrhythmias or sudden death continues to be explored (Bourke, 1991). If sustained arrhythmias are inducible in this way, there is a significant risk of spontaneous ventricular tachycardia or sudden death, but the positive predictive accuracy is again low. Those with negative responses to stimulation have a low incidence of spontaneous ventricular arrhythmias; however, most studies so far have found the positive predictive accuracy to be low enough so that it is not justified to utilize this expensive test routinely (Dhingra, 1991). In patients with spontaneous sustained ventricular tachycardia after myocardial infarction, EPS allows selection of appropriate antiarrhythmic therapy, which will reduce the incidence of recurrence.

The development of automatic implantable defi-brillators has permitted their use in patients who have had one or more spontaneous recurrences of sustained ventricular tachycardia or fibrillation despite appropriate antiarrhythmic therapy.

C. Beta-Adrenergic-blocking Agents: These drugs decrease myocardial oxygen demand and cardiac work; are antihypertensive and antiarrhythmic; and inhibit sympathetic impulses to the heart. There have now been a substantial number of placebo-controlled, double-blind intervention trials with both cardioselective and noncardioselective beta-adrenergic-blocking drugs. The largest trials are the Norwegian Multicenter Study Group (1981), using timolol, and the Beta Blocker Heart Attack Study Group (1981) in the USA, using propranolol. Taken as a whole, the results are impressive in showing that life is prolonged by these drugs. Combining results in 15 beta-blocker versus placebo trials, overall mortality was reduced by 22%, sudden death by 33%, nonsudden death by 20%, and nonfatal reinfarction by 20% with beta-blocker therapy (Frishman, 1991). There is no agreement on when the drugs should be started after the infarction and for how long they should be continued. Unless there are contraindications, disturbing side effects, or the patient is in a very low risk group, serious consideration should be given to the use of such drugs about 10 days after the onset of the myocardial infarction. The patients most likely to benefit from beta-adrenergic-blocking drugs are those who have had electrical or mechanical complications during acute myocardial infarction (Yusuf, 1985).

Beta-blocking drugs may be as effective as antiarrhythmic therapy chosen by electrophysiologic study. In 115 patients with symptomatic sustained ventricular tachyarrhythmias whose arrhythmias were inducible by programmed electrical stimulation, patients were randomized to a group whose antiarrhythmic therapy was guided by the electrophysiologic study and a group who received metoprolol. In a follow-up of 2 years, the incidence of recurrent nonfatal arrhythmias and sudden death combined was virtually the same in both groups—46% for the electrophysiologic group and 48% for the metoprolol group (Steinbeck, 1992).

D. Anti-Platelet-Aggregating Agents: Platelet aggregation is thought to be a factor in the development of atherosclerosis and acute coronary thrombosis; drugs that inhibit platelet aggregation have been used in various trials (Willard, 1992).

The Aspirin Myocardial Infarction Study Research Group (1980) found that although aspirin interferes with platelet aggregation, it does not reduce the total mortality rate in patients with a history of myocardial infarction. One-fourth of patients receiving aspirin developed symptoms of gastritis or gastric erosion. Aspirin is used in survivors of acute myocardial infarction, often in combination with dipyridamole or more recently with streptokinase (ISIS-2 Collaborative Group, 1988). A new large-scale trial of aspirin for primary prevention, using physicians in the USA as subjects, has demonstrated the effectiveness of 325 mg of aspirin every other day (Steering Committee of the Physicians' Health Study Research Group, 1989). The combination of aspirin and dipyridamole has been used in two so-called Paris trials. The second trial showed a reduction in mortality rate, but the results might be due to the aspirin. Of seven prospective, randomized, placebo-controlled clinical trials of aspirin therapy after myocardial infarction, six have shown a decrease in mortality with aspirin (Frishman, 1991).

E. Prevention of Recurrent Myocardial Infarction or Death: Physician-supervised exercise programs increase the physical work capacity of patients and improve morale. There is no convincing evidence that exercise decreases the likelihood of recurrence of myocardial infarction or the mortality rate. Exercise improves the coronary risk profile, decreasing the blood pressure, triglycerides, and body fat, improving glucose tolerance, and increasing high-density lipoproteins (HDL) (Fletcher, 1990; Fletcher, 1992). Despite the subjective and objective improvement seen in some patients following exercise rehabilitation, the claims for increased survival are premature (Shaw, 1981; Council on Scientific Affairs, 1981; Rechnitzer, 1983). The large number of subjects needed as well as the necessity for follow-up for long periods precludes a definitive controlled trial of exercise for cardiac rehabilitation. A meta-analysis of the randomized, controlled trials showed a benefit that appears to be related to exercise. The incidence of reinfarction is not reduced, but sudden death may be reduced (Oldridge, 1988).

The age-adjusted overall ischemic heart disease mortality rate declined by 20% in the USA between 1968 and 1976 (Figure 8–36) (Stamler, 1984). Improved survival was reported in both sexes, in all age groups, and in all major ethnic groups. The cause of the decline may be due to vigorous attempts to manage risk factors. These include (1) identification and treatment of hypertension; (2) efforts to reduce cigarette smoking; (3) extensive availability and use of coronary care units; (4) efforts to encourage a prudent diet to decrease serum lipids and weight; (5) supervised exercise training; and (6) extensive use of coronary bypass surgery.

Special efforts should be made to educate the patient with known coronary disease and the patient's family about the disease, emphasizing the importance of cooperating with the physician in the vigorous treatment of complex ventricular arrhythmias and the use of drugs to improve left ventricular function. Family members should be instructed generally regarding resuscitation and take courses on the technique.

The patient and family should have emergency telephone numbers readily available. The family should be urged to call for medical assistance at the

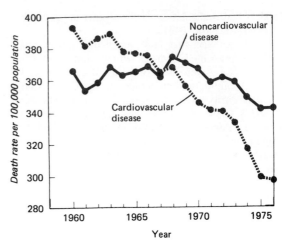

Figure 8–36. Cardiovascular and noncardiovascular mortality rates, 1960–1976. (Reproduced, with permission of the American Heart Association, Inc, from Levy RI: Progress toward prevention of cardiovascular disease: A 30-year retrospective. Circulation 1979;60:1555.)

first symptom and bring the patient to a coronary care unit at the first sign of acute myocardial infarction or prolonged chest distress.

The physician should consider the use of beta-adrenergic-blocking drugs for long-term treatment (see above) unless the patient has a contraindication to their use. A number of therapeutic trials have shown that several of these agents (timolol, metoprolol, propranolol, and alprenolol) decrease the likelihood of sudden death and nonfatal myocardial infarction and are associated with lower mortality rates.

It is not yet clear what the ultimate role of newly approved antiarrhythmic drugs will be in preventing sudden death syndrome or myocardial infarction.

F. Anticoagulants: Long-term use of anticoagulants to prevent thromboembolic complications has been recommended by some for at least 20 years, and the risks and benefits have been argued. The treatment is difficult, and benefits seem marginal. Deaths due to thromboembolic complications are infrequent in patients with acute myocardial infarction or chronic coronary disease, possibly because of early ambulation and rehabilitation programs. Patients at particular risk of thromboembolism due to prolonged cardiac failure or a history of venous thromboses should be considered for long-term anticoagulant treatment. Patients with mural thrombus demonstrated by two-dimensional echocardiography should be anticoagulated (Dinerman, 1989). Bleeding from various sites in the body is the most important complication of the treatment and may require hospitalization or may even be fatal. The ease with which a stable prothrombin time can be achieved with oral anticoagulants is an important factor in the decision to use the treatment.

G. Coronary Heart Surgery: See below.

CORONARY HEART SURGERY

In 1967, Favaloro and Effler revolutionized treatment of the patient with coronary artery disease by introducing the saphenous vein bypass surgical procedure. Over the past 23 years, the use of surgical procedures for revascularization of the heart has increased exponentially. The coronary bypass procedure—in which the obstructed coronary artery is bypassed by inserting the saphenous vein into the aorta proximal to the coronary arteries and beyond the obstruction distally or, alternatively, by anastomosing the internal mammary artery to a point distal to the obstructed artery has become one of the most frequent surgical procedures done in the USA. In 1988, the number of bypass operations was 141.8 per 100,000 in the USA, or over 300,000 cases per year. Endarterectomy is done in a minority of cases.

With the introduction of percutaneous transluminal coronary angioplasty (PTCA), increasingly the uncomplicated one-vessel and now two-vessel disease patients are being treated with PTCA, leaving the three-vessel disease patients and the complicated patients for bypass surgery.

Results of Coronary Bypass Surgery

A. Relief of Angina Pectoris: Bypass surgery is now performed extensively for double- and triple-vessel disease. Most patients with single-vessel disease are revascularized by PTCA. Relief of angina of effort occurs in 70–80% of patients. The surgical mortality rate of bypass surgery in stable angina is now 1–3%. The mortality rate is higher if the operation is an emergency or the patient is over 70 years of age, has unstable angina, or requires resection of a ventricular aneurysm, replacement of the mitral valve, or closure of an acquired ventricular septal defect. The mortality rate is higher also in women, in part because of late referral for bypass surgery (Khan, 1991).

B. Improvement in Survival and Prevention of Myocardial Infarction: The three major trials of coronary saphenous vein bypass surgery versus medical management of patients with symptomatic coronary artery disease are the Veterans Administration Randomized Trial (Murphy, 1977), the European Randomized Trial (European Coronary Surgery Study Group, 1980), and the Coronary Artery Surgical Study (CASS), 1983. Despite problems with each of these studies, it is from these trials and their follow-up data that a great deal of our present thinking about the value of coronary artery surgery is derived.

The benefit in survival over medical management is unequivocally proved in the symptomatic patient with a significant left main coronary artery lesion, in patients with left ventricular dysfunction and three-vessel disease; survival is probably also increased in patients with two-vessel disease and decreased left ventricular function, especially those with significant proximal left anterior descending coronary arterial lesions (Kirklin, 1991).

A significant number of patients with angina who achieved relief after operation had recurrence of angina at a rate of 5% per year, which is not surprising because coronary artery disease is progressive. Also not surprising is that over a 5- to 10-year period, especially with saphenous vein grafts, the benefit of surgery is lost and the medical and surgical survival curves approach each other—probably because of disease progression in the native coronary artery and deterioration of the saphenous vein bypass graft. In the Veterans Administration Cooperative Study, the benefits of coronary bypass surgery on survival, symptoms, and postinfarction mortality were transient and lasted less than 11 years. There was no reduction in the incidence of myocardial infarction. The loss of effectiveness was probably due to progression of the coronary disease and saphenous vein graft closure (VA Coronary Artery Bypass Surgery Cooperative Study Group, 1992). With better long-term patency of the internal mammary artery as a graft, we must wait to see if survival benefit of surgical over medical management continues to dissipate with time (Varnauskas, 1988).

In the prevention of myocardial infarction, none of the randomized studies convincingly show that surgery is better than medical management; however, the benefit of surgery over medical management is clear when survival is used as an end point. The more severe the extent of coronary artery disease, the greater the comparative benefit of surgery over medical management; and the more severe the left ventricular dysfunction, as long as ischemia is present, the greater the comparative benefit of surgery.

The decreased operative risk of bypass surgery in the past 5 years has been due to improved anesthetic and surgical techniques, myocardial protection during surgery, and better pre- and postoperative care. Studies have shown that the probability of early postoperative cardiac death is less after operations performed in the most recent era compared with those done in earlier years (Califf, 1989).

Objective improvement occurs in about half of these patients. Electrocardiography shows less evidence of ischemia induced by graded exercise. Resting left ventricular function as measured by ejection fraction is usually not changed after surgery. Occasionally, there will be dramatic improvement if patients with acute ischemic syndromes are studied postoperatively at a time when myocardial "stunning" (Scott, 1992) is no longer present. Careful pre- and postoperative studies have shown a slight improvement in resting ejection fraction in patients with stable angina who were revascularized (Dilsizian, 1988), suggesting preoperative subclinical myocardial ischemia.

With exercise, there is increased left ventricular

contractility with improved ejection fraction and improved left ventricular wall motion in patients who preoperatively had impaired segmental left ventricular walls—especially if the graft to the myocardial segment remains patent following surgery. Most patients have sufficient subjective improvement so that they can return to work. Relapse may occur as a result of occlusion of the previously patent graft when a patient appears to be improving.

The long-term effectiveness of saphenous vein bypass surgery in patients who have had a good technical result and a patent graft is now being reported (Varnauskas, 1988; VA Coronary Bypass Cooperative Study Group, 1992). The return of angina is the most prevalent of the postoperative ischemic events. If angina returns early after surgery, it is due to incomplete revascularization or to early closure of grafts, usually related to technical problems at the time of surgery. Angina occurring later is a reflection of narrowing or closure of one or more grafts, progression of disease in the native vessels, or both. Summarizing the results of most large series, the return of angina occurs at a linearized rate of 4–5% per year. In one large study, angina had returned in 37% of patients by 10 years; whether more frequent use of the internal mammary artery either as a pedicle graft or as a free graft will change this outcome is not yet well studied.

Perioperative myocardial infarction is an important risk factor for later death. Its incidence appears to be decreasing as intraoperative myocardial protection improves. Early studies indicated a rate of 5%, but the latest reports are about 2.5%. In the CASS study, surgery or medical management was associated with no differences in death (or late myocardial infarction) as an outcome in the entire group with three-vessel disease; however, in many large series of bypass patients, for the first 5 years after surgery, 95% are free of myocardial infarction. By 10 years after surgery, 15%—and by 15 years 35%—have had another infarction (Kirklin, 1991).

Long-term survival after bypass surgery is dependent on preoperative left ventricular function as well as freedom from intraoperative myocardial damage. In one series, the mortality rate was 12% at 5 years, 25% at 10 years, and 40% at 15 or more years after surgery (Kirklin, 1991), which represents a linearized rate of between 2% and 3% per year. As in the return of angina postoperatively, events appear to accelerate after the first 5 years.

Long-term graft patency is still a major limitation of saphenous vein grafts. Diffuse intimal hyperplasia is universally found in grafts in place over 1 year. Later atherosclerotic changes occur progressively, so that in one study graft occlusions increased steadily from 8% early to 20% at 5 years and 41% at 10 years. Disease was absent in all grafts after placement but increased to 38% in 5 years and 75% at 10 years (Fitzgibbon, 1991). Other studies have shown similar attrition rates of grafts where only half are patent at

10 years, an attrition rate of 5–7% per year (Campeau, 1984). Patency rates of grafts to larger coronary arteries are higher than those to smaller vessels, perhaps because of the better run-off. Arm veins and synthetic conduits have a still lower patency rate.

The highest patency rate is seen with internal mammary arteries used as conduits, especially when they are anastomosed to the left anterior descending coronary artery. Patency after 10 years has been reported to be 95% (Loop, 1986). It is not known whether other arterial grafts such as the gastroepiploic artery will be as good. The use of aspirin at the time of surgery and after has been shown to improve graft patency (Goldman, 1989; Gavaghan, 1991).

Surgical treatment is indicated when there is severe stenosis of the left main coronary artery; 2- to 3-year survival rates are higher for surgically treated than for medically treated groups (85–90% vs 65–69%) (Chaitman: Am J Cardiol, 1981; CASS Principle Investigators and Their Associates, 1983). Surgical treatment is most beneficial for patients in whom left main stenosis exceeds 75% and in whom there is three-vessel disease and abnormal left ventricular function. In the CASS study reported by Zimmern (1982), long-term survival is possible despite total occlusion of the left main coronary artery, although in groups of patients, bypass surgery improved survival rates. There were significant lesions of the other major coronary arteries in about 60% of patients in both groups.

The CASS study (1983) was designed to determine whether coronary revascularization when the patient is first seen resulted in better survival than if revascularization were postponed until medical management had failed to control the angina. This randomized study found that the annual surgical mortality rate was only 1.4% and the mortality rate in the medically treated group only 1.6%—considerably less than in any of the medically treated control groups in previous trials. This low mortality rate could be a function of modern medical therapy or of the fact that the patients with more severe angina pectoris were deleted by the design of the study. Only some of the patients received beta-adrenergic-blocking agents, and none received calcium entry-blocking drugs. Angina was relieved in 80–90% of patients. The results show that there is no difference in survival rates or the development of myocardial infarction between surgical patients and medical patients in whom the angina is well controlled medically, even though they had multivessel disease or previous myocardial infarction. However, the study did not include patients with significant left main artery stenosis or those at high risk with grade III or grade IV angina (angina of increasing severity per Canadian Cardiovascular Society gradings [Campeau, 1976]), unstable angina, or postmyocardial infarction angina. It is clear that angina pectoris refractory to medical therapy is a prime indication for surgery, but indications for surgery in high-risk patients with diseases other than left main coronary stenosis were not provided by the CASS report.

Subgroup analysis of patients in the CASS study with reduced ejection fraction and three-vessel disease showed that the operated patients had a better prognosis than those treated medically. The European Randomized Trial showed that patients with three-vessel disease and normal ejection fractions had a small benefit in survival if operated upon rather than treated medically.

Indications for revascularization are present when the comparative benefit of surgery is greater than that of medical management. On medical management, the time-related survival is dependent in part on the number of diseased vessels. Because the time-related survival after bypass surgery is only weakly affected by the number of diseased vessels, comparative surgical benefit increases in proportion to the number of diseased vessels (Myers, 1989; Califf, 1989).

The greater the number of vessels with proximal stenosis, the greater the comparative benefit of surgery (Myers, 1989). A proximal stenosis in the left anterior descending coronary artery particularly increases the comparative surgical benefit (Varnauskas, 1988).

Left ventricular function is the most important determinant of prognosis. The more severe the left ventricular dysfunction, the greater the comparative benefit from surgery, even though early and late mortality rates are higher in those with poor function than in those with good function.

Given the above facts, the patient most likely to benefit from revascularization is the one who, if another ischemic event occurs, will be left with poor left ventricular function. This would include patients with good left ventricular function and a large volume of potentially ischemic muscle as well as those with previous infarction who had decreased left ventricular function and a small amount of ischemic myocardium at risk. In either case, the next event will leave the patient with poor left ventricular function. Those with scarred myocardium and severe left ventricular function who have no reversible ischemia do not benefit from revascularization (Norris, 1981).

C. Factors Influencing Operative Results: The surgical results, including the operative deaths that occur, are influenced by the presence of acute myocardial necrosis at surgery; by the presence of previous myocardial infarction with segmental abnormalities of left ventricular motion; by increased left ventricular end-diastolic volume and pressure; by impaired left ventricular function, such as a decreased ejection fraction; and by the number of procedures performed at one operation. When end-diastolic volume is increased (especially if the patient has cardiac failure) or if the ejection fraction is less than 35%, the operative mortality rate is higher. If surgery is done after an acute myocardial infarction, there is a pro-

gressive fall in mortality rate if the bypass is done after the first week. The mortality rate stabilizes at about 30–60 days. As a result, elective surgery is usually delayed at least 1–2 months following an acute myocardial infarction, unless the patient is at high risk (angina or ischemia on treadmill tests with a low double-product [heart rate × systolic blood pressure]) or had transient congestive heart failure during the acute infarction, when there is a large amount of reversible ischemia.

The availability of a skilled cardiac surgeon with a well-trained, efficient team and adequate diagnostic and therapeutic facilities is necessary if bypass surgery is performed for incapacitating angina in patients with good left ventricular function. Coronary angiograms of high quality are essential in preparation for coronary bypass surgery. The presence of severe disease is not sufficient to justify surgery; the patient must also have arteries that supply viable myocardium and that can be bypassed.

Complications of Coronary Bypass Surgery

The adverse results that have followed bypass surgery include the following:

(1) Intraoperative myocardial infarction in 2.5–5% of patients, manifested by new Q waves, the development of increased MB CK, and positive pyrophosphate isotope scans.

(2) A surgical mortality rate of approximately 1–3%, which rises to 10% if additional procedures are required.

(3) Increased complications if a distal segment satisfactory for anastomosis has not been found preoperatively by coronary angiography and the surgeon finds poor distal vessels at operation.

(4) Early (within 1 year) occlusion of about 10% of the grafts, often related to technical problems or a relatively low blood flow at the time of the grafting.

(5) Progression of coronary disease postoperatively. There is some evidence that progression of stenoses is greater in the proximal portion of bypassed arteries than in arteries that have been untouched (Hwang, 1990).

(6) Late occlusion of bypass graft. If, in addition to progression of a partially stenosed artery, the graft applied distally to the stenosis becomes occluded, the patient is then worse off, develops more left ventricular dysfunction and more segmental contraction disorders, and may have more severe angina.

(7) Persistence of exercise-induced ventricular premature beats even when ventricular scars and ventricular aneurysms are resected. There is no convincing evidence that either the incidence or the type of arrhythmia is altered by revascularization.

(8) Decrease of collateral circulation that occurs after grafting and deterioration with respect to heart failure and chest pain over a period of years.

Management After Myocardial Revascularization

After revascularization, the object of treatment is to return the patient as rapidly as possible to normal; this includes facilitating complete recovery from the operation, promoting early long-term patency of the grafts, controlling risk factors as completely as possible, and detecting and treating recurrent myocardial ischemia should it develop.

The care of the patient in the immediate postoperative period is beyond the scope of this book; however, meticulous attention to pulmonary toilet, prevention of atelectasis, and prevention of pneumonia are essential, as is early ambulation. Progressive rehabilitation can return the patient to full activity within 6–8 weeks after surgery. Periods of time in which the patient is anxious and depressed are not unusual. During these periods, the patient can be assured that this is a common temporary state. A support group of patients who have recently had open heart surgery can be most helpful to the patient and family. Progressive increases in exercise, the most easily performed being walking, are important. The rate at which progression of activity occurs must depend on the patient's physical state, ventricular function, and other factors. Formal rehabilitation programs can be helpful (Fletcher, 1992). The patient should be urged to return to normal activity, including employment, as soon as possible. Return to normal activity after 6–8 weeks is expected.

Graft patency, especially of saphenous vein grafts, is enhanced up to 1 year by starting aspirin 6 hours after surgery, when it is given through the nasogastric tube (Goldman, 1989). Aspirin is most helpful in the small grafts with poor run-off, whereas the large grafts even without aspirin are more likely to remain patent. Graft patency may be enhanced by control of risk factors, especially cholesterol (Solymoss, 1988; Blankenhorn, 1987). Control of risk factors such as smoking, hypertension, cholesterol and triglycerides, obesity, diabetes, and sedentary life-style is very important. Evidence suggests that lowering cholesterol can markedly reduce progression of coronary artery and saphenous vein bypass graft disease.

Follow-up of the patient to detect the presence of continued ischemia due to graft closure or the presence of ungrafted vessels is important. Many cardiologists do stress tests with or without a radionuclide perfusion study some time after revascularization; this may be especially important if the patient had only silent ischemia preoperatively. There is evidence that although angina is markedly reduced after surgery, the prevalence of silent ischemia is just as great after surgery as it was preoperatively (Weiner, 1991). In many patients after bypass surgery, ST segment depression occurs at greater amounts of exercise and at greater double-products (systolic blood pressure × heart rate) than preoperatively. Although the recommendation is to treat ischemia, either silent or expressed as angina, with nitrates and beta-blocking drugs, the benefit of this course of action is unclear. Patients who are revascularized because of angina uncontrolled by medical management are not exercised if they remain asymptomatic until 6 months to 1 year has passed. Thereafter, the exercise study is repeated if symptoms occur or every 2–3 years if the patient remains asymptomatic.

If the patient develops angina or shows signs of severe ischemia on the exercise study, coronary arteriography should be done. The CT scan with contrast can determine patency of saphenous vein bypass grafts with a high degree of accuracy (Brundage, 1983) but does not identify grafts with high-grade obstruction. The indications for repeat revascularization are similar to those that indicated the first operation. If revascularization is necessary, angioplasty should be done if possible. If angioplasty is not possible or not advisable given the coronary disease, reoperation should be considered. The early risks of a second bypass operation are about twice those of the first, mostly related to the increased prevalence of unfavorable risk factors. A few patients will have a third and, rarely, a fourth operation (Loop, 1990).

PERCUTANEOUS TRANSLUMINAL CORONARY ANGIOPLASTY (PTCA)

In 1977, Andreas Gruentzig in Zurich performed the first PTCA, adapting a concept of Charles Dotter. The technique consists of passing a balloon-tipped catheter over a guidewire through a catheter into the coronary artery. The guidewire is slipped past the lesion in the coronary artery and the balloon-tipped catheter is passed over the wire, positioning the collapsed balloon at the level of the lesion. The balloon is then inflated with diluted contrast medium under 5–20 atm of pressure. Pathologic and experimental studies have indicated that this Samsonian technique decreases the degree of obstruction by fracturing the fibrous cap of the lesion and separating the plaque from the artery, creating a dissection. The arterial wall also stretches, but for the most part it then recoils. The injury stimulates factors that lead to "healing," and the plaque is remodeled over time, resulting in lesser degrees of obstruction. Unfortunately, especially if the media of the vessel is injured, intimal migration of smooth muscle cells is stimulated, leading to intimal hyperplasia, which is the cause of early restenosis, the major unsolved problem in PTCA. In addition, cracking of the fibrous plaque can lead to platelet adhesion and aggregation, fibrin deposition, and formation of a thrombus occluding the vessel, resulting in severe ischemia.

Estimates of the number of PTCA procedures done in the United States in 1990 exceed 300,000, with an approximately equal number done in the rest of the world. This technique is therefore as important an advance in the treatment of coronary artery disease as was coronary artery bypass approximately 10 years earlier.

When first introduced, PTCA was confined to dilating short, uncalcified, concentric lesions in a single vessel. In the 15 years since that time, the technology in the design of the equipment, involving the guiding catheters, the guidewires, and the balloons, has changed markedly: Stiff guidewires are now capable of penetrating older occlusions; flexible guidewires can be steered to reach previously inaccessible lesions; low-profile balloons on trackable catheters can be inflated to 15–20 atm without breaking; catheters with multiple holes and lumens large enough to allow perfusion to the distal vessel permit prolonged inflations (10–30 minutes) without signs of ischemia; and active perfusion systems permit blood and other perfusates, such as hemoglobin-based blood substitutes, to be infused at rates up to 55 mL/min to prevent myocardial infarction and to permit transport of patients with unstable arteries to surgery.

The equipment and personnel required to perform these procedures exceed the requirements of the ordinary diagnostic catheterization laboratory. High-resolution fluoroscopic and cineangiographic x-ray equipment and single- and biplane equipment for angled views allowing for three-dimensional imaging and digital processing of images have all improved the results and safety of PTCA. Full anesthesia and emergency resuscitation equipment is immediately necessary as well as—for all patients except those who would not under any circumstances be candidates for open heart surgery—some mechanism for surgical availability in case acute and unremitting ischemia develops.

Complications of PTCA depend on the age, sex, and physical condition of the patient; on left ventricular function; on whether the subserved myocardium is protected by collaterals; and on the type of lesion—whether it is long, calcified, eccentric, or occurring at branches. The "ideal" lesion is proximal but not at the ostium. In the young patient with good ventricular function, the complication rate should be minimal. In a patient with multivessel disease, calcification, long lesions, or poor left ventricular function, the complication rate is higher.

Overall, the complication rates are relatively low and consist of development of an acute ischemic syndrome in up to 5% of patients; emergency coronary artery bypass in 2–3% (up to 5–10% in complicated cases); myocardial infarction in 2–5%, non-Q wave infarctions being more prevalent than Q wave infarctions; and death in 0.5–3% depending on the age of the patient, the extent of the disease, and the degree of ventricular dysfunction (Roubin, 1990). Rupture of the artery is quite unusual.

Current Indications for PTCA

The indications for angioplasty have changed markedly since its introduction. The American Col-

lege of Cardiology/American Heart Association Task Force suggests that, as with other medical procedures, the decision to do PTCA must be based on the physician's evaluation of the risk/benefit ratio (Ryan, 1988). Patients who benefit from PTCA may include those with single-vessel disease, when PTCA is possible because of the angiographic appearance of the lesion; or those with multivessel disease, especially when the lesion responsible for the severe ischemia has been identified. The usual recommendation is to perform PTCA on this lesion and postpone PTCA on other lesions until the danger of acute occlusion has passed. PTCA is indicated in patients with acute myocardial infarction who are seen within 6 hours and who are not candidates for thrombolysis. PTCA is the preferred treatment for acute myocardial infarction with cardiogenic shock or severe failure. In a study of 81 patients with cardiogenic shock complicating acute myocardial infarction, revascularization by angioplasty predominantly was associated with a 56% in-hospital survival compared with an 8% survival with medical management. At a mean of 21 months' follow-up, this survival benefit persisted, with a 50% late survival in those revascularized versus a 2% survival of those treated medically. The most benefit was obtained when revascularization was done within 24 hours (Moosvi, 1992).

The benefits of PTCA are relief of angina pectoris (stable or unstable), reduction in the hospital stay for unstable angina, resolution of spontaneous or exercise-induced myocardial ischemia, and postponement of coronary artery bypass surgery. Other benefits—and especially advantages over bypass surgery—are under active investigation.

Results of Angioplasty

In patients with stable angina, a success rate over 90% is reported in most series, where success is defined as leaving the patient with a less than 50% obstruction. In one prospective study of over 400 patients, 85% were free of angina 5 years after initial PTCA (Talley, 1988). With multivessel disease, the results are not as good, but in one large study of over 1000 patients with two-vessel disease and almost 200 with three-vessel disease, clinical success was achieved in 85% of patients with two-vessel disease and 87% with three-vessel disease. In this study, success was defined as relief of at least one obstruction, usually the culprit lesion—or the lesion responsible for the acute ischemia—and no major complications (Roubin, 1987). Although complete revascularization by PTCA is a goal, complete revascularization is usually not achieved. The main reason is the relatively low success in dilating chronic complete obstruction and the reluctance to angioplasty lesions with 50–70% obstruction (Bourassa, 1992).

Overall, angiographic success is achieved in 80–90% of patients, with emergency coronary bypass required in 3–6% and myocardial infarction occurring in 3–5% (Q wave infarction in 2%). Mortality rates in most series are from 0.5% to 3.0%. In general, there is less success when the lesion is at the ostium of the vessel. One can most effectively dilate occlusions in saphenous vein bypass grafts when the obstruction is at the anastomosis with the coronary artery; next most effectively when the obstruction is in the body of the graft; and least effectively when it is at the anastomosis in the aorta.

Persisting Problems With PTCA

After angioplasty, the patient is usually given heparin for 48 hours, aspirin and nitrates, and frequently calcium channel blockers—all for the purpose of preventing thrombus formation and arterial spasm. Immediately after angioplasty, the prevention of acute occlusion and precipitation of an acute ischemic syndrome is the most important unsolved problem. This occurs in the catheterization laboratory or later that same day or night in 5–10% of cases. With acute occlusion, all advantages of PTCA over surgery are lost. The patient has a 25% chance of having a Q wave infarction, and the mortality rate in emergency bypass surgery varies from 3% to 10%. The patient who survives has all the problems in recovery that are associated with coronary artery bypass surgery. On precipitation of an acute occlusion, most patients are returned to the catheterization laboratory and reangiogrammed. Thrombolytic agents can be used in an attempt to lyse thrombi, as can heparin, vasodilators, and prolonged inflation of an angioplasty balloon with a salvage perfusion catheter or stents to tack down the occluded flap of intima. If reocclusion occurs, the perfusion catheter can be left in place across the obstruction and the patient taken to surgery. The patient can be supported with left heart bypass, percutaneously instituted balloon counterpulsation, or a coronary sinus retroperfusion catheter to supply oxygenated blood to the myocardium retrogradely.

Certainly, the most important chronic problem with angioplasty is restenosis. Restenosis is really an exaggeration of the healing process and, therefore, probably occurs to some extent in all patients. It is more likely to occlude the vessel if the original angioplasty result is suboptimal or if the vessel is very small. The greater the injury inflicted by the balloon catheter, the more vigorous the reparative and proliferative process. This intimal proliferative process occurs against a background of suboptimal dilation, residual thrombus, intimal flaps, and vessel wall recoil. The incidence varies from 20% to 40% (Leimgruber, 1986; Ellis, 1989) and is probably highest when angioplasty is undertaken for lesions in the proximal left anterior descending coronary artery.

Twenty percent of patients with restenosis have no symptoms and are discovered only if repeat angiography is done. When angina recurs within weeks (up to 4 months) after angioplasty, restenosis is the usual mechanism. When the angina occurs later, it is usu-

ally due to progression of atherosclerotic disease, usually at another location in the native coronary artery. Although vasodilators, anticoagulants, and antiplatelet agents are all used after angioplasty, there is no evidence that any of these drugs prevent restenosis. Better understanding of the biology of the healing process after damage to the arterial wall and of the nature of the growth factors stimulated will eventually lead to techniques to prevent restenosis (Ellis, 1989; Talley, 1988). On the average, 30% of patients may be expected to have recurrence within 4–6 months after PTCA, and 25% will need an additional revascularization procedure. After restenosis, it is possible to do a second and even a third angioplasty with prolonged success (Dimas, 1992). If multivessel disease is present, coronary artery bypass grafting is probably a better option.

Recanalizing total occlusions is another limitation of PTCA. Techniques to recanalize these vessels to maintain patency over the long term is one of the ongoing problems. Initial success rates for occlusions believed to be less than 6–8 weeks old are about 50–75%, down to 20% for occlusions over 3 months old (Roubin, 1990). To attack this problem, atherectomy devices may be most useful. Various technologies, including hot wires, rotational and mechanical abrasive devices, laser energy, and radiofrequency devices, are being evaluated.

The role of PTCA versus bypass surgery is being examined actively. The obvious advantages of PTCA are its easier acceptance by patients, the shortened time in the hospital, and the shorter convalescence time at home after the procedure. For one procedure, PTCA is less expensive than surgery, but the recurrence rates in angioplasty guarantee a second or even third procedure, so that the costs are no different.

Patients with left main coronary lesions and lesions at ostia are all better treated by surgery. Old bypass grafts are not amenable to angioplasty and should be treated by surgery (Parisi, 1992). Multivessel disease is being actively investigated by multicentered trials comparing PTCA with bypass surgery. The technique of using PTCA only to dilate the "culprit" lesion in patients with multivessel disease is also being investigated.

A number of prospective randomized trials comparing PTCA with bypass surgery are under way. A single trial from the Veterans Administration—the Angioplasty Compared to Medicine Study (ACME) trial—has been reported (Parisi, 1992). These investigators compared angioplasty with medical management and found in a 6-month follow-up that there was no difference in mortality rate or myocardial infarction but that PTCA offers earlier and more complete relief of angina. They also found that PTCA costs more and is associated with a higher percentage of complications than medical management.

The other trials comparing PTCA with bypass surgery have acronyms such as BARI (Bypass Angioplasty Revascularization Investigation), CABRI (Coronary Angioplasty Bypass Revascularization Investigation), EAST (Emory Angioplasty Surgery Trial), GABI (German Angioplasty Bypass Intervention Trial), and RITA (Randomized Interventional Treatment of Angina). The results of these trials are forthcoming. New technologic advances designed to remove obstructive material from the vessel itself are being developed, and these in general fall under the rubric of "atherectomy" devices. Three mechanical atherectomy devices are currently under clinical investigation:

(1) A directional atherectomy device using a rotation cylinder that pushes the shavings into a nosecone.

(2) The transluminal extraction atherectomy device, in which a rotating, cutting mechanical blade minces the tissue, which is extracted through the catheter by a suction system.

(3) Rotablator atherectomy, in which a device consisting of a rotating abrasive bullet-shaped burr spinning at 150,000 rpm liquefies the obstructive plaque into a colloidal suspension containing particles less than 5 μm in size which is washed through the capillary bed.

In general, these catheters are bulky and difficult to steer, and restenosis seems to occur at a rate similar to that observed following balloon angioplasty; however, the devices can be successful at ostial occlusions where angioplasty is not successful and also where the lesions are calcified.

Three types of laser devices, which deliver ultrashort pulses to prevent unwanted thermal energy, are currently being investigated: the pulsed eximer laser, the CO_2 laser, and the Nd:YAG laser. The energy is directed by the use of a coaxial guidewire system, and perforation of the vessel is a danger.

At least five different stents are being developed to provide a rigid, open structure that can be endothelialized but still maintain the lumen: the balloon-expandable coil; balloon-expanded, slotted tubes; self-expanding mesh; and the self-expanding Z-stent. These devices are undergoing clinical trials, and their ultimate usefulness is not known.

REFERENCES

Overview of Coronary Heart Disease

Braunwald E (editor): *Heart Disease: A Textbook of Cardiovascular Medicine,* 3rd ed. Saunders, 1988.

Chatterjee K et al (editors): *Cardiology: An Illustrated Text/Reference.* Lippincott/Gower, 1991.

Soto B, Russell RO Jr, Moraski RE: *Radiographic Anatomy of the Coronary Arteries: An Atlas.* Futura, 1976.

Pathogenesis of Atherosclerotic Coronary Heart Disease

AHA Committee: Risk factors and coronary disease: A statement for physicians. Circulation 1980;62:449A.

AHA Nutrition Committee: Dietary guidelines for healthy American adults: A statement for physicians and health professionals. Circulation 1988;77:721A.

Bassenge E, Busse R: Endothelial modulation of coronary tone. Prog Cardiovasc Dis 1988;30:349.

Bernstein MJ: Lowering blood cholesterol to prevent heart disease. JAMA 1985;253:2080.

Brensike JF et al: Effects of therapy with cholestyramine on progression of coronary atherosclerosis: Results of the NHLBI Type II Coronary Intervention Study. Circulation 1984;69:313.

Brown MS, Goldstein JL: Familial hypercholesterolemia: Genetic, biochemical and pathophysiological aspects. Adv Intern Med 1975;20:273.

Brown MS et al: Prenatal diagnosis of homozygous familial hypercholesterolaemia: Expression of a genetic receptor disease in utero. Lancet 1978;1:526.

Brundage BH: Computed tomography: A new view of cardiovascular disease. Prim Cardiol 1983;9(7):57.

Case RB et al: Type A behavior and survival after acute myocardial infarction. Multicenter Post-Infarction Research Group. N Engl J Med 1985;312:737.

Castelli WP: Epidemiology of coronary heart disease: The Framingham study. Am J Med 1984;76:4.

Davies MJ, Thomas AC: Plaque fissuring: The cause of acute myocardial infarction, sudden ischaemic death, and crescendo angina. Br Heart J 1985;53:363.

DeWood MA et al: Prevalence of total coronary occlusion during the early hours of transmural myocardial infarction. N Engl J Med 1980;303:897.

Dole WP: Autoregulation of the coronary circulation. Prog Cardiovasc Dis 1987;29:293.

East C, Grundy SM, Bilheimer DW: Normal cholesterol levels with lovastatin (mevinolin) therapy in a child with homozygous familial hypercholesterolemia following liver transplantation. JAMA 1986;256:2843.

Falk E: Plaque rupture with severe pre-existing stenosis precipitating coronary thrombosis: Characteristics of coronary atherosclerotic plaques underlying fatal occlusive thrombi. Br Heart J 1983;50:127.

Findings from the aspirin component of the ongoing Physicians' Health Study: Preliminary report. N Engl J Med 1988;318:262.

Forrester JS et al: A perspective of coronary disease seen through the arteries of living man. Circulation 1987;75:505.

Frick MH et al: Helsinki Heart Study: Primary prevention trial with gemfibrozil in middle-aged men with dyslipidemia: Safety of treatment, changes in risk factors, and incidence of coronary heart disease. N Engl J Med 1987;317:1237.

Fuller JH et al: Coronary-heart-disease risk and impaired glucose tolerance: The Whitehall study. Lancet 1980;2:373.

Fuster V et al: The pathogenesis of coronary artery disease and the acute coronary syndrome. N Engl J Med 1992;326:Part 1:242, Part 2:310.

Goldstein JL, Kita T, Brown MS: Defective lipoprotein receptors and atherosclerosis: Lessons from an animal counterpart of familial hypercholesterolemia. N Engl J Med 1983;309:288.

Goldstein JL et al: Hyperlipidemia in coronary heart disease: I. Lipid levels in 500 survivors of myocardial infarction. J Clin Invest 1973;52:1533.

Gordon DJ et al: Habitual physical activity and high-density lipoprotein cholesterol in men with primary hypercholesterolemia: The Lipid Research Clinics Coronary Primary Prevention Trial. Circulation 1983;67:512.

Grundy SM: HMG-CoA reductase inhibitors for treatment of hypercholesterolemia. N Engl J Med 1988;319:24.

Hagman M et al: Factors of importance for prognosis in men with angina pectoris derived from a random population sample: The Multifactor Primary Prevention Trial, Gothenburg, Sweden. Am J Cardiol 1988;61:530.

Hamby RI: Hereditary aspects of coronary artery disease. Am Heart J 1981;101:639.

Havel RJ, Goldstein JL, Brown MS: Lipoproteins and lipid transport. In: *Metabolic Control and Disease,* 8th ed. Bondy PK, Rosenberg LE (editors). Saunders, 1980.

Havel RJ et al: Lovastatin (mevinolin) in the treatment of heterozygous familial hypercholesterolemia: A multicenter study. Ann Intern Med 1987;107:609.

Kannel WB, Sorlie P: Some health benefits of physical activity: The Framingham study. Arch Intern Med 1979;139:857.

Kannel WB et al: Optimal resources for primary prevention of atherosclerotic diseases. Circulation 1984;70:157A.

Klocke FJ: Measurements of coronary blood flow and degree of stenosis: Current clinical implications and continuing uncertainties. J Am Coll Cardiol 1983;1:31.

Kottke BA et al: Apolipoproteins and coronary artery disease. Mayo Clin Proc 1986;61:313.

Kromhout D, Bosschieter EB, de Lezenne Coulander C: The inverse relation between fish consumption and 20-year mortality from coronary heart disease. N Engl J Med 1985;312:1205.

Kuo PT: Lipoproteins, platelets, and prostaglandins in atherosclerosis. (Editorial.) Am Heart J 1981;102:949.

Leon AS: Physical activity levels and coronary heart disease: Analysis of epidemiologic and supporting studies. Med Clin N Am 1985;69:3.

Levy RI et al: The influence of changes in lipid values induced by cholestyramine and diet on progression of coronary artery disease: Results of the NHLBI type II coronary intervention study. Circulation 1984;69:325.

Lipid Research Clinics Program: The Lipid Research Clinics Coronary Primary Prevention Trial results. I. Reduction in incidence of coronary heart disease. II. The relationship of reduction in incidence of coronary heart disease to cholesterol lowering. JAMA 1984;251:351, 365.

Lober PH: Pathogenesis of coronary sclerosis. Arch Pathol 1953;55:357.

Lovastatin Study Group II: Therapeutic response to lovastatin (mevinolin) in nonfamilial hypercholesterolemia: A multicenter study. JAMA 1986;256:2829.

Lown B, Graboys TB: Sudden death: An ancient problem newly perceived. Cardiovasc Med 1977;2:219.

Manninen V et al: Lipid alterations and decline in the incidence of coronary heart disease in the Helsinki Heart Study. JAMA 1988;260:641.

Maseri A, Chierchia S, L'Abbate A: Pathogenetic mechanisms underlying the clinical events associated with atherosclerotic heart disease. Circulation 1980;62:V-3.

Maseri A, Parodi O, Fox KM: Rational approach to the medical therapy of angina pectoris: The role of calcium antagonists. Prog Cardiovasc Dis 1983;25:269.

Mizuno K et al: Angioscopic evaluation of coronary artery thrombi in acute coronary syndrome. N Engl J Med 1992;326:287.

Morales AR, Romanelli R, Boucek RJ: The mural left anterior descending coronary artery, strenuous exercise and sudden death. Circulation 1980;62:230.

Multiple Risk Factor Intervention Trial Research Group: Multiple Risk Factor Intervention Trial: Risk factor changes and mortality results. JAMA 1982;248:1465.

Peto R et al: Randomised trial of prophylactic daily aspirin in British male doctors. Br Med J 1988;296:313.

Phillips AN et al: Parental death from heart disease and the risk of heart attack. Eur Heart J 1988;9:243.

Pitt B et al: Prostaglandins and prostaglandin inhibitors in ischemic heart disease. Ann Intern Med 1983;99:83.

Ragland DR, Brand RJ: Type A behavior and mortality from coronary heart disease. N Engl J Med 1988;318:65.

Rath M et al: Detection and quantification of lipoprotein(a) in the arterial wall of 107 coronary bypass patients. Arteriosclerosis 1989;9:579.

Rechnitzer PA et al: Relation of exercise to the recurrence rate of myocardial infarction in men: Ontario Exercise-Heart Collaborative Study. Am J Cardiol 1983;51:65.

Rosenman RH et al: Multivariate prediction of coronary heart disease during 8.5 year follow-up in the Western Collaborative Group Study. Am J Cardiol 1976;37:903.

Ross R, Glomset JA: The pathogenesis of atherosclerosis. (Part 1.) N Engl J Med 1976;195:369.

Ross R: Atherosclerosis: A problem of the biology of arterial wall cells and their interactions with blood components. Arteriosclerosis 1981;1:293.

Ross R: The pathogenesis of atherosclerosis: An update. N Engl J Med 1986;314:488.

Royal College of General Practitioners' Oral Contraception Study: Further analyses of mortality in oral contraceptive users. Lancet 1981;1:541.

Ruderman NB, Haudenschild C: Diabetes as an atherogenic factor. Prog Cardiovasc Dis 1984;26:373.

Salonen JL et al: Leisure time and occupational physical activity: Risk of death from ischemic heart disease. Am J Epidemiol 1988;127:87.

Schaefer EJ, Levy RI: Pathogenesis and management of lipoprotein disorders. N Engl J Med 1985;312:1300.

Schmidt SB et al: Lipoprotein and apolipoprotein levels in angiographically defined coronary atherosclerosis. Am J Cardiol 1985;55:1459.

Schwartz SM, Ross R: Cellular proliferation in atherosclerosis and hypertension. Prog Cardiovasc Dis 1984;26:355.

Shaw LW: Effects of a prescribed supervised exercise program on mortality and cardiovascular morbidity in patients after a myocardial infarction: The National Exercise and Heart Disease Project. Am J Cardiol 1981;48:39.

Slack J, Nevin NC: Hyperlipidaemic xanthomatoses. I. Increased risk of death from ischaemic heart disease in first degree relatives of 53 patients with essential hyperlipidaemia and xanthomatosis. J Med Genet 1968;5:4.

Slack J: Risks of ischaemic heart-disease in familial hyperlipoproteinaemic states. Lancet 1969;2:1380.

Slone D et al: Risk of myocardial infarction in relation to current and discontinued use of oral contraceptives. N Engl J Med 1981;305:420.

Stamler J, Stamler R: Intervention for the prevention and control of hypertension and atherosclerotic diseases: United States and international experience. Am J Med 1984;76(2A):13.

Swan HJC et al: Catheterization of the heart in man with use of a flow-directed balloon-tipped catheter. N Engl J Med 1970;283:447.

ten Kate LP et al: Familial aggregation of coronary heart disease and its relation to known genetic risk factors. Am J Cardiol 1982;50:945.

Vane JR: Prostaglandins and the cardiovascular system. (Editorial.) Br Heart J 1983;49:405.

von Schacky C: Prophylaxis of atherosclerosis with marine omega-3 fatty acids: A comprehensive strategy. Ann Intern Med 1987;107:890.

Waller BF, Palumbo PJ, Roberts WC: Status of the coronary arteries at necropsy in diabetes mellitus with onset after age 30 years: Analysis of 229 diabetic patients with and without clinical evidence of coronary heart disease and comparison to 183 control subjects. Am J Med 1980;69:498.

Weksler BB et al: Differential inhibition by aspirin of vascular and platelet prostaglandin synthesis in atherosclerotic patients. N Engl J Med 1983;308:800.

Williams RB Jr: Refining the type A hypothesis: Emergence of the hostility complex. Am J Cardiol 1987;60:27J.

Working Group on Management of Patients With Hypertension and High Blood Cholesterol: National Education Programs Working Group report on the management of patients with hypertension and high blood cholesterol. Ann Intern Med 1991;114:224.

Yusuf S, Wittes J, Friedman L: Overview of results of randomized clinical trials in heart disease: II. Unstable angina, heart failure, primary prevention with aspirin, and risk factor modification. JAMA 1988;260:2259.

Latent Coronary Heart Disease

Cohn PF, Kannel WB (editors): Recognition, pathogenesis, and management options in silent coronary artery disease. Circulation 1987;75:II-1.

Deanfield JE: Holter monitoring in assessment of angina pectoris. Am J Cardiol 1987;59:18C.

Fleg JL et al: Prevalence and prognostic significance of exercise-induced silent myocardial ischemia detected by thallium scintigraphy and electrocardiography in asymptomatic volunteers. Circulation 1990;81:428.

Gibson RS: Comparative analysis of the diagnostic and prognostic value of exercise ECG and thallium-201 scintigraphic markers of myocardial ischemia in asymptomatic and symptomatic patients. Cardiol Clin 1989;7:565.

Gordon DJ et al: Predictive value of the exercise tolerance test for mortality in North American men: The Lipid Research Clinics Mortality Follow-Up Study. Circulation 1986;74:252.

Josephson RA et al: Can serial exercise testing improve the prediction of coronary events in asymptomatic individuals? Circulation 1990;81:20.

Mark DB et al: Painless exercise ST deviation on the treadmill: Long-term prognosis. J Am Coll Cardiol 1989;14:885.

McHenry PL et al: The abnormal exercise electrocardiogram in apparently healthy men: A predictor of angina pectoris as an initial coronary event during long-term follow-up. Circulation 1984;70:547.

Multiple Risk Factor Intervention Trial Research Group: Exercise electrocardiogram and coronary heart disease mortality in the Multiple Risk Factor Intervention Trial. Am J Cardiol 1985;55:16.

Rifkin RD, Parisi AF, Folland E: Coronary calcification in the diagnosis of coronary artery disease. Am J Cardiol 1979;44:141.

Sudden Death

The Cardiac Arrhythmia Suppression Trial (CAST) Investigators: Preliminary report: Effect of encainide and flecainide on mortality in a randomized trial of arrhythmia suppression after myocardial infarction. N Engl J Med 1989;321:406.

Cobb LA, Werner JA, Trobaugh GB: Sudden cardiac death. 1. A decade's experience with out-of-hospital resuscitation. Mod Concepts Cardiovasc Dis 1980;49:31.

Cobb LA et al: Report of the American Heart Association Task Force on the Future of Cardiopulmonary Resuscitation. Circulation 1992;85:2346.

Cobb LA et al: Resuscitation from out-of-hospital ventricular fibrillation: 4 years follow-up. Circulation 1975;52:III-223.

Davies MJ: Pathological view of sudden cardiac death. Br Heart J 1981;45:88.

DiMarco JP, Haines DE: Sudden cardiac death. Curr Probl Cardiol 1990;15:183.

el-Sherif N et al: Prognostic significance of the signal-averaged ECG depends on the time of recording in the postinfarction-period. Am Heart J 1989;118:256.

Goldstein S et al: Characteristics of the resuscitated out-of-hospital cardiac arrest victim with coronary heart disease. Circulation 1981;64:977.

James TN (editor): Sudden cardiac death: 15th Bethesda Conference. J Am Cardiol 1985;5:1B.

Josephson ME et al: Electrophysiologic and hemodynamic studies in patients resuscitated from cardiac arrest. Am J Cardiol 1980;46:948.

Kannel WB, Thomas HE Jr: Sudden coronary death: The Framingham study. Ann NY Acad Sci 1982;382:3.

Kuller LH: Sudden death: Definition and epidemiologic considerations. Prog Cardiovasc Dis 1980;23:1.

Lown B: Mental stress, arrhythmias and sudden death. (Editorial.) Am J Med 1982;72:177.

Meissner MD et al: Relation of acute antiarrhythmic drug efficacy to left ventricular function in coronary artery disease. Am J Cardiol 1988;61:1050.

Mirowski M: The automatic implantable cardioverter-defibrillator: An overview. J Am Coll Cardiol 1985;6:461.

Montgomery WH, Donegan J, McIntyre K (editors): Proceedings of the 1985 National Conference on Standards and Guidelines for Cardiopulmonary Resuscitation and Emergency Cardiac Care. Circulation 1986;74:IV-1.

Moosvi AR et al: Effect of empiric antiarrhythmic therapy in resuscitated out-of-hospital cardiac arrest victims with coronary artery disease. Am J Cardiol 1990;65:1192.

Morady F et al: Electrophysiologic testing in the management of survivors of out-of-hospital cardiac arrest. Am J Cardiol 1983;51:85.

Myers A, Dewar HA: Circumstances attending 100 sudden deaths from coronary artery disease with coroner's necropsies. Br Heart J 1975;37:1133.

Scheinman MM: Nonpharmacologic treatment of life-threatening cardiac arrhythmias. Cardiovasc Rev Rep 1988;9:27.

Troup PJ: Implantable cardioverters and defibrillators. Curr Probl Cardiol 1989;14:673. (Erratum in 1990;15:119.)

Verzoni A et al: Prognostic significance and evaluation of late ventricular potentials in the first year after myocardial infarction: A prospective study. PACE 1989;12:41.

Weaver WD, Cobb LA, Hallstrom AP: Ambulatory arrhythmias in resuscitated victims of cardiac arrest. Circulation 1982;66:212.

Wellens HJ, Brugada P, Bar FW: The role of intraventricular conduction disorders in precipitating sudden death. Ann NY Acad Sci 1982;382:136.

Wilber DJ et al: Out-of-hospital cardiac arrest: Use of electrophysiologic testing in the prediction of long-term outcome. N Engl J Med 1988;318:19.

Angina Pectoris; Variant (Prinzmetal's) Angina (Coronary Spasm), Syndrome X

Alison HW et al: Coronary anatomy and arteriography in patients with unstable angina pectoris. Am J Cardiol 1978;41:204.

Bemiller CR, Pepine CJ, Rogers AK: Long-term observation in patients with angina and normal coronary arteriograms. Circulation 1973;47:36.

Bertolet BD, Pepine CJ: The vascular endothelium is a key to undertaking coronary spasm and syndrome X. Curr Opin Cardiol 1991;6:496.

Bott-Silverman C, Heupler FA Jr: Natural history of pure coronary artery spasm in patients treated medically. J Am Coll Cardiol 1983;2:200.

Brinker JA: Selection of a contrast agent in the cardiac catheterization laboratory. Am J Cardiol 1990;66:26F.

Califf RM et al: Importance of clinical measures of ischemia in the prognosis of patients with documented coronary artery disease. J Am Coll Cardiol 1988;11:20.

Epstein SE, Quyyumi AA, Bonow RO: Myocardial ischemia: Silent or symptomatic. N Engl J Med 1988;318:1038.

Fellows CL, Weaver WD, Greene HL: Cardiac arrest associated with coronary artery spasm. Am J Cardiol 1987;60:1397.

Hirshfeld JW Jr: Cardiovascular effects of iodinated contrast agents. Am J Cardiol 1990;66:9F.

Mark DB et al: Clinical characteristics and long-term survival of patients with variant angina. Circulation 1984;69:880.

Maseri A (editor): The concept of the total ischemic burden. (Symposium.) Am J Cardiol 1987;59:1C.

Maseri A, Chierchia S: Coronary artery spasm: Demonstration, definition, diagnosis, and consequences. Prog Cardiovasc Dis 1982;25:169.

Maseri A: Role of coronary artery spasm in symptomatic and silent myocardial ischemia. J Am Coll Cardiol 1987;9:249.

Morris JJ Jr (editor): Medical management of silent ischemia and myocardial infarctions. A symposium. Am J Cardiol 1988;61:1B.

Prinzmetal M et al: Angina pectoris. 1. A variant form of angina pectoris. Am J Med 1959;26:375.

Reagan K et al: Double-blind study of a new nonionic contrast agent for cardiac angiography. Radiology 1988;167:409.

Rozanski A et al: Mental stress and the induction of silent myocardial ischemia in patients with coronary artery disease. N Engl J Med 1988;318:1005.

Schroeder JS et al: Prevention of cardiovascular events in variant angina by long-term diltiazem therapy. J Am Coll Cardiol 1983;1:1507.

Stone PH, Goldschlager N: Left main coronary artery disease: Review and appraisal. Cardiovasc Med 1979;4:165.

Toyo-oka T et al: Increased plasma level of endothelin-1 and coronary spasm induction in patients with vasospastic angina pectoris. Circulation 1991;83:476.

Voelker W et al: Long-term clinical course of patients with angina and angiographically normal coronary arteries. Clin Cardiol 1991;14:307.

Walling A et al: Long-term prognosis of patients with variant angina. Circulation 1987;76:990.

Weiner DA et al: Significance of silent myocardial ischemia during exercise testing in patients with coronary artery disease. Am J Cardiol 1987;59:725.

Noninvasive & Invasive Studies

American Medical Association Council on Scientific Affairs Magnetic Resonance Imaging Panel: Magnetic resonance imaging of the cardiovascular system: Present state of the art and future potential. JAMA 1988;259:253.

Armstrong WF: Echocardiography in coronary artery disease. Prog Cardiovasc Dis 1988;30:267.

Armstrong WF: Exercise echocardiography: Ready, willing and able. (Editorial.) J Am Coll Cardiol 1988;11;1359.

Beller GA, Gibson RS: Sensitivity, specificity, and prognostic significance of noninvasive testing for occult or known coronary disease. Prog Cardiovasc Dis 1987;29:241.

Berger BC et al: Effect of coronary collateral circulation on regional myocardial perfusion assessed with quantitative thallium-201 scintigraphy. Am J Cardiol 1980;46:365.

Berman DS: Technetium-99m myocardial perfusion imaging agents and their relation to thallium-201: A symposium. Am J Cardiol 1990;66:1E.

Brown BG, Bolson EL, Dodge HT: Quantitative computer techniques for analyzing coronary arteriograms. Prog Cardiovasc Dis 1986;28:403.

Bruce RA: Exercise testing for evaluation of ventricular function. N Engl J Med 1977;296:671.

Bruce RA et al: Enhanced risk assessment for primary coronary heart disease events by maximal exercise testing: 10 years' experience of Seattle Heart Watch. J Am Coll Cardiol 1983;2:565.

Bruschke AVG et al: The anatomic evolution of coronary artery disease demonstrated by coronary arteriography in 256 nonoperated patients. Circulation 1981;63:527.

Camici P, Ferrannini E, Opie LH: Myocardial metabolism in ischemic heart disease: Basic principles and application to imaging by positron emission tomography. Prog Cardiovasc Dis 1989;32:217.

Chaitman BR et al: Angiographic prevalence of high-risk coronary artery disease in patient subsets (CASS). Circulation 1981;64:360.

Cheitlin MD: Finding the high-risk patient with coronary artery disease. JAMA 1988;259:2271.

Crawford MH, Amon KW, Vance WS: Exercise 2-dimensional echocardiography: Quantitation of left ventricular performance in patients with severe angina pectoris. Am J Cardiol 1983;51:1.

Davis K et al: Complications of coronary angiography from the Collaborative Study of Coronary Artery Surgery (CASS). Circulation 1979;59:1105.

Demer LL et al: Assessment of coronary artery disease severity by positron emission tomography: Comparison with quantitative arteriography in 193 patients. Circulation 1989;79:825.

Detrano R, Froelicher VF: Exercise testing: Uses and limitations considering recent studies. Prog Cardiovasc Dis 1988;31:173.

Detrano R, Gianrossi R, Froelicher V: The diagnostic accuracy of the exercise electrocardiogram: A meta-analysis of 22 years of research. Prog Cardiovasc Dis 1989;32:173.

Detrano R et al: Exercise-induced ST segment depression in the diagnosis of multivessel coronary disease: A meta analysis. J Am Coll Cardiol 1989;14:1501.

Edwards WD, Tajik AJ, Seward JB: Standardized nomenclature and anatomic basis for regional tomographic analysis of the heart. Mayo Clin Proc 1981;56:479.

Ellestad MH, Wan MKC: Predictive implications of stress testing: Follow-up of 2700 subjects after maximum treadmill stress testing. Circulation 1975; 51:363.

Epstein SE: Implications of probability analysis on the strategy used for noninvasive detection of coronary artery disease: Role of single or combined use of exercise electrocardiographic testing, radionuclide cineangiography and myocardial perfusion imaging. Am J Cardiol 1980;46:491.

Gianrossi R et al: Exercise-induced ST depression in the diagnosis of coronary artery disease: A meta-analysis. Circulation 1989;80:87.

Grossman W (editor): Cardiac Catheterization and Angiography, 3rd ed. Lea & Febiger, 1986.

Guidelines for clinical use of cardiac radionuclide imaging, December 1986: A report of the American College of Cardiology/American Heart Association Task Force on Assessment of Cardiovascular Procedures (Subcommittee on Nuclear Imaging). J Am Coll Cardiol 1986;8:1471.

Guidelines for coronary angiography. A report of the American College of Cardiology/American Heart Association Task Force on Assessment of Diagnostic and Therapeutic Cardiovascular Procedures (Subcommittee on Coronary Angiography). Circulation 1987;76: 963A.

Hewson EG et al: The prevalence of abnormal esophageal test results in patients with cardiovascular disease and unexplained chest pain. Arch Intern Med 1990; 150:965.

Hollenberg M et al: Treadmill score quantifies electrocardiographic response to exercise and improves test accuracy and reproducibility. Circulation 1980;61:276.

Kussmaul WG et al: Accuracy of subjective and computer-assisted assessments of angiographic left ventricular regional wall width. Cathet Cardiovasc Diagn 1990;20:153.

Lam JY et al: Safety and diagnostic accuracy of dipyridamole-thallium imaging in the elderly. J Am Coll Cardiol 1988;11:585.

Lipton MJ et al: Clinical applications of dynamic computed tomography. Prog Cardiovasc Dis 1986;28:349.

Martin CM, McConahay DR: Maximal treadmill exercise electrocardiography: Correlations with coronary arteriography and cardiac hemodynamics. Circulation 1972;46:956.

McNeer JF et al: The role of the exercise test in the evaluation of patients for ischemic heart disease. Circulation 1978;57:64.

Moss AJ: The Multicenter Postinfarction Research Group: Risk stratification and survival after myocardial infarction. N Engl J Med 1983;309:331.

Picano E, Lattamzi F: Dipyridamole echocardiography: A new window on coronary artery disease. Circulation 1991;(Suppl II):III−19.

Proudfit W et al: Prognosis of 1000 young women studied by coronary angiography. Circulation 1981;64: 1185.

Ranhosky A, Kempthorne-Rawson J: The safety of intravenous dipyridamole thallium myocardial perfusion imaging: Intravenous Dipyridamole Thallium Imaging Study Group. Circulation 1990;81:1205.

Richter JE, Bradley LA, Castell DO: Esophageal chest pain: Current controversies in pathogenesis, diagnosis and therapy. Ann Intern Med 1989;110:66.

Schroeder JS et al: Provocation of coronary spasm with ergonovine maleate: New test with results in 57 patients undergoing coronary arteriography. Am J Cardiol 1977;40:487.

Segar DS et al: Dobutamine stress echocardiography: Correlation with coronary lesion severity as determined by qualitative angiography. J Am Coll Cardiol 1992;19:1197.

Sobel BE, Ter-Pogossian MM, Geltman EM: Positron emission tomography in cardiac evaluation. Hosp Pract (Nov) 1981;16:93.

Stanford W et al: Sensitivity and specificity of assessing coronary bypass graft patency with ultrafast computed tomography: Results of a multicenter study. J Am Coll Cardiol 1988;12:1.

Tanenbaum JR et al: Detection of calcific deposits in coronary arteries by ultrafast computed tomography and correlation with angiography. Am J Cardiol 1989;63:870.

Villanueva-Meyer J et al: Simultaneous assessment of left ventricular wall motion and myocardial perfusion with technetium-99m-methoxy isobutyl isonitrile at stress and rest in patients with angina: Comparison with thallium-201 SPECT. J Nucl Med 1990;31:457

Weiner DA, McCabe CH, Ryan TJ: Identification of patients with left main and three vessel coronary disease with clinical and exercise test variables. Am J Cardiol 1980;46:21.

Zijlstra F et al: Which cineangiographically assessed anatomic variable correlates best with functional measurements of stenosis severity? A comparison of quantitative analysis of the coronary cineangiogram with measured coronary flow reserve and exercise/redistribution thallium-201 scintigraphy. J Am Coll Cardiol 1988;12:686.

Treatment & Prognosis of Stable Angina

Abrams J: A symposium: Third North American Conference on Nitroglycerine Therapy. Am J Cardiol 1992;70:43B

Agatston AS et al: Quantification of coronary artery calcium using ultrafast computed tomography. J Am Coll Cardiol 1990;15:827.

AHA Nutrition Committee: Dietary guidelines for healthy American adults: A statement for physicians. Circulation 1988;77:721A.

Antiplatelet Trialists' Collaboration: Secondary prevention of vascular disease by prolonged antiplatelet treatment. Br Med J 1988;296:320.

Blankenhorn DH et al: Beneficial effects of combined colestipol-niacin therapy on coronary atherosclerosis and coronary venous bypass grafts. JAMA 1987;257:3233. (Erratum: 1988;259:2698.)

Böhm M , Schwinger RH, Erdmann E: Different cardiodepressant potency of various calcium antagonists in human myocardium. Am J Cardiol 1990;65:1038.

Brown G et al: Regression of coronary artery disease as a result of intensive lipid-lowering therapy in men with high levels of apolipoprotein B. N Engl J Med 1990;323:1289.

Buchwald H et al: Effect of partial ileal bypass surgery on mortality and morbidity from coronary heart disease in patients with hypercholesterolemia: Report of the Program on the Surgical Control of the Hyperlipidemias (POSCH). N Engl J Med 1990;323:946.

The Cardiac Arrhythmia Suppression Trial (CAST) Investigators: Preliminary report: Effect of encainide and flecainide on mortality in a randomized trial of arrhythmia suppression after myocardial infarction. N Engl J Med 1989;321:406.

Cashin-Hemphill L et al: Beneficial effects of colestipol-niacin on coronary atherosclerosis: A 4-year follow-up. JAMA 1990;264:3013.

Chatterjee K, Rouleau JL, Parmley WW: Medical management of patients with angina: Has first-line management changed? JAMA 1984;252:1170.

Chatterjee K: Role of nitrates in silent myocardial ischemia. Am J Cardiol 1987;60(Suppl):18H.

deGraaf JC et al: Nitric oxide functions as an inhibitor of platelet adhesion under flow conditions. Circulation 1992;85:2284.

Frank CW, Weinblatt E, Shapiro S: Angina pectoris in men: Prognostic significance of selected medical factors. Circulation 1973;47:509.

Gage JE et al: Vasoconstriction of stenotic coronary arteries during dynamic exercise in patients with classic angina pectoris: Reversibility by nitroglycerin. Circulation 1986:73:865.

Goldman GJ, Pichard AD: The natural history of coronary artery disease: Does medical therapy improve the prognosis? Prog Cardiovasc Dis 1983;25:513.

Grover SA et al: The benefits of treating hyperlipidemia to prevent coronary heart disease. JAMA 1992;267:816.

Grundy SM: Cholesterol and coronary heart disease: A new era. JAMA 1986;256:2849.

Grundy SM, Vega GL: Causes of high blood cholesterol. Circulation 1990;81:412.

Grundy SM: HMG-CoA reductase inhibitors for treatment of hypercholesterolemia. N Engl J Med 1988;319:24.

Jafri SM et al: Medical therapy after acute myocardial infarction. Curr Probl Cardiol 1991;16:591.

Kane JP, Malloy MJ: Treatment of hyperlipidemia. Ann Rev Med 1990;41:471.

Kane JP et al: Regression of coronary atherosclerosis during treatment of familial hypercholesterolemia with combined drug regimens. JAMA 1990;264:3007.

Klimt CR, Knatterud GL, Stamler J: Persantine-Aspirin Reinfarction Study: Part II. Secondary coronary prevention with Persantine and aspirin. J Am Coll Cardiol 1986;7:251.

Malloy MJ et al: Complementarity of colestipol, niacin, and lovastatin in treatment of severe familial hypercholesterolemia. Ann Intern Med 1987;107:616.

Margolis JR et al: The diagnostic and prognostic significance of coronary artery calcification: A report of 800 cases. Radiology 1980;137:609.

Maseri A, Parodi O, Fox KM: Rational approach to the medical therapy of angina pectoris: The role of calcium antagonists. Prog Cardiovasc Dis 1983;25:269.

Michaelson SP et al: Recurrent myocardial infarction with normal coronary arteriography. N Engl J Med 1977;297:916.

Mitrovic V et al: Effects of the calcium antagonist, isradipine, and nifedipine on resting and exercise haemodynamics and the neurohumoral system in patients with stable chronic angina. Eur Heart J 1990;11:454.

Multiple Risk Factor Intervention Trial Research Group: Multiple Risk Factor Intervention Trial: Risk factor changes and mortality results. JAMA 1982;248:1465.

Ornish D et al: Can lifestyle changes reverse coronary heart disease? The Lifestyle Heart Trial. Lancet 1990;336:129.

Packer M et al: Hemodynamic consequences of combined beta-adrenergic and slow calcium channel blockade in man. Circulation 1982;65:660.

Parker JO: Nitrate therapy in stable angina pectoris. N Engl J Med 1987;316:1635.

Peduzzi P, Hultgren HN: Effect of medical vs surgical

treatment on symptoms in stable angina pectoris: The Veterans Administration Cooperative Study of Surgery for Coronary Arterial Occlusive Disease. Circulation 1979;60:888.

Peto R et al: Randomised trial of prophylactic daily aspirin in British male doctors. Br Med J 1988;296:313.

Prihoda JS, Illingworth DR: Drug therapy of hyperlipidemia. Curr Probl Cardiol 1992;17:551.

Ramee SR et al: Percutaneous angioscopy during coronary angioplasty using a steerable microangioscope. J Am Coll Cardiol 1991;17:100.

Ridker PM et al: Low-dose aspirin therapy for chronic stable angina: A randomized, placebo-controlled clinical trial. Ann Intern Med 1991;114:835.

Ruberman W et al: Ventricular premature complexes in prognosis of angina. Circulation 1980;61:1172.

Sheldon WC et al: Surgical treatment of coronary artery disease: Pure graft operations, with a study of 741 patients followed 3–7 yr. Prog Cardiovasc Dis 1975;18:237.

Sixty Plus Reinfarction Study Research Group: A double blind trial to assess long term oral anticoagulant therapy in elderly patients after myocardial infarction. Lancet 1980;2:989.

Smith P et al: The effect of warfarin on mortality and reinfarction after myocardial infarction. N Engl J Med 1990;323:147.

Stamler J, Stamler R: Intervention for the prevention and control of hypertension and atherosclerotic diseases: United States and international experience. Am J Med 1984;76(2A):13.

Steering Committee of the Physicians' Health Study Research Group: Final report on the aspirin component of the Ongoing Physicians' Health Study. N Engl J Med 1989;321:129.

Stern S, Tzivoni D: Ventricular arrhythmias, sudden death, and silent myocardial ischemia. Prog Cardiovasc Dis 1992;35:19.

Stone PH et al: Comparison of propranolol, diltiazem, and nifedipine in the treatment of ambulatory ischemia in patients with stable angina: Differential effects on ambulatory ischemia, exercise performance, and anginal symptoms: The ASIS Study Group. Circulation 1990;82:1962.

Thadani U, Whitsett T, Hamilton SF: Nitrate therapy for myocardial ischemic syndrome: Current perspectives including tolerance. Curr Probl Cardiol 1988;13:731.

Theron HDT, Lambert CR, Pepine CJ: Videodensitometry versus digital calipers for quantitative coronary angiography. Am J Cardiol 1990;66:1186.

Tobis JM et al: Intravascular ultrasound imaging of human coronary arteries in vivo: Analysis of tissue characterizations with comparison to in vitro histological specimens. Circulation 1991;83:913.

Yusuf S et al: Overview of results of randomized clinical trials in heart disease, unstable angina, heart failure, primary prevention with aspirin, and risk factor modification. JAMA 1988;260:2259.

Unstable Angina Pectoris

Ambrose JA, Fuster V: Thrombolytic therapy in unstable angina. Curr Opinion Cardiol 1989;4:499.

Ambrose JA et al: Angiographic evaluation of coronary artery morphology in unstable angina. J Am Coll Cardiol 1986;7:472.

Aroesty JM et al: Medically refractory unstable angina pectoris. II. Hemodynamic and angiographic effects of intraaortic balloon counterpulsation. Am J Cardiol 1979;45:883.

Brown CA et al: Prospective study of medical and urgent surgical therapy in randomizable patients with unstable angina pectoris: Results of in-hospital and chronic mortality and morbidity. Am Heart J 1981;102:959.

Bugiardini R et al: Angiographic morphology in unstable angina and its relation to transient myocardial ischemia and hospital outcome. Am J Cardiol 1991;67:460.

Cairns JA et al: Aspirin, sulfinpyrazone, or both in unstable angina: Results of a Canadian multicenter trial. N Engl J Med 1985;313:1369.

Chierchia S et al: Impairment of myocardial perfusion and function during painless myocardial ischemia. J Am Coll Cardiol 1983;3:924.

Cohen M, Fuster V, Chesebro JH: Unstable angina: Aspirin and anticoagulants. Curr Opinion Cardiol 1989;4:510.

Conti CR et al: Unstable angina pectoris: Morbidity and mortality in 57 consecutive patients evaluated angiographically. Am J Cardiol 1973;32:745.

de Feyter PJ et al: Coronary angioplasty for unstable angina: Immediate and late results in 200 consecutive patients with identification of risk factors for unfavorable early and late outcome. J Am Coll Cardiol 1988;12:324.

Gazes PC et al: Preinfarctional (unstable) angina: A prospective study: Ten-year follow-up. Circulation 1973;48:331.

Gold HK et al: A randomized, blinded, placebo-controlled trial of recombinant human tissue-type plasminogen activator in patients with unstable angina pectoris. Circulation 1987;75:1192.

Golino P et al: Divergent effects of serotonin on coronary-artery dimensions and blood flow in patients with coronary atherosclerosis and control patients. New Engl J Med 1991;324:641.

Jaffee AS et al: Abnormal technetium-99m pyrophosphate images in unstable angina: Ischemia versus infarction? Am J Cardiol 1979;44:1035.

Lewis HD Jr et al: Protective effects of aspirin against acute myocardial infarction and death in men with unstable angina: Results of a Veterans Administration Cooperative Study. N Engl J Med 1983;309:396.

Lichstein E et al: Relation between beta-adrenergic blocker use, various correlates of left ventricular function and the chance of developing congestive heart failure: The Multicenter Diltiazem Post-Infarction Research Group. J Am Coll Cardiol 1990;16:1327.

Luchi RJ, Scott SM, Deupree RH: Comparison of medical and surgical treatment for unstable angina pectoris: Results of a Veterans Administration Cooperative Study. N Engl J Med 1987;316:977.

Maseri A, Parodi O, Fox KM: Rational approach to the medical therapy of angina pectoris: The role of calcium antagonists. Prog Cardiovasc Dis 1983;25:269.

Mulcahy R et al: Natural history and prognosis of unstable angina. Am Heart J 1985;109:753.

Olsson G, Ablad B, Ryden L: Long-term cardiovascular effects of metoprolol therapy: A review article. J Clin Pharmacol 1990;30:S118.

Patterson DLH: Management in unstable angina. Post-grad Med J 1988;64:271.

Rentrop KP et al: Effects of intracoronary streptokinase and intracoronary nitroglycerin infusion on coronary angiographic patterns and mortality in patients with acute myocardial infarction. N Engl J Med 1985;311:1457.

Roberts KB et al: The prognosis for patients with new-onset angina who have undergone cardiac catheterization. Circulation 1983;68:970.

Russel RO Jr et al: Unstable angina pectoris. National Cooperative Study Group to Compare Surgical and Medical Therapy: II. In-hospital experience and initial follow-up results in patients with one, two and three vessel disease. Am J Cardiol 1978;42:839.

Russel RO Jr et al: Unstable angina pectoris. National Cooperative Study Group to Compare Surgical and Medical Therapy: III. Results in patients with S–T segment elevation during pain. Am J Cardiol 1980;45:819.

Russel RO Jr et al: Unstable angina pectoris. National Cooperative Study Group to Compare Surgical and Medical Therapy. IV. Results in patients with left anterior descending coronary artery disease. Am J Cardiol 1981;48:517.

Sherman CT et al: Coronary angioscopy in patients with unstable angina pectoris. N Engl J Med 1986;315:913.

Theroux P et al: Aspirin, heparin, or both to treat acute unstable angina. N Engl J Med 1988;319:1105.

Wallis DE et al: Safety and efficacy of esmolol for unstable angina pectoris. Am J Cardiol 1988;62:1033.

Weiner DA et al: Value of exercise testing in determining the risk classification and the response to coronary artery bypass grafting in three-vessel coronary artery disease: A report from the Coronary Artery Surgery Study (CASS) registry. Am J Cardiol 1987;60:262.

Weintraub RM et al: Medically refractory unstable angina pectoris. I. Long-term follow-up of patients undergoing intraaortic balloon counterpulsation and operation. Am J Cardiol 1979;43:877.

Williams RE et al: Angiographic morphology in unstable angina pectoris. Am J Cardiol 1988;62:1024.

Acute Myocardial Infarction

Ahnve S et al: Limitations and advantages of the ejection fraction for defining high risk after acute myocardial infarction. Am J Cardiol 1986;58:872.

Beller GA: Current status of nuclear cardiology techniques. Curr Probl Cardiol 1991;16:445.

Berger HJ, Gottschalk A, Zaret BL: Dual radionuclide study of acute myocardial infarction: Comparison of thallium-201 and technetium-99m stannous pyrophosphate imaging in man. Ann Intern Med 1978;88:145.

DeWood MA et al: Coronary arteriographic findings soon after non-Q-wave myocardial infarction. N Engl J Med 1986;315:417.

DeWood MA et al: Prevalence of total coronary occlusion during the early hours of transmural myocardial infarction. N Engl J Med 1980;303:897.

Forrester JS, Diamond GA, Swan HJC: Correlative classification of clinical and hemodynamic function after acute myocardial infarction. Am J Cardiol 1977;39:-137.

Gibson RS et al: Prediction of cardiac events after un-complicated myocardial infarction: A prospective study comparing predischarge exercise thallium-201 scintigraphy and coronary angiography. Circulation 1983;68:321.

Gibson RS et al: Value of early two dimensional echocardiography in patients with acute myocardial infarction. Am J Cardiol 1982;49:1110.

Hoit BD et al: Myocardial infarction in young patients: An analysis by age subsets. Circulation 1986;74:712.

Isner JM: Right ventricular myocardial infarction. JAMA 1988;259:712.

Johns JA et al: Quantification of acute myocardial infarct size by nuclear magnetic resonance imaging. J Am Coll Cardiol 1990;15:143.

Johnson LL et al: Antimyosin imaging in acute transmural myocardial infarctions: Results of a multicenter clinical trial. J Am Coll Cardiol 1989;13:27.

Kannel WB, Abbott RD: Incidence and prognosis of unrecognized myocardial infarction: An update on the Framingham study. N Engl J Med 1984;311:1144.

Klein LW, Helfant RH: The Q-wave and non-Q wave myocardial infarction: Differences and similarities. Prog Cardiovasc Dis 1986;29:205.

Klocke FJ: Measurements of coronary blood flow and degree of stenosis: Current clinical implications and continuing uncertainties. J Am Coll Cardiol 1983;1:31.

Liberthson RR et al: Atrial tachyarrhythmias in acute myocardial infarction. Am J Med 1976;60:956.

Lorell B et al: Right ventricular infarction: Clinical diagnosis and differentiation from cardiac tamponade and pericardial constriction. Am J Cardiol 1979;43:465.

Maseri A et al: Mechanisms and significance of cardiac ischemic pain. Prog Cardiovasc Dis 1992;35:1.

Morrison J et al: Correlation of radionuclide estimates of myocardial infarction size and release of creatine kinase-MB in man. Circulation 1980;62:277.

Pantridge JF, Webb SW, Adgey AAJ: Arrhythmias in the first hours of acute myocardial infarction. Prog Cardiovasc Dis 1981;23:265.

Peels CH et al: Usefulness of two-dimensional echocardiography for immediate detection of myocardial ischemia in the emergency room. Am J Cardiol 1990;65:687.

Pell S, Fayerweather WE: Trends in the incidence of myocardial infarction and in associated mortality and morbidity in a large employed population, 1957-1983. N Engl J Med 1985;312:1005.

Puleo PR et al: Early diagnosis of acute myocardial infarction based on assay for subforms of creatine kinase-MB. Circulation 1990;82:759.

Roberts R: Recognition, pathogenesis, and management of non-Q-wave infarction. Mod Concepts Cardiovasc Dis 1987;56:17.

Scheinman MM (editor): Cardiac Emergencies. Saunders, 1984.

Silverman KJ et al: Value of early thallium-201 scintigraphy for predicting mortality in patients with acute myocardial infarction. Circulation 1980;61:996.

Slater KD et al: Outcome in suspected acute myocardial infarction with normal or minimally abnormal admission electrocardiographic findings. Am J Cardiol 1987;60:766.

Sobel BE et al: Detection of remote myocardial infarction in patients with positron emission transaxial tomography and intravenous 11C-palmitate. Circulation 1977;55:853.

Solomon HA, Edwards AL, Killip T: Prodromata in acute myocardial infarction. Circulation 1969;40:463.

Swan HJC et al: Catheterization of the heart in man with use of a flow-directed balloon-tipped catheter. N Engl J Med 1970;283:447.

Swan HJC et al: Hemodynamic spectrum of myocardial infarction and cardiogenic shock: A conceptual model. Circulation 1972;45:1097.

Weiss ES et al: Evaluation of myocardial metabolism and perfusion with positron-emitting radionuclides. Prog Cardiovasc Dis 1977;20:191.

Yusuf S: Routine medical management of acute myocardial infarction: Lessons from overview of recent randomized controlled trials. Circulation 1990;82(Suppl II):II–117.

Course & Complications in Acute
Myocardial Infarction

AIMS Trial Study Group: Effect of intravenous APSAC on mortality after acute myocardial infarction: Preliminary report of a placebo-controlled clinical trial. Lancet 1988;1:545.

Applegate RJ, Dell'Italia LJ, Crawford MH: Usefulness of two-dimensional echocardiography during low-level exercise testing early after uncomplicated acute myocardial infarction. Am J Cardiol 1987;60:10.

Asinger RW et al: Incidence of left-ventricular thrombosis after acute transmural myocardial infarction: Serial evaluation by two-dimensional echocardiography. N Engl J Med 1981;305:297.

Baciewiez PA et al: Late follow-up after repair of left ventricular aneurysm and (usually) associated coronary bypass grafting. Am J Cardiol 1991;68:193.

Baim DS (editor): Interventional cardiology: 1987. (Symposium.) Am J Cardiol 1988;61:1G.

Bates RJ et al: Cardiac rupture: Challenge in diagnosis and management. Am J Cardiol 1977;40:429.

Battler A et al: The initial chest x-ray in acute myocardial infarction: Prediction of early and late mortality and survival. Circulation 1980;61:1004.

Bolooki H: Surgical treatment of complications of acute myocardial infarction. JAMA 1990;263:1237.

Bosch X et al: Early postinfarction ischemia: Clinical, angiographic, and prognostic significance. Circulation 1987;75:988.

Campbell RW, Murray A, Julian DG: Ventricular arrhythmias in first 12 hours of acute myocardial infarction: Natural history study. Br Heart J 1981;46:351.

Cohn LH: Surgical management of acute and chronic cardiac mechanical complications due to myocardial infarction. Am Heart J 1981;102:1049.

Dressler W, Leavitt SS: Pericarditis after acute myocardial infarction: Relapses over period of twenty-eight months. JAMA 1960;173:1225.

Drobac M et al: Ventricular septal defect after myocardial infarction: Diagnosis by 2-dimensional contrast echocardiography. Circulation 1983;67:335.

Faxon DP et al: The influence of surgery on the natural history of angiographically documented left ventricular aneurysm: The Coronary Artery Surgery Study. Circulation 1986;74:110.

Forman MB et al: Determinants of left ventricular aneurysm formation after anterior myocardial infarction: A clinical and angiographic study. J Am Coll Cardiol 1986;8:1256.

Fraker TD, Wagner GS, Rosati RA: Extension of myocardial infarction: Incidence and prognosis. Circulation 1979;60:1126.

Gatewood RP Jr, Nanda NC: Differentiation of left ventricular pseudoaneurysm from true aneurysm with two dimensional echocardiography. Am J Cardiol 1980;46:869.

George BS: Percutaneous cardiopulmonary support in patients with coronary artery disease: A critical review. Cor Art Dis 1991;2:661.

Gibson RS et al: Prognostic significance and beneficial effect of diltiazem on the incidence of early recurrent ischemia after non-Q-wave myocardial infarction: Results from the Multicenter Diltiazem Reinfarction Study. Am J Cardiol 1987;60:203.

Grube E, Redel D, Janson R: Non-invasive diagnosis of a false left ventricular aneurysm by echocardiography and pulsed Doppler echocardiography. Br Heart J 1980;43:232.

Herfkens RJ, Brundage BH, Lipton MJ: Cardiovascular applications of computed tomography. Cardiovasc Rev Rep 1983;4:979.

Higgins CB et al: False aneurysms of the left ventricle: Identification of distinctive clinical, radiographic, and angiographic features. Radiology 1978;127:21.

Hockings BE et al: Effectiveness of amiodarone on ventricular arrhythmias during and after acute myocardial infarction. Am J Cardiol 1987;60:967.

Kaul S: Echocardiography in coronary artery disease. Curr Probl Cardiol 1990;15:233.

Kereiakes DJ, Ports TA: Intra-aortic balloon counterpulsation and the diagnosis and management of surgical complications of acute myocardial infarction. In: *Cardiac Emergencies.* Scheinman MM (editor). Saunders, 1984.

Keren A et al: Natural history of left ventricular thrombi: Their appearance and resolution in the posthospitalization period of acute myocardial infarction. J Am Coll Cardiol 1990;15:790.

Lavie CJ, Gersh BJ: Mechanical and electrical complications of acute myocardial infarction. Mayo Clin Proc 1990;65:709. (Erratum in 1990;65:1032.)

Lemery R et al: Prognosis in rupture of the ventricular septum after acute myocardial infarction and role of early surgical intersection. Am J Cardiol 1992;70:147.

McNeer JF et al: Hospital discharge one week after acute myocardial infarction. N Engl J Med 1978;298:229.

Nishimura RA et al: Early repair of mechanical complications after acute myocardial infarction. JAMA 1986;256:47.

Nishimura RA et al: Papillary muscle rupture complicating acute myocardial infarction: Analysis of 17 patients. Am J Cardiol 1983;51:373.

Pfeffer MA et al: Effect of captopril on progressive ventricular dilatation after anterior myocardial infarction. N Engl J Med 1988;319:80.

Ritter WS et al: Permanent pacing in patients with transient trifascicular block during acute myocardial infarction. Am J Cardiol 1976;38:207.

Scanlon PJ et al: Urgent surgery for ventricular septal rupture complicating acute myocardial infarction. Circulation 1985;72:II–185.

Scheidt S et al: Mechanical circulatory assistance with the intraaortic balloon pump and other counterpulsation devices. Prog Cardiovasc Dis 1982;25:55.

Scheinman MM, Gonzalez RP: Fascicular block and acute myocardial infarction. JAMA 1980;244:2646.

Schuster EH, Bulkley BH: Early post-infarction angina: Ischemia at a distance and ischemia in the infarct zone. N Engl J Med 1981;305:1101.

Smyllie J et al: Diagnosis of ventricular septal rupture after myocardial infarction: Value of colour flow mapping. Br Heart J 1989;62:260.

Stratton JR, Resnick AD: Increased embolic risk in patients with left ventricular thrombi. Circulation 1987;75:1004.

Volpi A et al: In-hospital prognosis of patients with acute myocardial infarction complicated by primary ventricular fibrillation. N Engl J Med 1987;317:257.

Weisman HF, Healy B: Myocardial infarct expansion, infarct extension, and reinfarction: Pathophysiologic concepts. Prog Cardiovasc Dis 1987;30:73.

Zipes DP et al: Sudden cardiac death: Neural-cardiac interactions. Circulation 1987;76:I–202.

Prevention, Treatment, & Prognosis in Acute Myocardial Infarction; Thrombolysis

American College of Physicians Health and Public Policy Committee: Thrombolysis for evolving myocardial infarction. Ann Intern Med 1985;103:463.

Anderson JL et al: Multicenter reperfusion trial of intravenous anisoylated plasminogen streptokinase activator complex (APSAC) in acute myocardial infarction: Controlled comparison with intracoronary streptokinase. J Am Coll Cardiol 1988;11:1153.

Antiplatelet Trialists' Collaboration: Secondary prevention of vascular disease by prolonged antiplatelet treatment. Br Heart J 1988;296:320.

Aspirin Myocardial Infarction Study Research Group: A randomized, controlled trial of aspirin in persons recovered from myocardial infarction. JAMA 1980;243:661.

Bassand JP et al: Multicenter trial of intravenous anisoylated plasminogen streptokinase activator complex (APSAC) in acute myocardial infarction: Effects on infarct size and left ventricular function. J Am Coll Cardiol 1989;13:988.

Becker LC, Ambrosio G: Myocardial consequences of reperfusion. Prog Cardiovasc Dis 1987;30:23.

Beller GA: Pharmacologic stress imaging. JAMA 1991;265:633.

Bode C et al: Efficacy of intravenous prourokinase and a combination of prourokinase and urokinase in acute myocardial infarction. Am J Cardiol 1988;61:971.

Braunwald E (editor): Modern thrombolytic therapy. (Symposium.) J Am Coll Cardiol 1987;10(Suppl B).

Cercek B et al: Time course and characteristics of ventricular arrhythmias after reperfusion in acute myocardial infarction. Am J Cardiol 1987;60:214.

Chatterjee K, Ports TA, Parmley WW: Nitroprusside: Its clinical pharmacology and application in acute heart failure. Pages 25–62 in: Vasodilator Therapy for Cardiac Disorders. Gould L, Reddy CV (editors). Futura, 1979.

Chazov EI et al: [Intracoronary administration of fibrinolysin in acute myocardial infarction.] Ter Arkh 1976;48(4):8. (In Russian.)

Chesebro JH et al: Thrombolysis in Myocardial Infarction (TIMI) Trial, Phase I: A comparison between intravenous tissue plasminogen activator and intravenous streptokinase: Clinical findings through hospital discharge. Circulation 1987;76:142.

de Bono DP: The European Cooperative Study Group trial of intravenous recombinant tissue-type plasminogen activator (rt-PA) and conservative therapy versus rt-PA and immediate coronary angioplasty. J Am Coll Cardiol 1988;12(Suppl A):20A.

de Gaetano G: Primary prevention of vascular disease by aspirin. Lancet 1988;1:1093.

DeBusk RF: Specialized testing after recent acute myocardial infarction. Ann Intern Med 1989;110:470.

DeBusk RF et al: Serial ambulatory electrocardiography and treadmill exercise testing after uncomplicated myocardial infarction. Am J Cardiol 1980;45:547.

DeWood MA et al: Medical and surgical management of early Q wave myocardial infarction: I. Effects of surgical reperfusion on survival, recurrent myocardial infarction, sudden death, and functional class at 10 or more years of follow-up. J Am Coll Cardiol 1989;14:65.

DeWood MA et al: Prevalence of total coronary occlusion during the early hours of transmural myocardial infarction. N Engl J Med 1980;303:897.

Fareed J et al: Pharmacological modulation of fibrinolysis by antithrombotic and cardiovascular drugs. Prog Cardiovasc Dis 1992;34:379.

Froelicher VF et al: Exercise testing of patients recovering from myocardial infarction. Curr Probl Cardiol 1986;11:369.

Flaherty JT: Role of nitrates in acute myocardial infarction. Am J Cardiol 1992;70:73B

Fletcher GF: Current status of cardiac rehabilitation. Curr Probl Cardiol 1992;17:147.

Fung AY et al: Value of percutaneous transluminal coronary angioplasty after unsuccessful intravenous streptokinase therapy in acute myocardial infarction. Am J Cardiol 1986;58:686.

Furberg CD, Friedewald WT, Eberlein KA (editors): Proceedings of the workshop on implications of recent beta-blocker trials for post-myocardial infarction patients. Circulation 1983;67:I–1.

Gibson RS: The diagnostic and prognostic value of exercise electrocardiography in asymptomatic subjects and stable symptomatic patients. Curr Opin Cardiol 1991;6:536.

Gibson RS et al: Prediction of cardiac events after uncomplicated myocardial infarction: A prospective study comparing predischarge exercise thallium-201 scintigraphy and coronary angiography. Circulation 1983;68:321.

Goldberg RJ et al: Outcome after cardiac arrest during acute myocardial infarction. Am J Cardiol 1987;59:251.

Grundy SM: HMG-CoA reductase inhibitors for treatment of hypercholesterolemia. N Engl J Med 1988;319:24.

Gruppo Italiano per lo Studio della Streptochinasi nell'Infarto Miocardico (GISSI): Long-term effects of intravenous thrombolysis in acute myocardial infarction: Final report of the GISSI study. Lancet 1987;2:871.

Gruppo Italiano per lo Studio della Sopravvivènza

nell'Infarto Miocardico (GISSI-2): A factorial randomised trial of alteplase versus streptokinase and heparin versus no heparin among 12,490 patients with acute myocardial infarction. Lancet 1990;336:65

Gunnar RM et al: Guidelines for the early management of patients with acute myocardial infarction: A report of the ACC/AHA Task Force on Assessment of Diagnostic and Therapeutic Cardiovascular Procedures (Subcommittee to Develop Guidelines for the Early Management of Patients With Acute Myocardial Infarction). J Am Coll Cardiol 1990;16:249.

Hjalmarson åA (editor): Göteborg Metoprolol Trial in Acute Myocardial Infarction. Am J Cardiol 1984;53:1D.

Hsia J et al: A comparison between heparin and low-dose aspirin as adjunctive therapy with tissue plasminogen activator for acute myocardial infarction: Heparin-Aspirin Reperfusion Trial (HART) Investigators. N Engl J Med 1990;323:1433.

Hutter AM et al: Nontransmural myocardial infarction: Hospital and late clinical course of patients with that of matched patients with transmural anterior and transmural inferior myocardial infarction. Am J Cardiol 1981;48:595.

International Study Group: In-hospital mortality and clinical course of 20,891 patients with suspected acute myocardial infarction randomized between alteplase and streptokinase with and without heparin. Lancet 1990;336:71.

I.S.A.M. Study Group: A prospective trial of intravenous streptokinase in acute myocardial infarction (I.S.A.M.): Mortality, morbidity, and infarct size at 21 days. N Engl J Med 1986;314:1465.

ISIS-2 (Second International Study of Infarct Survival) Collaborative Group: Randomised trial of intravenous streptokinase, oral aspirin, both, or neither among 17,187 cases of suspected acute myocardial infarction. Lancet 1988;2:349.

ISIS-4 Collaborative Group Fourth International Study of Infarct Survival: Protocol for a large simple study of the effects of oral mononitrate, of oral captopril, and of intravenous magnesium. Am J Cardiol 1991;68:87D.

ISIS-1 (First International Study of Infarct Survival) Collaborative Group: Randomized trial of intravenous atenolol among 16,027 cases of suspected myocardial infarction: ISIS-I. Lancet 1986;2:57.

Jugdutt BI, Warnica JW: Intravenous nitroglycerin therapy to limit myocardial infarct size, expansion, and complications: Effect of timing, dosage and infarct location. Circulation 1988;78:906. (Erratum in 1989;79:1151.)

Kahn JK et al: Results of primary angioplasty for acute myocardial infarction in patients with multivessel coronary artery disease. J Am Coll Cardiol 1990;16:1089.

Kennedy JW et al: The Western Washington Intravenous Streptokinase in Acute Myocardial Infarction Randomized Trial. Circulation 1988;77:345.

Kennedy JW et al: The Western Washington Randomized Trial of Intracoronary Streptokinase in Acute Myocardial Infarction: A 12-month follow-up report. N Engl J Med 1985;312:1073.

Kern MJ: Intra-aortic balloon counterpulsation. Cor Art Dis 1991;2:649.

Kotler TS, Diamond GA: Exercise thallium-201 scintigraphy in the diagnosis and prognosis of coronary artery disease. Ann Intern Med 1990;113:684.

Krone RJ: The role of risk stratification in the early management of a myocardial infarction. Ann Intern Med 1992;116:223.

Lee L et al: Multicenter registry of angioplasty therapy of cardiogenic shock: Initial and long-term survival. J Am Coll Cardiol 1991;17:599.

Lo YS, Lesch M, Kaplan K: Postinfarction angina. Prog Cardiovasc Dis 1987;30:111.

MacMahon S et al: Effects of prophylactic lidocaine in suspected acute myocardial infarction: An overview of results from the randomized, controlled trials. JAMA 1988;260:1910.

MacMahon S et al: Reduction in major morbidity and mortality by heparin in acute myocardial infarction. (Abstract.) Circulation 1988;78:II–28.

Marder VJ, Sherry S: Thrombolytic therapy: Current status. (2 parts.) N Engl J Med 1988;318:1512, 1585.

Mark DB: Identification of acute myocardial infarction patients suitable for early hospital discharge after aggressive interventional therapy: Results from the Thrombolysis and Angioplasty in Acute Myocardial Infarction Registry. Circulation 1991;83:1186

Mark DB, Hlatky MA, Pryor DB: The exercise treadmill test in patients recovering from an acute myocardial infarction. In: *Acute Coronary Care in the Thrombolytic Era.* Califf RM, Mark DB, Wagner GS (editors). Year Book, 1988.

Marmor A, Sobel BE, Roberts R: Factors presaging early recurrent myocardial infarction ("extension").Am J Cardiol 1981;48:603.

Massie BM, Chatterjee K: Medical therapy for pump failure complicating acute myocardial infarction. In: *Cardiac Emergencies.* Scheinmann MM (editor). Saunders, 1984.

Matthay MA, Chatterjee K: Bedside catheterization of the pulmonary artery: Risks compared with benefits. Ann Intern Med 1988;109:826.

Meinertz T et al: The German multicenter trial of anisoylated plasminogen streptokinase activator complex versus heparin for acute myocardial infarction. Am J Cardiol 1988;62:347.

Mickelson JK et al: Antiplatelet antibody [7E3F(ab')$_2$] prevents rethrombosis after recombinant tissue-type plasminogen activator-induced coronary artery thrombolysis in a canine model. Circulation 1990;81:617.

Moss AJ, Bigger JT Jr, Odoroff CL: Postinfarct risk stratification. Prog Cardiovasc Dis 1987;29:389.

Moss AJ: The Multicenter Postinfarction Research Group: Risk stratification and survival after myocardial infarction. N Engl J Med 1983;309:331.

Moyé LA, Pfeffer MA, Braunwald E: Rationale, design and baseline characteristics of the Survival and Ventricular Enlargement trial: The SAVE Investigators. Am J Cardiol 1991;68:70D.

Muller JE et al: Myocardial infarct extension: Occurrence, outcome, and risk factors in the Multicenter Investigation of Limitation of Infarct Size. Ann Intern Med 1988;108:1.

National Heart Foundation of Australia Coronary Thrombolysis Group: Coronary thrombolysis and myocardial salvage by tissue plasminogen activator given up to 4 hours after onset of myocardial infarction. Lancet 1988;1:203.

Neuhaus KL et al: Intravenous recombinant tissue plasminogen activator (rt-PA) and urokinase in acute myocardial infarction: Results of the German Activator Urokinase Study (GAUS). J Am Coll Cardiol 1988;12:581.

Nicod P et al: Late clinical outcome in patients with early ventricular fibrillation after myocardial infarction. J Am Coll Cardiol 1988;11:464.

O'Neill W, Topol EJ, Pitt B: Reperfusion therapy of acute myocardial infarction. Prog Cardiovasc Dis 1988;30:235.

Olmsted WL, Groden DL, Silverman ME: Prognosis in survivors of acute myocardial infarction occurring at age 70 years or older. Am J Cardiol 1987;60:971.

O'Rourke RA: Noninvasive and invasive testing after myocardial infarction. Curr Probl Cardiol 1991;16:727.

Pfeffer MA, Braunwald E: Ventricular remodelling and unloading following myocardial infarction: A symposium. Am J Cardiol 1991;68:1D.

Pfeffer MA et al: Effect of captopril on mortality and morbidity in patients with left ventricular dysfunction after myocardial infarction. N Engl J Med 1992;327:669.

Popma JJ, Topol EJ: Adjuncts to thrombolysis for myocardial reperfusion. Ann Intern Med 1991;115:34.

PRIMI Trial Study Group: Randomized double-blind trial of recombinant pro-urokinase against streptokinase in acute myocardial infarction. Lancet 1989;1:863.

Reis SE, Gottlieb SO: Prognostic implications of transient asymptomatic myocardial ischemia as detected by ambulatory electrocardiographic monitoring. Prog Cardiovasc Dis 1992;35:77.

Ritchie JL et al: Ventricular function and infarct size: The Western Washington Intravenous Streptokinase in Myocardial Infarction Trial. J Am Coll Cardiol 1988;11:689.

Roberts R: Adjunctive therapies in thrombolysis: A symposium. Am J Cardiol 1991;67:1A.

Rodriguez LM et al: Incidence and timing of recurrences of sudden death and ventricular tachycardia during antiarrhythmic drug treatment after myocardial infarction. Am J Cardiol 1992;69:1403.

Rogers WJ et al: Selective versus routine predischarge coronary arteriography after therapy with recombinant tissue-type plasminogen activator, heparin and aspirin for acute myocardial infarction: TIMI II Investigators. J Am Coll Cardiol 1991;17:1007.

Ross AM: Acute myocardial infarction: Thrombolysis and angioplasty. (Symposium.) Circulation 1987;76(Suppl 2):II-1.

Rothbaum DA et al: Emergency percutaneous transluminal coronary angioplasty in acute myocardial infarction: A 3 year experience. J Am Coll Cardiol 1987;10:264.

Rouleau JL et al: Activation of neurohumoral systems following acute myocardial infarction. Am J Cardiol 1991;68:80D.

Ryan TJ: Revascularization for acute myocardial infarction: Strategies in need of revision. Circulation 1990;82:II-110.

Satler LF et al: Late angiographic follow-up after successful coronary arterial thrombolysis and angioplasty during acute myocardial infarction. Am J Cardiol 1987;60:210.

Scheidt S et al: Mechanical circulatory assistance with the intraaortic balloon pump and other counterpulsation devices. Prog Cardiovasc Dis 1982;25:55.

Schlant RC et al: The natural history of coronary heart disease: Prognostic factors after recovery from myocardial infarction in 2789 men: The 5-year findings of the Coronary Drug Project. Circulation 1982;66:401.

Schulman SP et al: Prognostic cardiac catheterization variables in survivors of acute myocardial infarction: A five year prospective study. J Am Coll Cardiol 1988;11:1164.

Shah PK, Swan HJC: Complications of acute myocardial infarction. In: *Cardiology,* vol 2. Parmley WW, Chatterjee K (editors). Lippincott, 1991.

Sharpe N et al: Early prevention of left ventricular dysfunction after myocardial infarction with angiotensin-converting-enzyme inhibition. Lancet 1991;337:872.

Sheehan FH et al: The effect of intravenous thrombolytic therapy on left ventricular function: A report on tissue-type plasminogen activator and streptokinase from the Thrombolysis in Myocardial Infarction (TIMI Phase I) trial. Circulation 1987;75:817.

Simoons ML et al: Thrombolysis with tissue plasminogen activator in acute myocardial infarction: No additional benefit from immediate percutaneous coronary angioplasty. Lancet 1988;1:197.

Sivarajan ES et al: Treadmill test responses to an early exercise program after myocardial infarction: A randomized study. Circulation 1982;65:1420.

Stein B, Roberts R: Current status of thrombolytic therapy in acute myocardial infarction. Tex Heart Inst J 1991;18:250.

Stone PH et al: Prognostic significance of location and type of myocardial infarction: Independent adverse outcome associated with anterior location. J Am Coll Cardiol 1988;11:453.

Swedberg K et al: Effects of the early administration of enalapril on mortality in patients with acute myocardial infarction: Results of the Cooperative New Scandinavian Enalapril Survival Study (CONSENSUS II). N Engl J Med 1992;327:678.

Tans AC, Lie KI, Durrer D: Clinical setting and prognostic significance of high degree atrioventricular block in acute inferior myocardial infarction: A study of 144 patients. Am Heart J 1980;99:4.

Thompson JA, Hess ML: The oxygen free radical system: A fundamental mechanism in the production of myocardial necrosis. Prog Cardiovasc Dis 1986;28:449.

Tiefenbrunn AJ: Clinical benefits of thrombolytic therapy in acute myocardial infarction. Am J Cardiol 1992;69:3A.

TIMI Research Group: Immediate vs delayed catheterization and angioplasty following thrombolytic therapy for acute myocardial infarction: TIMI II A results. JAMA 1988;260:2849.

TIMI Study Group: Comparison of invasive and conservative strategies after treatment with intravenous tissue plasminogen activator in acute myocardial infarction: Results of the Thrombolysis in Myocardial Infarction (TIMI) phase II trial. N Engl J Med 1989;320:618.

Topol EJ, Califf RM (editors): Myocardial reperfusion 1988: Practical considerations. A symposium. J Am Coll Cardiol 1988;12:1A.

Topol EJ et al: A randomized controlled trial of intravenous tissue plasminogen activator and early intravenous heparin in acute myocardial infarction. Circulation 1989;79:281.

Topol EJ et al: A randomized trial of immediate versus delayed elective angioplasty after intravenous tissue plasminogen activator in acute myocardial infarction. N Engl J Med 1987;317:581.

Turpie PGC et al: Comparison of high-dose with low-dose subcutaneous heparin to prevent left ventricular mural thrombosis in patients with acute transmural anterior myocardial infarction. N Engl J Med 1989;320:352.

Van de Werf F et al: Coronary thrombolysis with recombinant single-chain urokinase-type plasminogen activator in patients with acute myocardial infarction. Circulation 1986;74:1066.

Van de Werf F, Arnold AER: Intravenous tissue plasminogen activator and size of infarct, left ventricular function, and survival in acute myocardial infarction. Br Heart J 1988;297:1374.

Verstraete M et al: Acute coronary thrombolysis with recombinant human tissue-type plasminogen activator: Initial patency and influence of maintained infusion on reocclusion rate. Am J Cardiol 1987;60:231.

Verstraete M et al: Randomised trial of intravenous recombinant tissue-type plasminogen activator versus intravenous streptokinase in acute myocardial infarction: Report from the European Cooperative Study Group for Recombinant Tissue-Type Plasminogen Activator. Lancet 1985;1:842.

Visser CA et al: Incidence, timing and prognostic value of left ventricular aneurysm formation after myocardial infarction: A prospective, serial echocardiographic study of 158 patients. Am J Cardiol 1986;57:729.

Wackers FJT et al: Quantitative radionuclide assessment of regional ventricular function after thrombolytic therapy for acute myocardial infarction: Results of Phase I Thrombolysis in Myocardial Infarction (TIMI) trial. J Am Coll Cardiol 1989;13:998.

Waters DD et al: Comparison of clinical variables and variables derived from a limited predischarge exercise test as predictors of early and late mortality after myocardial infarction. J Am Coll Cardiol 1985;5:1.

Wilcox RG et al: Trial of tissue plasminogen activator for mortality reduction in acute myocardial infarction: Anglo-Scandinavian Study of Early Thrombolysis (ASSET). Lancet 1988;2:525.

Williams DO et al: One-year results of the Thrombolysis in Myocardial Infarction Investigation (TIMI) Phase II Trial. Circulation 1992;85:533.

Young FE, Nightingale SL, Temple RA: The preliminary report of the findings of the aspirin component of the ongoing Physicians' Health Study: The FDA perspective on aspirin for the primary prevention of myocardial infarction. JAMA 1988;259:3158.

Yusuf S et al: Beta blockade during and after myocardial infarction: An overview of the randomized trials. Prog Cardiovasc Dis 1985;27:335.

Yusuf S et al: Effect of intravenous nitrates on mortality in acute myocardial infarction: An overview of the randomised trials. Lancet 1988;1:1088.

Zaret BL et al: Assessment of global and regional left ventricular performance at rest and during exercise after thrombolytic therapy for acute myocardial infarction: Results of the Thrombolysis in Myocardial Infarction (TIMI) II Study. Am J Cardiol 1992;69:1.

Chronic (Established) Coronary Heart Disease

Aberg A et al: Declining trend in mortality after myocardial infarction. Br Heart J 1984;51:346.

Aspirin Myocardial Infarction Study Research Group: A randomized, controlled trial of aspirin in persons recovered from myocardial infarction. JAMA 1980;243:661.

Beta-Blocker Heart Attack Study Group: The β-blocker heart attack trial. JAMA 1981;246:2073.

Blumenthal JA et al: Comparison of high- and low-intensity exercise training early after acute myocardial infarction. Am J Cardiol 1988;61:26.

Bonow RO et al: Exercise-induced ischemia in mildly symptomatic patients with coronary-artery disease and preserved left ventricular function: Identification of subgroups at risk of death during medical therapy. N Engl J Med 1984;311:1339.

Bourke JP et al: Routine programmed electrical stimulation in survivors of acute myocardial infarction for prediction of spontaneous ventricular tachyarrhythmias during follow-up: Results, optimal stimulation protocol and cost-effective screening. J Am Coll Cardiol 1991;18:780.

Burkart F et al: Effect of antiarrhythmic therapy on mortality in survivors of myocardial infarction with asymptomatic complex ventricular arrhythmias: Basel Antiarrhythmic Study of Infarct Survival (BASIS). J Am Coll Cardiol 1990;16:1711.

Califf RM et al: Outcome in one-vessel coronary artery disease. Circulation 1983;67:283.

Campeau L et al: The relation of risk factors to the development of atherosclerosis in saphenous-vein bypass grafts and the progression of disease in the native circulation: A study 10 years after aortocoronary bypass surgery. N Engl J Med 1984;311:1329.

The Cardiac Arrhythmia Pilot Study (CAPS) Investigators: Effects of encainide, flecainide, imipramine and moricizine on ventricular arrhythmias during the year after acute myocardial infarction. Am J Cardiol 1988;61:501.

Case RB et al: Type A behavior and survival after acute myocardial infarction. The Multicenter Post-Infarction Research Group. N Engl J Med 1985;312:737.

Chatterjee K, Rouleau JL: Hemodynamic and metabolic effects of vasodilators, nitrates, hydralazine, prazosin, and captopril in chronic ischemic heart failure. Acta Med Scand [Suppl] 1981;651:295.

Council on Scientific Affairs: Physician-supervised exercise programs in rehabilitation of patients with coronary heart disease. JAMA 1981;245:1463.

Dhingra RC: Electrophysiologic studies during acute myocardial infarction: Do they prognosticate? (Editorial.) J Am Coll Cardiol 1991;18:789.

Dinerman J et al: Myocardial infarction: Short- and long-term use of anticoagulants. Curr Opin Cardiol 1989;4:540.

Dunn RF et al: Comparison of thallium-201 scanning in idiopathic dilated cardiomyopathy and severe coronary artery disease. Circulation 1982;66:804.

Dwyer EM et al: Nonfatal cardiac events and recurrent infarction in the year after acute myocardial infarction. The Multicenter Post-Infarction Research Group. J Am Coll Cardiol 1984;4:695.

Epstein SE, Palmeri ST, Patterson RE: Evaluation of patients after acute myocardial infarction: Indications for cardiac catheterization and surgical intervention. N Engl J Med 1982;307:1487.

Fletcher GT et al: Exercise standards. A statement for health professionals from the American Heart Association. Circulation 1990;82:2286.

Frishman WH: Secondary prevention with β-adrenergic blockers and aspirin in ischemic heart disease. Curr Opin Cardiol 1991;6:367.

Fuster V, Cohen M, Chesebro JH: Usefulness of aspirin for coronary artery disease. Am J Cardiol 1988;61:637.

Fuster V et al: Platelet-inhibitor drugs' role in coronary artery disease. Prog Cardiovasc Dis 1987;29:325.

Gibson RS et al: Prediction of cardiac events after uncomplicated myocardial infarction: A prospective study comparing predischarge exercise thallium-201 scintigraphy and coronary angiography. Circulation 1983;68:321.

Graham I et al: Natural history of coronary heart disease: A study of 586 men surviving an initial acute attack. Am Heart J 1983;105:249.

Hutter AM Jr et al: Nontransmural myocardial infarction: A comparison of hospital and late clinical course of patients with that of matched patients with transmural anterior and transmural inferior myocardial infarction. Am J Cardiol 1981;48:595.

Klimt CR et al: Persantine-Aspirin Reinfarction Study. Part II. Secondary coronary prevention with Persantine and aspirin. J Am Coll Cardiol 1986;7:251.

Klocke FJ: Measurements of coronary blood flow and degree of stenosis: Current clinical implications and continuing uncertainties. J Am Coll Cardiol 1983;1:31.

Kostis JB et al: Prognostic significance of ventricular ectopic activity in survivors of acute myocardial infarction: BHAT Study Group. J Am Coll Cardiol 1987;10:231.

Lim JS, Proudfit WL, Sones FM Jr: Left main coronary arterial obstruction: Long-term follow-up of 141 nonsurgical cases. Am J Cardiol 1975;36:131.

Marcus FI et al: Mechanism of death and prevalence of myocardial ischemic symptoms in the terminal event after acute myocardial infarction: Multicenter Postinfarction Research Group. Am J Cardiol 1988;61:8.

Mock MB et al: Survival of medically treated patients in the Coronary Artery Surgery Study (CASS) registry. Circulation 1982;66:562.

Nademanee K, Singh BN: Effects of sotalol on ventricular tachycardia and fibrillation produced by programmed electrical stimulation: Comparison with other antiarrhythmic agents. Am J Cardiol 1990;65:53A

Norwegian Multicenter Study Group: Timolol-induced reduction in mortality and reinfarction in patients surviving acute myocardial infarction. N Engl J Med 1981;304:801.

Oldridge NB et al: Cardiac rehabilitation after myocardial infarction: Combined experience of randomized clinical trials. JAMA 1988;260:945.

Oliver MF et al: WHO Cooperative Trial on primary prevention of ischaemic heart disease with clofibrate to lower serum cholesterol: Final mortality follow-up. Report of the Committee of Principal Investigators. Lancet 1984;2:600.

O'Rourke RA: Noninvasive and invasive testing after myocardial infarction. Curr Probl Cardiol 1991;16:721.

Pantely GA, Bristow JD: Ischemic cardiomyopathy. Prog Cardiovasc Dis 1984;27:95.

Pell S, D'Alonzo CA: Immediate mortality and 5-year survival of employed men with first myocardial infarction. N Engl J Med 1964;270:915.

Persantine-Aspirin Reinfarction Study Research Group: Persantine and aspirin in coronary heart disease. Circulation 1980;62:449.

Proudfit WL et al: Fifteen year survival study of patients with obstructive coronary artery disease. Circulation 1983;68:986.

Raymond R et al: Myocardial infarction and normal coronary arteriography: A 10 year clinical and risk analysis of 74 patients. J Am Coll Cardiol 1988;11:471.

Rechnitzer PA et al: Relation of exercise to the recurrence rate of myocardial infarction in men: Ontario Exercise-Heart Collaborative Study. Am J Cardiol 1983;51:65.

Ruberman W et al: Ventricular premature complexes in prognosis of angina. Circulation 1980;61:1172.

Sanz G et al: Determinants of prognosis in survivors of myocardial infarction: A prospective clinical angiographic study. N Engl J Med 1982;306:1065.

Schuster EH, Bulkley BH: Ischemic cardiomyopathy: A clinicopathologic study of 14 patients. Am Heart J 1980;100:506.

Shaw LW: Effects of a prescribed supervised exercise program on mortality and cardiovascular morbidity in patients after a myocardial infarction: The National Exercise and Heart Disease Project. Am J Cardiol 1981;48:39.

Steinbeck G et al: A comparison of electrophysiologically guided antiarrhythmic drug therapy with beta-blocker therapy in patients with symptomatic, sustained ventricular tachyarrhythmias. N Engl J Med 1992;327:987.

Steinberg JS et al: Predicting arrhythmic events after acute myocardial infarction using the signal-averaged electrocardiogram. Am J Cardiol 1992;69:13.

Stone PH et al: Prognostic significance of the treadmill exercise test performance 6 months after myocardial infarction. J Am Coll Cardiol 1986;8:1007.

Visser CA et al: Echocardiographic-cineangiographic correlation in detecting left ventricular aneurysm: A prospective study of 422 patients. Am J Cardiol 1982;50:337.

Weiner DA et al: Comparison of coronary artery bypass surgery and medical therapy in patients with exercised-induced silent myocardial ischemia: A report from the Coronary Artery Surgery Study (CASS) Registry. J Am Coll Cardiol 1988;12:595.

Weiss JN et al: Ventricular arrhythmias in ischemic heart disease. Ann Intern Med 1991;114:784.

Wenger NK, Marcus FI, O'Rourke RA (editors): Cardiovascular disease in the elderly. J Am Coll Cardiol 1987;10:1A.

Wenger NK: Rehabilitation of the coronary patient: Status 1986. Prog Cardiovasc Dis 1986;29:181.

White HD et al: Left ventricular end-systolic volume as the major determinant of survival after recovery from myocardial infarction. Circulation 1987;76:44.

Willard JE et al: The use of aspirin in ischemic heart disease. N Engl J Med 1992;327:175.

Yusuf S, Furberg CD: Effects of calcium channel blockers on survival after myocardial infarction. (Editorial.) Cardiovasc Drugs Ther 1987;1:343.

Yusuf S et al: Beta blockade during and after myocardial infarction: An overview of the randomized trials. Prog Cardiovasc Dis 1985;27:335.

Coronary Heart Surgery & Coronary Angioplasty

Barratt-Boyes BG et al: The results of surgical treatment of left ventricular aneurysms: An assessment of the risk factors affecting early and late mortality. J Thorac Cardiovasc Surg 1984;87:87.

Blackshear JL, O'Callaghan WG, Califf RM: Medical approaches to prevention of restenosis after coronary angioplasty. J Am Coll Cardiol 1987;9:834.

Bourassa MG et al: Strategy of complete revascularization in patients with multivessel coronary artery disease (A report from the 1985–1986 NHLBI PTCA registry.) Am J Cardiol 1992;70:174.

Califf RM et al: The evolution of medical and surgical therapy for coronary artery disease: A 15-year perspective. JAMA 1989;261:2077.

Campeau L: Grading of angina pectoris. (Letter.) Circulation 1976;54:522.

CASS Principal Investigators and Their Associates: Coronary Artery Surgery Study (CASS): A randomized trial of coronary artery bypass surgery: Survival data. Circulation 1983;68:939.

Chaitman BR et al: Angiographic prevalence of high-risk coronary artery disease in patient subsets (CASS). Circulation 1981;64:360.

Chaitman BR et al: Effect of coronary bypass surgery on survival patterns in subsets of patients with left main coronary artery disease: Report of the Collaborative Study in Coronary Artery Surgery. Am J Cardiol 1981;48:765.

Chokshi SK, Meyers S, Abi-Mansour P: Percutaneous transluminal coronary angioplasty: Ten years' experience. Prog Cardiovasc Dis 1987;30:147.

Cohen M, Packer M, Gorlin R: Indications for left ventricular aneurysmectomy. Circulation 1983;67:717.

Cote G et al: Percutaneous transluminal angioplasty of stenotic coronary artery bypass grafts: 5 years' experience. J Am Coll Cardiol 1987;9:8.

Detre K: Effect of bypass surgery on survival in patients in low- and high-risk subgroups delineated by the use of simple clinical variables. Circulation 1981;63:1329.

Detre K et al: Percutaneous transluminal coronary angioplasty in 1985-1986 and 1977-1981: The National Heart, Lung, and Blood Institute Registry. N Engl J Med 1988;318:265.

Dilsizian V et al: The effect of coronary artery bypass grafting on left ventricular systolic function at rest: Evidence for preoperative subclinical myocardial ischemia. Am J Cardiol 1988;61:1248.

Dimas AP et al: Repeat coronary angioplasty as treatment for restenosis. J Am Coll Cardiol 1992;19:1310.

Douglas JS Jr et al: Percutaneous transluminal coronary angioplasty in patients with prior coronary bypass surgery. J Am Coll Cardiol 1983;2:745.

Ellis SG et al: Importance of stenosis morphology with estimation of restenosis risk after elective coronary angioplasty. J Am Coll Cardiol 1989;63:30.

Epstein SE et al: Strategy for evaluation and surgical treatment of the asymptomatic or mildly symptomatic patient with coronary artery disease. Am J Cardiol 1979;43:1015.

European Coronary Surgery Study Group: Prospective randomised study of coronary artery bypass surgery in stable angina pectoris: Second interim report. Lancet 1980;2:491.

Favaloro RG et al: Direct myocardial revascularization by saphenous vein graft. III: Present operative techniques and indications. Ann Thorac Surg 1970;10:97.

FitzGibbon EM et al: Coronary bypass graft fate: Long-term angiographic study. J Am Coll Cardiol 1991;17:1075.

Frye RL et al: Randomized trials in coronary artery bypass surgery. Prog Cardiovasc Dis 1987;30:1.

Gavaghan TP et al: Immediate postoperative aspirin improves vein graft patency early and late after coronary artery bypass graft surgery. Circulation 1991;83:1526.

Gibson RS et al: Prospective assessment of regional myocardial perfusion before and after coronary revascularization surgery by quantitative thallium-201 scintigraphy. J Am Coll Cardiol 1983;3:804.

Goldman S et al: Saphenous vein graft patency 1 year after coronary artery bypass surgery and effects of antiplatelet therapy: Results of a Veterans Administration Cooperative Study. Circulation 1989;80:1190.

Hall RJ et al: Coronary artery bypass: Long-term follow-up of 22,284 consecutive patients. Circulation 1983;68:II—20.

Holmes DR Jr et al: The effect of medical and surgical treatment on subsequent sudden cardiac death in patients with coronary artery disease: A report from the Coronary Artery Surgery Study. Circulation 1986;73:1254.

Hwang MH et al: Progression of native coronary artery disease at 10 years: Insights from a randomized study of medical versus surgical therapy for angina. J Am Coll Cardiol 1990;16:1066.

Kent KM et al: Improved myocardial function during exercise after successful percutaneous transluminal coronary angioplasty. N Engl J Med 1982;306:441.

Khan SS, Matloff JM: Surgical revascularization in women. Curr Opin Cardiol 1991;6:904.

King SB III: Current status of percutaneous transluminal coronary angioplasty. Cardiovasc Rev Rep 1988;9:27.

Kirklin JW, Blackstone EH, Rogers WJ: The plights of the invasive treatment of ischemic heart disease. J Am Coll Cardiol 1985;5:158.

Kirklin JW et al: ACC/AHA Task Force on Assessment of Diagnostic and Therapeutic Cardiovascular Procedures (Subcommittee on Coronary Artery Bypass

Graft Surgery): Guidelines and indications for coronary artery bypass graft surgery. J Am Coll Cardiol 1991;17:543.

Leimgruber PP et al: Restenosis after successful coronary angioplasty in patients with single-vessel disease. Circulation 1986;73:710.

Loop FD et al: Influence of the internal-mammary-artery graft on 10-year survival and other cardiac events. N Engl J Med 1986;314:1.

Loop FD et al: Reoperation for coronary atherosclerosis: Changing practice in 2509 consecutive patients. Ann Surg 1990;212:378.

Lytle BW et al: Replacement of aortic valve combined with myocardial revascularization: Determinants of early and late risk for 500 patients, 1967-1981. Circulation 1983;68:1149.

McBride W, Lange RA, Hillis LD: Restenosis after successful coronary angioplasty: Pathophysiology and prevention. N Engl J Med 1988;318:1734.

Moosvi AR et al: Early revascularization improves survival in cardiogenic shock complicating acute myocardial infarction. J Am Coll Cardiol 1992;19:907.

Murphy ML et al: Treatment of chronic stable angina: A preliminary report of survival data of the randomized Veterans Administration Cooperative Study. N Engl J Med 1977;297:620.

Murray GC, Beller GA: Cardiac rehabilitation following coronary artery bypass surgery. Am Heart J 1983;105:1009.

Myers WO et al: Improved survival of surgically treated patients with triple vessel coronary artery disease and severe angina pectoris: A report from the Coronary Artery Surgery Study (CASS) registry. J Thorac Cardiovasc Surg 1989;97:487.

Norris RM et al: Coronary surgery after recurrent myocardial infarction: Progress of a trial comparing surgical with nonsurgical management for asymptomatic patients with advanced coronary disease. Circulation 1981;63:785.

Parisi AF, Folland ED, Hartigan P: A comparison of angioplasty with medical therapy in the treatment of single-vessel coronary artery disease: Veterans Affairs ACME Investigators. N Engl J Med 1992;326:10.

Passamani E et al: A randomized trial of coronary artery bypass surgery: Survival of patients with a low ejection fraction. (CASS) N Engl J Med 1985;312:1665.

Pigott JD et al: Late results of surgical and medical therapy for patients with coronary artery disease and depressed left ventricular function. J Am Coll Cardiol 1985;5:1036.

Roubin GS: Status of percutaneous transluminal coronary angioplasty. Curr Probl Cardiol 1990;15:721.

Roubin GS et al: Event free survival after successful angioplasty in multivessel coronary artery disease. (Abstract.) J Am Coll Cardiol 1987;9:15A.

Ryan TJ: Guidelines for percutaneous transluminal coronary angioplasty: A report of the American College of Cardiology/American Heart Association Task Force on Assessment of Diagnostic and Therapeutic Cardiovascular Procedures (Subcommittee on Percutaneous Transluminal Coronary Angioplasty). Circulation 1988;78:486.

Schaff HV et al: Survival and functional status after coronary artery bypass grafting: results 10 to 12 years after surgery in 500 patients. Circulation 1983;68:II-200.

Scott BD, Kerber RE: Clinical and experimental aspects of myocardial stunning. Prog Cardiovasc Dis 1992;35:61.

Selzer A: Preventive intervention in coronary artery disease. Primary Cardiol 1983;9:14.

Solymoss BC et al: Late thrombosis of saphenous vein coronary bypass grafts related to risk factors. Circulation 1988;78:I-140.

Talley JD, Hurst JW, King SB 3d: Clinical outcome 5 years after attempted percutaneous transluminal coronary angioplasty in 427 patients. Circulation 1988;77:820.

Varnauskas E, and the European Coronary Surgery Study Group: Twelve-year follow-up of survival in the Randomized European Coronary Surgery Study. N Engl J Med 1988;319:332.

Veterans Administration Coronary Artery Bypass Surgery Cooperative Study Group: Eleven year survival in the Veterans Administration randomized trial of coronary bypass surgery for stable angina. N Engl J Med 1984;311:1333.

Veterans Administration Coronary Artery Bypass Surgery Cooperative Study Group: Eighteen-year follow-up in the Veterans Affairs Cooperative Study of Coronary Artery Bypass Surgery for Stable Angina. Circulation 1992;86:121.

Vigilante GJ et al: Improved survival with coronary bypass surgery in patients with three-vessel coronary disease and abnormal left ventricular function: Matched case-control study in patients with potentially operable disease. Am J Med 1987;82:697.

Waldo AL et al: Diagnosis and treatment of arrhythmias during and following open heart surgery. Med Clin North Am 1984;68:1153.

Weiner DA et al: Prevalence and prognostic significance of silent and symptomatic ischemia after coronary bypass surgery: A report from the Coronary Artery Surgery Study (CASS) randomized population. J Am Coll Cardiol 1991;18:343.

Weiner DA et al: The role of exercise testing in identifying patients with improved survival after coronary artery bypass surgery. J Am Coll Cardiol 1986;8:741.

Whalen RE et al: Survival of coronary artery disease patients with stable pain and normal left ventricular function treated medically or surgically at Duke University. Circulation 1982;65:II-49.

Zimmern SH et al: Total occlusion of the left main coronary artery: The Coronary Artery Surgery Study (CASS) experience. Am J Cardiol 1982;49:2003.

Systemic Hypertension

Essential or primary hypertension is sustained elevated arterial pressure of unknown cause—as contrasted with secondary hypertension, where the cause is known. An etiologic classification is presented in Table 9–1. The criteria for the diagnosis of hypertension are arbitrary, because the arterial pressure is a continuous variable, rises with age, and varies from one occasion of measurement to another. Some authorities consider hypertension to be present when the diastolic pressure consistently exceeds 100 mm Hg in a person over age 60 or consistently exceeds 90 mm Hg in a person under that age. The Joint National Committee Report (1988) defines hypertension as a consistent elevation of blood pressure greater than 140/90 mm Hg. The vascular complications of hypertension are thought to be due to the raised arterial pressure and associated atherosclerosis of major arterial circuits.

Hypertension uncommonly has its onset before age 20 or after age 55, though the frequency is higher if one uses different criteria for children, eg, pressure exceeding the 90th percentile for age. Hypertension in young people is commonly due to chronic glomerulonephritis, renal artery stenosis, coarctation of the aorta, or pyelonephritis.

Transient elevations of blood pressure caused by excitement, apprehension, or exertion and the purely systolic elevation of blood pressure in elderly people caused by decreased compliance (increased stiffness) in their major arteries do not constitute hypertensive disease if the estimated mean blood pressure is less than 107 mm Hg (140/90). The pulse pressure is defined as the systolic pressure minus the diastolic pressure. The mean pressure as defined here is an approximation computed as follows:

$$\text{Diastolic blood pressure} + \frac{\text{Pulse pressure}}{3} = \text{Mean pressure}$$

However, predominant or isolated systolic elevation exceeding 160–180 mm Hg is a significant aortic (rather than arteriolar) disease reflecting either (1) atherosclerosis or (2) medial hypertrophy with collagen deposition without atherosclerosis, causing decreased compliance of the aorta, and the prognosis is therefore correspondingly less good than if both systolic and diastolic pressure are normal (see below). Both aortic and arteriolar processes may coexist.

Hypertension is an important preventable cause of cardiovascular disease. Epidemiologic studies have shown that only a small percentage of the hypertensive population is receiving effective antihypertensive therapy. Education of both physicians and patients is necessary so that hypertensive individuals can be identified and treated; to establish the concept that treatment is a lifelong process; and to emphasize that compliance with the treatment program is essential to an effective result.

Table 9–1. Etiology and classification of hypertension.

Primary (essential) hypertension: Hypertension of undetermined cause

Secondary hypertension: Hypertension due to—
1. Renal disease
   Renal arterial disease (renal artery stenosis due to atherosclerosis or fibromuscular hyperplasia), aneurysm, embolism, and infarction
   Renal parenchymal disease (acute and chronic glomerulonephritis), pyelonephritis, polycystic renal tuberculosis, pericapsular hemorrage, and subsequent scarring from trauma
   Renal tumors (Wilms' tumor, renin-producing tumors)
   Arteritis (polyarteritis nodosa, neurofibromatosis, and nonspecific)
2. Endocrine disorders:
   Cushing's syndrome
   Acromegaly
   Primary aldosteronism
   Pheochromocytoma
3. Coarctation of the aorta
4. Enzymatic defects (congenital adrenal hyperplasia):
   Enzymatic defect of 17α-hydroxylation, leading to amenorrhea due to overproduction of cortisol precursors
   Enzymatic defects of 11β-hydroxylation
5. Neurologic disorders: Increased intracranial pressure from brain tumors, cardiovascular accident, quadriplegia
6. Drug-induced hypertension:
   Prolonged administration of corticosteroids
   Excessive use of desoxycorticosterone and salts of 5α-fluoro compounds in the treatment of postural hypotension
   Use of amphetamines or excessive thyroxine
   Chronic licorice ingestion, producing pseudoaldosteronism
   Use of oral contraceptive agents
   Cyclosporine in transplant patients
   Cocaine (crack) abuse
7. Hypercalcemia from any cause
8. Neurogenic, possibly psychogenic, disorders
9. Deficiency of vasodilating tissue enzymes (speculative): prostaglandins, kallikrein, endothelium-derived relaxing factor, renal medullary tissue

EPIDEMIOLOGIC STUDIES OF THE PREVALENCE OF HYPERTENSION

There is no sharp dividing line between normotension and hypertension; when one plots the blood pressure at different ages in a large healthy population, the distribution curve does not demonstrate two distinct populations. Hypertension is a quantitative deviation from normal. As a result, the criteria for the diagnosis of hypertension must be regarded as arbitrary; this has caused confusion in the literature because different authors use different numbers to diagnose hypertension.

Epidemiologic studies indicate that about 15–20% of adults in the USA have blood pressures above 160/95 mm Hg, the upper limits of borderline according to WHO criteria. The percentage falls to 5% if a diastolic pressure of 105 mm Hg is used as the cutoff point. Insurance companies consider 140/90 mm Hg to be the upper limits of normal, as does the 1988 Report of the Joint National Committee. The Framingham epidemiologic study, published over the past 10–15 years, classified patients between 140/90 and 160/95 mm Hg as borderline hypertensives.

Prospective studies have shown that without treatment, hypertension increases the incidence of cardiac failure, coronary heart disease, hemorrhagic and thrombotic stroke, renal failure, peripheral artery disease, dissection of the aorta, and death. The morbid events have a higher incidence with increasing age even in a treated group (Veterans Administration Cooperative Study Group on Antihypertensive Agents, 1967, 1972). Preventing or reversing hypertensive complications by antihypertensive therapy is a major public health concern. This has led to intensive efforts to screen populations in various ways for the presence of hypertension. One must be cautious in extrapolating screening pressures, because about half of the individuals singled out in this way will be found to be "normal" on subsequent examinations.

Age & Hypertension

Hypertension is regarded as uncommon before age 20, though this view may not be completely justified because physicians have used adult criteria to determine normality in adolescents. Secondary hypertension is often found in young people: coarctation of the aorta, chronic glomerulonephritis, pyelonephritis, renal artery stenosis, endocrine disorders, cocaine abuse, and raised pressure from oral contraceptive agents must all be considered in this age group.

The mean blood pressure rises with age in most Western populations but not in all individuals in the population groups. In normal subjects, the greatest rise occurs between birth and age 20, when the average systolic pressure may increase from 80 to 120 mm Hg. There is then a slow increase in pressure until ages 35–45, when the rate of rise becomes

greater, and many individuals cross over into a range that is arbitrarily defined as high blood pressure. The systolic pressure may then continue to rise more slowly, not only because of decreased compliance of the aorta as a feature of aging but presumably also because of familial or genetic factors. The diastolic pressure follows the systolic rise up to about age 50, when the rise with age becomes less steep. Blood pressure distribution according to sex and age in the entire city of Bergen, Norway, has been tabulated by Humerfelt (1963). Blood pressure in childhood requires different guidelines (de Man, 1991), as do those in the very old (Heikinheimo, 1990).

The rise in pressure with age in various epidemiologic studies is greater in persons who gain the most weight and consume a high-salt and low-potassium diet (especially black women), in those with a low Ca^{2+} diet, in persons who have a family history of hypertension, in populations that habitually eat a diet very high in salt (eg, in northern Japan), and in persons who have personality or emotional factors that increase blood pressure. Populations that ingest a diet very low in sodium (< 70 mmol/d; 1.61 g/d) infrequently develop an increase in blood pressure with advancing age. Plasma norepinephrine increases and plasma renin decreases with age. Systemic vascular resistance also increases with age, and in patients with systolic hypertension, cardiac output decreases.

The roles of these various factors have not been adequately studied in populations that show a rise in pressure with age compared with those that do not. About 30% of the rise in pressure with age is due to genetic factors and the remainder to environmental factors whose nature has not been precisely determined. The relative significance of genetic and environmental factors varies in different individuals.

Race & Hypertension

The high prevalence and severity of hypertension in blacks—especially black women who have gained considerable weight—has been documented in many studies. Furthermore, the death rate from hypertension in blacks is greater than that in whites, though this may be a function of decreased access to treatment rather than an inherent susceptibility to hypertension. In the Veterans Administration Study (1967), black and white patients did equally well with treatment and equally badly without it. There may be genetic differences—blacks tend to have low plasma renin levels, a decreased ability to excrete a high sodium load, and there may be other factors. Psychosocial factors (suppressed hostility, low socioeconomic status), decreased potassium and calcium intake, increased salt intake, and family instability have all been thought to play a role (Anderson NB, 1989). There are few data to indicate that the prognosis with mild hypertension is worse in blacks than in whites. The higher mortality rate from hypertension in blacks is to a great extent due to their greater likelihood of having severe hypertension with cardiac failure or malignant hypertension, perhaps owing to lack of early adequate treatment.

Cigarette smoking raises the blood pressure; its role in the epidemiology of hypertension is unclear, but the adverse impact of smoking on coronary disease in hypertensives is well documented (Mancia: Managing coronary, 1990).

PATHOPHYSIOLOGY OF ESSENTIAL HYPERTENSION

Mean arterial pressure is the product of the systemic vascular resistance and the mean cardiac output. As a result, either an increase in cardiac output or an increase in systemic vascular resistance can raise the blood pressure; both factors in this relationship are constantly changing throughout the course of a day. Blood pressure is not a static physiologic feature but a variable one in all individuals, both normal and hypertensive, from one occasion of measurement to another.

Normal blood pressure is maintained by complex mechanisms made up of many interacting regulatory forces acting on cardiac output and peripheral resistance (see below).

As one proceeds along the cardiovascular system from the cardiac "pump" to the capacitance vessels (the veins), the arterial pressure drop is greatest at the precapillary resistance vessels (the arterioles); it is chiefly the caliber of these vessels that controls the systemic vascular resistance.

Many physiologic mechanisms are brought into play to maintain the blood pressure within a normal range. Functional and structural changes in the resistance vessels (arterioles) are brought about by many influences: increased smooth muscle contraction; baroreceptor reflexes sending afferent impulses to the medulla and hypothalamic centers; other influences on these centers resulting in efferent autonomic discharge; blood volume; humoral and neurogenic influences from the kidneys and endocrine organs; effects of the renin-angiotensin-aldosterone system; and local effects of tissue renin-angiotensin, endothelium-derived relaxing and constricting factors, prostaglandins, kinins, adenosine, serotonin, and atrial natriuretic factor. Intrinsic autoregulation also operates to control arteriolar caliber independently of sympathetic adrenergic stimuli. Transient elevations of blood pressure due to physiologic decrease in the caliber of arterioles should not be confused with sustained or established hypertension. Such transient factors as anxiety, emotion, fear, noise, pain, anger, cold, an unfamiliar or threatening environment, exercise, or tachycardia can increase the arterial pressure either by increasing cardiac output or as a result of arteriolar vasoconstriction, raising the systemic vascular resistance. The control systems influencing these various factors and the dominant role of the kidneys have both positive and negative feedback loops. The complex interrelationships of the factors have been analyzed by Guyton (1989) and others.

As indicated in the discussion of atherosclerosis, the physiologic functions of prostaglandins and thromboxanes are the subject of active research (Figure 8–6). The vasodilating action of prostacyclin (PGI^2) and the vasoconstricting action of thromboxane (TXA^2), which modulate blood flow within the kidney and thereby influence blood pressure, are of considerable interest. Prostaglandins increase the release of renin and are involved in the regulation of glomerular filtration, renal blood flow, and the excretion of electrolytes. Figure 8–6 depicts the pathway for biosynthesis and metabolism of prostaglandins.

The circadian rhythm of blood pressure in both normal subjects and hypertensive patients may be due to impulses from the central nervous system. As a rule, blood pressure is lowered during sleep and begins to rise immediately before or after awakening (Figure 9–1).

The various components of the regulatory systems controlling the blood pressure interact in a complex manner, being both independent and interdependent. The primary cause of essential hypertension is unknown, but some disorder of the kidneys, regulation of body fluid volume, and blood flow to the tissues must be involved, leading to a raised systemic vascular resistance (Davidman, 1984). The kidney is considered to play the most important role in the pathogenesis of hypertension, influenced by various factors discussed below. Numerous hypotheses regarding the etiology of hypertension have been championed, but none have been universally accepted as primary. Extensive investigations are continuing.

THE ROLE OF GENETIC FACTORS

Hypertension tends to aggregate in families; the ratio of genetic to environmental factors in the hypertensive population at large is thought to be about 30% and 70%, respectively. Genetic and environmental factors—as well as the influence of neurogenic and humoral factors—all interact in a multifactorial complex affecting the blood pressure. The correlation coefficient of blood pressure levels is 0.50–0.60 in identical twins, 0.25 in nonidentical twins, less between parents and children and least between adoptive children and their adoptive parents and between unrelated adults (Williams, 1990; 1991). Multiple genes are involved. Environmental factors of consequence have largely been limited to "psychosocial" abnormalities and salt (sodium chloride), calcium,

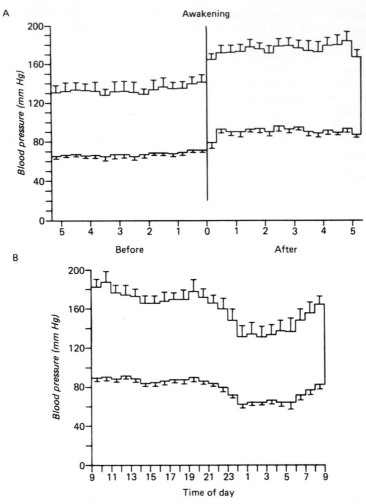

Figure 9–1. Mean systolic and diastolic pressures in 14 untreated hypertensive subjects. **A:** Data analyzed with respect to the moment of waking as recorded by the patients, in 20-minute intervals for a 5-hour period up to the moment of waking, and for a 5-hour period subsequent to waking. **B:** Data analyzed in hourly intervals over the 24-hour period. (Redrawn and reproduced, with permission, from Floras JS et al: Arousal and the circadian rhythm of blood pressure. Clin Sci Mol Med 1978;55[Suppl 4]:395s.)

and potassium intake; these may be in part genetic in origin. Alcohol, caffeine, and weight gain have been implicated but are less important in the majority of patients with hypertension, though obesity in early life has been found to be a predictor of subsequent hypertension (Stamler, 1991; Hall, 1992). The environmental influences act on a substrate of inherited susceptibility to hypertension.

Cellular Ionic Fluxes & Membrane Transport of Ions

These fluxes and membrane abnormalities are thought to be the expression of various specific genes. They determine the flow of ions such as sodium, chloride, potassium, calcium, and magnesium across cell membranes in the body, altering, in hypertension, the intra- and extracellular concentrations of the ions in response to neurogenic or humoral influences (Ives, 1989). For example, the concentration of Na^+-K^+ ATPase, the sodium pump, has been found to be decreased in patients with essential hypertension and in experimental hypertensive animals; the decreased enzyme may result from a postulated circulating inhibitor of the sodium pump that has not been identified. By a complex cascade of actions, the reduced sodium pump activity leads to an increase in intracellular sodium; this in turn leads to a rise in intracellular free calcium concentration via a sodium-calcium exchange mechanism (Haddy, 1983; Hilton, 1986). Combined with other factors, increased intracellular free calcium ion results in arterial and venous vasoconstriction (increased systemic vascular resistance) and decreased compliance of the aorta and the major arteries (Shepherd, 1990). Calcium entry-blocking drugs used in the treatment of hypertension reverse these actions and lessen the blood pressure and improve the distensibility of the aorta and its branches; this is thought to support the conceptual framework noted above.

Sodium-Lithium Countertransport (Na^+-Li^+ CT)

Another ion flux said to be a genetic marker and a risk factor in hypertension is the sodium-lithium countertransport (Weder, 1991). The countertransport is enhanced in some cases of essential hypertension, leading to increased intracellular sodium and calcium with consequences similar to those resulting from decreased sodium pump activity. This countertransport is increased, especially in hypertensives in whom the specific recessive gene for the ion transport is identified; furthermore, normotensives with high Na^+-Li^+ CT who carried the gene developed hypertension significantly more often than did those with low Na^+-Li^+ CT. There is, however, a significant overlap in the countertransport flux between unselected hypertensive and normotensive individuals (Hunt, 1991).

Calcium Transport Defects

Calcium transport defects have been noted in patients with hypertension and are presumably genetic in origin. A substantial number of hypertensive patients ingest less calcium yet excrete a larger amount of calcium in their urine than do normotensive controls. Serum calcium is low in some hypertensive patients, especially elderly individuals with low plasma renin levels. Calcium plays a fundamental role in vascular smooth muscle contraction, with resulting vasoconstriction; it has been proposed that a calcium regulatory abnormality may occur in essential hypertension (Wadsworth, 1990).

High sodium chloride intake in salt-sensitive, spontaneously hypertensive (SHR-S) rats raises the blood pressure, and the response is prevented when calcium is supplemented in the rats' diet; no such effect occurs in spontaneously normotensive Wistar-Kyoto (WKY) rats or in salt-resistant (SHR-R) rats. Central neural sympatholytic mechanisms are hypothesized to explain the preventive effect of calcium (Oparil, 1990).

The ionic flux alterations are usually not found in secondary hypertension, so they probably reflect cellular membrane expression of various genes in essential (primary) hypertension; their role in possibly initiating the disease is far from clear.

Insulin Resistance

Insulin resistance, hyperinsulinemia, lipid abnormalities, glucose intolerance, and obesity have been noted in hypertensive patients; insulin may be the underlying trigger, and its role is being actively investigated (Slater, 1991; Hall, 1992; Reaven, 1991). The reduction of glucose uptake is thought to be genetically determined. It has been proposed that hyperinsulinemia or a defect in skeletal muscle insulin action enhances efferent sympathetic outflow from the central nervous system and may be a risk factor for atherosclerosis (Ferrari, 1990; Natali, 1991). Significant correlations have been found occasionally between the diastolic blood pressure and insulin levels in the blood. Insulin independently affects many of the factors influencing the regulation of blood pressure. In one study of the development of hypertension in a 10-year follow-up of middle-aged men, elevated plasma levels of insulin (both fasting and in a glucose tolerance test) suggested that insulin resistance may be predictive (Skarfors, 1991).

Potassium Cation Abnormalities

Dietary intake of potassium is low in some hypertensive patients, especially in blacks. Increasing the potassium intake may lower the blood pressure in these patients. An experimental low-potassium diet (16 mmol/d) raised the pressure in hypertensives (Krishna, 1991). The mechanism is unclear. It has been observed that primitive peoples normally eat a low-sodium, high-potassium diet (as has been estimated for early humans)—in contrast to the relatively high-sodium, low-potassium diet eaten by some contemporary groups of people.

NEUROGENIC FACTORS: The Role of Baroreceptors

A primary immediate neural defense mechanism that responds to acute increases or decreases of arterial pressure is the function of the **baroreceptors** in the carotid sinus and the aortic arch. Neural firing (inhibitory) from receptors in the walls of these vessels is increased when the arterial pressure rises and is reduced when the pressure falls. The receptors are sensitive to mean pressure and to the rate of change of pressure; these initiate a reflex baroreceptor response affecting the blood pressure and the heart rate, reestablishing the original situation (see Figure 9–2 and Chapter 1).

There has been much speculation about the role of baroreceptors in the pathogenesis of hypertension. Early enthusiasm lessened when it was found that denervation of the baroreceptors or section of the baroreceptor nerves produced tachycardia and slight, highly variable, unstable neurogenic hypertension. It is now believed that the arterial baroreceptors, while important in buffering acute changes in pressure, are not the mechanism responsible for long-term control of arterial pressure. The response of the baroreceptors is reset at a higher level in hypertension; normal blood pressure is not then restored by this neurogenic response. If the blood pressure is then raised further, neurogenic impulses from the vasomotor center lower the pressure at this new, elevated set pressure, indicating that the buffering mechanism has been set at a

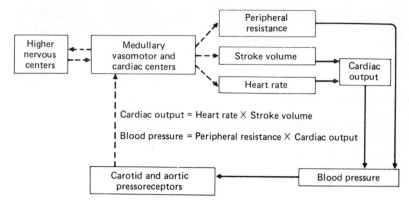

Figure 9–2. Blood pressure is sensed by the pressoreceptors, which send impulses to the central nervous system. The central nervous system sends impulses to motor fibers of the sympathetic and parasympathetic nervous system. When pressure at the receptor rises or falls, it is reflexly corrected by an alteration of heart rate, stroke volume, and peripheral resistance. Dotted lines indicate neural connections. (Reproduced, with permission, from Scher AM: Control of arterial blood pressure. In: *Physiology and Biophysics*, 20th ed, vol 2. Ruch TC, Patton HD [editors]. Saunders, 1974.)

higher level. The sensitivity of the baroreflex can be determined by noting the change in heart rate following injection of agents that increase blood pressure. Baroreceptor reflex control in hypertension has been found to be reduced (Sleight, 1991; Matsukawa, 1991; Parmer, 1992).

THE ROLE OF SALT, BODY FLUID VOLUME, & THE KIDNEY

Salt and body fluid volume and the influence of the kidney in their homeostasis have long been thought to be perhaps intimately involved in the pathogenesis of hypertension (NHLBI Workshop, 1991). Salt intake influences intracellular calcium and other ionic fluxes, and, as will be discussed later, interrelates with increased activity of the sympathetic nervous system and the renin-angiotensin-aldosterone system. The etiologic importance of sodium intake and hypertension has been debated for years. Although there are some salt-sensitive individuals in whom an increased salt intake results in a raised blood pressure—as it does in salt-sensitive Dahl rats (Dahl-S) and in the spontaneous hypertension rats of Okamoto (SHR-S)—most hypertensive patients are not salt-sensitive. Sodium chloride rather than sodium alone is the compound responsible for the rise in pressure resulting from salt loading in hypertensives who are salt-sensitive. The chloride ion also is important because other sodium salts, such as sodium citrate and sodium nitrate, do not have this effect or have it to a lesser degree (Kurtz, 1987). Potassium salts, such as potassium chloride and potassium bicarbonate, do not raise the blood pressure in hypertensives, so both sodium and chloride are important—but sodium is more important.

The role of sodium chloride has been assessed by experimental and clinical studies in which sodium chloride intake has been manipulated and by the difference in the prevalence of hypertension in population epidemiologic surveys in different countries. Populations with low average (< 60 mmol/d) sodium intakes (Brazilian Indians, some African tribes) infrequently have hypertension and do not experience a rise in blood pressure with age, as do most individuals in Western societies. Population groups who habitually ingested large amounts of salt daily ($> 300–500$ meq Na^+ per day)—as did the Northern Japanese in the past—have a higher prevalence of hypertension than do those with low or normal salt intake (150–250 meq/d). Of course, these populations have lifestyles and factors other than their salt intake that can affect the likelihood of hypertension. Furthermore, when individuals from a low-salt-intake population move to an area where their salt intake is increased, they develop elevated blood pressure in the same way as the local inhabitants. In a large multicentered intercountry study, the prevalence of hypertension was correlated—but not strongly—with the average level of salt intake (INTERSALT Cooperative Research Group, 1988; Stamler, 1989).

Selective inbreeding of rats through multiple generations has produced one strain of rats in which all develop hypertension as they mature and another strain in which none do. The best-studied are the Okamoto spontaneous hypertensive strain (SHR) and the Wistar-Kyoto nonhypertensive strain (WKY). The former have also been bred to be salt-resistant (SHR-R) or salt-sensitive (SHR-S). The SHR-S rats show a considerable increase in arterial blood pressure when they are ingesting a diet high in salt, whereas the SHR-R and the WKY rats do not. Other similar strains of rats have been developed, such as the Dahl salt-sensitive (DL-S) and the Dahl salt-resistant (DL-R) rats.

Hypertensive patients have been classified as being salt-sensitive or salt-resistant in their response to high-salt diets, but the criteria have been variable and conflicting. Patients with hypertension may substantially lower their blood pressure when on diuretic regimens or very strict low-salt diets. The fall in blood pressure in hypertensives taking intermediate low-sodium diets (< 100 meq/d) have only a slight reduction in blood pressure. The most striking example of the benefit of a diet very low in salt is the rice-fruit diet of Kempner—even accelerated hypertension was reversed when the Kempner diet was maintained over a period of time. However, most patients found it too difficult to continue on this rigid diet.

The kidney is the major organ controlling sodium balance and fluid volume and their relationship to hypertension. Hypertensives, as compared to normotensives, raise their arterial pressure, excrete more salt, and increase their urinary volume when an acute sodium load is given to susceptible individuals. This is presumably a genetic characteristic and is called pressure natriuresis (Firth, 1990). The increased excretion of salt and water as the pressure is raised is thought to be necessary to preserve body fluid volume. Another hypothesis of the mechanism by which the kidney influences hypertension is that the kidney, by a genetic fault, fails to excrete sodium normally because it has fewer nephrons and by increased reabsorption of sodium in the distal renal tubule (Brenner, 1988). This increases the extracellular fluid volume, which then presumably causes the brain (probably the hypothalamus) to secrete a putative circulating natriuretic substance to restore normal fluid volume. Salt loading stimulates sympathetic efferent arteriolar vasoconstriction, especially in the kidney, which raises the blood pressure (see next section). Such a possible chain of events involving the kidney and body fluid volume homeostasis leads to hypertension; however, the supposed circulating natriuretic hormone has never been identified (Guyton, 1989; de-Wardener, 1991). A coexistent hypothesis is that autoregulation of increased peripheral flow, by enhanced contraction of vascular smooth muscle, raises the blood pressure and returns the blood flow to normal (Ledingham, 1989).

The kidney-body fluid and autoregulation hypotheses have not been universally accepted as etiologic but have stimulated much thought and experimentation. Many hypertensive patients do not have a raised extracellular volume; this has been explained by noting that whatever initiates hypertension may be different from what maintains it. For example, in young individuals with borderline or early hypertension, hemodynamic studies demonstrate an elevated cardiac output with a normal systemic vascular resistance, while in established hypertension the cardiac output is normal or slightly decreased and the systemic vascular resistance is raised (Lund-Johansen, 1991). The elevated cardiac output, often with tachycardia, in young hypertensives with early disease results from increased sympathetic drive from the central nervous system (anterior hypothalamus or vasomotor center), which causes arteriolar and venous constriction, resulting in increased venous return to the heart (increased preload) and a higher heart rate, stroke volume, and, thus, cardiac output.

THE ROLE OF THE CENTRAL NERVOUS SYSTEM

The blood pressure is highly variable from one time to another during the day, as is clearly shown by ambulatory out-of-office recordings. Apart from exercise, the major cause of this variability is the daily assortment of "psychosocial" stimuli. The magnitude of this neurohormonal response is thought to be genetically linked. The importance of the central nervous system in the possible initiation of hypertension has been championed by Folkow (1987) and Henry (1990). Various studies in experimental hypertensive animals have demonstrated the effects of "psychosocial stress" on the heart rate, cardiac output, and systemic vascular resistance secondary to constriction of the afferent renal arterioles. Stress receptors in the cerebral cortex lead to stimulation of hypothalamic nuclei that have connections to the higher centers in the cortex and to the nucleus solitarius and result in a central sympathetic neural outflow to the viscera, including the kidney. A high-salt diet in young SHRs worsens the severity of the hyperkinetic response and significantly raises the plasma norepinephrine (Oparil, 1989). Hypertensive patients given mental tasks that evoke an emotional response (eg, mental arithmetic) or stressful stimuli in experimental animals (eg, air pressure to the head of SHR induce renal arteriolar vasoconstriction and increase efferent renal sympathetic nerve activity, which increase the cardiac output, pulse rate, and blood pressure. These central neural effects are more obvious when combined with a high-salt diet (DiBona, 1991). In a British Whitehall study relating grade of employment to mortality, a low employment grade was associated with a higher mortality rate, possibly related to "monotonous work, low control and low satisfaction" (Marmot, 1991). Oft-repeated emotional stimuli, often related to "psychosocial" situations, may, because of repeated episodes of arteriolar vasoconstriction, cause arteriolar muscle hypertrophy and a decreased arteriolar lumen, leading ultimately to a permanently raised peripheral resistance to blood flow. A considerably raised cardiac output, by autoregulation (arteriolar vasoconstriction whenever the peripheral blood flow is increased, thus restricting excessive blood-flow to the tissues), sets in motion the compensatory adaptive arteriolar vasoconstriction. However, not all patients with a high cardiac output develop these arteriolar changes; examples are arteriovenous fistulae or beriberi.

THE ROLE OF THE SYMPATHETIC NERVOUS SYSTEM

Increased activity of the sympathetic nervous system has been frequently implicated as a possible etiologic factor in the pathogenesis of hypertension (Abboud, 1982). Efferent renal sympathetic nerve traffic affects many functional aspects of the kidney that regulate blood pressure, body fluid volume, and sodium balance (DiBona, 1989; Folkow, 1987, 1989). Arteriolar vasoconstriction causing a raised resistance to blood flow is the fundamental hemodynamic abnormality in established hypertension. Psychosocial experiences influence the central nervous system to respond by stimulating the sympathetic efferent outflow to the viscera—especially the kidney—possibly enhanced by a genetic susceptibility, increased sodium chloride intake, and insulin resistance.

Borderline or early hypertensives in young individuals often have emotional instability, increased heart rate and cardiac output, a variably increased blood pressure, a raised plasma norepinephrine concentration, and elevated sympathetic nerve activity by microneurography (Anderson EA, 1989; Julius, 1990, 1991). Hemodynamically, they have afferent renal arteriolar vasoconstriction. In contrast to these younger individuals, plasma norepinephrine is usually normal in established hypertension; the hemodynamic effect of adrenergic efferent arteriolar constriction in the kidney may not be reflected in an increased plasma norepinephrine. Only a small amount of synthesized norepinephrine overflows into the plasma; it may have a considerable local effect on the kidney without raising the plasma concentration. The local tissue concentration of norepinephrine and that in the plasma are not equivalent. Later, at a time when the obvious hyperactivity present in early hypertension is no longer present, young hypertensives develop structural arteriolar abnormalities in the kidney that sustain the elevated arterial pressure in chronic established hypertension.

In mild or moderate hypertension, even when the plasma norepinephrine is normal, increased sympathetic nerve activity in muscles can be demonstrated by recording electrical potential changes by microneurography (microelectrodes are introduced into peripheral nerves through the skin). Microneurography has shown bursts of sympathetic nerve activity of increased amplitude in hypertensive patients associated with environmental stresses, such as a high-salt diet or the alerting reaction to mental stress (Esler, 1990; Mark, 1990).

Drugs (such as hexamethonium) that block postganglionic neurons or sympathetic ganglia and the sometimes dramatic falls in blood pressure in malignant hypertension following extensive surgical sympathectomy further support the role of the neurogenic component in hypertension.

The sympathetic nervous system exerts potent influences on the kidney by constricting the afferent arterioles. This stimulates renin release, with the formation of angiotensin (see below). Increased tubular reabsorption of sodium then follows the secretion of aldosterone from the adrenals, which reduces the excretion of sodium and the volume of urine. The renal effects are an example of the complex interactions involving the sympathetic nervous system, sodium, angiotensin, aldosterone, fluid volume, calcium, and other factors in the regulation of the blood pressure. Vasopressin (arginine vasopressin; AVP), another potent vasoconstrictor, is also stimulated by the sympathetic nervous system. Plasma levels and the pressor effects of AVP are reduced by beta-adrenergic-blocking drugs.

Sympathetic nervous system hyperactivity has been noted in individuals in stressful occupations; "job strain" has been related to hypertension and to increased left ventricular mass (Schnall, 1990). In contrast, nuns in a secluded order, when compared with laywomen with equivalent blood pressures and urinary sodium concentrations at baseline and who gained weight similarly, were found after a 20-year follow-up not to have developed hypertension nor a rise in blood pressure as they grew older, whereas the laywomen had the usual blood pressure rise with age seen in Western societies. It is thought that this was owing to the tranquil lifestyle of the nuns that by inference resulted in less sympathetic activity from the central nervous system (Timio, 1988).

THE ROLE OF NEUROHUMORAL FACTORS (Renin, Angiotensin, Aldosterone)

Renin, a proteolytic enzyme, is secreted by the juxtaglomerular cells surrounding the afferent arterioles near the vascular pole of the kidney in response to a "signal." It is hypothesized that the signal is related to stretching of the afferent arteriole or to decreased "effective" blood volume or to decreased sodium content of the nearby macula densa of the distal tubule. Renin then acts on a substrate in the plasma (α_2-globulin), producing the decapeptide angiotensin I, which is then acted upon by a converting enzyme in the lung to form the octapeptide angiotensin II, which is a potent pressor substance. Angiotensin II, by an effect on the zona glomerulosa of the adrenal cortex, increases the secretion of aldosterone, which results in sodium and water retention by its action on the distal renal tubule, thus restoring blood volume. By negative feedback, the secretion of renin is then reduced until equilibrium results (Figure 9–3).

The complex factors affecting renin levels and regulating renin release from the kidney are important in hypertension, and there is considerable evidence supporting the concept of regulation by the nervous system and the autonomic sympathetic amines. The

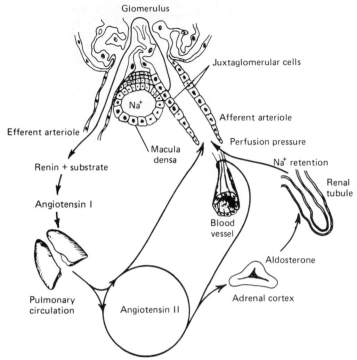

Figure 9–3. Feedback regulation of renin release. Several feedback loops are shown. An increase in angiotensin II concentration results in decreased renin secretion by increased sodium retention, resulting in increased extracellular fluid volume; direct negative feedback; increased blood pressure through the central nervous system; increased blood pressure through direct systemic vasoconstriction; and direct sodium effects on the macula densa. (Reproduced, with permission of the American Heart Association, from Haber E: The role of renin in normal and pathological cardiovascular homeostasis. Circulation 1976;54:849.)

mechanisms regulating renin release can be classified as **intrarenal,** which include (1) alteration of sensing by the afferent arteriole of changes in the renal perfusion pressure, (2) the influence of an alleged sodium receptor in the macula densa, which senses changes in the sodium concentration in the distal tubule, and (3) prostaglandins; **autonomic factors,** including the effects of catecholamines and nervous impulses via the renal nerves; and **humoral effects** of electrolytes, vasopressin, angiotensin, and adrenergic impulses from the higher cerebral centers. Renin exists in the plasma in an inactive prorenin form and in an active renin form.

There is considerable evidence that the area postrema has an active function in central cardiovascular control, including regulation of the blood pressure. Electrical stimulation of this area increases sympathetic outflow in a fashion similar to what happens when angiotensin II is infused into the central arteries. Ablation of this area reduces sympathetic outflow—in contrast to ablation of the nucleus solitarius, which causes severe hypertension (Ferrario, 1991).

Angiotensin is actively involved in the short- and long-time vasoconstriction that raises the blood pres-

sure; stimulates the synthesis of aldosterone from the zona glomerulosa of the adrenal gland, causing renal reabsorption of sodium from the distal tubules; decreases sodium excretion; and increases body fluid volume, which may be involved in the secretion of the putative circulating natriuretic hormone from the hypothalamus. The renin-angiotensin-aldosterone (RAA) system, by influencing renal excretory function and renal retention of sodium and water, has an important effect on renal pressure natriuresis to maintain normal sodium and water balance. Angiotensin activates the sympathetic nervous system as well as the secretion of aldosterone, causing vasoconstriction of the efferent arteriole of the kidney (Kaneko, 1991).

In a random group of hypertensive patients taking an unrestricted sodium diet, about 25% will have low, 60% normal, and about 15% high plasma renin concentrations, depending on age and on the severity of the hypertension as defined in different ways by different authorities. The mechanism of low-renin hypertension is unclear. Many such patients do not have increased body fluid or raised total exchangeable sodium. Low plasma renin is more common in blacks and in older patients. High plasma renin is usually associated with severe or accelerated hypertension and is probably the result of renal arteriolar damage except in young hypertensives with early disease.

The RAA system, while its primary role in essential hypertension is uncertain, plays a dominant role in the hypertension of renal artery stenosis (see below under Secondary Hypertension). Plasma renin is usually high in severe or accelerated hypertension, in which secondary hyperaldosteronism often occurs. The inverse relationship between serum sodium and plasma renin results in elevated plasma renin activity with sodium or volume depletion, as during diuretic therapy. Further evidence of the importance of the RAA system in hypertension is revealed in the excellent antihypertensive effect of drugs that inhibit the system (converting enzyme inhibitor agents).

The RAA system is the predominant humoral factor in the regulation of blood pressure and in the control of sodium and body fluid balance. The latter is influenced mainly by the secretion of aldosterone from the adrenal gland; however, the sympathetic nervous system enhances the RAA system and thus also influences sodium and water homeostasis.

THE ROLE OF LOCAL VASCULAR FACTORS IN HYPERTENSION

It has been established that the endothelium of small arteries and arterioles secretes vasoactive substances— some vasoconstrictive, such as renin, angiotensin, endothelin, and serotonin, whereas others are vasodilating, such as prostacyclin, PGE_2, kallikrein, and endothelium-derived relaxing factor (nitric oxide) (Dzau, 1989; Bohr, 1991). Deficiency of vasodilator peptides has only rarely been demonstrated in patients with hypertension; urinary kallikrein is decreased— perhaps as a result of a genetic defect in the renal synthesis of the vasodilator bradykinin. Synthesis of PGI_2 and PGE_2 is enhanced by stressful situations, responding to increased activity of the RAA system and the adrenergic nervous systems; they react with kinins and cause protective vasodilation (McGiff, 1991).

A balance between vasoconstrictor and vasodilator substances determines the ultimate effect of the local vascular factors. Angiotensin in the vessel walls of various organs, including the kidney and the brain, plays a significant physiologic role, distinct from plasma angiotensin, in causing increased systemic vascular resistance (Shepherd, 1990). It is inhibited by converting enzyme inhibitors just as is plasma angiotensin.

THE ROLE OF ATRIAL NATRIURETIC FACTOR

Increased pressure or stretch of the right atrial wall induces atrial cells to secrete a peptide hormone, atrial natriuretic factor (ANF). Injection of this substance causes a rapid increase in the urinary excretion of sodium and water and higher rates of glomerular filtration and of renal blood flow, reversing the effects of angiotensin and aldosterone. Plasma ANF is usually similar in normotensive and hypertensive populations, though in some studies it was found to be raised in hypertensive patients. Usually there is no significant relationship between plasma levels and the blood pressure. An exception may be made in the case of preeclampsia (see Chapter 22), in which ANF concentration is high even though the plasma volume is lower than in normal pregnancy. It is doubtful that ANF has a primary role in the initiation of hypertension, but it represents a regulatory hormonal mechanism to aid homeostasis in such conditions as cardiac and renal failure with salt and water overload, in which plasma ANF is elevated (Athanassopoulos, 1991). ANF is not the putative natriuretic factor discussed earlier.

THE ROLE OF VASOPRESSIN (AVP) (Antidiuretic Hormone [ADH])

Arginine vasopressin (AVP) is synthesized in the hypothalamic nuclei, and fibers containing AVP are found centrally, in the pituitary gland, and in the spinal cord. These fibers innervate areas such as the nucleus solitarius that influence sympathetic outflow and so are involved in cardiovascular regulation (Berecek, 1990). Vasopressin is a powerful vasopressor and antidiuretic hormone that interacts with the sympathetic nervous system. Plasma levels of vasopressin have been found to be elevated in low-and normal-renin hypertensive patients, and the levels then became normal after treatment with nonselective beta-blocking agents such as oxprenolol (Os, 1986). Vasopressin decreases water excretion (antidiuretic) and may increase the blood pressure by this volume increase as well as by its arteriolar vasoconstrictor effect. Its action may be direct or by potentiation of a similar action by catecholamines. Vasopressin is generally considered not to be a direct cause of initiation of hypertension.

PREVALENCE & DEVELOPMENT OF HYPERTENSION

National surveys have found the prevalence of hypertension to be approximately 20% of the adult population. Elevated arterial pressure has clearly been shown to be a major factor in the enhanced incidence and mortality rate of cardiac failure, malignant hypertension with renal failure, hemorrhagic and thrombotic stroke, coronary heart disease with angina pectoris and myocardial infarction, dissection of the aorta, and peripheral vascular disease.

The adverse effects of hypertension have led to efforts at primary prevention with emphasis on predictors of a raised blood pressure noted in early life, especially in those with a positive family history of hypertension. These include weight gain, high-salt diet, high Na^+ and low K^+ dietary intake, high saturated fat, excessive alcohol use (Stamler, 1991; Mockrin, 1991), and early increase in left ventricular mass (Deveraux, in Mockrin, 1991).

The prevalence and clinical course depends greatly on the criteria by which one diagnoses hypertension, the presence and severity of associated risk factors for atherosclerosis, and whether or not the patient has had adequate therapy. Hypertension has been classified as mild, moderate, and severe depending on whether the diastolic pressure is 90–104 mm Hg, 105–114 mm Hg, or over 115 mm Hg, respectively. In malignant hypertension the diastolic pressure is usually over 130 mm Hg and often as high as 140 mm Hg. The WHO classification considers pressures less than 140/90 mm Hg to be normal, 140/90–160/95 to be borderline, and greater than 160/95 to be definite hypertension.

If pressures greater than 160 mm Hg are associated with diastolic pressures less than 90 mm Hg, the condition is called **isolated systolic hypertension.** Whether one uses a diastolic pressure of 90, 95, or 100 mm Hg influences considerably the prevalence of hypertension, because most patients with hypertension have mild disease, about 40% of diastolic pressures falling in the range of 90–100 mm Hg. The lower the cutoff point, the greater will be the prevalence of hypertension (Joint National Committee, 1988).

Because of the increased morbidity and mortality rates in patients diagnosed as having hypertension, it is essential to establish its sustained presence before making the diagnosis. Arterial pressure is variable from one measurement to another and may exceed normal limits on some occasions and be below normal on others. Various authorities characterize this as borderline hypertension while others call it mild hypertension.

The blood pressure should be taken with the patient relaxed, in a warm room, and allowed 5–10 minutes of rest before the pressure is taken. All details of the proper technique of measurement should be strictly followed (Frohlich, 1988; Joint National Committee, 1988; O'Brien, 1985, 1990). Several pressures should be taken at the initial visit with the numbers averaged if the pressure exceeds 140/90 mm Hg. The patient should return for at least three individual measurements on different occasions to establish the diagnosis, because the patient may in fact have what has

been called "white coat" hypertension referable to the stress of the medical environment and the presence of the physician (Pickering, 1990). It may be necessary to obtain repeated blood pressure measurements over a period of weeks to reach a confident conclusion about the patient's pressure. Multiple readings increase the reliability of the blood pressure findings.

Ambulatory blood pressure recorders have been developed utilizing semiautomatic, automatic, or intra-arterial techniques. These have been used increasingly in recent years because of the observation that ambulatory recordings are usually (80% of cases) lower than office readings, are obtained during the usual activities of the patient, show less variability, are more reproducible, permit sleep pressures, and provide many more readings. Ambulatory pressures have been shown to be more closely correlated with the presence of target organ damage and with the development of clinical events than are office or casual readings (Meyer-Sabellek, 1990).

Ambulatory Blood Pressures

Evidence that ambulatory blood pressures provide a more reliable estimate of the morbidity or mortality than office pressures can be found in papers by Sokolow (1966), Perloff (1983, 1989), Mancia (Ambulatory, 1990), and Parati (1987) and in a book by Pickering (1991). There are many monitors now on the market, and one should verify the accuracy of the apparatus before using it to diagnose hypertension when transient, borderline, or mild elevations of pressure are found in the office environment or when there is an unexplained substantial difference between office pressures and expected target organ damage. In moderate to severe hypertension, when the office pressures are substantially raised, ambulatory pressures are usually not required for diagnosis because the importance of the pressures obtained and the need for therapy are clear. In borderline or mild hypertension, however, the physician needs to be assured that hypertension is established before starting treatment. There are as yet inadequate data to determine what pressure obtained by daytime ambulatory readings should be considered "normal"; data currently available suggest that an average reading of 130–135/80–85 mm Hg may be the upper limits of normal. Age is important, because in most Western societies the blood pressure rises variably with age; pressures considered normal in the age group 20–30 are infrequently found in patients over the age of 65. Automatically recorded ambulatory recordings permit the recording of sleep blood pressures; there are data to suggest that the usual fall in pressure during sleep may not occur or is lessened in some individuals, which appears to be an adverse prognostic sign. What has been called the "hypertensive load" has been noted in some studies (Kain, 1964); the percentage of readings throughout the 24 hours that exceed 140/90 mm Hg correlates well with the presence of target organ damage (Zachariah, 1991). Variability of the blood pressure can be computed in 24-hour readings; opinion differs as to whether variability influences prognosis. More data are needed. Separate averages are usually computed for daytime and nighttime pressures; there is variability, even beat-to-beat, during both time intervals. In one study, the ambulatory pressures during 24 hours averaged 118/72 mm Hg, 124/78 mm Hg during the day, and 106/61 mm Hg during the night—a difference of 18/17 mm Hg. A meta-analysis of 23 studies showed similar numbers (Staessen, 1991). There are marked differences in daytime ambulatory pressures in healthy individuals in various age groups; the 95th percentile averages varied from 114/88 mm Hg in the age group under 30 years to 150/98 mm Hg in the decade 40—49 (O'Brien, 1991). Intra-arterial invasive ambulatory pressures (the Oxford system) have been obtained; however, the usual 24-hour ambulatory monitoring is not invasive and obviously more desirable in clinical practice. Intra-arterial recordings have the advantage of not disturbing the patient during the frequent noninvasive cuff recordings, are valuable in research, but usually only two or three occasions of measurement are obtained (Mancia: Ambulatory, 1990; Meyer-Sabellek, 1990).

Significance of Ambulatory Blood Pressures

For all of this century, the traditional evaluation of the clinical significance of an elevated blood pressure was based on the office or casual blood pressure reading. Office pressures have served us relatively well, and a number of studies have shown increased morbidity and mortality in groups of patients in whom office pressures progressively rise (Build and Blood Pressure Study, 1959; Sokolow, 1961; Kannel, 1974). It was observed in our 1961 study that some patients with considerably elevated pressure did well (though the majority did not), and, conversely, that patients whose pressures were only slightly raised (though they usually did well) occasionally developed vascular complications early in their course. Similarly, Freis (Veterans Administration Cooperative Study Group on Antihypertensive Agents, 1967, 1970) found that although patients with diastolic pressures exceeding 105 mm Hg had a significantly lower incidence of vascular complications in the treated as compared with the control group, approximately two-thirds of the placebo group did not develop vascular complications during the period of observation despite the elevated diastolic pressure. Further, about one-third of patients receiving antihypertensive therapy continued to have elevated office diastolic pressures yet continued to do well clinically. This was interpreted as suggesting that even partial treatment was beneficial; an alternative explanation might be that this third of patients whose office diastolic pressure remained elevated despite good clinical results

represent patients whose ambulatory pressures might have been lower. Is it a coincidence that in our studies comparing office with ambulatory pressures, about a third of the total sample of patients had ambulatory blood pressures less than 140/90 mm Hg despite a raised office pressure? The office pressures in the Veterans Administration Study therefore might not have been representative of what the average daytime pressures were. The variable prognosis based on office pressures was the impetus for our development of ambulatory pressures obtained during a patient's usual activities—away from the physician and the medical environment (Hinman, 1962; Kain, 1964). The phenomenon of the pressor role of the physician and the elevated office pressures with lower ambulatory pressures was emphasized (Sokolow, 1966); more recently, it has been termed "white-coat hypertension," presumably related to behavioral factors related to the alerting or alarm reaction described years ago (Pickering, 1990). The physician's office and the authoritative figure of the physician are potent emotional stimuli that arouse anxiety and elevation of the blood pressure. Insufficient data are available to determine whether so-called white-coat hypertension is truly benign or whether the prognosis may still prove to be somewhat adverse. Follow-up data are required to answer the question; in the meantime, we are treating patients based on the office pressures but perhaps less vigorously than if both the office and the ambulatory pressures were elevated.

In a group of patients it was found that the ambulatory pressure was lower than the office pressure in 78%; however, the correlations between the two were significant, being 0.67 for systolic and 0.65 for diastolic pressure. The disparity between the ambulatory and the office pressures increased as the office pressure rose among groups of patients with an equivalent office blood pressure. Those with a large disparity ("low ambulatory blood pressure") had less target organ damage than did those with a small disparity. The average daily ambulatory blood pressure correlated more closely with the degree of target organ damage than did office pressures (Sokolow, 1966). The most useful data from ambulatory pressures are the average daytime and nighttime pressures and the "pressure load" and perhaps the variability of the pressure. When the average pressure is compared with the five highest readings throughout the day or the five lowest readings of the day, the correlation is 0.95. The average blood pressure load can be estimated by determining the percentage of readings throughout the day that exceed 140/90 mm Hg or the median pressure for the day. It is clear that the average ambulatory pressure is a better gauge of the load on the cardiovascular system than is the office pressure. Ambulatory blood pressure recordings are now used widely in the United States and abroad, though questions still remain regarding normal values and prognostic information and implications. The procedure is expensive and not universally reimbursable by third-party payers.

CLINICAL EVALUATION OF THE PATIENT WITH HYPERTENSION

The initial evaluation is designed to establish the presence of hypertension, to determine the status of the organs (target organs) that are affected by an elevated pressure, and to carefully evaluate the presence and degree of additional atherosclerotic risk factors. With the availability of effective contemporary pharmacologic and other means of treatment, recognition and management of treatable atherosclerotic risk factors other than hypertension are important. These include cigarette smoking, hyperlipidemia, diabetes mellitus, excessive use of alcohol, and psychosocial and emotional factors that influence the blood pressure. Hyperlipidemia is the most important risk factor, and one should not rely solely on hypercholesterolemia but should determine the high-density and low-density lipoproteins and the triglycerides (see Chapter 8). With the early use of antihypertensive agents and attention to risk factors, deaths formerly caused by cardiac failure, stroke, renal failure, and malignant hypertension are now much less frequent than in the days prior to effective pharmacologic therapy. Coronary heart disease and stroke are the two most common causes of death in mild and moderate hypertension today; this emphasizes the need for *comprehensive* treatment of the hypertensive patient. A medical history and laboratory data will disclose the presence of coronary risk factors. In addition, one should seek evidence for the presence of abnormalities of the heart, brain, kidney, and peripheral arteries in the patient's past history and by current evaluation (see below). A long duration of hypertension should make finding target organ damage more likely. A history of previous therapy for hypertension should be obtained—not only to determine the responses to whatever therapeutic agents were used but also because it gives the physician some insight into the matter of compliance if the patient has stopped treatment. Factors such as salt, potassium, calcium, and fat intake, the use of alcohol and tobacco, whether the patient is sedentary or habitually exercises, and, if possible, a record of the weight of the patient over the previous 10–20 years should be obtained. A record of medications the patient is taking or may have used in the past is valuable. Some medications, such as oral contraceptives, corticosteroids, or other drugs that may influence the blood pressure, should not be overlooked, such as cyclosporine in transplant patients or drugs that are known to stimulate the sympathetic nervous system; they may adversely affect the blood pressure. The 1988 Report of the Joint National Committee is valuable in providing information on the evaluation and treatment of hypertension.

Phases in the Development of Hypertension

There are many problems in identifying patients with hypertension, including systematic biases and the normal variability of the blood pressure. In the Charlottesville Blood Pressure Survey, for example, 20% of over 12,000 adults were initially classified as hypertensive, yet after repeated blood pressure measurements, only 9% were found to have sustained hypertension (Carey, 1976). Variability of the blood pressure, not only from one time of measurement to another but from beat to beat, has been demonstrated by intra-arterial pressure recordings. The major factors influencing variability are the level of pressure, the intensity of physical activity, negative affect, and the systolic variability resulting from progressive impairment of carotid sinus and aortic baroreflexes, as in older patients. Emotional states and the circumstances of measurement, whether in the physician's office, at work, at home, or during ambulatory recording, influence the blood pressure and diagnosis of hypertension.

A. Early Phase: In "labile" hypertension, the blood pressure is raised on some occasions but not on others; however, even in moderate or severe hypertension, the blood pressure level fluctuates, and the term should probably no longer be used as a way of characterizing borderline hypertension. Lability of blood pressure is greater in younger individuals, often resulting from increased cardiac output with or without increased systemic vascular resistance owing to excessive sympathetic adrenergic impulses arising in the central nervous system (the cortex, hypothalamus, or medullary centers). Emotional factors cause neurohumoral discharges from the higher cortical centers, which then increase sympathetic adrenergic excitation impulses, which then raise arterial pressure by vasoconstriction of the arterioles.

Variable hypertension is clearly related to age. Sustained hypertension is that which is present at almost all determinations, infrequently falling below 140/90 mm Hg except during sleep.

B. Established Hypertension: In between younger hypertensive patients with raised cardiac output and older hypertensive patients with established hypertension who have a normal cardiac output but a raised systemic vascular resistance are middle-aged individuals who may have both increased systemic vascular resistance and cardiac output.

Pulse Pressure

Both systolic and diastolic pressures are raised in the usual case of hypertension; the difference between them (the pulse pressure) depends not only upon age but upon whether the major component of the raised pressure is due to an increase in cardiac output or peripheral resistance or to decreased compliance of the aorta and central arteries. Increased pulse pressure does not necessarily signify a raised mean blood pressure. It can result from decreased compliance of the aorta and not from increased mean pressure unless the diastolic pressure exceeds 90 mm Hg. A wide pulse pressure is most apt to occur in early, fluctuating hypertension of young people with a raised output or in the elderly person with perhaps only a slight increase in diastolic pressure but with a greater increase in systolic pressure owing to a less distensible aortic and arterial bed. Actuarial data indicate that both systolic and diastolic pressures are important with respect to mortality, but it is often difficult to separate their effects because the correlation between them is so high, being on the order of $r = 0.7$.

Isolated Systolic Hypertension

Systolic hypertension is usually defined as a systolic pressure above 160 mm Hg and a diastolic pressure less than 90 mm Hg in individuals over age 65. Depending on cutoff points, such as a systolic pressure of 140 or 160 mm Hg and a diastolic pressure of 80, 90, or 95 mm Hg, the prevalence varies from 63% in whites if the pressure is over 140/90 mm Hg to 44% if over 160/95 mm Hg, but the prevalence is only 6.8% if one uses 160/80 mm Hg as a criterion (Working Group on Hypertension in the Elderly, 1986). The increased systolic pressure in epidemiologic studies begins to rise at about age 55 and then increases more steeply to age 80. The diastolic pressure levels off at about age 60 and may even decrease slightly. Various studies have demonstrated that the mortality rate in hypertensive patients is as closely related to systolic as to diastolic pressure, which means that the traditional emphasis solely on diastolic pressure is not valid. The mortality rate is increased in isolated systolic hypertension, perhaps because most cases (excluding conditions such as complete atrioventricular block, severe bradycardia, arteriovenous fistulas, thyrotoxicosis, and aortic insufficiency) are due to decreased distensibility and elasticity (increased rigidity) of the central aorta and its branches as a result of atherosclerosis or degenerative medial hypertrophy, often with collagen or calcific deposits. Atherosclerosis, being a generalized disorder, is apt to be present elsewhere if it occurs in the aorta, and so the mortality rate can be expected to be greater than in persons who do not have aortic atherosclerosis. If the diastolic pressure is greater than 90 mm Hg, the systemic vascular resistance is apt to be elevated, and therefore the hypertension is not isolated systolic hypertension. The mean pressure is estimated to be 113 mm Hg if the blood pressure is 160/90 mm Hg, but 127 mm Hg if one uses 160/95 mm Hg as the cutoff point (elevated from a normal of

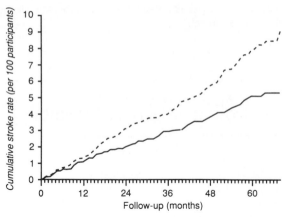

Figure 9–4. Cumulative fatal plus nonfatal stroke rate per 100 participants in the active treatment (solid line) and placebo (broken line) groups during the Systolic Hypertension in the Elderly Program. (Reproduced, with permission, from SHEP Cooperative Research Group: Prevention of stroke by antihypertensive drug treatment in older persons with isolated systolic hypertension: Final results of the Systolic Hypertension in the Elderly Program [SHEP]. JAMA 1991;265:3255. Copyright © 1991 by American Medical Association.)

107 mm Hg) (140/90 mm Hg). The raised mean pressure at the higher diastolic pressure suggests a raised peripheral vascular resistance (Working Group on Hypertension in the Elderly, 1986). Elderly patients with isolated systolic hypertension have a high prevalence of left ventricular hypertrophy (Pearson, 1991) and stroke (Ueda, 1988; SHEP Cooperative Research Group, 1991).

The mean pressure is the best index of the significance of a predominantly or purely systolic elevation of blood pressure with respect to the diagnosis of essential hypertension. The load on the left ventricle is increased if the systolic pressure is raised.

Cardiovascular complications (cardiac failure and especially stroke) have an increased incidence in isolated systolic hypertension, similar to that of hypertension in general. For years, treatment of this condition was debated and often not given. The SHEP study, recently completed, demonstrated significant benefit (especially in the prevention of stroke) with antihypertensive therapy (Figure 9–4). Valuable reviews of isolated systolic hypertension in the elderly are those of Staessen (1990), Robertson (1989), and Hollenberg (Am J Med 1991).

The essential effect of aging consists of decreased distensibility and enlargement of the aorta. Because the raised systolic pressure "compensates" for the decreased aortic distensibility (compliance), antihypertensive drugs may cause a decreased cardiac output, with weakness or faintness resulting from decreased perfusion of the vital organs. If medication is given, it should be given cautiously and in low doses, with careful observation of its effects. (See Treatment of Essential Hypertension, below.)

"Pseudohypertension" may occur in elderly patients because the sclerotic brachial artery resists compression by the blood pressure cuff; it can be diagnosed if the artery distal to the compressed cuff is palpable but no pulsation can be felt (Osler's test) (Kuwajima, 1990).

Mortality Rates Associated With Untreated Hypertension

Actuarial data gathered during a large insurance study dealing with almost 4 million lives and 100,000 deaths—as well as the Framingham Study—show that the mortality rate rises with increasing blood pressure (Figures 9–5 and 9–6) (Build and Blood Pressure Study, 1959; Kannel, 1974; Levy, 1990). There is no sharp dividing line below which the mortality rate is unaffected and above which it is increased. There were progressive excessive morbidity and mortality rates as blood pressure rose in the large group studied by the insurance companies, especially in younger individuals (the excess mortality rate is less in older subjects). The physician should think not in terms of hypertension or normotension ("either-or") but of the actual level of the blood pressure, both systolic and diastolic, in relationship to age. Data from many sources show that age is a major factor in determining the importance of the degree of deviation that any pressure represents and is of prognostic significance at any given level of blood pressure. A systolic pressure of 160 mm Hg, for example, would be in the 95th or 98th percentile for a 25-year-old but in the 50th percentile for a 60-year-old. The actuarial data from insurance companies likewise show the im-

portance of age and the much greater likelihood of a fatal outcome over a period of years in younger individuals as compared with older ones with similar pressures. The mortality rate is higher in males, perhaps because of the increased incidence of coronary disease (Figure 9–6).

CLINICAL FINDINGS

The clinical, laboratory, and radiologic findings relate to (1) the height of the blood pressure; (2) the involvement of "target organs," such as the heart, brain, kidneys, eyes, and peripheral arteries; (3) the presence of vascular complications, such as left ventricular hypertrophy, cardiac failure, myocardial infarction, cerebral infarction, cerebral hemorrhage, microalbuminuria or renal insufficiency, atherosclerosis elsewhere, and dissection of the aorta; (4) evidence of secondary "curable" hypertension; and (5) the presence and degree of atherosclerotic risk factors.

Symptoms

Primary hypertension early in its course is usually an asymptomatic disorder compatible with well-being for many years. Vague symptoms of nonspecific headache, dizziness, fatigue, and pounding of the heart may be present in hypertensive patients (often only after patients learn that they have the condition) but are no more frequent than in some groups of patients with normotension. The frequency of vague symptoms that resemble those seen in psychoneurotic disorders has led investigators to conclude that these nonspecific symptoms in patients with mild hypertension are functional in origin and not organic. Screening of adult population groups often reveals the blood pressure to be elevated in vigorous subjects who have no symptoms whatever.

A. Headaches: When hypertension is more severe—especially if it is the accelerated variety (with rapid rise in pressure and hemorrhages or exudates in the fundi, considered premalignant)—throbbing suboccipital headaches are common, worse in the morning and subsiding during the day. In malignant hypertension with visual disturbances, the headaches can be severe and difficult to relieve except by blood pressure reduction. In contrast with the typical suboccipital, throbbing hypertensive headache, the usual tension headache is more apt to be frontal and nonthrobbing; the differentiation may be difficult.

B. Left Ventricular Hypertrophy and Heart Failure: Left ventricular hypertrophy is an adaptive response to the raised blood pressure and increased systemic vascular resistance. It may be diagnosed by electrocardiography or echocardiography, and there may be impaired left ventricular diastolic function, even if systolic function is normal. When left ventricular dilation and early left ventricular failure occur

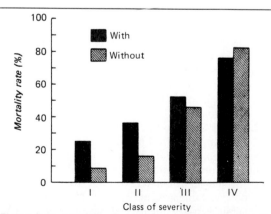

Figure 9–5. Mortality rates of hypertensive patients with and without atherosclerotic complications. Severity classes I–IV are described in the article and indicate progressively increasing severity of vascular complications. (Reproduced, with permission of the American Heart Association, from Sokolow M, Perloff D: The prognosis of essential hypertension treated conservatively. Circulation 1961;23:697.)

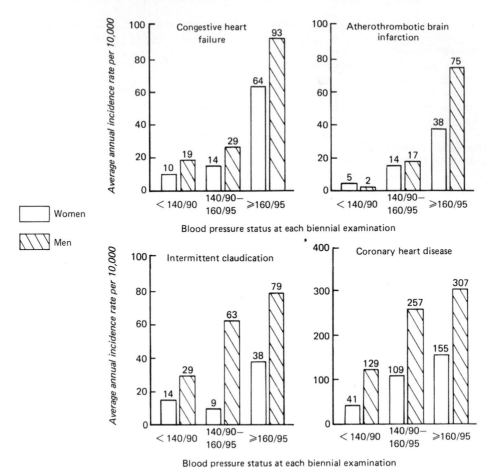

Figure 9–6. Average annual incidence of cardiovascular disease according to blood pressure status at each biennial examination, men and women 55–64, 16-year follow-up: Framingham Study. (Source: Framingham Monograph No. 26.) (Reproduced, with permission, from Kannel WB: Role of blood pressure in cardiovascular morbidity and mortality. Prog Cardiovasc Dis 1974;17:5.)

in patients with compensatory cardiac hypertrophy, symptoms include progressively more severe dyspnea on exertion, paroxysmal nocturnal dyspnea, and orthopnea (see Chapter 10). If coronary heart disease is also present, as it commonly is, patients may complain of angina pectoris or may develop myocardial infarction. Left ventricular failure resulting from the combination of increased afterload and work of the left ventricle due to hypertension and to associated coronary heart disease is frequent and makes a precise distinction between causative factors difficult. Cardiac failure does not usually occur from modest elevations of blood pressure alone. When the raised blood pressure is greater—and particularly when it occurs abruptly, as in malignant hypertension—cardiac failure may occur in the absence of coronary heart disease and is rapidly reversed when the blood pressure is lowered. Hypertensive patients with cardiac hypertrophy often develop symptoms and signs of cardiac failure if the sodium intake is abruptly

increased, as with ingestion of baking soda, Alka-Seltzer, or a high-sodium diet; these patients often respond rapidly to treatment. Cardiac failure is an uncommon cause of death in the well-managed patient unless it follows the complications of myocardial infarction.

C. Renal Symptoms: Although nephrosclerosis is a common finding on pathologic examination (by either necropsy or renal biopsy), renal failure is not common unless hypertension is accelerated, malignant, inadequately treated, or untreated. Early evidence of renal impairment is revealed by quantitative microalbuminuria. Patients with severe hypertension may develop nocturia or, more rarely, intermittent hematuria. In nonaccelerated cases, renal blood flow and the glomerular filtration rate may be decreased, but renal failure and azotemia are infrequent. If accelerated or malignant hypertension occurs, however, necrotic lesions in the arterioles and narrowed interlobular arteries may significantly decrease the renal blood flow and glomerular filtration rate; renal function may deteriorate rapidly over a period of weeks or months.

The most common cause of death in malignant hypertension is renal failure; determination of renal function is essential in all patients with hypertension, because it is important to lower the blood pressure before renal failure has occurred (see Course and Prognosis, below).

D. Central Nervous System Symptoms: Older patients with hypertension and associated cerebral and carotid artery atherosclerosis may develop any of the clinical manifestations that might be expected from the pathologic findings. Patients may develop severe headache, confusion, coma, convulsions, blurred vision, transient neurologic signs, ataxia, or neurologic deficit due to cerebral edema, infarction, or hemorrhage. If the blood pressure rises abruptly, acute cerebral symptoms may develop such as somnolence, coma, confusion, or convulsions, collectively known as hypertensive encephalopathy—presumably due to cerebral edema—and these may be quickly reversed with rapidly acting antihypertensive agents. Cerebral blood flow autoregulation is shifted upward in hypertension; the upper limit, if exceeded, leads to vasodilation, exudation of fluid, and cerebral edema (Strandgaard, 1989). More commonly, however, when these severe cerebral symptoms develop, a vascular accident has occurred rather than cerebral edema.

Acute interruption of the blood supply to a localized area of the brain causes a focal neurologic deficit (stroke). The most common type is thrombotic cerebral infarction, which may be manifested by a "lacuna" stroke (see later); the least common is cerebral embolus; and intermediate in frequency is cerebral hemorrhage from rupture of a berry aneurysm or a Charcot-Bouchard microaneurysm of one of the small arteries of the brain. Subarachnoid hemorrhage may also occur. Impaired blood supply may be either intra- or extracranial and may occur at a variety of sites in any of the extracranial arteries, especially the internal carotid, basilar, and vestibular arteries. The intracranial sites for atherosclerosis are chiefly the middle cerebral artery and the circle of Willis (Figure 9–7).

E. Claudication: When atherosclerosis involves the aorta and the arteries of the lower extremities, patients may present with intermittent claudication, and hypertension is only noted incidentally.

F. Chest Pain: As indicated under heart failure (above), coronary heart disease frequently complicates hypertension (see Chapter 8). Hypertension accelerates atherosclerosis of the coronary arteries, especially if patients have concomitant lipid abnormalities. Coronary disease is uncommon in population groups with serum cholesterol concentrations under 140–160 mg/dL despite the presence of hypertension. Patients may develop angina pectoris or

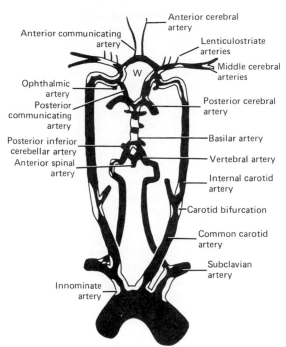

Figure 9–7. Major vascular lesions in stroke. Shown are the extracranial and intracranial arteries supplying blood to the brain as well as to the circle of Willis (W) and its principal branches. The main locations of atherosclerosis of the cerebral vessels are the carotid bifurcation and takeoff of the branches from the aorta and of the innominate and subclavian arteries. (Courtesy of LC McHenry, Jr.) (Reproduced, with permission, from Cooper ES, West JW: Hypertension and stroke. Cardiovasc Med 1977;2:429.)

myocardial infarction; chest pain may not be due to dissection of the aorta but to angina pectoris and myocardial ischemia. Severe chest pain radiating to the back, followed by interruption of the arterial supply to the head, neck, back, and lower extremities, occurs after dissection of the aorta. Hypertension may be noted only incidentally in patients who present with severe chest pain simulating acute myocardial infarction or with acute aortic insufficiency from proximal dissection of the aorta.

Signs

The physical signs in hypertension are related to the height of the blood pressure, its underlying cause, its duration and severity, the presence and degree of involvement of the target organ, and complications resulting from vascular involvement.

A. Blood Pressure: Varying levels of blood pressure on different occasions of measurement are the rule in hypertension. Many patients with elevated pressures on the first examination have normal or lower pressures on subsequent ones; this is especially true in isolated systolic hypertension.

The patient should be relaxed, comfortably warm, and unhurried, and the physician's routine should include allowing the patient to adjust to the examining room. The pressure must be taken in both arms to avoid discrepancies caused by atherosclerosis of the subclavian artery; the arm in which the pressure is to be taken on subsequent occasions should be noted, especially if there is a discrepancy between them. Pressure in the legs should be determined at least on the initial examination to exclude coarctation of the aorta.

Accurate technique in taking the blood pressure is essential, and nurses, field workers, and others must be carefully instructed in placement of the rubber bag over the artery and the speed of inflation and deflation; the size of the arm cuff should be appropriate to the circumference of the upper arm (O'Brien, 1985). Guidelines for determining the blood pressure in children can be found in de Man (1991).

The body position of the patient is also important; when the patient sits, the diastolic pressure may increase over recumbent levels. The systolic pressure may stay the same or occasionally may fall slightly in the standing position, but it may increase in the sitting position. If the patient is hypovolemic as a result of administration of diuretics or has postural hypertension from antihypertensive agents interfering with adrenergic transmission, the systolic and diastolic pressures may be considerably lower in the sitting and

standing positions than in recumbency; the sitting position is preferred for serial readings. In autonomic insufficiency, postural hypotension is accompanied by little or no tachycardia, in contrast to the tachycardia that occurs in postural hypotension due to hypovolemia. This helps identify the cause of hypotension if that should occur.

Because of the transient rise in pressure that occurs with the stress of the examination in the sometimes threatening environment of the doctor's office, a raised pressure (unless it is very high) must be present on at least three different occasions of measurement before one considers the pressure to be representative. Sometimes the pressure is so variable that it is elevated on one occasion but well within the normal range on another; this may occur in 10–20% of individuals during any short period of time. It then becomes necessary to obtain frequent office, home, or ambulatory blood pressure readings over a period of weeks or even months or to have readings taken by a nurse in the office under relaxed circumstances without the doctor being present. Ambulatory monitoring of the blood pressure, once normal values are established, may resolve the dilemma quickly and help define when treatment is desirable (Pickering, 1992).

1. Home measurement and ambulatory blood pressure recordings– The patient or a member of the patient's family can be taught to take blood pressure readings at home with simple blood pressure

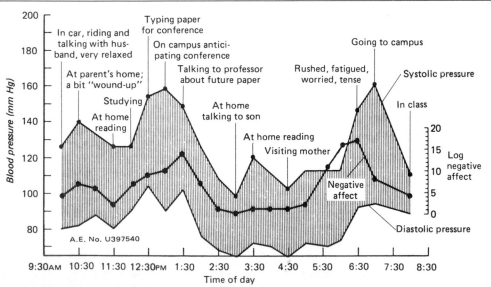

Figure 9–8. Serial blood pressure obtained with ambulatory blood pressure recordings correlated with patient's activities and emotions. The negative affect scale was derived from the patient's serial entries on an adjective checklist coincident with each blood pressure recording. The peak blood pressure readings, both systolic and diastolic, occurred when the patient was on the university campus where she returned after a lapse of many years in order to get her PhD. Each time she was on the campus, the negative affect was greater. She admitted that she really did not want to get her PhD. (Reproduced, with permission, from Sokolow M et al: Preliminary studies relating portably recorded blood pressures to daily life events in patients with essential hypertension. Bibl Psychiatr 1970;144:164. S Karger AG, Basel.)

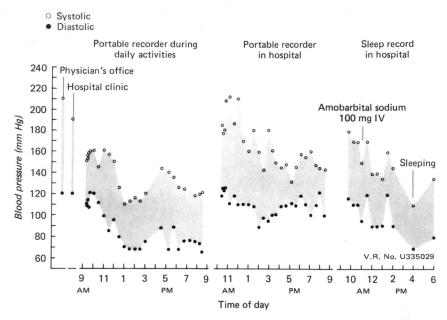

Figure 9–9. Ambulatory blood pressure recordings in a patient who had normal pressures during his daily activities but elevated pressures when in the hospital clinic. When he was put to sleep in the hospital with intravenous sodium amobarbital, his pressures were similar to those during his outside activities.

devices, usually at rest in the sitting position. Home readings in relaxed circumstances are usually more uniform than ambulatory pressures taken throughout the day at work, in social situations, etc. Systolic and diastolic pressures taken three or four times a day can be averaged into weekly mean pressures. Mean blood pressures so obtained are reliable not only in establishing the presence of hypertension but also in providing a baseline to evaluate treatment. Home blood pressures are lower than office pressures but higher than ambulatory ones (Pickering, 1991). The expense of ambulatory pressures makes home pressures a reasonable alternative. These ancillary techniques are usually needed only when raised pressures are mild to moderate (< 180/105 mm Hg). Examples of the use of ambulatory blood pressure monitoring are shown in Figures 9–8 and 9–9. Table 9–2 shows office and ambulatory pressures related to severity of hypertension.

Table 9–2. Ambulatory and office mean systolic and diastolic blood pressures related to degree of severity of hypertensive complications.[1]

Class or Grade of Severity[2]	Overall Severity	Severity of Individual Complications		
		Odular Funduscopic Abnormalities	Left Ventricular Hypertrophy	Cardiac Enlargement
Ambulatory (mm Hg)				
0	137/82	139/83	147/89	155/94
I	150/91	152/92	161/99	
II	165/101	171/105	168/100	162/98
III	192/124	207/128	198/128	171/114
Office (mm Hg)				
0	148/94	154/96	158/99	170/104
I	167/101	167/102	178/108	
II	181/112	183/113	187/111	181/110
III	206/125	237/131	220/129	177/116

[1] Reproduced, with permission, from the American Heart Association, Inc., Sokolow M et al: Relationship between the level of blood pressure measured casually and by portable recorders and severity of complications in essential hypertension. Circulation 1966;34:279.
[2] Classes of severity are graded 0–III depending on the presence and degree of changes in the fundi, ECG, chest film, and renal function. Class 0 denotes no abnormalities other than a raised blood pressure. (For further details see Sokolow & Perloff, 1961.)

Even when office blood pressures are more than moderately raised, an occasional patient will have essentially normal readings at home when pressures are taken by someone other than a physician or when pressures are recorded by a portable apparatus. Prolonged recording with intra-arterial or automatic devices, especially during sleep, is valuable in assessing hypertension and may demonstrate a marked decrease in pressures in the early morning hours (Figure 9–1). Ambulatory pressures are particularly helpful in mild to moderate hypertension. Target organ damage is more frequent when ambulatory as well as office pressures are raised, indicating the need for pharmacologic therapy (see below).

B. Signs in Target Organs: Particular emphasis should be placed on the following signs in assessing involvement of the target organs affected by hypertension or its vascular complications.

1. Retina– One should note particularly the degree of narrowing or irregularity of the arterioles and the presence of arteriovenous defects ("nicking" or "nipping"), flame-shaped or circular hemorrhages or fluffy cotton-wool exudates, or papilledema with blurring of the temporal edge or elevation of the optic disk. Keith, Wagener, and Barker (1939) have classified the retinal changes (called Keith-Wagener changes) as follows:

KW I	Minimal arteriolar narrowing, irregularity of the lumen, and increased light reflex.
KW II	More marked narrowing with focal spasm, more marked irregularity, and arteriovenous nicking with changes in course and distention of the vein as it crosses the arteriole. The arteriole and the venule travel in the same sheath, and when there is thickening of the arteriole it compresses the venule.
KW III	In addition to the arteriolar changes noted previously, multiple flame-shaped hemorrhages and fluffy "cotton wool" exudates are scattered throughout the retinas. These are due to localized axon swellings and swollen nerve fibers in avascular areas (Figure 9–10). Hard, very small, sharply defined translucent exudates are due to exudation in a different part of the retina, are of lesser significance, and do not indicate acute arteriolar damage.
KW IV	Any of the above with the addition of papilledema with blurring of the temporal side of the optic disk and elevation of the disk.

Blurring of the nasal edge of the disk alone is not necessarily due to papilledema. Old, healed papilledema in the absence of current elevation of the disk margins is often revealed by the presence of small collateral vessels crossing the edge of the disk.

"Benign" hypertension is the rule when KW I and

KW II are present, whereas KW III and KW IV are associated with accelerated or malignant hypertension. When malignant hypertension develops abruptly with only a short history of hypertension, patients may have hemorrhages, exudates, or papilledema in the absence of arteriolar changes or arteriolar nicking.

The Keith-Wagener classification has some deficiencies, particularly in the differentiation of hypertensive from atherosclerotic changes in KW I and II and in the interpretation of single hemorrhages and "hard" exudates. The two processes, hypertension and atherosclerosis, are independent entities, but hypertension accelerates atherosclerosis. When the arterioles are narrowed and irregular and compress the venules, the findings are a combination of the two pathologic processes and are not due to hypertension alone; therefore, arteriovenous nicking indicates the presence of atherosclerosis and, by inference, a longer duration of the hypertensive process. The fundal changes of accelerated hypertension are an urgent indication for immediate and vigorous antihypertensive therapy.

Retinopathy is more common in diabetics who also have an elevated blood pressure, suggesting the need for rigorous antihypertensive treatment that may reduce the incidence of retinopathy in these patients.

2. Heart– Examination of the heart and blood vessels may reveal evidence of left ventricular hypertrophy, left ventricular failure, or involvement of the various arteries by atherosclerosis. Raised systemic vascular resistance increases the afterload on the left ventricle, and, depending upon the stage of the disease, the heart may show concentric hypertrophy or combined hypertrophy and dilation. Although left ventricular hypertrophy is initially compensatory—reducing wall stress—and beneficial following the development of hypertension with raised systemic vascular resistance, progressive left ventricular hypertrophy reaches a point at which the increased left ventricular mass no longer is able to compensate for the raised arterial pressure, so its contractile ability deteriorates, leading to the development of left ventricular failure. Combined hypertrophy and dilation represent the earliest evidence of left ventricular failure.

Left ventricular wall thickness and left ventricular mass as determined by echocardiography are the best signs of left ventricular hypertrophy. The upper limit of normal for left ventricular wall thickness at autopsy is usually considered to be 1.5 cm, whereas heart weight is related to total body weight and is greater in men than in women. Heart weight exceeding 400 g is abnormal in either sex, though 360 g is usually considered the upper limit of normal.

As shown by Traube in the late 19th century, the best bedside sign of left ventricular hypertrophy is a left ventricular heave, a localized sustained lift of the left ventricular impulse. When the carotid pulse is felt

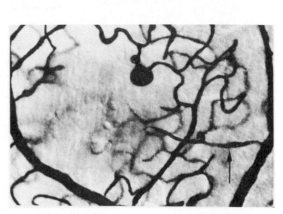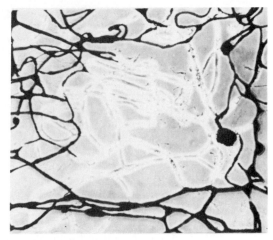

Figure 9–10. *Left:* Retina of a patient with malignant hypertensive retinopathy, showing a cotton-wool spot. The capillaries within the affected area have failed to become injected, whereas the capillaries at the margin are dilated and show aneurysmal formation. Swollen nerve fibers may be seen in the avascular area. The terminal arteriole (arrow) showed hyalin lipid occlusion. (Injected with India ink; stain: oil red 0; × 90.) *Right:* Retina of a patient with malignant hypertensive retinopathy, showing a cotton-wool spot. The retina has been digested, revealing that capillaries are present within the uninjected zone; they appear patent and consist of simple basement membrane tubes without endothelial cells or pericytes. (Injected with India ink; × 130.) (Reproduced, with permission, from Ashton N: Pathophysiology of retinal cotton-wool spots. Br Med Bull 1970;26:143.)

together with the point of maximal impulse, normally the PMI falls before the carotid pulse. In the supine position, if the PMI is maintained beyond the carotid pulse, left ventricular hypertrophy is present. Because concentric hypertrophy is the rule prior to dilation and left ventricular failure, the heart is not displaced to the left unless cardiac failure is present. The decreased distensibility of the thick left ventricle commonly produces a presystolic gallop (S_4); this does not indicate cardiac failure but is a sign of decreased left ventricular compliance. The presence of a left ventricular heave and an S_4 indicates established left ventricular hypertrophy and usually long-standing disease.

If the patient has been untreated or inadequately treated with antihypertensive agents, there may be evidence of left and right heart failure with chronic passive congestion of the liver. (Some mechanisms leading to hypertensive heart failure are illustrated in Figure 9–11). Diastolic dysfunction (not in the figure) with "stiff heart syndrome" and decreased compliance of the left ventricle may cause heart failure independent of or additive to systolic dysfunction (see Chapter 10). This is present in about one-third of the elderly hypertensive patients with congestive heart failure.

Left ventricular hypertrophy may be prevented or reversed by antihypertensive therapy. Left ventricular

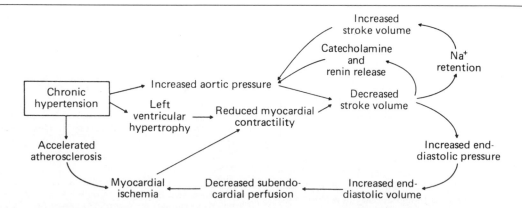

Figure 9–11. Some mechanisms initiated by hypertension that may lead to left ventricular decompensation. Vicious circles tend to aggravate the problem. (Redrawn and reproduced, with permission, from Cohn JN et al: Hypertension and the heart. Arch Intern Med 1974;133:969.)

hypertrophy is an important prognostic sign. Assessment of left ventricular mass by echocardiography is the most sensitive clinical method of determining left ventricular hypertrophy; the ECG is highly specific but less sensitive. Left ventricular hypertrophy is a significant precursor of congestive heart failure, coronary heart disease, ventricular arrhythmias, and sudden death (Tarazi, 1987; Siegel, 1990; Frohlich, 1989; Koren, 1991). Its presence makes antihypertensive treatment more urgent. Although there is a relatively poor correlation between left ventricular hypertrophy and *office* blood pressures, there is a more significant relationship between left ventricular mass, left ventricular hypertrophy determined by electrocardiography, and *ambulatory* pressures. Hypertension is a major predisposing risk factor for atherosclerosis; coronary heart disease and stroke are the two most common causes of death in hypertensive patients. Angina, myocardial infarction, and cerebral ischemic syndromes may be the presenting or predominant clinical features. Coronary reserve is diminished, and microvascular abnormalities may explain angina in the absence of overt coronary lesions on angiography (Dellsperger, 1990; Brush, 1988; Tarazi, 1987). Exercise and dipyridamole-thallium-201 scintigraphy may detect myocardial ischemia in asymptomatic patients with left ventricular hypertrophy (Tubau, 1989; Houghton, 1992).

3. Arteries and veins– Hypertension induces arterial and arteriolar disease, predominantly in the arterioles and interlobular arteries of the kidney but also in the larger arteries of the body. Early in the course of hypertensive disease, the arterioles and arteries are histologically normal, because the rise in pressure is due to functional vasoconstriction with decreased arteriolar caliber and not to structural change. Later on, the renal arterioles demonstrate medial hypertrophy and intimal fibrous thickening, resulting in a lower lumen-to-wall ratio and raised systemic vascular resistance even at full vasodilation. Arterioles throughout the body are affected to various degrees, but in almost all cases of established hypertension the renal arterioles show the structural changes of nephrosclerosis (Figure 9–12).

The larger arteries are usually spared in established hypertension until atherosclerosis develops as an independent process accelerated by the hypertension. When this occurs, the arterial lesions show no distinguishing feature that separates atherosclerosis accelerated by hypertension from atherosclerosis that develops independently of hypertension. The lesions may appear in the aorta, the coronary arteries (Table 9–3), the arteries to the lower extremities, and the arteries of the neck and brain. Deposition of collagen and calcium in the media of the large arteries may occur in older patients independently of atherosclerosis and cause increased stiffness and decreased compliance resulting in enhanced pulse pressure, and isolated systolic hypertension.

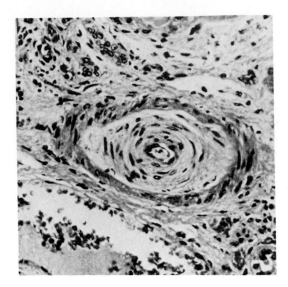

Figure 9–12. Cellular intimal hyperplasia (proliferative endarteritis or endarteritis fibrosa) in an interlobular renal artery (H&E; × 220). (Reproduced, with permission, from Kincaid-Smith P, McMichael J, Murphy EA: The clinical course and pathology of hypertension with papilloedema [malignant hypertension]. Q J Med 1958;27:117.)

Atherosclerosis of the aorta aggravates medial necrosis, which is more common in hypertensive atherosclerotic disease, and patients may develop aortic medial changes and even dissection, pathologically indistinguishable from cystic medial necrosis in Marfan's syndrome.

The jugular venous pulse is usually normal in the absence of right ventricular failure; the carotid pulses are usually normal in volume and upstroke unless the patient has coarctation of the aorta, in which case the carotid pulse is unusually prominent and jerky. The presence of bruits over the carotid artery should always be sought as a possible clue to the presence of atherosclerotic disease of the internal carotid arteries. The presence of pulmonary rales is valuable in recognizing early left ventricular failure. If the failure is

Table 9-3. Coronary arteriosclerosis in hypertensive and nonhypertensive patients.[1]

Grade of Coronary Artery Disease (Left Artery)	Percentage of Patients in Each Grade	
	Hypertensives (152 Cases)	Nonhypertensives (146 Cases)
None	11.2	71.2
Slight to moderate	50.6	26.0
Severe	38.1	2.8
Thrombus	21.0	0

[1] Modified from Bell ET, Clawson BJ: Primary (essential) hypertension: A study of 420 cases. Arch Pathol 1928;5:939. Reproduced, with permission, from Heptinstall RH: Relation of hypertension to changes in the arteries. Prog Cardiovasc Dis 1974;17:25.

more obvious and more severe, pulsus alternans may be noted. Particular note should be made of the volume and character of all the pulses and their symmetry on the two sides. This serves not only to demonstrate coarctation of the aorta if the pulses of the lower extremities are weak and delayed as compared with those of the radial arteries but also to provide a baseline in the event the patient develops chest pain, with variation in the various pulses suggesting aortic dissection. Bruits should be sought, especially over the femoral and popliteal arteries, to determine the presence of atherosclerosis of these vessels. Bruits should also be sought in the epigastrium and in the flanks, since they may suggest renovascular hypertension. Examination of the abdominal aorta may reveal an aneurysm as a complication of concomitant atherosclerosis.

Coarctation of the aorta is strongly suggested by weak or delayed femoral pulses in comparison with the radial pulses, a basal systolic ejection murmur transmitted to the interscapular area, and palpable collateral intercostal arteries along the posterior-inferior rib margins and scapular borders. The carotid pulse is unusually prominent and jerky. Careful palpation below each rib posteriorly should be done in a search for pulsating intercostal arteries, which are prominent in coarctation of the aorta and serve as collateral vessels to arteries below the coarcted site. (See also Chapter 11.)

4. Kidneys– Long-standing hypertension produces progressive renal nephrosclerosis with tubular atrophy, progressive scarring of the glomeruli, and slight shrinkage of the size of the kidney. Unless malignant hypertension supervenes, the clinical findings of renal failure are uncommon; however, the kidneys are somewhat small and granular, with a thin cortex.

When the hypertension is more severe or occurs rapidly, the interlobular arteries of the kidney become involved, and there may also be focal necrosis of the renal arterioles (Figure 9–13). This combination of abnormalities impairs renal blood flow and glomerular filtration rate, which in turn increases the secretion of renin and the production of angiotensin, further impairing renal function. This sequence of events is common in accelerated or malignant hypertension, in which fibrinoid necrosis of arterioles, especially of the kidney, occurs.

Polycystic kidneys are suspected if the kidneys are large and easily palpable, especially in the presence of long-standing hypertension, when the kidneys would be expected to be small.

5. Brain– In long-standing hypertension, so-called Charcot-Bouchard microaneurysms (Figure 9–14) may develop in the small arteries of the brain; rupture of these small aneurysms is responsible for cerebral hemorrhage that commonly interrupts the course of long-standing hypertension. MRI may reveal small, deep infarcts of the brain (lacunae), which may present as stroke or be clinically silent. Lacunae were

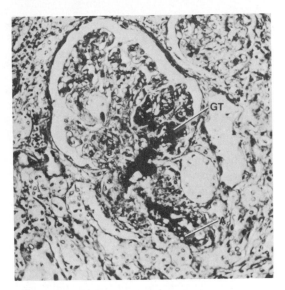

Figure 9–13. Fibrinoid necrosis in an afferent arteriole (A) extending into the glomerular tuft (GT) (Mallory's azo carmine; × 180). (Reproduced, with permission, from Kincaid-Smith P, McMichael J, Murphy EA: The clinical course and pathology of hypertension with papilloedema [malignant hypertension]. Q J Med 1958;27:117.)

found in almost half of elderly (> 70 years) patients; the silent lesions were more closely related to ambulatory than to office pressures as well as to the presence of left ventricular hypertrophy (Shimada, 1990).

In addition, the brain may show atherosclerotic occlusion or thrombosis in the internal carotid, basilar, or vertebral artery system as well as thrombosis in the vessels of the circle of Willis. Cerebral infarction may then occur and may become hemorrhagic if hemorrhagic transformation results or if anticoagulants

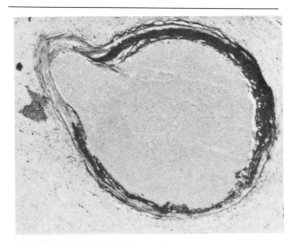

Figure 9–14. Cross section of Charcot-Bouchard microaneurysm showing plasma insudation of wall (PTAH; × 90). (Reproduced, with permission, from Russell RW: How does blood pressure cause stroke? Lancet 1975;2:1283.)

are used. Cerebral hemorrhage entering the cerebral ventricles may also result from rupture of microaneurysms.

6. Central nervous system– Examination for evidence of residual neurologic deficit from previous cerebral infarction may be fruitful. There may be a positive Babinski or Hoffman reflex, hemiparesis, hemiplegia, or hemianopia. The presence of ataxia may indicate involvement of the posterior-inferior cerebellar artery.

7. Endocrine dysfunction– The patient should be examined for signs suggesting any of several types of endocrine abnormalities. Cushing's syndrome is suspected if one observes central truncal obesity, hirsutism, acne, purple striae, moon facies, and thin skin with ecchymoses. Primary aldosteronism is suggested by muscular weakness, hypoactive deep tendon reflexes, and diminished or absent vasomotor circulatory reflexes. Pheochromocytoma is suspected if an attack of headache, sweating, palpitations, and a markedly increased blood pressure is induced by an examination over the upper abdomen that presses on a tumor. Almost all patients with pheochromocytoma are symptomatic.

Laboratory Findings

Laboratory investigations are designed to determine the involvement of any of the target organs affected by hypertension and to recognize evidence of secondary hypertension.

A. Urinalysis: Urinalysis is usually normal until renal impairment occurs, when the specific gravity may become low and mild proteinuria may appear. In malignant hypertension, there may be substantial hematuria and proteinuria, approaching values suggesting nephrosis. A low fixed specific gravity suggests advanced renal parenchymal disease or the hypokalemic nephropathy of primary aldosteronism. The presence of granular or red cell casts and hematuria suggests glomerulonephritis. The presence of pyuria favors chronic pyelonephritis, but if advanced renal failure is present, the microscopic appearance of the urinary sediment is often not helpful in diagnosis. In connective tissue disorders, such as lupus erythematosus, the urine sediment may show red cells, white cells, and casts of all types at the same time (Krupp, 1943).

A fresh, clean voided urine specimen should be examined for bacteria. If organisms are found, the specimen should be cultured and quantitative bacterial counts performed to establish the presence of cystitis or chronic pyelonephritis. If no organisms are found but other features of the history are suggestive of urinary tract infection, cultures should be repeated, because the bacilluria in chronic pyelonephritis may be intermittent.

B. Blood Chemistry: In advanced renal parenchymal disease, the serum creatinine and blood urea nitrogen are elevated, and anemia associated with advanced azotemia may be present. In aldosteronism, the serum or plasma urea nitrogen and serum creatinine are usually normal; renal function is not severely impaired, but the serum potassium is low, and serum sodium and bicarbonate are increased.

It is usually not necessary to order more sensitive renal function studies if the serum creatinine and blood urea nitrogen are normal; however, if the serum urea nitrogen approaches 20 mg/dL or the serum creatinine is 1.3 mg/dL or above, it is wise to determine the creatinine clearance as a measure of the glomerular filtration rate, because the latter may be reduced even though the serum creatinine may be within the normal range.

Electrocardiographic Findings

A. Left Ventricular Hypertrophy: The ECG is the most readily available specific means of establishing the presence of left ventricular hypertrophy, though echocardiographic determination of left ventricular mass is more sensitive. The ECG is often abnormal when there is no left ventricular heave and when the chest x-ray shows no left ventricular enlargement. The ECG reflects hypertrophy and not dilation (except perhaps in advanced left ventricular hypertrophy), whereas the chest x-ray reveals enlargement rather than hypertrophy. The earliest electrocardiographic sign of left ventricular hypertrophy is increased voltage of the QRS complexes in the left ventricular leads. As hypertrophy continues, the T waves become of lower amplitude, and this change is followed by slight depression of the ST segment; later, the ST segment depression is more marked and associated with asymmetrically inverted T waves in the left ventricular leads. In the fully developed pattern, the left ventricular QRS voltage is high and the ST segment in these leads is depressed, with a convex contour followed by an asymmetrically inverted T wave. Table 9–4 sets forth the electrocardiographic criteria for the diagnosis of left ventricular hypertrophy in adults. Some authorities use only abnormal QRS voltage to define left ventricular hypertrophy and do not include the ST–T (repolarization) abnormalities, thus eliminating the more advanced degrees of left ventricular hypertrophy. This weakens the electrocardiographic diagnosis of left ventricular hypertrophy; ST–T abnormalities, in conjunction with high QRS voltage, indicate a greater degree of left ventricular hypertrophy and should be included in the criteria for left ventricular hypertrophy. Myocardial ischemia must be considered when ST–T abnormalities are present; myocardial ischemic ST–T changes have been found by stress electrocardiography or Holter monitoring, and coronary angiographic lesions have been noted in about half of asymptomatic hypertensive patients who have voltage and repolarization electrocardiographic abnormalities. Microvascular coronary disease and decreased coronary vasodilator reserve has also been found in advanced

Table 9–4. Criteria for electrocardiographic diagnosis of left ventricular hypertrophy in adults over 30 years of age.

Standard limb leads
(1) Voltage $R_1 + S_3 = 25$ mm or more.
(2) RST_1 depressed 0.5 mm or more.
(3) T_1 flat, diphasic, or inverted, particularly when associated with (2) and a prominent R wave.
(4) T_2 and T_3 diphasic or inverted in the presence of tall R waves and findings in (2).
(5) T_3 greater than T_1 in the presence of left axis deviation and high voltage QRS complex in leads I and III.

Precordial leads
(1) $RV_5 + SV_1$ more than 35 mm.
(2) Tallest R + deepest S more than 45 mm.
(3) Voltage of R wave in V_5 or V_6 exceeds 26 mm.
(4) RST segment depressed more than 0.5 mm in V_4, V_5, or V_6.
(5) A flat, diphasic, or inverted T wave in leads V_{4-6} with normal R and small S waves and findings in (2).
(6) Ventricular activation time in V_5 or V_6 = 0.06 s or more, especially when associated with a tall R wave.

Unipolar limb leads
(1) RST segment depressed more than 0.5 mm in aVL or aVF.
(2) Flat, diphasic, or inverted T wave, with an R wave of 6 mm or more in aVL or aVF and findings in (1).
(3) Voltage of R wave in aVL exceeds 11 mm.
(4) Upright wave in aVR.

left ventricular hypertrophy and may explain impaired coronary perfusion and myocardial ischemia (Dellsperger, 1990; Houghton, 1992). The ST–T changes in leads V_5 and V_6 owing to left ventricular hypertrophy may normalize with treatment of the hypertension; this is uncommon if the ST–T abnormalities are caused by chronic coronary disease. Examples of the development and regression of the electrocardiographic changes in left ventricular hypertrophy are shown in Figures 9–15 and 9–16. Patients with increased left ventricular volume may not have the typical electrocardiographic signs of left ventricular hypertrophy, because dilation of the left ventricle decreases the left ventricular QRS voltage but not the ST–T changes in advanced left ventricular hypertrophy.

B. Electrocardiographic Differentiation From Coronary Disease: In myocardial ischemia (see Chapter 8), the ST segment when depressed is horizontally depressed and the T wave when inverted is symmetrically inverted with or without ST depression. The characteristic ST–T changes in advanced left ventricular hypertrophy include depressed ST and asymmetrically inverted T waves and occur only in leads reflecting left ventricular potentials. The in-

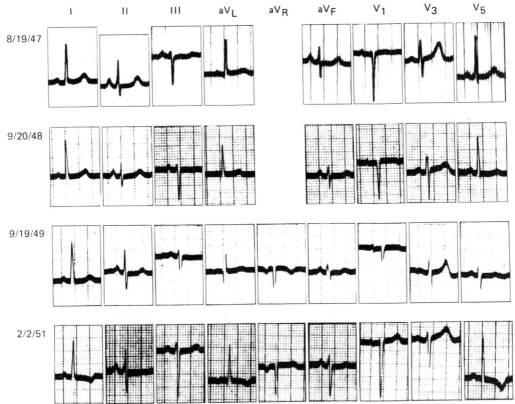

Figure 9–15. Progressive ST–T abnormalities in leads I, aVL, and V5 between 1947 and 1951 in a 53-year-old woman with left ventricular hypertrophy. Serial chest x-rays showed no change in the size of the heart during this period. (Reproduced, with permission, from Grubschmidt HA, Sokolow M: The reliability of high voltage of the QRS complex as a diagnostic sign of left ventricular hypertrophy in adults. Am Heart J 1957;54:689.)

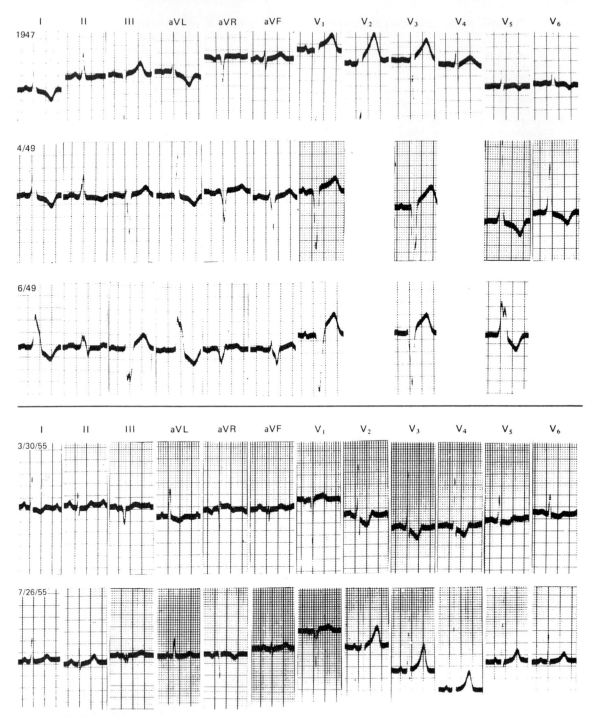

Figure 9–16. Top: Hypertensive cardiovascular disease and angina pectoris in a 73-year-old man. Cardiac enlargement 32%. Note progression from left ventricular hypertrophy to incomplete left bundle branch block to complete left bundle branch block with a wide monophasic QRS complex in lead I. **Bottom:** Malignant hypertension on 3/30/55 reversed to almost normotensive levels on 7/26/55 following unilateral nephrectomy in a 62-year-old man. Complete return of ST–T changes in leads V_{2-6} to normal in 4 months.

verse of this pattern is present in leads to the right of the transitional zone—ie, in the right precordial leads, the ST segment is elevated and there is a tall, asymmetrically elevated T wave. This is in contrast to myocardial ischemia, in which the ST and T abnormalities seen in the left ventricular leads (V_{4-6}) may involve V_2 and V_3 as well, crossing the transitional zone. The ECG may also reveal evidence of previous myocardial infarction with classic Q waves or ischemic ST segments. In patients with long-standing hypertension, especially if there have been multiple episodes of myocardial ischemia, peripheral left ventricular conduction defects may be present with slurred QRS complexes, usually with a QRS duration less than 0.12 s. Even with advanced left ventricular hypertrophy, the frontal plane axis rarely exceeds −30 degrees; when the axis is farther to the left, in the range of −45 degrees, a left anterior fascicular block is superimposed and the axis change is not due to the left ventricular hypertrophy per se. Progressive abnormalities may include incomplete and complete left bundle branch block.

C. Effect of Drugs on ECG: In hypertensive patients receiving diuretic agents with resultant hypokalemia, sagging nonspecific ST segments and prominent U waves may be present similar to those found in primary aldosteronism. If the patient has been receiving digitalis, the characteristic sagging ST segments of digitalis and the decreased QT interval resulting from shortening of the action potential may also be present. Other drugs also influence the ECG, but these two are the most common.

Imaging Studies

A. Plain Chest Film: The plain chest film may be completely normal despite hypertension if the concentric hypertrophy has not led to dilation. The convex rounding of the left ventricle seen especially on lateral views may allow the radiologist to suspect the presence of concentric hypertrophy, but it is not until left ventricular dilation has occurred that enlargement of the left ventricle will be confirmed. The chest x-ray may show notching of the ribs in coarctation of the aorta, but this finding is rarely present before the late teen years. If there is left ventricular failure, pulmonary venous engorgement can be seen with or without diversion of blood to the upper lobes, and pleural effusion is also present. In the acute pulmonary edema of hypertension, there may be "bat's wing" densities or fluid in the interlobar spaces. The aortic knob may be enlarged and the descending aorta dilated out of proportion to the patient's age, suggesting the presence of associated aortic atherosclerosis. If the widening is excessive, chronic dissection of the aorta may be suspected; this may be confirmed by imaging techniques, transesophageal echocardiography, or aortography. (For examples of chest x-rays, see Chapter 1.)

B. Intravenous Urograms: Excretory urography may provide evidence of possible renal vascular or renal parenchymal disorders as causes of hypertension.

C. Echocardiographic Findings: Echocardiography is the most sensitive aid in the recognition of left ventricular hypertrophy in hypertension. There are significant correlations among various echocardiographic measurements, radiologic estimates of heart volume, and electrocardiographic evidence of left ventricular hypertrophy. The presence of left ventricular dilation may allow the left ventricular thickness to remain normal, but the left ventricular mass will be increased.

CONSEQUENCES OF UNTREATED HYPERTENSION

The prognosis of untreated hypertension with respect to mortality in hypertension is related to the age, race, and sex of the patient; the height of the blood pressure; abnormalities of the fundi, ECG, and chest x-ray; and the presence or absence of atherosclerotic complications when the patient is first seen; and the presence or absence of significant risk factors for atherosclerosis. Figures 9–4, 9–5, 9–6, 9–17, and 9–18 illustrate the relationships of the vascular complications and the mortality rate to these various factors (Sokolow, 1961; Kannel, 1974). The mortality rate is considerably lower in developing rural communities, perhaps in part because of the lower levels of serum cholesterol in these populations. Similar low mortality data are found in some African countries where hypertension is relatively benign and does not increase the incidence of coronary

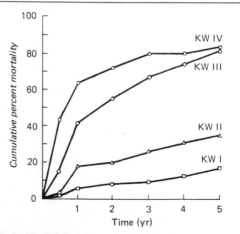

Figure 9–17. Relationship of mortality rate and initial fundal classification in hypertensive patients. (Reproduced, with permission of the American Heart Association, from: Sokolow M, Perloff D: The prognosis of essential hypertension treated conservatively. Circulation 1961;23:697.)

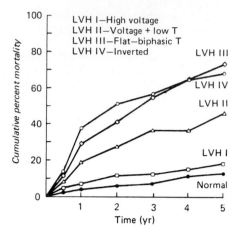

Figure 9–18. Relationship of mortality rate and initial degree of left ventricular hypertrophy (ECG) in hypertensive patients. (Reproduced, with permission of the American Heart Association, from Sokolow M, Perloff D: The prognosis of essential hypertension treated conservatively. Circulation 1961;23:697.)

disease; the combination of hypertension and abnormal plasma lipids apparently is required. Acute coronary events are uncommon in these developing areas but more common in urban communities with more affluent patients.

Complications

Most complications of hypertensive disease and their treatment are discussed elsewhere in this book (left ventricular hypertrophy, cardiac failure, microalbuminuria and renal insufficiency, malignant hypertension, hemorrhagic stroke, myocardial infarction, transient ischemic attacks, cerebral infarction). Hypertension is one of the most important of the known risk factors for the development of cardiovascular disease. Hypertensive encephalopathy and aortic dissection are discussed below. In general, the presence of a significant complication may warrant hospitalization so that patients can be given appropriate treatment for severe hypertension. Ancillary methods of treatment should not be neglected, such as that for cardiac failure, aspirin or other anticoagulants, surgical correction of the carotid artery lesion in transient ischemic attacks, and surgery in aortic dissection. Treatment of the elevated blood pressure is usually of less importance than treating other problems in patients with angina pectoris, myocardial infarction, or atherosclerosis of the iliofemoral circulation with intermittent claudication. After a follow-up of 18 years, 105 cerebral infarctions occurred in the Framingham Study, only ten of which occurred in normotensive persons. Hypertension is the most common and most important precursor of cerebral infarction in stroke (Kannel, 1974, 1976). The pressure may be high in hemorrhagic stroke and hypertensive encephalopathy

with neurologic deficit; these patients should have their blood pressure lowered cautiously, as described in the section on malignant hypertension. Borderline hypertension in early adult life often is associated with a risk of established hypertension and coexists with other coronary risk factors; it requires careful follow-up (Julius, 1990).

Mild Hypertension

The average patient with mild to moderate hypertension is asymptomatic; the only abnormality is the rise in arterial pressure. The patient may complain of nonspecific headache or dizziness, but these have been shown to fluctuate with the emotional state and are unrelated to the height of the blood pressure in benign hypertension. Visual symptoms are absent or unrelated to the blood pressure.

Ambulatory blood pressure recordings may demonstrate "normal" blood pressures in some patients who have a pressor response to the physician and the medical environment. With equivalent office pressures, patients whose ambulatory pressures are low have a better prognosis than those patients in whom both office and ambulatory pressures are elevated.

Moderate Hypertension

Prognostic studies in untreated patients have shown that headaches and dizziness have no adverse prognostic significance unless they are associated with accelerated hypertension or with other evidence of neurologic disorder. When hypertension persists without treatment (as it almost always does), the patient may remain asymptomatic, but examination may reveal evidences of target organ damage (see above). The development of vascular abnormalities such as left ventricular hypertrophy or retinal arteriolar changes presages the development of clinical events and is an adverse prognostic sign (Sokolow, 1961; Perloff, 1983, 1989).

If there is no accelerated phase, the first symptoms may reflect the development of left ventricular failure or stroke.

Hypertensive Encephalopathy & Crisis

This syndrome results from a rapid, considerable rise in blood pressure, causing increased vascular permeability and cerebral edema, resulting in an acute neurologic clinical state that may be rapidly reversible if treated early and vigorously but may develop into malignant hypertension if not managed promptly. The patient complains of severe headache, confusion, impaired vision, restlessness, and perhaps focal neurologic signs. There may be cotton-wool patches in the retina or early papilledema, and the differentiation from malignant hypertension may be difficult. Rapid but graduated reduction of blood pressure usually reverses the process before complications develop in the kidney and heart.

Table 9–5. Symptoms marking onset of malignant phase of hypertension in 104 cases.[1]

Symptom	Number of Cases
Visual impairment	79
Acute headache	6
Gross hematuria	5
Visual impairment and gross hematuria	3
Acute cardiac failure	1
Gastrointestinal upset with nausea, vomiting, and epigastric pain	1
Undetermined due to vagueness of symptoms	9

[1] Reproduced, with permission, from Schottstaedt, MF, Sokolow M: The natural history and course of hypertension with papilledema (malignant hypertension). Am Heart J 1953;45:331.

Malignant Hypertension

Malignant hypertension is a syndrome characterized by a rapidly rising blood pressure (diastolic pressure usually in excess of 130–140 mm Hg), regardless of the cause of the initial hypertension. The initial symptoms are usually visual disturbances associated with papilledema, hemorrhage, and exudate in the fundi; severe suboccipital headaches and weakness; and gross hematuria (Table 9–5). Unless effective antihypertensive therapy is given promptly, there may be severe visual loss, and death usually occurs in less than a year due to uremia, heart failure, or cerebral hemorrhage (Table 9–6). With contemporary treatment, the prognosis of malignant hypertension and hypertensive crises (KW III or KW IV) has dramatically improved, with 5-year survivals in the 50–70% range; in one study it was maintained for 10 years, depending on the grade of retinopathy, (Houston, 1989; Perry, 1966). (See below under Treatment.) Pathologic changes are seen in the arterioles and in the small interlobular arteries (Figures 9–10 and 9–14). The kidney is progressively destroyed by ischemic atrophy of the nephrons, with decrease in glomerular filtration rate and renal blood flow because of fibrinoid necrosis of the arterioles and cellular intimal proliferation of the interlobular arteries. Some patients with pathologically proved fibrinoid necrosis do not have papilledema, but they usually have hemorrhages or exudates in the fundi. Prognostic studies have shown that the 3- to 5-year mortality rate is essentially indistinguishable in untreated patients with KW III fundi as compared with those who have KW IV fundi; both represent accelerated hypertension, KW IV being more severe. In treated patients (see below), the prognosis for patients with KW III fundal changes is better than that of those with KW IV changes.

Examination of the retina for evidence of accelerated hypertension is necessary in all hypertensive patients, because the early stages of the malignant phase may be essentially asymptomatic—though severe headache, acute visual disturbances, and gross hematuria are the usual presenting manifestations. The rapid rise in blood pressure may cause cardiac failure and renal failure within a month, and treatment to lower the blood pressure is therefore urgent. Patients seen early with evidence of accelerated or malignant hypertension may have normal renal function and even absence of proteinuria. This rapidly progresses, however, to malignant hypertension with proteinuria and azotemia and then finally to renal failure. For this reason, treatment is essential before the development of renal failure (Schottstaedt, 1952; Kincaid-Smith, 1959).

Malignant hypertension is a quantitatively more severe form of hypertension, and prevention is more effective than treatment of the established or advanced disease. Accelerated or malignant hypertension is rare in effectively treated hypertensive patients. If no treatment is given, the mortality rate in 1 year is 80% and in 2 years it approaches 100%.

Development of Clinical Manifestations of Atherosclerosis

The patient may develop a symptom indicating atherosclerotic involvement in one of the major vessels. Most common is the development of angina pectoris or acute myocardial infarction, though the first manifestation may be intermittent claudication, transient ischemic cerebral attacks, or even cerebral infarction or cerebral hemorrhage.

Development of Cardiac Disease

A. Hypertensive Heart Failure and Left Ventricular Hypertrophy: In a large series of patients

Table 9–6. Cause of death in relation to initial severity of hypertension[1,2]

Severity of Hyper-tension	Total Number Deaths	Cardiac Failure	"Hypertensive" Causes		Coronary Thrombosis	Cerebro-vascular Accident	Aortic Dissection	Noncardio-vascular Causes
			Uremia	Malignant Hyper-tension				
KW 1 and II	32	2	0	1	8	11	0	10
KW III and IV	121	19	9	17	25	41	3	7

[1] In an additional 8 patients, cause of death was unknown.
[2] Reproduced, with permission, from the American Heart Association, Inc., Sokolow, M, Perloff D: The prognosis of essential hypertension treated conservatively. Circulation 1961;23:697.

followed prospectively for an average of 61/2 years, the prevalence of left ventricular hypertrophy increased as blood pressure increased, and the mortality rate doubled in men when compared with men who had normal ECGs at the outset (Dunn, 1990). Because hypertension is a common cause of heart failure and an important risk factor in accelerating coronary atherosclerosis—and because it is responsible in part for at least half of all deaths from heart failure and for almost all cases of cerebral hemorrhage (Kannel, 1974)—the most important means of preventing cardiovascular disease is to identify and treat hypertension before complications develop. Cardiac failure in hypertension—in the absence of myocardial infarction—is almost always preceded by left ventricular hypertrophy with increased left ventricular mass. Cardiovascular complications occur twice as often and death ten times as often if increased left ventricular mass by echocardiography is present (Koren, 1991).

It is difficult to separate the effects of hypertension and coronary heart disease in causing heart failure when they coexist in the same patient. Cardiac failure is frequent, however, in young adults with coarctation of the aorta and hypertension who do not have coronary disease. The importance of treating the elevated blood pressure and the coarctation in such cases should be readily apparent.

Before the advent of antihypertensive therapy, heart failure was responsible for death in 50% of patients with hypertension. Heart failure is now uncommon in well-treated hypertensives. Paroxysmal or nocturnal dyspnea with or without angina or myocardial ischemia is often the result of hypertension. Once left ventricular failure with paroxysmal dyspnea or pulmonary edema has occurred, the prognosis for life in untreated patients is poor (see Chapter 10) (see also Table 9–6).

B. Effect of Hypertension on Coronary Disease: Coronary artery disease associated with hypertension is commonly present without development of hypertensive heart failure. The evidence supporting the role of hypertension in accelerating coronary heart disease has been corroborated by pathologic data and by the prospective studies of the Framingham group (see Chapter 8). Bell and Clawson (1928) found that severe coronary disease was ten times more common in an autopsied group of patients who had hypertension during life than in a normotensive group (Table 9–3). They also showed a high correlation between the severity of atherosclerosis in the cerebral, carotid, and basilar-vertebral arteries and the systolic blood pressure.

Since the purely hypertensive complications of a raised pressure are prevented or reversed by antihypertensive therapy, the atherosclerotic complications predominate and are the most common cause of disability and death in treated hypertensive patients. Atherosclerotic arterial disease in all its manifestations—cerebral infarction, cerebral hemorrhage, and carotid and extremity atherosclerosis—is particularly prevalent in the hypertensive population, but coronary artery disease has the same manifestations in nonhypertensive atherosclerotic patients as in hypertensive patients.

Dissection of the Aorta

Aortic dissection is a tear through the intima into the media of the aortic wall anywhere from the proximal ascending aorta to the distal aorta beyond the left subclavian artery. Blood then dissects distally and proximally. It is often unrecognized, especially in pregnant women; hypertension is the most important precursor of dissection; Marfan's syndrome is next in importance. Early diagnosis is essential so that treatment can be started to lower the pressure, decrease the rate of rise of left ventricular pressure and left ventricular contraction, and prevent dissection and obstruction of major branches of the aorta and rupture into the pericardial or pleural cavities. Without treatment, acute aortic dissection has an extremely high fatality rate, though 10–15% of patients may have a chronic course. The current status of diagnosis and treatment is summarized by DeSanctis (1987), Gerson (1990), and Glower (1990). The onset is acute in 90% of cases, with severe instantaneous chest pain radiating to the neck, jaw, back, or abdomen, combined with evidence of varying or sequential obstruction of the branches of the aorta and diminished or absent pulses from the carotids to the femoral arteries. The abrupt development of chest pain, aortic insufficiency, diminished or absent pulses, or the appearance of signs of "sympathectomy" on one side and of neurologic deficit with cerebral symptoms should make one think of dissection of the aorta. The pain may be differentiated from that of acute myocardial infarction by its instantaneous onset with maximum severity, the absence of central pulses, and the presence of hypertension despite pain or even shock. Neurologic symptoms and signs occur in about 15% of patients. In rare instances, the dissection is painless or relatively so.

The diagnosis, location, and extent of the dissection can be best established by supravalvular aortography, transesophageal color Doppler echocardiography, CT scans, and MRI (Adachi, 1990), though it can be strongly suspected clinically and radiologically (Figures 9–19 and 9–20).

Aortic dissection has been classified as type I, which involves the proximal ascending aorta and aortic arch, at times extending distally to the iliac arteries; type II, which involves only the ascending aorta and is sometimes combined with type I and called proximal dissection; and type III, which involves only the distal aorta beyond the left subclavian artery. Types I and II can involve the support of the aortic valve, causing aortic insufficiency and heart failure, and are more serious than type III. The pathogenesis

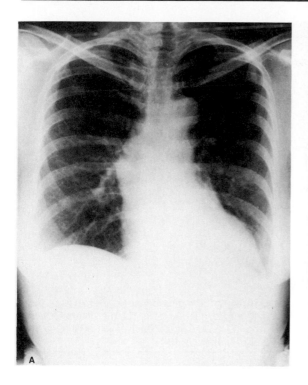
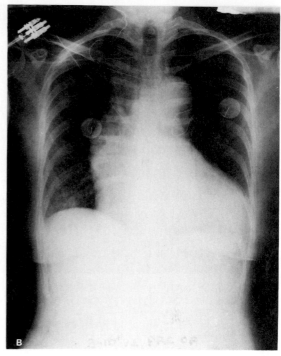
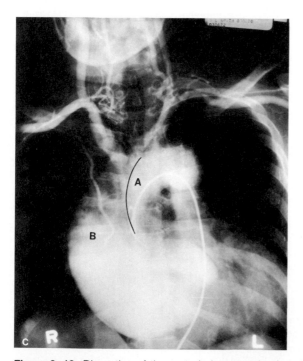
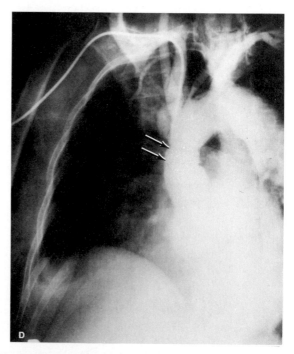

Figure 9–19. Dissection of the aorta in hypertension in a 52-year-old man with severe chest pain. ***A:*** 3/6/72—Plain chest film predissection showing dilated ascending aorta in asymptomatic patient. ***B:*** 3/10/72—Preoperative plain chest film postdissection after sudden severe chest pain showing massive dilation of the ascending and descending aorta with striking changes since A. ***C:*** 3/7/72—Aortogram showing the true channel (A) and the aneurysmal sac (B), partially filled with contrast medium. The dark line shows the separation between the true and false channels. ***D:*** 3/28/72—Postoperative angiogram after resection of the ascending aorta and aneurysmal sac and insertion of a Dacron graft (arrows) from the ascending aorta. Pathologic focal degeneration of media and intimal fibrosis.

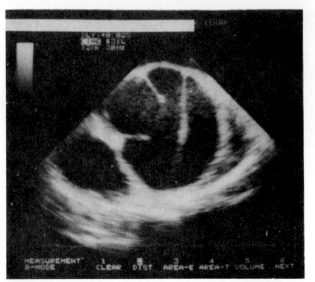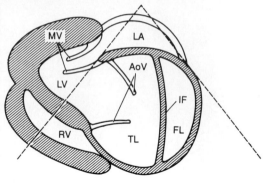

Figure 9–20. Echocardiogram showing the intimal flap, as clearly visualized by transesophageal examination. (MV, mitral valve; LV, left ventricle; LA, left atrium; AoV, aortic valve; IF, intimal flap; RV, right ventricle; TL, true lumen; FL, false lumen.) (Reproduced, with permission, from Adachi H et al: Early diagnosis and surgical intervention of acute aortic dissection by transesophageal color flow mapping. Circulation 1990;82[Suppl IV]:IV-19.)

of dissection is illustrated in Figure 9–21. Types I and II are often classified and treated as proximal (type A), while type III is known as distal dissection (type B).

In proximal dissection, the mortality rate is high; aortic insufficiency may occur, and the aorta may rupture into the pericardium or pleura. After immedi-ate lowering of the blood pressure with intravenous antihypertensive agents, sodium nitroprusside or tri-methaphan combined with a beta-adrenergic drug such as propranolol (to decrease the left ventricular rate of pressure rise, or dP/dt) and establishment of the diagnosis, surgical treatment is recommended.

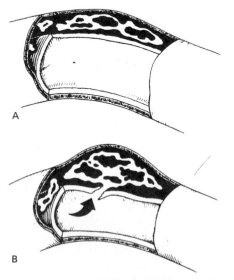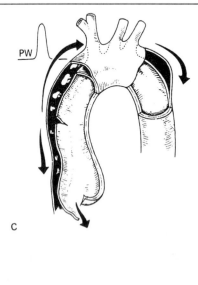

Figure 9–21. Diagrammatic representation of pathogenesis of aortic dissection. *A:* Cystic medial necrosis in the aortic wall sets the stage. *B:* Combined forces acting on the aortic wall result in the intimal tear, directing aortic bloodstream into the diseased media. *C:* Resulting dissecting hematoma is propagated by the pulse wave (PW) produced by each myocardial contraction. (Reproduced, with permission, from Wheat MW: Treatment of dissecting aneurysms of the aorta: Current status. Prog Cardiovasc Dis 1973;16:87.)

With surgical treatment, survival may be as high as 80–85% (Haverich, 1985; Glower, 1990).

Distal dissection may be monitored in the intensive care unit and treated medically with drugs that both lower the arterial pressure and reduce the force of left ventricular contraction and ejection into the weakened aorta. Severe pain is relieved promptly once the arterial pressure has been reduced to the lowest possible level compatible with adequate perfusion of the vital circuits of the body. Intensive antihypertensive therapy prior to definitive diagnostic studies includes sodium nitroprusside or trimethaphan (Arfonad) infusion combined with intravenous beta-blocking agents. Nifedipine, 10–20 mg sublingually or orally, or enalapril intravenously can be substituted after the blood pressure is controlled in order to avoid cyanide toxicity (Crawford, 1990). Surgical treatment is reserved for the patient who fails to respond or develops complications such as extension of the dissection, vascular compromise of organs or limbs, or saccular aneurysm. When intensive intravenous hypertensive therapy is used, the renal output must be carefully monitored and not allowed to decrease below 20 or 30 mL/h.

The prognosis for untreated aortic dissection is poor (Figure 9–22). When the dissection is confined to the distal aorta, medical antihypertensive treatment permits most patients to survive without operation. With reduction in operative mortality rates, there is an increasing tendency to send even distal dissections

to surgery. In proximal aortic dissections, the prognosis is poor with medical treatment alone because of the risks of aortic insufficiency, cardiac failure, rupture into the pericardium, or progression of the dissection. With surgical treatment of proximal dissections, the mortality rate in 2 weeks has decreased from 80% to 10–15% (Glower, 1990). Medical treatment should be continued following surgery in order to prevent a subsequent tear and to control the complications of hypertension. Transesophageal echocardiography is valuable in follow-up of either medical or surgical treatment (Mohr-Kahaly, 1989).

DISEASES & DISORDERS ASSOCIATED WITH SECONDARY HYPERTENSION

Secondary hypertension may result from a variety of known diseases or disorders—in contrast to primary or essential hypertension.

Prevalence of Secondary Hypertension

The frequency of secondary hypertension in the hypertensive population at large has apparently been considerably overestimated, presumably because most of the reported studies have dealt with hospitalized patients. In randomly selected patients, the prevalence is now considered to be 1–5%—unless the patient has severe hypertension, in which case the prevalence is higher. The vigor with which diagnostic investigations for secondary hypertension are conducted obviously influences the frequency with which it is found. A higher percentage of renal artery stenosis amenable to surgery can be found if aggressive search for secondary causes, as by renal angiography, is performed in patients with severe hypertension (see below).

RENAL DISEASE

1. RENAL ARTERY STENOSIS

The most common cause of significant renal artery stenosis is atherosclerosis, followed by fibromuscular hyperplasia; small renal artery; small kidney; and miscellaneous lesions, including thrombosis, aneurysm, and fibrosis. Atherosclerosis occurs in older patients with severe disease of recent onset that is often resistant to treatment. Fibromuscular hyperplasia occurs in younger individuals—usually females—with milder disease.

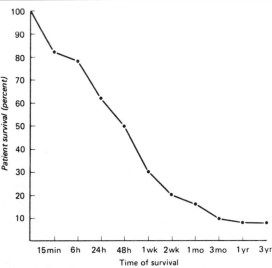

Figure 9–22. Graphic illustration of the length of survival of 963 patients with acute aortic dissection who were not treated. (Reproduced, with permission, from Wheat MW: Treatment of dissecting aneurysms of the aorta: Current status. Prog Cardiovasc Dis 1973;16;87; as modified from Anagnostopoulos CE, Prabhaker MJS, Kittle CF: Aortic dissections and dissecting aneurysms. Am J Cardiol 1972;30:263.)

The case for a primary role for the renin-angiotensin-aldosterone (RAA) system was strengthened with the demonstration of a marked increase in plasma renin within a few minutes after ligation of the renal artery in a dog. Barger (1979) further established the role of the RAA system by showing the marked decrease in blood pressure when converting enzyme inhibitors were given and then withdrawn in these experimental dogs. In humans with severe hypertension secondary to renal artery stenosis, plasma renin is usually elevated, but in mild to moderate hypertension, the plasma renin is usually normal.

The kidney has been shown to produce antihypertensive factors that counteract the effects of constricting one renal artery in the dog. When the uninvolved kidney is removed, the rise in blood pressure is more brisk and more sustained, indicating that the normal kidney has an antihypertensive function. Vasodilator lipid and tissue substances such as kinins, prostaglandins, and nitric oxide are present in the kidney and may counteract the RAA factors that elevate blood pressure. Decreases in prostaglandin E, prostacyclin, or kallikrein-bradykinin all have been considered possible pathogenetic factors. There may be a local homeostatic balance between agents that tend to increase arteriolar vasoconstriction and those that produce vasodilation; vasoconstriction may occur when this balance is disturbed.

Clinical Findings

There are no distinctive symptoms that separate primary hypertension from secondary hypertension due to renal artery stenosis. Factors that favor a diagnosis of renal vascular hypertension are a negative family history of hypertension; recent onset of hypertension; the presence of a systolic or diastolic epigastric bruit transmitted to the flanks; severe hypertension, especially if recent and difficult to control; accelerated or malignant hypertension; hypertension appearing for the first time after age 50; and significant x-ray findings (see below).

Laboratory Screening Examinations

None of the traditional screening tests such as intravenous urograms, measurement of differential renal function by the Howard-Stamey test, or differential renal vein renin levels reliably predict the results of renal angioplasty or renal artery surgery. These tests have a significant number of both false-positive and false-negative results. Plasma renin, when low, is of value in excluding significant renal artery stenosis.

Imaging Studies

A. Intravenous Urography: Rapid-sequence intravenous urography suggests renal artery stenosis if it shows one kidney to be shorter than the other by 1.5 cm or more, with delayed appearance, hyperconcentration, and delayed emptying of the contrast me-

dium. The test is infrequently used today except upon urologic indications because of its expense, occasional adverse reactions, and the frequency of false-negative results.

B. Radioisotopic Kidney Studies: A variety of isotopes have been tried but are infrequently used, because of technical difficulties and frequent false-

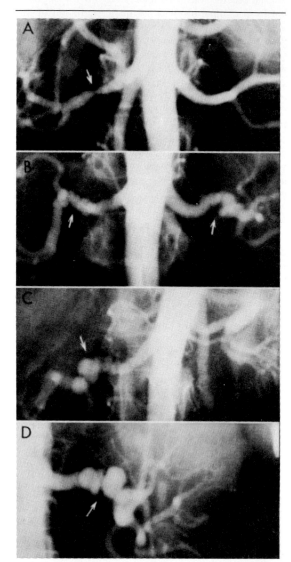

Figure 9–23. Renal aortograms of fibromuscular hyperplasia of the renal arteries. **A** and **D,** unilateral; **B** and **C,** bilateral. In **C,** the disease on the left is obscured by the tortuous overlapping vessel; upright arteriograms or studies with the patient in deep inspiration would have better defined the lesion on the left. In **B,** the pathologic changes extend into the branches of the main renal arteries, and in **C** and **D,** aneurysms are present. (Reproduced, with permission, from Palubinskas AJ, Perloff D, Wylie EJ: Curable hypertension due to renal artery lesions. Radiologia Clinica 1964;33:207. S Karger AG, Basel.)

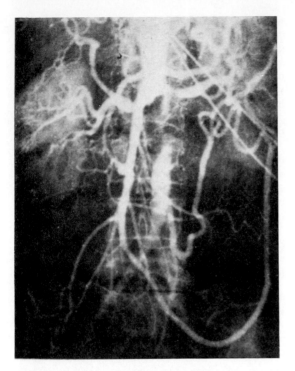

Figure 9–24. Aortogram of a 46-year-old woman. Complete obstruction of the abdominal aorta and stenosis of the proximal portion of the left renal artery were found at operation to be due to atherosclerosis. (Reproduced, with permission of the American Heart Association, from Perloff D et al: Hypertension secondary to renal artery occlusive disease. Circulation 1961;24:1286.)

positive and false-negative results. However, captopril, by exaggerating the decreased blood flow from a stenotic renal artery, reduces the uptake of isotope renography and has been used with some success, though this technique is also associated with some errors in accuracy when judged by renal arteriography. Captopril plus isotope renography has the advan-

tage of establishing the functional significance of an arteriographic stenotic lesion (Pickering, Circulation 1991; Mann, 1991).

C. Renal Angiography: If there are no contraindications, anatomic visualization by percutaneous renal angiography is the recommended definitive study when renal artery stenosis is strongly suspected on the basis of the history, clinical findings, or isotope renogram (Figures 9–23 and 9–24; Table 9–7) (Carmichael, 1986). If stenosis is present, one can then consider other studies to establish its functional significance. In addition to conventional arteriography, selective techniques may evaluate branch renal artery stenosis (Schambelan, 1974).

Treatment & Prognosis

Treatment consists of medical management as in essential hypertension and revascularization either by renal percutaneous transluminal angioplasty (RPTA) or by surgery. Because the surgical mortality rate is higher in patients who have angina, a history of myocardial infarction, or extensive cerebral vascular disease, the initial treatment of choice is RPTA unless the lesion is ostial or peripheral.

A. Renal Percutaneous Transluminal Angioplasty (RPTA): (Figure 9–25.) When renal artery stenosis is significant, proximal, noncalcific, discrete, and nonostial—especially in patients in whom the surgical resection risk is considerable—RPTA should be promptly employed, not only to correct the elevated blood pressure but to preserve or improve renal function. Cure or significant improvement occurs in about 80% of patients with fibromuscular hyperplasia and 60–70% of patients with atherosclerotic stenosis. There may be restenosis in some patients, but this can be corrected by repeat dilation, as in coronary artery stenosis (see Chapter 8) (Canzanello, 1989).

Renal function deteriorates if renal artery stenosis is severe, complete, or bilateral. In one study, renal angioplasty was technically successful in 82%, and

Table 9–7. Frequency of major occlusive renal artery disease in relation to clinical indications for arteriography.[1]

	Patients with Abnormal Arteriogram		Patients with Normal Arteriogram		Total Patients
	Number	Percent	Number	Percent	Cases
Aortoiliac atherosclerosis	60	73	22	27	82
Onset of hypertension over age 50	33	70	15	30	48
Epigastric bruit	108	64	59	36	167
KW III or IV fundi	28	52	26	48	54
Abnormal intravenous pyelogram	94	41	132	59	226
Recent onset of hypertension	70	40	101	60	171
Recent increase in hypertension	31	37	51	63	82
Onset of hypertension under age 20	7	13	46	87	53
Hypertension without other indications	4	10	35	90	39

[1] Reproduced, with permission, from Sokolow M et al: Current experiences with renovascular hypertension. In: *Proceedings of the International Club on Arterial Hypertension.* Expansion Scientifique Française, 1966.

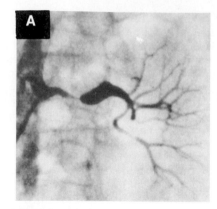

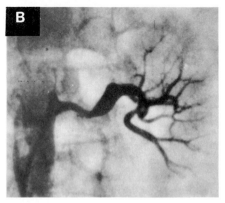

Figure 9–25. Results of renal percutaneous transluminal angioplasty shown by selective renal arteriogram of the left renal artery. ***A:*** Renal artery before the dilation procedure, showing subtotal stenosis and poststenotic dilation. ***B:*** After withdrawal of the dilation catheter, the renal artery shows moderate residual stenosis. (Reproduced, with permission, from Grüntzig A et al: Treatment of renovascular hypertension with percutaneous transluminal dilation of a renal-artery stenosis. Lancet 1978;1:801.)

58% of the successful procedures had a beneficial effect in patients with significant azotemia. Although renal dialysis was required in some cases, renal failure would have been progressive if renal vascularization had not been done (Sos, 1991). The same principle holds for surgical revascularization to preserve renal function (Novick, 1991).

B. Surgical Treatment:

1. Selection of patients– Surgical treatment is now recommended when RPTA is not feasible or has failed for patients with severe hypertension who have a functionally significant renovascular lesion, especially if renal function is unilaterally impaired. Although many patients have bilateral disease, the functional significance of the more impaired side can often be determined. Improvement in renal function is an important objective of renal revascularization in severe hypertensives with strongly suspected renal artery stenosis. Renal failure may be the presenting

feature in atherosclerotic renovascular disease. Surgical revascularization in atherosclerotic renovascular disease had a surgical mortality rate of only 2%; 40% of patients were cured, 51% were improved, and renal function was improved or stabilized in 89% (Novick, 1991). Following surgical resection, there may be a significant postoperative incidence of neurologic deficits, myocardial ischemia or infarction, or arrhythmias.

2. Repair of distal artery– As is true of atherosclerosis generally, disease may appear initially in any portion of the arterial circuit and not be demonstrable elsewhere. Nephrectomy is inadvisable in the presence of fibromuscular hyperplasia, since the disease is often bilateral or, even if not bilateral at the outset, may develop in a few years in the opposite kidney. This consideration is not so important in atherosclerotic disease if the kidney is atrophic and nonfunctioning and the disease is unilateral.

3. Results of surgical repair in general– The results of surgical treatment vary with the cause—being better when fibromuscular hyperplasia is present (Lawrie, 1989; Novick, 1991). About half of patients with atherosclerotic renovascular hypertension have diastolic pressures less than 100 mm Hg following surgical repair; the figure is closer to 75% in patients with fibromuscular hyperplasia. One-fourth to one-half of the patients, especially with atherosclerotic disease, require some antihypertensive therapy following surgical treatment. The prognosis following revascularization depends on whether renal function is preserved and whether the blood pressure is lowered by the procedure. Some patients with atherosclerotic renal stenosis require additional vascular procedures involving the aorta or aortic-femoral-atrial reconstruction. The operative mortality rate is higher in these cases, but long-term benefit occurs in the majority of survivors (Lawrie, 1989).

2. RENAL PARENCHYMAL LESIONS

Acute and chronic glomerulonephritis, chronic pyelonephritis, lupus erythematosus, polycystic kidney disease, and scarring from old trauma probably are the most common causes of secondary hypertension due to renal parenchymal factors.

Prior to the phase of renal failure, the diagnosis of acute glomerulonephritis can be strongly suspected from the history of poststreptococcal proteinuria, edema, or hypertension with associated hematuria and red cell casts. It can also be discovered by accidentally finding hematuria or proteinuria in a healthy young adult; by uncovering a history of pyelonephritis or lupus erythematosus; by finding bacteria and white cells in the urine; by finding evidence of renal or ureteral stone; or by uncovering a family history of early death from uremia and hypertension due to polycystic kidneys. Hypertension occurs in 50–75%

of patients with polycystic disease of the kidneys, presumably because renal ischemia and increased plasma renin activity result from cystic pressure (Chapman, 1990). The presence of polycystic kidneys can be established by an intravenous urogram demonstrating large polycystic kidneys. Urinalysis, urine culture, renal function studies, and serologic studies to rule out hyperparathyroidism, lupus erythematosus, or diabetes are helpful ancillary measures. Additional studies may include a retrograde urogram with determination of ureteral reflux during cystoscopy in patients with pyelonephritis, renal arteriograms, and renal biopsy.

When renal failure has occurred, the urinary sediment and the degree of proteinuria may be similar in primary hypertension in the malignant phase and in chronic renal parenchymal disease.

The accelerated form of hypertension that occurs in the late stages of renal disease further aggravates the deterioration of renal function, and efforts to lower the blood pressure are essential regardless of the cause. Control of the high blood pressure prolongs life and delays the onset of renal failure; when the latter occurs, dialysis or renal transplantation is indicated.

3. ARTERITIS

Connective Tissue Disorders (Polyarteritis Nodosa, Lupus Erythematosus) (See also Chapter 20.)

A wide variety of systemic diseases may cause vasculitis that results in hypertension. The pathologist, therefore, may find evidence of scleroderma, polyarteritis nodosa, lupus erythematosus, rheumatoid arthritis, or nonspecific arteritis. The pathologic features may be predominantly in the arterioles, may extend to the small interlobular arteries of the kidney, or may involve the major arteries in the body leading to the consequences that follow all varieties of vascular obstruction. In addition, there may be cardiac hypertrophy, cerebral hemorrhage, aortic dissection, and fundal changes or necrotizing lesions in the kidney following malignant hypertension.

Connective tissue disorders such as polyarteritis nodosa are often associated with vasculitis of the interlobular arteries and of the arterioles of the kidneys and are associated with hypertension in about half of cases. The hypertension may be severe, and, rarely, the patient may present with the malignant phase. The disease is often generalized, involving many body systems, and the hypertension may merely be part of a generalized systemic disease.

Renovascular lesions are common in lupus erythematosus, but hypertension is much less common than in polyarteritis nodosa. Other forms of arteritis of nonspecific cause may also induce hypertension

and subsequent renal failure when the lesions involve the kidney.

Treatment is with corticosteroids and conventional antihypertensive drugs. Other immunosuppressive drugs may be of value as well.

Recklinghausen's Disease (Neurofibromatosis)

Some authorities have argued that pheochromocytoma is frequent in Recklinghausen's disease. However, the major findings are vascular lesions of the small- to medium-sized arteries with decreased or obliterated lumens, microaneurysm formation, and intimal proliferation. The vascular lesions of neurofibromatosis are different from those of polyarteritis nodosa and do not show perivascular infiltration or necrosis. Arteriography may demonstrate small aneurysms in various larger tributaries of the gastrointestinal tract arteries, as can also be seen in polyarteritis. Hypertension can occur—as it may in any condition associated with renal arteritis—and the mechanism probably involves the renin-angiotensin-aldosterone system.

ENDOCRINE DISORDERS

1. CUSHING'S SYNDROME & DISEASE

Cushing's syndrome is probably a more common cause of hypertension than primary aldosteronism. Although the terms "Cushing's syndrome" and "Cushing's disease" have been used interchangeably, they should be distinguished. The term "Cushing's disease" originally denoted a primary tumor of the anterior pituitary causing bilateral adrenal hyperplasia and hypercortisolism. Because the pituitary tumor often could not be identified, the oversecretion of cortisol and the bilateral adrenal hyperplasia then were called Cushing's syndrome. The original "disease" designation has been validated by recent advances in CT and MRI that confirm the primacy of a pituitary tumor in these cases. It was subsequently learned that a benign adenoma of the adrenal and ectopic ACTH-producing tumors (eg, bronchogenic carcinoma) could also cause the ectopic hypercortisolism. The symptoms of Cushing's disease are also simulated by a syndrome induced by exogenous administration of corticosteroids or ACTH for a wide variety of diseases.

The advent of microsurgery of the anterior pituitary has shown that most cases of hypercortisolism are due to a tumor (often microscopic) of the basophilic or chromophobic cells of the anterior pituitary (Cushing's disease) or to an adenoma of the adrenal gland (Cushing's syndrome); idiopathic bilateral adrenal hyperplasia is now considered rare. It is speculated that some cases of Cushing's syndrome are hypothalamic in origin, with the anterior pituitary stimulated by excess hypothalamic-releasing factor.

Hypertension is a common accompaniment of Cushing's syndrome, though most patients present primarily to an endocrinologist because of a characteristic appearance with "moon" facies, central truncal obesity, muscular weakness, ecchymoses with thin skin, purple striae, increased acne, hirsutism, and perhaps osteoporosis. Hypertension may be mild or severe, but malignant hypertension is rare.

Clinical Findings

A. Symptoms and Signs: The diagnosis of Cushing's syndrome is suspected from the clinical features, but most patients with obesity, hirsutism, and round, bloated facies do not have Cushing's disease.

B. Laboratory Findings: Because cortisol is increased several times above normal values, sodium and water may be retained, with increased extracellular fluid volume. The pathogenesis of hypertension in Cushing's syndrome is not established but is probably due to this increased salt and water retention, increased vascular responsiveness to pressor agents, or increased plasma renin substrate. In pure cortisol excess, plasma renin and aldosterone are normal, as is the serum potassium.

Both cortisol and ACTH levels are elevated in Cushing's disease with pituitary hypercortisolism; increased ACTH stimulates the adrenal cortex to secrete more cortisol. In addition, one can determine the morning plasma 17-hydroxycorticosteroid (17-OHCS) levels after suppression of ACTH by giving the patient 1 mg of dexamethasone and a sedative [phenobarbital, 100 mg, or flurazepam, 15–30 mg] at bedtime the night before. Normal individuals usually suppress the plasma 17-OHCS from the normal value of 10–20 μg/dL to less than 5 μg/dL, whereas patients with Cushing's disease rarely suppress from elevated values of 15–40 μg/dL to less than 10 μg/dL (Ann Intern Med, 1976). However, the test is not infallible; some patients do not respond to the corticoids as anticipated. In Cushing's syndrome due to adrenal adenoma, increased cortisol production suppresses the hypothalamic-pituitary axis and reduces the level of ACTH. The diagnosis is further supported when plasma cortisol is not suppressible by dexamethasone (Kaye, 1990). Petrosal sinus sampling for ACTH, when the central-to-peripheral vein values have a ratio of 2:1, is the best test to differentiate Cushing's disease from ectopic sources of ACTH (Klibanski, 1991).

C. Imaging Studies: The radiologic diagnosis of pituitary tumors is difficult, and in most cases standard skull films are normal. The use of CT scans or MRI increases the frequency of positive findings.

Adrenal tumors are usually large and associated with atrophy of the surrounding as well as the contralateral adrenal. Preoperative lateralization of the

tumor is not always successful, though it has been considerably improved by MRI. If this fails, it is always necessary to expose and explore both adrenal glands. Sampling of blood from both adrenal veins and adrenal venography may be helpful in localizing the tumor, but the adrenal scan is simpler and should be employed first. If carcinoma of the adrenal is suspected, arteriography may be helpful, because the tumor is vascular.

Treatment

Once the diagnosis of Cushing's disease is made and exogenous administration of corticosteroids or ACTH excluded, a search should be made for ectopic ACTH-producing tumors or an adrenal adenoma. If either of these tumors is identified (see above), surgical resection is the treatment of choice. If neither is present and Cushing's disease is diagnosed, transsphenoidal resection of the pituitary under microscopic visualization is the preferred treatment in adults (Mampalam, 1988), and the results have been very satisfactory, with a low (~1%) mortality rate and rare cases of permanent diabetes insipidus. The statistical results of microsurgery in childhood Cushing's disease are uncertain. Irradiation of the anterior pituitary and cryosurgery, formerly used in treatment, have been superseded.

Chemotherapy with cyproheptadine or mitotane with or without pituitary irradiation has been reported to have achieved favorable results in a few cases.

If ectopic ACTH-producing tumors cannot be resected, metyrapone can be tried to inhibit the synthesis of cortisol.

Prognosis

Without treatment, the symptoms and signs of the syndrome become progressively worse, although the hypertension may be controlled by antihypertensive therapy. If hypertension is overlooked because other findings dominate the clinical picture, complications of hypertension such as cardiac failure and cerebral or renal vascular disease may develop and cause death.

2. ACROMEGALY

Acromegaly is caused by excessive production of growth hormone by specific cells of the anterior pituitary gland. The disorder is associated with hypertension in about one-third of patients, though other clinical and metabolic consequences are more common. Symptoms include early complaints of fatigue, paresthesias, amenorrhea, arthralgia, and headache. Later symptoms include increasing size of the hat, gloves, and shoes; visual disturbances that develop insidiously over a period of years; decreased libido; and excessive perspiration, with warm, moist hands. On examination, there may be progressive mandibular enlargement, as shown by serial photographs;

large tongue; increased soft tissue over the heels, hands, and feet; widening spaces between the teeth; hypertension; and, sometimes, goiter. Radiologically, enlargement and ballooning of the sella turcica can be recognized. The hypertension is rarely severe, and treatment is directed at the acromegaly per se.

The diagnosis can be established on immunoassay by finding a high serum growth hormone (GH) level (10–15 ng/mL) that falls below 2 ng/mL 1–2 hours after oral administration of 100 g of glucose. Another sensitive test finding is an elevated plasma insulin-like growth factor I, a measure of excess GH (Klibanski, 1991). About 10% of patients have a lower than expected serum GH concentration, and in these patients abnormal growth hormone regulation by the hypothalamus is thought to be the cause. It is still not certain how many cases of acromegaly are due to an independent pituitary tumor and how many are due to abnormality of the hypothalamic growth hormone-releasing factor, which then induces pituitary hyperfunction. Contrast-enhanced (with gadolinium) MRI may demonstrate an enlarged sella and a pituitary mass (Klibanski, 1991).

Treatment

Treatment now consists of transsphenoidal microsurgery of the pituitary tumor in Cushing's disease. However, if the tumor is large, encroaching on the optic chiasm and the third ventricle, open surgical resection may be required. Irradiation of the pituitary is disappointing as judged by the fall in serum growth hormone, perhaps because the disease is far-advanced before irradiation is undertaken. Serum concentrations above 15 ng/mL may persist for several years, and reoperation may be necessary. Chemotherapy with the somatostatin analogue octreotide (100–300 mg subcutaneously three times daily) rapidly decreases growth hormone and reverses cardiac failure, if present, and decreases plasma volume (Chanson, 1990). Bromocriptine (5–20 mg three times daily) activates dopamine receptors in the brain and reduces growth hormone production; the effects are usually transient. Complete clinical remission is uncommon.

3. PRIMARY ALDOSTERONISM

Primary aldosteronism is usually due to oversecretion of aldosterone by an adenoma of the adrenal. It is a relatively uncommon cause of hypertension (1–2% of cases). Some patients (20–25%) have bilateral adrenal hyperplasia rather than adenoma (70–80%), and these patients have a milder variety of aldosteronism (Biglieri, 1982). Patients with primary adenoma excrete greater amounts of aldosterone in the urine and have lower plasma renin and serum potassium levels than do patients with aldosteronism secondary to bilateral adrenal hyperplasia.

The laboratory diagnosis of hypertension due to mineralocorticoid oversecretion is summarized by Biglieri (1982, 1991). In the discussion of these conditions, we rely heavily on his work.

Aldosteronism itself is not the cause of the hypertension, because aldosterone levels may be much higher in conditions in which hypertension is absent, such as normal pregnancy, cirrhosis of the liver, and Addison's disease.

Adenomas may be relatively small (1–2 cm in diameter) and difficult to find at surgery; are golden yellow in appearance; and are associated with normal or hyperplastic adrenal tissue surrounding the tumor. This is in contrast to Cushing's syndrome, in which the gland surrounding a tumor is atrophic and the opposite adrenal may also be hypoplastic.

Clinical Findings

The clinical features of primary aldosteronism are often no different from those of essential hypertension; occasionally, symptoms related to potassium depletion, such as nocturia, polyuria, fatigue, paresthesias, or postural hypotension, may predominate. One now rarely sees the paralysis due to extremely low potassium reported in the early literature. Aldosteronism is more frequent in women under 40 years of age; hypertension is usually mild to moderate; retinopathy is usually grade I or grade II; and malignant hypertension is rare. Hypertensive complications, such as cardiac failure, are uncommon. If there is severe hypokalemic alkalosis, the patients may have autonomic insufficiency with postural hypotension without tachycardia. In suspected cases, the initial screening test is a determination of serum potassium.

A. Serum Potassium: If the serum potassium is consistently above 4 meq/L on a normal sodium intake, the likelihood of a primary aldosterone-producing adenoma is sufficiently remote that no further studies are indicated. The serum potassium may be normal if the patient is taking a low-sodium diet, because potassium excretion at the sodium-potassium exchange site in the distal tubule is reduced; patients should therefore be taking a normal-sodium diet before serum electrolytes are measured. If the serum potassium is less than 4 meq/L—and especially (in the absence of diuretic therapy) if it is less than 3.5 meq/L—the 24-hour urine potassium and serum potassium should be determined on a normal-sodium diet of approximately 100–150 meq/d. In primary aldosterone-producing adenomas, serum potassium falls over a period of 5 days if the patient has been placed on a high-sodium diet. If the 24-hour urine potassium exceeds 30 meq/L in the presence of a serum potassium less than 3.5 meq/L (especially if the serum potassium falls as a result of the high sodium intake), further biochemical studies such as plasma aldosterone and renin are indicated to exclude aldosteronism. If primary aldosteronism accounts for the hypokalemia and increased potassium excretion in the urine, there should also be salt and water retention and increased extracellular and plasma volume, associated with decreased circulatory reflexes and lack of hypertension overshoot following the Valsalva maneuver (Biglieri, 1982).

B. Evaluation of Low Serum Potassium in Hypertensive Patients: When potassium excretion is increased by diuretics in antihypertensive therapy, sodium is excreted as well, producing the combination of a low serum potassium and a low serum sodium (130–135 meq/L). In addition, mild alkalosis is present, with serum bicarbonate in the range of 25–32 meq/L. If serum sodium is increased (144–149 meq/L) and serum bicarbonate is also increased (35–39 meq/L) in these patients with low serum potassium, primary aldosteronism becomes more likely.

C. Plasma Renin: Plasma renin values are very low or nil in aldosteronism because the increased blood volume (see negative feedback loop in Figure 9–3) decreases renal renin secretion. If the plasma concentration is normal or high, primary aldosteronism is excluded as a cause of hypokalemia. A low plasma renin level is even more significant if it remains low following upright posture and the use of potent diuretics, which stimulate renin secretion in the normal individual but which may not do so in the presence of the hypervolemia secondary to increased aldosterone production. If the plasma renin level remains low, especially after provocative maneuvers to increase it, plasma and urinary aldosterone values should be determined. Interpretation of the plasma renin concentration may be doubtful unless the conditions of testing are rigidly controlled. This is best done in the hospital and consists of control of sodium and potassium intake, avoidance of antihypertensive drugs, ambulation for 4 hours before the sample is taken, and sodium depletion with diuretics on the day of the test to make certain that plasma renin does not respond to these maneuvers and remains suppressed. These tests are done only in special laboratories that have facilities to measure the hormone accurately.

D. Plasma Aldosterone: Increased plasma aldosterone with clinical and laboratory evidence of excess aldosterone production may be due either to the presence of an isolated adrenal adenoma or to bilateral adrenal hyperplasia. Adenoma is suspected if the plasma aldosterone fails to increase in the upright posture, as it does in hyperplasia, or if an iodine 131 iodocholesterol scintiscan or a CT scan localizes a tumor in one of the adrenals.

Desoxycorticosterone has no effect on adenoma; ie, it does not suppress the production of aldosterone from the tumor, as it does in indeterminate aldosteronism (hyperplasia).

E. Adrenal Scan: Most cases of adrenal adenoma can be identified and localized by an adrenal scintiscan or more definitively by CT scan, MRI, or abdominal ultrasound. It is important to attempt to localize the adenoma so the surgeon will know which adrenal is involved.

Treatment & Prognosis

If bilateral renal hyperplasia rather than adenoma is the cause, the patient should be treated with antihypertensive therapy, including spironolactone (the aldosterone antagonist), rather than bilateral adrenalectomy, because of the high prevalence of persistent hypertension and the need for replacement therapy after adrenalectomy. Spironolactone (300 mg/d in divided doses for 1 month, followed by smaller doses) usually corrects both the serum potassium and the hypertension. In adenoma, resection of the adrenal tumor is required and promptly decreases aldosterone production and restores the serum potassium to normal, but hypertension is "cured" in only 60–70% of cases. Because of this relatively low "cure" rate in mild aldosteronism due to hyperplasia, when the blood pressure, serum potassium, and hypervolemia can be corrected by spironolactone, medical rather than surgical treatment can be considered.

Without surgery, however, the symptoms of adenoma can only be partially controlled by medical treatment, and surgical removal is required. The serum potassium usually falls to less than 2.5–3 meq/L after thiazide therapy in unsuspected cases of aldosteronism, leading to hypokalemic symptoms of fatigue, nocturia, arrhythmia, and nephropathy; these are corrected by spironolactone. Failure to control blood pressure leads to cardiac and cerebral complications found in other types of hypertension. Postural hypotension may be a problem because of a defect in circulatory reflexes.

4. SECONDARY ALDOSTERONISM

Secondary hyperaldosteronism is much more common than the primary form and is usually due to accelerated or severe hypertension, which, by reducing renal blood flow, initiates the production of angiotensin, which in turn increases the secretion of aldosterone. Patients with secondary aldosteronism are liable to have elevated plasma renin concentrations as well—in contrast to the expected low plasma renin in primary aldosteronism. This difference is critical in distinguishing the two entities. The serum potassium may be low in both secondary and primary aldosteronism, but the serum sodium is not elevated in secondary as it is in primary aldosteronism. The serum sodium is rarely less than 140 meq/dL in primary cases, and it may be as high as 155 meq/dL. When the blood pressure is reduced by antihypertensive agents (but not spironolactone), secondary aldosteronism is reduced, and the serum potassium may rise to normal even though oral diuretics tend to increase the plasma renin. The "effective" blood volume is raised in both types of aldosteronism but is reduced in patients with cirrhosis of the liver or Addison's disease, conditions in which renin levels may be very high. Secondary aldosteronism may occur in renal artery stenosis because of the increased secretion of renin, with resulting increased plasma and urinary aldosterone.

Treatment

Vigorous antihypertensive therapy lowers the blood pressure, causing secondary aldosteronism to disappear.

5. PHEOCHROMOCYTOMA

Pheochromocytoma is a dramatic but rare tumor. It arises anywhere in the chromaffin system (the remnant of the fetal neural crest) that synthesizes epinephrine and norepinephrine. The overwhelming majority occur in the adrenal medulla, but these tumors may occur in chromaffin cells in the abdomen, the periaortic area, the organ of Zuckerkandl, and, rarely, in the thorax and bladder wall (Figure 9–26). They are often multiple and familial and rarely may be associated with other endocrinopathies such as Sip-

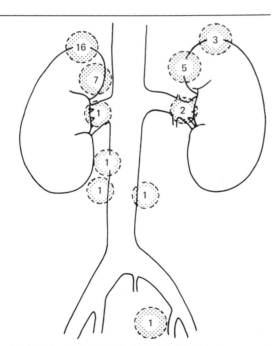

Figure 9–26. Illustrations of the sites of occurrence of pheochromocytoma in 34 patients, with the number of tumors found at various locations indicated with the circles. (Adapted and reproduced, with permission, from Zelch JV, Meaney TF, Belhobek GH: Radiologic approach to the patient with suspected pheochromocytoma. Radiology 1974;111:279.)

ple's disease (multiple parathyroid adenomas) or Recklinghausen's disease (neurofibromatosis); most patients have no associated endocrinopathy. These tumors are usually benign, but about 10% are malignant and require treatment with radiation therapy and chemotherapy.

It is important to recognize pheochromocytoma promptly, because successful excision of the tumor is curative in almost all of the benign tumors and prevents the severe hypertensive crises that may cause myocardial infarction, fatal ventricular arrhythmias, or cerebral hemorrhage. Manger (1977) presents a valuable review.

Tumors vary in the relative amounts of norepinephrine and epinephrine they secrete, and the clinical signs may vary depending on which catecholamine is secreted.

Clinical Findings

A. Symptoms and Signs: The most typical clinical features are those associated with an abrupt surge of catecholamine secretion, causing pallor, sweating, palpitations, headache, and anxiety, usually all occurring together in association with an abrupt rise in systolic and diastolic pressures.

1. Cause of attacks– The attacks may be spontaneous or precipitated by changes in posture, pressure on the abdomen, procedures such as intravenous urograms or renal arteriograms, or anesthesia. Pheochromocytoma should be excluded before invasive studies for other causes of hypertension are ordered, because of the hazard of precipitating a severe attack. (*Note:* Intravenous phenoxybenzamine must be available for emergency use [Figure 9–27].) One or another of these symptoms (but not all together) may be present in anxiety attacks, and most patients referred with a diagnosis of possible pheochromocytoma have transient rises in pressure associated with anxiety. If epinephrine is the amine secreted, flushing rather than pallor is characteristic, and the patient is more tremulous. In rare instances, precursors of norepinephrine may be secreted, and hypotension is occasionally found when dopamine is secreted in large amounts. The hypertension may be intermittent but is usually sustained, with intermittent superimposed rises in conjunction with paroxysmal symptoms. Malignant hypertension with papilledema occurs more frequently in pheochromocytoma than in Cushing's syndrome or aldosteronism.

2. Symptoms during attacks– The rise in blood pressure may be severe, and during attacks in young people, diastolic pressures of 150 mm Hg are not unusual. The high, abrupt rises in pressure may cause patients to present with myocardial ischemia or infarction, stroke, ventricular arrhythmias, cardiac failure, or several of these complications.

When pheochromocytoma occurs in the urinary bladder, the hypertensive crises may be induced by

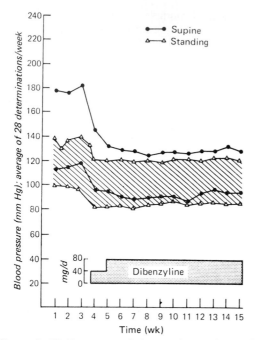

Figure 9–27. Response of the supine and standing blood pressure to treatment with phenoxybenzamine (Dibenzyline) in a patient with malignant pheochromocytoma. Note that the marked orthostatic fall in blood pressure present in the pretreatment period is reduced after therapy is begun. (Reproduced, with permission, from Engelman K, Sjoerdsma A: Chronic medical therapy for pheochromocytoma: A report of four cases. Ann Intern Med 1964;61:231.)

Table 9–8. Normal range of catecholamine and metabolite concentrations.[1,2]

Urine
Catecholamines:[3]
Norepinephrine: 10–70 μg/24 h
Epinephrine: 0–20 μg/24 h
Normetanephrine and metanephrine: < 1.3 mg/24 h
Vanillylmandelic acid: 1.8–9.0 mg/24 h
Dopamine: < 200 μg/24 h
Blood
Catecholamines: < 1 μg/L
Adrenal medulla
Norepinephrine: 0.04–0.16 mg/g
Epinephrine: 0.22–0.84 mg/g

[1] Reproduced, with permission, from Melmon KL: Catecholamines and the adrenal medulla, In: *Textbook of Endocrinology*, 5th ed. Williams RH (editor), Saunders, 1974.
[2] Since the values obtained in different laboratories vary considerably, only a general range can be given.
[3] In most patients with pheochromocytomas, total catecholamine excretion is > 300 μg/d.

diagnosis by demonstrating short peaks of elevated pressure coincident with the episodic symptoms (Mancia, 1979). Not only is measurement of plasma norepinephrine a most useful diagnostic test, but plasma measurements at different venous sites may help localize the tumor.

1. VMA determination– Determination of vanillylmandelic acid (VMA), one of the products of catecholamine metabolism, is a screening test that is available in most laboratories. Clofibrate gives false-negative results, but the spectrophotometric assay is not affected by common foods such as bananas, coffee, or vanilla desserts, which do affect the less precise calorimetric test (now rarely used). Normal VMA excretion is less than 7 mg/24 h but may be five to ten times this amount in pheochromocytoma. Methyldopa does not interfere with assay for VMA, but it does interfere with assay for total urinary catecholamine excretion.

2. Metanephrine– Determination of other metabolites, notably metanephrine on a single voided specimen, has been shown to be simple, sensitive, and highly reliable, with the distinct advantage of not requiring a 24-hour specimen. The upper limits of normal for the assay are 1 μg per milligram of creatinine in the urine. Single voided urine specimens from 500 hypertensive patients contained 0.35 ± 0.35 (2 SD) μg of metanephrine per milligram of creatinine, with a range of 0.06–1.18 μg/mg of creatinine, whereas in pheochromocytoma, spot specimens were 1–100 μg/mg of creatinine (Kaplan, *Clinical Hypertension*, 1990). Chlorpromazine produces falsely high readings, but no diet or obesity drugs or antihypertensive drugs interfere with the test. This assay may be positive when the VMA assay is negative, but the reverse is rarely true.

3. Imaging studies– CT scan or MRI may demonstrate the tumor. MIBG (metaiodobenzylguanidine) using iodine 123 or iodine 131 specifically lo-

urination, or the patient may have asymptomatic hematuria. The crises occur immediately with voiding and rapidly subside in a few minutes. A review of 35 previously reported cases and a well-studied individual case are offered by Raper (1977).

B. Laboratory Findings: The laboratory diagnosis of pheochromocytoma in patients who have a characteristic history usually can be accomplished by assay of catecholamine or its metabolites such as metanephrine in the 24-hour urine specimen. Table 9–8 shows the normal range of catecholamine and metabolite concentrations in the urine and blood.

Plasma norepinephrine concentrations of 2.5–5 μg/L, in contrast to the normal 0.25–1 μg/L, occur in patients with pheochromocytoma. Most of the norepinephrine released at the adrenergic nerve ending is reabsorbed, metabolized, or taken up again by the axon terminal. That which escapes into the circulation, while much higher than normal, is only a small fraction of the amount that is released. The sudden release of norepinephrine into the circulation in hypertensive crises in patients with pheochromocytoma produces dramatic effects. In patients with brief episodes of catecholamine release, prolonged intraarterial blood pressure recordings may establish the calizes in the adrenal tissue or in tumors of the neuroectodermal crest, and pheochromocytomas may therefore be readily identified by uptake of adrenal-specific radioisotopes. The method is particularly valuable when there are extra-adrenal tumors (Hattner, 1984).

4. Urine tests– Urinary assay of the free catecholamines norepinephrine and epinephrine is infrequently used in screening, since these substances are technically more difficult to measure and may be increased in the urine, causing false-positive results if the patient has been receiving bronchodilators, nasal sprays, or drugs such as tetracycline or chlorpromazine that produce urinary fluorescence. Methyldopa also interferes with the catecholamine test but not the VMA test. In the absence of interfering drugs, the plasma catecholamines, when abnormally high, are more sensitive than the urinary metabolites in the diagnosis of pheochromocytoma (Bravo, 1979).

5. Pharmacologic tests– Combined glucagon stimulation and clonidine suppression tests are promising; the former is highly specific but not sensitive; the latter is the reverse. The diagnosis of pheochromocytoma can be excluded if both tests are negative (Grossman, 1991). Histamine, by inducing outpouring of catecholamines from the tumor, may produce a hypertensive crisis with arrhythmia, myocardial ischemia, or even death, and is rarely performed today.

Treatment

Because the increased secretion of catecholamines results in hypertension and reduced plasma volume in many instances, alpha-adrenergic-blocking drugs (combined with beta-adrenergic-blocking drugs agents in order to inhibit the peripheral actions of the catecholamines) must be used whether ultimate treatment is medical or surgical.

A. Medical Treatment: Give phentolamine, 10–30 mg orally every 4–6 hours, or phenoxybenzamine, 10–50 mg orally twice daily, to control both blood pressure and blood volume before technical procedures that may cause marked rises or falls in pressure are done to localize the tumor (Figure 9–27). During such acute hypertensive episodes, in order to avoid myocardial ischemia or arrhythmias, patients should be given phentolamine, 1–5 mg intravenously every 5–10 minutes, until the pressure falls and is stabilized. If severe tachycardia or other arrhythmias occur, 1–2 mg of propranolol can be given intravenously over a 10-minute period followed by 20 mg orally every 6 hours. When intravenous phentolamine is given, patients are best placed in the Fowler position so they can be shifted swiftly to the supine position if pressure falls excessively. Intravenous phentolamine stops attacks dramatically; this drug should be available for all diagnostic procedures that might liberate catecholamines and induce an attack.

B. Surgical Treatment: If surgery is contemplated, careful examination of the head and neck, chest fluoroscopy, chest x-rays, intravenous urograms with tomography, and scans with MIBG (see above) should be carried out to localize the tumor.

Surgical excision of the tumor is the treatment of choice, after suitable preparation with alpha-adrenergic-blocking agents (see above) to restore the blood volume and lower the blood pressure, as well as daily propranolol (10–40 mg three times daily) to control tachycardia and arrhythmias. Before it was recognized that it was important to control the blood volume preoperatively, the intraoperative course was characterized by marked rises in pressure due to surgical manipulation, and a fall to hypotensive levels when the tumor was excised. Phentolamine should be available for immediate intravenous use for the former and norepinephrine and volume expanders for the latter.

Prognosis

As indicated above, acute hypertensive crises may precipitate ventricular arrhythmias and myocardial or cerebral ischemia or infarction. These are not prevented by the usual antihypertensive therapy, and patients with acute crises are therefore at considerable risk from these complications.

In patients with sustained hypertension without acute severe hypertensive episodes, conventional antihypertensive therapy may lower the blood pressure without affecting the basic mechanism of increased secretion of catecholamine. Incidentally discovered adrenal masses during CT or MRI are common but usually are not hormonally significant; when such masses are discovered, biochemical screening is indicated to exclude pheochromocytoma and primary aldosteronism; one should also search for clinical features characteristic of these disorders. If the mass becomes larger on serial follow-up, surgical exploration may be considered.

COARCTATION OF THE AORTA
(See also Chapter 11.)

Coarctation in adults consists of a localized narrowing or constriction in the region of the ligamentum arteriosum and is often associated with a bicuspid aortic valve. The patient may present with hypertension or with a basal systolic ejection murmur that is crescendo-decrescendo when due to the bicuspid aortic valve or late systolic when it occurs at the coarcted site. Rarely, patients present with intermittent claudication of the legs. The patient is usually male, and coarctation can be suspected from mildly to moderately elevated blood pressure, increased pulsations of the carotid arteries, and delayed, weak, or absent pulsations in the femoral arteries and arteries distal to them. If there is doubt about whether the pulses are delayed and weak in the legs, the blood pressure should be taken in the legs; if there is still doubt, pressures can be obtained in the arms and legs before and after exercise. Exercise aggravates the disparity between the pressures in the upper and lower extremities. If the patient is past puberty, pulsating collateral intercostal arteries below the margins of the ribs posteriorly may be found. Coarctation varies in severity, but by early adult life the patient almost always has signs of left ventricular hypertrophy, and the chest x-ray may show scalloping of the ribs as a result of the enlarged collateral intercostal arteries.

Treatment & Prognosis

Anatomic correction is required for all but the mildest cases of coarctation, and repair can usually be achieved safely in early childhood and even in infancy. Transluminal angioplasty has been used with increasing frequency and some success. However, aneurysms of the aorta or pulmonary artery and rupture of the aorta have occurred. Some authorities recommend angioplasty only if the stenosis has recurred following surgery. The surgical mortality rate of repair of coarctation is less than 3%. The risk is higher if surgery is delayed until the 40s, when coronary heart disease may be superimposed and the sclerotic aorta results in increased operative complications.

Without treatment, coarctation usually leads to death by the 40s; the patient dies of cardiac failure, ruptured cerebral aneurysm, infective endarteritis, or aortic dissection.

The incidence of persistent hypertension following repair of a coarctation is now 5–10%. If surgery is delayed until after age 20, complications of the hypertension may still follow.

ENZYMATIC DEFECTS
(Congenital Adrenal Hyperplasia)

Rare conditions causing inherited congenital adrenal hyperplasia were not considered hypertensive disorders until recently. They are due to enzymatic defects in the synthesis of cortisol and are treated with cortisol.

1. 17α-HYDROXYLASE DEFICIENCY

Some patients with amenorrhea and hypertension have a 17-αhydroxylase deficiency that blocks the synthesis not only of cortisol from cholesterol and pregnenolone but also of androgens (androsterone) and estrogens (17α-hydroxyprogesterone) by the adrenal gland. As a result, secondary sex characteristics fail to develop at puberty, and women present with amenorrhea. By positive feedback, the decreased cortisol stimulates the pituitary gland to secrete excessive amounts of ACTH, which in turn stimulates the adrenal to produce increased deoxycorticosterone, causing mineralocorticoid excess with hypertension and hypokalemia (Biglieri, 1981).

Treatment with moderate doses of cortisol diminishes excessive ACTH secretion and consequently the amount of deoxycorticosterone secreted, correcting the hypokalemia and hypertension. The initial dosage of cortisol should be low and cautiously increased.

2. 11β-HYDROXYLASE DEFICIENCY

Cortisol precursors are raised, and synthesis of cortisol is decreased also in 11β-hydroxylase deficiency. The patient presents with hypertension, normal to low serum potassium, decreased plasma renin activity, and often low plasma aldosterone (Biglieri, 1981). Serum 11-deoxycortisol and deoxycorticosterone are elevated. Excessive deoxycorticosterone causes hypertension and hypokalemia in 11β- and 17α-hydroxylase deficiency.

Treatment consists of oral cortisol, which by negative feedback halts the increased ACTH secretion; the resulting decreased deoxycorticosterone corrects the hypokalemia and hypertension. As with 17α-hydroxylase deficiency, cautious administration of cortisol is advised.

HYPERTENSION DUE TO ORAL
CONTRACEPTIVE AGENTS

There is an association between the use of oral contraceptive agents and the development of hypertension. In many instances the rise in pressure is slight, but in a few patients severe or even malignant hypertension has resulted. There is some evidence that individuals who develop hypertension have either a family history of hypertension or a history of preeclampsia-eclampsia. The rise in pressure is often gradual, and the incidence of hypertension is greater over a period of years than during the first 6 months of use of the agent. The elevated pressure falls gradually even weeks to several months after oral contraceptives are stopped.

The mechanism by which the oral contraceptive agents produce hypertension is not certain. The most generally accepted hypothesis is that it is caused by the considerable rise in renin substrate that follows the use of the estrogen-progesterone agents.

Oral contraceptive agents increase plasma renin and aldosterone as well as renin substrate. When hypertension is associated with a raised plasma aldosterone as well as a raised plasma renin, primary aldosteronism is excluded, but oral contraceptive agents must be considered in females. Screening of female hypertensives by determining plasma renin and aldosterone levels may make it unnecessary to stop the oral contraceptive agents for several months, as is otherwise necessary in order to determine this possible etiologic role in the hypertension (Oparil, 1981).

A *rising* blood pressure, however, calls for cessation of oral contraceptives and use of an alternative method of contraception.

The Royal College of General Practitioners in England (1977) indicates that there is an increased mortality rate from circulatory diseases in women who have used oral contraception, with the risk increasing with age, smoking, the size of the estrogen dose, and the duration of use. The English study may be influenced by the large number of physicians and the small number of deaths in relation to the total number of women involved in the study. Further prospective studies are in progress, especially with agents that contain smaller amounts of estrogens.

TREATMENT OF ESSENTIAL HYPERTENSION

One of the major advances in cardiology in the past 35 years has been the development and widespread use of effective antihypertensive agents. The introduction of ganglionic-blocking agents such as hexamethonium for the treatment of severe hypertension in 1950 was the beginning of a new era in the management of hypertension and showed for the first time that blood pressure could be lowered safely, that the elevated pressure was not essential for adequate perfusion of vital organs (as had been supposed by some), and that the dire consequences of the hypertension, such as the malignant phase, could be reversed or prevented. Compounds with different mechanisms of action have been developed that usually can be taken without seriously interfering with the patient's accustomed mode of life. The decrease in mortality rate—about 40% in the past 20 years—has been dramatic in the more severe varieties of hypertension and its complications. The availability of effective drugs makes it important to find the large numbers of people with unrecognized hypertension who can benefit from therapy.

Why Should Hypertension Be Treated? Benefits of Treatment

Hypertension per se should be treated because vascular abnormalities and their complications occur whether raised blood pressure is primary or secondary. The importance of associated coronary risk factors and the benefits of treating them and the hypertension have been analyzed (Kaplan, 1990; Stamler, 1991; Kannel, 1991; National Education Programs Working Group, 1991). Any drug regimen that brings the blood pressure down into the normal range will prevent and reverse the malignant phase of hypertension, improve cardiac failure, decrease the mortality rate from dissection of the aorta, prevent hemorrhagic stroke, and prolong life.

Clinical Trials of Antihypertensive Therapy

Effective antihypertensive drug therapy has conclusively demonstrated the therapeutic value of lowering the blood pressure. The Veterans Administration Study (1967, 1970), utilizing a diuretic, reserpine, and hydralazine was the first of a number of randomized, double-blind studies that established the contemporary approach to the treatment of hypertension (Tables 9–9, 9–10, and 9–11). A series of subsequent trials, including the Australian Therapeutic Trial (1980), the Medical Research Council Trial (1985), the Helgeland Oslo study (1980); Amery, for the European Working Party Trial in the Elderly (1991); the Hypertension Detection and Follow-up Program (1988), the Multiple Risk Factor Intervention Trial (1990), Rutan (1988), and others all demonstrated decreased blood pressure, decreased stroke, prevention or reversal of cardiac failure, and improved mortality rates and—but little or no reduction of coronary heart disease. The trials varied in the blood pressure cutoff points at which to begin therapy, the drugs used, and whether the hypertension was mild to moderate or severe. Smaller studies

Table 9–9. Incidence of morbid events with respect to level of prerandomization blood pressure.[1]

| Prerandomization Blood Pressure (mm Hg) | Control Group | | | Treated Group | | | Percent Effectiveness |
| | Patients Randomized | Patients With "Morbid Event" | | Patients Randomized | Patients With "Morbid Event" | | |
		Number	Percent		Number	Percent	
Systolic < 165	98	15	15.3	108	10	9.3	40
Systolic 165+	96	41	42.7	78	12	15.4	64
Total	194	56		186	22		
Diastolic 90–104	84	21	25.0	86	14	16.3	35
Diastolic 105–114	110	35	31.8	100	8	8.0	75
Total	194	56		186	22		

[1] Reproduced, with permission, from Veterans Administration Cooperative Study Group on Antihypertensive Agents: Effects of treatment on morbidity in hypertension. JAMA 1970;213:1143. Copyright © American Medical Association.
[2] Morbid events include hypertensive complications such as heart failure, cerebral hemorrhage, accelerated or malignant hypertension, or dissection of the aorta.

Table 9–10. Effect of treatment on mortality rate and major cardiovascular complications. (After Veterans Administration Cooperative Study Group, 1970.)[1]

Diastolic Blood Pressure (mm Hg)	Placebo				Treated				Follow-Up Period (Years)
			Complications				Complications		
	No.	Deaths	No.	%	No.	Deaths	No.	%	
115–129	70	4	27	38.6	73	0	1	1.4	1.6
90–114	194	19	56	29	186	8	22	11.8	3.3

[1] Reproduced, with permission, from Nagle R: The prognosis of hypertension, Practitioner (July) 1971;207:52.

showed benefit in severe and malignant hypertension (Joint National Committee, 1988; Cutler, 1989; Perry, 1966).

Good antihypertensive therapy is also effective in preventing recurrence of stroke in patients who have recovered from a previous stroke. The recurrence rate of stroke was 16%, 32%, or 55% when the blood pressure control was good, fair, or poor, respectively (Beevers, 1973). Furthermore, decline in the occurrence or recurrence of stroke has been the most beneficial effect of antihypertensive treatment in all therapeutic trials of hypertension.

Many studies have shown that malignant hypertension, cardiac failure, and hemorrhagic stroke are rare in the effectively treated hypertensive patient and that when malignant hypertension and cardiac failure develop in an untreated or inadequately treated hypertensive patient, lowering the blood pressure will reverse these complications. Whether lowering the blood pressure will prevent late atherosclerotic complications such as cerebral infarction, coronary heart disease, or atherosclerosis of the peripheral arteries is

still an unanswered question. Some studies suggest that treatment of hypertension decreases the incidence of clinical coronary disease (Joint National Committee, 1988), and it is possible that agents used in therapy that increase serum lipids (diuretics, beta-adrenergic blockers) may have prevented a decline in coronary events. It has also been suggested that asymptomatic coronary disease present in some of the hypertensive patients treated in the trials may have prevented beneficial effects from becoming obvious. Atherosclerosis develops over a period of years, and most of the therapeutic trials have been too short to demonstrate the effectiveness of therapy.

The age of the patient when therapy is begun also influences the incidence of morbid events. In the Veterans Administration study (1972) (Table 9–11), the incidence of morbid events in the placebo control group almost tripled in patients over 50 when compared with those under 50. In the treated group, complications (morbid events) still occurred in the older group, but their incidence was significantly less than in the untreated group. Therapeutic trials are still un-

Table 9–11. Incidence of assessable events by age and diagnostic category in the VA study.[1]

Diagnostic Category	Age (Years)						Total Events	
	< 50		50–59		60+			
	C	T	C	T	C	T	C	T
Cerebrovascular accident	5	1	5	1	10	3	20	5
Congestive heart failure	1	0	1	0	9	0	11	0
Accelerated hypertension or renal damage	5	0	2	0	0	0	7	0
Coronary artery disease[2]	4	4	4	2	5	5	13	11
Atrial fibrillation	0	2	0	1	2	0	2	3
Aortic dissection	0	0	1	0	1	0	2	0
Other[3]	0	0	1	0	0	3	1	3
Total morbid events	15	7	14	4	27	11	56	22
Diastolic > 124 mm Hg	15	0	3	0	2	0	20	0

Abbreviations: C = control group; T = treated group.

[1] Modified and reproduced, with permission, from the American Heart Association, Inc., Veterans Administration Cooperative Study Group on Antihypertensive Agents: Effects of treatment on morbidity in hypertension. 3. Influence of age, diastolic pressure, and prior cardiovascular disease; further analysis of side-effects. Circulation 1972;45:991.
[2] Myocardial infarction or sudden death.
[3] Includes in treated group one patient terminated because of hypotensive reactions, one death from ruptured atherosclerotic aneurysm, and one patient with second-degree heart block. Control group includes one patient with left bundle branch block.

der way in various parts of the world to test the hypothesis that effective antihypertensive therapy in mild hypertensives in whom asymptomatic coronary disease can be excluded—begun at a younger age, in smaller doses, using different antihypertensive agents that do not elevate the serum lipids or have other adverse metabolic effects—will decrease, delay, or prevent atherosclerosis.

Not only has effective treatment reduced mortality rates, but the severity of hypertension has declined. Malignant hypertension is now uncommon (except when atherosclerotic renal artery stenosis is present); left ventricular mass is decreased by most antihypertensive drugs; progressive rise in the level of blood pressure is prevented; uremia is now infrequent as a complication of hypertension; and the inexorable progression of renal dysfunction in such conditions as diabetic nephropathy is now slowed (Parving, 1990). Coronary artery disease with angina pectoris and myocardial infarction is now the most common cause of death in hypertensive individuals; stroke is now the second most common cause of death, but the mortality rate has decreased 40–50% in the past 20 years. Ambulatory recordings of blood pressure have proved more accurate and more helpful in the evaluation, treatment, and possibly in the prediction of outcome in hypertension.

BASIC PRINCIPLES OF TREATMENT

When to Treat Hypertension

Considerable care must be taken to establish the diagnosis of hypertension before instituting treatment, because treatment is usually a lifelong process. Treatment is rarely urgent in the absence of severe or accelerated hypertension. Hypertension can never be diagnosed on the basis of pressures obtained on a single day, because more than a third of individuals fail to sustain elevated levels. Established hypertension must be differentiated from transient elevation of blood pressure caused by excitement, apprehension, exertion, or the systolic elevation of blood pressure that occurs in elderly people as a result of increased stiffness of the aorta or at any age as a result of a raised cardiac output, increased cardiac contraction, or increased stroke output from a slow ventricular rate.

There is no single point at which all physicians will agree that antihypertensive treatment is required. In addition, if one uses as a criterion diastolic pressures of 105 mm Hg or more, the prevalence of hypertension in the adult population falls from 20% to about 5%, thus decreasing the number of patients requiring treatment.

Hypertension can be considered a continuum, progressing from (1) the earliest manifestations of transient occasional rises of blood pressure, to (2) asymptomatic established hypertension without vascular abnormalities or complications, to (3) the presence of vascular abnormalities alone without complications, to (4) the presence of vascular complications, and finally to (5) death. At what point along the continuum one decides to institute treatment depends on the presence of associated risk factors for coronary disease and the philosophy and conviction of the physician that the benefits warrant the difficulties of lifelong treatment with antihypertensive agents.

When Should Drug Treatment Be Initiated?

The major dilemma regarding when drug treatment should be initiated concerns patients whose diastolic pressure is in the range of 90–100 mm Hg (most hypertensives); when the diastolic pressure exceeds 100 mm Hg, the decision to treat is clear. Large therapeutic trials found that patients in the lower group had only a modest decrease in cardiovascular morbidity or mortality. If the diastolic pressure is consistently less than 95 mm Hg and there are minimal or no significant risk factors for atherosclerosis, the patient can be observed closely and treated with nonpharmacologic methods.

The younger the individual, the more significant is any given level of blood pressure, so that a pressure that might be in the 50th percentile in the sixth decade would be in the 90th or 95th percentile in an individual in the third decade, with a corresponding doubled or tripled mortality rate over a period of 20–30 years. Although it has not been proved that treating borderline hypertension prevents the development of atherosclerosis, the Framingham Study showed that the development of coronary disease is more frequent in borderline hypertensive than in normotensive individuals (see Figure 9–6).

Significance of Vascular Abnormalities & Vascular Complications (Target Organ Damage)

"Target organ" damage refers to that found in organs most likely to be damaged by an elevated blood pressure—the heart, brain, kidneys, eyes, and peripheral arteries. The development of vascular complications ("clinical events") is clearly related to the presence of prior vascular abnormalities (fundal, echocardiographic, or electrocardiographic abnormalities but no symptoms), even when comparable degrees of elevation of blood pressure are present. Insurance company data and data from other sources have shown that for any given elevation of blood pressure, the likelihood of cardiac failure and death is much greater when either left ventricular hypertrophy or abnormalities of the arterioles of the retina are present (Sokolow, 1961). For this reason, the presence of asymptomatic target organ damage warrants therapy in mild hypertension because the measured blood pressure at any given time may not be representative of the average value, as determined by ambulatory methods.

Evaluation of Blood Pressure Elevation

From the foregoing, it follows that one should identify hypertension early in its course because it is often asymptomatic, which means that the first manifestation may be a complication, and if the condition is not recognized until later, damage to the arterioles, arteries, and target organs may have already occurred. Treatment should not be delayed until clinical vascular complications have appeared. The first complication may be one that carries permanent morbidity or a high mortality rate, eg, cardiac failure, malignant hypertension, aortic dissection, or hemorrhagic stroke. These complications, unfortunately, are commonly seen in untreated hypertensives, especially in patients who have not received optimum medical therapy or have discontinued therapy. For these reasons, vigorous efforts are now being made to make certain that the blood pressure is measured and recorded in every patient who enters the health care system for any reason. A high percentage of patients with elevated blood pressure in screened populations have normal pressures in the doctor's office. The current standard of what constitutes normal blood pressure is based on resting office pressures.

Even if the pressure is raised in the doctor's office, one must be certain that the elevated pressure is not transient. For example, one needs measurements on at least three separate occasions even if the diastolic pressure varies between 100 and 120 mm Hg. If diastolic pressures are so variable that they are 90–100 mm Hg on one occasion but less than that 90 mm Hg on another, it may be necessary to take readings over a period of months before concluding that the patient is indeed an established hypertensive who needs pharmacologic lifelong therapy. If the pressures are highly variable on different occasions, they can be taken by the patient or a family member at home, or by a nurse in the office. Ambulatory pressures can be obtained by utilizing a portable blood pressure recorder (see Figures 9–8, 9–9, and 9–28). In almost 30% of cases, even patients with consistently elevated office pressures will have normal pressures after several days of hospitalization for other reasons. The average drop in blood pressures in these patients is about 20–

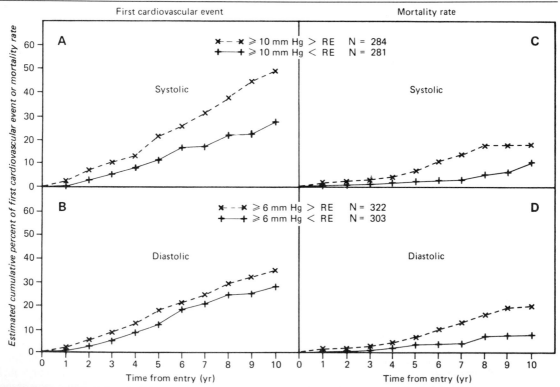

Figure 9–28. Estimated cumulative 10-year incidence of first clinical cardiovascular event *(A, B)* and cardiovascular mortality rate *(C, D)* among patients classified according to differences between observed and predicted blood pressures. The latter are derived from the regression equation (RE) for the regression of ambulatory on office pressures. $P = \leq.005$ for *A, B, C, D.* (Redrawn, modified, and reproduced, with permission, from Perloff D, Sokolow M, Cowan R: The prognostic value of ambulatory blood pressure. JAMA 1983;249:2792. Copyright © 1983 by American Medical Association.)

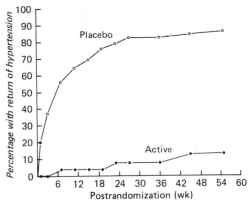

Figure 9–29. Return of hypertension after stopping treatment. Cumulative percentage of patients attaining diastolic blood pressure of 95 mm Hg or higher on two successive clinic visits is shown on the ordinate. Time after randomization is shown on the abscissa. At 6 weeks after randomization, 51% of the placebo group demonstrated 95 mm Hg, and at 6 months 82% of the placebo group had reached this level. (Reproduced, with permission of the American Heart Association, from: Veterans Administration Cooperative Study Group on Antihypertensive Agents: Return of elevated blood pressure after withdrawal of antihypertensive drugs. Circulation 1975;51:1107.)

vinced that this particular patient will benefit from treatment even after the potential side effects of the drug regimen have been considered, the patient must then be educated regarding treatment, and every responsible effort must be made to see to it that the patient continues in treatment indefinitely. In the Veterans Administration Study (1975), hypertension returned, usually by 6 months, in 85% of patients in whom treatment was deliberately stopped (Figure 9–29).

The decision to begin antihypertensive therapy requires careful judgment and thorough discussion with the patient and should never by undertaken lightly. Once begun, treatment should be continued without interruption, modified if necessary, along with treatment of other risk factors of atherosclerosis.

Treat According to Severity

In the average patient with mild (diastolic pressures 90–104 mm Hg) or moderate hypertension (diastolic pressures 105–114 mm Hg), it is preferable to begin with low doses and to gradually increase the dosage or substitute or add drugs of the same or a different class. More rapid control is needed when the patient has accelerated hypertension, encephalopathy, or cardiac failure or in similar urgent circumstances. The physician must estimate the urgency of the role of the elevated blood pressure and choose drugs accordingly. Even when it is urgent to lower the pressure quickly, one must not act precipitously, since too rapid a fall in pressure can precipitate acute central nervous system or renal complications.

In mild to moderate disease, one should begin with drugs of modest potency in low dosage given once or twice daily in order to avoid toxic side effects that might discourage the patient. If a drug of one class is ineffective or causes unacceptable side effects, another drug of the same class or of a different class

30 mm Hg depending on the age of the patient and the height of the pressure; the significance of this difference is not known, but it may result from removing the patient from his or her "stressful" ordinary life to the more "protected" environment of the hospital. The blood pressure-lowering effects of nonpharmacologic treatment are modest.

When the physician has taken an adequate number of readings under appropriate conditions and is con-

Table 9–12. Effects of different antihypertensive agents on coronary risk factors.[1]

	Diuretic	Beta Blockade	Alpha Blockade	Calcium Blockade	ACE Inhibition
Blood pressure	+	+	+	+	+
Total cholesterol	–	NS	+	NS	NS
HDL cholesterol	NS	—	NS	NS	NS
Glucose intolerance	–	–	+	NS	+
Hyperinsulinemia	–	–	+	NS	+
Physical activity	NS	–	+	NS	NS
Left ventricular hypertrophy	–	+	+	+	+

[1] Reproduced, with permission, from Kaplan NM: Changing hypertension treatment to reduce the overall cardiovascular risk. J Hypertens 1990;8(Suppl 7):S175.

Key:
+ = improvement
– = aggravation
NS = not significant

Table 9–13. Favorable and adverse factors in the choice of antihypertensive drugs.

	Favorable	Adverse
Diuretics	Low cost, usually few symptoms, can be combined with other agents; valuable in cardiac failure and excess-volume states; effective in low-renin states (elderly, blacks).	Volume depletion, metabolic abnormalities (hypokalemia, lipid abnormalities, impaired glucose tolerance, raised uric acid). Worsens gout, diabetes mellitus, perhaps fosters arrhythmias; impotence.
Beta-blockers	Benefits associated angina, hypertrophic cardiomyopathy, recurrent myocardial infarction, migraine, arrhythmias. Useful in younger hyperkinetic patients.	Induces bronchospasm; fatigue; decreased mental acuity; decreased exercise tolerance; decreased renal blood flow, bradycardia, nasal congestion, lipid abnormalities, decreased symptoms and slowed recovery from hypoglycemia in diabetics receiving insulin, worsens claudication, CNS nocturnal symptoms, abrupt discontinuation syndrome, impotence.
ACE inhibitors	Valuable in congestive heart failure. No lipid abnormalities, fatigue, or CNS symptoms. Slows renal impairment in diabetic nephropathy. Decreases left ventricular mass.	First-dose angioedema; cough; rash; proteinemia and neutropenia if large doses (captopril); may cause renal failure in bilateral, severe renal artery stenosis; minor taste change; should not be used in pregnancy; expensive.
Calcium entry-blocking drugs	Coronary and cerebral vasodilator; decreases left ventricular mass; helpful in hypertrophic cardiomyopathy; useful in elderly and in blacks; no CNS symptoms; useful for Raynaud's disease, arrhythmias and claudication; lipids not affected.	Constipation (especially verapamil and diltiazem); headache, edema, flushing (nifedipine); AV block (verapamil) but useful in supraventricular tachycardia mostly verapamil). If patient has heart failure, do not combine with beta-blocker. Care with cardiac failure. Expensive.
Central α_2-adrenergic receptor agonist drugs	Cardiac output and lipids unchanged; no reflex sympathetic response to vasodilation.	Slow mental responses; sedation; fluid retention; dry mouth; rebound hypertension if drug stopped abruptly (clonidine); postural hypotension; autoimmune disease (methyldopa); hepatic abnormalities; AV conduction defects may occur; bradycardia.
Alpha-adrenergic receptor-blocking drugs	No lipid abnormalities or reflex sympathetic response to vasodilation. No metabolic or CNS abnormalities. Cardiac output unaffected. Relaxes urinary bladder sphincter and helps in prostatism.	First-dose hypotension; fluid retention; sedation; dry mouth; decreased alertness; rebound hypertension if drug stopped abruptly (clonidine); postural hypotension; autoimmune disease (methyldopa); hepatic test abnormalities. AV conduction defects may occur with bradycardia.
Peripheral adrenergic inhibitors	Effective and inexpensive (reserpine); low-dose (0.1 mg); can be combined with diuretics. Low cost.	Mental depression with larger doses; fluid retention; nasal congestion; peptic ulcer (reserpine in larger doses); abrupt diarrhea and exercise hypotension (guanethine); retrograde ejaculation.
Direct vasodilators	Potent (minoxidil); can be used IM or IV (hydralazine); when combined with reserpine, is useful in children.	Lupus syndrome and immune disease if > 200 mg/d (hydralazine); hirsutism; fluid retention (minoxidil); tachycardia; headache; reflex sympathetic stimulation with tachycardia; raised cardiac output with hydralazine. Do not use in dissecting aorta. Does not reverse left ventricular mass.

may be substituted or added; dosage should be individually titrated to obtain the desired effect (< 90 mm Hg diastolic) without adverse responses. All therapy must be individualized, depending on the response of the patient and the presence of associated conditions that may make the choice of a class of drugs favorable or adverse (see Tables 9–12 and 9–13). The objective of treatment is to use as few agents as possible with the fewest possible side effects and to reduce the blood pressure permanently without interfering too much with the patient's life-style. The availability of a number of drugs with different mechanisms of ac-

tion allows the physician to use trial and error to obtain an effective combination of agents with which the patient can live comfortably. Forcing the patient to accept unpleasant side effects usually leads to discouragement and noncompliance, especially if the patient was asymptomatic before therapy. The drugs are used orally except in compelling situations, when parenteral therapy is used in combination with oral therapy.

The purpose of therapy is to prevent complications and enhance survival. The immediate objective is to achieve a sitting office diastolic pressure of less than

90 mm Hg or a systolic pressure less than 140 mm Hg. A pressure of 150/100 mm Hg is acceptable if untoward side effects make a lower pressure difficult to achieve, especially in patients with severe hypertension at the outset or in patients over age 70. The physician should assess the patient's social, emotional, economic, and environmental problems in all cases, especially if the response to treatment is poor. The strategy of comprehensive care includes education of the patient and an effort to make treatment as convenient and acceptable as possible to ensure compliance with long-term management. Treatment must be individualized, with minimal doses (for example) in frail elderly people.

GENERAL NONPHARMACOLOGIC THERAPEUTIC MEASURES

General measures include a diet low in salt and saturated fats, an adequate K^+ and Ca^{2+} intake, exercise and a low-calorie for weight reduction if overweight, measures to promote physical fitness and encourage relaxation, cessation of cigarette smoking, and avoidance of excessive alcohol use. Risk factors for atherosclerosis not susceptible to intervention include a family history of hypertension and its complications, black racial background, and male sex. However, adherence to nonpharmacologic measures may prevent the development of hypertension in persons thought to be susceptible to the disease because of genetic predisposition and environmental factors (see also Pathophysiology) (National Education Programs, 1991; Kaplan, 1991).

Cigarette smoking, hypercholesterolemia, high serum concentrations of LDL cholesterol or low concentrations of HDL cholesterol, evidence of target organ damage (especially left ventricular hypertrophy), and a sedentary lifestyle should be the focus of aggressive management, either alone in borderline hypertension or combined with pharmacologic therapy when that is indicated. An increased left ventricular mass on echocardiography improves prediction of subsequent hypertension in normal persons (de Simone, 1991).

A large NIH study of nonpharmacologic interventions in persons with high normal diastolic pressures (80–89 mm Hg) found that weight reduction (losing 3.9 kg) and reduction of sodium intake (by 44 mmol/d) lowered the systolic pressure by 2.9 mm Hg and the diastolic pressure by 2.3 mm Hg. Whether these modest declines in blood pressure have prognostic significance is not known. Some of these subjects may have had borderline hypertension, because a few required antihypertensive therapy during the 18-month follow-up (Trials of Hypertension, 1992). Other references regarding exercise in hypertension are World Hypertensive League, 1991; Stamler, 1989; and Oberman, 1990.

Weight reduction is recommended not only because it may infrequently reduce the blood pressure to normal but also because obesity aggravates and increases the likelihood of diabetes and insulin resistance, marginally increases the likelihood of coronary heart disease, and detracts from the patient's sense of well-being.

Moderate physical activity is encouraged not only for its effect on weight loss and general sense of well-being but also because moderate exercise modestly decreases the systemic vascular resistance. Advocates of physical exercise as a preventive measure against the complications of coronary artery disease believe that physical fitness decreases the likelihood of fatality if the patient does develop acute myocardial infarction.

Cigarette smoking increases not only the incidence of coronary heart disease but also the likelihood of ventricular fibrillation and sudden death—especially if the patient has left ventricular hypertrophy or concomitant coronary artery disease. Hypertensive patients should be urged to stop smoking.

There is no evidence that moderate amounts of alcohol, coffee, or tea are harmful to hypertensive patients; in fact, they may be helpful by virtue of their relaxant effects. Excessive use of alcohol, however, is undesirable because it increases the serum triglyceride concentration and may produce alcoholic cardiomyopathy. In a patient whose cardiac afterload is already increased by raised blood pressure, alcohol may favor the development of cardiac failure or arrhythmias. The combination of hypertensive heart disease, coronary heart disease, and alcoholic cardiomyopathy is particularly unfavorable.

Treatment with antihypertensive drugs may be added if the diastolic pressure is less than 95 mm Hg and associated coronary risk factors are present. If repeated observations indicate diastolic pressure greater than 100 mm Hg, pharmacologic antihypertensive therapy should be started.

Relaxation, Meditation, or Biofeedback Therapy

A variety of methods have been used over the years to relax hypertensive patients. Before the days of effective antihypertensive drug therapy, sedation, progressive relaxation, psychotherapy, frequent vacations, and attention to the environment were all used with only marginal benefit. More recently, transcendental meditation, biofeedback, yoga exercises, and other methods of relaxation have been explored in an effort to combat the environmental increase in systemic vascular resistance and cardiac output that occurs with the stresses of modern life. In a group of 20 hypertensive patients who went through a professionally supervised program of transcendental meditation, no significant change in blood pressure occurred after 6 months (Pollack, 1977), though some subjects had a greater sense of well-being. We have been unimpressed by reports of long-term, meaningful beneficial effects of biofeedback training on blood pressure, and in the absence of data solidly demonstrating its value we rely on antihypertensive agents rather than on psychologic or nonpharmacologic methods as the primary means of treating hypertension.

ANTIHYPERTENSIVE DRUG TREATMENT

Goals & General Aspects

The object of hypertensive therapy is to lower the blood pressure to 140/90 mm Hg or less for as much of the day as possible—consistent with the patient's cooperation and the absence of disabling side effects—to prevent complications, to prevent progressive rise of the blood pressure level, and to improve survival rates. In mild disease, good control is achieved with a single drug in about half of patients. For older patients with impaired cerebral or coronary circulation in whom it is important to avoid excess hypotension or rapid changes in pressure, one should accept a diastolic pressure of 100 mm Hg if lowering the pressure further produces cerebral or anginal symptoms. The lower limit of autoregulation is higher in hypertension; cerebral hypoperfusion may occur if the pressure is reduced below this limit (Strandgaard, 1989). In uncooperative patients with poor compliance, or in patients who find it difficult to take medication more than once a day, the physician should prescribe a long-acting drug that can be taken once daily or accept partial control of the blood pressure if insisting on more frequent medication would cause the patient to abandon therapy altogether. If cardiac failure is present, one should avoid a drug or combinations of drugs that have negative inotropic effects (beta-blockers plus verapamil). The response to therapy should be determined not only by office pressure readings but by some variety of stationary home or ambulatory portable recordings to obtain more representative pressures; these pressures are used to determine therapy until prospective studies prove that nonoffice recordings are better prognostically.

The physician must first determine how urgent it is to lower the blood pressure and then choose accordingly oral or parenteral treatment, the drugs and doses to be initiated, the frequency with which they should be repeated, and the speed with which the blood pressure should be brought under control. The presence of coexisting conditions as well as other coronary risk factors should be evaluated and treatment provided as indicated; the effects of different antihypertensive agents on these factors influence the physician's choice of drugs (Table 9–12) (Kaplan, 1990). The physician must also balance the beneficial response of the blood pressure to treatment against side effects that may interfere with treatment; this may require

adjustment of dosage or change to a different therapeutic agent. The costs of medications, visits to the physician, and laboratory tests must also be considered. Treatment is empiric but should be individualized. By consideration of favorable and adverse effects and by trial and error, one arrives at the drug or combination of drugs that will lower the blood pressure while interfering as little as possible with the patient's life and work, taking into account all aspects of the patient's medical condition (asthma, cardiac failure, etc) (Tables 9–13 and 9–14).

There has been considerable difference of opinion about the so-called J effect—an increased mortality rate in patients in whom the diastolic pressure has been lowered to 80–85 mm Hg or less. Some authors believe, however, that lowering the diastolic blood pressure below 85–90 mm Hg is unwise if the patient has known coronary disease (Cruikshank, 1990; Farnett, 1991; Samuelsson, 1990; Fletcher, 1992).

Choice of Initial Drug Treatment

The choice of the class of drug used for initial therapy is based on a number of factors, including the cost, the patient's age, the presence of associated diseases (eg, cardiac or renal failure, gout, diabetes, asthma, arrhythmias), the patient's life-style, requirements for mental alertness, and side effects that may have occurred from previous therapy (eg, hypokalemia or gout from diuretics; bradycardia, bronchoconstriction, nasal congestion, mental slowing, or sexual dysfunction from beta-blocking therapy). If the first drug selected is ineffective, one can increase the dose, but doing so may enhance adverse effects. Alternatively—especially when the first drug is poorly tolerated—one can change to a second drug with a different mechanism of action. In mild hypertension, after good control of the blood pressure has been achieved for at least a year, dosages can be decreased in stepwise fashion or the drug can be stopped completely (see later), though in most cases the blood pressure will rise again; it can then be reinstituted at a lower dose.

Standard drug treatment in the past followed a "stepped-care approach" of increasing potency and variety of drugs. In the USA, patients were usually given a diuretic agent such as a thiazide initially. If the response was inadequate or if side effects occurred that were disturbing to either the patient or the physician, second and third drugs such as the beta-blockers, adrenergic inhibitors, or vasodilators were added. In Europe, patients were often given beta-blockers as the initial drug to which diuretics and, if necessary, vasodilators were subsequently added. These and similar combinations have reduced the incidence of stroke and heart failure and lowered the mortality rate by 40–50%. However, several of the recent multicenter therapeutic trials have emphasized the side effects from these agents that interfered with the quality of life or had adverse metabolic effects

Table 9–14. Oral antihypertensive medications.[1]

	Initial Daily Dosage	Usual Daily Range	Adverse Effects and Other Comments
Diuretics			
Bendroflumethiazide	2.5 mg	2.5–5 mg once daily	Hypokalemia, hypomagnesemia hyperglycemia, hyperuricemia (even gout), photosensitivity rash, sexual dysfunction, increased cholesterol levels, increased LDL. Nitrogen retention especially in elderly patients.
Chlorthalidone	12.5–2.5 mg	12.5–50 mg once daily	
Hydrochlorothiazides	12.5–50 mg	12.5–50 mg once daily	
Indapamide	2.5 mg	2.5–5 mg once daily	
Metolazone	2.5 mg	2.5–5 mg once daily	
Other thiazides	Various	Various	
Potassium-sparing agents			
Amiloride	5 mg	5–10 mg once daily	Hyperkalemia; with triamterene, gynecomastia, renal stones, and raised serum creatinine.
Spironolactone	25 mg	50–100 mg once daily	
Triamterene	25 mg	50–100 mg once daily	
Combination agents			
Dyazide	1³/₄–2 capsules	1–4 capsules in 1 or 2 doses ¹/₂–2 tablets	
Maxzide	¹/₂ tablet	¹/₂–2 tablets	
Moduretic	¹/₂ tablet		
Beta-blockers			
Acebutolol	400 mg daily	400–800 mg daily	Bradycardia, nasal congestion, fatigue, bronchospasm, sleep disturbances, cold extremities, sexual dysfunction, dizziness, headache, raised triglycerides, increased LDL, decreased HDL cholesterol, sodium retention, left ventricular failure.
Atenolol	25 mg once daily	50–100 mg once daily	
Betaxolol	5–10 mg once daily	10–20 mg once daily	
Carteolol	2.5 mg once daily	2.5–5 mg once daily	
Labetalol (α and β)	100 mg twice daily	100–400 mg twice daily	
Metoprolol	100 mg daily	40–120 mg twice daily	
Nadolol	20 mg once daily	40–80 mg twice daily	
Penbutolol	10 mg once daily	20 mg once daily	
Pindolol	5 mg twice daily	5–20 mg twice daily	
Propranolol	20–40 mg twice daily	40–120 mg twice daily	
Timolol	5 mg twice daily	10–20 mg twice daily	
ACE inhibitors			
Benazepril	5–10 mg once daily	20–40 mg once daily	With large doses of captopril, proteinuria and neutropenia; rare with low doses and not with enalapril; angioneurotic edema, cough, hypotension, renal failure, skin rash, and taste disturbance. May aggravate impaired renal function.
Captopril	12.5–25 mg twice daily	25–100 mg in 2 or 3 doses	
Enalapril	2.5–5 mg once daily	5–40 mg in 1 or 2 doses	
Fosinopril	5–10 mg once daily	20–60 mg once daily	
Lisinopril	5–10 mg once daily	10–40 mg once daily	
Quinapril	10 mg once daily	10–30 mg once daily	
Ramipril	2.5 mg once daily	5–10 mg once daily	
Calcium entry blockers			
Bepridil	200 mg once daily	200–300 mg once daily	SA and AV conduction defects, particularly with verapamil, and tachycardia, particularly with nifedipine; peripheral edema and hypotension especially with nifedipine; bradycardia, particularly with verapamil, headache, skin rash. Slow-release form of verapamil now available.
Diltiazem	30 mg 3 times daily	90–180 mg twice daily	
Diltiazem SR	90 mg once daily	90–120 mg twice daily	
Felodipine	5–10 mg once daily	10–20 mg once daily	
Isradipine	2.5 mg twice daily	2.5–10 mg twice daily	
Nicardipine	10 mg twice daily	20–40 mg twice daily	
Nifedipine XL	10 mg capsule	10–30 mg twice daily	
Nimodipine	30 mg once daily	30–90 mg once daily	
Nitrendipine	30 mg twice daily	60 mg twice daily	
Verapamil	5–10 mg once daily	10–40 mg once daily	
Verapamil SR	40–80 mg twice daily 90 mg once daily	120–360 mg in 2 doses 180–240 mg once daily	
Central-acting alpha adrenergic agonists			
Clonidine	0.1 mg twice daily	0.25–0.3 mg twice daily	Lethargy, dry mouth, sexual dysfunction; fever, hemolytic anemia, hepatitis with methyldopa; rebound hypertension with clonidine. Transcutaneous formulation available with clonidine.
Clonidine TTS Patches	3.5 mg patch once weekly (0.1 mg once daily)	10.5 mg patch once weekly (0.3 mg once daily)	
Guanabenz	4 mg twice daily	4–16 mg twice daily	
Guanfacine	1 mg	1–3 mg	
Methyldopa	250 mg twice daily	250 mg–1 g twice daily	
Alpha adrenergic receptor inhibitors			
Doxazosin	1 mg bedtime	1–8 mg once daily	Postural hypotension, especially with first dose; headache and palpitation; fluid retention; fatigue; sedation; dry mouth.
Prazosin	0.5–1 mg bedtime	3–7.5 m twice daily	
Terazosin	1 mg (long-acting)	1–5 mg	

(continued)

Table 9–14. (*Continued*)

	Initial Daily Dosage	Usual Daily Range	Adverse Effects and Other Comments
Adrenergic neuronal inhibitors			
Guanadrel	2.5–5 mg twice daily	10–30 mg twice daily	Depression, peptic ulcer with reserpine; postural hypotension especially with exercise with guanethidine.
Guanethidine	10 mg	25–50 mg daily	
Reserpine	0.05–0.1 mg	0.1–0.25 mg daily	
Arteriolar dilators			
Hydralazine	10–25 mg twice daily	25–100 mg twice daily	Headache, palpitations, tachycardia, angina; lupus if hydralazine exceeds 200 mg/d. Marked fluid retention and hirsutism with minoxidil. Do not use in aortic dissection.
Minoxidil	2.5–5 mg	5–20 mg twice daily	

[1] New drugs, new long-acting preparations, and new pharmaceutical formulations are being rapidly developed and approved by the FDA. Professional sources such as *Physician's Desk Reference* (annual publication updated quarterly) and *Facts and Comparisons* (annual volume; loose-leaf edition updated monthly) as well as the manufacturers' information services and marketing programs should be consulted frequently for new information.

and might have been responsible for the slight increase in mortality rate seen in vigorously treated patients. For example, diuretics induce metabolic and hemodynamic changes such as hypokalemia, decreased glomerular filtration rate and renal blood flow, hyperuricemia, hyperglycemia, and hyperlipidemia. Beta-blockers can aggravate asthma and induce bradycardia, atrioventricular conduction defects, lethargy, cold extremities and Raynaud's syndrome, cardiac failure, impotence, and vivid, unpleasant dreams. These side effects led to the use of newer therapeutic agents for initial therapy that have different mechanisms of action (see Tables 9–13 and 9–14).

Two additional classes of drugs are now available that are well tolerated with relatively few side effects and good therapeutic potency: the angiotensin-converting enzyme (ACE) inhibitors and the calcium entry-blocking agents.

Thus, the physician now has a choice of at least four major classes of drugs for the initial treatment of hypertension. In addition, three other classes of antihypertensive drugs may be given for initial treatment in the event of intolerance or contraindications to the four major initiating drugs. These include the central adrenergic inhibitors such as clonidine, peripheral alpha-adrenergic-blocking drugs such as prazosin, and direct vasodilators such as hydralazine. Table 9–14 lists the classes of drugs now available for treatment as well as some drug combinations.

All of the classes of drugs mentioned above have been advocated for initial monotherapy. Each class of drug has advantages and disadvantages, depending on the individual evaluation of the patient. Table 9–13 describes the factors influencing the choice of a drug in particular circumstances. Instead of increasing the dosage of the initial drug to its maximum before adding a second drug, it is more desirable to use two drugs in low dosage. This increases tolerability of the drugs, reduces side effects, and improves the blood pressure response.

SPECIFIC ANTIHYPERTENSIVE DRUGS

Drugs used in the treatment of hypertension vary in dosage, potency, side effects, mechanism of action, route of administration, and cost. The available drugs are summarized in Tables 9–13, 9–14, and 9–15 (see also Joint National Committee, 1988).

Oral Diuretic Agents

The thiazides are the prototype of this group of drugs, which act initially by depleting the body of sodium, potassium, and fluid volume and later by decreasing the systemic vascular resistance. They effectively reduce mortality rates and the incidence of stroke but have only minimal or no effect on reducing myocardial ischemia. The decrease in left ventricular mass is less than with other agents such as ACE inhibitors or calcium entry blockers.

The sodium, potassium, chloride, and water losses may be substantial over the first few days and then tend to diminish. Early in the course of treatment, hypovolemia may be associated with dizziness, weakness, nausea, cramps, and postural hypotension; later, the plasma volume and extracellular volume return almost to normal (reduced about 3–5%), and postural hypotension is uncommon. The dose-response curves are such that maximum diuretic effect occurs with about 100 mg of hydrochlorothiazide, given as a single dose. Thiazides increase the tubular reabsorption of urate, raising plasma uric acid, which in susceptible individuals may cause acute gout attacks.

Hypokalemia is a major problem associated with

Table 9–15. Treatment of hypertensive crises (adult dosages).[1]

Drug	How Supplied	Initial Dose and Route	Onset of Action	Duration of Action (Before Repeat Dose)
PARENTERAL ADMINISTRATION				
Adrenergic inhibitors				
Methyldopa (Aldomet)	250 mg/5 mL ampule	250–500 mg IV	2–4 hours	4–12 hours
Trimethaphan camsylate[2] (Arfonad)	500 mg/10 mL ampule	1–4 mg/min IV	Seconds to minutes	As long as infused
Reserpine (Serpasil)	5 mg/2 mL (also 10 mL) ampule	0.5–1 mg IM or IV bolus, slowly	2–6 hours	6–12 hours
Propranolol[3] (Inderal)	1 mg/1 mL	1 mg IV bolus, slowly	Minutes	4–6 hours
Labetalol				
Normodyne Trandate	20 mL vials or 40 mL multidose vials or ampules (for slow infusion, diluted to 250 mL)	20–80 mg IV slowly (over 1 minute) every 10 minutes, followed by 2 mg/min IV infusion.[4]	5–10 minutes	10 minutes for bolus injection
Vasodilators				
Diazoxide[2] (Hyperstat)	300 mg/20 mL ampule	50–300 mg IV rapidly	1–5 minutes	5–12 hours
Hydralazine (Apresoline)	20 mg/1 mL ampule	5–10 mg IV or IM bolus, slowly	15–30 minutes	1–4 hours
Sodium nitroprusside (Nipride)	50 mg/5 mL vial	0.5–8 µg/kg/min IV by infusion of D_5W, not by direct injection	Immediate; can ↑ infusion rate every 5–10 minutes as needed	As long as infused
Nitroglycerin	Intravenous	0.5–10 µg/kg/min IV	1–3 minutes	As long as infused
Diuretics				
Furosemide (Lasix)	20 mg/2 mL ampule	40–80 mg IV bolus	15–30 minutes	8–12 hours
Ethacrynate sodium (Edecrine)	50 mg/50 mL vial	50 mg IV bolus	15–30 minutes	8–12 hours
Calcium entry blockers				
Nicardipine (Cardene)	Intravenous	5 mg IV/h, ↑ by 1–2.5 mg/h every 15 minutes, up to 15 mg/h	1–5 minutes	3–6 hours
ORAL ADMINISTRATION				
Nifedipine (Adalat, Procardia)	Capsules	10–20 mg	5–15 minutes	3–5 hours
Clonidine (Catapres)	Tablets	0.2 mg initially, then 0.1 mg/h; maximum, 7 mg		6–8 hours
Captopril (Capoten)	Tablets	6.5–25 mg	15–30 minutes	4–6 hours

[1] New drugs, new long-acting preparations, and new pharmaceutical formulations are being rapidly developed and approved by the FDA. Professional sources such as *Physician's Desk Reference* (annual publication updated quarterly) and *Facts and Comparisons* (annual volume; loose-leaf edition updated monthly) as well as the manufacturers' information services and marketing programs should be consulted frequently for new information.
[2] Requires closely monitored supervision and titration for proper dosage.
[3] The prototype of beta-adrenergic blocking drugs. See text for others.
[4] Be alert for bronchial constriction, heart block, and orthostatic hypotension (1988 National Report).
[5] Photosensitive. Must be protected from light.

the use of diuretics. It is due to impaired reabsorption of potassium (K^+) at the sodium-potassium exchange site, where aldosterone causes increased secretion of potassium and reabsorption of sodium. The magnitude of the decrease in serum K^+ is variable but averages about 0.6 meq/L (10–15%) in patients receiving 50 mg/d of hydrochlorothiazide. For this reason, smaller doses of hydrochlorothiazide are now recommended (12.5–25 mg/d, increased to 50 mg/d only if necessary). It takes 60–80 meq/d of potassium (given as 10% KCl elixir) to raise the serum potassium to the pretreatment value (Schwartz, 1974). Total potassium in the body may be normal when the serum potassium is reduced, and patients may have a substantial loss of total body potassium with a normal serum potassium. The acid-base equilibrium influences the intra- and

Table 9–16. Average serum electrolytes after 6–8 weeks' treatment with 50 mg hydrochlorothiazide or 100 mg ethacrynic acid daily.[1]

Treatment Group	Sodium (meq/L)	Potassium (meq/L)	Chloride (meq/L)	Bicarbonate (meq/L)	Urea (mg/dL)	Uric Acid (mg/dL)
Control	143.9	4.3	103.3	27.5	29.8	5.3
Hydrochlorothiazide	137.8	3.7	95.4	29.0	32.0	7.2
Ethacrynic acid	139.4	3.8	98.0	27.9	41.1 (31.8)[2]	7.0

[1] Reproduced, with permission, from Dollery CT, Parry EHO, Young DS: Diuretic and hypotensive properties of ethacrynic acid: A comparison with hydrochlorothiazide. Lancet 1964;1:947.
[2] This figure is the average after eliminating the results on one patient whose blood urea rose to 155 mg/dL on ethacrynic acid.

extracellular balance of potassium, and if there is a tendency to alkalosis, the serum potassium may fall. Table 9–16 shows the average serum electrolytes after 6–8 weeks of treatment with diuretics. In the Veterans Administration Study (1967), the serum potassium levels on the initial, first, and second annual examinations showed that most patients after 1–2 years had levels exceeding 3.5 meq/L but that 20% were between 2.5 and 3.5 meq/L. The electrolyte response to a diuretic is enhanced by bed rest; the urine volume and sodium excretion in normal individuals when they are in bed is of the same order of magnitude as when they are up and about and receiving a diuretic. During bed rest, water and sodium excretion doubles, but K^+ excretion does not change. The increased reabsorption of uric acid in the proximal tubule leads to raised serum uric acid, which in individuals with a history of gout may cause acute gout that can be prevented by the use of probenecid or allopurinol. Infrequently, glucose reabsorption in the proximal tubule is also increased, and patients with a susceptibility to diabetes may develop hyperglycemia. The average increase in fasting blood sugar after 2 years of diuretic therapy was about 9 mg/dL (Murphy, 1982); changes between 6 and 14 years were not striking. When thiazides were withdrawn for 7 months, the average reduction in fasting blood glucose was 10% and in the 2-hour postprandial value 25% (Murphy, 1982).

The hemodynamic changes that occur during long-term therapy have been described by Lund-Johansen (1991). If the dosage of diuretics is excessive, the patient may develop severe hyponatremia and dehydration with hypovolemia, but this is uncommon if the thiazides and not the loop diuretics (eg, furosemide) are used in moderate doses. The potassium loss makes digitalis toxicity more likely, so that particular care must be taken to avoid hypokalemia if digitalis is also being used. Hypokalemia is more common when dietary potassium is low, sodium intake is high, and laxatives are used frequently. If the serum potassium falls below 3.5 meq/L on ordinary doses of thiazides, the possibility of primary hyperaldosteronism should be considered.

If symptoms of hypokalemia develop (polyuria, nocturia, muscle weakness, and fatigue) or if digitalis is prescribed, potassium-sparing diuretics such as spironolactone, amiloride, or triamterene may be added to the thiazides or other diuretics such as chlorthalidone, furosemide, bendroflumethiazide, and metolazone, provided renal function is adequate and the patients do not take oral potassium supplements. Spironolactone may induce gynecomastia by altering the metabolism of testosterone; triamterene may result in impaired renal function. In a cooperative study in patients over 60 years of age who received both hydrochlorothiazide, 25 mg daily, and triamterene, 50 mg daily, there was a progressive rise in serum creatinine (Amery, 1991). The rise in serum creatinine correlated significantly with the fall in systolic blood pressure and with the rise in serum uric acid. Further studies are required to determine the hazards of triamterine in elderly patients.

Patients with hypokalemia and symptoms who are not being given potassium-sparing drugs should be placed on a high-potassium diet (Table 9–17) or potassium supplements. (Enteric-coated potassium sup-

Table 9–17. Foods helpful in addition to normal diet to supplement potassium (K^+) intake.[1]

Quantities of foods to supply approximately 0.5 g (500 mg) (13 meq) of potassium (K^+)
1 cup tomato juice[1]
1 cup low-sodium tomato juice, prune juice
1¼ cups orange juice, tangerine juice, orange-grapefruit juice, grapefruit juice
1 medium-sized banana
7–8 dates
4 figs
7 large prunes
½ cup raisins (dark)
6 apricots (fresh)
½ cantaloupe
1 cup broccoli
¾ cup winter squash
10 brussels sprouts, cooked
1 large white potato
1 large sweet potato
⅓ cup lentils (dry)
1½ cups raw cauliflower
4 tbsp nonfat milk powder[2]
1½ cups nonfat milk[2]

[1] Courtesy of California Heart Association.
[2] High in potassium but also high in sodium.

plements should be avoided because of their propensity for producing ulceration of the small intestine.) Liquid potassium preparations are unpleasant to take. If hypokalemia occurs at levels of 3–3.5 meq/L, oral potassium supplements of 40–80 meq/d in divided doses should be prescribed unless renal failure is present. Alternatively, the physician can prescribe potassium-sparing drugs such as amiloride, spironolactone, or triamterene (see Table 9–14); when these are used, the patient should stop potassium supplements and avoid a high-potassium diet.

Used alone, oral diuretic agents suffice in many cases to lower the pressure satisfactorily, though some authorities prefer to begin with beta-adrenergic-blocking drugs because of the side effects of diuretics. In the elderly, other drugs may be equally effective; the choice depends on associated conditions, life-styles, and tolerance (Tjoa, 1990). Approximately 40% of patients with borderline or mild hypertension with diastolic pressures of 90–110 mm Hg respond satisfactorily to diuretics alone; the average reduction in blood pressure with hydrochlorothiazide is about 20 mm Hg systolic and 10–15 mm Hg diastolic. Since the need to lower the pressure is not urgent, thiazides should be started in low dosage, eg, 12.5–25 mg of hydrochlorothiazide once daily, the lower amount being used in patients who are elderly, are receiving digitalis, or have a clinical condition in which an unexpectedly large diuresis of water, sodium, and potassium would be precarious. Response to the thiazides begins to be evident within a few days, and by 2 weeks one can be fairly certain whether the dosage used is adequate. If not, it can be increased by increments to a maximum single dose of 50 mg. A dosage of 50 mg once a day is usually sufficient if diuretics alone are going to be effective in lowering the blood pressure. If a month of thiazide therapy does not lower the blood pressure to the desired level, adding or substituting a second drug is indicated. The effects of diuretics are additive to that of other drugs; therefore, the dosage of diuretic should be decreased or the new drug given in smaller amounts. If oral diuretics are added to an already stabilized regiment because of sodium retention or inadequate control of hypertension, the dose of the basic drug should be reduced about 50% before the diuretic is added to avoid excessive fall in pressure. Diuretics increase total serum cholesterol and LDL and decrease HDL cholesterol. The question has been raised whether these lipid effects may be responsible for the failure of antihypertensive therapeutic trials to decrease ischemic coronary events. Most trials have included diuretic or β-adrenergic-blocking drugs or both, and both have adverse lipid effects.

Beta₁-Adrenergic-Blocking Drugs

These drugs block the β_1-adrenoceptors, thus decreasing sympathetic effects on the circulation. They lower the blood pressure effectively and decrease the plasma renin concentration, pulse rate, and cardiac output. They lessen the likelihood of arrhythmias or angina if the patient is receiving vasodilators or has concomitant coronary heart disease. However, beta-blockers may cause adverse side effects if the patient has a history of asthma, Raynaud's phenomenon, left ventricular failure, bradycardia, or ventricular conduction defects or if vigorous mental or physical activity is required.

Beta-adrenergic-blocking agents reduce systolic and diastolic blood pressure by reducing the heart rate both at rest and after exercise by about 25% and the cardiac index during exercise by about 15%; systemic vascular resistance shows no change or may rise slightly. These drugs should be used with caution if combined with another drug that has a negative inotropic action. Renal blood flow and the glomerular filtration rate may fall slightly. In addition to their beta-blocking activities, beta-blockers decrease renin release and systemic vascular resistance.

Because beta-blocking drugs neutralize the reflex tachycardia and increase in cardiac output that follow administration of vasodilator drugs, they are particularly effective when combined with diuretic and vasodilator drugs. They may mask the tachycardia and sweating and other warning signs of hypoglycemia in diabetics receiving insulin, especially while these patients are fasting. Suitable precautions should be taken. Propranolol (or other beta-blockers) may cause Raynaud's phenomenon in cold weather, bradycardia, asthma, hypotension, syncope, left ventricular failure, and occasionally central nervous system symptoms such as lethargy, depression, and intense dreams.

The approved beta-adrenergic-blocking agents and their dosages are noted in Table 9–14. They should be started at a low dose and titrated to a well-tolerated effective one. Atenolol and nadolol may have significant clinical advantages in that they are effective with once-daily dosing. Atenolol and metoprolol do not cross the blood-brain barrier and therefore result in fewer central nervous system side effects. All beta-adrenergic-blocking agents have similar effects in the treatment of hypertension but differ with respect to dosage, duration of effect, lipid solubility and entry into the brain, intrinsic sympathomimetic activity, and cardioselectivity for β_1 receptors. Lipid-soluble agents are said to cause more adverse central nervous system effects because they enter the brain. Cardioselective agents have predominant effects on β_1 receptors and little effect on β_2 receptors and are therefore more advantageous in the treatment of angina and arrhythmias but more apt to worsen bronchospasm. Intrinsic sympathomimetic activity or partial agonist activity has an advantage in causing less bradycardia, less fall in cardiac output with exercise and thus better exercise tolerance, and perhaps less blockage of β_2 receptors in asthma; however, drugs with intrinsic sympathomimetic activity (eg, pindolol) should be avoided in patients with dissecting aorta because of their agonist activity. The pharmacologic characteristics are noted in Tables 8–4 and 8–5. A drug with intrinsic sympathomimetic activity and a weak agonist effect (eg, pindolol) may cause less bradycardia; however, the beta-blocking effect is predominant. All of the beta-adrenergic-blocking drugs are more effective when combined with a diuretic.

The beta-adrenergic-blocking drugs in moderate dosages produce an average fall of mean blood pressure of about 20 mm Hg (range, 10–40 mm Hg), and there is an increasing tendency, especially in Europe, to begin therapy with these drugs rather than with the diuretic. If a diuretic has been given with inadequate response, a beta-blocker can be used as a second drug. Excessive doses may cause postural hypotension and mental slowing, and the decrease in cardiac output may be significant, especially in patients with impending or actual left ventricular failure. An ultra-short-acting intravenous beta-blocker (esmolol) is available; it is cardioselective and useful in supraventricular tachycardia and peri- and postoperative hypertension (Sonnenblick, 1985).

Combined Alpha- & Beta-Adrenergic Blocking Agents (Labetalol)

A combination that blocks both adrenergic systems may offer significant advantages in some patients. Beta-receptor blockade counteracts the reflex increase in heart rate and cardiac output produced by other vasodilating agents such as hydralazine, and alpha blockade counteracts the vasoconstriction and increase in systemic vascular resistance; however, postural hypotension may occur. Labetalol can be used either orally (200–800 mg/d) or, in hypertensive crises, intravenously, 20–40 mg initially over 2 minutes followed by, if necessary, additional boluses of 40 mg every 10 minutes to the desired diastolic level, usually above 110 mm Hg. Mean arterial blood pressure is reduced by about 20% and systemic vascular resistance by about 15%. If angina pectoris is present, it may be relieved, because the beta-blocking potency counteracts reflex tachycardia.

ACE Inhibitors

Angiotensin-converting enzyme (ACE) inhibitors inhibit the conversion of angiotensin I to angiotensin II, thus decreasing concentrations of the latter and increasing the concentration of renin. Angiotensin II is a potent pressor agent; it increases sympathetic drive and catecholamine activity; stimulates the secretion of aldosterone, which results in salt and water retention; and may decrease renal function, especially in either bilateral renal artery stenosis or stenosis of the renal artery of a single functioning kidney (see Secondary Hypertension). The ACE inhibitors counteract these actions, lower the blood pressure in hy-

pertensive patients, and inhibit the degradation of bradykinin and stimulate the local synthesis of prostaglandins. Hemodynamically, ACE inhibitors cause a fall in arterial pressure, a decrease in systemic vascular resistance, a slight rise in cardiac output, and some improvement in renal function. The fall in blood pressure may be considerable if patients are sodium- or volume-depleted or are receiving beta-adrenergic-blocking drugs; ACE inhibitors should be used with considerable caution in such circumstances.

All ACE-inhibiting drugs approved by the FDA have similar mechanisms of action. They are all approximately equal in effectiveness but vary in their duration of action as well as their degree of vasodilation and, in the case of captopril, effect on AV conduction (Williams, 1988). Captopril and nifedipine have the shortest durations of action; enalapril is intermediate in duration of action; and fosinopril, benazepril, ramipril, and lisinopril have the longest duration of action (Anderson, 1991; Robertson, 1987; Rotmensch, 1988). The ACE inhibitors are active not only in the circulation but also in the vascular endothelium, especially of the brain and kidney. The vascular endothelium and vascular walls demonstrate ACE activity and explain why nephrectomized patients may continue to have low circulating angiotensin. Angiotensin inhibitors reverse the stimulating effect of angiotensin on the central nervous system, decreasing systemic vascular resistance and blood pressure. The hemodynamic effects of the various ACE inhibitors are similar; they have the advantage that they do not produce reflex tachycardia and have no adverse metabolic effects, as do some other antihypertensive agents. The long-acting compounds can be given once daily instead of twice daily, as is required of the other drugs of this class. All of the drugs decrease left ventricular mass if it is raised.

Adverse effects result chiefly from the vasodilating action of the drugs, which may cause headache, flushing, and edema. Disturbing, dry irritating cough occurs in about 5–10% of patients. Faulty taste discrimination and rash may occur. Angioedema is uncommon but may occur on initiating treatment and require immediate treatment with intravenous antihistamines and corticosteroids. In patients with unilateral renal artery stenosis, the drugs can be used if the opposite kidney is normal, but this is often difficult to determine. If the patient has severe or malignant hypertension, one should consider evaluating the renal arteries prior to using ACE inhibitors. A patient who has bilateral renal artery stenosis or renal artery stenosis of a single functioning kidney may develop azotemia and renal failure. Glomerular capillary pressure is maintained by efferent arteriolar contraction in the hypertensive state. In diabetics with hypertension, dilation of the efferent arterioles by ACE inhibitors is beneficial: By preventing glomerular capillary hypertension, the progression (if present) of albuminuria and impaired renal function is retarded (Mimran, 1989). Patients with high plasma renin should be started with a low-dose ACE inhibitor. Hypovolemia should be corrected before ACE inhibitors are introduced; diuretics can be stopped several days before and blood volume restored. ACE inhibitors are said to be less effective in blacks, but the data are conflicting. In addition to decreasing left ventricular mass, the drugs improve left ventricular diastolic function. In general, although the blood pressure-lowering effects of the ACE inhibitors and calcium blockers are similar to other antihypertensive drugs, the sense of well-being and the quality of life are better with ACE inhibitors (with the exception of the cough) and with the calcium blockers (with the exception of the constipation) (see later).

Comparison of therapeutic effectiveness with other antihypertensive drugs is difficult because of differences in the patient populations studied and the questions of comparable dosage. The data are conflicting (Schrader, 1990; Beevers, 1991).

The doses of the various drugs of this class (as well as other antihypertensive oral medications) are tabulated in Table 9–14. If the beneficial effect on the blood pressure is inadequate with monotherapy of the ACE inhibitors, one can add a small dose of diuretic or calcium-entry-blocking drugs (Beevers, 1991).

Calcium Entry-Blocking Agents

As with ACE inhibitors, there has been a profusion of articles and symposia on the use of these agents in the treatment of hypertension. New drugs of this class are being introduced with some frequency. The calcium ion is intimately involved in muscle contraction in various organs of the body, including the blood vessels. Drugs of this class that block entry of calcium into the cells have been effective and well tolerated; these include verapamil, diltiazem, nifedipine, isradipine, nimodipine, nitrendipine, and nicardipine. There is also accumulating evidence that calcium-entry-blocking agents are antiatherosclerotic, slow the progression of early atherosclerotic lesions, inhibit the migration of muscle cells into an injured intima, and improve renal function and cerebral function following cerebral ischemia (Oparil, 1991). They are all similarly effective in the treatment of hypertension but differ in their atrioventricular conduction and selective vasodilation characteristics (Kaplan, 1989). They specifically inhibit the flow of calcium ion into the myocardial cell cytoplasm, thus decreasing Ca^{2+} availability to the contractile mechanism, resulting in vasodilation and a fall in blood pressure. A number of agents are now available in slow-release preparations, having a long-acting effect. Because the drugs are potent vasodilators, they are particularly valuable when hypertension is associated with angina or coronary spasm. Nifedipine is the most potent vasodilator. Drugs of this class reduce systemic vascular resistance, slightly increase the cardiac output without significant change in renal function, increase the glomerular filtration rate and renal blood flow, and lower renal resistance. With the exception of nifedipine, they produce little if any reflex tachycardia or sodium retention, but they do have side effects associated with vasodilation, such as peripheral edema, hypotension, headache, flushing, and dizziness. The vasodilating action of diltiazem is intermediate between that of verapamil and that of nifedipine. Verapamil has the added action of inhibiting sinoatrial and atrioventricular conduction, causing bradycardia or AV block; it should not be used when these conduction defects are present or if they develop. The combination of digoxin and verapamil is especially potent in accentuating the bradycardia and atrioventricular block. Constipation is an important side effect of the calcium-entry-blocking agents; verapamil may be the most constipating of the drugs of this class. Metabolic abnormalities do not occur with calcium entry blockers, which is a distinct advantage. Drugs of this class are effective despite variations of age, renin activity, or race. The longer-acting drugs can be given once daily, as can long-acting formulations of verapamil, diltiazem, and nifedipine as well.

The calcium entry-blocking drugs have a negative inotropic action and should be used with caution in patients with early left ventricular failure in order to prevent the development of more severe congestive heart failure. They should be used with caution with other agents that have negative inotropic action, such as beta-blockers. In addition to reversing increased left ventricular mass, the drugs improve diastolic filling (Grossman, 1988; Phillips, 1991).

Several of the drugs in this class can be given intravenously. For example, diltiazem can be given as an intravenous infusion at an initial rate of less than 10 $\mu g/kg/min$, which reduces severe hypertension about 25%; atrioventricular block may occur (Onoyama, 1988). Nicardipine, being water-soluble, is effective as an intravenous infusion in severe hypertension. It can be given at a rate of 4–15 mg/h until a satisfactory fall in blood pressure has occurred. The infusion is then maintained for 6–24 hours with an infusion of 6–8 mg/h (Wallin, 1988; Clifton, in Parmley, 1989).

Nifedipine, as with other members of the class, can be given orally or sublingually in hypertensive crises. Nifedipine capsules, 5–20 mg, may lower the pressure dramatically within 30 minutes; significant hypotension may occur, and close observation is mandatory.

Centrally Acting Alpha-Adrenergic Agonists

Alpha-adrenergic agonists act in the brain stem, stimulating α_2 receptors that inhibit sympathetic activity. Drugs of this class include clonidine, methyldopa, guanabenz, and guanfacine (Table 9–14). The drugs are effective clinically in lowering the blood pressure, but the side effects (unpleasant dry mouth, lethargy, bradycardia, constipation, postural hypotension, and rebound or "discontinued" hypertension (if the drugs are stopped abruptly) have prevented them from achieving widespread popularity for initial therapy. In addition to the central mechanisms noted above, sympathetic activity is also reduced by peripheral mechanisms (Dollery, 1988). The sedative effect of the drugs is particularly disturbing to patients who must be mentally alert in their work or avocation. The absence of adverse metabolic actions is a favorable factor.

Clonidine can be started at a dosage of 0.1 mg and gradually titrated upwards. The average daily dose is about 0.5–0.6 mg. Low-dose clonidine (75 μg twice daily), alone or combined with a low dose of chlorthalidone (15 mg), resulted in a fall in diastolic blood pressure to less than 90 mm Hg in 69% of a large series of patients and prevented an adverse rise in pressure, such as occurred in patients receiving placebo (Clobass Study Group, 1990). Transdermal clonidine (TTS) in patches of 3.5 cm^2 (equivalent to a dose of 0.1 mg)—to a maximum of 10.5 cm^2 (0.3 mg/d)—is effective for a week; however, contact dermatitis under the patch occurs in about one-third of patients. Pretreatment of the skin with steroid cream or spray may decrease the adverse local effects. In one study, when compared with verapamil-SR, transdermal clonidine was equally effective and compliance was better (Burris, 1991).

Methyldopa is effective and can be used parenterally. It is especially valuable in pregnancy and in patients with impaired renal function, because renal blood flow is maintained and cardiac output is increased. It can be used in patients with acute nephritis. The side effects are similar to those of clonidine but include impotence and the infrequent occurrence of hemolytic anemia and other immune complex disease. Because of the availability of other compounds in this and other classes, methyldopa has been used less frequently in recent years.

Guanabenz is equally effective, is short-acting, and has side effects equivalent to those of clonidine; guanfacine, however, while equally effective, is longer-acting than either clonidine or guanabenz and can be given once daily instead of twice daily. It causes less somnolence and less severe withdrawal or discontinuation syndrome upon sudden cessation of the drug. There seem to be definite advantages to guanfacine, but further experience is needed. The alpha-adrenergic agonists lower total and LDL cholesterol and raise HDL cholesterol; they can also be used in patients with bronchospasm and claudication (Wilson, 1986).

α_1-Adrenergic Receptor Blockers

Prazosin, the prototype of this class of drugs, is a moderately effective vasodilator that relaxes smooth muscle by blocking the α_1-adrenergic postsynaptic receptors. Newer drugs such as terazosin and doxazosin have a longer duration of action than prazosin and can be given once daily (Table 9–14). Because they dilate both the arterial and venous circulations, they are of value when hypertension is associated with cardiac failure. Plasma volume increases in most cases and may require associated diuretic therapy.

The actions of the various α_1-adrenergic blockers are similar. Their advantages over some antihypertensive agents include beneficial effects on plasma lipids (they lower total cholesterol and LDL cholesterol and raise HDL cholesterol), and they can be useful in patients with bronchospasm, claudication, and prostatism (Kirby, 1989). The initial dose of any of the three drugs should be small (eg, 0.5 mg of prazosin, 1 mg of doxazosin or terazosin), especially if the patient is volume-depleted, and should be given at bedtime because of the possibility of postural hypotension. Given in divided doses, they can be gradually increased to tolerance, depending on the patient's response; the maximum daily dosage varies from 6 to 15 mg of prazosin, 4 mg of terazosin, and 16 mg of doxazosin (Khoury, 1991; Tomoda, 1989; Ames, 1989). Side effects include postural hypotension, dizziness, fatigue, headache, drowsiness, general lack of energy, and sexual dysfunction. Tolerance to prazosin may develop in some patients.

Peripheral Adrenergic-Inhibiting Agents

Reserpine also has a central action and has been used for many years, originally in psychiatric clinics. Because of the large doses previously used, mental depression followed, at times resulting in suicide. As a result, the drug fell out of favor; however, when given in small doses (0.05–0.1 mg/d), reserpine rarely produces mental depression, and in the Veterans Administration Study of 1970, the combination of reserpine, oral diuretics, and hydralazine significantly benefited patients whose diastolic pressure exceeded 105 mm Hg.

Guanethidine, a postganglionic neuronal-blocking agent, was valuable in the early days of the treatment of malignant hypertension. Since other compounds with fewer side effects are now available, it is used infrequently today. It is long-acting; oral doses can be started at 10–20 mg once daily and titrated upward at weekly intervals. Diuretic therapy may counteract the sodium retention and permit a smaller dose. Guanethidine has the disadvantage of taking 3–5 days to be eliminated if overdose occurs. It should not be used with reserpine or methyldopa.

Guanadrel is a postganglionic sympatholytic agent that depletes norepinephrine from storage sites and lowers the blood pressure significantly, as does guanethidine. The glomerular filtration rate and renal blood flow fall when the patient stands. The drug has no adverse metabolic consequences or impairment of exercise tolerance. It decreases serum cholesterol and triglycerides (Darga, 1991).

Direct Arteriolar Dilators

Hydralazine, the prototype of this class of drugs, can be used orally, intramuscularly, or intravenously. It decreases systemic vascular resistance by acting directly on the smooth muscle of arteries and arterioles. It raises cardiac output, which may result in side effects of palpitation, angina, headache, and reflex tachycardia. These can be prevented by first administering beta-blocking drugs, reserpine, or methyldopa. The side effects are less frequent when the dose is initially small (10–25 mg) and gradually increased to 100 mg twice daily. If this dose is exceeded, a syndrome simulating lupus erythematosus may occur, with fever, arthritis, positive LE cells, and antinuclear antibodies in the serum. These reverse when the drug is stopped. In children with acute glomerulonephritis with severe hypertension, 5–15 mg of hydralazine may be combined with 1–5 mg of reserpine intramuscularly.

Minoxidil is a powerful vasodilator of this class. It may reduce the blood pressure significantly when all of the conventional drugs mentioned above fail to do so (Figure 9–30). It has the adverse effects shared by all vasodilator drugs, but sodium retention is more marked, and it has the unusual side effect of hirsutism, which limits its use in women. The drug is a useful addition to the oral therapeutic protocol in severe hypertension, especially if there is beginning impairment of renal function. Minoxidil is begun in small doses of 2.5–5 mg/d and may be given two or three times daily, with gradually increasing titration to a maximum dosage of 20 mg/d.

Diazoxide

Diazoxide is a parenteral vasodilator that acts directly on the smooth muscle of the arterioles. When given in a bolus dose intravenously, it lowers the blood pressure within minutes and lowers systemic vascular resistance about 25%. The fall in pressure persists for many hours, with a gradual rise following the initial rapid fall. The hemodynamic effects also include an increase in heart rate, cardiac index, and left ventricular ejection rate. Hypotension occurs infrequently, especially if one starts with a dose such as 50–75 mg instead of 300 mg and repeats the dose at intervals of 5–10 minutes until the desired antihypertensive effect is achieved. If diazoxide is used repeatedly, sodium and water retention may occur and require diuretics.

There is a dose-response relationship to the use of diazoxide in hypertensive children. A dose of 2–3 mg/kg is a reasonable one. Table 9–18 describes drugs used in the treatment of acute severe hypertension in children.

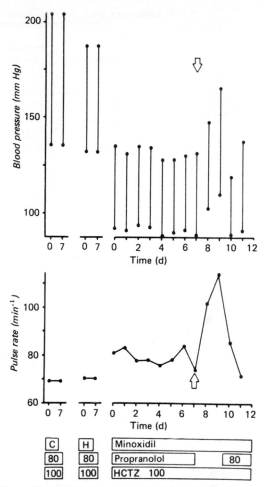

Figure 9–30. Blood pressure and heart rate data are summarized from one patient during the control period (C),the hydralazine period (H), and the minoxidil period. The effect of withdrawing propranolol (arrows) is shown by the increase in blood pressure and heart rate. (HCTZ, hydrochlorothiazide.) (Reproduced, with permission of the American Heart Association, from: Gottlieb TB, Katz FH, Chidsey CA III: Combined therapy with vasodilator drugs and beta-adrenergic blockade in hypertension: A comparative study of minoxidil and hydralazine. Circulation 1972;45:571.)

Diazoxide is valuable in hypertensive urgencies because of its effectiveness, rapid onset, and long duration of action and because monitoring usually is required only for the first 15 or 20 minutes to make certain that excess hypotension has not occurred. Like hydralazine, it can be given intermittently in severe hypertension when potent oral therapy is being titrated. The major side effect, other than the possibility of excess hypotension, is hyperglycemia, and like other vasodilators, including hydralazine and minoxidil, it increases renin secretion.

Table 9–18. Pharmacologic therapy of acute severe hypertension in children.[1]

Drug	Administration	Starting Dose	Onset of Action (min)	Duration (h)	Mechanism
Reserpine	IM	0.07 mg/kg	60–120	4–6	Postganglionic depletion of catecholamines
Hydralazine hydro- chloride	IM or IV	0.2 mg/kg	10–30	3–6	Vasodilation
Diazoxide	IV (push)	2–3 mg/kg	1–3	4–12	Vasodilation
Sodium nitroprus- side	IV (infusion)	60 mg/L (0.03–0.5 mg/min)	$\frac{1}{2}$–1	Length of infusion	Vasodilation
Trimethaphan cam- sylate	IV (infusion)	1 g/L (1–10 mg/min)	$\frac{1}{2}$–1	Length of infusion	Sympathetic ganglionic blocker
Ethacrynic acid, furosemide	IV	0.5–1.0 mg/kg	10–20	2–4	Blocks tubular reab- sorption of sodium and chloride, smooth muscle vasodilation

[1] Reproduced, with permission, from McLain LG: Therapy of acute severe hypertension in children. JAMA 1978;239:755.

FAILURE TO CONTROL HYPERTENSION

About 90–95% of all cases of mild to moderately severe hypertension can be managed with the drugs listed above. If the blood pressure is not controlled, one should suspect that the patient is not taking the medication properly or is taking too much salt. The entire regimen should then be reviewed. Substitution of drugs of a different class or addition of one or more drugs of a different class may be required. The use of other medications—nonsteroidal anti-inflammatory agents, corticosteroids, contraceptive pills, over-the-counter cold remedies, etc—should be considered for their possible neutralizing or aggravating effects on the antihypertensive regimen. Alternatively, there may be a substantial disparity between office and home or ambulatory readings, or the cuff of the blood pressure apparatus may be too narrow for the patient's arm. It is also possible that an accelerated or malignant phase has supervened—often because of poor compliance with treatment (see next section)—or that a new process such as renal artery stenosis, progressive renal damage, or pyelonephritis, has developed. Patients who have failed to respond to the full therapeutic regimen listed above—as well as patients who have acute hypertensive encephalopathy, malignant hypertension, acute pulmonary edema or severe cardiac or renal failure, aortic dissection, hemorrhagic stroke with a markedly raised blood pressure, or episodic rises in pressure suggesting pheochromocytoma—should be hospitalized. In some cases, if the patient is uncontrollable on medications as an outpatient, a trial period of hospitalization may be useful. This removes the patient from the surrounding social and work environment, which may be contributing pressor influences interfering with the antihypertensive drugs, and allows close monitoring of treatment of the blood pressure and, if necessary, the use of parenteral medication.

TREATMENT OF MALIGNANT HYPERTENSION OR HYPERTENSIVE CRISES

The hallmark of malignant hypertension is papilledema, but retinal hemorrhages and exudates (KW III) indicate accelerated hypertension and can be considered premalignant and warrant the same vigorous treatment. After the patient is hospitalized, preferably in an intensive care facility, the vigor of therapy depends on the clinical severity of the malignant hypertension. A hypertensive *emergency* exists when the blood pressure must be reduced within 1 hour. Hypertensive *urgency* exits when pressure can be reduced over several hours. Some patients with malignant hypertension are critically ill, with diastolic pressures exceeding 150 mm Hg and imminent or existing acute target organ damage; their blood pressure should be lowered within hours. Other patients, early in the course of the malignant phase, may have much less commanding symptoms; therapy can then be given orally or parenterally but intermittently, with the objective of lowering the pressure within a few days (Houston, 1989; Calhoun, 1990).

The importance of the prompt reduction of the pressure in patients with malignant hypertension is shown in Figure 9–31. The data demonstrate the great improvement in survival of patients with malignant hypertension given modern therapy (40% survival after 12 years, as compared to nil in the days before effective treatment was available) but also show that 12-year survival occurs only in the cases of

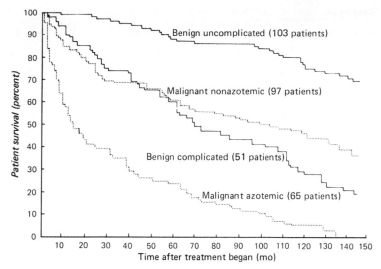

Figure 9–31. Percentage of surviving patients in each group for every month after inception of therapy. (Reproduced, with permission, of the American Heart Association, from: Perry HM Jr et al: Studies on the control of hypertension. 8. Mortality, morbidity, and remission during 12 years of intensive therapy. Circulation 1966;33:958.)

nonazotemic malignant hypertension in whom the blood pressure is lowered before renal failure occurs. In patients with malignant hypertension in whom renal failure and azotemia were present when the patient was first treated, the 12-year survival rate was nil, although the 6-year survival rate was still 20%—in contrast to the average survival of 8 months in the days before modern therapy was available (Schottstaedt, 1952; Perry, 1966). Dialysis treatment will probably improve the figures.

The pressure should not be lowered to normal immediately, because this may produce neurologic deficit or oliguria; it is wiser to give smaller doses to lower the diastolic pressure to about 115–120 mm Hg and observe whether this pressure is tolerated without neurologic symptoms or evidence of decreased cardiac output with oliguria. Autoregulation of cerebral blood flow occurs at higher pressures in hypertensives than in normotensives. Autoregulation fails if the blood pressure rises too high or falls below the lower limit of mean pressure of about 120 mm Hg. This results in vasodilation of cerebral arterioles and cerebral edema at high levels or cerebral hypoperfusion at low levels of pressure. Therapy can then be continued or increased to lower the pressure to 110 mm Hg diastolic for a day or so before gradually bringing it down to 100 mm Hg. It should be reemphasized that the great potency of the parenteral drugs is a distinct hazard. An intra-arterial blood pressure monitor or close supervision by nurse and physician, and a controlled infusion pump system are necessary when potent intravenous therapy is given in hypertensive emergencies utilizing such drugs as nitroprusside or nitroglycerin. Start with the smallest possible dose

and increase or decrease the rate of infusion if needed. A modest fall in pressure is satisfactory at first (approximately 20–25%); a greater fall can be achieved later, after it is demonstrated that this can be tolerated without untoward symptoms (Calhoun, 1990; Houston, 1989; Garcia, 1987).

Parenteral drugs that can be used in malignant hypertension and other hypertensive emergencies are listed in Table 9–15 along with route of administration, initial dose, time of onset, and duration of action. The choice of treatment in various causes of hypertensive emergencies is shown in Table 9–19. When the more potent drugs such as nitroprusside sodium and nitroglycerin are used, the blood pressure is lowered in a matter of seconds or minutes, but the hazard of overshooting the mark and producing severe hypotension is also greater. The choice of drugs depends upon the physician's own experience and the availability of constant surveillance, as is necessary with infusions of nitroprusside sodium or nitroglycerin. The rate of infusion must be carefully titrated to avoid excessive hypotension and should be decreased as soon as possible after the blood pressure falls. When the blood pressure has been stabilized at a level of diastolic 100–110 mm Hg, the infusion rate can be slowed and oral agents begun. As soon as practical, the infusion should be stopped and oral therapy resumed (see below). If the clinical care facilities do not permit careful, constant supervision of the infusion in a coronary care or intensive care unit, it is safer to give boluses of diazoxide, 50–75 mg rapidly intravenously, which lowers the pressure in minutes but may last for hours and can be repeated. If the situation is less urgent, 5–10 mg of hydralazine intra-

Table 9–19. Types of hypertensive emergencies and treatment recommendations.[1]

Type of Emergency	Recommended Treatment	Drugs to Avoid
Hypertensive encephalopathy	Sodium nitroprusside, labetalol, diazoxide	β-Antagonists, methyldopa, clonidine
Cerebral infarction	No treatment, sodium nitroprusside, labetalol	β-Antagonists, methyldopa, clonidine
Intracerebral hemorrhage, subarachnoid hemorrhage	No treatment, sodium nitroprusside, labetalol	β-Antagonists, methyldopa, clonidine
Myocardial ischemia, myocardial infarction	Nitroglycerin, labetalol, calcium antagonists, sodium nitroprusside	Hydralazine, diazoxide, minoxidil
Acute pulmonary edema	Sodium nitroprusside and loop diuretic, nitroglycerin and loop diuretic	Hydralazine, diazoxide, β-antagonists, labetalol
Aortic dissection	Sodium nitroprusside and β-antagonist, trimethaphan and β-antagonist, labetalol	Hydralazine, diazoxide, minoxidil
Eclampsia	Hydralazine, diazoxide, labetalol, calcium antagonists[2]	Trimethaphan, diuretics, β-antagonists
Acute renal insufficiency	Sodium nitroprusside, labetalol, calcium antagonists	β-Antagonists, trimethophan
Grade III or grade IV KW funduscopic changes[3]	Sodium nitroprusside, labetalol, calcium antagonists	β-Antagonists, clonidine, methyldopa
Microangiopathic hemolytic anemia	Sodium nitroprusside, labetalol, calcium antagonists	β-Antagonists

[1] Reproduced, with permission, from Calhoun DA, Oparil S: Treatment of hypertensive crisis. (Current Concepts.) N Engl J Med 1990;323:1177.
[2] Because of the potential risk to the fetus, reserve for patients with eclampsia that is refractory to treatment with other agents.
[3] Grade III changes include exudates and hemorrhage; grade IV changes, papilledema.

muscularly or intravenously can also be given intermittently and without such close supervision. Intramuscular hydralazine acts in 15–30 minutes and may persist for hours. Methyldopa, 250–500 mg, can be given intramuscularly or intravenously, but this drug usually takes 2–4 hours before its effect becomes obvious (up to 6 hours in renal failure); and although it is effective in some patients, it may not lower the pressure in severe hypertensive emergencies. In less urgent situations, oral therapy can be used (see below).

In dissecting aorta, hemorrhagic stroke with high arterial pressure, and severe acute left ventricular failure, sodium nitroprusside or trimethaphan, together with beta-blockers, are the drugs of choice initially; potent oral drugs can be substituted later. If sodium nitroprusside is used, beta-blockers must be added to decrease the force of cardiac contraction.

The presence of impaired renal function should not deter the physician from lowering the pressure, though drugs that decrease the renal blood flow should be avoided. Temporary renal dialysis may be required if the serum creatinine exceeds 4–5 mg/dL. In the presence of impaired renal function, thiazide diuretics are less effective, and a loop diuretic should be used instead. At times, high doses are necessary. Calcium entry-blocking agents, ACE inhibitors, and vasodilators (eg, hydralazine, prazosin, clonidine, or methyldopa) are effective in the presence of impaired renal function, do not reduce renal blood flow, and can be used alone or in combination after the blood pressure is brought under control with parenteral therapy.

Oral Therapy

Whenever possible in hypertensive emergencies, intravenous therapy should be used. In hypertensive urgencies, intravenous therapy can be used, but if there is no target organ damage, oral therapy can be started. Two of the most frequently effective drugs during the acute phase are sublingual or oral nifedipine, 10 mg, repeated if necessary in an hour, or clonidine. The latter can be given in a dosage of 0.1–0.2 mg initially followed by 0.05–0.1 mg every hour for a total dose of 0.6–0.7 mg, followed by chronic therapy (Anderson, 1986; Calhoun, 1990) (Figure 9–32).

Renal Failure & Dialysis

If renal failure is present and the patient is receiving intermittent renal dialysis, therapy should be rigorous to lower the pressure. If the patient's serum creatinine is less than 4 mg/dL—indicating moderate renal failure—and if the patient is not receiving dialysis and is not oliguric, vigorous therapy may prevent the need for hemodialysis. If the patient is receiving

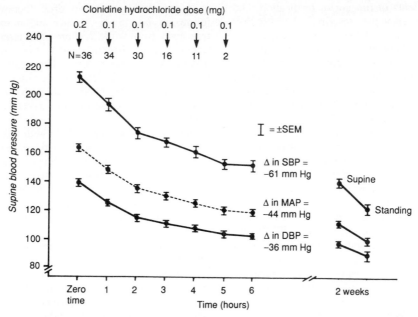

Figure 9–32. Blood pressure response to clonidine loading. N, number of patients receiving dose of clonidine at each hour of protocol; SBP, systolic blood pressure; DBP, diastolic blood pressure; MAP, mean arterial pressure (diastolic plus one-third of pulse pressure. (Reproduced, with permission, from Anderson RJ et al: JAMA 1981;246:848—as reproduced in Anderson RB, Reed WG: Current concepts in treatment of hypertensive urgencies. Am Heart J 1986;111:211. Copyright © 1981 by American Medical Association.)

hemodialysis, lowering the pressure will often gradually reduce the required frequency of hemodialysis. Renal dysfunction is greatly aggravated by severe hypertension, and lowering the blood pressure is an essential aspect of the treatment in this situation, utilizing renal dialysis if necessary until the renal interlobular arteriolar lesions can heal.

Follow-Up Evaluation

After the blood pressure is brought under control with potent parenteral medication, the beneficial antihypertensive effect can be maintained with more moderate oral therapy. Once the malignant phase is reversed by antihypertensive therapy, the patient often reverts to benign hypertension and can be controlled for years with oral drugs. The serum creatinine, which may rise modestly during the first 2–3 weeks after antihypertensive therapy is started, gradually falls, and 6 months later it is usually lower than when the patient was first seen with malignant hypertension. Impaired renal function persists, however, and the serum creatinine and creatinine clearance may stabilize at a low or moderately high level. The inability to completely restore renal function to normal once it has reached a certain point of impairment is one of the main reasons why prompt vigorous antihypertensive therapy should be given to patients with accelerated hypertension.

FOLLOW-UP THERAPY OF ESSENTIAL HYPERTENSION

The patient being treated with oral therapy of mild to moderate disease as well as the patient discharged from the hospital after treatment for severe or malignant hypertension should be seen approximately once a week as an outpatient until the situation is stabilized and an acceptable therapeutic program has been achieved. The frequency of visits can gradually be decreased, but in all but the mildest cases patients should be seen at intervals of 3–6 months even after they are well controlled to be certain they are taking their medication and that the response to therapy is maintained. Circumstances in the patient's life, renal artery stenosis, acute pyelonephritis, or unknown factors may worsen the hypertension even when the patient is on therapy. The patient must be encouraged to communicate with the physician whenever new or untoward symptoms appear and should be warned frequently against stopping medication without consulting the physician. Uncontrolled hypertension as well as the rebound or discontinuation effect may occur when antihypertensive agents are abruptly stopped; this is especially true with the centrally acting drugs, such as clonidine. In patients with coronary disease, severe angina may occur with abrupt cessation of beta-adrenergic-blocking agents. It is common for patients to run out of medication, and they often do not renew the prescription because they are free of symptoms and the drugs are expensive. This problem should be anticipated and prevented by full discussion with frequent reinforcement. Before assuming that antihypertensive therapy is inadequate, especially if the patient has previously been well controlled on the same medication, the possibility of noncompliance should be considered.

Ambulatory blood pressure recording may reveal better control of blood pressure than was thought from office readings alone (see above). A 10-year prospective study demonstrated that the prognosis for the development of vascular complications with target organ damage and for survival was better when ambulatory pressures were significantly lower than average office pressures (Perloff, 1983, 1989) (Figure 9–28). In some cases, hospitalization may allow a more adequate estimate of the effectiveness of treatment and has the added advantage of removing the patient from a perhaps stressful environment that may be raising the blood pressure.

At each medical visit, the blood pressure should be determined and the patient questioned regarding medication, life events, and the appearance of new or untoward symptoms that may suggest a change in the course of the disease. Specific search should be made for any evidence of involvement or worsening of the target organs; in particular, examination of the fundi, heart, neurologic status, and peripheral vessels should be made at each visit. At approximately yearly intervals, repeat electrocardiography, possibly echocardiography, renal function studies, and chest x-rays are desirable. If the patient is taking oral diuretic agents, serum potassium, uric acid, plasma glucose, and serum creatinine should be measured every 6–12 months. The effect of upright posture should be noted at each visit, not only with drugs that interfere with sympathetic transmission but also with oral diuretic agents, because postural hypotension may occur if hypovolemia is excessive. If the patient is receiving spironolactone, amiloride, or triamterene, serum potassium should be checked more frequently, and the ECG should be repeated frequently to exclude hyperkalemia; the patient taking these medications must be repeatedly admonished not to take oral potassium supplementation. If renal function is impaired, potassium-sparing drugs should not be used.

Serial assessment of left ventricular mass and diastolic function is helpful in determining response to treatment.

Management of Patient Compliance

Studies on patients' compliance with the treatment program have shown that this is a difficult problem not entirely solved by free drugs, ready access to physicians, education of patients regarding hypertension, and better education of physicians about the need for antihypertensive drug therapy. Frequent follow-up visits are a nuisance and an expense, take time away from work, and are often emotionally disturbing, so that patients tend to find excuses not to make or keep appointments. The attitude of the patient toward the physician or the clinic is important; long waits for care, short visits with the physicians, and expensive prescriptions adversely influence compliance.

Nurse practitioners may help with this problem by making more time available for the patient, including a discussion of personal problems. A social worker can function in somewhat the same way by developing a relationship in which the patient feels free to discuss personal and socioeconomic problems, and clinical volunteers can often assist with the less severe or complicated cases.

Every large clinic should provide some means whereby patients can obtain clear answers to questions about their disease, the drugs they are taking, and their personal concerns. If the physician does not provide this service, an experienced clinical pharmacist or nurse should do so and discuss the mechanism of action and problems concerning drugs, including possible interactions with drugs prescribed for other disorders.

It appears well established that nurse practitioners, supervised closely by physicians, can do routine follow-up examinations for patients whose hypertension is adequately controlled. The nurse practitioner can be taught to examine the fundi, listen to the heart for gallop rhythm, and examine for rales in the lungs and changes in the arterial pulses. Industrial nurses have also been used effectively in hypertension clinics in large factories. The use of such nurses in private practice has not been studied in sufficient detail to permit conclusions whether it would be feasible.

A concerned physician who acknowledges the patient as a partner in the therapeutic enterprise will have minimal problems with patient compliance.

Can Therapy Be Discontinued if Blood Pressure Becomes Normal on Treatment?

This question has been studied by a number of investigators, and the general conclusion is that with infrequent exceptions, moderate to severe hypertension requires antihypertensive therapy for life because hypertension returns when the drugs are stopped. In mild hypertension, however, after the blood pressure has been normal for several years, about 5–20% of patients remain normotensive when antihypertensive therapy is discontinued (Fletcher, 1988). A Veterans Administration Study (1975) (Figure 9–29) indicated that there is a gradual recurrence of hypertension over a period of 3–9 months in 82% of patients with mild to moderate disease when antihypertensive therapy is stopped. More rarely, the pressure may begin to rise within the first month, especially if the patient has had severe disease before therapy has begun. If the pressure remains normal for 18 months to 2 years, the recurrence rate is low.

The hazard of stopping therapy is that there may be a rebound phenomenon, with intense vasoconstriction and tachycardia, which may then be more difficult to reverse even if the same regimen used for successful control is restarted. In patients with severe hypertension before treatment, there have been reports of strokes or myocardial infarction within weeks after stopping therapy. When the physician decides to stop treatment, it should be done gradually with close follow-up.

With the exception of stopping therapy for a short time to do specialized studies to exclude secondary hypertension, we ordinarily do not stop therapy unless the patient has become normotensive for 1–2 years and had mild hypertension originally. At first, an attempt can be made in stepwise fashion to reduce dosage or decrease the number of drugs prescribed. It is not often that therapy can be stopped permanently, even though some patients (see above) remain normotensive for 1–2 years on no medication. The likelihood of the blood pressure remaining normal in all but the mildest cases is sufficiently small that if one attempts to stop therapy, close observation should be maintained to make certain the patient does not have a high-pressure rebound. Patients should be informed about what is being done so that they will maintain close contact with the physician and not be lost to follow-up.

REFERENCES

Abboud FM: The sympathetic system in hypertension: State-of-the-art review. Hypertension 1982;4(Suppl II):208.

Adachi H et al: Early diagnosis and surgical intervention of acute aortic dissection by transesophageal color flow mapping. Circulation 1990;82(Suppl IV):19.

Amery A et al (editors): The European Working Party on High Blood Pressure in the Elderly. Am J Med 1991;90(Suppl 3A).

Ames RP et al: Effectiveness of doxazosin in systemic hypertension. Am J Cardiol 1989;64:203.

Anderson EA et al: Elevated sympathetic nerve activity in borderline hypertensive humans: Evidence from direct intraneural recordings. Hypertension 1989;14:177.

Anderson NB et al: Hypertension in blacks: Psychosocial and biological perspectives. J Hypertens 1989;7:161.

Anderson RJ et al: Once-daily fosinopril in the treatment of hypertension. Hypertension 1991;17:636.

Anderson RJ, Reed WJ: Current concepts in treatment of hypertensive urgencies. Am Heart J 1986;111:211.

Ashida T et al: Effects of nifedipine SR and enalapril on office, home and ambulatory blood pressure in "white-coat" systemic hypertension. Am J Cardiol 1990;66:498.

Athanassopoulos G, Cokkinos DV: Atrial natriuretic factor. Prog Cardiovasc Dis 1991;33:313.

Australian Therapeutic Trial in Mild Hypertension: Report by the Management Committee. Lancet 1980;1:1261.

Barger AC: The Goldblatt Memorial Lecture. Part I: Experimental renovascular hypertension. Hypertension 1979;1:447.

Beevers DG et al: Antihypertensive treatment and the course of established cerebral vascular disease. Lancet 1973;1:1407.

Beevers DG et al: Comparison of lisinopril versus atenolol for mild to moderate essential hypertension. Am J Cardiol 1991;67:59.

Bell ET, Clawson BJ: Primary (essential) hypertension: A study of 420 cases. Arch Pathol 1928;5:939.

Berecek KH, Swords BH: Central role of vasopressin in cardiovascular regulation and the pathogenesis of hypertension. Hypertension 1990;16:213.

Biglieri EG: Adrenocortical components in hypertension. Cardiovasc Rev Rep 1982;3:734.

Biglieri EG: Enzymatic disorders and hypertension. Clin Endocrinol Metab 1981;10:453.

Biglieri EG: Spectrum of mineralocorticoid hypertension: Clinical conference. Hypertension 1991;17:251.

Bohr DF, Dominiczak AF, Webb RC: Pathophysiology of the vasculature in hypertension. Hypertension 1991;18:69.

Bravo EL et al: Circulating and urinary catecholamines in pheochromocytoma: Diagnostic and pathophysiologic implications. N Engl J Med 1979;301(Suppl):682.

Brenner BM, Garcia DL, Anderson S: Glomeruli and blood pressure: Less of one, more the other? Am J Hypertens 1988;1:335.

Brown MA, Whitworth JA: Hypertension in human renal disease. (Editorial review.) J Hypertens 1992;10:701.

Brunner HR, Mancia G (editors): Ambulatory blood pressure and cardiovascular risk factors. Satellite Symposium to the Fifth European Meeting on Hypertension, 13 June 1991, Venice, Italy. J Hypertens 1991;9(Suppl):S1.

Brunner HR, Waeber B (editors): *Ambulatory Blood Pressure Recording*. Raven Press, 1992.

Brush JE Jr et al: Angina due to coronary microvascular disease in hypertensive patients without left ventricular hypertrophy. N Engl J Med 1988;319:1302.

Build and Blood Pressure Study, vol 1. (Chicago) Society of Actuaries, 1959.

Burris JF et al: Therapeutic adherence in the elderly: Transdermal clonidine compared to oral verapamil for hypertension. Am J Med 1991;91(Suppl 1A):22.

Calhoun DA, Oparil S: Treatment of hypertensive crisis. N Engl J Med 1990;323:1177.

Canzanello VJ et al: Percutaneous transluminal renal angioplasty in management of atherosclerotic renovascular hypertension: Results in 100 patients. Hypertension 1989;13:163.

Cappucio FP, MacGregor GA: Does potassium supplementation lower blood pressure? A meta-analysis of published trials. J Hypertens 1991;9:465.

Carey RM et al: The Charlottesville Blood-Pressure Survey: Value of repeated blood-pressure measurements. JAMA 1976;236:847.

Carmichael DJS et al: Detection and investigation of renal artery stenosis. Lancet 1986;1:667.

Cesana G et al: Ambulatory blood pressure normalcy: The PAMELA Study. J Hypertens;9(Suppl):S17.

Chanson P et al: Cardiovascular effects of the somatostatin analog octreotide in acromegaly. Ann Intern Med 1990;113:921.

Chapman AB et al: The renin-angiotensin-aldosterone system and autosomal dominant polycystic kidney disease. N Engl J Med 1990;323:1091.

Chobanian AV (editor): The role of calcium antagonists in hypertension. Symposium. Am J Cardiol 1992;69:1E.

Clobass Study Group: Low-dose clonidine administration in the treatment of mild or moderate essential hypertension: Results from a double-blind placebo-controlled study (Clobass). J Hypertens 1990;8:539.

Collins R et al: Blood pressure, stroke and coronary heart disease. Part 2. Short-term reductions in blood pressure: Overview of randomised drug trials in their epidemiological context. Lancet 1990;335:827.

Cowley AW Jr: The concept of autoregulation of total blood flow and its role in hypertension. Am J Med 1980;68:906.

Crawford ES: The diagnosis and management of aortic dissection. JAMA 1990;254:2537.

Cruickshank JM: Benefits and potential harm of reducing high blood pressure—The J-curve phenomenon. Prim Cardiol 1990;16:19.

Cutler JA, MacMahon SW, Furberg CD: Controlled clinical trials of drug treatment for hypertension. A review. Hypertension 1989;13(Suppl I):36.

Dahlöf B, Pennert K, Hansson L: Reversal of left ventricular hypertrophy in hypertensive patients: A meta-analysis of 109 treatment studies. Am J Hypertens 1992;5:95.

Darga LL et al: Comparison of the effects of guanadrel sulfate and propranolol on blood pressure, functional capacity, serum lipoproteins and glucose in systemic hypertension. Am J Cardiol 1991;67:590.

Davidman M, Opsahl J: Mechanisms of elevated blood pressure in human essential hypertension. Med Clin North Am 1984;68:301.

de Man SA et al: Blood pressure in childhood: Pooled findings of six European studies. J Hypertens 1991;9:109.

de Simone G et al: Echocardiographic left ventricular mass and electrolyte intake predict arterial hypertension. Ann Intern Med 1991;114:202.

Dellsperger KC, Marcus ML: Effects of left ventricular hypertrophy on the coronary circulation. Am J Cardiol 1990;65:1504.

DeSanctis RW et al: Aortic dissection. N Engl J Med 1987;317:1060.

deWardener HE: Kidney, salt intake, and Na^+, K^+-ATPase inhibitors in hypertension. The 1990 Corcoran lecture. Hypertension 1991;17:830.

DiBona GF: Stress and sodium intake in neural control of renal function in hypertension. Hypertension 1991;17(Suppl III):2.

DiBona GF: Sympathetic nervous system influences on the kidney. Role of hypertension. Am J Hypertens 1989;2(Suppl):119S.

Dollery CT: Advantages and disadvantages of alpha$_2$-adrenoceptor agonists for systemic hypertension. Am J Cardiol 1988;61(Suppl D):1D.

Doyle AE (editor): Angiotensin-conferting enzyme (ACE) inhibition: Benefits beyond blood pressure control. Am J Med 1992;92(Suppl 4B):1S.

Dunn FG et al: Left ventricular hypertrophy and mortality in hypertension: An analysis of data from the Glasgow Blood Pressure Clinic. J Hypertens 1990;8:775.

Dzau VJ, Safar ME: Large conduit arteries in hypertension: Role of the vascular renin-angiotensin system. Circulation 1988;77:947.

Dzau VJ: Multiple pathways of angiotensin production in the blood vessel wall: Evidence, possibilities, and hypothesis. J Hypertens 1989;7:933.

Dzau VJ: Significance of vascular renin-angiotensin pathway. (Editorial.) Hypertension 1986;8:553.

Esler M, Lambert G, Jennings G: Increased regional sympathetic nervous activity in human hypertension: Causes and consequences. J Hypertens 1990;8(Suppl 7):53.

Farnett L et al: The J-curve phenomenon and the treatment of hypertension. Is there a point beyond which pressure reduction is dangerous? JAMA 1991;265:489.

Ferrari P, Weidmann P: Editorial review: Insulin, insulin sensitivity and hypertension. J Hypertens 1990;8:491.

Ferrario CM, Averill DB: Do primary dysfunctions in neural control of arterial pressure contribute to hypertension? Hypertension 1991;18(3 Suppl):I38.

Firth JD, Raine AEG, Ledingham JGG: The mechanism of pressure natriuresis: Editorial review. J Hypertens 1990;8:97.

Fletcher AE, Bulpitt CJ: How far should blood pressure be lowered? N Engl J Med 1992;326:251.

Fletcher AE, Franks PJ, Bulpitt CJ: The effect of withdrawing antihypertensive therapy: A review. J Hypertens 1988;6:431.

Folkow B: Psychosocial and central nervous influences in primary hypertension. Circulation 1987;76(Suppl I):10.

Folkow B: Sympathetic nervous control of blood pressure: Role in primary hypertension. Am J Hypertens 1989;2(Suppl):103S.

Frishman W: Clinical pharmacology of the new beta-adrenergic blocking drugs: Part 2. Physiologic and metabolic effects. Am Heart J 1979;97:797.

Frohlich ED (chairman) et al: Recommendations for human blood pressure determination by sphygmomanometers: Report of a special task force appointed by the Steering Committee, American Heart Association. Hypertension 1988;11(Suppl A):209.

Frohlich ED (editor): A symposium: American Heart Association Prevention Conference II—Hypertension. Hypertension 1991;18(Suppl I).

Frohlich ED (editor): Hypertension—The heart and the kidney. A symposium. Am J Cardiol 1987;60(Suppl I).

Frohlich ED: Left ventricular hypertrophy, cardiac diseases and hypertension: Recent experiences. J Am Coll Cardiol 1989;14:1587.

Garcia JY Jr, Vidt DG: Current management of hypertensive emergencies: Review. Drugs 1987;34:263.

Genest J et al (editors): *Hypertension: Physiopathology and Treatment,* 2nd ed. McGraw-Hill, 1983.

Gerson P (editor): Aortic dissection: A special section of the Texas Heart Institute Journal. Tex Heart Inst J 1990;17:253.

Gifford RW: Management of hypertensive crisis. JAMA 1991;266:829.

Glower DD et al: Comparison of medical and surgical therapy for uncomplicated descending aortic dissection. Circulation 1990;82(Suppl IV):39.

Grossman E et al: Glucagon and clonidine testing in the diagnosis of pheochromocytoma. Hypertension 1991;17:733.

Grossman E et al: Systemic and regional hemodynamic and humoral effects of nitrendipine in essential hypertension. Circulation 1988;78:1394.

Guyton AC: Dominant role of the kidneys and accessory role of whole-body autoregulation in the pathogenesis of hypertension. Am J Hypertens 1989;2:575.

Haddy FJ: Abnormalities of membrane transport in hypertension. Hypertension 1983;5(Suppl V):66.

Hall JE et al: Obesity-associated hypertension. Hyperinsulinemia and renal mechanisms. Hypertension 1992;18(Suppl I):I–45.

Hall JE, Mizelle HL, Woods LL: The renin-angiotensin system and long-term regulation of arterial pressure. J Hypertens 1986;4:387.

Hall WD: Hypertension in the elderly with a special focus on treatment with angiotensin-converting enzyme inhibitors and calcium antagonists. Am J Cardiol 1992;69:33E.

Hattner RS et al: Scintigraphic detection of pheochromocytomas using metaiodo-(I-131)-benzylguanidine. Noninvas Med Imag 1984;1:105.

Haverich A et al: Acute and chronic aortic dissections—Determinants of long-term outcome for operative survivors. Circulation 1985;72(Suppl II):22.

Hedblad B, Janzon L: Hypertension and ST segment depression during ambulatory electrocardiographic recording: Results from the Prospective Population Study "Men Born in 1914" From Malmö, Sweden. Hypertension 1992;20:32

Heikinheimo RJ et al: Blood pressure in the very old. J Hypertens 1990;8:361.

Helgeland A: Treatment of mild hypertension: A five year controlled drug trial: The Oslo study. Am J Med 1980;69:725.

Henry JP, Grim CE: Psychosocial mechanisms of primary hypertension. J Hypertens 1990;8:783.

Hilton PJ: Cellular sodium transport in essential hypertension. N Engl J Med 1986;314:222.

Hinman AT, Engel BT, Bickford AF: Portable blood pressure recorder: Accuracy and preliminary use in evaluating intradaily variations in pressure. Am Heart J 1962;63:663.

Hollenberg N, Frohlich ED, Schwartz A (editors): Diversity and potential: Calcium antagonists in the 1990s. Symposium. Am J Hypertens 1991;4(Suppl):393S.

Hollenberg NK (editor): Hypertension in an aging population: Problems and opportunities. Am J Med 1991;90(Suppl 4B).

Hollister AS, Inagami T: Atrial natriuretic factor and hypertension: A review and metaanalysis. Am J Hypertens 1991;4:850.

Houghton JL et al: Morphologic, hemodynamic and coronary perfusion characteristics in severe left ventricular hypertrophy secondary to systemic hypertension and evidence for nonatherosclerotic myocardial ischemia. Am J Cardiol 1992;69:219.

Houston MC: Pathophysiology, clinical aspects, and treatment of hypertensive crises. Prog Cardiovasc Dis 1989;32:99.

Humerfelt SB: An epidemiological study of high blood pressure. Acta Med Scand 1963;407(Suppl).

Hunt SC et al: A prospective study of sodium-lithium countertransport and hypertension in Utah. Hypertension 1991;17:1.

Hypertension Detection and Follow-Up Program Cooperative Group: Persistence of reduction in blood pressure and mortality of participants in the Hypertension Detection and Follow-Up Program. JAMA 1988;259:2113.

INTERSALT Cooperative Research Group: INTERSALT: An international study of electrolyte excretion and blood pressure: Results for 24 hour urinary sodium and potassium excretion. Br Med J 1988;297:319.

Ives HE: Ion transport defects and hypertension. Where is the link? Hypertension 1989;14:590.

Joint National Committee: The 1988 report of the Joint National Committee on Detection, Evaluation, and Treatment of High Blood Pressure. Arch Int Med 1988;148:1023.

Julius S et al: Hyperkinetic borderline hypertension in Tecumseh, Michigan. J Hypertens 1991;9:77.

Julius S et al: The association of borderline hypertension with target organ changes and high coronary risk. Tecumseh Blood Pressure Study. JAMA 1990;264:354.

Kain HK, Hinman AT, Sokolow M: Arterial blood measurements with a portable recorder in hypertensive patients: 1. Variability and correlation with "casual" pressures. Circulation 1964;30:882.

Kaneko Y, Laragh JH (editors): New developments in angiotensin converting enzyme inhibitory action. (Symposium.) Am J Hypertens 1991;4(Suppl):1S.

Kannel WB, McGee D, Gordon T: A general cardiovascular risk profile: The Framingham Study. Am J Cardiol 1976;38:46.

Kannel WB: Role of blood pressure in cardiovascular morbidity and mortality. Prog Cardiovasc Dis 1974;17:5.

Kannel WB: Role of blood pressure in the development of congestive heart failure. N Engl J Med 1972;287:782.

Kannel WB: The clinical heterogeneity of hypertension. Am J Hypertens 1991;4:283.

Kaplan NM: *Clinical Hypertension,* 5th ed. Williams & Wilkins, 1990.

Kaplan NM: Calcium entry blockers in the treatment of hypertension: Current status and future prospects. JAMA 1989;262:817.

Kaplan NM: Changing hypertension treatment to reduce the overall cardiovascular risk. J Hypertens 1990;8(Suppl 7):175.

Kaplan NM: Long-term effectiveness of nonpharmacological treatment of hypertension. Hypertension 1991;18(Suppl I):I–153.

Kaye TB, Crapo L: The Cushing syndrome: An update on diagnostic tests. Ann Intern Med 1990;112:434.

Keith NM, Wagener HP, Barker ND: Some different types of essential hypertension: Their course and prognosis. Am J Med Sci 1939;197:332.

Khoury AF, Kaplan NM: α-Blocker therapy of hypertension: An unfulfilled promise. JAMA 1991;266:394.

Kincaid-Smith P, McMichael J, Murphy EA: The clinical course and pathology of hypertension with papilledema (malignant hypertension). Q J Med 1958;27:117.

Kirby RS: Alpha-adrenoceptor inhibitors in the treatment of benign prostatic hyperplasia. Am J Med 1989;87(Suppl 2A):26.

Klibanski A, Zervas NT: Diagnosis and management of hormone-secreting pituitary adenomas. N Engl J Med 1991;324:822.

Koren MJ et al: Relation of left ventricular mass and geometry to morbidity and mortality in uncomplicated essential hypertension. Ann Intern Med 1991;114:345.

Kostis JB: Angiotensin-converting enzyme inhibitors: Emerging differences and new compounds. Am J Hypertens 1989;2:57.

Krakoff LR (editor): Calcium channel blockers in cardiovascular disease: Current concepts and new clinical findings. (Symposium.) Am J Hypertens 1990;3(Suppl):289S.

Krishna GG, Kapoor SC: Potassium depletion exacerbates essential hypertension. Ann Intern Med 1991;115:77.

Krishna GG, Miller E, Kapoor S: Increased blood pressure during potassium depletion in normotensive men. N Engl J Med 1989;320:1177.

Krupp MA: Urinary sediment in visceral angiitis (periarteritis nodosa, lupus erythematosus, Libman-Sacks disease): Quantitative study. Arch Intern Med 1943:71:54.

Kurtz TW, Al-Bander HA, Morris RC Jr: "Salt-sensitive" essential hypertension in men. Is the sodium ion alone important? N Engl J Med 1987;317:1043.

Kuwajima I et al: Pseudohypertension in the elderly. J Hypertens 1990;8:429.

Laragh JH: The renin system and four lines of hypertension research: Nephrone heterogeneity, the calcium connection, the prorenin vasodilator limb, and plasma renin and heart attach. (Dahl Memorial Lecture.) Hypertension 1992;20:267.

Laragh JH, Brenner BM: *Hypertension: Pathophysiology, Diagnosis, and Management.* 2 vols. Raven Press, 1990.

Lawrie GM et al: Renovascular reconstruction: Factors affecting long-term prognosis in 919 patients followed up to 31 years. Am J Cardiol 1989;63:1085.

Ledingham JM: Autoregulation in hypertension: A review. J Hypertens 1989;7(Suppl 4):97.

Lees KR: The dose-response relationship with angiotensin converting enzyme inhibitors: Effects on blood pressure and biochemical parameters. J Hypertens 1992;10(Suppl 5):S3.

Levy D et al: Prognostic implications of echocardiographically determined left ventricular mass in the Framingham Heart Study. N Engl J Med 1990;332:1561.

Lindholm LH: Cardiovascular risk factors and their interactions in hypertensives. J Hypertens 1991;9(Suppl 3):S3.

Lund-Johansen P: Twenty-year follow-up of hemodynamics in essential hypertension during rest and exercise. Hypertension 1991;18(Suppl):54S.

Mampalam TJ, Tyrrell JB, Wilson CB: Transsphenoidal microsurgery for Cushing disease: A report of 216 cases. Ann Intern Med 1988;109:487.

Mancia G (editor): Managing coronary heart disease risk in hypertensive smokers. (Symposium.) J Hypertens 1990;8(Suppl 5).

Mancia G et al: Ambulatory blood pressure monitoring in the evaluation of antihypertensive treatment. Am J Med 1989;87(Suppl 6B):64.

Mancia G et al: Prolonged intra-arterial blood-pressure recording in diagnosis of phaeochromocytoma. Lancet 1979;2:1193.

Mancia G: Ambulatory blood pressure monitoring: Research and clinical applications. J Hypertens 1990;8 (Suppl 7):1.

Manger WM, Gifford RW Jr: *Pheochromocytoma.* Springer, 1977.

Manger WM, Peart WS (editors): First Irvine H. Page International Hypertension Research Symposium: The Page mosaic. Hypertension 1991;18(Suppl):1.

Mann SJ et al: Captopril renography in the diagnosis of renal artery stenosis: Accuracy and limitations. Am J Med 1991;90:30.

Mark AL: Regulation of sympathetic nerve activity in mild human hypertension. J Hypertens 1990;8(Suppl 7):67.

Marmot MG et al: Health inequalities among British civil servants: The Whitehall II Study. Lancet 1991;337:1387.

Marshall JJ, Kontos HA: Endothelium-derived relaxing factors. A perspective from in vivo data. Hypertension 1990;16:371.

Matsukawa T et al: Reduced baroreflex changes in muscle sympathetic nerve activity during blood pressure elevation in essential hypertension. J Hypertens 1991;9:537.

McGiff JC, Carroll MA, Escalante B: Arachidonate metabolites and kinins in blood pressure regulation. Hypertension 1991;18(Suppl):150S.

McMahon S et al: Blood pressure, stroke, and coronary heart disease: Part I. Prolonged experiences in blood pressure: Prospective observational studies corrected for the regression dilution bias. Lancet 1990;335 765.

Medical Research Council Working Party: MRC trial of treatment of mild hypertension: Principal results. Br Med J 1985;291:97.

Melby JC: Diagnosis of hypercholesterolemia. Endocrinol Metab Clin North Am 1991;20:247.

Meyer-Sabellak WA (editor): International Consensus Conference on Indirect Ambulatory Blood Pressure Monitoring. J Hypertens 1990;8(Suppl 6).

Mimran A, Ribstein J: Angiotensin converting enzyme inhibitors and renal function. J Hypertens 1989;7(Suppl 5):3.

Mimran A, Ribstein J: Antihypertensive therapy in

renal disease and transplantation. J Hypertens 1992;10(Suppl 5):S79.

Mockrin MJ, Horan MJ (editors): Symposium: Predictors of hypertension. Proceedings of a workshop. Am J Hypertens 1991;4:585S.

Mohr-Kahaly S et al: Ambulatory follow-up of aortic dissection by transesophageal two-dimensional and color-coded Doppler echocardiography. Circulation 1989;80:24.

Multiple Risk Factor Intervention Trial Research Group: Mortality rates after 10.5 years for participants in the Multiple Risk Factor Intervention Trial (MRFIT). JAMA 1990;263:1795.

Murphy MB et al: Glucose intolerance in hypertensive patients treated with diuretics: A fourteen-year follow-up. Lancet 1982;2:1293.

Myers MG, Reeves RA: White coat phenomenon in patients receiving antihypertensive therapy. Am J Hypertens 1991;4:844.

Natali A et al: Impaired insulin action on skeletal muscle metabolism in essential hypertension. Hypertension 1991;17:170.

National Education Programs Working Group: Working Group on Management of Patients with Hypertension and High Blood Cholesterol: National Education Programs Working Group Report on the Management of Patients with Hypertension and High Blood Cholesterol. Ann Intern Med 1991;114:224.

National Heart, Lung and Blood Institute Workshop on Salt and Blood Pressure. Hypertension 1991;17(Suppl I).

Novick AC et al: Trends in surgical revascularization for renal artery disease: Ten years' experience. JAMA 1987;257:498.

Novick AC: Management of renovascular disease. A surgical perspective. Circulation 1991;83(Suppl I):167.

O'Brien E et al: Twenty-four-hour ambulatory blood pressure in men and women aged 17 to 80 years: The Allied Irish Bank Study. J Hypertens 1991;9:355.

O'Brien E, Fitzgerald D, O'Malley K: Blood pressure measurement: Current practice and future trends. Br Med J 1985;290:729.

O'Brien E, O'Malley K: Blood pressure measurement. J Ir Coll Phys Surg 1990;19:281.

Oberman A et al: Pharmacologic and nutritional treatment of mild hypertension: Changes in cardiovascular risk status. Ann Intern Med 1990;112:89.

Okamoto K (editor): *Spontaneous Hypertension: Its Pathogenesis and Complications.* Igaku Shoin, 1972.

Onoyama K et al: Effect of a drip infusion of intravenous diltiazem on severe systemic hypertension. Curr Ther Res 1988;43:361.

Oparil S et al: Central mechanisms of hypertension. Am J Hypertens 1989;2:474.

Oparil S et al: Dietary Ca^{2+} prevents NaCl-sensitive hypertension in spontaneously hypertensive rats by a sympatholytic mechanism. Am J Hypertens 1990;3 (Suppl):179S.

Oparil S, Calhoun DA: The calcium antagonists in the 1990s. An overview. Am J Hypertens 1991;4(Suppl): 396S.

Oparil S: Hypertension and oral contraceptives. J Cardiovasc Med 1981;6:381.

Oren S et al: Immediate and short-term cardiovascular effects of fosinopril, a new angiotensin-converting enzyme inhibitor, in patients with essential hypertension. J Am Coll Cardiol 1991;17:1183.

Os I et al: Increased plasma vasopressin in low renin essential hypertension. Hypertension 1986;8:506.

Parati G et al: Relationship of 24-hour blood pressure mean and variability to severity of target-organ damage in hypertension. J Hypertens 1987;5:93.

Parmer RJ, Cervenka JH, Stone RA: Baroreflex sensitivity and heredity in essential hypertension. Circulation 1992;85:497.

Parmley WW (editor): A Symposium: Clinical experience with a second generation calcium antagonist—nicardipine, a vasoselective agent. Am J Cardiol 1989;64:16.

Parving H-H: The impact of hypertensive and antihypertensive treatment on the course and prognosis of diabetic nephropathy. J Hypertens 1990;8(Suppl 7):187.

Patel R, Ansari A, Grim CE: Prognosis and predisposing factors for essential malignant hypertension in predominantly black patients. Am J Cardiol 1990;66: 868.

Pearson AC et al: Echocardiographic evaluation of cardiac structure and function in elderly subjects with isolated systolic hypertension. J Am Coll Cardiol 1991;17:422.

Perini C, Müller FB, Bühler FR: Suppressed aggression accelerates early development of essential hypertension. J Hypertens 1991;9:499.

Perloff D et al: Prognostic value of ambulatory blood pressure measurements: Further analyses. J Hypertens 1989;7(Suppl 3):3.

Perloff D, Sokolow M, Cowan R: The prognostic value of ambulatory blood pressure. JAMA 1983;249:2792.

Perloff D, Sokolow M, Cowan R: The prognostic value of ambulatory blood pressure monitoring in treated hypertensive patients. J Hypertens 1991;9(Suppl 1): S33.

Perloff D, Sokolow M: Ambulatory blood pressure and assessment of cardiovascular risk. In: *Ambulatory Blood Pressure Recording.* Brunner HR, Waeber B (editors). Raven Press, 1992.

Perloff D, Sokolow M: Ambulatory blood pressure: The San Francisco experience. J Hypertens 1990;8(Suppl 6):105.

Perry HM Jr et al: Studies on the control of hypertension. 8. Mortality, morbidity, and remission during 12 years of intensive therapy. Circulation 1966;33:958.

Phillips RA et al: Normalization of left ventricular mass and associated changes in neurohormones and atrial natriuretic peptide after 1 year of sustained nifedipine therapy for severe hypertension. J Am Coll Cardiol 1991;17:1595.

Pickering G: *High Blood Pressure,* 2nd ed. Churchill, 1968.

Pickering TG et al: The role of behavioral factors in white coat and sustained hypertension. J Hypertens 1990;8(Suppl 7):141.

Pickering TG: *Ambulatory Monitoring and Blood Pressure Variability.* Science Press, 1991.

Pickering TG: Diagnosis and evaluation of renovascular hypertension: Indications for therapy. Circulation 1991;83(Suppl I):147.

Pickering TG: The Ninth Sir George Pickering Memorial Lecture: Ambulatory monitoring and the definition of hypertension. J Hypertens 1992;10:401.

Pollack AA et al: Limitations of transcendental meditation in the treatment of essential hypertension. Lancet 1977;1:71.

Pool JL et al: Controlled multicenter study of the antihypertensive effects of lisinopril, hydrochlorothiazide, and lisinopril plus hydrochlorothiazide in the treatment of 394 patients with mild to moderate essential hypertension. J Cardiovasc Pharmacol 1987;9(Suppl 3):S36.

Position of beta blockers in present and future therapy of systemic hypertension. June 24–29, 1990, Montreal, Quebec, Canada. Am J Cardiol 1991;67(Suppl B):1B.

Predictors of Hypertension Workshop: Mockrin MJ, Horan MJ (editors): Symposium: Predictors of hypertension. Proceedings of a workshop. Am J Hypertens 1991;4:585S.

Pringle SD et al: Pathophysiologic assessment of left ventricular hypertrophy and strain in asymptomatic patients with essential hypertension. J Am Coll Cardiol 1989;13:1377.

Raper AJ et al: Pheochromocytoma of the urinary bladder: A broad clinical spectrum. Am J Cardiol 1977;40:820.

Reaven GM: Insulin resistance, hyperinsulinemia, and hypertriglyceridemia in the etiology and clinical course of hypertension. Am J Med 1991;90(2A):7S.

Reef EG, Sullivan JM: Alpha- and beta-adrenergic blockade in the treatment of hypertension. Cardiovasc Rev Rep 1991;May:61.

Robertson JIS (editor): A symposium: Ramipril—A new angiotensin converting enzyme inhibitor. Symposium. Am J Cardiol 1987;59(Suppl D).

Robertson JIS: Hypertension and its treatment in the elderly. Clin Exper Hypertens [Part A] 1989;11(5–6):779.

Rotmensch HH, Vlasses PH, Ferguson RK: Angiotensin-converting enzyme inhibitors. Med Clin North Am 1988;72:399.

Royal College of General Practitioners' Oral Contraception Study: Mortality among oral-contraceptive users. Lancet 1977;2:727.

Rutan GH et al: Mortality associated with diastolic hypertension and isolated systolic hypertension among men screened for the Multiple Risk Factor Intervention Trial. Circulation 1988;77:504.

Samuelsson OG et al: The J-shaped relationship between coronary heart disease and achieved blood pressure level in treated hypertension: Further analyses of 12 years of follow-up of treated hypertensives in the Primary Prevention Trial of Gothenburg, Sweden. J Hypertens 1990;8:547.

Schambelan M et al: Selective renal-vein sampling in hypertensive patients with segmental renal lesions. N Engl J Med 1974;290:1153.

Schnall PL et al: The relationship between "job strain," workplace diastolic blood pressure, and left ventricular mass index: Results of a case-control study. JAMA 1990;263:1929.

Schottstaedt MF, Sokolow M: The natural history and course of hypertension with papilledema (malignant hypertension). Am Heart J 1952;45:331.

Schrader J et al: Comparison of the antihypertensive efficiency of nitrendipine, metoprolol, mepindolol and enalapril using ambulatory 24-hour blood pressure monitoring. Am J Cardiol 1990;66:967.

Schulman SP et al: The effects of antihypertensive therapy on left ventricular mass in elderly patients. N Engl J Med 1990;322:1350.

Schwartz AB, Swartz CD: Dosage of potassium chloride elixir to correct thiazide-induced hypokalemia. JAMA 1974;230:702.

Setaro JF, Black HR: Refractory hypertension. N Engl J Med 1992;327:543.

SHEP Cooperative Research Group: Prevention of stroke by antihypertensive drug treatment in older persons with isolated systolic hypertension. Final results of the Systolic Hypertension in the Elderly Program (SHEP). JAMA 1991;265:3255.

Shepherd JT: Increased systemic vascular resistance and primary hypertension: The expanding complexity. J Hypertens 1990;8(Suppl 7):15.

Shimada K et al: Silent cerebrovascular disease in the elderly. Correlation with ambulatory pressure. Hypertension 1990;16:692.

Siegel D et al: Risk of ventricular arrhythmias in hypertensive men with left ventricular hypertrophy. Am J Cardiol 1990;65:742.

Skarfors ET, Lithell HO, Selinus I: Risk factors for the development of hypertension: A 10-year longitudinal study in middle-aged men. J Hypertens 1991;9:217.

Slater EE: Insulin resistance and hypertension. Hypertension 1991;18(Suppl I):I–108.

Sleight P: Role of the baroreceptor reflexes in circulatory control, with particular reference to hypertension. Hypertension 1991;18(Suppl):31S.

Sokolow M, Ball RE: Factors influencing conversion of chronic atrial fibrillation with special reference to serum quinidine concentration. Circulation 1956;14:568.

Sokolow M et al: Preliminary studies relating portably recorded pressures to daily life events in patients with hypertension. In: Psychosomatics in Essential Hypertension. Koster M, Musaph H, Visser P (editors). Karger, 1970.

Sokolow M et al: Relationship between level of blood pressure measured casually and by portable recorders and severity of complications in essential hypertension. Circulation 1966;34:279.

Sokolow M, Perloff D: The prognosis of essential hypertension treated conservatively. Circulation 1961;23:697.

Sonnenblick EH (editor): A symposium: Esmolol—an ultrashort-acting intravenous beta blocker. Am J Cardiol 1985;56(Suppl F).

Sos TA: Angioplasty for the treatment of azotemia and renovascular hypertension in atherosclerotic renal artery disease. Circulation 1991;83(Suppl I):162.

Staessen J, Amery A, Fagard R: Isolated systolic hypertension in the elderly: Editorial review. J Hypertens 1990;8:393.

Staessen JA et al: Mean and range of the ambulatory pressure in normotensive subjects from a meta-analysis of 23 studies. Am J Cardiol 1991;67:723.

Stamler J et al: INTERSALT study findings: Public health and medical care implications. Hypertension 1989;14:570.

Stamler J: Blood pressure and high blood pressure. Aspects of risk. Hypertension 1991;18(Suppl I):I–95.

Strandgaard S, Paulson OB: Cerebral blood flow and its pathophysiology in hypertension. Am J Hypertens 1989;2:486.

Tarazi RC (editor): The heart and coronary vessels in hypertension. Circulation 1987;75(Suppl I).

Taylor SH (editor): Clinical settings for selective alpha-adrenergic receptor inhibition: Rationale and management strategies. Proceedings of a symposium. Am J Med 1989;87(Suppl 2A). .

Timio M et al: Age and blood pressure changes: A 20-year follow-up study in nuns in a secluded order. Hypertension 1988;12:457.

Tjoa HI, Kaplan NM: Treatment of hypertension in the elderly. JAMA 1990;264:1015.

Tomoda F et al: Hemodynamic and endocrinological effects of a new selective α_1-blocking agent, terazosin, in patients with essential hypertension. Results of long-term treatment. Am J Hypertens 1989;2:834.

Treasure T, Raphael MJ: Investigation of suspected dissection of the thoracic aorta. Lancet 1991;338:490.

Trials of Hypertension Prevention Collaborative Research Group: The effects of nonpharmacologic interventions on blood pressure of persons with high normal levels: Results of the Trials of Hypertension Prevention, Phase I. JAMA 1992;267:1213.

Tubau JF et al: Usefulness of thallium-201 scintigraphy in predicting the development of angina pectoris in hypertensive patients with left ventricular hypertrophy. Am J Cardiol 1989;64:45.

Ueda K et al: Prognosis and outcome of elderly hypertensives in a Japanese community: Results from a long-term prospective study. J Hypertens 1988;6:991.

Veterans Administration Cooperative Study Group on Antihypertensive Agents: Effects of treatment on morbidity in hypertension. 1. Results in patients with diastolic blood pressure averaging 115 through 129 mm Hg. JAMA 1967;202:1028.

Veterans Administration Cooperative Study Group on Antihypertensive Agents: Effects of treatment on morbidity in hypertension. 2. Results in patients with diastolic blood pressures averaging 90 through 114 mm Hg. JAMA 1970;213:1143.

Veterans Administration Cooperative Study Group on Antihypertensive Agents: Effects of treatment on morbidity in hypertension. 3. Influence of age, diastolic pressure, and prior cardiovascular disease: Further analysis of side-effects. Circulation 1972;45:991.

Veterans Administration Cooperative Study Group on Antihypertensive Agents: Return of elevated blood pressure after withdrawal of antihypertensive drugs. Circulation 1975;51:1107.

Wadsworth RM: Calcium and vascular reactivity in ageing and hypertension. J Hypertension 1990;8:975.

Wallin JD et al: Intravenous nicardipine for the treatment of severe hypertension. Am J Med 1988;85:331.

Weber MA (editor): Hypertension: Meeting therapeutic challenges, providing effective management. Symposium. Am J Med 1991;91(Suppl 1A):15.

Weder AB et al: Red blood cell lithium-sodium countertransport in the Tecumseh Blood Pressure Study. Hypertension 1991;17:652.

Williams GH: Converting-enzyme inhibitors in the treatment of hypertension. N Engl J Med 1988;319:1517.

Williams RR et al: Are there interactions and relations between genetic and environmental factors predisposing to high blood pressure? Hypertension 1991;18(Suppl I):I–29.

Williams RR et al: Multigenic human hypertension: Evidence for subtypes and hope for haplotypes. J Hypertens 1990;8(Suppl 7):39.

Wilson MF et al: Comparison of nguanfacine versus clonidine for efficacy, safety and occurrence of withdrawal syndrome in step-2 treatment of mild to moderate essential hypertension. Am J Cardiol 1986;57(Suppl E):43E.

Working Group on Hypertension in the Elderly: Statement on hypertension in the elderly. JAMA 1986;256:270.

World Hypertensive League: Physical exercise in the management of hypertension: a consensus statement. J Hypertens 1991;9:283.

Zachariah PK et al: Age-related characteristics of ambulatory blood pressure load and mean load pressure in normotensive subjects. JAMA 1991;265:1414.

Zachariah PK, Sheps SG, Smith RL: Clinical use of home and ambulatory blood pressure monitoring. Mayo Clin Proc 1989;64:1436.

10

Cardiac Failure

DEFINITIONS

The heart has two primary functions: to provide cardiac output sufficient to meet all physiologic and metabolic demands and to generate arterial pressures sufficient to perfuse the organs. Cardiac failure can be broadly defined as a state in which the heart fails to meet the varying oxygen and metabolic needs of the body under differing circumstances, or a state in which cardiac output (the ability of the heart to pump blood) is reduced relative to the metabolic demands of the body, assuming the existence of adequate venous return. The definition is arbitrary and controversial, because the phenomena of heart failure are complex and incompletely understood.

Cardiac failure may be present in the resting state or may appear only with excessive stress. It is easily recognized in its later stages, when symptoms and signs due to pulmonary or systemic venous congestion, increased ventricular volume and diastolic pressure, and decreased cardiac output are present.

In patients with heart disease, transient cardiac failure may be induced by any of the acute precipitating events listed below. When the precipitating event subsides with time or is cured by appropriate treatment, the patient's cardiac status may return to its previous asymptomatic state.

The diagnosis of cardiac failure, like that of any other disease, depends upon its definition, which varies with different authorities. The distinction must be maintained between the presence of heart disease and the presence of cardiac failure, and the latter should be perceived as a continuum from (1) recognition of the presence of cardiac disease, to (2) a preclinical phase in which hemodynamic abnormalities but not symptoms may be present, and finally to (3) an overt clinical phase in which it is obvious to all that cardiac failure is present.

The heart fails ("decompensates") when various compensatory mechanisms are excessive (eg, salt and water retention, increased systemic vascular resistance) or when cardiac hypertrophy, raised atrial pressure, ventricular dilation, and increased force of contraction (see below) are inadequate to maintain the function of a diseased heart whose work load has been increased.

Initially, either the left or, less commonly, the right ventricle may fail; ultimately, however, especially after salt and water retention occurs, combined left and right failure (congestive failure) is the rule.

CAUSES OF HEART FAILURE

The causes of ventricular failure can be summarized as follows:

(1) Intrinsic myocardial disease: Coronary heart disease, cardiomyopathy, infiltrative diseases such as hemochromatosis, amyloidosis, sarcoidosis, and myocarditis.
(2) Excess work load:
  (a) Increased resistance to ejection (pressure load): Hypertension, stenosis of aortic or pulmonary valves, hypertrophic cardiomyopathy.
  (b) Increased stroke volume (volume load): Aortic insufficiency, mitral insufficiency, tricuspid insufficiency, congenital left-to-right shunts.
  (c) Increased body demands ("high-output failure"): Thyrotoxicosis, anemia, pregnancy, arteriovenous fistula.
(3) Iatrogenic myocardial damage:
  (a) Drugs such as doxorubicin (Adriamycin) or disopyramide.
  (b) Radiation therapy for mediastinal tumors or Hodgkin's disease.

Factors Precipitating Failure

In at least half of cases, demonstrable precipitating disease or factors that increase the work load of the heart are present, and these factors should be sought in every patient with cardiac failure. They include arrhythmias, respiratory infection, myocardial infarction, pulmonary embolism, rheumatic carditis, thyrotoxicosis, anemia, excessive salt intake, corticosteroid administration, pregnancy, the stopping of medications, and excessive or rapid administration of parenteral fluids. Fever may aggravate failure (as in acute myocardial infarction) but does not cause it de novo.

Heart failure may occur in patients with normally functioning hearts that are subjected to excessive loads. The clearest example of this is systemic arteriovenous fistula. Even in otherwise healthy young

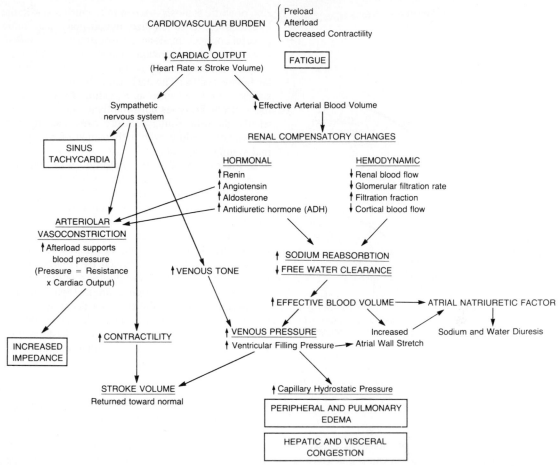

Figure 10–1. Pathophysiology of congestive heart failure. Decreased cardiac output leads to changes mediated by the renal compensatory and sympathetic nervous systems. Raised venous pressure results in peripheral and pulmonary edema and hepatic and visceral congestion.

people, a large fistula can produce heart failure; in older people, thyrotoxicosis, severe anemia, beriberi, or Paget's disease of bone may cause heart failure even though cardiac output is high.

HEMODYNAMIC & PATHOPHYSIOLOGIC FEATURES OF HEART FAILURE* (Figure 10–1)

Compensatory Mechanisms

The compensatory mechanisms by which the heart responds to an increased load include the following: (1) Concentric hypertrophy (hypertrophy without dilation) provides larger contractile cells. (2) Increased fiber length or dilation increases the force of contrac-

---

*The derived indices used in this chapter are discussed in Chapter 4.

tion, as shown by the Frank-Starling law (Figure 10–2). (3) Neurohumoral activation, including activation of the sympathetic nervous system, the renin-angiotensin system, endothelin, and the release of antidiuretic hormone, is characteristic of congestive heart failure. Activation of the sympathetic nervous system occurs early, before symptoms are present (Mancia, 1990; Francis, 1990). Increased sympathetic nervous system activity increases the force of contraction at any fiber length without increasing the filling pressure, stimulates the renin-angiotensin-aldosterone system, and raises the heart rate and the systemic vascular resistance to maintain arterial pressure. The renin-angiotensin system, in turn, has been shown to amplify catecholamine release from nonadrenergic nerve endings, thereby augmenting vascular tissue responses to sympathetic activation (Hirsch, 1990). Venous tone increases with sympathetic nervous system activity. Production of endothelin and antidiuretic hormone (vasopressin) increases. With

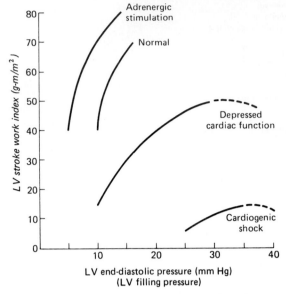

Figure 10–2. Family of Frank-Starling curves showing relation of force of contraction (left ventricular stroke work index) to fiber length or pressure (left ventricular end diastolic pressure or filling pressure). (Modified and reproduced, with permission, from Swan HJC, Parmley WW: Congestive heart failure. In: *Pathologic Physiology: Mechanisms of Disease,* 5th ed. Sodeman WA Jr, Sodeman WA [editors]. Saunders, 1974.)

left and right atrial stretch and increased pressure, atrial natriuretic factor is released, causing natriuresis and diuresis.

A. Hypertrophy and Compliance: Concentric hypertrophy is most apt to occur when the load placed on the heart is due to increased resistance to ejection with increased impedance, characteristically seen in aortic stenosis and hypertension. Early in the course of the disease, the only cardiac abnormality that can be identified is left ventricular hypertrophy, recognized both clinically and by echocardiography and electrocardiography (see Chapter 9). The increased thickness causes a decrease in the distensibility, or compliance, of the left ventricle, so that diastolic filling is slowed and the left ventricular end-diastolic pressure is raised, with a normal left ventricular volume; the raised filling pressure is required to augment left ventricular output in accordance with the Frank-Starling principle. The raised left ventricular end-diastolic pressure does not necessarily imply ventricular failure but occurs whenever compliance is decreased, as in the cardiac states noted above or in hypertrophic or infiltrative cardiomyopathy. It also occurs early in acute myocardial infarction, when the infarcted area becomes stiff and less distensible. The decreased compliance of the left ventricle results in a more forceful atrial contraction, which is the basis for an S_4 gallop. Later—eg, in patients with hyperten-

sion or aortic stenosis—when left ventricular volume increases (because cardiac hypertrophy and more forceful contraction alone are insufficient to compensate), the left ventricular early, mid-, and end-diastolic pressures rise even further, and left ventricular failure occurs. The early diastolic increase of resistance to filling causes an S_3 gallop. In some cases, the ventricle becomes noncompliant and the left ventricular diastolic filling pressure rises, causing congestive heart failure even with normal or nearly normal systolic function.

B. Increased Stroke Volume and Failure: When the increased cardiac load is due to increased stroke volume, typically represented by aortic insufficiency, the increased stretch increases fiber length and so increases the force of left ventricular contraction as demonstrated by the Frank-Starling principle. As the stretch increases, left ventricular volume increases, as can be demonstrated by enlargement of the heart on the plain film of the chest or the echocardiogram or by left ventricular angiography. In these circumstances, distensibility is not decreased, and it is common to find an increased left ventricular volume with normal left ventricular end-diastolic pressure and normal or increased cardiac output. When left ventricular performance declines in the later stages of this type of lesion (as well as in so-called congestive cardiomyopathy), the ejection fraction falls from its normal value of 60–70% and may be as low as 10–20% in very severe failure. The left ventricular ejection fraction is best determined by left ventricular angiography and the right ventricular ejection fraction by radionuclide angiography, although echocardiography provides an estimate. In general, patients tolerate increased volume load better than increased resistance load even though left ventricular wall tension and myocardial oxygen consumption increase when the heart is dilated and enlarged (law of Laplace). (See Figure 1–27 for definition and details.)

C. Increased Sympathetic Stimulation: Increased sympathetic stimulation can be demonstrated in patients with cardiac failure by increased levels of catecholamines in blood and urine and by depletion of norepinephrine in cardiac tissue, notably atrial appendages removed at operation. Several investigators have demonstrated the importance of the sympathetic nervous system in improving cardiac contractility in cardiac failure and have noted its exhaustion in failure, probably associated with down-regulation of beta-adrenergic receptors. Beta-adrenergic blocking agents in the usual dosages may worsen or precipitate ventricular failure by decreasing the sympathetic support to the heart. Compensatory increased sympathetic stimulation as well as increased angiotensin II, increased vasopressin, and perhaps increased endothelin all may excessively raise systemic vascular resistance; the enhanced afterload is the basis for using vasodilators in therapy.

Pathophysiology of Decompensation

Early in the course of various cardiac diseases, the compensatory mechanisms are adequate to maintain a normal cardiac output and normal intracardiac pressures at rest and after exercise. Hypertrophy may be recognized by physical examination, electrocardiography, or echocardiography; when ventricular dilation occurs, cardiac enlargement can be seen on the plain chest film. Compensated heart disease becomes "decompensated" as ventricular volume and filling pressures of the respective ventricles increase, although a raised filling pressure may be due to decreased compliance rather than to ventricular failure early in the course of the disease. This is known as diastolic dysfunction and can be the primary cause of increased left ventricular filling pressure and pulmonary congestion in a significant proportion of patients in congestive heart failure. Diastolic dysfunction is particularly common in elderly patients with hypertension and in patients with myocardial ischemia due to coronary artery disease.

As the filling pressure increases, hydrostatic pressure exceeds colloid osmotic pressure at the capillary level, and pulmonary venous congestion occurs. When the lymphatics can no longer adequately remove the excess fluid, interstitial and then alveolar edema of the lungs occurs, resulting in symptoms of left ventricular failure, with dyspnea, exertional cough, orthopnea, paroxysmal nocturnal dyspnea, and pulmonary edema when the disease involves the left ventricle. Raised venous pressure, hepatomegaly, dependent edema, and ascites occur when failure involves the right ventricle (congestive or right ventricular failure). Cardiac output may be normal at this phase, especially at rest, but may be decreased on exercise; as stroke volume diminishes on exercise, tachycardia returns the minute cardiac output to normal. The arteriovenous oxygen difference widens as blood flow decreases to nonessential vascular systems. When the ventricular filling pressure is increased—especially when ventricular compliance is decreased—atrial hypertrophy increases the force of atrial systole and thereby aids filling; loss of this so-called "atrial kick" can decrease the cardiac output when atrial fibrillation occurs.

High-Output Failure

Although cardiac failure is usually associated with low cardiac output, especially with exercise, it may occur when output is greater than normal, because the heart cannot maintain the high output necessitated by the underlying cause. Tissue demands for oxygen may require increased cardiac output; this may occur in severe anemia, acute beriberi, thyrotoxicosis, Paget's disease, and large arteriovenous fistula or during extreme exertion in hot, humid climates. Systemic vascular resistance is decreased in these conditions, although the high output in thyrotoxicosis is probably due also to a combination of the effects of thyroxin and catecholamines on the heart. Greatly decreased systemic vascular resistance causes large amounts of blood to pass from the arteries to the veins, increasing the venous return and hence the cardiac output. Vasodilation initially decreases relative arterial blood volume and causes the kidney to activate the renin-angiotensin-aldosterone system; this results in renin release and increased aldosterone production, causing salt and water retention and blood volume expansion. Pulmonary and systemic venous congestion follows, resulting in the clinical syndrome of heart failure. Management of the condition is that of the underlying cause (eg, arteriovenous fistula).

The hemodynamic effects of high-output states vary considerably with the underlying state of the myocardium. Thus, a relatively minor "high output" factor such as anemia may be of much greater importance in an older patient with degenerative heart disease than in a younger person. In addition, the "high-output" load may increase the demand of oxygen by the myocardium relative to supply and cause anginal pain rather than heart failure.

Pathophysiologic Mechanisms of Salt & Water Retention

Increased sodium and water retention secondary to aldosterone production leads to an increase in blood volume, which, by raising the hydrostatic pressure in the capillaries, leads first to interstitial edema and then to transudation of fluid into tissues that have decreased tissue pressure, such as the subcutaneous tissues. As a result, edema of the ankles and lower extremities occurs when the patient is ambulatory and edema of the sacral area when the patient is recumbent. Symptoms such as dyspnea and edema are aggravated by salt and water retention and are reversed by the use of diuretics and low-sodium diets.

If sodium is restricted, moderate water intake does not add to sodium retention, as it does with free sodium intake. Water intake need not be restricted if sodium intake is restricted, unless dilutional hyponatremia is present. In severe heart failure, antidiuretic hormone is elevated, decreasing free water clearance. With atrial stretch, atrial natriuretic factor is released. Both of these can contribute to dilutional hyponatremia.

CLINICAL FINDINGS

When a patient with any type of heart disease—congenital, valvular, hypertensive, coronary, metabolic, etc—develops symptoms and signs of cardiac

Table 10–1. Criteria for diagnosis of congestive heart failure (left and right).[1,2]

Major criteria
  Paroxysmal nocturnal dyspnea or orthopnea
  Dyspnea and cough on exertion
  Neck vein distention
  Rales
  Cardiomegaly
  Acute pulmonary edema
  S_3 gallop
  Increased venous pressure > 16 cm water
  Hydrothorax
Minor criteria
  Ankle edema
  Night cough
  Hepatomegaly
  Pleural effusion
  Vital capacity reduced by one-third from maximum
  Tachycardia (rate of ≥ 120/min)
Major or minor criterion
  Weight loss ≥ 4.5 kg in 5 days in response to treatment

[1] Adapted and reproduced, with permission, from McKee PA et al: The natural history of congestive heart failure: The Framingham Study. N Engl J Med 1971;285:1441.
[2] For establishing a definite diagnosis of congestive heart failure, 2 major or one major and 2 minor criteria must be present concurrently.

failure, the findings are usually not specific for any particular etiologic category. Symptoms and signs of pulmonary or systemic venous congestion, increased cardiac volume, and diastolic pressure combined with decreased cardiac output, raised venous pressure, and evidences of salt and water retention clearly indicate that cardiac failure has occurred. With left heart failure, left atrial pressure increases and, in turn, increases the afterload on the right ventricle, ultimately resulting in right heart failure. Left heart failure is the most common cause of right heart failure.

In patients with congenital heart disease, pulmonary heart disease, endocarditis involving the valves on the right side, right ventricular infarction, primary pulmonary hypertension, or obstructive diseases of the lungs, raised venous pressure, enlarged tender liver, and systemic edema indicate that cardiac disease has progressed to right-sided congestive failure. This is also true when pulmonary hypertension complicates mitral stenosis, and right heart failure and tricuspid regurgitation follow.

The criteria for diagnosis of congestive heart failure are listed in Table 10–1.

Left Ventricular Failure

Left ventricular failure is most commonly due to coronary heart disease, dilated cardiomyopathy, hypertension, or valvular heart disease, usually aortic valvular disease. Less common causes are mitral valve disease, hypertrophic cardiomyopathy, left-to-right shunts, and congenital heart lesions. Infective endocarditis may lead to left ventricular failure. Left ventricular failure may also occur in various connective tissue disorders, thyrotoxicosis, severe anemia, arteriovenous fistula, myocarditis, beriberi, and myocardial involvement by tumors or granulomas.

Left ventricular failure may occur acutely with fluid overload, as may happen with too rapid infusion of large amounts of blood or saline in patients with minimal evidence of left ventricular failure prior to infusion. It may result abruptly from ventricular or atrial arrhythmias associated with a rapid ventricular rate, severe anemia, acute leukemia, or abrupt slowing of the ventricular rate, as in atrioventricular block. Drugs such as beta-adrenergic blockers, disopyramide, and verapamil, especially in combination, have a negative inotropic effect and may cause left ventricular failure by removing sympathetic drive to the heart. These drugs should be used with caution in patients with incipient left ventricular failure.

A. Symptoms:

1. Dyspnea– The increased fluid in the tissue spaces causes dyspnea, at first on effort and then at rest, by stimulation of stretch receptors in the lung and chest wall and by increased work of breathing. The work of breathing is greater because of the increased stiffness of the lungs, and the patient is aware of difficulty in breathing. Transudation of fluid into the alveoli superimposes cough on dyspnea of effort, and this combination is suggestive of left ventricular failure. The symptoms are usually progressive, and the earliest manifestation is shortness of breath on exertion that previously caused no difficulty. As pulmonary engorgement progresses, less and less activity brings on dyspnea and cough, until both are present even when the patient is at rest.

2. Orthopnea– Shortness of breath in recumbency is precipitated by the increase in pulmonary engorgement owing to autotransfusion of fluid accumulated in the lower part of the body during upright posture. It is promptly relieved by propping up the head or trunk. Orthopnea can be accompanied by nocturnal cough on lying down. When the pulmonary blood volume is thus increased, the patient characteristically goes to sleep without difficulty but awakens several hours later with dyspnea (paroxysmal nocturnal dyspnea).

3. Paroxysmal nocturnal dyspnea– Paroxysmal nocturnal dyspnea with cough usually develops in a setting of progressive dyspnea on exertion and orthopnea, but it may appear at any time and may be the first manifestation of left ventricular failure in severe hypertension, aortic stenosis or insufficiency, or myocardial infarction. It also occurs in patients with tight mitral stenosis, but in this condition it is due to pulmonary venous congestion from obstruction at the mitral valve rather than left ventricular failure. Paroxysmal nocturnal dyspnea or cough may be associated with inspiratory and expiratory wheezing due to bronchospasm (so-called cardiac asthma). Depending upon the amount of fluid that accumulates in the lungs, the patient with paroxysmal nocturnal dyspnea may awaken with dyspnea that lasts only a few minutes and is relieved by sitting or standing or that progresses rapidly into an alarming episode of pulmonary edema.

4. Acute pulmonary edema– Rapidly rising pulmonary capillary pressure causes gross transudation of fluid into the alveoli, resulting in acute pulmonary edema that causes the patient to sit up in bed gasping for breath. The patient is also cold, pale, anxious, and profusely sweating. With increase in pulmonary congestion, perfusion of blood through nonventilated alveoli causes a right-to-left shunt with progressive decrease in arterial Po_2. The patient may become cyanotic, cough up frothy white or pink sputum, and be fearful of imminent death. Patients may ignore progressive dyspnea on exertion, but they rarely ignore acute pulmonary edema. Most attacks subside gradually in 1–3 hours, possibly because of the upright position as well as the progressive decrease in cardiac output. With increasing work of breathing, there is progressive fatigue, hypoventilation, increase in arterial Pco_2, and hypoxemia and respiratory failure. In some instances, the left ventricle rapidly weakens, leading to shock and death. Left atrial pressure has been shown to rise to 50 or 60 mm Hg during episodes of pulmonary edema.

Heroin administration is one of the common causes of pulmonary edema; the mechanism of action is presumably increased capillary permeability. This results in arterial hypoxemia and acidosis, which can be quite marked. The arterial Po_3 is usually less than 40 mm Hg in the presence of pulmonary edema, and the pH hovers around 7.15.

5. Interpretation of dyspnea– When dyspnea on exertion is the only symptom, its interpretation is often difficult, especially when the patient is obese and in poor physical condition (see Chapter 2).

a. Patients in poor physical condition almost never have orthopnea or paroxysmal nocturnal dyspnea, and the dyspnea is rarely progressive over a short period of time as it is when left ventricular failure develops in aortic stenosis or coronary disease.

b. Pulmonary causes of dyspnea such as chronic bronchitis, pulmonary fibrosis, and asthmatic bronchitis are more difficult to differentiate because the wheezing of left ventricular failure due to bronchospasm may simulate that of asthma. However, the patient with chronic lung disease usually gives a history of smoking, long-standing cough, or sputum production and frequent episodes of purulent bronchitis in winter. Cough is often present in the absence of dyspnea.

c. Moderate to severe anemia may also produce exertional dyspnea.

d. Advanced age, debility, extreme obesity, ascites due to any cause, abdominal distention due to gastrointestinal disease, or advanced stages of pregnancy may produce orthopnea in the absence of heart disease.

e. Patients with neurocirculatory asthenia or anxiety states with psychophysiologic cardiovascular reactions may suffer from sighing respirations simulating dyspnea.

6. Fatigue– Exertional fatigue and weakness due to reduced cardiac output are late symptoms and disappear promptly with rest. Severe fatigue rather than dyspnea is the chief complaint of patients with mitral stenosis who have developed pulmonary hypertension and low cardiac output.

7. Nocturia as a symptom of edema– Nocturia may represent excretion of edema fluid accumulated during the day and increased renal perfusion in the recumbent position; it reflects the decreased work of the heart at rest and often the effects of diuretics given during the day. It may also be due to noncardiac causes.

B. Signs: Evidence of the primary disease responsible for the failure, eg, hypertension or aortic stenosis, is almost always present. In some instances of severe failure due to aortic stenosis, the murmur may be absent or difficult to hear because of the decreased velocity of ejection and reduced cardiac output.

Evidence of so-called primary disease is at times misleading. For example, because of the compensatory systemic vasoconstriction that occurs in any condition with reduced cardiac output via the baroreceptor mechanism, blood pressure may be modestly or even markedly raised in patients with cardiac failure due to any cause; one should therefore be cautious in defining the disease as hypertensive heart failure unless the blood pressure remains elevated after the failure is relieved by treatment.

1. Enlargement of heart– In the presence of symptoms of cardiac failure, hypertrophy or dilation of the left ventricle is usually found on examination and confirmed by evidence of left ventricular hypertrophy on the ECG and left ventricular enlargement on the x-ray or echocardiogram. Left ventricular dilation may be absent if diastolic dysfunction is the cause of the heart failure.

2. Ventricular heave– The best clinical sign of left ventricular hypertrophy is a left ventricular heave at the apex of the heart. The heave is a localized, sustained, systolic outward motion of the left ventricular impulse that differs from the hyperdynamic left ventricular impulse of exertion, anxiety, or regurgitant valve disease and from the right ventricular heave of right ventricular hypertrophy. The latter is more diffuse, is felt over the center of the chest, and causes apical retraction rather than a lift during systole. The point of maximal impulse (PMI) normally collapses before the carotid arterial pulse. If the PMI is sustained longer than the simultaneously palpated carotid arterial pulse, left ventricular hypertrophy is probably present.

3. Third heart sound– (See Chapter 3.) When there is increased left ventricular volume, an exaggerated third heart sound is often heard during the rapid inflow phase of ventricular filling. The S_3 gallop is related to a sudden decrease in the rate of left ventricular filling early in diastole.

4. Fourth heart sound– Decreased compliance of the left ventricle with resultant forceful contraction of the left atrium causes a fourth heart sound or atrial gallop that may be felt or seen.

5. Rales or "crackles"– Rales in the lungs may be absent at rest and even early in the episode of nocturnal dyspnea, when transudation occurs into the tissue spaces and not into the alveoli; on the chest x-ray, pulmonary edema can be seen even in the absence of rales. Later, however, when alveolar fluid appears, the rales are loud and generalized; frothy, bubbling fluid may be obvious all over the lungs. Pleural effusion may occur, almost always with concomitant right heart failure.

6. Cheyne-Stokes respiration– Cheyne-Stokes respiration is commonly seen in advanced cardiac failure (see Chapter 3).

7. Tachycardia– As the stroke volume decreases, tachycardia compensates to maintain the minute cardiac output; it is usually present in cardiac failure.

8. Pulsus alternans– (See Chapter 3.)

C. Electrocardiographic and Chest X-Ray Findings: The ECG is usually more sensitive than the chest x-ray but less sensitive than two-dimensional echocardiograms in demonstrating chamber hypertrophy. Occasionally, the ECG may be normal or minimally abnormal when the echocardiogram shows concentric left ventricular hypertrophy in aortic stenosis. When dilation predominates over hypertrophy, the chest x-ray may show enlargement, whereas the ECG may show little or no abnormality. The ECG also may be confusing, with nonspecific manifestations of associated effects of treatment with digitalis or diuretics (hypokalemia) or with superimposed coronary disease. An apparent discrepancy in the specific chamber that is hypertrophied or enlarged on the chest x-ray as compared to the ECG usually means that both chambers are involved, although the ECG is less likely to give an erroneous picture when the abnormality is clear-cut.

D. Echocardiographic Findings: Echocardiography is both sensitive and specific for an increased left ventricular mass. A valuable sign of severe left ventricular failure is a wide E point separation between excursion of the anterior mitral valve leaflet and the ventricular septum, as shown in Figure 10–3 (Massie: Mitral-septal separation, 1977).

Right Ventricular Failure

Right ventricular failure is usually secondary to chronic left ventricular failure but may occur alone. Other causes of right ventricular failure are tight mitral stenosis with pulmonary hypertension, pulmonary valve stenosis, cor pulmonale due to chronic lung disease, primary pulmonary hypertension with tricuspid insufficiency, right ventricular infarction, and congenital diseases such as Eisenmenger's complex and pulmonary hypertensive ventricular or atrial septal defects. Tricuspid or mitral valve stenosis may produce systemic venous congestion similar to that of right ventricular failure. In this case, the congestion is due to obstruction at the valve rather than to right

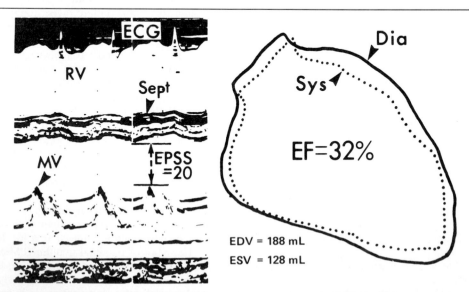

Figure 10–3. Echocardiogram of patient with alcoholic cardiomyopathy demonstrating a decreased ejection fraction of 32%, a large end-diastolic volume, and a wide separation between the anterior portion of the mitral valve leaflet and the ventricular septum. (EF, ejection fraction; EDV, end-diastolic volume; ESV, end-systolic volume; MV, mitral valve; RV, right ventricle; Sept, septum; EPSS, end [E] point of mitral valve separated from septum; Sys, systole; Dia, diastole.) (Reproduced, with permission, from Massie BM et al: Mitral-septal separation: A new echocardiographic index of left ventricular function. Am J Cardiol 1977;39:1008.)

ventricular failure, unless there is another, more proximal obstruction (eg, tricuspid valve stenosis with more proximal mitral stenosis). Another cause of right ventricular failure is involvement of the pulmonary and tricuspid valves by infective endocarditis or carcinoid.

A. Symptoms: The dominant symptoms of right ventricular failure are those of systemic venous congestion—in contrast to left ventricular failure, in which symptoms of pulmonary venous congestion predominate. Pulmonary symptoms are rare unless there is associated left ventricular failure or unless right ventricular failure is due to chronic lung disease. Paroxysmal nocturnal dyspnea is uncommon.

1. Fatigue– The patient may complain of fatigue as cardiac output is reduced.

2. Dependent edema– Edema of the ankles may occur when the patient is up and about; edema of the sacral area, flanks, and thighs when in bed.

3. Liver engorgement– If right ventricular failure occurs rapidly, as when atrial fibrillation develops in tight mitral stenosis, congestion of the liver with distention of its capsule may result, causing right upper quadrant pain which has often been confused with that of cholecystitis or other abdominal disease.

4. Anorexia and bloating– Hepatic and visceral engorgement secondary to the raised venous pressure may cause anorexia, bloating, and other nonspecific gastrointestinal symptoms.

B. Signs: Evidence of the underlying disease is usually found when specifically sought, although special investigations may be necessary.

1. Right ventricular hypertrophy– In primary right ventricular failure, right ventricular hypertrophy can be diagnosed on the basis of right ventricular heave and right atrial gallop rhythm by auscultation.

2. Right ventricular heave– Usually present are a right ventricular heave over the lower central chest; a right-sided S_4 gallop, a right-sided S_3 gallop, or both; a loud pulmonary second sound at the base of the heart; and increased jugular venous pressure with systolic pulsations of tricuspid insufficiency are usually present. Right-sided events, including S_4, S_3, and tricuspid insufficiency murmurs, are frequently increased in intensity with inspiration.

3. Right atrial gallop– A right-sided S_3 is often heard, especially when right ventricular failure is due to increased resistance to right ventricular outflow, as in pulmonary stenosis or pulmonary hypertension.

4. Murmurs– If the underlying disease is congenital or valvular, characteristic murmurs will be heard, although in some patients with Eisenmenger's syndrome with severe pulmonary hypertension and a balanced shunt flow, no murmurs may be heard. Murmurs of pulmonary and tricuspid regurgitation may be heard in primary pulmonary hypertension and chronic lung disease.

5. Chronic pulmonary signs– If right ventricular failure is secondary to chronic lung disease, there will be evidence of decreased distensibility of the lungs, rales, rhonchi, wheezes, a prolonged expiratory phase, and signs of chronic bronchitis.

6. Jugular pulse– The jugular venous pulse will demonstrate the pulsating systolic wave of tricuspid insufficiency (which may also be palpated over the liver, with systolic expansion of the liver); Presystolic a waves may be prominent when there is decreased compliance of the right ventricle and raised right atrial pressure. The a waves are also prominent in pulmonary stenosis with right ventricular failure and in tricuspid stenosis. The venous pressure rises further when the physician exerts right upper quadrant pressure, and the right atrial pressure may be raised as much as 5 mm Hg by this maneuver (hepatojugular reflux). The systolic jugular venous pulse of tricuspid insufficiency is often associated with a pansystolic murmur over the xiphoid, often accentuated by inspiration and associated with a right-sided S_4 gallop, S_3 gallop, or both, also louder on inspiration.

7. Pulmonary second sound– The pulmonary second sound is accentuated if there is pulmonary hypertension but may be fainter, with a wider split from A_2, if pulmonary stenosis is mild to moderate, and absent in severe pulmonary stenosis.

8. Pitting edema– Pitting edema of the ankles, lower extremities, and back is found in established right ventricular failure. Initially, the dependent edema caused by right heart failure usually subsides overnight. Eventually, it fails to subside with initial bed rest and may even increase during recumbency.

9. Ascites– Ascites is rarely prominent unless right ventricular failure has been neglected or obstructive lesions such as constrictive pericarditis, tricuspid stenosis, or cardiac tamponade are present. In constrictive pericarditis, the jugular venous pressure is raised, but there is no clinical evidence of tricuspid insufficiency; in fact, the dominant wave seen in the neck may be a prominent y descent.

10. Hydrothorax (pleural and pericardial effusion)– Hydrothorax is common in congestive heart failure, occurring in about a third of severe cases. It is more common in biventricular than in left ventricular failure alone and more apt to occur in the right pleural space than in the left; bilateral hydrothorax is less common. Some authorities believe that isolated left hydrothorax should make one consider other conditions such as pulmonary infarction, pericarditis, or a subdiaphragmatic condition such as pancreatitis, but well-documented isolated left hydrothorax has often been reported. Fluid may accumulate in any serous cavity (eg, the pericardial and peritoneal cavities—the latter more apt to result from tricuspid stenosis or constrictive pericarditis). Rapid changes in the heart shadow should make one think of pericardial effusion rather than cardiac enlargement.

The mechanism of hydrothorax is not clearly understood. Pleural effusion may be related to the fact that the systemic veins interfere with fluid absorption from the pleura when systemic venous pressure is elevated. Pleural effusion is common with right-sided congestive heart failure but is uncommon in acute pulmonary edema without right heart failure. It may also occur when swelling of the liver leads to engorged lymphatics, which may penetrate the diaphragm en route to the thoracic duct.

C. Electrocardiographic Findings:

1. Left ventricular pattern– If the ECG shows predominant left ventricular hypertrophy, it is likely that right ventricular failure is not the primary disorder but is secondary to left-sided failure.

2. Right ventricular pattern– Right ventricular hypertrophy is almost always found in congenital heart disease (eg, pulmonary stenosis) although combined hypertrophy may be found when ventricular septal defect produces cardiac failure. Right ventricular hypertrophy is also marked in primary pulmonary hypertension or pulmonary hypertensive mitral stenosis, but it is usually slight in clinically significant chronic cor pulmonale.

3. Right axis deviation and right ventricular hypertrophy– See Figures 11–16 and 11–20.

4. P waves– Prominent P waves in leads II and III and a dominant peaked anterior P wave in V_1 and V_2 indicate right atrial abnormality, usually hypertrophy, which is often a clue to the presence of chronic cor pulmonale—in contrast to mitral stenosis, in which the P waves are wide and slurred and posteriorly (negatively) directed in V_1, indicating left atrial abnormality, usually hypertrophy.

High-Output Failure

Arteriovenous fistula is an uncommon cause of heart failure and may be congenital or acquired. The congenital variety may be due to congenital arteriovenous angioma, often involving a limb. Acquired fistulas are due to trauma (including surgical trauma), usually involving the larger arteries of the limbs. They occur following surgery and may be visceral (eg, following nephrectomy) or musculoskeletal (eg, after laminectomy). The condition may be insidious, and the fistula may not be clinically obvious.

Arteriovenous fistulas are created surgically in patients with renal disease in order to facilitate hemodialysis. Although such arteriovenous shunts are well tolerated by patients with normal hearts, they may cause heart failure in older patients with associated heart lesions. In high-output failure due to other causes such as severe anemia, Paget's disease of bone, thyrotoxicosis, or beriberi, the factor responsible for the failure is usually less obvious.

A. Symptoms: Dyspnea on exertion, edema of the ankles, and fatigue are indistinguishable from the same symptoms occurring in other patients with heart failure.

B. Signs: It is the physical signs of high output failure that provide the clue to diagnosis. The cardinal sign is tachycardia that is disproportionate to the degree of failure and associated with a hyperdynamic cardiac impulse and clinical evidence of cardiac enlargement. Venous pressure is often elevated, and the pulse pressure is widened. A systolic ejection mur-

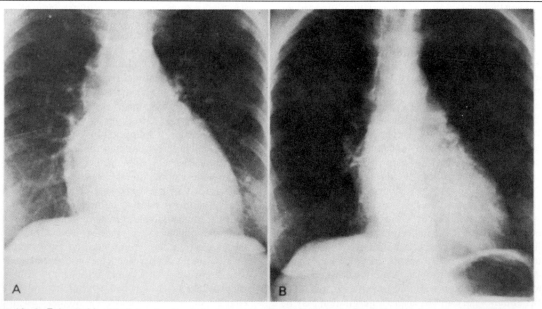

Figure 10–4. Enlarged heart and pulmonary venous congestion in a patient with high-output cardiac failure due to an end-to-side cephalic vein-radial artery fistula **(A)** before and **(B)** after banding of the vein. One month after banding, the heart has become smaller, and pulmonary venous congestion has improved. (Reproduced, with permission, from Anderson CB et al: Cardiac failure and upper extremity arteriovenous dialysis fistulas. Arch Intern Med 1976;136:292.)

mur may be heard at the base, resulting from increased stroke volume. In large arteriovenous fistulas, occlusion increases peripheral resistance, raises systemic arterial pressure, and causes a reflex bradycardia via the baroreceptor reflexes (Branham's sign). If this sign is positive, the fistula is large enough to be a potential cause of heart failure; however, a negative sign does not exclude arteriovenous fistula as a cause of failure. A hidden fistula should be searched for in any case of unexplained heart failure when a large heart and tachycardia are present. Examination of the patient should include listening for continuous bruits over the abdomen, extremities, and back. If the fistula is in a limb, the extremity may be larger than normal and warm and may show marked varicosities. Infection of the fistula may lead to infective endarteritis.

C. Radiologic, Electrocardiographic, and Echocardiographic Findings: Cardiac enlargement is usually seen on the chest x-ray, and the ECG or echocardiogram may show evidence of left ventricular hypertrophy (Figure 10–4).

Acute Heart Failure

When cardiac failure is acute, the clinical picture is different in different disorders, as described in other chapters.

IMAGING STUDIES OF THE HEART

Plain Films

Plain film posteroanterior and lateral views of the chest may provide the first evidence of cardiac failure.

A. Heart Shadow: The film is usually abnormal, with hypertrophy and enlargement of the involved chamber, although the heart may not be enlarged if the patient has concentric hypertrophy (as in aortic stenosis or hypertension) or coronary heart disease.

B. Pulmonary Congestion: The pulmonary pattern may be helpful in confirming chamber enlargement and in distinguishing between left and right ventricular failure. In left ventricular failure, as the resistance of the pulmonary arteries of the lower lobes increases, blood is redistributed to the arteries of the upper lobes, where resistance is lower (Figures 10–4 to 10–6), as can be seen on the plain film when the left atrial pressure rises to 20–25 mm Hg. The same pattern occurs in the pulmonary venous congestion of mitral stenosis, owing to the pressure on small vessels and airways by interstitial fluid.

In pulmonary hypertension, the pulmonary artery is dilated. In severe (especially primary) pulmonary hypertension, the main and central pulmonary arteries may be enlarged, with abrupt reduction in the caliber of the more peripheral pulmonary arteries. There is no evidence of pulmonary venous engorgement such as occurs in right ventricular failure and no evidence

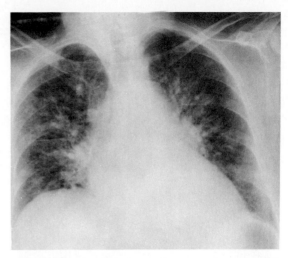

Figure 10–5. Posteroanterior chest x-ray in a man with acute pulmonary edema due to left ventricular failure. Note the bat's wing density, cardiac enlargement, increased flow to upper lobes, and pulmonary venous congestion.

of redistribution of blood such as occurs in left ventricular failure.

When fluid accumulates in the interlobular septa, horizontal Kerley B lines at the angles of the lateral lower lobes can be seen that reflect such fluid. Fluid may be localized in the interlobular spaces, simulating a tumor mass. Interstitial fluid may surround vessels and small airways, causing fuzziness of the borders and "cuffing." Fluid entering the airways and alveoli results in the alveolar pattern characteristic of pulmonary edema.

Attempts have been made to estimate left atrial pressure on the basis of signs of pulmonary venous congestion on the plain film, but the reliability of this method is only about 60%, chiefly because of the lag in appearance and disappearance of the findings in the chest film.

C. Pleural Effusion: In chronic left ventricular failure with raised pulmonary venous pressure, there may be small right- or left-sided pleural effusions, usually the former. Large effusions are usually due to right heart failure.

D. Calcification: Calcification of the mitral or aortic valve or in the pericardium or coronary arteries may be the clue to diagnosis.

E. Aorta: Examination of the aorta is often rewarding. If it is diffusely dilated, it suggests hypertensive disease; but if only the proximal aorta is dilated, especially if it can be seen within the heart shadow, it strongly suggests aortic stenosis. Fine eggshell calcification of the proximal aorta suggests aortitis, commonly due to syphilis (see Chapter 20); if the aorta is widely dilated proximally and in the arch but not distally, the question of dissection must be

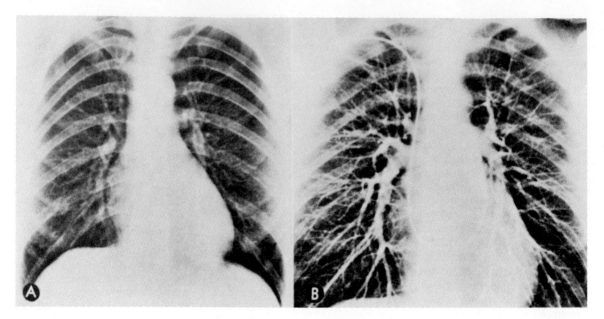

Figure 10–6. Chest x-rays and pulmonary arterial angiograms demonstrating that the vessels to the upper lobes are larger and more numerous than those to the lower lobes with hilar indistinction. *A:* Chest x-ray. *B:* Pulmonary arterial angiogram. (Reproduced, with permission, from Turner AF, Lau FYK, Jacobson G: A method for the estimation of pulmonary venous and arterial pressures from the routine chest roentgenogram. Am J Roentgenol 1972;116:1.)

resolved by further studies. A localized aneurysm may also be demonstrated. The aorta may be small compared to the main pulmonary artery in patients with atrial septal defect or mitral stenosis. All of the congenital anomalies that may affect the aorta or its branches may be seen.

F. Rib Notching: Notching of the ribs may be the first sign of coarctation of the aorta in a patient with hypertension (see Chapter 11).

G. Left Atrial Study: Careful study of the left atrium is often helpful. Disproportionate left atrial enlargement, as in mitral stenosis or mitral regurgitation, may lead to a search for calcification of the mitral valve, echocardiographic studies, and careful physical examination. With left ventricular enlargement, the left atrium may be enlarged proportionately.

H. Other Findings: Chest films often show unexpected findings such as acute inflammatory disease of the lungs, pneumothorax, malignant tumors, or hilar nodes of lymphoma or sarcoidosis. In patients presenting with severe dyspnea, carcinomatous lymphatic spread in the lungs may occasionally lead to the diagnosis of carcinoma of the stomach or other organs.

Echocardiographic Studies

The two-dimensional echocardiogram may demonstrate left or right ventricular hypertrophy or increased chamber size. The left or right atrium may also be enlarged. The extent of systolic ventricular motion may be decreased, demonstrated by lessened fractional shortening of the ventricular chamber. E-point septal separation may be seen. Quantitative estimates of ventricular volumes and ejection fraction can be obtained. Opening of the mitral or aortic valve (or both) may be decreased, as may be motion of the aortic root—all consistent with a decreased stroke volume. Doppler examination can demonstrate mitral or tricuspid valve insufficiency. The primary cause of the heart failure can also at times be demonstrated, (eg, aortic or mitral stenosis, ventricular aneurysm, a flail mitral valve with ruptured chordae tendineae, vegetations, or infective endocarditis).

With diseases causing diastolic dysfunction and failure (eg, hypertrophic cardiomyopathy), ventricular hypertrophy may be seen. If failure is due primarily to diastolic dysfunction, the left ventricle may not be dilated, and systolic motion of the ventricle may be normal. Doppler echocardiography may demonstrate changes related to decreased compliance, such as a considerable increase in velocity during atrial contraction compared to that of early left ventricular filling.

Radioisotope Studies

Radionuclide angiography can estimate left and right ventricular volumes; the difference between diastolic and systolic volumes represents ventricular stroke volume. The ejection fraction can be estimated and is closely correlated with the measurement obtained by left ventriculography. With failure, one or both ventricles may be dilated, with decreased ejection fraction. Sophisticated computer programs allow volume loops to be drawn and the rate of ventricular filling measured; this reflects diastolic ventricular compliance.

LABORATORY FINDINGS

Red and white cell counts, hemoglobin, packed cell volume, and sedimentation rate are normal in uncomplicated heart failure. Polycythemia may occur in chronic cor pulmonale (see Chapter 19). Urinalysis often discloses significant proteinuria and granular casts. The blood urea nitrogen may be elevated out of proportion to the level of the serum creatinine because of reduced renal blood flow, but the urine specific gravity is high in the absence of primary renal disease. Serum sodium, potassium, chloride, and HCO_3- are within normal limits in the usual case of congestive heart failure before diuretics are used. Specific tests should be made for any suspected unusual causes of heart failure, such as thyrotoxicosis, infective endocarditis, syphilis, connective tissue disease, and pheochromocytoma.

DIFFERENTIAL DIAGNOSIS

Cardiac failure must be distinguished from all conditions associated with dyspnea, cough, pulmonary venous congestion, venous pressure elevation, decreased cardiac output, cardiac enlargement, or peripheral edema. These clinical findings occur in a wide variety of conditions that can be conveniently discussed in groups, as in the following paragraphs.

Noncardiac & Nonthoracic Conditions Simulating Cardiac Failure

Examples include the dyspnea and fatigue of obesity, of sedentary individuals, and of emotional states with hyperventilation, and the edema that occurs as a result of thrombophlebitis or of prolonged sitting in people with varicose veins or elderly people with poor skin turgor. In these conditions, there are usually no objective signs of heart disease such as significant murmurs, friction rub, gallop rhythm, cardiac enlargement, or raised venous pressure. Cardiac diagnostic procedures—noninvasive or invasive—reveal no abnormalities of the cardiovascular system. At times these symptoms and signs from noncardiac causes occur in patients with known cardiac disease. As indicated in the introductory paragraphs, the presence of cardiac disease does not imply that all of the patient's symptoms and signs are due to cardiac failure.

Cardiac failure must be diagnosed on the basis of symptoms and signs combined with noninvasive and invasive techniques discussed in this chapter.

Lung Disease & Acute Respiratory Tract Infections Presenting With Respiratory Symptoms

These entities are discussed in Chapter 19. Right heart failure may occur in chronic lung disease (cor pulmonale), but many patients with chronic lung disease with chronic bronchitis, emphysema, etc, have dyspnea and cough for many years without abnormality of the heart. Patients with acute respiratory symptoms may have acute infections of the bronchi or lungs associated with fever and other symptoms and signs of acute illness. The differential diagnosis, including clinical and pulmonary function studies, is discussed in Chapter 19. Most helpful in chronic lung disease is the long history of chronic cough and sputum production, dyspnea, and wheezing, combined with clinical findings of poor lung expansion and chronic wheezes and rales. Also helpful are a history of cigarette smoking or of repeated respiratory infections in the absence of cardiac enlargement, gallop rhythm, ventricular heaves, or raised venous pressure. Venous pressure becomes elevated when right heart failure complicates chronic lung disease, but pulmonary symptoms are present for many years without this objective finding. Pulmonary function studies aid in the diagnosis of specific chronic lung diseases, and hemodynamic studies reveal increases of pressure in the pulmonary artery and the right heart with no abnormality in the left heart. When both right and left heart failure are present, the differentiation may be difficult.

In pulmonary disease without cardiac involvement, there is no dilation or altered wall motion of either ventricle. If pulmonary disease results in elevated pulmonary vascular resistance and pulmonary hypertension, the right ventricle may become dilated and hypokinetic. Two-dimensional echocardiography can be helpful in imaging both ventricles, but in the presence of chronic pulmonary disease it is often technically difficult to obtain a good study; radionuclide angiography can be very helpful.

Massive Pulmonary Embolism

Pulmonary embolism may produce symptoms similar to those of cardiac failure. Acute right ventricular failure may follow massive pulmonary embolism with or without the development of acute pulmonary infarction, as noted on chest x-ray. Acute right ventricular failure may also follow pulmonary hypertension associated with signs of acute right ventricular overload, with physical signs of pulmonary hypertension and evidence on the ECG of right ventricular dilation rather than systemic venous congestion. More precise diagnosis is provided by the combination of chest x-ray, pulmonary radioisotope scan, and pulmonary angiography (see Pulmonary Embolism).

Diseases of the Pericardium & Myocardium

Pericarditis and myocarditis due to various causes are discussed at length in Chapters 18 and 17, respectively. The most important distinguishing feature of congestive cardiomyopathy with cardiac failure is raised left ventricular filling pressure relative to the right side. Findings of pericarditis such as pericardial friction rub can be diagnostic. Echocardiography is helpful in recognizing and quantifying the presence of pericardial effusion, which may not be suspected clinically.

TREATMENT OF CARDIAC FAILURE

Table 10–2. Principles of treatment of cardiac failure. These are discussed in sequence in the text that follows.

1. Verify the diagnosis and estimate the urgency of treatment.
2. Reduce the energy requirement of the heart.
3. Reduce sodium intake unless diuretics have been given.
4. Correct arrhythmias.
5. Provide adequate but not excessive diuresis.
6. Identify and treat unsuspected acute myocardial processes.
7. Treat operable conditions that increase the load on the heart or interfere with left ventricular function.
8. Treat extracardiac factors.
9. Digitalize adequately.
10. Treat systemic diseases affecting the heart.
11. Withdraw offending drugs affecting the heart.
12. Control ascites and effusions.
13. Treat with vasodilators.
14. Add inotropic agents if necessary.
15. Consider intra-aortic balloon counterpulsation.
16. Provide emergency treatment of severe heart failure or acute pulmonary edema according to cause and severity.
17. Consider cardiac transplantation.

Cardiac failure may be of any degree of severity ranging from mild evidence of left ventricular failure, with increasing dyspnea on accustomed effort, to an emergency characterized by severe pulmonary edema, markedly reduced cardiac output, and an urgent threat to life. Treatment therefore varies from a calm, conservative approach with nonurgent methods to urgent emergency measures, depending upon the judgment of the physician.

The objectives of treatment are to remove the cause, increase the force and efficiency of myocardial contraction, decrease abnormal raised systemic vascular resistance, and reduce the abnormal retention of sodium and water. The patient shares a significant responsibility in the management of the disease, because treatment is long-term and involves restriction in diet and activity and the reliable use of cardiac drugs.

Identify, treat, and if possible eliminate the factor precipitating the cardiac failure, eg, infection (especially respiratory), pulmonary infarction, overexertion, increased sodium intake, medication, arrhythmias—particularly with rapid ventricular rates (eg, atrial fibrillation)—myocardial infarction, and anemia. The rationale for drug therapy in congestive heart failure can best be understood by consideration of the pathophysiology of compensatory mechanisms set in motion by a perceived decrease in cardiac output. The clinical picture of congestive heart failure results from overuse of these neural and hormonal compensations. Excessive sodium and water retention resulting in elevation in capillary hydrostatic pressure and net increases in lung water can be reduced by use of

diuretics and preload reducing or vasodilating agents. The decreased stroke volume can be increased by inotropic agents, which moves the heart to a steeper ventricular function curve, resulting in a higher stroke volume for any given left ventricular volume. Another way of increasing stroke volume is to reduce the increased impedance to ejection, which is elevated in congestive heart failure. This can be accomplished with arteriolar vasodilators or so-called afterload reducing drugs. There is also evidence that the excessive renin-angiotensin activation is beneficially counteracted by converting enzyme-inhibitor drugs, yielding a benefit beyond that of simple afterload reduction. It is presently believed that when congestive heart failure is evident, the patient should be treated with a combination of drugs from all three of the drug groups mentioned.

The principles governing the treatment of cardiac failure are outlined in Table 10–2 and will be elaborated below.

VERIFY THE DIAGNOSIS & ESTIMATE THE URGENCY OF TREATMENT

Determination of the cardiac disease causing heart failure is essential, since the cause often determines therapy. In congestive heart failure in patients with aortic stenosis, diuretics and digitalis may be helpful, but surgery or balloon valvuloplasty should not be delayed.

Dyspnea, edema, fatigue, and other findings may

not be due to cardiac failure even in patients with known heart disease. Careful questioning, taking into account the patient's intelligence, cooperation, understanding of language, and the possible effects of statements or diagnoses made by previous physicians, is always required.

The urgent treatment of pulmonary edema is discussed at the end of this chapter.

REDUCE THE ENERGY REQUIREMENT OF THE HEART

This is achieved by restricting physical and psychologic activity. Even modest activity induces sodium retention, tachycardia, and increased oxygen demands.

Rest

Physical and mental rest may be the most important aspect of treatment of early cardiac failure when cardiac reserves are reduced because compensatory mechanisms are beginning to falter and compensated heart disease is starting to "decompensate." The patient may be asymptomatic and have sufficient cardiac reserve to supply tissue oxygen needs at rest but not when stress is imposed. Many patients with mild cardiac failure improve dramatically with no treatment other than rest in bed, although if failure is more severe, other forms of therapy may be required. Rest not only decreases the work of the heart; recumbency decreases the stimulus to aldosterone production induced by erect posture, and sodium diuresis may result. About one-third of patients with left ventricular failure will respond with sodium and water diuresis and recover from cardiac failure with bed rest alone.

The duration of the period of physical and mental rest depends upon the severity of the heart failure, the age of the patient, and the cause of the underlying heart disease leading to failure, but even in the mildest cases the physician usually errs in allowing the patient to resume activity too early. Attention to the domestic, economic, and social situation of the patient is important; it obviously does no good to prescribe bed rest or rest in a chair if the patient has to do the marketing, cook and clean house, and care for the family. Mobilization of social service agencies, home care assistance programs, and all family resources is often helpful. A major flaw in treatment is an insufficient period of rest before the patient returns to the accustomed routine of stressful activities.

Reassurance

Dyspnea due to cardiac failure is a frightening experience. A reassuring and realistically optimistic attitude on the part of the physician and the judicious use of sedatives are important features of management.

REDUCE SODIUM INTAKE UNLESS DIURETICS HAVE BEEN GIVEN

Sodium in any form aggravates the peripheral manifestations of cardiac failure. Sodium excretion in patients with cardiac failure is usually decreased, and if the failure is severe it may be markedly decreased. When diuretics are used in adequate doses, strict sodium restriction is usually not necessary unless cardiac failure is severe or the patient has severe sodium retention such as occurs in chronic constrictive pericarditis. It is usually sufficient to avoid added salt in the diet, but patients must be warned about the sodium content of medications such as Alka-Seltzer or baking soda and foods high in sodium such as potato chips, pretzels, salted nuts, etc. The severity of sodium restriction should be adjusted according to the severity of cardiac failure and the effectiveness of diuretic therapy.

CORRECT ARRHYTHMIAS

Intermittent disturbances of rhythm may include paroxysmal atrial fibrillation or flutter, frequent ventricular premature beats or ventricular tachycardia, complete atrioventricular block, junctional rhythms due to digitalis toxicity, and sick sinus syndrome. Either rapid or slow heart rates may be deleterious. Rapid heart rates decrease diastolic filling time and impair coronary perfusion and may produce myocardial ischemia, decreasing the total cardiac output when stroke volume cannot be increased. An irregular rapid ventricular rate is more harmful than a regular rate, because systolic ejection is more profoundly disturbed by the irregular ventricular filling and subsequent response. When the ventricular rate is slow and the stroke output cannot be increased sufficiently to maintain an adequate minute volume output, patients may develop cardiac failure as well as impaired cerebral perfusion independently of episodes of syncope or Stokes-Adams attack. Rapid ventricular rates continuing for days or weeks can themselves, even in the absence of underlying heart disease, produce congestive heart failure. One of the best animal models for congestive heart failure is produced by pacing-induced tachycardia in the dog.

The prevention and treatment of arrhythmias and of atrioventricular block may be crucial in the management of cardiac failure and are discussed at length in Chapters 14 and 15. Disturbances in rhythm and conduction may not be fully appreciated, because they may be paroxysmal or nocturnal. In patients with paroxysmal nocturnal dyspnea, the precipitating role of the arrhythmia may not be recognized without continuous monitoring of the ECG. With slow ventricular rates, artificial endocardial pacemakers may be required to induce a more rapid rate.

PROVIDE ADEQUATE BUT NOT EXCESSIVE DIURESIS

Physiology & Pharmacology

The treatment of cardiac failure was revolutionized in the late 1950s by the development of oral thiazide diuretic agents. About 40% of patients with cardiac failure will fail to respond to bed rest and digitalis and will require diuretic therapy to overcome the hypervolemia of cardiac failure.

A. Sodium Reabsorption in Cardiac Failure: Although the major physiologic event in cardiac failure is loss of the pumping action of the heart, failure of this function leads to hemodynamic changes in the kidneys, resulting in secondary retention of salt and water due to decreased cardiac output and glomerular filtration rate, increased aldosterone secretion, and other less well defined causes, which in turn leads to the congestive phenomena of the lungs and extremities that we call left and right heart failure, respectively. Although cardiac output is maintained adequately at rest in many patients as cardiac disease

progresses, there comes a time when additional stresses such as exercise, emotion, or tachycardia fail to elicit an adequate increase in cardiac output, resulting in renal hemodynamic changes leading to increased renal tubular reabsorption of sodium. Renal tubular reabsorption of sodium is an important mechanism in regulation of isotonicity and volume of the extracellular fluids. The kidney responds to decreased cardiac output, especially with stress, by increased retention of sodium and water. This may be lifesaving in the event of hemorrhage but is deleterious in the presence of cardiac failure, causing pulmonary and systemic venous congestion and many of the more distressing clinical symptoms and signs of cardiac failure.

B. Diuretic Therapy: The increased sodium and water retention resulting from decreased cardiac output and consequently decreased glomerular filtration rate in cardiac failure can be counteracted by the diuretic agents. See Figure 10–7 for sites of action of various diuretics. Sodium is filtered at the glomerulus, where it enters the proximal renal tubule as part

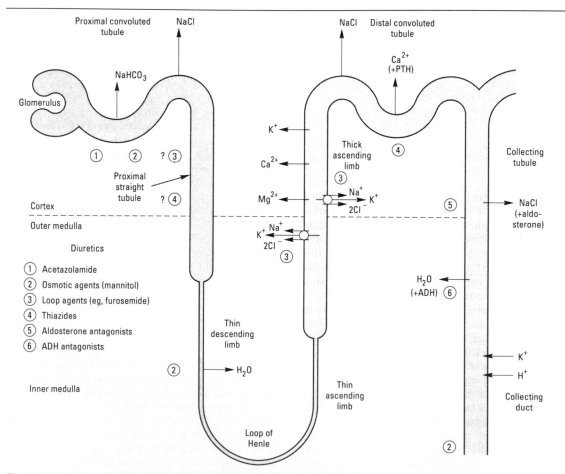

Figure 10–7. Sites of action of diuretics in the tubules. (Reproduced, with permission, from Katzung BG [editor]: *Basic and Clinical Pharmacology,* 5th ed. Appleton & Lange, 1992.)

of the protein-free ultrafiltrate fluid that begins its passage down the renal tubule. Drugs may promote sodium excretion in the urine by increasing the amount of sodium filtered at the glomerulus. The tubular fluid then proceeds down the distal convoluted tubule to the so-called sodium potassium exchange site at the end of the tubule, which is under the influence of aldosterone. The amount of potassium exchanged for sodium depends upon the amount of sodium in the tubular fluid delivered to this distal tubular site; it is greater when the sodium in the diet is high or when decreased reabsorption of sodium follows the use of thiazide or loop diuretics. As a result, a drug that prevents reabsorption of sodium as it passes along the tubule increases the excretion of potassium as well as sodium, and loss of both ions is the physiologic result of the diuretic agents. Increased diuresis of sodium is what is desired; increased diuresis of potassium is not desired and may produce hypokalemia—usually mild, with serum potassium infrequently below 3 meq/L.

C. Excessive Sodium Loss With Diuresis: However, with large doses of diuretic agents (especially the potent loop diuretics), when the amount of generalized edema due to salt and water retention is great, diuresis may be excessive, ie, the patient may lose such large quantities of salt and water in a matter of days that sodium depletion and hypovolemia replace sodium retention and hypervolemia. With hypovolemia, the reduction in left ventricular volume is such that the decreased stroke volume falls, further reducing the minute cardiac output. The patient may then become lethargic, restless, and sleepy, have postural hypotension and muscle cramps, and become severely ill. Hypovolemia can be suspected clinically if the jugular venous pulsations can no longer be seen even in the supine position, when postural hypotension occurs, and when the BUN rises out of proportion to the rise in serum creatinine. The physician must then liberalize the sodium intake and stop the diuretics until a balance has been restored. To prevent excessive hypovolemia, diuresis should be started with milder diuretics in small doses—eg, hydrochlorothiazide, 12.5–25 mg/d—and the dose increased only when it is certain that diuresis is not adequate with the smaller dose.

D. Counteracting Potassium Loss: In patients in whom significant hypokalemia results from the diuretic therapy, a high-potassium diet containing fresh fruits and vegetables, especially bananas, oranges, tomato juice, and other foods shown in Table 9–17, is helpful. The average fall in serum potassium in patients receiving 50 mg of hydrochlorothiazide twice daily was 0.62 meq/L. A daily potassium supplement of 60 meq 10% KCl elixir was required to restore the original level in most patients (Schwartz, 1974). If the serum potassium is still low, agents such as spironolactone—which is a competitive antagonist of aldosterone—or amiloride or triamterene—neither of

which is an aldosterone antagonist—can be used to decrease the amount of potassium exchanged for sodium at the distal sodium-potassium exchange site. Spironolactone by itself is a weak sodium diuretic, but when given in combination with other diuretics it decreases the loss of potassium and so prevents hypokalemia. If, however, the patient has impaired renal function with oliguria or is receiving potassium supplements, serum potassium may rise progressively and hyperkalemia, with resulting severe cardiac conduction defects, may follow. In the presence of normal urine output and normal renal function, spironolactone rarely produces hyperkalemia because of the built-in defense system whereby an increase in serum potassium increases the secretion of aldosterone. However, if spironolactone, amiloride, or triamterene is used, serum potassium must be monitored frequently and frequent ECGs obtained so that an early rise in serum potassium or the appearance of high peaked T waves will not be missed. When the serum potassium increases to 5 or 6 meq/L, the drugs should be stopped; levels over 8 meq/L are extremely dangerous and must be avoided because of the cardiac effects.

Renal stones and possibly interstitial renal changes have developed in patients receiving triamterene; further study is required to determine the effect of the drug on the kidney.

Clinical Use of Diuretics

The prototype class of oral diuretic agents is the thiazide group of drugs typified by chlorothiazide and hydrochlorothiazide (see Chapter 9 for additional details about drugs and dosages).

A. Indications for Oral Diuretics:

1. Treatment of mild edema– When edema is minimal or the evidence of left ventricular failure is slight, bed rest and sodium restriction may be adequate to effect diuresis.

2. Treatment of more severe failure– When cardiac failure is more severe, diuretic therapy is needed unless absolute bed rest and restriction of sodium intake to 300 mg/d are ordered. These restrictions on activity and diet are undesirable, and most patients with cardiac failure are not given strict low-sodium diets. Moderate restriction of sodium (no added salt in the diet) and small doses of a diuretic will usually reverse the salt and water retention that occurs with moderate cardiac failure. Because diuretics increase renin-angiotensin release, which if excessive is thought to be harmful in congestive heart failure, it is recommended that diuretics never be the sole drug used in treatment but that they be used with a converting enzyme inhibitor as an afterload-reducing agent.

B. Drugs and Dosages:

1. Thiazide diuretics– The initial dose of the thiazide diuretics is 12.5–25 mg of hydrochlorothiazide once daily, increased to 50 mg daily. The dose-response characteristics of the thiazides are such that the maximum response occurs at a dosage of 100 mg; therefore, no single dose larger than 100 mg should be given. When the thiazides are given orally, the onset of action is about 1 hour, the peak effect is reached in about 4 hours, and the duration of action varies, sometimes extending into the next 24-hour period. The patient should be weighed nude before breakfast each day. Diuretics can be given as necessary to maintain a steady dry weight. The drug should be given intermittently (every other day or twice a week if possible) to allow for restoration of losses of potassium and sodium; if the patient can be held at a steady dry weight without symptoms with a diuretic given twice a week, side effects are rare. Long-acting diuretics (chlorthalidone, metolazone) are discussed in Chapter 9.

2. Loop diuretics (furosemide, ethacrynic acid, bumetanide)– If cardiac failure is severe or renal failure is present and if diuresis does not occur with the use of moderately potent drugs such as the thiazides, the more potent loop diuretics can be used. These agents act on the ascending limb of the loop of Henle and will cause continued excretion of sodium when doses of furosemide up to 500 mg are given. Effectiveness depends on the size of the individual dose rather than the total daily dose. Furosemide and ethacrynic acid can be started at 40 mg/d and bumetanide at 0.5–1 mg/d. The dose can be gradually increased and then given twice daily if necessary, depending upon the severity of heart failure and the presence of renal failure. Oral loop diuretics have the same onset of action, peak effect, and duration of action as the oral thiazides (see above). When loop diuretics are given intravenously, as in the management of acute pulmonary edema, there may be significant diuresis within 15–30 minutes. Even before diuresis begins, there is a drop in pulmonary venous pressure, because intravenous furosemide also has preload-reducing properties. Because thiazides and loop diuretics act at different levels of the nephron, when either alone is ineffective the combination may restore effective diuresis.

3. Spironolactone, amiloride, and triamterene– These diuretics counteract the action of aldosterone at the distal tubule Na^+-K^+ exchange site (spironolactone by competitive antagonism). They rarely are used alone but are combined with thiazide or loop diuretics to diminish potassium loss. They should not be used in the presence of oliguria or renal failure because of the hazard of hyperkalemia (see Chapter 9). Acetazolamide, acidifying drugs, aminophylline, and osmotic diuretics are rarely useful in cardiac failure.

Toxicity of Diuretics

In addition to sodium depletion and hypokalemia (discussed above), chronic hypovolemia produced by the diuretics as well as by direct action of the diuretics on the renal tubule may result in 20–30% increases of serum creatinine and uric acid and occasionally of plasma or serum glucose. Patients with a history of gout may develop acute gouty arthritis, and the dosage of thiazides must be reduced or the patient must be given uricosuric drugs such as probenecid or allopurinol. Diabetes mellitus is rarely induced in individuals with no history of the disease, but in patients with diabetes, hyperglycemia induced by diuretics may require increasing doses of insulin. The slight increases in serum creatinine, uric acid, and serum glucose and the associated hypokalemia usually cause no symptoms and are reversible when the agents are discontinued. The long-term hazards of these biochemical changes are not known, especially in patients with underlying impairment of renal function; however, there have been no reports of their deleterious effects on the kidney or other organs, even after almost 20 years of use.

Metabolic Alkalosis

Additional electrolyte and water disturbances that may occur in patients with cardiac failure treated with diuretic agents include hypokalemic and hypochloremic alkalosis. An increase in serum bicarbonate compensates for the loss of chloride and hydrogen ions, because both hydrogen and potassium are exchanged in the distal tubule for sodium. Chloride and potassium replacement can be accomplished with potassium chloride.

Dilutional Hyponatremia

Dilutional hyponatremia may occur in treated cardiac failure, especially when water intake is increased. In contrast to patients who develop depletional hyponatremia due to sodium depletion resulting from excessive diuresis, patients with dilutional hyponatremia (including those with equivalent degrees of hyponatremia, sometimes to as low as 110 meq/L) continue to have an increased total body burden of sodium and generalized edema despite low serum sodium. The use of hypertonic saline, which is valuable in depletional hyponatremia, may worsen cardiac failure in dilutional hyponatremia because the total body sodium is already increased. The patient may be ill, thirsty, and weak, and treatment consists of decreasing the water intake to about 500–700 mL/d and giving furosemide if necessary. As excess body water is lost through the skin and lungs, the balance between sodium and water is restored and the serum sodium gradually rises.

In depletional hyponatremia, the specific gravity of the urine is usually high; in dilutional hyponatremia, urine specific gravity is low because of decreased solute excretion.

Caution With Diuretic Therapy

Diuretic therapy should be used with caution in patients who are receiving digitalis, because hypokalemia increases the hazard of digitalis toxicity. Diuretics should be used intermittently whenever possible and in the smallest effective dose, and digitalis should be given cautiously, with frequent observations including determinations of serum digitalis levels. Not only may hypokalemia and digitalis interact to increase digitalis toxicity, but the sicker cardiac patients may have decreased appetite and take less potassium in their diet, aggravating the situation. In these circumstances, small doses of spironolactone can be added if oliguria or renal failure is not present; patients should be observed for the hyperkalemia that may then result. Hirsutism and enlarged breasts, which can be very painful, may also occur. In the presence of renal failure, the loop diuretics are effective, whereas the thiazides are not; spironolactone should be avoided in renal failure, especially if there is oliguria. The loop diuretics are not recommended for the treatment of moderate cardiac failure if adequate diuresis can be achieved with the milder diuretics such as the thiazides.

IDENTIFY & TREAT UNSUSPECTED ACUTE MYOCARDIAL DISORDERS

The cause of cardiac failure is often unsuspected unless one specifically seeks it out by using appropriate investigative techniques. The principle often-unsuspected disorders are listed in Chapter 17. Acute dyspnea may mask the chest discomfort of acute myocardial infarction or be present without chest discomfort. The fever of infective endocarditis may be low-grade and intermittent. Murmurs may be minimal, and preexisting cardiac disease may be unsuspected, especially in drug addicts. Acute nephritis with salt and water retention may be entirely unsuspected unless one examines the urine, takes the blood pressure, and thinks of the possibility. Acute pericardial effusion must be distinguished from cardiac dilation not only because unrecognized tamponade may be life-threatening but also because the cause of the effusion must be determined and specific therapy given as needed. To help in identifying the underlying cause of the congestive heart failure and because congestive heart failure may be partly or even predominantly due to diastolic ventricular dysfunction, an echocardiogram should always be obtained in patients with heart failure. (For further details see Chapters 9, 15, 16, 17, and 20.)

TREAT OPERABLE CONDITIONS THAT INCREASE THE LOAD ON THE HEART OR INTERFERE WITH LEFT VENTRICULAR FUNCTION.

This should be done after maximal improvement has been achieved on medical treatment. Obviously, emergency situations must always be dealt with first, but the ideal management of cardiac failure is to identify and remove the cause of ventricular dysfunction if that is possible. Medical treatment of cardiac failure per se is a temporizing measure that does not reach the underlying cause. Operative procedures may also be palliative but in many instances can be semicurative and result in dramatic improvement.

Conditions potentially treatable by means of operation should be evaluated while the patient is responding to bed rest and medical treatment. (See other chapters for surgical treatment of individual diseases.)

TREAT EXTRACARDIAC FACTORS

Extracardiac factors that increase the work of the heart include fever; anemia; acid-base, electrolyte, and endocrine abnormalities; hypoxia; and obesity, among many others. These factors increase the heart rate and myocardial oxygen demand; may decrease coronary blood flow and produce myocardial ischemia; may lead to the development of cardiac arrhythmias, with resulting impairment of coronary perfusion and production of myocardial ischemia; and may aggravate or induce toxicity from therapeutic agents such as digitalis when hypokalemia is present. Cardiac failure induced by such extracardiac factors should be treated in accordance with the principles outlined in this chapter. At the same time, the underlying extracardiac factors should also be treated with appropriate measures.

DIGITALIZE ADEQUATELY

In addition to rest, diuretics, management of arrhythmias, and the other approaches discussed above, treatment with digitalis should be started.

Digitalis has been one of the major medical resources in the treatment of cardiac failure. There are a wide variety of digitalis-like preparations, but digitalis is the generic term for any compound containing a steroid glycoside ring, a lactone ring, and a sugar residue. In recent years, the longer duration of action of digitoxin has caused it to be used less frequently than digoxin, a purified glycoside with shorter duration of action. Digoxin is overwhelmingly the digitalis preparation most frequently used in the USA and other parts of the world, in some places under different names. Table 10–3 lists the dosages and methods of administration of parenteral glycoside preparations that are available for clinical use.

Although newer inotropic agents and vasodilators are being used with greater frequency in patients with cardiac failure (see below), digitalis compounds have the advantages of many years of experience and established effectiveness, both in the presence of sinus rhythm and in atrial fibrillation. Digitalis is most ef-

Table 10–3. Parenteral cardiac glycoside preparations: Average adult doses and methods of administration.[1]

Glycoside and Preparations Available	Dose		Rapid Method of Administration	Speed; Maximum Action and Duration
	Digitalizing	Maintenance		
Deslanoside, 2-mL ampules, 0.4 mg	8 mL (1.6 mg)	0.2–0.4 mg (1–2 mL)	1.2 mg (6 mL) IV or IM and follow with 0.2–0.4 mg (1–2 mL) IV or IM every 3–4 hours until effect is obtained.	1–2 hours; duration, 3–6 days.
Digoxin, 2-mL ampules, 0.25 mg/mL	1.5 mg (6 mL)	0.125–0.75 mg (1–3 mL)	0.5–1 mg (2–4 mL) IV and 0.25–0.5 mg (1–2 mL) in 3–4 hours; then 0.25 mg (1 mL) every 3–4 hours until effect is obtained.	1–2 hours; duration, 3–6 days.

[1]Check manufacturers' descriptive literature. Dosage sizes of tablets and ampules change from time to time.

fective in patients with chronic cardiac failure and is less effective in patients with acute cardiac failure, acute myocardial infarction, severe primary cardiomyopathy, acute rheumatic carditis, and chronic lung disease. The value of digitalis in chronic cardiac failure with sinus rhythm has been controversial, and some authors have not found it efficacious; others have (DiBianco, 1989). Furthermore, withdrawal and readministration of digitalis have often demonstrated improved hemodynamics (Arnold, 1980). Lee (1982) found digoxin effective in about half the patients with severe chronic cardiac failure and sinus rhythm. In a double-blinded placebo and digoxin cross-over study, digoxin was found to decrease symptoms and increase exercise capacity and ejection fraction compared with placebo (Guyatt, 1988). Furthermore, digoxin has been found to have an independent beneficial hemodynamic effect when given with captopril in congestive heart failure (Gheorghiade, 1989). It is rarely effective in acute failure such as occurs in acute myocardial infarction. Digoxin is more effective in patients with atrial fibrillation than in those with sinus rhythm, because it decreases atrioventricular conduction and slows the ventricular rate in addition to its direct inotropic action.

Indications for Administration
(See also Chapter 15.)

(1) Atrial fibrillation or flutter with a rapid ventricular rate.

(2) Cardiac failure with sinus rhythm or atrial fibrillation.

(3) Supraventricular paroxysmal tachycardia.

(4) Prevention of paroxysmal atrial or junctional arrhythmias in patients in whom quinidine has failed or is not tolerated.

(5) Maintenance therapy to prevent recurrence of cardiac failure in patients who have received digitalis initially for cardiac failure.

Mechanism of Action

The use of beta-adrenergic blocking agents does not interfere with the inotropic action of digitalis, and

this apparently rules out the sympathetic nervous system as the mediator of its inotropic effect. Digitalis is bound to sites on the membrane of heart muscle cells, where it may affect the net uptake of potassium, sodium, and calcium. Digitalis inhibits Na^+-K^+ ATPase at the cellular membrane, resulting in an increase in intracellular Na^+, which through the Na^+-Ca^{2+} exchanger increases the intracellular Ca^{2+}. Increased availability of calcium ions, enhancing cardiac contraction, is thought to be the basic mechanism by which digitalis acts to increase the force and velocity of contraction.

Digitalis has a potent electrophysiologic action that results in increased automaticity of the secondary pacemakers in the atrioventricular nodal junction, in the atrioventricular nodal-His bundle junction, and of secondary pacemakers throughout the Purkinje system responsible for the ectopic rhythms that are a sign of digitalis toxicity. Digitalis has complicated effects on the atrium because it has direct effects on the atrial muscle and indirect effects on the autonomic nervous system. Digitalis slows the impulse conduction velocity in the specialized conduction tissues and increases the velocity in the working cardiac muscle. This slowed conduction in the atrioventricular node is beneficial in atrial fibrillation because it decreases the number of impulses per minute reaching the ventricles. However, atrial fibrillation occurring in patients with Wolff-Parkinson-White syndrome can have marked increases in the ventricular rate if given digitalis, because of the increased conduction velocity in the working cardiac muscle that comprises the bypass tract. Ventricular tachycardia or fibrillation may then occur (see Chapter 14).

Pathophysiologic & Hemodynamic Effects

The effects of digitalis described above on the isolated cardiac muscle fiber in vitro must be distinguished from the clinical effects in the patient with cardiac failure or myocardial ischemia. Hemodynamic studies in patients who are in manifest heart failure have shown that digitalis increases cardiac output, decreases right atrial and peripheral venous pressure, decreases the filling pressure of the left ventricle, and increases the urinary excretion of sodium and water, thereby correcting some of the hemodynamic and metabolic abnormalities in cardiac failure. There is evidence that digitalis produces marked sympathoinhibitory actions in humans with heart failure, perhaps resulting from afferent activation of low- or high-pressure baroreceptor mechanisms (Ferguson, 1989). These clinical effects are not uniform, however, and digitalis is less effective in the presence of acute myocarditis, myocardial ischemia, high output cardiac failure, pulmonary or systemic venous congestion resulting from mechanical defects, and some cases of diffuse extensive primary cardiomyopathy or ischemic cardiomyopathy. It is possible that the stage of hemodynamic alteration in cardiac failure affects the response to digitalis and that this may explain the minimal hemodynamic benefit seen in some patients. Digitalis is more effective in the presence of atrial fibrillation with a rapid ventricular rate, because its ability to block conduction through the atrioventricular node decreases the ventricular rate and improves coronary perfusion. Better ventricular filling during diastole decreases left atrial pressure and pulmonary venous congestion. The effect of slowing the ventricular rate is particularly advantageous in the presence of obstructive lesions such as mitral stenosis.

Pharmacokinetics

A. Effect of Drug: As is true of all drugs, the various digitalis preparations may have different clinical effects depending upon the rate of absorption, the amount of body fluid in which the drug is distributed,

its bioavailability, the renal function, the rate of metabolic degradation, thyroid function, and the mode of excretion—all of which may differ in different patients, so that no one dosage schedule is suitable for all patients. The bioavailability of digitalis—the amount absorbed and available to the body—was recognized as a cause of unpredictable blood levels and clinical effectiveness. The result has been that the FDA now includes dissolution rates as a part of the criteria for acceptance of all digoxin and other preparations.

B. Physiologic Factors: A number of studies have been published on the kinetics of digoxin and other digitalis preparations (Smith, 1984). Absorption rates vary with the speed of dissolution of the tablets and are enhanced by sluggish gastrointestinal motility and hypothyroidism and decreased by the concomitant use of nonabsorbable drugs or antacids; rates are increased by hyperthyroidism and the use of elixir as compared to tablet digoxin preparations. In patients with normal renal function, the mean half-life of digoxin (the time required for the digoxin in the body to decrease by 50%) is about 36 hours, but the range is wide and the standard deviation is about 8 hours. In contrast, the half-life of digitoxin is 4–6 days. The renal excretion of digoxin depends on the glomerular filtration rate; the dose of drug must be decreased in patients with impaired renal function and reduced glomerular filtration rate to prevent accumulation with high serum levels and toxicity. Figure 10–8 relates the blood urea nitrogen level to the clearance of digoxin, reflecting the delayed clearance in the presence of poor renal function.

Radioisotope studies have shown that when digoxin is given to patients who have not received dig-

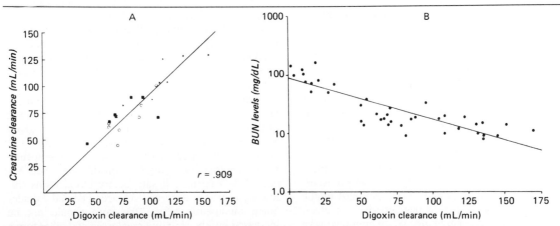

Figure 10–8. *A:* Relationship of creatinine clearance to digoxin clearance in donors before (x) and after (o) unilateral nephrectomy and in recipients (s) of these kidneys. The correlation coefficient, R = .909, is highly significant. (Reproduced, with permission, from Doherty JE, Flanigan WJ, Dalrymple GV: Tritiated digoxin. 17. Excretion and turnover times in normal donors before and after nephrectomy and in the paired recipient of the kidney after transplantation. Am J Cardiol 1972;29:470.) ***B:*** Relationship of blood urea nitrogen (BUN) to the clearance of digoxin. The higher the BUN Level, the lower the digoxin clearance. (Reproduced, with permission, from Doherty JE: Digitalis glycosides: Pharmacokinetics and their clinical implications. Ann Intern Med 1973;79:229.)

italis in the past few days, a daily dose leads to a steady-state serum digoxin level in 6–9 days. If renal function is normal, a loading or saturation dose is considered unnecessary unless rapid digitalization is desired. A daily dose of digoxin given for four to five half-lives of digoxin results in a steady-state plateau of serum digoxin even if the dose is continued indefinitely. The drug is bound tightly to the tissues and so is not removed by dialysis or by open heart bypass procedures.

Serum Digoxin Levels

Radioimmunoassay techniques have permitted accurate and reliable measurement of serum digoxin and digitoxin levels, which can be correlated with the dose of the drug and the clinical effects (Smith, 1984). Serum digitoxin levels are 5–15 times greater than serum digoxin levels. Mixtures of different digitalis glycosides cannot be evaluated by radioimmunoassay.

Age, renal function, thyroid status, and interference with absorption by noncardiac drugs have all been shown to influence the serum digoxin level. About three-fourths of an oral dose of digoxin is absorbed from the gastrointestinal tract, and patients who have reached a steady state with daily maintenance doses of the drug achieve a new peak within 3 hours of administration of the next oral dose of digoxin, with the level beginning to rise within an hour. Because about one-third of the body stores of digoxin is excreted daily (assuming that renal function is normal) and because the half-life of digoxin is about 112 days, the effects of digoxin will be dissipated in 4–5 days (four to five half-lives) after the drug is stopped.

In general, levels under 2 ng/mL are not likely to be associated with digitalis toxicity, whereas levels greater than 3 ng/mL are quite likely to be associated with toxic effects. Judgment is required in attempting to use the serum level as an isolated indication of toxicity (Smith, 1984). Verapamil also raises serum digoxin levels. The factor most often neglected in patients receiving digitalis who develop digitalis toxicity is renal function. In patients with renal failure the half-life of digoxin is prolonged, resulting in toxic serum levels unless smaller doses of the drug are given (Figure 10–8). Thyroid abnormalities, electrolyte and acid-base balance, the severity and nature of the underlying heart disease, the patient's age and renal function, and the patient's compliance with therapy are other important factors. Serum levels must be interpreted in the light of all of the factors that might influence toxicity, including interactions with other drugs the patient may be taking. When quinidine was given to patients receiving digoxin, the serum digoxin levels approximately doubled. The mean volume of distribution and the rate of renal clearance of digoxin are reduced during quinidine administration (Smith, 1984). Serum digoxin levels must be interpreted with caution in the presence of abnormalities of serum potassium. Elevated serum levels and manifestations of digitalis toxicity are apt to occur when ordinary doses of digoxin are given to patients with low serum potassium.

Serum levels are particularly helpful in patients who are unable to give a clear clinical history, especially of preceding digitalis administration, and in patients who fail to respond to the drug or seem to become toxic with only average doses of digoxin. Serum levels should be obtained roughly 6–8 hours after the last dose (Smith, 1984).

When serum levels are unusually low following average doses of digoxin (< 0.5 ng/mL), the possibility of patient noncompliance must be considered or the possibility that the medication is not being taken as specifically instructed.

Administration of Digoxin

A. Average Situation: In the average patient with mild to moderate cardiac failure in whom digitalization is not urgent, digoxin can be given orally in an average maintenance dose of 0.25 mg/d. If the patient is old or has impaired renal function, hypothyroidism, or hypokalemia, the dose should be halved, eg, 0.125 mg/d. No saturation or loading dose is required. If after 7–10 days a therapeutic effect has not been obtained (relief of cardiac failure, slowing of the ventricular rate, diuresis and weight loss), serum digoxin levels should be measured to be certain that the patient is absorbing or taking the drug and that an adequate serum level has been achieved. If the serum level is low (< 0.8–1.2 ng/mL) and clinical improvement has not occurred, the daily dose can be increased to 0.375 mg/d for 7–10 days and the serum digoxin level again determined. If the level is still low, the maintenance dose can be increased to 0.5 mg/d. Some patients require 0.75 mg/d to produce clinical benefit without toxicity. In general, when digitalis is given, all other factors that might have a bearing on digitalis toxicity (hypokalemia, ischemia, hypoxia) should be stabilized so that a maintenance dose can be established that will be safe over a prolonged period.

If the clinical situation is more urgent, with increasing dyspnea and orthopnea, give 0.25 or 0.5 mg of digoxin every 6 hours until 1.5 mg has been given and then maintain the level with 0.25 mg every 8–12 hours until the appearance of evidence of therapeutic benefit or toxicity or until serum digoxin levels exceed 2.5–3 ng/mL. If satisfactory blood levels following a proper dose are not accompanied by adequate therapeutic effect, the dose should not be increased but the situation reassessed and other forms of treatment used (see below). As already noted, the clinical response to digitalis is not uniformly good, especially in severe cardiac failure or when failure is due to extracardiac, mechanical, or inflammatory causes. About 20% of patients given digoxin in general hospitals develop signs of toxicity, perhaps because they continue to receive progressive increments of digoxin after failing to respond to usually adequate doses.

B. Emergency Situation: When it is necessary to obtain a digitalis effect within hours, as in pulmonary edema; or when symptomatic atrial fibrillation occurs postoperatively; or in the presence of mitral stenosis; or when the rapid ventricular rate produces dyspnea, angina, or cerebral impairment, intravenous therapy can be given, eg, digoxin, one-third to one-half of the total (1–1.5 mg) digitalizing dose every 2–4 hours, decreasing the dose by half when the ventricular rate begins to slow. At that time, oral digoxin therapy should then be instituted to avoid toxicity, which is more likely to occur when frequent doses of digoxin are administered intravenously.

Criteria of Adequate Digitalization

Digitalis is administered until a therapeutic effect is achieved (eg, relief of cardiac failure or slowing of the ventricular rate in atrial fibrillation), or until anorexia or arrhythmia appears (the earliest toxic effect). In atrial fibrillation, slowing of the ventricular rate to less than 80/min after mild exercise such as five or six sit-ups is usually sufficient evidence that digitalis is blocking atrial impulses in the atrioventricular node.

The most characteristic changes on the ECG following administration of digitalis are depressed sagging ST segments in a direction opposite to that of the major QRS deflection in the lead involved (Figure 10–9). Later, especially if the serum levels are higher, the PR interval may be prolonged as partial atrioventricular block develops and the QT interval shortens as the duration of the action potential decreases. ST–T changes cannot be used as criteria of digitalis toxicity but merely of digitalis effect because they do not correlate positively with toxic symptoms or other manifestations such as arrhythmia; furthermore, they may persist after the serum levels fall to zero. Typical ST–T changes are helpful, however, in alerting the physician to the possibility that the patient has been receiving digitalis without knowing it.

Digitalis Toxicity

A detailed discussion of digitalis toxicity and an extensive bibliography can be found in Smith (1984).

A. Symptoms: In patients with cardiac failure who are otherwise in a relatively stable state, the first manifestation of digitalis toxicity is usually anorexia or mild nausea. Vomiting occurs later. To detect this change one must obtain a clear history of appetite before beginning digitalis therapy. If the patient is seen before each dose and the drug stopped when anorexia or mild nausea develops, more important manifestations of toxicity can be avoided, and the gastrointestinal symptoms will subside in 24 hours. Other symptoms are neurologic (eg, confusion) and ocular (the perception of yellow color around lights, scotomas).

B. Electrocardiographic Changes: The most common important myocardial manifestation of digitalis toxicity is cardiac arrhythmia that results from enhanced automaticity and decreased conduction in the specialized automatic cells in the atria and ventricles and in the atrioventricular node. The combination leads to reentry as well as ectopic rhythms (Table 10–4). Ventricular premature beats are the most common arrhythmia occurring as a result of digitalis overdosage, but they do not usually progress to ventricular tachycardia or fibrillation unless early warnings are ignored, large doses are used, or high serum levels result from impaired renal function or other factors previously discussed.

Paroxysmal atrial tachycardia with block is probably the next most common arrhythmia; the pacemaker focus of the atrial arrhythmia is often the junctional tissue at the atrial-atrioventricular nodal junction. This arrhythmia is rarely seen in the absence of associated diuretic therapy with hypokalemia—in contrast to the ventricular arrhythmias and atrioventricular block that occur even when diuretics are not used (Figure 15–3).

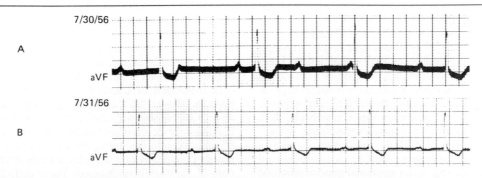

Figure 10–9. A: Complete atrioventricular block due to digitalis toxicity in a 60–year-old man given potassium chloride, 10 g orally daily. **B:** Partial atrioventricular block with PR interval of 0.4 s in 24 hours. Note the sagging ST segment and short QT interval due to digitalis.

Table 10–4. Frequency of various digitalis-induced arrhythmias in 10 series with a total of 631 patients.[1]

	Number of Series	Number of Arrhythmias		
Ventricular arrhythmias		470 (71%)		
Ventricular premature beats			420	
Bigeminy	9			150
Multifocal	4			121
Not specified	4			79
Other (frequent, unifocal, occasional, etc)	3			70
Ventricular tachycardia	7		50	
Atrioventricular block		194 (29%)		
First-degree	7		87	
Second-degree	10		58	
Wenckebach	3			4
Third-degree	6		37	
Unspecified	2		12	
Atrial arrhythmias		177 (26%)		
Atrial fibrillation	9		80	
With slow rate	2			21
Paroxysmal atrial tachycardia with block	7		59	
Atrial premature beats	4		27	
Atrial flutter	4		11	
Sinoatrial arrhythmias		85 (13%)		
Sinus tachycardia	3		29	
Sinus bradycardia	4		27	
With nodal escape	1			11
Sinus arrest	2		11	
Sinoatrial block	3		7	
Wandering pacemaker	3		11	
Atrioventricular dissociation	4	65 (9.8%)		
Atrioventricular nodal arrhythmias		47 (7%)		
Nodal tachycardia			32	
Nodal rhythm	2		11	
Nodal premature beats	1		4	

[1] Reproduced, with permission, from Fisch C: Treatment of arrhythmias due to digitalis. J Indiana State Med Assoc 1967;60:146.

Atrioventricular block is the third most common disturbance in rhythm in digitalis toxicity, and this is directly related to decreased conduction in the atrioventricular node, which is a cardinal electrophysiologic effect of digitalis. The atrioventricular block is usually slight, consisting only of prolongation of the PR interval, but in more severe toxicity, complete atrioventricular block may occur (Figure 10–9).

Digitalis also slows conduction in the sinoatrial node, and sinoatrial block with a shift in the pacemaker to the atrioventricular junction or to the lower atrium may result; digitalis excess must always be considered when sinoatrial abnormalities are present. Atrioventricular dissociation (see Chapter 14), with the atria and ventricles beating independently, is commonly the result of digitalis excess and is due to a combination of atrioventricular block and enhanced pacemaker activity in the junctional regions proximal or distal to the atrioventricular node. The atrioventricular dissociation may be intermittent, owing to a combination of only a partial defect in conduction and the fortuitous occurrence of P waves when the ventricles are not refractory. Atrioventricular dissociation may be due to acceleration of a subsidiary pacemaker in the junctional region even when the dominant sinus pacemaker is not unduly depressed or atrioventricular block present. So-called nonparoxysmal atrioventricular junctional tachycardia due to enhanced acceleration of the junctional pacemaker can occur with or without complete atrioventricular dissociation by chance capture of the ventricles, since atrioventricular block is not present.

C. Influence of Cardiac Disease on Arrhythmias or Symptoms of Toxicity: The extent and type of the underlying cardiac disease influence the likelihood of development of toxicity from digitalis. Changing conditions during the course of the cardiac illness may precipitate digitalis toxicity even if the dose of the drug is unchanged. These include hypokalemia resulting from diuretic therapy, hypoxia, and decreases in renal function that may follow hypovolemia or decreased cardiac output. Toxicity may therefore occur not because the drug is given incorrectly or in excessive doses but because there are other factors that must be recognized and managed.

D. Cardiac Disease Producing Arrhythmias: Cardiac arrhythmias in patients with cardiac failure do not always imply digitalis toxicity but may occur even when digitalis is not given. This is particularly true in heart failure associated with coronary heart disease, when ventricular arrhythmias may be the composite result of (1) localized ischemia; (2) variable and disproportionate duration of action potentials in adjacent fibers, with disparate refractory periods; and (3) variable conduction because of patchy myocardial fibrosis, leading to reentry or ectopic arrhythmias. The presence of arrhythmia, therefore, must not be assumed to be due to digitalis toxicity, especially at the onset of digitalis administration or if the patient is on a stable maintenance dose of digitalis when first seen.

Cardiac arrhythmias often disappear when cardiac failure is appropriately treated. Clinical judgment based on experience and careful analysis of all of the clinical findings, including serum digoxin levels, may warrant the conclusion that cardiac failure and not digitalis excess is the cause of the arrhythmia. If the reverse is the case and digitalis toxicity is strongly suspected and confirmed by serum digoxin levels, digitalis and diuretics must be stopped and the patient observed closely. If renal function is adequate and the serum potassium level is normal, digitalis-induced arrhythmias usually subside within 2–3 days.

Treatment of Digitalis Toxicity

A. Initial Measures: The obvious initial step is to stop digitalis and diuretics and identify and treat conditions that increase the likelihood of digitalis toxicity: hypokalemia, hypoxia, myocardial ischemia, hypovolemia, and impaired renal function. It is usually sufficient to stop the digitalis and diuretics and observe the patient closely if there are no life-threatening arrhythmias with rapid ventricular rates, such as ventricular tachycardia or multifocal ventricular premature beats occurring early in diastole, or if these arrhythmias do not induce myocardial ischemia or hypotension or make the cardiac failure worse. If rapid ventricular arrhythmias induce severe hemodynamic abnormalities or threaten ventricular fibrillation, intravenous potassium should be infused under close supervision (not given by bolus injection) at a rate of 10–20 meq/h unless the patient has hyperkalemia, severely impaired renal function, or atrioventricular block. A common method is to give 50–100 meq/L of potassium chloride in 5% dextrose or saline at a slow rate of 0.25–0.35 meq/min. If the situation is less urgent, potassium can be given orally in a dosage not to exceed 80 meq in 4–6 hours, unless the patient has the contraindications noted above for intravenous use.

B. Alternative Measures: With ventricular tachycardia, if potassium is ineffective or cannot be used, the most effective drug is phenytoin or propranolol (or its equivalent), with quinidine or lidocaine in reserve. The dosages are phenytoin, 3–5 mg/kg intravenously; or propranolol, 0.5–2 mg intravenously at a rate of 0.5 mg/min, repeated in 1–2 hours; or quinidine gluconate, 0.8 g in 500 mL dextrose, 1 mL/min; or lidocaine, 1 mg/kg intravenously every 1–5 minutes followed by an infusion of 0.5–2 mg/min.

C. Monitoring of ECG With Potassium: When potassium is given by infusion, the ECG should be monitored continuously and serum potassium levels determined. Oral therapy should be given when the infusion is stopped. The need for potassium is less urgent in the presence of atrioventricular block, and in such circumstances the drug should be used intravenously with considerable caution.

D. Temporary Pacemaker: If complete atrioventricular block is present with a slow ventricular rate—and especially if it is associated with an accelerated junctional tachycardia—a temporary endocardial pacemaker should be introduced prior to the use of drugs that depress escape pacemakers to avoid ventricular standstill and a Stokes Adams attack.

E. Electrical Cardioversion: Great caution must be exercised in the use of electrical cardioversion in the presence of ectopic rhythms that may be due to digitalis toxicity, whether atrial or ventricular. Digitalis enhances the susceptibility of the myocardium to electric shock, and ventricular fibrillation may result. If the arrhythmia is life-threatening, atrial pacing with overdrive suppression of the ectopic foci is probably the treatment of choice if intravenous drug therapy as outlined above is ineffective.

F. Digoxin Immune Fab (DIFAB): Digoxin Immune fab antigen binding fragments (DIFAB) are extremely effective in the treatment of potentially life-threatening digoxin or digitoxin intoxication. The dosage is variable depending on the body burden of the digitalis. It is administered intravenously through a membrane filter over 30 minutes. Each vial contains 40 mg of DIFAB that will bind 0.6 mg of digoxin. In urgent situations, one can give 20 vials (800 mg) intravenously, but tables are available and should be consulted for calculating the dose (consult the Physicians' Desk Reference). In general, DIFAB should be given if digoxin blood level exceeds 10 ng/mL or if healthy adults have taken 10 mg digoxin or if children have taken 4 mg (Smith, 1984).

A multicenter study of the treatment of 150 cases of life-threatening digitalis intoxication with digoxin-specific Fab antibody fragments was reported (Antman, 1990). Eighty percent had resolution of all signs and symptoms of digitalis toxicity, 10% improved, and 10% showed no response. The median time to response after termination of the Fab infusion was 19 minutes, and 75% had some evidence of response by 1 hour. Fourteen patients (9%) had adverse events, mostly hypokalemia or exacerbation of heart failure. A recent report of over 700 patients treated with Fab reported only a 50% complete response to treatment, with a 24% partial response. Recrudescent toxicity occurred in 2.8% and was mainly due to giving too small a dose of antibody (Hickey, 1991).

Prevention of Toxicity

Prevention of toxicity is obviously superior to treatment of toxicity. Digitalis toxicity is least in the following circumstances: (1) when the drug is used in patients in whom hypokalemia, hypoxia, and other factors influencing the half-life of the drug and hence its serum level are known and treated before the drug is used; (2) when digoxin is used in the smallest maintenance dose likely to be effective in the light of the total clinical picture; (3) when the patient during digitalization is seen daily prior to the next dose and early manifestations of toxicity are carefully sought; (4) when rapid digitalization and rapid diuretic therapy are avoided unless the clinical situation is urgent; and (5) when oral rather than parenteral preparations are used unless the indications for parenteral therapy are clear.

TREAT SYSTEMIC DISEASES AFFECTING THE HEART (See Chapter 17.)

Myxedema

Myxedema may result in a large "quiet" heart (poor pulsations), with myocardial dilation and edema between the fibers, or pericardial effusion or a mixture of both. Myxedema is a slowly progressive disease with subtle signs that may be missed (see Chapter 17).

Hyperthyroidism

Hyperthyroidism may not be obvious, especially in the apathetic form in older people. Cardiac failure is uncommon in younger people with thyrotoxicosis; more commonly, the increased secretion of thyroxine unmasks preexisting cardiac disease, usually coronary heart disease, and is more common in patients over 40 years of age. As a result, the response to treatment with radioiodine or thyroidectomy is not as dramatic as the treatment of myxedema heart with thyroxine; nevertheless, substantial benefits accrue from treatment of the hyperthyroidism (see Chapter 17).

Connective Tissue Disorders

Lupus erythematosus and other disorders in this group should be specifically sought because the acute vasculitis and hypertension often respond to corticosteroid therapy.

Pericardial Effusion

This must be considered because tamponade may occur, although it is not common.

Thiamine Deficiency

Beriberi heart disease is uncommon except in chronic alcoholics who eat poorly and in inhabitants of areas where famine is severe. In patients with borderline thiamine nutritional status, cardiac failure may develop when food intake is abruptly reduced or if an increased requirement for thiamine develops, such as in a febrile illness.

When chronic thiamine deficiency has resulted in chronic cardiac failure, cardiac output is reduced rather than increased, and there is no evidence of increased flow to the extremities; the clinical picture resembles that of the low output state which occurs in congestive cardiomyopathy due to alcohol.

Anemia

Severe anemia, whether from blood loss, blood dyscrasias, or acute leukemia, may result in cardiac dilation, with evidence of generalized cardiac failure such as systemic and pulmonary venous congestion, functional regurgitation of the mitral and tricuspid valves, and rarely, if the anemia is quite severe, dilation of the aortic ring associated with an aortic diastolic murmur. Less severe anemia can produce or aggravate cardiac failure if the patient has underlying heart disease of any kind—coronary, hypertensive, or rheumatic; the decreased oxygen-carrying capacity of the hemoglobin and the increased cardiac output demanded by the anemia may precipitate cardiac failure. When anemia develops slowly, as in untreated pernicious anemia, it may be quite severe before dyspnea or other evidence of cardiac failure develops.

When blood even in the form of packed red cells is given for severe anemia, especially in the presence of cardiac failure, the patient should be closely monitored by inspection of the venous pulse, by examination of the lung bases for rales, and by auscultation for the development of gallop rhythm. The patient should be recumbent during the infusion of blood so that if fluid overload results in pulmonary edema with acute dyspnea, the patient can sit up, abruptly decreasing the pulmonary blood volume. Blood should be given slowly.

Inadvertent Rapid Administration of Sodium

The principles outlined above pertaining to administration of blood apply as well to infusions containing sodium. Acute pulmonary venous congestion and left ventricular failure may develop postoperatively in patients without intrinsic cardiac disease if intravenous saline or blood is given too rapidly, as may happen in patients with borderline compensation or chronic cardiac disease in whom intravenous saline is given for any reason. Saline solution should be given slowly and with the same precautions as when blood is given, and the physician should consider whether dextrose and water or 0.5 N saline would serve as well.

Diseases Being Treated
With Adrenal Corticosteroids

Corticosteroid therapy, especially with sodium-retaining steroids such as 9α-fluorinated compounds for postural hypotension due to autonomic insufficiency, may lead to salt retention and hypertension, increasing both the load on the heart and the extracellular volume, which may in turn lead to cardiac failure. Parenteral corticosteroids sometimes given for arthritis may unobtrusively cause iatrogenic Cushing's syndrome, with hypertension, salt and water retention, and left ventricular failure, especially in patients with underlying heart disease.

Polycythemia Vera

This is an uncommon cause of cardiac failure. The increased circulating red cell mass increases blood viscosity and impairs coronary perfusion. The diagnosis is suggested by the high red blood cell count and confirmed by the finding of a high total red cell mass with normal oxygen saturation, thus excluding chronic lung disease and secondary polycythemia.

Pulmonary Embolism

Pulmonary emboli often precipitate congestive heart failure in patients with heart disease, and the abrupt development of cardiac failure in a patient with known heart disease should prompt a search for unsuspected pulmonary emboli. Recurrent pulmonary emboli—even very small ones—may over a period of months or years cause diffuse obstructive pulmonary arterial disease and severe pulmonary hypertension. The episodes may not have been recognized, and the presenting picture is of primary pulmonary hypertension with right ventricular hypertrophy and right ventricular failure. If recurrent pulmonary emboli are recognized, anticoagulant therapy or appropriate venous ligation may prevent recurrent episodes and pulmonary hypertension.

WITHDRAW OFFENDING DRUGS
AFFECTING THE HEART

Obtain a history of the use of medications that may cause cardiac damage or depression (see Chapter 17). Excessive sedation may not be obvious in patients taking several drugs, and some may not even know what drugs they are receiving.

Beta-Adrenergic Blocking Drugs

These compounds are probably the most frequent offenders because they are given for a wide variety of disorders, such as arrhythmias, angina, hypertension, and hypertrophic cardiomyopathy; when given to patients with incipient left ventricular failure, they may produce florid ventricular failure in hours or days. Inappropriate use of beta-adrenergic blocking drugs must be considered in every patient with cardiac failure, particularly when the onset is abrupt.

Quinidine

Quinidine has a negative inotropic action, but cardiac failure is likely to be induced only in patients with chronic cardiac disease and atrial fibrillation who are not given digitalis before quinidine. In this circumstance, the ventricular rate may rise to 150/min or more, resulting in cardiac failure as decreased diastolic filling impairs coronary perfusion. Cardiac failure was the most common manifestation of quinidine "toxicity" in the early days of its use, when digitalis was not given first, but it is now rare.

Calcium Entry-Blocking Drugs

Verapamil is the calcium blocker with the greatest negative inotropic action, diltiazem has less effect, and nifedipine has the least effect. Cardiac failure may worsen if verapamil is used, especially in combination with disopyramide or beta adrenergic blocking drugs.

Antileukemic Agents

Daunorubicin or doxorubicin (Adriamycin) may produce cardiomyopathy and cardiac failure, especially when given in combination with other cytotoxic agents. This toxic effect is dose-related ($\approx$ 500 mg) and associated with manifestations of cardiac toxicity such as changes on the ECG prior to the development of cardiac failure (see Chapter 17).

Disopyramide

This antiarrhythmic agent has a substantial negative inotropic action. About half of patients who have previously been in cardiac failure will have a recurrence when disopyramide is used. This does not occur in patients with no history of cardiac failure.

Emetine

Emetine given for amebiasis may produce electrocardiographic evidence of myocardial toxicity, but cardiac failure is rare.

Corticosteroids
See Chapter 17.

Spironolactone

In patients with impaired renal function who are receiving spironolactone, especially those who are taking potassium salts as well, hyperkalemia may develop, with resulting cardiac conduction defects and idioventricular rhythms that may induce cardiac failure. Conduction defects, however, are more common.

Digitalis

Digitalis may produce ectopic rhythms by increasing automaticity and favoring reentry arrhythmias, which may lead to cardiac failure. Similarly, it may uncommonly produce complete atrioventricular block, and the slow ventricular rate in patients with borderline compensation may result in cardiac failure.

Phenothiazines & Tricyclic Antidepressants That Have a "Quinidine-Like" Action

These drugs may cause arrhythmias and cardiac failure, especially if underlying heart disease is present and failure is precipitated by the arrhythmias.

CONTROL ASCITES & EFFUSIONS

Thoracocentesis and abdominal paracentesis are not often required today because of the potency of the newer diuretics such as furosemide. However, large amounts of fluid in the pleural and abdominal cavities may cause severe distress, and fluid retained in cavities under increased pressure may itself, by uncertain mechanisms, trigger retention of salt and water. Removing the fluid mechanically not only makes the patient more comfortable by relieving dyspnea and abdominal distress but may also induce sodium diuresis.

TREAT WITH VASODILATORS

An important advance in the treatment of heart disease has been the use of vasodilators (to decrease the raised systemic vascular resistance) in the treatment of cardiac failure.

Vasodilators were first used in severe heart failure during acute myocardial infarction or cardiomyopathy, with the response monitored in the coronary care unit (see Chapter 8). Patients with left ventricular failure and cardiogenic shock who have low cardiac output and a high left ventricular filling pressure (> 20 mm Hg) often improve when impedance to left ventricular output, elevated systemic vascular resistance, or afterload is reduced by vasodilator therapy. The striking benefit from intravenous nitroprusside, illustrated in Figure 10–10, led to the use of other vasodilators. The acute short-term benefits (decreased left ventricular filling pressure and increased cardiac output) followed by diuresis and clinical improvement also occur with chronic oral therapy (Chatterjee, 1983).

Drugs induce vasodilation by several different mechanisms. Hemodynamic studies have shown that some vasodilators (hydralazine, minoxidil, calcium entry-blocking drugs) act directly on the smooth muscle of the arterioles, decreasing the afterload. Nitrates act by releasing endothelium-derived relaxing factor, now identified as nitric oxide, from the endothelium and decrease the preload by dilating the venous capacitance bed primarily. Prazosin, trimazosin, and doxazosin reduce the afterload by blocking postsynaptic alpha-adrenergic receptors. Captopril, en-

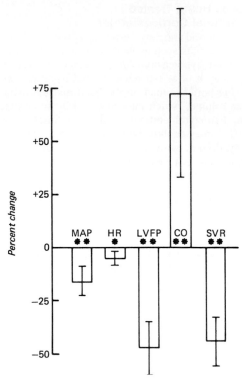

Figure 10–10. Average percentage change from control values during intravenous infusion of sodium nitroprusside in 18 patients with intractable heart failure. Vertical lines represent the standard error of the mean. (MAP, mean arterial pressure; HR, heart rate; LVFP, left ventricular filling pressure; CO, cardiac output; SVR, systemic vascular resistance. $**P < .001$; $*P < .01$.) (Reproduced, with permission, from Guiha NH et al: Treatment of refractory heart failure with infusion of nitroprusside. N Engl J Med 1974;291:587.)

alapril, and lisinopril (and other converting enzyme inhibitors) inhibit the conversion of angiotensin I to angiotensin II and thus as a second benefit decrease the angiotensin II and decrease the production of catecholamines. Vasodilator drugs may act at sites other than their dominant one; eg, nitrates may also decrease afterload, and prazosin and angiotensin-converting enzyme inhibitors decrease both preload and afterload. The choice of vasodilators depends on whether the predominant hemodynamic abnormality is raised left ventricular filling pressure or decreased cardiac output. Drugs that predominantly decrease preload are valuable in the former instance; those that decrease afterload are best in the latter instance. Vasodilators should be used cautiously if the arterial pressure is low. These agents can be given in combination with positive inotropic agents.

Figure 10–11 shows the beneficial hemodynamic effects of isosorbide dinitrate; there is a marked increase in venous capacitance and a more modest rise

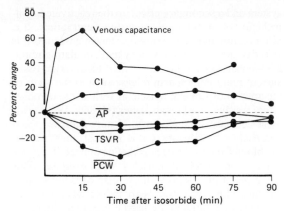

Figure 10–11. Effect of isosorbide dinitrate on five hemodynamic parameters over the course of 90 minutes. These data represent the mean percentage change from control values in 12 patients. A substantial increase in venous capacitance is seen at 5 minutes, with peak effect at 15 minutes. All other hemodynamic parameters have peak effect at 15–30 minutes. After 75 minutes, these effects are markedly reduced. (AP, mean arterial blood pressure; CI, cardiac index; PCW, mean pulmonary capillary wedge pressure; TSVR, total systemic vascular resistance.) (Reproduced, with permission, from Gray R et al: Hemodynamic and metabolic effects of isosorbide dinitrate in chronic congestive heart failure. Am Heart J 1975;90:346.)

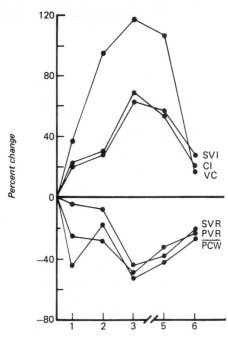

Figure 10–12. Hemodynamic changes after application of nitroglycerin ointment to the skin of a patient with severe mitral regurgitation. (CI, cardiac index; PCW, mean pulmonary capillary wedge pressure; PVR, pulmonary vascular resistance; SVI, stroke volume index; SVR, systemic vascular resistance; VC, venous capacitance.) (Reproduced, with permission, from Taylor WR et al: Hemodynamic effects of nitroglycerin ointment in congestive heart failure. Am J Cardiol 1976;38:469.)

in cardiac index. Decrease in cardiac size demonstrated by x-ray substantiates further the long-term benefit of oral nitrate therapy in severe cardiac failure. Figure 10–12 indicates that nitroglycerin ointment is also effective; transdermal slow-release patches are often preferred to the ointment. Recent evidence suggests a large variation in the amount of nitroglycerin absorbed from patches. Tachyphylaxis may occur with nitroglycerin usage; this can be avoided by allowing a nitrate-free period by removing nitroglycerin patches for 12-hour periods during each 24 hours. Isosorbide is better used three times a day to allow a nitrate-free period.

Vasodilator therapy in mitral and aortic incompetence reduces the regurgitant flow, improves the systolic emptying of the left ventricle, and thus increases the forward ejection fraction. Decreased left ventricular size reduces left ventricular wall tension and so improves left ventricular performance. This may benefit patients with mitral and aortic regurgitation and cardiac failure.

In Figure 10–13, the effects of vasodilator drugs are projected onto the family of Frank-Starling curves after adrenergic stimulation and in shock. It can be seen that the combination of nitrates and hydralazine (decreasing both preload and afterload) is more effective than either alone in decreasing left ventricular filling pressure and increasing the cardiac index and

stroke work index (Massie: Hemodynamic advantage, 1977).

A Veterans Administration Cooperative Study (the V-Heft-1 Trial), a double-blinded, placebo-controlled trial of hydralazine-isordil versus prazosin, was reported in patients with chronic congestive heart failure and moderate symptoms (NYHA II and III) treated with diuretics and digitalis (Cohn, 1986). There was a highly significant (34%) reduction in 2-year mortality rates in the group treated with the hydralazine-isordil combination compared with the placebo-treated group; there was no difference between the prazosin-treated group and the group receiving placebo. This study provided the first evidence that patients with chronic congestive heart failure could have improved survival on therapy with a vasodilating drug. In a later study, more symptomatic NYHA IV patients with chronic congestive heart failure were treated in a double-blinded, placebo-controlled trial with enalapril versus placebo in patients already treated with digitalis and diuretics. There was a highly significant 40% reduction in mortality rate by the end of 6 months and 31% at 1 year.

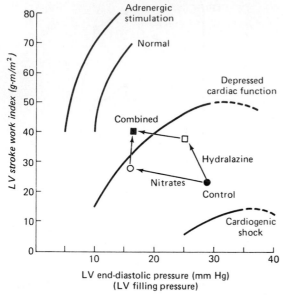

Figure 10–13. Effect of nitrates and hydralazine, alone and combined, on left ventricular performance in 12 patients with severe chronic cardiac failure projected onto the family of Frank-Starling left ventricular performance curves of Figure 10–2. (Adapted and reproduced, with permission, from Massie B et al: Hemodynamic advantage of combined oral hydralazine and nonparenteral nitrates in the vasodilator therapy of chronic heart failure. Am J Cardiol 1977;40:79.)

All the reduction in mortality was in the patients with progressive heart failure. No difference was seen in the incidence of sudden death; there was evidence of increased survival of the enalapril group compared with those taking other vasodilators (CONSENSUS Trial Study Group, 1987).

Another study randomized patients with chronic congestive heart failure receiving digitalis and diuretics who had moderate symptoms (NYHA II and III) and ejection fractions of 35% or less to enalapril compared with placebo (SOLVD Investigators, 1991). A second Veterans Administration trial (V-Heft-II: Cohn, 1991) randomized patients with chronic congestive heart failure on treatment with digitalis and diuretics who were mildly to moderately symptomatic (94% NYHA II and III) to an enalapril group and hydralazine-isordil group (Cohn, 1991). At 2 years, there was a highly significant reduction in mortality rate of 25% in the enalapril group compared with the hydralazine-isordil group. The reduction was greatest in the less symptomatic patients and was attributed to a reduction in the incidence of sudden death.

These studies provide excellent evidence that converting enzyme inhibitors have an advantage over other types of vasodilators, perhaps because of their beneficial effect on the activated renin-angiotensin

system and a secondary effect on the reactivated sympathetic system found in congestive heart failure. It is also possible that the renin-angiotensin antagonism is effective not only in the kidney and circulating renin-angiotensin system but also at the local target-tissue sites of renin-angiotensin release such as the walls of the arteries of skeletal muscle as well as the coronary artery, cardiac, and renal tissues (Hirsch, 1990). This local decrease in angiotensin II may decrease vasoconstriction locally where it is greatest, thus increasing blood flow to the organs that most need it, eg, the kidneys and skeletal muscles with exercise. This could result in increases in exercise capacity seen in patients with congestive heart failure when converting enzyme inhibitors are used compared with direct smooth-muscle dilators, such as hydralazine.

Drugs, Dosages, & Routes of Administration
(See also Tables in Chapters 8 and 9.)

A. Sodium Nitroprusside (Nipride): Sodium nitroprusside is supplied as a powder in vials containing 50 mg for intravenous use. Solutions with 500–1000 mL of dextrose in water must be prepared immediately before administration, should not be given after 4 hours, and should be given alone without other medication. The intravenous solution should be wrapped in aluminum foil to protect it from light and given by microdrip regulator to allow precise measurement of the rate of flow. Administration of infusion of sodium nitroprusside is begun at a rate of 16 μg/min and the infusion rate increased at intervals of 3–5 minutes until the pulmonary capillary wedge pressure is reduced to 18 mm Hg or below or becomes stable—provided the systolic blood pressure remains above 100 mm Hg. Some patients respond much more sensitively over a wide range of flow (16–200 μg/min), and the drip rate must be individualized accordingly. The drug works in seconds, and its effects dissipate rapidly when the drip is turned off. Side effects of nausea and sweating occur if blood pressure is lowered too rapidly.

B. Intravenous Nitroglycerin: Intravenous infusion of nitroglycerin is begun at a rate of 5 μg/min and is increased by 3–5 μg every 3–5 minutes. The same precautions about systolic pressure apply as with sodium nitroprusside. The average maximal rate of infusion is about 50 μg/min.

Intravenous vasodilator therapy for acute heart failure should only be given when patients can be monitored closely (as in the coronary care unit) and hypotension can be avoided or treated. If sodium nitroprusside is used for prolonged periods, serum thiocyanate levels should be monitored to avoid toxicity. Thiocyanate is a metabolite of sodium nitroprusside, and toxicity may occur from elevated levels of this compound (300 nmol/dL) (Vesey, 1976).

Abrupt cessation of intravenous nitroprusside may cause a rebound rise in left ventricular filling pressure and a fall in cardiac output. It is best to reduce the rate of infusion slowly and add oral vasodilators when it is decided to stop intravenous nitroprusside.

C. Isosorbide Dinitrate: Give 10–40 mg orally or 5–15 mg sublingually three times a day. This drug is an effective agent in improving left ventricular performance at rest and with moderate exercise, but not at maximum exercise (Franciosa, 1979).

D. Topical Nitrates (Nitroglycerin Ointment [Nitrol] and Transdermal Nitrates): Nitroglycerin ointment (Figure 10–12) is usually applied to the skin of the chest or abdomen, and the dose is determined by the size of the ointment strip applied to the skin. The beginning dose is usually 15 mg, or about 11/2 inch of the ointment strip. This is particularly valuable in patients with nocturnal angina or dyspnea, because the duration of action is 3–6 hours. Left ventricular filling pressure may decrease by about one-third and cardiac index may increase by about one-fourth in patients with heart failure managed in this way. Use of transdermal nitroglycerin, 5–30 mg in a slow-release patch, may supersede use of topical ointment because the patch is easier to use and is effective for 8–12 hours, whereas the ointment is effective for only 3–6 hours. To avoid tachyphylaxis, a 12-hour nitrate-free period should be allowed between uses of nitroglycerin patch or ointment.

E. Hydralazine: (See Chapter 9.) Begin with 25 mg and 2.5 mg, respectively, and gradually increase the dose, depending on the patient's response, to 25–75 mg and 5–20 mg, three times daily, respectively. Hydralazine together with isordil has proved effective for both short- and long-term treatment of chronic cardiac failure, with an increase in stroke volume and cardiac output and a decrease in pulmonary arterial wedge pressure at rest and during exercise (Massie: Hemodynamic advantage, 1977). Long-term alpha-receptor blockade with terazosin, 1–3 mg/d, has improved exercise ability and hemodynamics (Weber, 1980), but with prazosin the lack of effect on survival in the V-Heft study has led to its not being used in heart failure.

Although hydralazine by itself successfully increases cardiac index in patients with congestive heart failure, treadmill exercise time is not increased. This is consistent with the hypothesis that the increase in cardiac input is due to increased flow to nonactive arteriolar beds. Since the increased flow is not to the active muscle beds, exercise tolerance is not increased. Treadmill time is increased with the angiotensin-converting enzyme inhibitor captopril, which suggests that vasodilators that have both preload and afterload activity do allow for increased exercise tolerance. In general, vasodilators that decrease pulmonary arterial wedge pressure increase exercise time.

F. Other Agents: Alpha-adrenergic blocking agents such as phentolamine (Regitine) can be infused intravenously at a rate of 10–40 mg/kg/min, or

used orally as for pheochromocytoma in a dosage of 50 mg four times daily. The left ventricular filling pressure can be reduced by a decrease in venous return and controlled hypotension by the monitored infusion of trimethaphan (Arfonad). Trimethaphan can be given as 0.5% solution (500 mg in 1 L of 5% glucose in water) by infusion pump and the dose adjusted so as not to lower the systolic pressure below 90 mm Hg.

G. Combined Preload and Afterload Reducing Drugs: A combination of nitrates and hydralazine is more effective than either alone. The same is true when nitrates are combined with prazosin or when captopril is combined with hydralazine (Massie, 1983). In cases of severe failure, left ventricular performance may be effectively augmented by a combination of sodium nitroprusside infusion and infusion of an inotropic agent such as dobutamine or by a combination of dopamine and intravenous nitroglycerin (Figure 10–14). The increase of pulmonary wedge pressure caused by dopamine is counteracted by the decrease caused by nitroglycerin.

H. Angiotensin-Converting Enzyme (ACE) Inhibitors (Captopril, Enalapril, and Lisinopril): The original angiotensin-converting enzyme inhibitor, captopril, has been given orally in the treatment of acute and chronic cardiac failure to reduce systemic vascular resistance and plasma aldosterone levels; the other ACE inhibitors are similar. Captopril reduces preload and afterload, maintains renal function, increases the cardiac index, and decreases the left ventricular filling pressure and diastolic volume (Kramer, 1983). Caution must be exercised because some patients have developed hypotension, a rise in BUN and creatinine, proteinuria, rash, and leukopenia after daily doses of 25–150 mg of the drug. Renal biopsy in some of these patients with proteinuria has shown glomerular membrane nephropathy. More data are required to determine the frequency and severity of these untoward effects.

Captopril should be started at the smallest dose, 6.25 mg. Starting doses of enalapril and lisinopril should also be small. The blood pressure should be monitored for hypotension, which is most likely to occur within 1–2 hours after the initial dose in patients with hypovolemia, hypoglycemia, or low serum sodium concentration. Enalapril and lisinopril have the advantages of being more potent, having a longer duration of action, and not producing the toxic manifestations of captopril (Baim, 1983; DiCarlo, 1983). Enalapril must be metabolized by the liver before the active calcium entry-inhibiting agent is released.

I. Calcium Entry-Blocking Agents: Although calcium entry-blocking agents—especially nifedipine—are vasodilators, they have not been shown to prolong survival and will, in addition, have a negative inotropic effect; they are not used in the treatment of congestive heart failure.

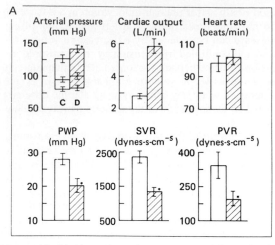
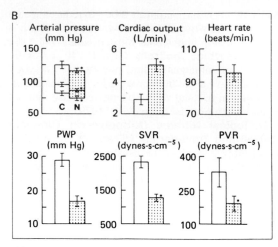

Figure 10–14. Hemodynamic response to dobutamine infusion **(A)** and to nitroprusside **(B)** in 12 cases of severe heart failure. (C, control period; D, dobutamine; N, nitroprusside.) Note marked increase in cardiac output, with only slight increase in systolic arterial pressure and decrease in pulmonary wedge pressure (PWP). Systemic vascular resistance (SVR) and pulmonary vascular resistance (PVR) decrease. (Reproduced, with permission, from Cohn JN, Franciosa JA: Selection of vasodilator, inotropic, or combined therapy for the management of heart failure. Am J Med 1978;65:181.)

J. Beta-Adrenergic Blocking Agents: Although beta-adrenergic blocking agents can precipitate heart failure in some patients, they have been shown (paradoxically) in some patients with severe congestive heart failure to be beneficial, both clinically and hemodynamically (Waagstein, 1989). The patients were started on a small dose of metoprolol (5 mg twice daily) and titrated gradually up to 50 mg three times daily. The goal was to reduce the heart rate to 50–70 beats per minute.

The mechanism of the improvement is not clear but could result from the benefits of a slower heart rate, diastolic filling, and myocardial oxygen consumption. There is also some evidence that there is an increase in ventricular beta-adrenergic receptors (up-regulation), which may result in a more normal response to sympathetic stimulation.

ADD INOTROPIC AGENTS
IF NECESSARY

Experience in coronary care units and intensive care units has shown that patients with acute myocardial infarction in cardiac failure with low output states as well as patients recovering from open heart surgery with low-output states often benefit from inotropic agents other than digitalis. Norepinephrine, isoproterenol, dobutamine (Leier, 1983), dopamine, and intravenous amrinone and milrinone have been used and are discussed in Chapter 8. The choice of drugs depends upon the status of the hemodynamic variables at the time, and as with the vasodilator agents, it is desirable to monitor these variables prior to treatment. Arterial pressure, left ventricular filling pressure, and cardiac output are the essential parameters to be monitored.

Norepinephrine & Isoproterenol

If the left ventricular filling pressure and cardiac index are within the normal range (LVFP, 12–15 mm Hg; CI[CO/m²], 2.5–3.5 L/min/m²) and hypotension due to vasodilation is the dominant presenting clinical feature, a drug such as norepinephrine, which acts chiefly as an alpha-adrenergic peripheral vasoconstrictor, can be used. If the left ventricular filling pressure is on the high side (> 15 mm Hg), norepinephrine may further increase the filling pressure and lead to pulmonary edema. Similarly, if the patient has moderate hypovolemia, continued use of vasopressor drugs such as norepinephrine will aggravate hypovolemia by disproportionate increase in venous constriction as compared to arteriolar constriction, with subsequent loss of fluid into the interstitial tissues.

Isoproterenol, by producing vasodilation, may aggravate hypotension, although it has a positive inotropic action. If hypotension is not present, it may simultaneously decrease left ventricular filling pressure and increase cardiac output. On the other hand, isoproterenol stimulates the heart and may induce ventricular premature beats and increase heart rate and myocardial oxygen consumption. As a result, myocardial ischemia may be induced.

Dopamine & Dobutamine

Dopamine hydrochloride (Intropin) and dobutamine (Dobutrex) (a relatively cardiospecific beta-adrenergic agent) have been found to be powerful inotropic agents useful in the treatment of cardiac failure, decreasing both preload and afterload (Goldstein, 1980; Leier, 1983). Dopamine is the immediate precursor in the synthesis of norepinephrine and stimulates dopaminergic receptors; it has the advantage that while it may increase cardiac output and decrease left ventricular filling pressure in low output cardiac failure, it does so in doses of less than 10 μg/kg/min without decreasing renal blood flow. Sodium and water diuresis, therefore, may be enhanced, especially when dopamine is used in conjunction with diuretics. The effects of dopamine depend upon its dose; because it is a beta-adrenergic agonist, it may produce tachycardia and ventricular arrhythmia as the dose is increased. In larger doses it also stimulates alpha-adrenergic receptors, and a raised blood pressure may result, whereas dobutamine does not have this effect. In smaller dosages ($<$ 10 μg/kg/min), dopamine usually does not cause tachycardia or raise the arterial pressure. As with vasodilator agents, dopamine should be started at a low rate of infusion, eg, 2–4 μg/kg/min, while the hemodynamic parameters are being monitored. The flow should be adjusted as with vasodilator agents, depending upon the hemodynamic response.

Dobutamine is a derivative of dopamine and has a striking effect on increasing the cardiac output, with only a slight increase in the heart rate and a moderate increase in the mean blood pressure and without important side effects. It can be given at a rate of 10 μg/kg/min and, like dopamine, can be combined with intravenous nitroprusside or nitroglycerin in critical situations. The infusion must be adjusted depending upon the clinical and hemodynamic response (Leier, 1983).

Dopamine and dobutamine have several problems that limit their usefulness. They increase heart rate and afterload, which increases myocardial oxygen demand and requires increased coronary blood flow, and are possibly arrhythmogenic and may increase mortality rates. Patients have been shown to develop rapid tolerance to many adrenergic agonists, perhaps because of decrease of active beta-adrenergic receptors. Digital ischemia with cyanosis and pain may occur as a result of vasoconstriction due to alpha-adrenergic stimulation from dopamine. Treatment consists of alpha-adrenergic blockade, such as the use of chlorpromazine intravenously. In a typical case, a 10-mg intravenous loading dose followed by an infusion at a rate of 0.6 mg/min (7.3 μg/kg/min) was given by Valdes (1976), with reversal of the digital ischemia within minutes. Other alpha-adrenergic blockers (eg, phentolamine, 50 mg) may be used alternatively.

Low cardiac output is common in the immediate period following cardiopulmonary bypass, and inotropic agents such as dopamine, dobutamine, intravenous amrinone and milrinone, and epinephrine may increase the cardiac index significantly. Other β1 agonists (eg, pirbuterol) as well as β2 agonists (pre-

nalterol and salbutamol) have undergone therapeutic trial in congestive heart failure. Unfortunately, they all cause β-receptor down-regulation and tachyphylaxis and are arrhythmogenic.

Amrinone & Milrinone

Amrinone is a synthetic positive inotropic drug used orally in dosages of 50–300 mg (Wynne, 1984). It is the prototype of the phosphodiesterase inhibitors. These drugs inhibit the enzyme that degrades cyclic adenosine monophosphate, thereby increasing the influx of calcium into the cell and the uptake of calcium into the sarcoplasmic reticulum. These actions result in an increase in calcium available for release to the contractile mechanism. Amrinone increases cardiac index, left ventricular ejection fraction, and effective renal plasma flow and decreases systemic vascular resistance. Despite its effectiveness with acute use in refractory cardiac failure, oral clinical use has been restricted because of the development of thrombocytopenia in about 20% of patients. Milrinone, an analogue of amrinone, is more potent; has some vasodilator effects as well as its dominant inotropic effects; and, to date, has not caused thrombocytopenia. It has a short half-life and must be given daily in multiple doses (Wynne, 1984). Although the short-term benefits of the two drugs are real, reports of their long-term effectiveness have shown no long-term beneficial effect, and there is evidence— possibly because of the increase in contractility or because of arrhythmogenesis—of a decrease in survival. Enoximone, a newer phosphodiesterase inhibitor, showed no long-term benefit when added to digitalis and diuretics and was attended by an increased mortality rate (Uretsky, 1990). It is not likely that these drugs will be useful in the chronic treatment of congestive heart failure.

CONSIDER INTRA-AORTIC BALLOON COUNTERPULSATION
See Chapter 7.

PROVIDE EMERGENCY TREATMENT OF SEVERE HEART FAILURE OR ACUTE PULMONARY EDEMA ACCORDING TO CAUSE & SEVERITY

Severe heart failure or acute pulmonary edema is often a grave emergency, and treatment varies depending upon the cause and severity. Morphine and rest in bed in the sitting position alone may suffice, although intravenous diuretics (see below) may also be required. Acute pulmonary edema may be treated with sublingual nitroglycerin, beginning with 0.4– 0.6 mg and repeating the dose every 10 minutes if necessary (Bussman, 1978), or with sublingual nifedipine, 10 mg. See also Chapters 8, 9, and 12. Blood pressure should be monitored to recognize and avoid hypotension. If the attack is due to ventricular tachycardia or to atrial fibrillation with a rapid ventricular rate and the patient has severe dyspnea or pulmonary edema, cardioversion should be instituted without delay.

Intravenous nitroglycerin is the treatment of choice in acute severe left ventricular failure with pulmonary edema and severe dyspnea (as in myocardial infarction), when the wedge pressure may be high but the cardiac output is essentially normal. When the cardiac output is reduced in the presence of a high wedge pressure, intravenous nitroprusside is preferable because it dilates both arterioles and venules, whereas intravenous nitroglycerin is primarily a venodilator.

A patient who fails to respond to bed rest, digitalis, and diuretics in the hospital—and antihypertensive therapy if hypertensive—should be monitored in a critical care unit. Continuous monitoring of the ECG and intra-arterial blood pressures is required, and a flow-directed catheter should be introduced to allow intracardiac pressures and cardiac output to be intermittently observed, ie, pulmonary artery diastolic pressure or preferably pulmonary capillary wedge pressure, cardiac output by the thermodilution method, and arterial blood gases. Special nursing care is required for continuous close observation.

The patient is sedated with morphine, 5–10 mg intravenously, and placed in the sitting position, which decreases the venous return to the heart—the equivalent of venesection—and may allow an increase in cardiac output. Intravenous furosemide is given in a dosage of 40–80 mg, and oxygen is given by face mask in high concentration (40–60%) and a high flow rate (6–8 L/min). Improvement should occur within an hour. Morphine relieves anxiety, depresses pulmonary reflexes, decreases pulmonary artery wedge pressure, and induces sleep. Relief from forceful respiration decreases the negative intrathoracic pressure and the venous return to the heart. Oxygen relieves hypoxia and dyspnea and decreases pulmonary capillary permeability. Positive pressure breathing for short periods may be of great value, especially if there is respiratory acidosis with impaired ventilation. Positive pressure breathing improves ventilation, removes CO_2, and decreases venous return to the heart. If the patient has severe impairment of cardiac output, positive pressure breathing should be used with caution because the cardiac output may fall further. If the patient has acute bronchospasm, aminophylline, 0.25–0.5 g infused slowly intravenously, is often helpful. In addition to decreasing the bronchospasm, it may increase the glomerular filtration rate, renal blood flow, and cardiac output as well as the urinary excretion of sodium and water.

If the patient is still dyspneic or has episodic increases in dyspnea and fails to respond to the treatment given above, parenteral vasodilator agents should be added. If the situation is critical and systolic pressure exceeds 100 mm Hg, an infusion of sodium nitroprusside can be started at a dosage of 8–16 μg/min and titrated to the response of the patient (see above and Chapter 8). Intravenous nitroglycerin can also be used (see above), depending on the cardiac output and systemic vascular resistance. If the situation is less critical, isosorbide dinitrate, 5–15 mg sublingually or 10–40 mg orally, can be used, and if the systolic pressure is not decreased below 100 mm Hg, sublingual nitroglycerin, 0.3–0.6 mg, or sublingual nifedipine, 10 mg, can be given. This is often helpful in acute pulmonary edema associated with hypertension. If the vasodilators just mentioned are not effective in relieving the dyspnea, one can add hydralazine, 50–75 mg orally or 2.5–10 mg intramuscularly, to dilate the arteriolar bed. The combination of nitrates and hydralazine produces both venous and arteriolar dilation and is more effective than either drug used alone. If the patient has acute hypertensive heart failure, captopril, 25 mg orally, enalapril, 5–10 mg orally, or nifedipine, 10 mg sublingually, may prove beneficial in 30–60 minutes. Venesection is infrequently used today unless the patient has acute pulmonary edema secondary to rapid intravenous infusion of sodium-containing fluids. Removal of 300–500 mL of blood is the most direct way of reducing the venous return to the heart and may decrease right atrial and peripheral venous pressure in low output cardiac failure. It should not be used if anemia is present.

If ventilation is impaired and acidosis is present, tracheal intubation may be helpful and further decrease the work of the heart.

If the patient does not promptly respond to the aggressive therapy described above, one should consider potentially curable causes of congestive heart failure that may require specific treatment directed at the cause, such as severe aortic stenosis, acute valvular insufficiency from infective endocarditis, severe mitral or pulmonary stenosis, severe thyrotoxicosis or myxedema heart disease, pericardial effusion, and the other conditions mentioned earlier in this chapter. One may also need to consider cardiac transplantation.

CARDIAC TRANSPLANTATION

When the patient continues to be functional class IV despite maximal medical management and aggressive consideration of surgical repair, cardiac transplantation is a widely available and successful therapy. With the development of frequent myocardial biopsies to detect early rejection and triple-drug therapy with cyclosporine, azathioprine, and corticosteroids for combating organ rejection, the long-term success of transplantation has been reflected in the exponential increase in the number of patients transplanted. By 1990, over 12,000 procedures had been performed worldwide according to the Registry of the International Society for Heart Transplantation (ISHT) (Fragomeni, 1988). In 1987 worldwide, 1441 heart transplants were performed in 128 centers—88% of them in the United States.

Presently, the perioperative mortality rate is approximately 10%, and the 1-year survival is 80–90% with a 3-year survival of between 75% and 80% worldwide. In a small number of cases, the actuarial 10-year survival is 72.7%, so it appears that long-term mortality is leveling out after 3 years (Fragomeni, 1990).

If survival were attended by a miserable quality of life, cardiac transplantation would be a failure as a clinical option. On follow-up of these patients, however, 90% are in functional class I, and 70% have returned to school or to work.

The limiting factor in cardiac transplantation is the scarcity of the donor organ. Since donor hearts are not immediately available, ventricular assist devices (VAD) have been developed to support the patient's circulation mechanically until a donor heart can be found. The simplest of these devices is the intra-aortic balloon counterpulsation pump. More efficient and more expensive VADs—external mechanical pumps that augment the failing natural heart—have been developed (Farrar, 1988). For this reason, patients considered for transplantation must be subject to the most scrupulous screening in order to provide the benefit of this procedure to the largest number of patients. The choice of patients for transplantation is not a simple matter and involves not only assessment of the patient's prognosis on continued medical management but social, emotional, ethical, and financial considerations as well. The indications for transplantation have broadened, but essentially the patients must have exhausted all methods of conventional therapy and still have a poor prognosis of only a 6–12 months of likely survival; must have no serious non-cardiac disease; and pulmonary vascular resistance must be less than 4 mm Hg/L/min (Wood units); and must be emotionally stable, have good home support, and be realistic and compliant. Patients undergoing heart transplantation are generally under 65 years of age.

Some patients who are class III or class IV may be satisfied with a totally sedentary life but still be at high risk of dying within 6 months, with demise frequently occurring as sudden death. It is therefore necessary to risk-stratify patients to identify those at greatest risk of early demise. There are clinical and laboratory parameters that identify such patients. For instance, functional class IV patients have a survival rate of 50% in 1 year (CONSENSUS Trial, 1987). Patients with poor ventricular function manifested by an ejection fraction of under 10% have a 6-month survival of 17% (Keogh, 1988). Exercise studies

measuring functional capacity by determining peak oxygen consumption (VO_{2max})—a function of peak cardiac output and tissue oxygen extraction—have been correlated with the functional class of the patient (Weber, 1985). Functional class I patients have a VO_{2max} of over 20 mL O_2/kg/min and functional class IV patients less than 10 mL O_2/kg/min. Patients with less than 10 mL O_2/kg/min VO_{2max} have a 30% 1-year survival rate (Massie, 1987). Other factors, such as plasma level of norepinephrine and electrophysiologic induction of sustained nonsuppressible ventricular tachycardia, also identify patients at high risk of early demise.

The postoperative course is difficult and requires, in addition to the immunosuppressive drugs mentioned above, frequent endomyocardial biopsies to detect early rejection. The commonest cause of death in cardiac transplant patients is infection (38%), with hypertension and cardiac complications (25%) and acute rejection (24%) less common (Fragomeni, 1990). Cyclosporine-induced hypertension resulting from renal arteriolar vasoconstriction and renal and hepatic dysfunction are all common. Complications from prolonged use of corticosteroids are well recognized. Between 35% and 40% of patients will have developed some degree of coronary arteriopathy by the third year after transplantation. This consists of intimal proliferation—frequently called "diffuse atherosclerosis"—involving the coronary vessels and even the intramural vessels and may be a form of chronic rejection.

Heart-lung and lung transplantation have lagged behind cardiac transplantation, but improved survival in recent studies has stimulated greater interest. By 1988, the ISHT had reported 388 heart-lung transplants, mainly for primary pulmonary hypertension, congenital heart disease, and Eisenmenger's syndrome. In 1988, the ISHT registry reported 219 patients operated on worldwide, with an actuarial survival of 71.2% at 2 months and 62.4% at 2 years. The late causes of death were, again, infection in 67% and organ rejection in 11% (Fragomeni, 1990). The major problem with lung transplantation is that there is no good way to monitor for early lung rejection.

In 15 patients with single-lung transplants, there were nine long-term survivors and excellent functional results (Toronto Lung Transplant Group, 1988). Both single- and double-lung transplantation are being extensively evaluated at present (Toronto Lung Transplant Group, 1988).

TOTALLY IMPLANTABLE ARTIFICIAL HEART

The totally implantable artificial heart is still being developed. The Jarvik heart was implanted in a small number of patients, all of whom lived for some time but died of infection and thromboembolism. The major problem with this heart is that the power source is external and requires percutaneous lines. When the problems of the artificial heart are overcome, it will be a major advance in the treatment of patients with terminal cardiac disease.

PROGNOSIS

The overall prognosis of the patient with congestive heart failure, or cardiac failure, has improved considerably in recent years because of the therapeutic advances discussed in the foregoing pages—especially the availability of oral diuretics, ACE inhibitors, vasodilators, inotropic agents, and surgical and medical treatment of underlying causes. However, it remains poor because treatment is often delayed until cardiac failure is far-advanced, ie, because treatable conditions such as hypertensive heart failure and valvular heart disease with heart failure are not recognized and treated early.

In moderate nonprogressive cardiac failure, the annual mortality rate is about 10–15%, whereas in severe progressive cardiac failure, the annual mortality rate is 50% or more. The prognosis is worse when left ventricular failure is associated with a left ventricular ejection fraction of less than 20%, disabling symptoms, and markedly decreased exercise tolerance. The prognosis is also worse when the cardiac failure is associated with hyponatremia or considerable elevation of the plasma norepinephrine. Patients die suddenly from cardiac arrhythmias as frequently as from pump failure, but there are no convincing data that antiarrhythmic therapy can prevent the sudden deaths. Nevertheless, when the ventricular arrhythmias in cardiac failure are symptomatic, vigorous treatment is recommended (see Chapter 15). Nonsustained ventricular tachycardia should be treated if the patient is symptomatic, but the data are controversial for asymptomatic patients, because the complications of therapy may be substantial and the therapeutic benefit may not be clear.

If treatment is decided upon, quinidine or procainamide is probably the best first choice. Mexiletine or tocainide can be tried if these are ineffective or poorly tolerated. Disopyramide should be avoided since it may worsen heart failure. Mexiletine and tocainide are less likely to worsen heart failure but have been used less because of side effects and proarrhythmic tendencies. Encainide and flecainide are extremely effective in eliminating premature ventricular contraction, but with depressed left ventricular function they have a very high proarrhythmic effect; they should be used only in sustained ventricular tachycardia. Amiodarone is the most effective drug but has a substantial level of toxicity (see Chapter 15); it may be used if the ventricular arrhythmia is symptomatic and produces hemodynamic deterioration (Massie, 1987). There is some evidence that a low dose, under 400 mg per day, has a low incidence of toxicity and may be effective in reducing death from arrhythmia.

At times, however, the basic cause (eg, ischemic cardiomyopathy or dilated cardiomyopathy) cannot be reversed, and treatment is therefore only palliative (Franciosa, 1983; Wilson, 1983; Massie, 1988).

REFERENCES

Definition & Causes

Braunwald E, Mock MB, Watson JT (editors): *Congestive Heart Failure: Current Research and Clinical Applications.* Grune & Stratton, 1982.

Kannel WB et al: Role of blood pressure in the development of congestive heart failure: The Framingham Study. N Engl J Med 1972;287:781.

Hemodynamics & Pathophysiology

Anderson FL et al: Myocardial catecholamine and neuropeptide Y depletion in failing ventricles of patients with idiopathic dilated cardiomyopathy: Correlation with β-adrenergic receptor downregulation. Circulation 1992;85:46.

Cannon PJ: The kidney in heart failure. N Engl J Med 1977;296:26.

Curtiss C et al: Role of the renin-angiotensin system in the systemic vasoconstriction of chronic congestive heart failure. Circulation 1978;58:763.

Drexler H et al: Alterations of skeletal muscle in chronic heart failure. Circulation 1992;85:1621.

Ferguson DW et al: Sympathoinhibitory responses to digitalis glycosides in heart failure patients: Direct evidence from sympathetic neural recordings. Circulation 1989;80:65.

Francis GS et al: Comparison of neuroendocrine activation in patients with left ventricular dysfunction with and without congestive heart failure: A substudy of the Studies of Left Ventricular Dysfunction (SOLVD). Circulation 1990;82:1724.

Frand UI, Shim CS, Williams MH Jr: Heroin induced pulmonary edema: Sequential studies of pulmonary function. Ann Intern Med 1972;77:29.

Grogan M et al: Left ventricular dysfunction due to atrial fibrillation in patients initially believed to have idiopathic dilated cardiomyopathy. Am J Cardiol 1992;69:1570.

Hirsch AT et al: Potential role of the tissue renin-angiotensin system in the pathophysiology of congestive heart failure. Am J Cardiol 1990;66:22D.

Katz SD et al: Impaired endothelium-mediated vasodilation in the peripheral vasculature of patients with congestive heart failure. J Am Coll Cardiol 1992;19:918.

Kienzle MG et al: Clinical, neurologic, and sympathetic

neural correlates of heart rate variability in congestive heart failure. Am J Cardiol 1992;69:761.

Leithe ME et al: Relationship between central hemodynamics and regional blood flow in normal subjects and in patients with congestive heart failure. Circulation 1984;69:57.

Little WC: Enhanced local dependence of relaxation in heart failure: Clinical implications. Circulation 1992;85:2326.

Mancia G: Neurohumoral activation in congestive heart failure. Am Heart J 1990;120:1532.

Mancini D et al: Contribution of skeletal muscle atrophy to exercise intolerance and altered muscle metabolism in heart failure. Circulation 1992;85:1364.

Mancini DM et al: Respiratory muscle function and dyspnea in patients with chronic congestive heart failure. Circulation 1992;86:909.

McMurray JJ et al: Plasma endothelium in heart failure. Circulation 1992;85:1374.

Minotti JR et al: Neurodiagnostic assessment of skeletal muscle fatigue in patients with congestive heart failure. Circulation 1992;86:903.

Packer M: The neurohumeral hypothesis: A theory to explain the mechanics of disease progression in heart failure. J Am Coll Cardiol 1992:20:248.

Parmley WW, Talbot L: Heart as a pump. In: *Handbook of Physiology—The Cardiovascular System I.* American Physiological Society, 1979.

Pearson AC et al: Assessment of diastolic function in normal and hypertrophied hearts: Comparison of Doppler echocardiography and M-mode echocardiography. Am Heart J 1987;113:1417.

Semigran MJ et al: Effects of atrial natriuretic peptide on myocardial contractile and diastolic function in patients with heart failure. J Am Coll Cardiol 1992;20:98.

Spinale FG et al: Changes in myocardial blood flow during development of and recovery from tachycardia-induced cardiomyopathy. Circulation 1992;85:717.

Staub NC: The pathogenesis of pulmonary edema. Prog Cardiovasc Dis 1980;23:53.

Stein L et al: Pulmonary edema during volume infusion. Circulation 1975;52:483.

Clinical Findings

Glower DD et al: Mechanical correlates of the third heart sound. J Am Coll Cardiol 1992;19:450.

Massie BM et al: Mitral-septal separation: New echocardiographic index of left ventricular function. Am J Cardiol 1977;39:1008.

Popp RL: M mode echocardiographic assessment of left ventricular function. Am J Cardiol 1982;49:1312.

Rackow EC et al: Relationship of colloid osmotic pressure and pulmonary capillary pressure to pulmonary edema. Cardiovasc Med 1978;3:407.

Wahr DW, Wang YS, Schiller NB: Left ventricular volumes determined by two-dimensional echocardiography in a normal adult population. J Am Coll Cardiol 1983;1:863.

Treatment

Abrams J: A reappraisal of nitrate therapy. JAMA 1988;259:396.

Abrams J: Use of nitrates in ischemic heart disease. Curr Probl Cardiol 1992;17:487.

Anderson JL et al: Efficacy and safety of sustained (48-hour) intravenous infusions of milrinone in patients with severe congestive heart failure: A multicenter study. J Am Coll Cardiol 1987;9:711.

Antman EM et al: Treatment of 150 cases of life-threatening digitalis intoxication with digoxin-specific Fab antibody fragments: Final report of a multicenter study. Circulation 1990;81:1774.

Arnold SB et al: Long-term digitalis therapy improves left ventricular function in heart failure. N Engl J Med 1980;303:1443.

Baim DS et al: Evaluation of a new bipyridine inotropic agent—milrinone—in patients with severe congestive heart failure. N Engl J Med 1983;309:748.

Bigger JT Jr (editor): Management of ventricular arrhythmias in patients with congestive heart failure. (A Symposium.) Am J Cardiol 1986;57(Suppl B).

Burke CM et al: Twenty-eight cases of human heart-lung transplantation. Lancet 1986;1:517.

Bussmann WD, Schupp D: Effect of sublingual nitroglycerin in emergency treatment of severe pulmonary edema. Am J Cardiol 1978;41:931.

Chatterjee K, Parmley WW: Vasodilator therapy for acute myocardial infarction and chronic congestive heart failure. J Am Coll Cardiol 1983;1:133.

Chatterjee K et al (The Captopril Multicenter Research Group I): A cooperative multicenter study of captopril in congestive heart failure: Hemodynamic effects and long-term response. Am Heart J 1985;110:439.

Cohn JN: Current therapy of the failing heart. Circulation 1988;78:1099.

Cohn JN, Swedberg K, Kjekshus J (editors): Advances in congestive heart failure. (Symposium.) Am J Cardiol 1988;62(Suppl A).

Cohn JN et al: Effect of vasodilator therapy on mortality in chronic congestive heart failure: Results of a Veterans Administration Cooperative Study. N Engl J Med 1986;314:1547.

Colucci WS, Wright RF, Braunwald E: New positive inotropic agents in the treatment of congestive heart failure: Mechanisms of action and recent clinical developments. (Two parts.) N Engl J Med 1986;314:290, 349.

DiBianco R et al: A comparison of oral milrinone, digoxin, and their combination in the treatment of patients with chronic heart failure. N Engl J Med 1989;320:677.

DiCarlo L et al: Enalapril: A new angiotensin converting enzyme inhibitor in chronic heart failure: Acute and chronic hemodynamic evaluations. J Am Coll Cardiol 1983;2:865.

Farrar DJ et al: Heterotropic prosthetic ventricles as a bridge to cardiac transplantation: A multicenter study in 29 patients. N Engl J Med 1988;318:333.

Fragomeni LS, Bonser RS, Kaye MP: Clinical results of heart and heart-lung transplantation. Prog Cardiovasc Dis 1990;33:97.

Fragomeni LS, Kaye MP: The Registry of the International Society for Heart Transplantation: Fifth Official Report—1988. J Heart Transplant 1988;7:249.

Franciosa JA, Cohn JN: Effect of isosorbide dinitrate on response to submaximal and maximal exercise in patients with congestive heart failure. Am J Cardiol 1979;43:1009.

Genton R, Jaffe AS: Management of congestive heart

failure in patients with acute myocardial infarction. JAMA 1986;256:2556.

Gheorghiade M et al: Comparative hemodynamic and neurohormonal effects of intravenous captopril and digoxin and their combinations in patients with severe heart failure. J Am Coll Cardiol 1989;13:134.

Gheorghiade M et al: Hemodynamic effects of intravenous digoxin in patients with severe heart failure initially treated with diuretics and vasodilators. J Am Coll Cardiol 1987;9:849.

Gheorghiade M, Zarowitz BJ: Review of randomized trials of digoxin therapy in patients with chronic heart failure. Am J Cardiol 1992;69:48G.

Goldstein RA, Passamani ER, Roberts R: A comparison of digoxin and dobutamine in patients with acute infarction and cardiac failure. N Engl J Med 1980;303:846.

Goodwin JF: Cardiac transplantation. Circulation 1986;74:913.

Gorlin R: Angiotensin-converting enzyme inhibitors in the treatment of congestive heart failure. Cardiovasc Rev Rep 1988;9:26.

Guyatt GH et al: A controlled trial of digoxin in congestive heart failure. Am J Cardiol 1988;61;371.

Hickey AR et al: Digoxin immune Fab therapy in the management of digitalis intoxication: Safety and efficacy results of an observational surveillance study. J Am Coll Cardiol 1991;17:590.

Hofflin JM et al: Infectious complications in heart transplant recipients receiving cyclosporine and corticosteroids. Ann Intern Med 1987;106:209.

Jamieson SW et al: Combined heart and lung transplantation. Lancet 1983;1:1130.

Kahan BD: Immunosuppressive therapy with cyclosporine for cardiac transplantation. Circulation 1987;75:40.

Keogh AM et al: Timing of cardiac transplantation in idiopathic dilated cardiomyopathy. Am J Cardiol 1988;61:418.

Kereiakes DJ, Ports TA: Intra-aortic balloon counterpulsation and the diagnosis and management of surgical complications of acute myocardial infarction. in: Cardiac Emergencies. Scheinman MM (editor). Saunders, 1984.

Kjekshus J et al: Effects of enalapril on long-term mortality in severe congestive heart failure. Am J Cardiol 1992;69:103.

Konstam MA et al: Effects of the angiotensin converting enzyme inhibitor enalapril on the long-term progression of left ventricular function in patients with heart failure. Circulation 1992;86:431.

Kramer BL, Massie BM, Topic N: Controlled trial of captopril in chronic heart failure: A rest and exercise hemodynamic study. Circulation 1983;67:807.

Kukin ML: Vasodilation therapy and survival in chronic congestive heart failure. J Am Coll Cardiol 1992;19:1360.

Lazar JM et al: Outcome and complications of prolonged intraaortic balloon counterpulsation in cardiac patients. Am J Cardiol 1992;69:955.

Lee DCS et al: Heart failure in outpatients: A randomized trial of digoxin versus placebo. N Engl J Med 1982;306:699.

Leier CV, Unverferth DV: Dobutamine. Ann Intern Med 1983;99:490.

LeJemtel TH et al: Systemic and regional hemodynamic effects of captopril and milrinone administered alone and concomitantly in patients with heart failure. Circulation 1985;72:364.

Levine AB, Levine TB: Patient evaluation for cardiac transplantation. Prog Cardiovasc Dis 1991;33:219.

Ljungman S et al: Renal function in severe congestive heart failure during treatment with enalapril. (The Cooperative North Scandinavian Enalapril Survival Study [CONSENSUS] Trial.) Am J Cardiol 1992;70:479.

McEnany T et al: Clinical experience with intra-aortic balloon pump support in 710 patients. Circulation 1977;56(Suppl III).

Massie BM: New trends in the use of angiotensin converting enzyme inhibitors in chronic heart failure. Am J Med 1988;84(Suppl 4A):36.

Massie B et al: Hemodynamic advantage of combined administration of hydralazine orally and nitrates nonparenterally in the vasodilator therapy of chronic heart failure. Am J Cardiol 1977;40:794.

Massie BM et al: Hemodynamic responses to combined therapy with captopril and hydralazine in patients with severe heart failure. J Am Coll Cardiol 1983;2:338.

Massie BM et al: Long-term oral administration of amrinone for congestive heart failure: Lack of efficacy in a multicenter controlled trial. Circulation 1985;71:963.

Miller RR et al: Differential systemic arterial and venous actions and consequent cardiac effects of vasodilator drugs. Prog Cardiovasc Dis 1982;24:353.

Mungall DR et al: Effects of quinidine on serum digoxin concentration: A prospective study. Ann Intern Med 1980;93:689.

O'Connell JB et al: Cardiac transplantation: Recipient selection, donor procurement, and medical follow-up: A statement for heart professionals from the Committee on Cardiac Transplantation of the Council on Clinical Cardiology, American Heart Association. Circulation 1992;86:1061.

Packer M: Vasodilator and inotropic therapy for severe chronic heart failure: Passion and skepticism. J Am Coll Cardiol 1983;2:841.

Packer M, Medina N, Yushak M: Role of the renin-angiotensin system in the development of hemodynamic and clinical tolerance to long-term prazosin therapy in patients with severe chronic heart failure. J Am Coll Cardiol 1986;7:671.

Packer M et al: Comparison of captopril and enalapril in patients with severe chronic heart failure. N Engl J Med 1986;315:847.

Packer M et al: Functional renal insufficiency during long-term therapy with captopril and enalapril in severe chronic heart failure. Ann Intern Med 1987;106:346.

Parmley WW: Pathophysiology and current therapy of congestive heart failure. J Am Coll Cardiol 1989;13:771.

Risöe C et al: Nitroprusside and reginal vascular capacitance in patients with severe congestive heart failure. Circulation 1992;85:997.

St. Goar F et al: Intracoronary ultrasound in cardiac transplant recipients: In vivo evidence of "angiographically silent" intimal thickening. Circulation 1992;85:979.

Scheidt S et al: Mechanical circulatory assistance with

the intraaortic balloon pump and other counterpulsation devices. Prog Cardiovasc Dis 1982;25:55.

Schwartz AB, Swartz CD: Dosage of potassium chloride elixir to correct thiazide-induced hypokalemia. JAMA 1974;230:702.

Smith TW (editor): *Digitalis Glycosides*. Grune & Stratton, 1986.

Smith TW et al: Digitalis glycosides: Mechanisms and manifestations of toxicity. (Three parts.) Prog Cardiovasc Dis 1984;26:413, 495; 27: 21.

Sturm JT et al: Treatment of postoperative low output syndrome with intraaortic balloon pumping: Experience with 419 patients. Am J Cardiol 1980;45:1038.

Toronto Lung Transplant Group: Experience with single-lung transplantation for pulmonary fibrosis. JAMA 1988;259:2258.

Uretsky BF et al: Multicenter trial of oral enoximone in patients with moderate to moderately severe congestive heart failure: Lack of benefit compared with placebo. Circulation 1990;82:774.

Vesey CJ, Cole PV, Simpson PJ: Cyanide and thiocyanate concentrations following sodium nitroprusside infusion in man. Br J Anaesth 1976;48:651.

Waagstein F et al: Long-term β-blockade in dilated cardiomyopathy: Effects of short- and long-term metoprolol treatment followed by withdrawal and readministration of metoprolol. Circulation 1989;80: 551.

Walker WG et al: Uses and complications of diuretic therapy: A symposium. Johns Hopkins Med J 1976;121: 194.

Walsh RW et al: Beneficial hemodynamic effects of intravenous and oral diltiazem in severe congestive heart failure. J Am Coll Cardiol 1984;3:1044.

Weber KT, Janicki JS: Cardiopulmonary exercise testing for evaluation of chronic cardiac failure. Am J Cardiol 1985;55(Suppl A):22.

Weber KT et al: Long-term vasodilator therapy with trimazosin in chronic cardiac failure. N Engl J Med 1980;303:242.

Wenger TL et al: Treatment of 63 severely digitalis-toxic patients with digoxin-specific antibody fragments. J Am Coll Cardiol 1985;5(Suppl A):118.

Whelton A (editor): Current trends in diuretic therapy. (Symposium.) Am J Cardiol 1986;57:1A.

Wynne J, Braunwald E: New treatment for congestive heart failure: Amrinone and milrinone. J Cardiovasc Med 1984;9:393.

Prognosis of Cardiac Failure

Baim DS et al: Survival of patients with severe congestive heart failure treated with oral milrinone. J Am Coll Cardiol 1986;7:661.

Bigger TJ Jr: Why patients with congestive heart failure die: Arrhythmias and sudden cardiac death. Circulation 1987;75(Suppl 4):28.

Cohn JN et al: A comparison of enalapril with hydralazine-isosorbide dinitrate in the treatment of chronic congestive heart failure. N Engl J Med 1991;325:303.

Cohn JN et al: Veterans Administration Cooperative Study on Vasodilator Therapy of Heart Failure: Influence of prerandomization variables on the reduction of mortality by treatment with hydralazine and isosorbide dinitrate. Circulation 1987;75(Suppl IV):49.

CONSENSUS Trial Study Group: Effects of enalapril on mortality in severe congestive heart failure: Results of the Cooperative North Scandinavian Enalapril Survival Study (CONSENSUS). N Engl J Med 1987;316: 1429.

Franciosa JA et al: Survival in men with severe chronic left ventricular failure due to either coronary heart disease or idiopathic dilated cardiomyopathy. Am J Cardiol 1983;51:831.

Likoff MJ, Chandler SL, Kay HR: Clinical determinants of mortality in chronic congestive heart failure secondary to idiopathic dilated or to ischemic cardiomyopathy. Am J Cardiol 1987;59:634.

Massie BM: Is neurohormonal activation deleterious to the long-term outcome of patients with congestive heart failure? J Am Coll Cardiol 1988;12:547.

Massie BM, Conway M: Survival of patients with congestive heart failure: Past, present, and future prospects. Circulation 1987;75(Suppl IV):11.

Packer M: Lack of relation between ventricular arrhythmia and sudden death in patients with chronic heart failure. Circulation 1992;85:I-50.

Packer M, Parmley WW (editors): Physiologic determinants of survival in congestive heart failure. (Symposium.) Circulation 1987;75(Suppl 4):IV-1.

Schocken DD et al: Prevalence and mortality rate of congestive heart failure in the United States. J Am Coll Cardiol 1992;20:301.

Setaro JF et al: Long term outcome in patients with congestive heart failure and intact systolic left ventricular performance. Am J Cardiol 1992;69:1212.

Stevenson LW et al: Poor survival of patients with idiopathic cardiomyopathy considered too well for transplantation. Am J Med 1987;83:871.

SOLVD Investigators: Effect of enalapril on survival in patients with reduced left ventricular ejection fractions and congestive heart failure. N Engl J Med 1991;325:293.

Wilson JR et al: Prognosis in severe heart failure: Relation to hemodynamic measurements and ventricular ectopic activity. J Am Coll Cardiol 1983;2:40

11 Congenital Heart Disease (With Special Reference to Adult Cardiology)

Congenital heart disease represents the largest share of pediatric cardiologic practice. Neonatal cardiology, which differs significantly from adult cardiology, is a subject of great current interest. Although it is reasonable to equate congenital heart disease in older children (6 years and over) with that seen in adults, it is not possible to devise a single description of the characteristics of congenital heart disease encompassing neonatal, infant, and adult disease. This chapter is confined to the clinical picture of congenital lesions as seen in adults and older children and does not purport to describe congenital heart disease as seen in infants.

Presentations of Congenital Heart Disease in the Adult

The internist or the cardiologist will see patients with congenital heart disease in a variety of settings.

A. Hemodynamically Minor Lesions: The importance of these lesions is that—

1. The diagnosis is missed or mistaken, eg, a right-sided aortic arch is misdiagnosed as a right parasternal mass.

2. The natural history of the lesion is important, eg, the development of infective endocarditis on a bicuspid aortic valve or the development of calcific degenerative changes and severe aortic stenosis later in life.

B. Hemodynamically Significant Lesions:

1. Undiagnosed lesions, eg, atrial septal defect, ventricular septal defect, patent ductus arteriosus.

2. Lesions that are at present inoperable, eg, ventricular septal defect and pulmonary hypertension, Eisenmenger's syndrome.

C. Surgically Palliated Lesions:

1. With physiologic improvement, eg, Blalock-Taussig shunt in tetralogy of Fallot and atrial-to-pulmonary artery shunt (Fontan procedure) in tricuspid atresia.

2. With anatomic physiologic correction, the largest number of patients seen, eg, patched interventricular septal defect, closed atrial defect, and corrected tetralogy of Fallot.

3. Above with complications at surgery, eg, pulmonary valve insufficiency, patch aneurysm, and calcification of conduit.

D. Surgically "Cured": Very few lesions can be said to be completely "cured." Ligated patent ductus arteriosus is one example. All other lesions have potential late complications for which the patient must be observed.

Causes of Congenital Heart Disease

The basic causes of congenital heart disease, which occurs in about 0.9% of live births, are unknown.

Definite genetic causes have been identified, eg, one gene abnormality in some families of patients with Marfan's disease. Another proved genetic abnormality is trisomy 21 (Down's syndrome). Other congenital occurrences are undoubtedly due to environmental causes and toxic substances that affect the developing embryo at a stage crucial to cardiac development and result in congenital heart disease. Peripheral pulmonary stenosis and patent ductus arteriosus are seen in babies of mothers with German measles during the first trimester.

In Western countries, the diagnosis is usually made in the first 5 years of life. The same spectrum of congenital lesions is seen in all parts of the world, and congenital abnormalities in other systems are seen in only about a third of cases. This pattern of involvement of the heart alone suggests that disturbances in the complex embryologic development of the heart account for most of the lesions. Congenital lesions are not confined to humans and are seen in virtually all mammals.

Classification of Congenital Heart Disease

A classification based on embryologic studies has limited use for adult patients. The clinical classification used in this book gives an indication of the relative frequency with which lesions are encountered after puberty.

Not all forms of congenital heart disease are described in this chapter. The commonest abnormality—bicuspid aortic valve—which occurs in about 2% of the population, is most relevant to aortic valve disease and is described in Chapter 13. Similarly, congenital mitral valve lesions are described with other forms of mitral disease in Chapter 12, and hyper-

Table 11–1. Classification of congenital heart disease.

Predominant left-to-right shunts
Examples:
 Atrial septal defects
 Ventricular septal defects
 Patent ductus arteriosus
Predominant right-to-left shunts (arterial desaturation)
Examples:
 Tetralogy of Fallot
 Ventricular septal defect, patent ductus arteriosus, atrial
  septal defect with pulmonary vascular disease
  (Eisenmenger's syndrome)
Valvular stenosis and atresia, and chamber atresia
Examples:
 Pulmonary valve stenosis
 Right ventricular hypoplastic syndromes
 Pulmonary atresia
Great-vessel anomalies, venous and arterial
Examples:
 Coarctation of the aorta
 Total anomalous pulmonary venous return
Transposition and inversions
Examples:
 Dextrocardia with situs inversus, "corrected"
 L-transposition of the great vessels
 Transposition of the great vessels

trophic obstructive cardiomyopathy is dealt with in Chapter 17 along with other types of cardiomyopathy. Rare congenital conditions that mimic valvular disease, such as cor triatriatum and sinus of Valsalva aneurysm, are also described in the valve disease chapters. Acquired ventricular septal defect is described under coronary artery disease in Chapter 8 rather than under ventricular septal defect.

The possible combinations of different forms of congenital heart lesions are legion, and they will be mentioned only in passing. Each heading in the classification covers a number of forms of disease that differ in severity, anatomic detail, and pathophysiology.

A useful anatomic-pathophysiologic classification is shown in Table 11–1. In this classification, all congenital cardiovascular lesions can be categorized in one or more groups. For example, tetralogy of Fallot can be classified in the right-to-left shunt and in the valvular stenosis groups. Furthermore, each pathophysiologic lesion can occur at one or more "levels" of the cardiovascular system: Left-to-right shunts can occur at the venous level, eg, anomalous pulmonary vein draining into the innominate vein or superior vena cava; at the atrial level, eg, atrial septal defect, ruptured sinus of Valsalva into the right atrium; at the ventricular level, eg, ventricular septal defect, ruptured sinus of Valsalva into the right ventricular outflow tract; or at the arterial level, eg, patent ductus arteriosus, aortopulmonary window.

Syndromes Due to Genetic Abnormalities

Several specific syndromes involve congenital cardiovascular lesions as common manifestations of genetically determined disease.

Marfan's syndrome is an autosomally dominant trait that involves mesodermal tissue. Its manifestations involve the eye and the skeleton, as well as the cardiovascular system. In the eye, myopia, dislocation of the lens, and retinal detachment are commonly seen. The skeletal abnormalities include long arms and legs and big hands and feet. The patient's arm span characteristically exceeds the patient's height. Arachnodactyly, kyphoscoliosis, and laxity of the joints are also seen. About a third of cases have congenital cardiovascular disease. Congenital abnormality of the media of the aorta, consisting of a decrease in the number of smooth muscle cells and fragmentation of elastic lamellae of the aortic media, leads to aortic dilation with aortic incompetence (Chapter 13) and aortic dissection (Chapter 9). Atrial septal defect is also associated with Marfan's syndrome.

Down's syndrome (trisomy 21) is a common form of mental retardation due to chromosomal abnormality. It has an incidence directly related to the age of the mother and occurs in more than 1% of births in 45-year-old women. Congenital heart disease occurs in about 20% of cases, the commonest lesions being ostium primum defect (see Atrial Septal Defect, below) and ventricular septal defect (p 352).

Turner's syndrome (primary ovarian agenesis) is confined to females and is due to the lack of one X chromosome. It causes infantilism, dwarfism, a web neck, cubitus valgus, and primary amenorrhea. The cardiovascular lesions associated with Turner's syndrome are coarctation of the aorta and pulmonary stenosis.

ATRIAL SEPTAL DEFECT

Atrial septal defect is the commonest and most important congenital heart lesion the cardiologist is likely to encounter in adults.

Anatomic Types

The clinical syndrome of atrial septal defect covers a wide range of lesions that are often clinically indistinguishable. The anatomic sites of the different types of defects are shown in diagrammatic form in Figure 11–1. The commonest form—**ostium secundum defect**—involves the center of the atrial septum in the area of the fossa ovalis. The next most common—**ostium primum defect**—involves the lower part of the septum above the atrioventricular valves. The valves themselves are not infrequently cleft, giving rise to incompetence of the mitral or tricuspid valves. An even more extensive form of the defect results in a **complete endocardial cushion defect,** in which there is also a ventricular septal defect and a common atrioventricular canal. This defect is seen in about 20% of persons with Down's syndrome. A third form of defect involves the upper part of the septum and is

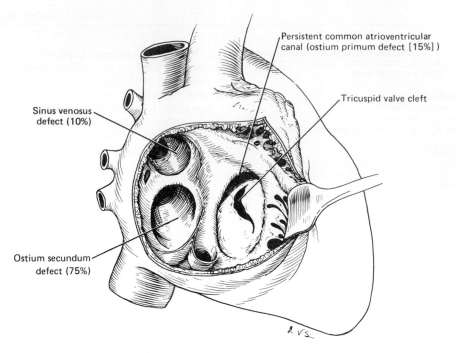

Anatomic features of atrial septal defects.

Cardinal features: *Left-to-right shunt into right atrium; high tricuspid flow; increased pulmonary blood flow; normal pulmonary arterial pressure.*

Variable factors: *Size of defect; size of shunt; anomalous venous drainage with sinus venosus defect; valve clefts with ostium primum defect.*

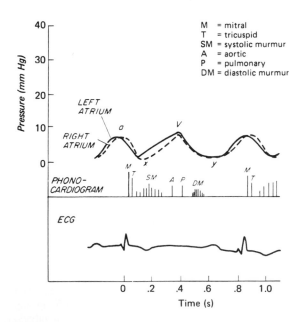

M = mitral
T = tricuspid
SM = systolic murmur
A = aortic
P = pulmonary
DM = diastolic murmur

Diagram showing auscultatory and hemodynamic features of atrial septal defect.

Chest x-ray of a patient with an ostium secundum atrial septal defect. The heart is large, with a prominent pulmonary artery (PA) and a small aorta.

Figure 11–1. Atrial septal defect. Structures enlarged: right atrium, right ventricle, pulmonary artery, and left atrium. Note small left ventricle and aorta.

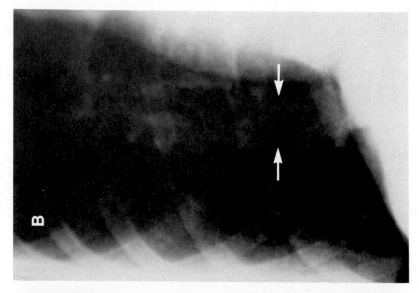

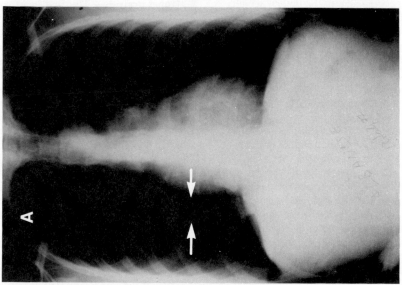

Figure 11–2. Scimitar vein syndrome. **A:** Chest x-ray, posteroanterior view, in a patient with total anomalous pulmonary venous drainage to the right lung. The arrows indicate the "scimitar" sign, which is the vertical anomalous pulmonary vein parallel to the right atrium. This anomalous vein drains the entire right lung into the vena cava at the level of the diaphragm. **B:** Detail of an angiogram of a patient with anomalous drainage of the right lung into the inferior vena cava. Note the opacified anomalous veins paralleling the right atrium (arrows).

known as **sinus venosus defect.** More unusually, it can be at the lower posterior part of the atrial septum near the inferior vena cava orifice. It is the most unusual of the types of atrial septal defects and is often associated with partial anomalous pulmonary venous drainage, usually drainage of the right upper lobe into the superior vena cava. A persistent left-sided superior vena cava and anomalous venous drainage into the coronary sinus or right atrium may occur. In most cases with anomalous venous drainage, there is also an atrial defect.

Partial or complete unilateral anomalous pulmonary venous drainage to the inferior vena cava gives rise to radiologic picture known as the **scimitar vein syndrome** (Figure 11–2). The "scimitar" is the anomalous pulmonary vein seen either along the right cardiac border or, in cases in which there is sequestered lung and rightward displacement of the heart, behind the cardiac silhouette. It is associated with thoracic abnormalities involving the lungs and chest wall.

Cardinal Features & Pathogenesis

The essential feature of atrial septal defect is a left-to-right shunt of pulmonary venous return into the right atrium that produces a high tricuspid flow and increased blood flow to the lungs, with a normal pulmonary arterial pressure. The severity of the lesion depends only in part on the size of the defect, which can limit the size of the shunt. Atrial septal defect is often not diagnosed in infancy or childhood. At birth, the right and left ventricles are equal in size and thickness, and right-to-left shunt via a patent foramen ovale can normally occur. Whenever an atrial septal defect is present, however, left-to-right shunting is minimal at birth. With the normal decrease in pulmonary vascular resistance that follows birth, the right ventricle becomes more compliant. It then fills more readily than the left ventricle, and as a result, left-to-right shunting becomes apparent. Most atrial septal defects are large enough (2×2 cm or more) to equalize pressures between the right and left atrium. Thus, the magnitude of the left-to-right shunt depends mainly on the filling characteristics of the right and left ventricles. The increased pulmonary flow is readily accepted by the pulmonary circulation, so that pulmonary arterial pressure is usually low. The presence of anomalous venous drainage does not affect the clinical picture, but the presence of associated mitral or tricuspid incompetence or a complete endocardial cushion defect makes the lesion more severe.

Clinical Findings

A. Symptoms and Signs: The diagnosis of atrial septal defect is easily missed, and the examiner must maintain a high index of suspicion if all cases are to be recognized.

About half of patients with atrial septal defect are asymptomatic when the diagnosis is made. Symptoms develop in 60% of patients by age 30. The lesion is often noted in early adult life, either on routine physical examination or (more often) on a chest x-ray. The commonest presenting symptom is dyspnea on exertion (65%), followed by palpitations due to atrial arrhythmia (20%), and chest pain, which is usually not anginal in nature. A spurious past history of rheumatic fever may be present (5%). In about 20% of adult cases, the diagnosis of atrial septal defect presents some difficulty, either because the patient is middle-aged and the possibility of a congenital lesion is not considered or because the clinical picture is atypical. In about half of these cases, the patient is in right heart failure when first seen and edema and ascites tend to be more prominent than dyspnea.

Patients with Marfan's syndrome or other skeletal abnormalities (eg, Ehlers-Danlos syndrome or arachnodactyly) may also have atrial septal defects.

1. Cardiac signs– The physical signs depend on the magnitude of pulmonary blood flow and the status of pulmonary vascular resistance. Increased right ventricular stroke volume produces a hyperdynamic right ventricular impulse with a visible and palpable pulse over the pulmonary artery in the second or third left intercostal space. A pulmonary systolic ejection murmur is almost always present because of increased flow through the pulmonary valve, but the murmur is often soft.

2. Heart sounds– The first heart sound is often loud because the tricuspid valve closes from a wide open position with right ventricular systole. There is relative tricuspid stenosis in atrial septal defect because the diastolic flow across the tricuspid valve is usually twice the normal value or more. In addition to the loud tricuspid first sound, there is often a right-sided third sound and a tricuspid diastolic murmur that becomes louder during inspiration. The presence of a midsystolic click suggests associated mitral valve prolapse.

The second heart sound is widely split in patients with atrial septal defect. The normal widening of the split with inspiration does not occur (Figure 11–3).

3. Mitral and tricuspid incompetence– In patients with ostium primum defects there may also be a hyperdynamic left ventricular impulse and a pansystolic apical murmur if mitral incompetence is present. Tricuspid incompetence also occurs with ostium primum defects, giving a pansystolic murmur that is best heard at the left lower sternal border. Incompetence of the atrioventricular valves can also occur in ostium secundum defects, especially when heart failure develops.

4. Pulse– The pulse is of normal or small amplitude, and the venous pressure is normal. A prominent V wave can be seen in the cervical veins at times, although the jugular venous pressure is rarely elevated. Atrial fibrillation commonly develops in about 10–20% of patients after age 40, and other varieties of atrial arrhythmia are also seen.

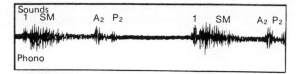

Figure 11–3. Ejection murmur (SM) and widely split second sound recorded at the upper left sternal border in a patient with atrial septal defect. (Courtesy of Roche Laboratories Division of Hoffman-La Roche, Inc.)

B. Electrocardiographic Findings: The ECG demonstrates the pattern of incomplete bundle branch block in 90% of individuals with an atrial septal defect (Figure 11–4).

In the 10% of patients in whom the ECG is normal, the diagnosis is more difficult. Left axis deviation in a patient with a right ventricular conduction defect (Figure 11–5) is strongly suggestive of ostium primum defect, but a normal or rightward axis does not rule out such a defect. If pulmonary hypertension develops, there will almost certainly be evidence of progressive right ventricular hypertrophy on the ECG. The presence of a tall secondary R wave in patients with conduction defects has been taken as evidence of right ventricular hypertrophy, but this sign may be due solely to the late depolarization of the right ventricular outflow tract.

C. Imaging Studies: The chest x-ray is of great importance in the diagnosis of atrial septal defect. The heart is usually enlarged in proportion to the pulmonary blood flow, and the main pulmonary artery and its branches are dilated and stand out in contrast to the aorta, which looks small (Figure 11–1). The right atrium is more prominent in this lesion than in any other except Ebstein's malformation, and

the right ventricle is also enlarged. A persistent left-sided superior vena cava is common in sinus venosus defects and can be seen on the chest x-ray (Figure 11–6).

Pulmonary plethora with increased lung markings due to enlarged pulmonary arteries and veins is common. These signs are due to increased pulmonary blood flow and are nonspecific.

D. Special Investigations:

1. Noninvasive techniques–

a. Echocardiography can be used to detect reduced or paradoxic movement of the ventricular septum as well as increased right ventricular size. These signs are indicative of increased right ventricular stroke volume, which suggests but does not specifically establish a diagnosis of atrial septal defect. Tricuspid or pulmonary incompetence can also cause this sign.

Atrial septal defects are not well seen in the conventional two-dimensional echocardiographic views. A subcostal approach intersects the atrial septum at a more favorable angle and improves the recognition of defects. Combination of two-dimensional echocardiography with Doppler studies can provide an estimate of the pulmonary-to-systemic flow ratio that correlates closely with values obtained at cardiac catheterization. The development of Doppler color flow mapping has increased the accuracy of ultrasonic diagnosis of atrial defects. This new technique allows the pattern and direction of flow through the defect to be seen (Figure 11–7).

The presence of an interatrial communication can usually be established by contrast echocardiography (see also Chapter 5).

Most often, the presence of an atrial septal defect and the magnitude of left-to-right shunt can be accurately diagnosed by Doppler echocardiography. In

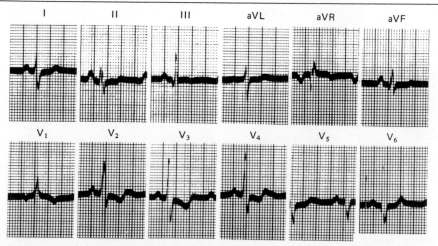

Figure 11–4. ECG from a 23-year-old woman with atrial septal defect proved by catheter. Widely split second sound and short systolic murmur at the base on phonocardiogram. Incomplete right bundle branch block with rsR in lead V$_1$. Right ventricular pressure ^{35}/₀.

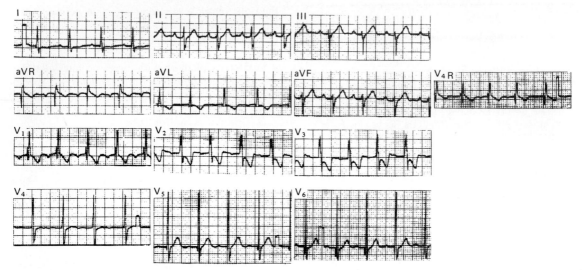

Figure 11–5. ECG of a patient with ostium primum defect showing left axis deviation and right bundle branch block. (Reproduced, with permission, from Chung EK: *Electrocardiography.* Harper & Row, 1974.)

this situation, as long as there is no question of the shunt size or the pulmonary vascular resistance, surgery can be undertaken without further study.

b. Radionuclear studies can be used to estimate the size of the left-to-right shunt. First-pass radioangiography with ^{99m}Tc, injected as a bolus and detected with a gamma camera, generates a time-activity curve, and computer-based deconvolution of the curve provides a measure of the pulmonary-to-systemic flow ratio. The difference between right and left ventricular stroke volumes can be determined from the ratio of counts leaving the left and right ventricles with each beat. Gated cardiac pool scan-

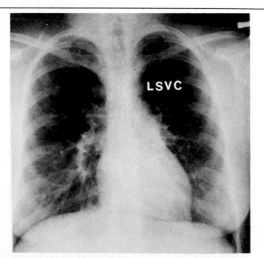

Figure 11–6. Chest x-ray of a 19–year-old woman with sinus venosus atrial septal defect with anomalous pulmonary venous drainage and a persistent left-sided superior vena cava (LSVC).

ning can also be used to measure the right ventricular ejection fraction.

2. Invasive techniques–

a. Cardiac catheterization is used in atrial septal defect to measure pulmonary and systemic blood pressure and flow and to pass the catheter through the atrial septal defect into the left atrium and ventricle. The chances of passing the catheter across an atrial defect are better if the study is performed using the femoral vein, but the pulmonary artery is more difficult to enter using the leg approach. The left and right atrial mean pressures usually appear to be equal, and the pressure difference across the defect is small and occurs mainly late in systole, before the *v* wave, as shown in Figure 11–8. These pressure fluctuations occur during the cardiac cycle and form the basis for paradoxic embolism seen in patients with atrial septal defects and even patent foramen ovale.

b. Pulmonary flow measurement– Pulmonary arterial oxygen saturation gives a rough indication of the size of pulmonary blood flow. Values between 80% and 85% indicate slightly increased flow; 85–90%, moderate increase; and over 90%, a large flow. The accuracy of pulmonary flow measurements falls as the size of the left-to-right shunt increases. The pulmonary arteriovenous oxygen difference becomes smaller, with the result that small errors in the measurement of oxygen content have a large effect on the calculated pulmonary flow.

c. Systemic flow measurement– Systemic output cannot be accurately measured in atrial septal defect because mixed venous oxygen content is difficult to measure. Some appropriately adjusted average value for superior and inferior vena caval oxygen contents must be selected to use as a value for a mixed venous sample. It is conventionally assumed

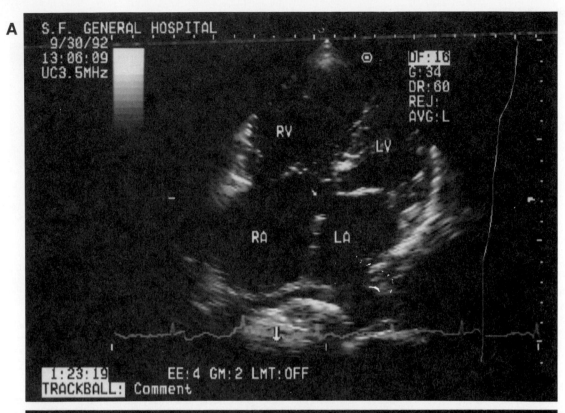

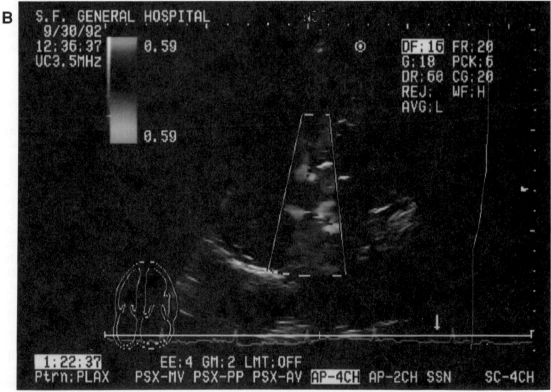

Figure 11–7. ***A:*** Two-dimensional echocardiogram of a 70-year-old man in the four-chamber view with a secundum interatrial septal defect. Pulmonary blood flow was twice the systemic blood flow. Small white arrow points to the defect. (RV, right ventricle; RA, right atrium; LA, left atrium; LV, left ventricle.) ***B:*** Color Doppler showing flow through the defect in the Doppler window.

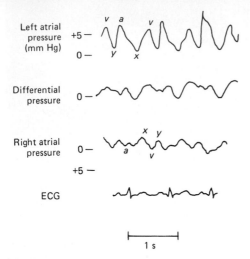

Figure 11–8. Simultaneous left and right atrial and differential pressure across an atrial septal defect. The pressure difference across the defect is greatest before the *v* wave. The right atrial pressure tracing is inverted because it is recorded by a differential manometer.

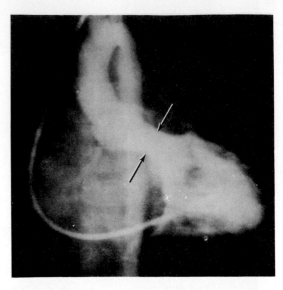

Figure 11–9. Left ventricular angiogram in a patient with ostium primum defect showing "gooseneck" deformity of the left ventricular outflow tract.(Courtesy of E Carlsson.)

that the mixed venous oxygen content is one-third of the superior vena caval content plus two-thirds of the inferior vena caval content. However, because of the large amount of highly saturated blood from the renal veins and incomplete mixing, the inferior vena cava saturation is falsely elevated and the calculated shunt underestimated. A more accurate estimation of the magnitude of the shunt is obtained if the mixed venous oxygen content is estimated by using the averaged two parts superior vena caval and one part inferior vena caval oxygen content. With age, the left ventricle becomes stiffer and less compliant. The resistance to filling in diastole is increased compared with the right ventricle, thereby increasing the left-to-right shunt.

Systemic blood flow tends to vary with age in patients with atrial septal defect. It is normal in young persons and decreases with age as atrial fibrillation and heart failure become more prevalent. The increase in pulmonary to systemic flow ratio with age is due as much to a decrease in systemic flow as to an increase in pulmonary flow. With age, the left ventricle becomes stiffer and less compliant. The resistance to filling in diastole is increased compared with the right ventricle, thereby increasing the left-to-right shunt.

d. Complete anatomic diagnosis of atrial septal defect cannot be established with certainty in all cases. Unexpected anomalies of pulmonary venous return may be overlooked. Recognition of ostium primum defects is important, since patching of the defect and mitral valve surgery may be needed instead of simple closure of the defect. Left ventricular angiography is the best means of diagnosing this lesion.

A "gooseneck" deformity of the left ventricular outflow tract is seen on a posteroanterior view of the ventricle (Figure 11–9). This narrowing of the outflow tract of the left ventricle is caused by an abnormal attachment of the anterior leaflet of the mitral valve to the ventricular septum.

e. Intracardiac pressure measurements in atrial septal defect are an important procedure. Right-sided pressures are usually lower than expected. Pressure differences between the right ventricle and the pulmonary artery are found in patients with markedly increased flow (flow gradient) and in patients with associated pulmonary stenosis.

Right and left atrial pressures may be raised in older patients in whom heart failure has occurred, but values over 15 mm Hg are uncommon when the two atria are in free communication. In small defects there may be a detectable mean pressure difference between the two atria. A raised left atrial pressure with a significant pressure difference between the two atria indicates a small atrial defect and associated mitral disease. This may be either congenital, as in ostium primum lesions, or acquired, as in Lutembacher's syndrome, where it is presumably rheumatic in origin.

f. Pulmonary vascular resistance should be measured in all patients with atrial septal defect. It is normally less that 2 mm Hg/L/min. It tends to be slightly raised (up to 3.5 mm Hg/L/min) in older patients with large shunts. A marked increase in resistance (7.5 mm Hg/L/min or more) constitutes a possible contraindication to surgery, and the decision whether or not to close the defect may be difficult.

Differential Diagnosis

A. Rheumatic Heart Disease: Atrial septal defect is likely to be misdiagnosed as rheumatic mitral valve disease with mixed mitral stenosis and incompetence. The combination of cardiac enlargement, systolic and diastolic murmurs arising at the atrioventricular valves, and atrial fibrillation in a middle-aged woman can easily be mistaken for a rheumatic lesion, and pulmonary plethora due to increased blood flow can be confused in the chest x-ray with pulmonary congestion. The presence of a large heart with only mild symptoms and the patient's ability to easily tolerate the onset of atrial fibrillation should suggest the possibility of an atrial defect.

B. Other Lesions: Small atrial septal defects may be confused with a normal heart especially in the presence of pectus excavatum. Idiopathic dilation of the pulmonary artery may also lead to confusion. Atrial septal defect is often difficult to diagnose during pregnancy. Many of the physical findings and radiographic features may be mimicked by the physiologic state seen in pregnancy, with high cardiac output and high diaphragm, making the heart seem enlarged.

Complications

A. Pulmonary Vascular Disease: Pulmonary vascular disease is the most important complication of atrial septal defect. In patients with ostium secundum defects, it is always acquired after puberty. In patients with ostium primum or sinus venosus defects with anomalous venous drainage, the congenital form of pulmonary hypertension (Eisenmenger's syndrome) occurs, in which a raised pulmonary vascular resistance develops in infancy or childhood and does not develop in later life. Acquired pulmonary hypertension is due to the long-term effects of increased pulmonary blood flow on the pulmonary vascular bed, and pulmonary thromboembolism may initiate or aggravate the condition, especially in pregnancy. The incidence of this form of pulmonary hypertension, sometimes called acquired Eisenmenger's syndrome, is decreasing with earlier and more accurate diagnosis of congenital heart disease, but it still occurs in about 5% of cases. This complication is not inevitable, occurring in only about 10% of adult patients with large atrial septal defects.

1. Symptoms and signs of pulmonary vascular disease– Increased dyspnea or cyanosis on exertion and intolerance of altitude are the commonest presenting symptoms. The patient may develop cyanosis and clubbing of the fingers, and polycythemia and increase in hematocrit are almost invariably found. There is usually a large *a* wave in the jugular venous pulse, and the heart is almost always greatly enlarged, with a prominent right ventricular heave. A pulmonary ejection click and a loud pulmonary valve closure sound are heard, and the second sound is closely split. The ECG shows right ventricular hypertrophy and often atrial fibrillation (Figure 11–10). Chest x-ray confirms cardiac enlargement and usually shows marked enlargement of the central pulmonary arteries. There is a progressive increase in the heart size and also in the size of the pulmonary arteries (Figure 11–11).

2. Cardiac catheterization– Cardiac catheterization shows pulmonary arterial hypertension and a pulmonary blood flow that is normal or only slightly increased. Right-to-left intracardiac shunting may be present at rest, with an arterial saturation of 85–95%,

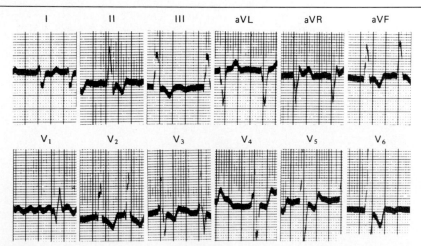

| I | II | III | aVL | aVR | aVF |

| V₁ | V₂ | V₃ | V₄ | V₅ | V₆ |

Figure 11–10. ECG of a 56–year-old woman with severe cardiac failure, pulmonary hypertension, and large atrial septal defect proved at autopsy. Tracing shows atrial fibrillation, right ventricular hypertrophy, and right ventricular conduction delay.

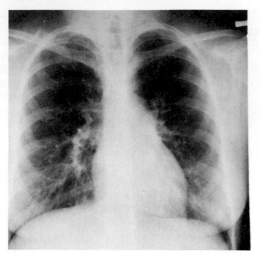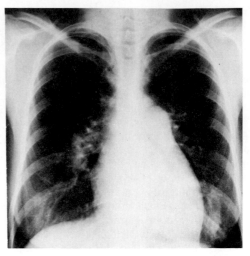

Figure 11–11. Serial chest x-rays taken 4 years apart in a 19-year-old patient with an atrial septal defect (sinus venosus) and systemic lupus erythematosus in whom severe pulmonary vascular disease developed. Heart size increased, and pulmonary arterial enlargement became more prominent.

or desaturation may develop during exercise. Accurate measurement of pulmonary vascular resistance—plus study of the effects of vasodilator drugs such as tolazoline or acetylcholine plus oxygen breathing—is needed to decide whether surgery is warranted. Closure of the defect is likely to be successful when the pulmonary vascular resistance does not exceed 7.5 mm Hg/L/min. Closure of the defect is usually not indicated if the arterial saturation is below 90%. The magnitude of the left-to-right shunt is a factor of almost equal importance. If the pulmonary blood flow is increased, closing the defect can reduce the load on

pulmonary circulation and reverse or halt the progress of pulmonary vascular disease. Surgery in advanced cases has a high mortality rate, and the results are poor because the "safety valve" of an actual or potential right-to-left shunt is removed.

B. Heart Failure: Heart failure is the other, almost equally important complication of atrial septal defect (Figure 11–12). It is usually seen in association with atrial fibrillation and is directly related to the age of the patient and the presence of a disease decreasing left ventricular compliance and interfering with the filling of the left ventricle. In some instances, heart

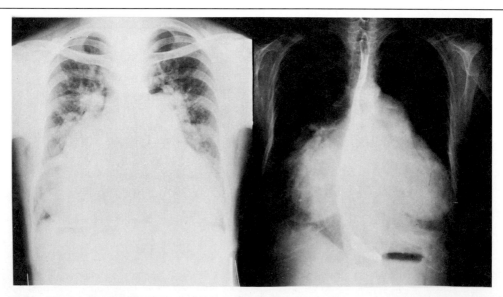

Figure 11–12. Chest x-ray with overpenetrated view and barium-filled esophagus in a patient with atrial septal defect in heart failure.

failure occurs in the absence of a left ventricular lesion. The mechanism of failure in these cases in obscure. It has been suggested that right ventricular dilation compromises left ventricular filling.

C. Atrial Arrhythmias: Atrial fibrillation and other atrial arrhythmias are common, especially atrial fibrillation after age 40 in the absence of surgical treatment. These arrhythmias are also related to the severity of the lesion and are less common in patients with small shunts. Restoration of sinus rhythm should be postponed until after surgery. Unfortunately, recurrence of atrial fibrillation even after closure of the atrial septal defect is common.

D. Other Complications: Infective endocarditis is rare in atrial septal defect. Patients with ostium primum defects are more prone to develop this complication than are those with other atrial septal defects, presumably because of valvular involvement.

Treatment

Surgery is the treatment of choice in patients with atrial septal defect

A. Closure of Defect: Closure of atrial defects is performed under direct vision during cardiopulmonary bypass. Ostium secundum defects can usually be sutured directly; the insertion of patches and baffles is likely to be needed only in ostium primum and sinus venosus defects. Although surgery almost always closes the atrial defect, residual defects may be overlooked, or the lesion may recur if stitches tear out postoperatively. Only rarely does a large left-to-right shunt recur.

B. Relocation of Pulmonary Veins: Relocation of pulmonary veins is needed in patients with partial anomalous venous drainage. The atrial septal defect can often be sutured in such a way as to provide a tunnel through which the anomalous venous flow can be redirected into the left atrium without actually transecting the anomalous vein.

C. Mitral Incompetence: Partial suture of valve clefts, especially in the mitral valve, is the treatment of choice in younger patients. It is especially important to avoid excessive closure of the cleft, since this shortens the anterior leaflet and frequently causes or aggravates mitral incompetence or may cause mitral stenosis. Residual mitral incompetence is common. Mitral valve replacement is reserved for older patients.

Indications & Contraindications to Surgery

Surgery is indicated in all patients with a pulmonary-to-systemic flow ratio of 2:1 or more. Smaller defects can safely be left open, especially when there is a significant pressure difference across the defect. Age is no bar to surgery. The operation is recommended for asymptomatic persons because it markedly reduces pulmonary blood flow in patients with large shunts and most patients will develop symptoms in middle age. If heart failure develops, the patient should receive medical treatment with digitalis and diuretics, and surgical correction should be undertaken when the patient's condition has stabilized. In patients whose vascular resistance is low, the mortality rate should be less than 1%. In patients with severe pulmonary vascular disease, the results of surgery are significantly worse, with a mortality rate of around 10%. Severe pulmonary vascular disease with shunt reversal is the principal contraindication to surgery. An attempt to restore sinus rhythm should be made about 6 weeks after operation in any patient with atrial fibrillation or flutter in whom arrhythmia persists. If atrial fibrillation persists the patient should be anticoagulated with warfarin.

Prognosis

The prognosis in atrial septal defect is good even without surgical treatment, and if operation is performed before symptoms develop, the patient should have a normal life expectancy. Patients with small defects who do not develop associated degenerative or atherosclerotic lesions in middle life may live long enough to die of another cause. The possibility of increasing left-to-right shunting with increasing age, the development of atrial fibrillation, and left ventricular disease are generally sufficient causes to advise surgery without waiting for signs of deteriorating cardiac function. The prognosis in ostium secundum lesions is better than that in ostium primum defects, and the development of pulmonary hypertension greatly worsens the prognosis.

Long-Term Results in Operated Cases

The long-term results after atrial septal defect closure are better than those after any other intracardiac operation. Since closure under direct vision became the rule, incomplete closure has become rare. Heart size may not return to normal if a large defect has been closed after puberty. The second heart sound may remain split and a systolic murmur may persist in spite of closure of the defect. The rsR′ pattern usually persists in the ECG, and the pulmonary arteries remain large on the chest x-ray.

Right ventricular function does not always return to normal, especially in patients in whom closure of the defect is carried out in adult life. Atrial arrhythmias usually persist or recur in older patients.

PULMONARY STENOSIS

All forms of obstruction to blood flow to the lungs associated with an intact ventricular septum are included under this heading. Thus, patients with valvular stenosis, infundibular stenosis (involving the part of the right ventricle distal to the crista supraventricularis), and pulmonary artery stenosis of all

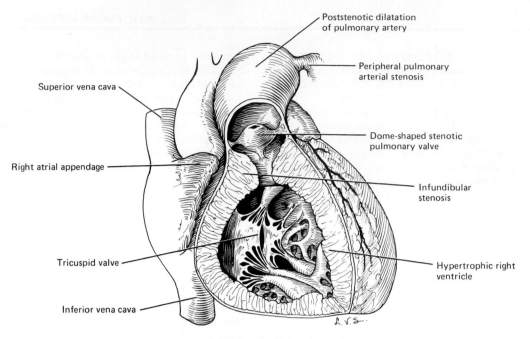

Anatomic features of pulmonary stenosis.

Cardinal features: *Reduction in pulmonary blood flow; right ventricular hypertrophy; murmur at the site of obstruction.*

Variable factors: *Severity of obstruction; site of obstruction: valvular, infundibular, or in pulmonary artery; patency of foramen ovale determines reversed interatrial shunt.*

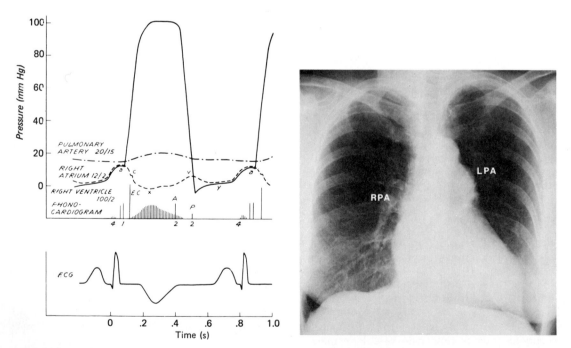

Diagram showing auscultatory and hemodynamic features of pulmonary stenosis. EC, ejection click; A, aortic; P, pulmonary.

Chest x-ray of a patient with severe pulmonary stenosis showing large left pulmonary artery (LPA). RPA, right pulmonary artery.

Figure 11–13. Pulmonary stenosis. Structures enlarged: right ventricle and sometimes pulmonary artery (poststenotic dilation).

degrees of severity are included, while Fallot's tetralogy and more complex lesions in which obstruction to the flow of blood to the lungs is associated with ventricular septal defect are described elsewhere.

Cardinal Features & Pathogenesis

The cardinal features of pulmonary stenosis include reduction in pulmonary blood flow, right ventricular hypertrophy, and a murmur at the site of obstruction. Among the variable factors that may be operating, the severity of obstruction influences the pulmonary blood flow and the extent of hypertrophy. Other factors are the site of obstruction (valvular, infundibular, or in the pulmonary artery) and the patency of the foramen ovale, which determines the presence of reversed interatrial shunt.

Pulmonary stenosis is a common form of congenital heart disease in adults mainly because this category includes patients with hemodynamically insignificant lesions. Two-thirds of adult cases are mild, and many could be classified as examples of idiopathic dilation of the pulmonary artery. Severe pulmonary valvular stenosis in the adult is rare. The spectrum of cases as shown in Figure 11–13 is wide because of differences in severity and of varying sites of obstruction.

Female patients with Turner's syndrome characterized by 45 rather than 46 chromosomes—or male patients with Noonan's syndrome—may have pulmonary stenosis. Amenorrhea in females, ocular hypertelorism, webbing of the neck, and short stature are seen in these syndromes. Peripheral pulmonary artery stenosis is one of the lesions commonly associated with maternal rubella.

Clinical Findings

A. Symptoms: Hemodynamically insignificant or mild pulmonary stenosis does not cause significant symptoms. Detection of a murmur during physical examination may cause the patient to become abnormally aware of the heart and develop noncardiac pain.

1. Dyspnea– While many patients with pulmonary stenosis are asymptomatic, dyspnea is the commonest presenting symptom in patients with moderate or severe pulmonary stenosis. Its origin is obscure, and the conventional explanation of cardiac dyspnea—pulmonary congestion and reduced lung compliance—is not applicable. Patients with pulmonary stenosis tend to hyperventilate during exercise, and inadequate perfusion of the exercising muscles is thought to provoke reflex ventilatory stimulation.

2. Dizziness and faintness on exertion, palpitations, and chest pain– These may rarely be the presenting symptoms in severe cases of pulmonary stenosis. The chest pain may be indistinguishable from that of angina of effort, and the fainting attacks are similar to the syncope on unaccustomed effort that occurs in patients with severe aortic stenosis.

3. Right heart failure– Right heart failure often occurs in early adult life in severe cases, and if the patient has not been seen previously, the diagnosis may be difficult when the patient presents in right heart failure with an extremely low cardiac output and little or no murmur.

B. Physical Signs: Cyanosis is seen only in severe cases. It may be peripheral and due to low cardiac output, or central and due to arterial desaturation as a result of reversed interatrial shunt through a patent foramen ovale. In this case, it may be associated with clubbing of the fingers and polycythemia.

The pulse is of small amplitude, and there is a prominent *a* wave in the jugular venous pulse in severe cases. In infants, the high pressure in the right atrium can blow open a patent foramen ovale, and cyanosis can occur. A right ventricular substernal heave is felt in moderate and severe cases. In infants, the high pressure in the right atrium can blow open a patent foramen ovale, and cyanosis can occur.

A systolic murmur is always present except in moribund patients. In cases of valvular stenosis, the duration of the murmur is a function of the severity of the lesion. In mild cases of valvular stenosis, the murmur is short and diamond-shaped on the tracing. It is preceded by an ejection click (Figure 11–14) whose intensity classically decreases on inspiration and increases on expiration. If the obstruction is infundibular, the murmur is longer and more like the pansystolic murmur of ventricular septal defect. In pulmonary artery stenosis, the murmur peaks later and resembles the murmur of aortic stenosis.

The loudness and timing of the pulmonary valve closure sound are valuable clues to the severity of valvular stenotic lesions. In mild cases, the second sound is normally or widely split, and the split moves normally with respiration. In moderately severe lesions, the pulmonary closure sound is delayed, occurring up to 0.1 s after aortic closure. It is also diminished in intensity because pulmonary blood flow tends to be low, but it still moves with inspiration (Figure 11–15). In severe cases, the pulmonary valve closure sound is inaudible, and even aortic closure may not be heard because the sound is buried in the long pulmonary systolic murmur that results from

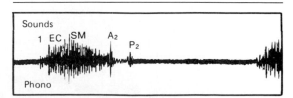

Figure 11–14. Typical phonocardiogram (recorded in third left interspace) in valvular pulmonary stenosis showing ejection click (EC), ejection murmur (SM), and late soft P$_2$. (Courtesy of Roche Laboratories Division of Hoffman- La Roche, Inc.)

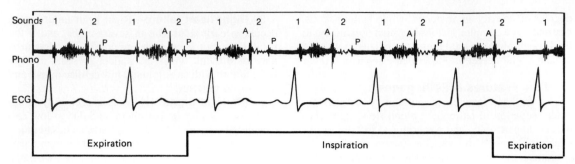

Figure 11–15. Phonocardiogram, showing ejection murmur and soft late P₂—later still on inspiration—in pulmonary stenosis. (Courtesy of Roche Laboratories Division of Hoffman-La Roche, Inc.)

prolonged contraction of the overloaded right ventricle. Pulmonary diastolic murmurs are uncommon before surgery, but pulmonary incompetence not infrequently follows valvotomy. In peripheral pulmonary artery stenosis the auscultatory findings can be confused with those of pulmonary hypertension because in both conditions pulmonary valve closure is usually loud and often palpable and the second sound is often split. The murmur of peripheral pulmonary artery stenosis is sometimes heard better or heard only in the axilla or in the back.

C. Electrocardiographic Findings: Right ventricular hypertrophy in pulmonary stenosis is proportionate to the severity of the obstruction to right ventricular outflow. In mild obstruction, the ECG shows only slight right ventricular dominance, whereas severe obstruction produces some of the most striking examples of right ventricular hypertrophy (Figure 11–16). In severe cases, tall, peaked P waves are evidence of right atrial enlargement, and right bundle branch block sometimes occurs.

D. Imaging Studies: In mild cases, the heart is of normal size. Even in moderate to severe cases, cardiac enlargement may be absent because hypertrophy of the right ventricle occurs at the expense of the cavity of the ventricle. If the patient develops right ventricular failure, however, cardiac enlargement involving the right ventricle and right atrium always occurs. The main pulmonary artery and left pulmonary artery are commonly enlarged when the lesion is valvular. Poststenotic dilation does not involve the right pulmonary artery, which is smaller and lies lower in the chest than the left pulmonary artery, as shown in Figure 11–13. Pulmonary arterial dilation is unrelated to the severity of stenosis, and in cases with insignificant lesions, the main pulmonary artery may be markedly dilated. In such cases a diagnosis of idiopathic dilation of the pulmonary artery is sometimes made, and it is not clear if a distinction can or should be made between hemodynamically insignificant pulmonary stenosis and idiopathic dilation of the pulmonary artery. In infundibular lesions, the pul-

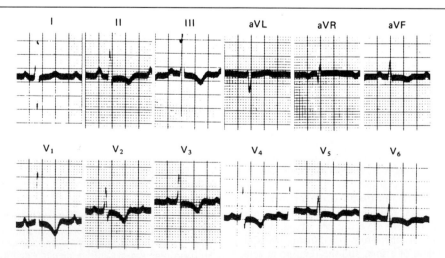

Figure 11–16. ECG of 25-year-old woman with pulmonary stenosis, patent interatrial septum, and cyanosis. Right ventricle, 1.5 cm; left ventricle, 1.1 cm. Normal coronary arteries. The tracing shows severe right ventricular hypertrophy.

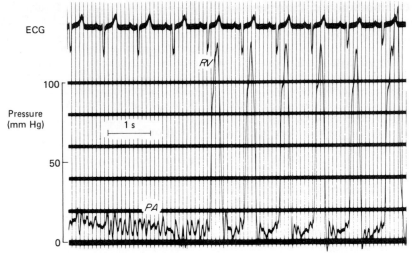

Figure 11–17. Pressure tracing showing withdrawal of a catheter across a stenotic pulmonary valve. (PA, pulmonary artery; RV, right ventricle.)

monary artery is not dilated, and the lesion is often associated with ventricular septal defect. Isolated infundibular stenosis is rarely seen. If the obstruction is severe, the configuration of the heart resembles that seen in Fallot's tetralogy with infundibular obstruction (seep 347). If the obstruction is in the pulmonary arteries, the main pulmonary artery is usually dilated. In any severe obstructive lesion, especially with right ventricular failure, the pulmonary blood flow is often reduced, and the lung markings are abnormally sparse.

E. Special Investigations:

1. Noninvasive techniques– Echocardiography is not always helpful in identifying the site of obstruction in pulmonary stenosis or in assessing its severity. The pulmonary valve is the most difficult valve to examine echographically, and the thickness of the valve does not always indicate the severity of the obstruction. However, it can be seen in the short-axis view, and even the doming of the pulmonary valve can be detected. Doppler studies can usually be used to estimate the pressure difference across the valve (see Chapter 4).

2. Invasive technique– The definitive technique for diagnosis and assessment of severity of pulmonary stenosis is cardiac catheterization. Measurement of pulmonary arterial and right ventricular pressures and pulmonary blood flow is needed to establish the diagnosis and severity of the stenosis. The anatomic site of the stenosis can usually be established by drawing the catheter from the pulmonary artery to the right atrium through the right ventricle and closely following the pressure changes. A sample tracing of pulmonary arterial and right ventricular pressures is shown in Figure 11–17. In patients with high infundibular lesions and those with both valvular and infu-

ndibular stenosis, angiography may be needed to establish the site of obstruction.

Differential Diagnosis

A. Atrial Septal Defect: Mild valvular lesions can resemble or be associated with an atrial septal defect. The systolic murmur and widely split second sound are common to both lesions.

B. Ventricular Septal Defect: Infundibular stenosis may be confused with a small ventricular septal defect because both lesions have a loud, long systolic murmur, best heard to the left of the sternum.

C. Pulmonary Hypertension: Pulmonary artery stenosis tends to be confused with primary pulmonary hypertension or with Eisenmenger's syndrome. The pressure in the main pulmonary artery is raised in these conditions, and the loud second heart sound and evidence of right ventricular overload are common to all of them.

D. Fallot's Tetralogy: When the pulmonary stenosis is moderate or severe and at the valvular or infundibular level, Fallot's tetralogy is the most important differential diagnosis. The ready fall in arterial oxygen saturation with exercise or amyl nitrite inhalation is perhaps the clearest point suggesting a diagnosis of Fallot's tetralogy.

Complications

A. Right Heart Failure: Right heart failure is an important late complication of moderate or severe pulmonary stenosis.

B. Infective Endocarditis: Infective endocarditis occurs in under 5% of cases of pulmonary stenosis and has a good prognosis because valvular damage is seldom severe, and pulmonary regurgitation—even severe regurgitation—is well tolerated over many years.

C. Valvular Calcification and Incompetence:
Valvular calcification and incompetence can occur
with advancing age and are more likely after
valvotomy.

D. Pulmonary Thrombosis and Embolism: Pulmonary thrombosis and embolism tend to occur in
severe cases in which pulmonary blood flow is reduced. They may cause an increase in pulmonary
vascular resistance in older patients. If this is the
case, surgical relief of the stenosis does not bring
complete relief.

Treatment

Insignificant and mild lesions run a benign course.
An example of a chest x-ray that was indistinguishable from another taken 30 years later is shown in
Figure 11–18. No treatment is needed, but the patient
should be followed and seen at intervals. Antibiotic
prophylaxis for the prevention of endocarditis (see
Chapter 16) is necessary in both idiopathic dilation of
the pulmonary artery and mild pulmonary stenosis,
even though this complication is rare.

Valvotomy is recommended when the pressure difference between the right ventricle and the pulmonary
artery is more than 60 mm Hg, with a normal pulmonary blood flow. With pressure differences in the
range of 40–60 mm Hg, other considerations such as
heart size, age, and associated lesions influence the
decision for or against surgery.

Percutaneous balloon valvuloplasty, using the technique devised by Grüntzig (see Chapter 6), has become the procedure of choice for valvotomy in valvular pulmonary stenosis. A balloon slightly greater in
diameter that the stenosed valve is inflated under
pressure in the valve for about 10 seconds on several
occasions. No ill effects have been reported, and success, as measured by reduction in right ventricular
pressure and increase in pulmonary artery pressure
with no change in cardiac output, is consistently reported. A similar technique can be used in peripheral
pulmonary artery stenosis.

Prognosis

The prognosis in pulmonary stenosis is directly related to the severity of the lesion. The mortality rate
associated with surgical valvotomy is very low. With
balloon valvuloplasty, the rate is also very low. The
truly long-term (30- to 40-year) prognosis of patients
operated on in infancy and childhood has yet to be
determined; however, the necessity to repeat valvotomy in pulmonary stenosis so far has been extremely
infrequent, and patients have done well over 20–30
years after surgery. The long-term outcome after balloon valvuloplasty is still unknown.

Long-Term Problems in Operated Cases

Failure to resect sufficient muscle may result in
residual obstruction; or conversely, excessive resection may weaken the outflow tract of the right ventricle and lead to aneurysm formation. Right ventricular
failure is the commonest long-term problem in patients with pulmonary stenosis and may occur as a
result of incomplete relief of obstruction or the
long-term effects of the pulmonary incompetence that
is almost inevitably produced by surgery. Pulmonary valve incompetence occurs after balloon valvuloplasty but is rarely severe. Calcification of the
pulmonary valve may occur with time, and since surgical treatment usually consists of opening up a
dome-shaped valve that bears no cusps, the valve is
inevitably abnormal after operation.

FALLOT'S TETRALOGY

Cardinal Features & Pathogenesis

The cardinal features of Fallot's tetralogy (Figure
11–19) are right ventricular hypertrophy, large ventricular septal defect, right ventricular outflow obstruction, and overriding aorta.

The ventricular septal defect is high in the membranous portion of the septum and large enough to
equalize the pressures in the right and left ventricles.
The right ventricular outflow tract obstruction can be
either valvular or infundibular or both, and the overriding of the aorta results in ejection of some right
ventricular blood directly into the aorta. In some
cases, an equivalent form of lesion occurs in which
both great vessels arise from the right ventricle, a
condition termed **double outlet right ventricle.** The
principal variable determining the severity of Fallot's

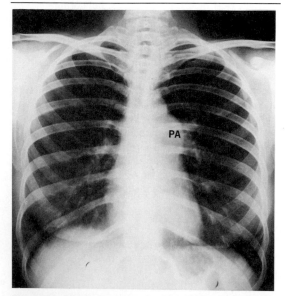

Figure 11–18. Chest x-ray of a 28-year-old woman with a
dilated pulmonary artery (PA). Another chest x-ray taken
30 years later showed no change in the size of the heart
or the pulmonary artery.

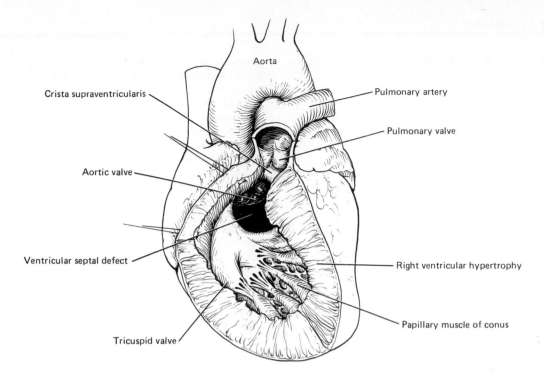

Anatomic features of Fallot's tetralogy. (Reproduced, with permission, from Way LW (editor): *Current Surgical Diagnosis & Treatment,* 8th ed. Appleton & Lange, 1988.

Cardinal features: *Right ventricular hypertrophy; large ventricular septal defect; right ventricular outflow obstruction; overriding aorta.*

Variable factors: *Severity of right ventricular outflow obstruction determines size of shunt and pulmonary blood flow; site of obstruction: valvular or infundibular or both.*

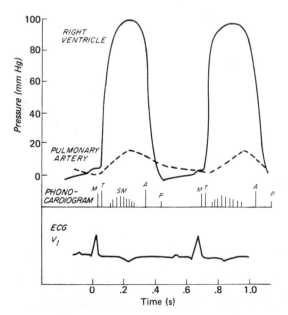

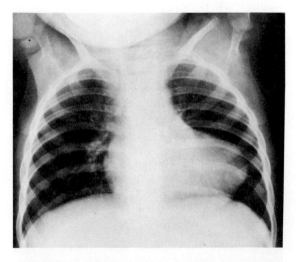

Diagram showing auscultatory and hemodynamic features of Fallot's tetralogy. M, mitral; T, tricuspid; SM, systolic murmur; A, aortic; P, pulmonary.

Chest x-ray of a child with Fallot's tetralogy showing a boot-shaped heart (coeur en sabot). (Courtesy of G Gamsu.)

Figure 11–19. Fallot's tetralogy. Structures enlarged: none in severe cases. Large aorta. Large right ventricle in mild cases.

tetralogy is the degree of right ventricular outflow obstruction. The site (valvular, infundibular, or both) of obstruction and the degree of overriding of the aorta play little part in determining the size of the pulmonary blood flow (the principal variable is outflow obstruction) because the right and left ventricular pressures are kept equal by the large ventricular defect.

The spectrum of cases of Fallot's tetralogy ranges from cases of pulmonary atresia in which no blood passes through the pulmonary valve to patients with low, moderate, and high pulmonary blood flow. In the mildest cases of pulmonary stenosis there is even a left-to-right shunt through the ventricular defect, and the pulmonary-to-systemic blood flow ratio may be more than 2:1.

The pathophysiologic features of Fallot's tetralogy can be due to two types of lesion. In some cases, right ventricular outflow tract obstruction is present from birth; the pulmonary valve ring and pulmonary arteries are small, or pulmonary atresia may be present. In other cases, infundibular pulmonary stenosis develops later in childhood in patients with a large ventricular septal defect. In these cases, the pulmonary valve ring and pulmonary arteries are normal or even enlarged. These anatomic considerations influence the results of surgery, which are better in patients with a larger pulmonary valve ring.

The most characteristic feature of the condition is the marked drop in arterial oxygen saturation that occurs with exercise.

The overall heart size in Fallot's tetralogy varies with the severity of the lesion. In the severest cases the heart is not enlarged; in fact, it may be smaller than normal. The aorta is usually large and may be right-sided. The right ventricle, although hypertrophied, is not large unless there is a left-to-right shunt. There may be poststenotic dilation of the pulmonary artery if the right ventricular obstruction is at the valve. The left pulmonary artery may be absent in Fallot's tetralogy, but this abnormality, like a right-sided aortic arch, may occur independently.

Clinical Findings

A. Symptoms:

1. Cyanosis at birth– In all but its mildest forms Fallot's tetralogy is detectable at birth when cyanosis (blue baby) is noted. Cyanosis on exercise always occurs, but clubbing of the fingers is not seen in milder cases.

2. Dyspnea– Patients with Fallot's tetralogy are always disabled by dyspnea. Some patients say that they are not short of breath, perhaps because they have never experienced normal exercise tolerance, and sometimes it is not until after the lesion has been treated surgically that they realize how short of breath they actually were.

3. Squatting– Adopting the squatting position for relief of dyspnea after exercise is almost patho-

gnomonic of Fallot's tetralogy in children. The mechanisms underlying the relief obtained from squatting are described in Chapter 2.

4. Other symptoms– Chest pain, arrhythmia, and congestive heart failure are rare in Fallot's tetralogy but are more commonly seen in adults than in children. Because the right ventricle never generates a systolic pressure higher than the systemic arterial pressure, the clinical picture is different from that of severe pulmonary stenosis, in which a right ventricular pressure above systemic level can cause chest pain and right heart failure.

B. Attacks of Faintness:
In some severe cases, especially with infundibular stenosis, the patient is subject to attacks of faintness and cyanosis. The patient seldom presents with these features initially, but they tend to occur later in the course of the disease. The mechanism of these attacks is infundibular muscular spasm, which reduces pulmonary blood flow. The right-to-left shunt increases, and the patient becomes progressively more hypoxic. Death may occur in the attack, but more commonly the episode is self-limited. These attacks rarely persist into adult life and respond to treatment with propranolol in 80% of cases.

C. Variability of Symptoms:
Because the resistance to blood flow to the lungs—the pulmonary stenosis—is usually fixed, the systemic resistance is of great importance. Systemic vasodilation due to muscular exercise, arterial hypoxia, fever, pregnancy, or increased environmental temperature tends to increase or produce right-to-left shunting. As a result, the clinical status of patients with Fallot's tetralogy tends to be unstable and varies from day to day with the weather and the patient's activity and environment.

D. Physical Signs:
The physical signs of Fallot's tetralogy vary widely according to the severity of the lesion.

The pulse is of normal volume because the systemic output is well maintained. The venous pressure is normal, with at most a small *a* wave visible in the neck.

The heart is quiet, with little right ventricular heave in severe cases. In milder cases with left-to-right shunts, there is a larger, more hyperdynamic right ventricle. The intensity and length of the ejection murmur arising from right ventricular outflow obstruction vary with the severity of the lesion. In pulmonary atresia or severe pulmonary stenosis, the pulmonary blood flow may be so small that there is no pulmonary systolic ejection murmur. In such cases an almost continuous murmur due to collateral bronchial blood flow or flow through a patent ductus arteriosus may be heard, especially over the back. In mild acyanotic cases, the murmur is long and loud. It may be pansystolic and arise from the ventricular septal defect in patients with a left-to-right shunt. Since the outflow obstruction is always severe enough to raise

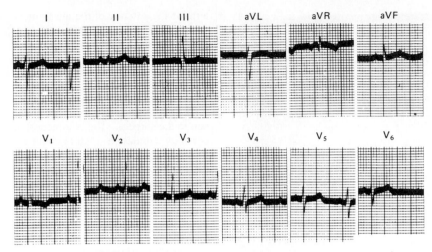

Figure 11–20. ECG of 7-year-old boy with Fallot's tetralogy showing right ventricular hypertrophy.

the right ventricular pressure to systemic levels, the pulmonary valve closure sound is usually inaudible. However, it can be detected by phonocardiography.

E. Electrocardiographic Findings: The ECG always shows some evidence of right ventricular hypertrophy in Fallot's tetralogy (Figure 11–20), but the changes may be surprisingly mild. In milder cases with a left-to-right shunt, there may be evidence of biventricular hypertrophy. P waves are seldom abnormal, and gross right ventricular hypertrophy of the type found in severe pulmonary stenosis is not seen. Left ventricular hypertrophy only occurs in patients with a large, palliative, surgically produced left-to-right shunt.

F. Imaging Studies:

1. Severe lesions– With severe pulmonary stenosis and reduced pulmonary blood flow, the left atrium and left ventricle are small; as a consequence, the overall heart size is reduced. The combination of right ventricular hypertrophy and infundibular stenosis gives the classic "coeur en sabot" (boot-shaped heart) radiologic picture, with the apex pointing upward and to the left (Figure 11–19). In severe cases, especially those with pulmonary atresia, increased bronchial collateral blood flow may give rise to a reticulated pattern of blood vessels in the lungs.

2. Milder lesions– In milder, acyanotic cases and those with valvular stenosis, the heart shadow is larger, and poststenotic dilation of the pulmonary artery is seen. In some cases with infundibular stenosis, the heart shadow may appear surprisingly normal, as shown in Figure 11–21. Normal lung fields—or even pulmonary plethora—are seen in the milder cases.

The finding of a right-sided aortic arch (Figure 11–22) is independent of the severity of the lesion.

G. Special Investigations:

1. Noninvasive techniques–

a. Hematocrit– The degree of polycythemia, as shown by the hematocrit, varies with the degree of arterial hypoxia and thus with the severity of the lesion. Hematocrit levels as high as 75–80% are seen, especially in adults.

b. Echocardiography– Two-dimensional echocardiographic examination of the heart is of particular value in establishing the diagnosis of Fallot's tetralogy. Two-dimensional echocardiography with Doppler can establish the diagnosis of tetralogy of Fallot most of the time. The four-chambered view can show the overriding aorta, and with angulation of the beam can show the drop-out and position of the ventricular septal defect (Figure 11–23). Doppler can reveal the abnormal flow across the ventricular septal defect and

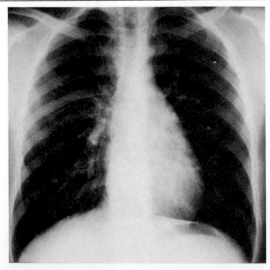

Figure 11–21. Chest x-ray of a 16-year-old boy with mild Fallot's tetralogy. The cardiac silhouette is almost normal in size and shape.

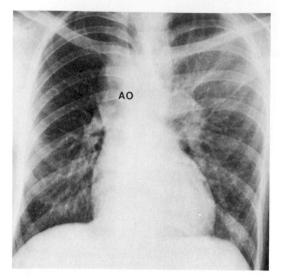

Figure 11–22. Chest x-ray of a man with Fallot's tetralogy with a Blalock-Taussig anastomosis. The aorta (AO) is right-sided.

termine the patency of the anastomosis that was produced. This may require retrograde arterial catheterization. In long-standing palliative shunts, calculation of the pulmonary vascular resistance is important.

Angiographic demonstration of right ventricular outflow obstruction, aortic anatomy, and the ventricular septal defect should also be carried out routinely.

The anatomy of the coronary circulation is important to the surgeon. The commonest anomalies of the coronary circulation, seen in about 10% of cases, are the presence of a single coronary ostium from which the whole coronary arterial system arises and the origin of the anterior descending branch from the right coronary artery rather than the left. A large conus branch is often present, and congenital aneurysms of the coronary arteries may be seen.

Differential Diagnosis

Fallot's tetralogy must be distinguished from pulmonary stenosis with reversed interatrial shunt. It is not always possible to make the distinction on clinical grounds, and two-dimensional echo-Doppler with contrast injection or even cardiac catheterization is often necessary to make the correct diagnosis.

Complications

Progressive polycythemia may lead to cerebral or pulmonary thrombosis. Cerebral embolism or abscess formation is sometimes seen as a result of paradoxic embolization from the right heart through the shunt. Infective endocarditis can occur at the site of the ventricular septal defect in mild cases, or on the pulmonary valve, or in both places. It is occasionally seen both before and after palliative surgery. Right heart failure with edema and raised venous pressure is rare except after surgery.

the high-velocity flow across the obstructive right ventricular-outflow tract. With pulsed Doppler, the exact site of the right ventricular outflow obstruction can be determined.

2. Invasive techniques– Cardiac catheterization is indicated before any surgical operation in patients with Fallot's tetralogy. The aim of the study is to measure the pulmonary arterial pressure and show that the right ventricular and aortic pressures are the same and to determine the site of the right ventricular outflow tract obstruction. In patients who have had palliative shunt operations, it is also important to de-

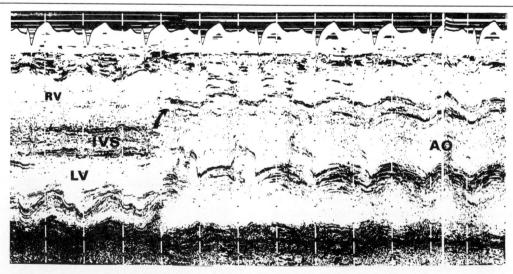

Figure 11–23. Echocardiogram showing aorta overriding ventricular septum in a patient with Fallot's tetralogy. (RV, right ventricle; IVS, interventricular septum; LV, left ventricle; AO, aorta.) (Courtesy of NB Schiller.)

Prevention

Antibiotic prophylaxis for the prevention of endocarditis (see Chapter 16) is necessary both before and after the operation.

Surgical Treatment

A. Palliative Surgery: Palliative surgery was introduced over 45 years ago with dramatic results. Blood flow to the lungs can be increased by anastomosis between the subclavian and pulmonary arteries (Blalock-Taussig operation), the descending aorta and the left pulmonary artery (Potts operation) or the ascending aorta and right pulmonary artery (Waterston operation). Patients with severe forms of Fallot's tetralogy benefited greatly from these operations, which resulted in lessening of cyanosis and marked improvement in exercise tolerance. Curative surgery, with complete repair of the defect, was accomplished in the 1950s and is now the treatment of choice.

B. Complete Repair: Complete repair is always indicated in adult patients. If the patient has reached adult life without surgery, the lesion is likely to be relatively mild, and complete correction should be comparatively easy, since the pulmonary vascular bed, left atrium, and left ventricle are probably capable of accepting a normal right ventricular output. The mortality rate of complete repair in adult patients is now less than 5%.

C. Complete Repair Following Palliative Surgery: If the patient has previously had a Blalock-Taussig or Potts operation, complete repair is still indicated. The operation may be more difficult because the shunt must be identified and closed, and the right ventricular outflow tract may be hypoplastic, or an aneurysm may have developed at the site of the anastomosis. Any patient with symptoms severe enough to have warranted palliative surgery in childhood would probably not have survived to adulthood without operation. A decision about the timing of complete operative repair is difficult, because the patient may be reasonably stable, leading a sheltered life, and unwilling to submit to a second life-threatening cardiac operation. Pulmonary vascular disease occurs most frequently in patients with Potts shunts and less often in patients with Blalock-Taussig anastomoses. However, on long-term follow-up, pulmonary vascular disease not uncommonly develops in either case.

Prognosis

The prognosis in untreated Fallot's tetralogy is poor, and only patients with mild lesions survive to adult life without surgery. The condition is not a static one, since progressive infundibular hypertrophy may develop and decrease the blood flow to the lungs. At the same time, the right-to-left shunt through the ventricular septal defect can increase, leading to cyanosis, clubbing, and polycythemia. Fallot's tetralogy is a severe condition, and even in its mild form the pulmonary stenosis must be considered severe because right ventricular pressure equals systemic pressure.

Long-Term Results in Operated Cases

The improvement in symptoms resulting from complete correction—or even palliative surgery—in Fallot's tetralogy is usually so dramatic that the patient is able to "lead a normal life." Though symptom-free, such patients often show considerable residual abnormalities. A residual systolic murmur may be present because of right-sided obstruction at the infundibular or valvular level. A diastolic murmur of pulmonary incompetence or aortic incompetence may develop, and echo-Doppler studies and cardiac catheterization usually show some evidence of abnormality, especially during exercise studies. Conduction abnormalities and arrhythmias may cause sudden unexpected death years after an otherwise satisfactory repair, especially in older patients. If an attempted complete correction is only partially successful, recatheterization and reoperation are indicated, because pulmonary hypertension, with a large left-to-right shunt through an open ventricular defect, may develop rapidly and lead to right heart failure or a permanent increase in pulmonary vascular resistance.

VENTRICULAR SEPTAL DEFECT

Ventricular septal defect is probably the commonest congenital cardiac defect present at birth. Only about 10% of cases of adult congenital heart disease, however, have a ventricular septal defect without any associated lesion. The explanation for the difference is that many if not most ventricular defects present in infancy spontaneously close; this is true even with large defects with huge left-to-right shunts that have caused heart failure in infancy.

Cardinal Features

The cardinal features of ventricular septal defect (Figure 11–24) are left-to-right shunt into the right ventricle, increased pulmonary blood flow, and usually a low pulmonary artery pressure. Variable features are the size of the defect (large or small), the site of the defect (membranous or muscular), the level of the pulmonary vascular resistance (see Eisenmenger's syndrome), and the presence or absence of associated aortic incompetence. Only a small number of ventricular defects occur in the muscular part of the septum, and these may be multiple. The size and site of the ventricular defect determine the size of the left-to-right shunt, which in turn determines the clinical picture. Associated aortic incompetence, seen with supracristal defects, causes further left ventricular enlargement. A left-to-right shunt at the ventricular

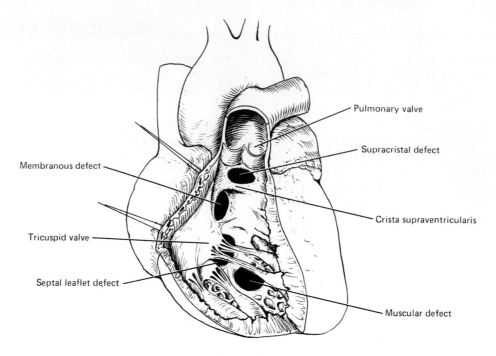

Anatomic location of ventricular septal defects. (Reproduced, with permission, from Way LW (editor): *Current Surgical Diagnosis & Treatment,* 8th ed. Appleton & Lange, 1988.

Cardinal features: *Left-to-right shunt into right ventricle; increased pulmonary blood flow; pulmonary arterial pressure usually low.*

Variable factors: *Size of defect; site of defect: membranous or muscular; associated aortic incompetence.*

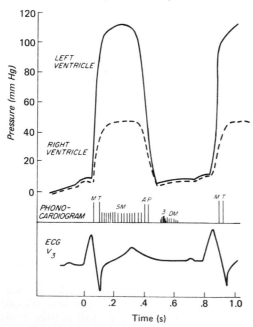

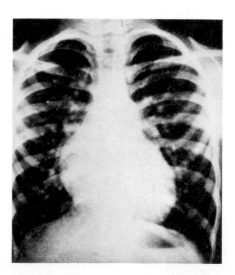

Diagram showing auscultatory and hemodynamic features of ventricular septal defect. M, mitral; T, tricuspid; SM, systolic murmur; A, aortic; P, pulmonary; DM, diastolic murmur.

Dilatation of the pulmonary artery and pulmonary plethora in a case of ventricular septal defect. (Reproduced, with permission, from Wood P: *Diseases of the Heart and Circulation,* 3rd ed. Lippincott, 1968.)

Figure 11–24. Ventricular septal defect. Structures enlarged: left atrium, left ventricle, and right ventricle.

level produces an increased flow through the left atrium, left ventricle, and right ventricle. The right atrium is the only chamber through which flow is normal.

The clinical spectrum of cases is wide, varying from maladie de Roger, in which a loud murmur and thrill are the only detectable abnormalities, to defects large enough to cause moderate pulmonary hypertension and large left-to-right shunts.

Clinical Findings

A. Symptoms and Signs: Symptoms in patients with ventricular septal defect depend on the size of the defect and the age of the patient. Small shunts cause no significant hemodynamic effects and are compatible with a normal life expectancy. Larger defects, with pulmonary to systemic flow ratios of 1.5:1 or more, may cause dyspnea after age 30, and large defects with flow ratios of 3:1 or more are rare in adults but are usually associated with dyspnea on exertion. There is usually a history of a heart murmur present since infancy.

The physical signs of ventricular septal defect are dominated by the loud pansystolic murmur and thrill that are present in the third and fourth left intercostal spaces inside the apex. In more than half of adult cases, these are the only abnormal physical signs. In patients with larger shunts, the pulse is jerky, resembling a miniature water-hammer pulse, and the cardiac impulse is hyperdynamic. The increased force of left ventricular contraction, which is associated with ejection of an increased stroke volume out through the aorta and also into the low-pressure right ventricle, causes a hemodynamic pattern similar to that seen in mitral incompetence.

The increased pulmonary blood flow causes increased flow through the mitral valve, which produces a third heart sound and a short apical diastolic flow murmur resulting from relative mitral stenosis.

B. Electrocardiographic Findings: The ECG is normal in more than half of adult cases. In patients with large left-to-right shunts, there is evidence of mild biventricular overload, with both tall R waves and deep S waves over the transitional zone leads, together with Q waves in the left ventricular leads. These findings are illustrated in Figure 11–25.

C. Imaging Studies: The chest x-ray shows a normal cardiac configuration if the shunt is small. Cardiac enlargement is proportionate to the size of the shunt. Since large left-to-right shunts are rare in adults, increased heart size, which typically involves the left atrium, both ventricles, and the pulmonary artery, is not often seen. Left atrial appendage enlargement is not seen in ventricular septal defect, even when the left atrium is enlarged.

Echocardiography (Figure 11–26) is particularly helpful in differential diagnosis. Although ventricular septal defect may be confused with certain conditions on physical examination, echocardiography reveals distinguishing features of these disorders, which include mitral incompetence, hypertrophic cardiomyopathy, infundibular stenosis, and ostium primum defects with mitral incompetence. Doppler echocardiography, especially with color flow mapping, can be used to determine the site of the defect and estimate the pressure drop across it.

Cardiac catheterization is indicated to confirm the diagnosis, especially if surgical treatment is contemplated. In patients with small defects, a left-to-right shunt may not be detectable from blood samples

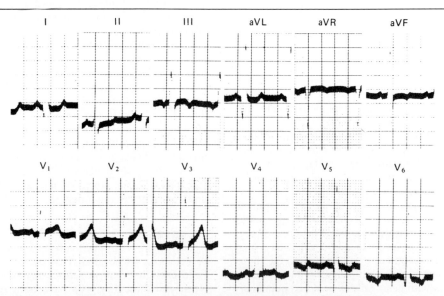

Figure 11–25. ECG of a 21-year-old man with ventricular septal defect proved by catheter; right ventricular pressure is $^{39}/_{6}$.

A

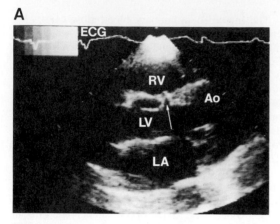

B

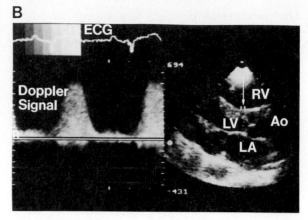

Figure 11–26. ***A:*** Two-dimensional echocardiograph showing long-axis view in a patient with ventricular septal defect marked by arrow. ***B:*** Echocardiograph and ultrasonic Doppler blood velocity signal demonstrating systolic flow through the ventricular septal defect. The arrow in B marks the position of the sample volume at the right ventricular end of the defect. (RV, right ventricle; LV, left ventricle; Ao, aorta; LA, left atrium.)

taken from the right heart chambers, and right-sided pressures are usually normal. Left ventricular injection of contrast material will establish the diagnosis.

Differential Diagnosis

Ventricular septal defect is readily confused on physical examination with mitral incompetence, infundibular stenosis, ostium primum defects with cleft mitral valves, and hypertrophic obstructive cardiomyopathy. All these lesions can cause a loud pansystolic murmur and thrill in the left chest. Echocardiography with Doppler easily distinguishes these lesions.

Complications

Infective endocarditis is the principal complication of ventricular septal defect. It occurs on the right ventricular wall at the point at which the jet stream of the shunt impinges on the endocardium. Since the infection is initially confined to the right heart and no valve is involved, the prognosis with treatment is good. Endocarditis occurs in about 5% of cases of uncomplicated ventricular septal defects and may recur.

Aortic incompetence occasionally occurs as an associated lesion, especially in patients with a supracristal defect. It is usually due to prolapse of an aortic valve cusp. It gives rise to a long diastolic murmur that, in conjunction with the pansystolic murmur of the ventricular defect, gives an almost continuous murmur. The aortic incompetence is usually moderate or severe and may develop as the patient grows. In some cases, prolapse of an aortic valve cusp may occlude the defect and diminish or abolish the shunt.

The total number of adult patients with ventricular septal defects with heart failure, acquired pulmonary hypertension, and atrial arrhythmias is much lower than in atrial septal defect, because so few patients

with large ventricular defects are seen in adult life. Almost all large ventricular septal defects will eventually develop pulmonary vascular disease and pulmonary hypertension. Systemic hypertension and coronary atherosclerosis may occur in older patients but do not cause the severe problems seen in patients with atrial septal defects, because the size of the left-to-right shunt is limited by the size of the defect and is relatively uninfluenced by the compliance of either ventricle.

Treatment

A. Medical Treatment: The need for antibiotic prophylaxis (see Chapter 16) and acute awareness of the possibility of infective endocarditis are important points to remember in treating patients with ventricular septal defect.

B. Surgical Treatment: Closure of the defect is indicated if the pulmonary/systemic flow ratio is 2:1 or greater. In patients with smaller shunts, endocarditis is the only hazard, and prophylaxis to prevent endocarditis is indicated; surgery is not. If endocarditis has occurred or recurred, closure is indicated even if the defect is small. The hazards of not operating on a ventricular defect are much less than those involved in leaving an atrial defect unclosed. Surgery is also required in patients with ventricular septal defect and aortic incompetence and can prevent the progression of aortic regurgitation.

Prognosis

The prognosis in uncomplicated ventricular septal defect in adults is good. Few patients have defects large enough to cause serious hemodynamic problems, and those few who have been recatheterized after 10 years of follow-up have shown no significant change in their status.

Long-Term Results in Operated Cases

Infants with ventricular septal defects large enough to cause heart failure and pulmonary hypertension in the first 5 years of life have been treated surgically for 30 years or more. Increasing numbers of these patients are now being seen in adult cardiology clinics. Pansystolic murmurs due to residual ventricular defects are not uncommon, but the defects are seldom sufficient to warrant reoperation. Residual pulmonary hypertension is less likely in those operated in the first 2 years of life, and left ventricular function is usually within normal limits, with resting pulmonary capillary wedge pressures at the upper limit of normal.

Aortic incompetence may persist or develop after surgery and is often progressive. Right bundle branch block is common, even after disclosure of the defect via the transatrial route, and right ventricular function is usually abnormal as assessed by radionuclear methods. Ventricular arrhythmias and sudden death are seen, even in patients with good hemodynamic results. Pulmonary vascular disease is not usually reversed, and many asymptomatic patients have high pulmonary arterial pressures and residual septal defects.

PATENT DUCTUS ARTERIOSUS

Persistent patency of the ductus arteriosus is the prime example of a congenital heart lesion resulting from persistence of the normal fetal circulation. It is a common finding in infants whose mothers had rubella during pregnancy.

Cardinal Features

Patent ductus arteriosus is the commonest form of aortopulmonary communication. The shunt is from the aorta at a point just distal to the left subclavian artery into the left pulmonary artery, as shown in Figure 11–27. Aortopulmonary window, in which there is a large communication between the proximal aorta and the main pulmonary artery, is a much rarer lesion that is clinically indistinguishable. The size of the aortopulmonary communication and the relative pulmonary-to-systemic vascular resistance determines the size of the left-to-right shunt.

Patent ductus arteriosus results in an increased flow through the left atrium and left ventricle and also through the aorta and pulmonary artery. Since flow is not increased through the right heart, the lesion loads only the left heart.

Patent ductus arteriosus is more than twice as common in females as in males, and the diagnosis is now usually made in infancy or childhood.

Clinical Features

A. Symptoms and Signs: In hemodynamically insignificant lesions, which constitute more than half of adult cases, the patient is asymptomatic. A murmur has sometimes been present since birth, but more commonly the diagnosis is made later in childhood. A false history of rheumatic fever is present in about 10% of cases. With a large left-to-right shunt, the principal symptom is dyspnea on exertion, with palpitation and chest pain much less frequently seen.

The only abnormality in more than half of cases is the typical "machinery" murmur, heard high in the left chest below the clavicle. It is loudest at the time of the second heart sound, as shown in Figure 11–27. The murmur is not necessarily continuous in infancy and may be mainly systolic up to age 5, perhaps because the pulmonary vascular resistance is high in infancy and the pressure difference between the aorta and pulmonary artery is less at this time. In patients with large left-to-right shunts, cardiac enlargement and a prominent hyperdynamic left ventricular impulse are found. In patients with the largest shunts, a wide pulse pressure and a collapsing pulse are seen because of the large left ventricular stroke volume and the rapid runoff of aortic blood into the low-pressure pulmonary circulation. Palpable pulmonary valve closure, reversed splitting of the second heart sound, and an apical diastolic murmur due to increased diastolic flow across the mitral valve are found in patients with large shunts. All of these features are seen also in aortopulmonary window; the only distinguishing feature—a murmur heard low down in the third or fourth left interspace—is not a reliable indication of the diagnosis.

B. Electrocardiographic Findings: Left ventricular hypertrophy in patent ductus arteriosus is related to the size of the shunt.

C. Imaging Studies: The heart is of normal size when the shunt is small. A prominent pulmonary artery shadow running up to a large aortic knob is the most distinguishing radiologic sign of patent ductus arteriosus. Pulmonary plethora with left atrial and left ventricular enlargement and a large ascending aorta are seen in patients with large shunts (Figure 11–27). The ductus may calcify in later life.

Two-dimensional echocardiography from the suprasternal notch provides the best noninvasive view of the ductus. Doppler studies demonstrate disturbed flow from the aorta into the pulmonary artery throughout the cycle (Figure 11–28). This may not distinguish a patent ductus from an aortopulmonary window or from anomalous drainage of a coronary artery into the pulmonary artery. Cardiac catheterization is indicated to confirm the presence of a left-to-right shunt at pulmonary arterial level and to measure the pulmonary and systemic pressure and flow. In right heart catheterization the aorta can be entered via the ductus in patients with large shunts. The characteristic position of the catheter is shown in Figure 11–29, and its passage down the descending aorta leaves no doubt about the diagnosis. Measurement of the pulmonary/systemic flow ratio is the best means of es-

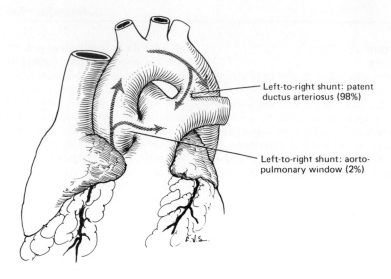

Left-to-right shunt: patent ductus arteriosus (98%)

Left-to-right shunt: aorto-pulmonary window (2%)

Anatomic sites of aortopulmonary defects.

Cardinal features: *Ductus distal to left subclavian artery; aorto-pulmonary window near root of aorta; left-to-right shunt; pulmonary arterial pressure usually low in patent ductus arteriosus.*

Variable factors: *Size of communication; size of left-to-right shunt.*

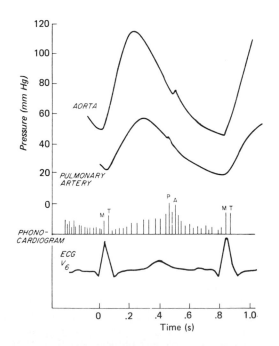

Diagram showing auscultatory and hemodynamic features of patent ductus arteriosus. The continuous murmur is loudest at the time of the second heart sound. M, mitral; T, tricuspid; P, pulmonary; A, aortic.

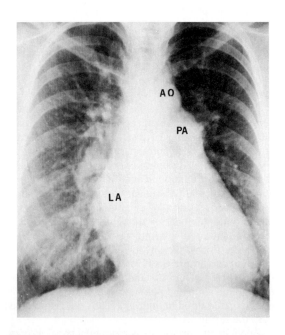

Chest x-ray of a patient with a large patent ductus arteriosus. The aorta (AO), pulmonary artery (PA), and left atrium (LA) are enlarged.

Figure 11–27. Patent ductus arteriosus and aortopulmonary window. Structures enlarged: left atrium and ventricle, aorta, and pulmonary artery.

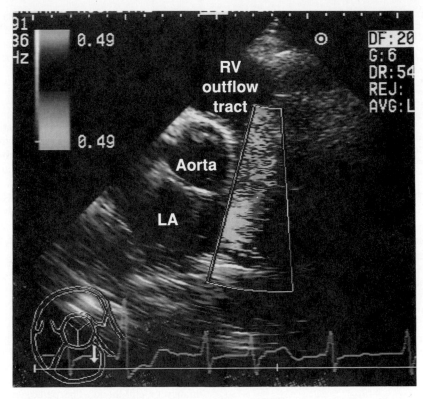

Figure 11–28. Short axis view at the aortic root level of two-dimensional Doppler echocardiogram. The patient is a 28-year-old woman with a patent ductus arteriosus. The Doppler window shows the mosaic cell of a continuous flow disturbance in the main pulmonary artery consistent with a patent ductus arteriosus. The picture was taken in diastole. (LA, left atrium.)

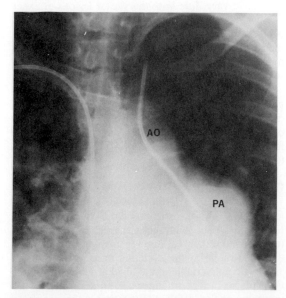

Figure 11–29. Chest x-ray showing the position of a cardiac catheter passing through a patent ductus arteriosus from the pulmonary artery (PA) to the aorta (AO).

tablishing the hemodynamic severity of the lesion. Ratios of 2:1 or more are found in moderate and severe lesions.

It has become customary to make absolutely certain of the site of the shunt by retrograde aortography. An injection of contrast material into the aortic arch with the patient in the left anterior oblique position will fill the pulmonary artery and outline the ductus.

Differential Diagnosis
(Table 11–2)

Patent ductus arteriosus can be differentiated from aortopulmonary window by cardiac catheterization and angiography. The other lesions that have to be distinguished are those causing continuous or near-continuous murmurs. A venous hum gives a continuous bruit heard above the clavicle that is abolished by pressing on the veins at the root of the neck to interfere with blood flow. The bruit is caused by local narrowing of the vein and is often influenced by posture. Aortic valve disease and ventricular septal defect with aortic incompetence cause murmurs that may be continuous but show two peaks, one in mid systole and the other in early diastole. The murmurs of pulmonary artery stenosis and increased collateral

Table 11–2. Causes of continuous murmurs.

- Patent ductus arteriosus
- Aortopulmonary window
- Coronary arteriovenous fistula
- Coronary cameral fistula
- Internal mammary-to-pulmonary artery fistula
- Rupture of sinus of Valsalva aneurysm to right atrium or right ventricle
- Anomalous coronary artery arising from the pulmonary artery
- Accessory coronary artery into pulmonary artery
- Pulmonary arteriovenous fistula
- Interventricular septal defect with aortic regurgitation
- Cervical venous hum
- Severe proximal pulmonary artery stricture
- Severe multiple peripheral pulmonary artery stenosis
- Severe multiple vessel obstruction with pulmonary embolism
- Aortic regurgitation and mitral regurgitation
- Vascular tumors
- Bronchial circulation

bronchial blood flow start late in systole and peak before the second sound. An accessory coronary artery draining into the pulmonary artery can also cause a continuous murmur heard in the same area as the murmur of a patent ductus arteriosus. The murmur may peak later in diastole than does the murmur of a patent ductus.

Complications

Infective endarteritis is an important but infrequent complication. The infection occurs on the low-pressure side of the shunt or where the jet of aortic blood impinges on the wall of the pulmonary artery.

The left recurrent laryngeal nerve runs in close proximity to the ductus. It may be subjected to pressure or cut at surgery, causing hoarseness.

Acquired pulmonary hypertension with increase in pulmonary vascular resistance occurs in patients with large left-to-right shunts. In most patients with pulmonary hypertension, the raised resistance is present from early infancy (see Eisenmenger's Syndrome, below).

Treatment

Triple ligation of a patent ductus arteriosus is recommended in all patients with left-to-right shunt in whom the diagnosis is confirmed. The operative mortality rate is negligible if the shunt is small. In older patients and those with large left-to-right shunts, the aortopulmonary communication is short and friable and may be calcified. The aortic wall may tear easily, and surgical closure can be extremely difficult, even with cardiopulmonary bypass. In such cases the mortality rate rises to about 10%. It is important to apply several ligatures to the ductus at surgery rather than simply tie it once.

Prognosis

The prognosis is good in mild cases. Surgery is prophylactic against infective endarteritis in hemo-

dynamically insignificant lesions. Endarteritis seldom threatens life, and it is only in the rare patient with a huge left-to-right shunt and in the patient with pulmonary vascular disease that life expectancy is less than normal.

Long-Term Results in Operated Cases

The long-term results in operated patients with patent ductus arteriosus are better than those with any other congenital heart lesion. Since the operation is extracardiac, conduction defects and arrhythmias are rare. The only important problem is recurrence of left-to-right shunt; it occurs in about 10% of cases in which a single ligature is used. If left-to-right shunt recurs several years after ligation, the acquired shunt lesion is much less well tolerated than the congenital shunt.

EISENMENGER'S SYNDROME

The term Eisenmenger's syndrome is used to describe pulmonary hypertension due to pulmonary vascular disease with reversed shunt. By definition, the pulmonary hypertension does not develop late in the course of the disease but has been present from early infancy or childhood. The pathogenesis of the pulmonary vascular obstruction is poorly understood.

It is convenient to group under the heading Eisenmenger's syndrome all patients with cardiac defects associated with pulmonary hypertension that has been present since early life, because pulmonary hypertension is responsible for the physical signs and determines the clinical course. Clinical features and clinical course vary little with the site of lesions or exact anatomic nature of the defects. In practice, the exact anatomic nature of the lesion in adults with Eisenmenger's syndrome may remain unproved until autopsy, and associated lesion defects can be present without changing the clinical picture.

Eisenmenger's syndrome accounts for about 7% of cases of adult congenital heart disease and is seen more commonly in females than in males. In about one-third of cases, ventricular septal defect is the only lesion that is associated with pulmonary hypertension.

Cardinal Features

The pulmonary arterial pressure is at or near systemic level, and the shunt is either bidirectional or right-to-left. The pulmonary vascular resistance is raised to more than 7.5 mm Hg/L/min and is often in the same range as the systemic vascular resistance. The principal variable is the level at which the shunt takes place. In **Eisenmenger's complex,** which is the prototype of the lesion, the location is the ventricle, as shown in Figure 11–30. Because Eisenmenger's original patient had a ventricular defect, the term

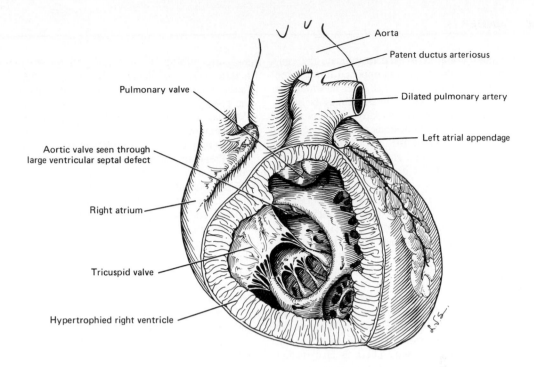

Anatomic features of Eisenmenger's complex.

Cardinal features: *Pulmonary hypertension at systemic level; communication(s) between right and left heart; bidirectional or right-to-left shunt; raised pulmonary vascular resistance.*

Variable factors: *Site of communication: Ventricle (Eisenmenger's complex), patent ductus arteriosus, aortopulmonary window, ostium primum defect, atrioventricular canal, truncus arteriosus transposition, single atrium, single ventricle, total anomalous venous drainage.* Not *present in ostium secundum defect.*

Diagram showing auscultatory and hemodynamic features of Eisenmenger's complex. M, mitral; T, tricuspid; EC, ejection click; SM, systolic murmur; A, aortic; P, pulmonary; DM, diastolic murmur.

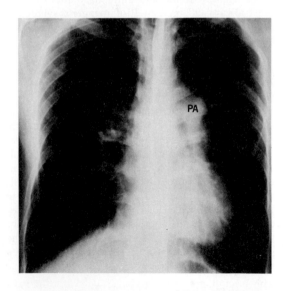

Chest x-ray of a patient with Eisenmenger's syndrome showing small heart and large pulmonary artery (PA) with oligemic lungs.

Figure 11–30. Eisenmenger's syndrome. Structures enlarged: right ventricle, right atrium, and pulmonary artery.

Eisenmenger's complex is used to indicate the ventricular nature of the defect, as opposed to the more general term Eisenmenger's syndrome, in which the defect may be at any level. The shunt may be at the aortopulmonary, atrioventricular, atrial, or ventricular level. Complex congenital lesions such as truncus arteriosus, transposition of the great arteries, single atrium or ventricle, or total anomalous venous drainage may be associated with the pulmonary hypertension.

It is thought that the Eisenmenger reaction, which is the development of severe pulmonary vascular disease, may occur in any form of congenital heart disease in which a large pulmonary blood flow, usually at high pressure, is present in fetal, neonatal, or infant life. Clues to the mechanism of development of this form of pulmonary hypertension must be sought in the neonatal period. The increased pulmonary vascular resistance results from a failure of the pulmonary vessels to increase in number by branching as the lung grows, so that the ratio of vessels to airways at any given level is decreased. There is also medial smooth muscle hypertrophy, and this smooth muscle extends farther out into the small vessels. There is also intimal hyperplasia related to the trauma of the high shear forces in the smaller vessels. These changes do not regress with elimination of the high shear and high flow by closure of the defect. In adult patients, the pulmonary vascular disease of Eisenmenger's syndrome is severe enough to rule out closure of the defect or defects.

The right ventricle and pulmonary artery are almost always enlarged in Eisenmenger's syndrome. The other chambers that may be enlarged depend on the site of the associated lesion or lesions.

Acquired Pulmonary Hypertension (Eisenmenger Reaction)

Pulmonary hypertension develops after puberty in some patients, usually those with large left-to-right shunts due to ostium secundum atrial septal defects. In these cases the term "atrial septal defect with pulmonary hypertension" or "acquired Eisenmenger syndrome" has been used. In extremely rare cases, pulmonary hypertension develops after puberty in patients with other lesions, eg, ventricular septal defect or patent ductus arteriosus. Acquired pulmonary hypertension tends to progress more rapidly than the pulmonary vascular lesions seen in Eisenmenger's syndrome.

Clinical Findings

A. Symptoms and Signs: Patients with Eisenmenger's syndrome are invariably disabled by dyspnea. A murmur or cyanosis is often said to have been present from infancy, and the absence of any history of severe illness in infancy or childhood is striking. Pneumonia, heart failure, feeding problems, and susceptibility to infection, which are common manifestations of large left-to-right shunts in infancy, are not encountered in retrospective reviews of the history of adults with Eisenmenger's syndrome. Whereas dyspnea is invariably present regardless of age, hemoptysis, palpitation, chest pain, and fainting attacks may be seen in adolescence and young adult life. Pregnancy is poorly tolerated, and spontaneous abortion is common.

The physical signs are those of pulmonary hypertension. Cyanosis and clubbing of the fingers may be present, and there is often a prominent *a* wave in the jugular venous pulse. There may be "differential" cyanosis in patients with a reversed shunt through a patent ductus arteriosus. The shunted blood passes preferentially to the lower part of the body via the ductus and descending aorta. Thus, there may be cyanosis and clubbing of the toes when the hands—especially the right hand—are pink and show no clubbing of the fingers (Figure 11–31). The difference is best seen when the systemic circulation has been subject to vasodilation, eg, after a hot shower or bath.

The heart is usually not much enlarged and is often quiet. A right ventricular heave may be present, and pulmonary valve closure is often palpable. There is usually a systolic ejection click, followed by a short systolic ejection murmur over the pulmonary artery and a loud single second heart sound. An early diastolic murmur of pulmonary incompetence (Graham Steell murmur) is common, and the clearest examples of this murmur are encountered in Eisenmenger's syndrome. Signs of congestive heart failure are seldom seen, but progressive cyanosis and polycythemia are common.

B. Electrocardiographic Findings: The ECG in patients with Eisenmenger's syndrome always shows right ventricular hypertrophy (Figure 11–32). In patients with atrioventricular canal defects, left axis deviation may be present even when pulmonary vascular resistance is markedly raised.

C. Imaging Studies: The main trunk and branches of the pulmonary artery are large, but the heart is usually only slightly enlarged (Figure 11–33). Evidence of slight pulmonary plethora may be present, and the sparseness of the peripheral pulmonary vessels may be difficult to recognize.

D. Special Investigations:

1. Noninvasive techniques– Following the level of the hematocrit is useful in assessing the progress of the disease. Echocardiography is helpful in determining the site of the shunt lesion.

With echo-Doppler, most often a jet of tricuspid insufficiency can be demonstrated that allows estimation of the pressure gradient from the right ventricle to the right atrium. If the venous pressure is added to this gradient, an accurate measure of the systolic pressure in the right ventricle and, in the absence of pulmonary stenosis, the pulmonary artery can be obtained.

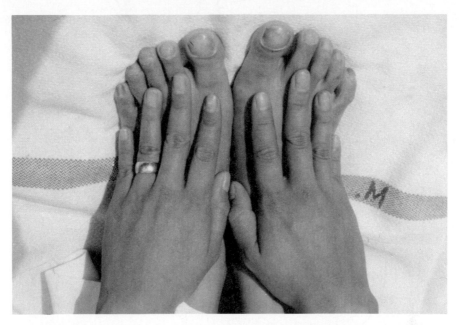

Figure 11-31. Hands and feet of a 30-year-old woman with a patent ductus arteriosus and severe pulmonary vascular disease resulting in large right-to-left shunt through the ductus. Note clubbed, cyanotic toes and pink, normal fingers.

2. Invasive techniques–

a. Cardiac catheterization is always required to establish the diagnosis and show that pulmonary arterial pressure is raised and that pulmonary vascular resistance is at about the same level as systemic resistance. A left-to-right shunt may be detectable from analysis of the oxygen content of samples of blood obtained from the right heart chambers, and the catheter may cross a septal defect at catheterization. When the defect is at the atrioventricular level, pulmonary arterial pressure may be less than systemic pressure.

b. Wedge pressure measurement is of great importance, since it is always possible that the patient has a curable lesion that can be identified in this way. The abruptly tapering peripheral pulmonary arteries of patients with Eisenmenger's syndrome may not permit the wedging of a conventional cardiac catheter. In such cases, a Swan-Ganz balloon catheter should be used, and the pressure in the pulmonary artery distal to the inflated balloon should be taken as an indirect measure of the pulmonary venous pressure.

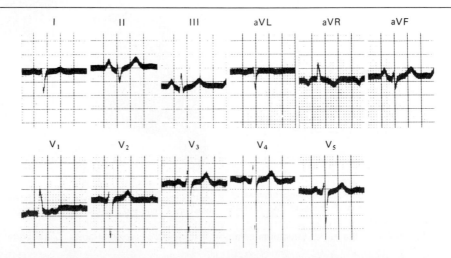

Figure 11–32. ECG of a 30-year-old man with Eisenmenger's syndrome showing right ventricular hypertrophy.

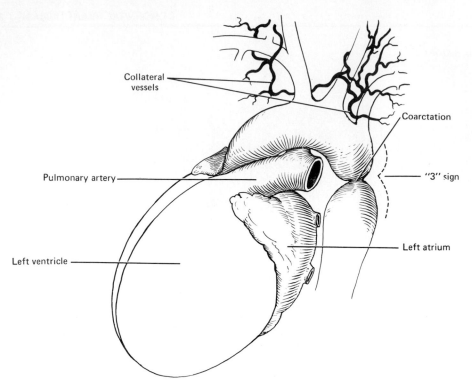

Anatomic features of coarctation of the aorta.

Cardinal features: *Obstruction distal to left subclavian artery; high pressure in proximal aorta; pressure drop across obstruction; poststenotic dilatation.*

Variable factors: *Severity of obstruction; size of collateral vessels; site in acquired lesions.*

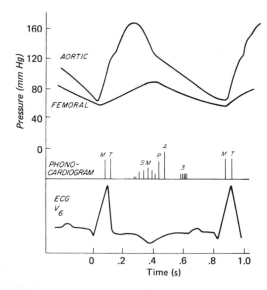

Diagram showing auscultatory and hemodynamic features of coarctation of the aorta. M, mitral; T, tricuspid; SM, systolic murmur; P, pulmonary; A, aortic.

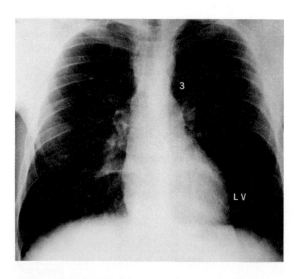

Chest x-ray of 19-year-old man with coarctation of the aorta showing "3" sign and slight left ventricular (LV) prominence.

Figure 11–33. Coarctation of the aorta. Structures enlarged: left ventricle, proximal aorta. Distal aorta: poststenotic dilation.

Differential Diagnosis

Eisenmenger's syndrome must be distinguished from pulmonary hypertension due to acquired lesions that raise left atrial pressure. Tight mitral stenosis is by far the commonest of these lesions, but rare lesions such as left atrial myxoma, cor triatriatum, and sclerosing mediastinitis with pulmonary venous obstruction may occur. Primary (idiopathic) and thromboembolic pulmonary hypertension should also be excluded because such conditions carry a worse prognosis than Eisenmenger's syndrome. The history of a murmur and cyanosis dating back to early childhood is of great help in identifying congenital lesions but is not always available. In some patients with severe acquired pulmonary hypertension, opening of the foramen ovale may cause right-to-left shunting and lead to an erroneous diagnosis of a congenital lesion. Peripheral pulmonary artery stenosis may also be a possible cause of the physical signs of increased pressure in the main pulmonary artery.

Complications

When patients with Eisenmenger's syndrome are recatheterized after 10–20 years, it is remarkable how few changes are found in the hemodynamic status of the patient. Similarly, clinical findings show little change occurring between adolescence and the third and fourth decades. Complications of progressive polycythemia, pulmonary thromboembolism, and pulmonary infarction tend to become more frequent with the passage of time, and serious hemorrhage from plexiform angiomatous lesions in the pulmonary arterial bed may be fatal. Infective endocarditis is rare, and atrial arrhythmias are uncommon. With polycythemia, there is a poorly defined tendency to excessive bleeding. This is usually minor, manifested by easy bruising, bleeding gums, petechiae, and hemoptysis. It is more frequent when the hematocrit is above 60% and tends to decrease when the hematocrit is lower.

Treatment

A. Medical Treatment: Anticoagulant therapy and phlebotomy have been recommended but have not been shown to have any significant effects on the course of the disease. At present, phlebotomy is recommended only for symptoms due to the hyperviscosity seen with polycythemia. These include headache, fatigue, faintness, dizziness, paresthesias, irritability, myalgia, and impaired mentation. In patients receiving multiple phlebotomies, it is important to make sure that iron deficiency does not occur, because iron-deficient erythrocytes form relatively rigid microcytes, thus increasing viscosity.

B. Surgical Treatment: If the pulmonary vascular resistance is equivalent to systemic vascular resistance with little or no left-to-right shunt, the surgical closure of intracardiac or extracardiac (ductus or aortopulmonary window) defects in patients with Eisen-

menger's syndrome is almost always contraindicated. In those patients, closure removes the "safety valve" of a right-to-left shunt and tends to convert the patient's status to that associated with primary pulmonary hypertension. If the patient survives the operation, right heart failure and early death are likely to follow.

In some cases it is difficult to be sure that the pulmonary vascular resistance is indeed so high that surgical correction of the defect is out of the question. In patients with obvious cyanosis and pulmonary vascular resistance at or near the level of systemic resistance, there is no question of surgical correction, but in some cases there is still some left-to-right shunt, the pulmonary arterial pressure may not be as high as the systemic (as in a patient with an atrioventricular defect), and the possibility exists that surgery might be helpful. The outlook is best in patients with aortopulmonary defects, especially patent ductus arteriosus, and worst in cases with ventricular septal defect. Heart-lung transplantation offers new hope in the treatment of Eisenmenger's syndrome. The patients are young, and the possibility of treating the heart and lung lesions with a single operation is attractive. This form of therapy is still in the experimental stage.

Prognosis

Life expectancy is significantly reduced in patients with Eisenmenger's syndrome, and few patients in their 40s and 50s are seen by physicians. The course of the disease is not one of steady progression, as in primary pulmonary hypertension, and in a sheltered environment patients can live for 20 years or more with surprisingly little disability or evidence of progression.

Long-Term Results in Operated Cases

Operation to close intracardiac defects is almost always contraindicated in patients with Eisenmenger's syndrome and, if performed, is associated with a high immediate mortality rate. In Eisenmenger's syndrome, pregnancy results in an increased maternal mortality rate and is associated with a high fetal loss; therefore, in the first trimester, therapeutic abortion should be advised.

COARCTATION OF THE AORTA

Cardinal Features & Pathogenesis

This obstructive aortic lesion, which is characteristically associated with hypertension in the upper half of the body, with lower pressure in the legs, is usually diagnosed in childhood. The obstruction almost invariably is in the aortic isthmus just distal to the origin of the left subclavian artery and at the level where the ductus arteriosus joins the descending aorta, as shown in Figure 11–33. The obstruction may rarely be at other sites in the aorta, eg, at the origin of the left subclavian artery. In such cases, it is important to compare the blood pressure in the right arm with that in the leg, since the left arm and the legs may be at the site of obstruction. Collateral vessels develop that tend to bypass the obstruction. The principal variables in the lesion are the severity of the obstruction, which varies from complete aortic atresia to slight narrowing, and the size of the collateral vessels. These can be so large that a minimal pressure difference is present between the ascending and descending aorta in a patient with complete aortic obstruction at the site of coarctation.

In coarctation of the aorta, the left ventricle is hypertrophied and enlarged in proportion to the severity of the lesion. The proximal aorta is distended, and there is a poststenotic dilation of the aorta distal to the obstruction.

Coarctation of the aorta is associated with a number of other left-sided congenital lesions, namely, bicuspid aortic valve (which may be present in up to 80% of patients with coarctation), patent ductus arteriosus, aortic stenosis or incompetence, ventricular septal defect, mitral stenosis, aortic or mitral atresia, and other hypoplastic left heart syndromes. Coarctation of the aorta represents about 5% of cases of adult congenital heart disease and is more common in males than in females by a factor of more than 2:1. Some clinically insignificant narrowing of the aorta at the isthmus of the aorta is common, even in the absence of hypertension.

Clinical Findings

A. Symptoms and Signs: Coarctation of the aorta produces few symptoms. The lesion is usually discovered by finding an abnormally high blood pressure or a systolic murmur. Dyspnea on exertion, headache, and throbbing in the head are sometimes seen. In older, untreated cases, intermittent claudication may occur. Left heart failure, with pulmonary congestion and edema, occurs late in the disease, even in cases presenting in adult life.

The diagnosis of coarctation of the aorta can be readily made on physical examination. The carotid arteries show well-marked, bounding pulsations resulting from the forceful ejection of the left ventricular stroke volume into the reduced capacity of the arterial bed. There is usually a prominent pulsation in the suprasternal notch. The level of arterial pressure varies considerably with the age of the patient, being higher in older persons. The pulse pressure in the arms is wide, whereas that in the legs is reduced. The femoral pulses may be absent in severe cases; if they are present, the characteristic sign of delay between the timing of the upstrokes of the radial and femoral pulses should be sought. The examiner should first locate the femoral pulse with one hand and then palpate the radial pulse to detect and time the difference

between the arrival of the two waves. The pulses are synchronous in subjects with normal hearts, whereas delays of 0.1 second are readily discernible in patients with coarctation. Collateral vessels are often present on the back. They are best detected by feeling the intercostal arteries under the ribs and the enlarged arteries around the scapula as the patient bends forward.

B. Cardiac Signs: The heart is often enlarged, with a prominent left ventricular heave. Two varieties of murmur in coarctation of the aorta can usually be distinguished. One arises from the aortic obstruction and is late systolic in timing and ejection in type. The other type is longer and more continuous and arises from the collateral vessels. Both are heard best in the back, the murmur due to coarctation usually being heard best between the scapulas, left of the spine. The aortic valve closure sound is loud, and a third heart sound and a short delayed diastolic murmur arising from the mitral valve are occasionally heard. An aortic systolic ejection click and a decrescendo diastolic murmur due to the bicuspid aortic valve will often be heard.

C. Hemodynamic Findings: In coarctation of the aorta, the left ventricle pumps into a restricted arterial bed. This accounts for the high arterial pressure and pulse pressure seen in the upper extremities. However, the hemodynamics of coarctation are not as simple as they seem, and mechanical factors cannot account for all the findings. There may be disproportionate left ventricular hypertrophy and unexplained high resting cardiac output. There is also a contribution from the renin-angiotensin system to the development and maintenance of the upper body hypertension.

D. Electrocardiographic Findings: Some degree of left ventricular hypertrophy is present in all but the mildest cases. The electrocardiographic changes may be out of proportion to the level of arterial pressure. This suggests that aortic stenosis or left ventricular disease may also be present. Left bundle branch block is sometimes seen in older patients, and atrial fibrillation may occur.

E. Imaging Studies: The characteristic radiologic sign is the so-called "3" sign in the region of the aortic knob. It is shown in Figure 11–33. The upper half of the 3 is formed by the origin of the left subclavian artery and the lower half by the poststenotic dilation of the aorta below the coarctation. Rib notching is another radiologic sign closely associated with coarctation. It is caused by the large collateral intercostal arteries that erode the inferior surfaces of the ribs. The sign, which may be absent in childhood, is not invariably present in adults and is more significant in the outer portions of the ribs, 10 cm or more from the costovertebral junction. Left ventricular enlargement with prominence of the ascending aorta is seen in most cases.

F. Special Investigations: Patients with coarcta-

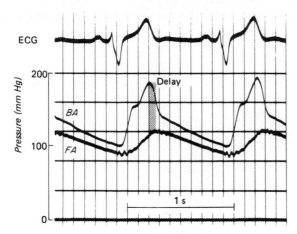

Figure 11–34. Pressure tracing above (BA) and below (FA) the site of obstruction in a patient with coarctation of the aorta. The delay of the peak systolic wave is indicated.

tion of the aorta present such a clear clinical picture that many are referred for surgical treatment without the need for special investigation. The pressure difference across the obstruction (Figure 11–34) can be measured reasonably accurately from indirect blood pressure levels in the right arm and leg. Aortography is recommended to estimate the length of the narrowed segment and to look for aneurysm formation at or near the coarctation. Transesophageal echocardiography can nicely demonstrate the location, severity, and length of the coarctation.

Differential Diagnosis

Coarctation of the aorta enters into the differential diagnosis of systemic hypertension (see Chapter 9). Minor forms of the lesion without systemic hypertension cause more problems in diagnosis, and when aortic stenosis or marked dilation of the ascending aorta coexists, coarctation may be difficult to detect. Acquired forms of coarctation may occasionally cause problems in diagnosis. When trauma ruptures the aorta, a hematoma may form that produces coarctation by external aortic compression.

Aortic obstruction due to aortitis (see Chapter 20) is another acquired lesion that can be confused with coarctation.

Complications

Subarachnoid hemorrhage due to rupture of a congenital aneurysm in the circle of Willis, aortic rupture and aortic dissection, and left ventricular failure were the common causes of death before surgical treatment became available. Infective endarteritis may occur at the site of coarctation or on the bicuspid aortic valve.

Treatment

If the lesion is hemodynamically significant, surgical resection of the coarcted area should always be

recommended. In the past, the ends of the cut aorta were sutured without the insertion of a graft. End-to-end anastomosis is now less common, and patch aortoplasty or graft insertion is often performed. Although the operation is relatively easy in childhood, it can be extremely difficult in older patients with larger collateral vessels and friable aortic tissue. Reoperation to deal with an inadequate previous repair presents serious problems. The mortality rate is higher in older patients, being approximately 10% in patients over age 30.

In patients with severe lesions, the sudden increase in perfusion pressure, especially of the gut and other abdominal organs, results in an acute postoperative rise in blood pressure and an arterial lesion that histologically resembles the arteritis of malignant hypertension or polyarteritis nodosa. Abdominal pain may be severe enough to warrant exploratory laparotomy. Antihypertensive medication with propranolol and expectant treatment are all that is required, and the lesions are short-lived. Paraplegia is another rare complication of surgery. Interference with the blood supply to the spinal cord at operation is responsible. This complication can also occur in patients who have not been operated on.

Nonsurgical treatment using percutaneous balloon dilation has been recently introduced for the relief of coarctation. It has been shown to be effective even in adult patients, but the incidence of local aneurysm formation seems to be increased. This approach may increase the frequency of the peculiar form of arteritis seen after relief of coarctation of the aorta.

Prognosis

The prognosis in coarctation of the aorta is good when surgical treatment is performed in childhood. Blood pressure does not always return to normal, especially if the lesion is not corrected until adult life, and left ventricular hypertrophy and a high output state may persist. The later development of aortic incompetence or stenosis (which occurs when the bicuspid aortic valve, so commonly associated with coarctation, calcifies in middle life) tends to worsen the prognosis.

Long-Term Results
in Operated Cases

Persistent hypertension in the upper part of the body is the most important long-term problem. It occurs most commonly in two groups of patients: those in whom surgery is performed in the first year of life, and those in whom repair is delayed until after the age of 30. Patients show a tendency to develop hypertension later in life, and only 20% of patients followed for 25 years or more were free of complications and had normal blood pressure. Other complications include restenosis or aneurysm formation at the site of repair.

Congestive heart failure, like persistent hyperten-

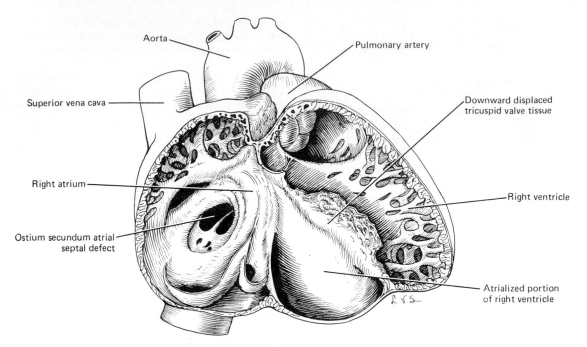

Aorta

Pulmonary artery

Superior vena cava

Downward displaced
tricuspid valve tissue

Right atrium

Right ventricle

Ostium secundum atrial
septal defect

Atrialized portion
of right ventricle

Figure 11–35. Anatomic features of Ebstein's malformation (Redrawn from the illustrations of Dr Frank H Netter, as printed in: Heart. Vol 5 of: *CIBA Collection of Medical Illustrations.* CIBA Pharmaceutical Company, 1969.)

sion, is more likely to occur in older patients in whom operation was performed in adult life. Cerebrovascular accidents are also correlated with postoperative hypertension and represent a significant problem, occurring in about 5% of operated patients.

A bicuspid aortic valve is commonly associated with coarctation of the aorta. Thus, valvular calcification with an aortic systolic murmur and the development of aortic valve disease in middle age are to be expected.

Infective endarteritis also remains a problem, and penicillin or amoxicillin prophylaxis for major dental work is still required in operated patients.

EBSTEIN'S MALFORMATION

This rare congenital malformation is illustrated in Figure 11–35 and represents about 1% of cases of adult congenital heart disease.

The basic abnormality is downward displacement of a portion of the tricuspid valve, with atrialization of a large part of the right ventricle. The septal and posterior leaflets of the tricuspid valve are usually involved. The principal variable is the presence or absence of an associated ostium secundum atrial septal defect. The atrialized portion of the ventricle hinders rather than helps the forward flow of blood, and the tricuspid valve is congenitally incompetent. The lesion is remarkably well tolerated and was first recognized clinically in a cyanotic form in patients who

also had an atrial septal defect. More acyanotic cases without atrial defects have come to be recognized, and it now appears that the lesion probably occurs more commonly without an atrial defect. Pulmonary blood flow is reduced, especially when right-to-left shunting through an atrial defect is present.

Clinical Findings

A. Symptoms and Signs: Dyspnea and fatigue are the commonest presenting symptoms. Atrial arrhythmias commonly cause palpitations, and right heart failure occurs with increasing age. The pulse is of small amplitude, and the venous pressure is usually raised in adult patients. Atrial fibrillation is usually present after age 20. The heart is quiet, with distant heart sounds. Systolic clicks are common and are due to displacement of the posterior cusp of the tricuspid valve during systole. There is usually a systolic murmur of tricuspid origin and wide splitting of the second heart sound. A short, scratchy diastolic murmur or third heart sound arising from the tricuspid valve is usually heard at the left sternal edge. The murmurs tend to increase in intensity during inspiration.

B. Electrocardiographic Findings: The ECG usually shows incomplete or complete right bundle branch block and a low voltage. Preexcitation (Wolff-Parkinson-White syndrome) is seen in about 20% of cases, and other atrial and ventricular arrhythmias are common.

C. Imaging Studies: The heart is large, with a well-defined border because its excursions are small.

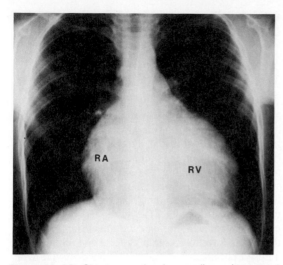

Figure 11–36. Chest x-ray showing cardiac enlargement involving the right atrium (RA) and right ventricle (RV) in a patient with Ebstein's malformation.

The lungs are oligemic and the pulmonary artery is not enlarged (Figure 11–36). The cardiac enlargement is all right-sided.

D. Special Investigations:

1. Noninvasive techniques– Echocardiography reveals delayed closure of the tricuspid valve coinciding with an early systolic click. There is rightward rotation of the heart, large excursions of the triscupid valve, and downward displacement of the entire valve mechanism. These findings are not specific and reflect marked right heart dilation. More specific changes are seen on two-dimensional studies (Figure 11–37) in which the abnormal position of the tricuspid valve is more clearly seen, and a definite diagnosis can usually be made.

2. Invasive techniques– Cardiac catheterization can confirm the diagnosis. Right-sided pressures are all about the same level, and it is difficult to tell from the pressure tracings whether the catheter is in the pulmonary artery, the distal right ventricle, the proximal right ventricle, the right atrium, or the superior vena cava. Because the atrialized part of the right

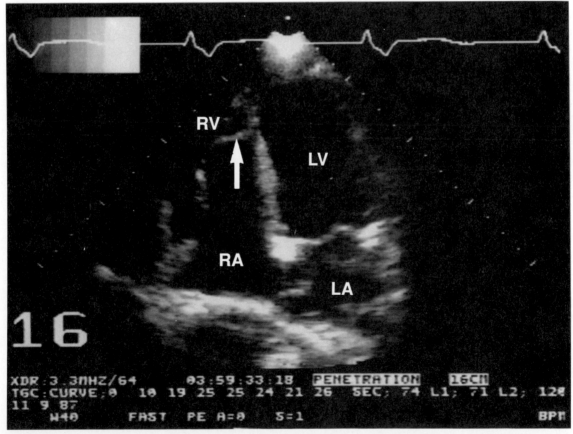

Figure 11–37. Two-dimensional echocardiogram in four-chamber view of a 60-year-old man with Ebstein's disease. Note the marked displacement of the septal leaflet (arrow) of the tricuspid valve deep into the right ventricle. (RV, right ventricle; RA, right atrium; LV, left ventricle; LA, left atrium.)

ventricle is depolarized like the right ventricle, a pull-back across the tricuspid valve in Ebstein's disease using an electrode catheter and monitoring the intra-cardiac electrogram and the intracardiac pressure simultaneously will show a change from right ventricular to right atrial pressure but no change in the electrogram. If this can be demonstrated, a diagnosis of Ebstein's disease can be made.

Angiocardiography with injection into the right atrium can demonstrate the tricuspid valve to be displaced into the right ventricle, but the two-dimensional echocardiogram is so much better in demonstrating this that angiocardiography is now rarely done.

Differential Diagnosis

Massive cardiac enlargement due to pericardial disease can usually be distinguished on the basis of the history. The cardiac enlargement will have developed recently, whereas in Ebstein's malformation there is a long history of heart disease. Severe right heart failure in patients with congenital pulmonary stenosis may produce a somewhat similar picture, and advanced rheumatic tricuspid valve disease can be recognized and ruled out because there will almost certainly be some associated mitral valve disease.

Complications

Atrial arrhythmias and right heart failure are sufficiently common to be considered as part of the disease rather than as complications. Sudden death is relatively common and attributed to arrhythmia.

Treatment

Plication of the right atrium, eliminating the atrialized portion of the ventricle, has been advocated. The operation is palliative and is certainly not indicated in mild forms of the condition. If tricuspid regurgitation is hemodynamically severe and compromising cardiac output, tricuspid valve replacement has been advocated. The results of surgical treatment are generally not excellent, but it is possible at the same time to surgically ablate the accessory atrioventricular pathways. If the patient has preexcitation and control of arrhythmia is a problem, surgery may be indicated for a dual purpose. Epicardial mapping is necessary, and the results of cutting accessory pathways are good when the pathway has been clearly identified (see Chapter 14). If tricuspid regurgitation is well tolerated and tricuspid valve replacement not in question, catheter ablation is the procedure of choice.

Prognosis

Patients with Ebstein's malformation have a reduced life expectancy and seldom reach age 50. Persons with milder forms of the disease can have an almost normal life span. Postoperative arrhythmias are common and probably account for the high incidence of sudden death.

MORE COMPLEX & COMBINED CONGENITAL HEART LESIONS

1. TRANSPOSITION OF THE GREAT ARTERIES

In transposition of the great arteries, the right ventricle pumps blood returning from the systemic veins into the aorta, while the left ventricle pumps arterialized blood from the pulmonary veins into the pulmonary artery (Figure 11–38). If the infant is to survive, there must be some form of septal defect or aortopulmonary communication to permit cross-circulation of the blood. The pulmonary blood flow is usually increased in infants with this lesion, and only those who have large septal defects and who develop a raised pulmonary vascular resistance survive without surgery.

If transposition of the great arteries is associated with pulmonary stenosis, the pulmonary vascular bed may be protected and the patient may present with a clinical picture resembling Fallot's tetralogy and benefit from a palliative Blalock-Taussig operation. If transposition is associated with tricuspid atresia, that lesion dominates the clinical picture.

Transposition of the great arteries with increased pulmonary blood flow is a relatively common lesion in infancy, and most patients die within the first year unless treated surgically. In early infancy, the patient's condition may deteriorate when the ductus arteriosus closes. In such cases, the surgical creation of

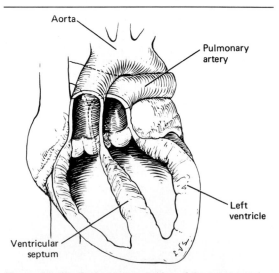

Figure 11–38. Typical transposition of the great arteries. The aorta arises from the morphologic right ventricle and is anterior to and slightly to the right of the pulmonary artery, which originates from the morphologic left ventricle. (Reproduced, with permission, from Way LW [editor]: *Current Surgical Diagnosis & Treatment,* 8th ed. Appleton & Lange, 1988.)

an atrial septal defect (Blalock-Hanlon operation) was first advocated. A more successful palliative procedure has been the Rashkind procedure—the "noninvasive" creation or enlargement of an atrial septal defect. A balloon catheter is passed into the left atrium and, after inflation, pulled forcefully back into the right atrium, tearing the septum. The procedure is surprisingly well tolerated.

The development of Mustard's operation for the correction of transposition has led to the increased survival of patients. The operation consists of excision of the atrial septum and insertion of a baffle made of pericardial tissue, which is sewn into the atrium to redirect the pulmonary venous flow to the mitral valve and the systemic venous return to the tricuspid valve.

The long-term results of this operation are still being evaluated. Their clinical status is far from normal, and problems often arise from failure of the baffle to grow. Baffle leaks are relatively uncommon, but obstruction to venous return from either the lungs or the systemic circulation (superior rather than inferior vena cava) is not uncommon, and second operations may be needed.

The extensive atrial surgery tends to disrupt the conduction system, and supraventricular arrhythmias (tachycardia or bradycardia) are common. Sudden death has been reported and has been attributed to arrhythmia. The ability of the embryologic right ventricle to support the systemic circulation has been questioned, and evaluation of the "systemic" right ventricle shows that its function is not that of the normal left ventricle. Occasional instances of the "systemic" right ventricle failing are reported. This has led to a more recent approach to correction—the Jatene procedure or arterial "switch" operation. In this operation, the main pulmonary artery is transected proximal to its bifurcation and anastomosed, end-to-side, to the ascending aorta. This directs arterialized blood from the lungs returning to the heart via the embryologic left atrium and ventricle to the systemic circulation. A valved conduit is then inserted to connect the embryologic right ventricle, carrying systemic venous return, to the pulmonary artery and lungs.

This operation makes the thicker, embryologic left ventricle supply the systemic flow and has given better results. The possibility of banding the pulmonary artery to induce hypertrophy in the weaker ventricle before correction has been recommended. The Jatene arterial switch operation is at present the procedure of choice.

2. CORRECTED TRANSPORTATION

In physiologically corrected transportation, the aorta arises from the embryonic right ventricle, whereas the pulmonary artery arises from the embry-

onic left ventricle. The term "corrected" indicates that unlike the situation in transposition of the great arteries, the systemic venous return goes to the lungs through the "anatomic" left ventricle, and the pulmonary venous blood passes to the aorta through the "anatomic" right ventricle. The atrioventricular valves are transposed so that the venous "tricuspid" valve is mitral in shape, and the systemic "mitral" valve has three cusps (Figure 11–39). The morphology of the ventricle can be accurately determined by two-dimensional echocardiography. The abnormality can be associated with almost any form of congenital heart disease, but ventricular septal defect, infundibular stenosis, Ebstein's displacement of the left-sided atrioventricular valve or tricuspid valve, and complete heart block are the lesions most commonly seen.

The exact positions of the origins of the great vessels in relation to one another can vary, but the aorta is commonly on the left, beside or in front of the pulmonary artery. The lesion can be seen in adult life and is presumably compatible with a normal life span if it is the sole abnormality. There are instances of congestive failure of the anatomic right ventricle, which acts as the systemic ventricle, suggesting that the anatomic right ventricle is not capable of sustaining the systemic circulation for 70 or 80 years.

Physiologically corrected transposition should be suspected in patients with congenital complete atrioventricular block. Because the aortic root and valve are in an anterior and left-sided position, the second heart sound is frequently loud in the second left interspace. Since the ventricles and their conduction systems are inverted, the ECG frequently shows reversed initial forces with a Q wave in V_1 and no Q wave in V_6. The chest radiograph may show a smooth convexity along the left upper margin of the cardiac silhouette due to the displaced ascending aorta.

Problems may occur during cardiac catheterization because it is difficult to enter the pulmonary artery. In such cases a Swan-Ganz balloon catheter will often float through the right ventricle and enter the pulmonary artery, making it possible to record the pulmonary arterial pressure, which, varies with the associated lesions.

The long-term problems in surgery treated cases mainly stem from conduction defects and arrhythmias.

3. TRUNCUS ARTERIOSUS

In truncus arteriosus, there is a single semilunar valve, because the embryonic truncus has not divided into a pulmonary trunk and aorta. The vessels to the lungs thus arise from the truncus (Figure 11–40). A ventricular septal defect is always part of this lesion. The level of pulmonary flow and pulmonary vascular resistance varies. Almost all patients who survive infancy have a raised pulmonary vascular resistance, or there is obstruction of the pulmonary arteries at their

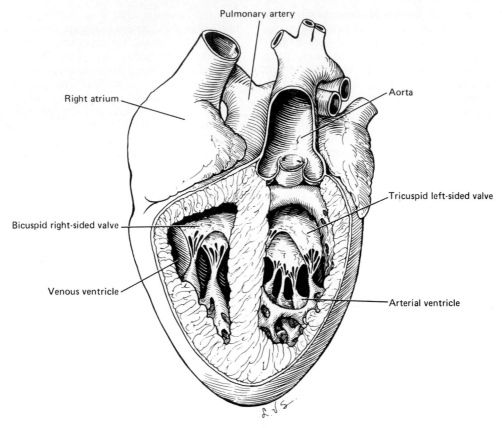

Pulmonary artery

Right atrium

Aorta

Tricuspid left-sided valve

Bicuspid right-sided valve

Venous ventricle

Arterial ventricle

Figure 11–39. Anatomic features of corrected transposition. The aorta arises in front and to the left of the pulmonary artery, but the great vessels are connected to the appropriate ventricles (aorta to arterial ventricle; pulmonary to venous ventricle). The right-sided atrioventricular valve is bicuspid (mitral); the left-sided atrioventricular valve has three cusps. (Redrawn from the illustration of Dr Frank H Netter, as printed in: Heart. Vol 5 of: *CIBA Collection of Medical Illustrations.* CIBA Pharmaceutical Company, 1969.)

origin from the truncus. The exact origin of the vessels supplying the lungs varies and has been used to classify patients into four types. This classification does not greatly influence the clinical picture, except that type IV, in which the blood supply to the lungs arises from bronchial vessels, is really pulmonary atresia and best considered to be a severe form of Fallot's tetralogy. In many cases, the common outflow valve has more than three cusps. This valve tends to be incompetent and causes a loud immediate diastolic murmur. The lesion can now be treated surgically by the Rastelli procedure (insertion of a valved conduit), provided that pulmonary vascular resistance is not too high and the vessels to the lungs are of an adequate size to receive the shunt. A plastic right ventricular prosthesis is interposed between the right atrium and the pulmonary arteries, which are removed from the aorta and sutured to the prosthesis. The ventricular defect is closed, and although the result is not a normal heart, the outcome is more favorable than it used to be. If the truncus valve is

severely incompetent, valve replacement is needed, which increases the surgical mortality.

The long-term results of the surgical treatment of truncus arteriosus are just beginning to be appreciated. Calcification and obstruction in the prosthesis may occur, and residual pulmonary hypertension is often a problem.

4. TRICUSPID ATRESIA

In cases of atresia of the tricuspid valve, there must be an atrial defect through which all the systemic venous return reaches the left heart (Figure 11–41). As a result, there is left ventricular hypertrophy that shows up clearly on the ECG as left ventricular dominance because the right ventricle is absent or not functional. Various associated lesions, especially transposition of the great arteries, may be present, and the origin of blood flow to the lungs is the principal variable. There may be associated pulmonary atresia

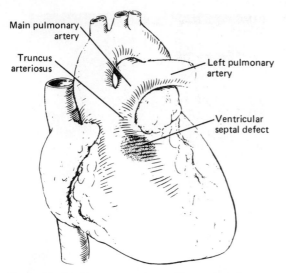

Figure 11–40. Truncus arteriosus. The main pulmonary artery arises from the truncus arteriosus downstream to the truncal semilunar valve. A ventricular septal defect is always present. (Modified and reproduced, with permission, from Way LW [editor]: *Current Surgical Diagnosis & Treatment,* 8th ed. Appleton & Lange, 1988.)

with reduced pulmonary blood flow, and there may be a ventricular septal defect through which an increased pulmonary blood flow reaches the lungs. If pulmonary atresia is present and blood flow is reduced (reaching the lungs via a patent ductus or bronchial vessels), a palliative Blalock-Taussig shunt may increase the pulmonary blood flow and increase the patient's life span. In rare cases, the tricuspid atresia is not complete, and there is a small underdeveloped right ventricle. In such patients, the characteristic finding of the lesion (left ventricular hypertrophy on the ECG) is still present.

Treatment

Effective palliation by means of Glenn's operation, anastomosing the superior vena cava to the right pulmonary artery, has increased the number of patients reaching adult life, but resistance to pulmonary blood flow may increase. Correction by Fontan's procedure involves connecting the right atrium to the pulmonary artery via a valved conduit or anastomosing the right atrium directly to the pulmonary artery, then closing the atrial septal defect. This operation is now being carried out in older patients who have had palliative surgery. The indications for this further surgery are

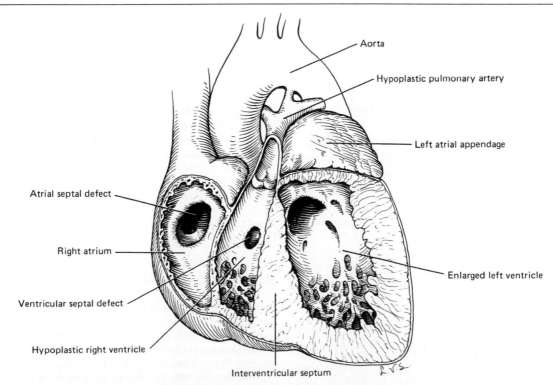

Figure 11–41. Tricuspid atresia, right-sided view.

not yet clear, and long-term results are not available. For unknown reasons, pulmonary arteriovenous fistulas in the lower lobes are prone to develop after Glenn and Fontan operations.

A serious postoperative problem in patients with the Fontan procedure has been the development of atrial arrhythmias, especially atrial tachycardia and flutter. This arrhythmia is difficult to treat with antiarrhythmic drugs and is associated with sudden death. If the arrhythmia is not controllable with drugs, ablation of the atrioventricular node can be performed together with insertion of a DDD pacemaker. If atrial arrhythmia continues, the pacemaker can be reprogrammed to a VVI pacemaker. (See Chapter 14.)

A modification of the Glenn and Fontan procedures has been advocated in order to remove the right atrium from the circulation entirely. In this operation, the inferior and superior vena cava are joined by constructing a tunnel in the right atrium and anastomosing this to the pulmonary artery, a bidirectional Glenn procedure. Whether this will eliminate the problem of atrial arrhythmias over the long term is not yet known.

5. TOTAL ANOMALOUS PULMONARY VENOUS DRAINAGE

In this lesion, all the blood returning from the lungs enters the right heart (Figure 11–42). There must of necessity be an atrial septal defect. The principal variable is the route taken by the pulmonary venous return, which is most commonly via a left-sided superior vena cava—or ascending common pulmonary

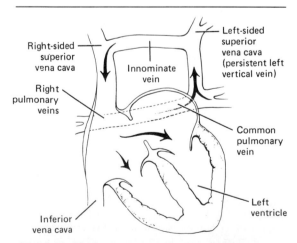

Figure 11–42. Common type of total anomalous pulmonary venous connection. The pulmonary veins connect to a persistent left-sided superior vena cava (left vertical vein), the innominate vein, and the right superior vena cava. (Reproduced, with permission, from Way LW [editor]: *Current Surgical Diagnosis & Treatment*, 8th ed. Appleton & Lange, 1988.)

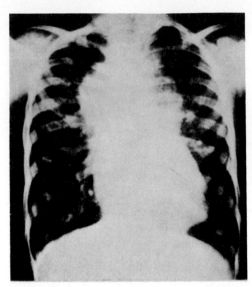

Figure 11–43. Chest x-ray showing typical "snowman" appearance owing to total anomalous pulmonary venous drainage into left innominate vein. (Reproduced, with permission, from Wood P: *Diseases of the Heart and Circulation,* 3rd ed. Lippincott, 1968.)

vein—to the innominate vein and thence to the right atrium via the normally placed right superior vena cava. The other common pattern seen in infancy is via the inferior vena cava below the diaphragm. The pulmonary blood flow and blood pressure vary, and the pulmonary venous return may be obstructed, leading to pulmonary venous congestion and edema. In this case, percutaneous balloon dilation of the obstruction may be beneficial. Obstruction to venous return is commoner when the anomalous pulmonary vein returns below the diaphragm. The variety of the lesion most commonly seen in older children is the pattern involving the innominate vein. The venous return is free, and there is usually raised pulmonary vascular resistance. In this lesion there is a characteristic chest x-ray picture called "snowman heart" (Figure 11–43). The upper circular shadow is the anomalous venous pathway that lies above the lower circular shadow formed by the rest of the heart.

CONGENITAL CONDUCTION DEFECTS

Congenital defects of the cardiac conduction system are described in Chapter 14. The most important are the Wolff-Parkinson-White syndrome and congenital complete atrioventricular block. Both lesions usually occur without associated congenital defects, but the former may be seen in association with Ebstein's anomaly and the latter with corrected transportation and ventricular septal defect. Conduction defects and arrhythmias are commonly a problem both early and late after extensive surgery for congenital heart disease.

CONGENITAL ABNORMALITIES OF THE CORONARY CIRCULATION

Anomalies of the coronary circulation are seen alone or in association with other lesions.

The commonest congenital coronary anomaly is that the left circumflex coronary artery originates from the right sinus of Valsalva and passes behind the aorta en route to its normal area of distribution. As common is the separate origin of the left circumflex and anterior descending coronary arteries from the left coronary sinus.

An important abnormality exists when the left coronary artery arises from the pulmonary artery. In this lesion, the blood flows through the anomalous vessel into the pulmonary artery, and a right-to-left shunt is seen. There is usually an electrocardiographic pattern of severe myocardial ischemia or infarction (Figure 11–44). Ligation of the abnormal vessel benefits the patient but does not cure the condition. Reanastomosis of the vessel to the aorta is the treatment of choice.

When the entire left coronary artery arises from the right sinus of Valsalva, it passes obliquely and posteriorly behind the right ventricular outflow tract. This oblique passage can make the orifice slit-like and cause obstruction. The lesion has been found in young persons who collapse and die suddenly, especially during exercise. When the right coronary artery arises from the left coronary sinus and passes anteriorly between the right ventricular outflow tract and the aorta, sudden death is less common than when the left coronary artery arises anomalously, though acute inferior wall myocardial infarction does occur in this lesion.

Coronary arteriovenous and arteriocameral fistulas are seen both as isolated lesions and in association with other lesions. The coronary arteries arise appropriately from the sinuses of Valsalva, and vessels enter a fistulous area, usually draining into the right atrium, right ventricle, or coronary sinus. The right coronary artery is more frequently involved than the left, and the patient presents with a continuous murmur over the lower precordium in a position unlike that seen with patent ductus arteriosus. Although fistula flow may be high, causing a large left-to-right shunt, it is often not sufficient to cause significant increase in pulmonary blood flow, and the diagnosis is usually made by angiography. On echocardiography, a fistula can be suspected if either the right or left coronary artery is seen to be large at its origin.

A more common form of coronary arteriovenous fistula is often seen at coronary angiography. An accessory coronary artery arises from the pulmonary artery, resulting in a fistulous connection between the normal coronary arteries and the main pulmonary artery. In some patients, this condition produces a continuous murmur, but in most patients it is silent. Few complications have been described in patients with these lesions, and their presence is ordinarily only detected at the time of coronary angiography.

ABNORMAL POSITION OF THE HEART

Cause of Abnormal Position of the Heart; Associated Conditions

Displacement of the heart interferes with physical examination more than it impairs function of the heart. Abnormalities on the ECG and chest x-ray due to displacement of the heart are also confusing and often suggest more serious abnormalities than are actually present.

Abnormal position of the heart may be due to congenital abnormalities, as in dextrocardia, or to absence of the left pericardium. It may be due to lung disease, which either pushes or pulls the heart and mediastinal contents to one side, or to abnormalities of the thoracic cage, which may be congenital or acquired. There may be associated congenital abnormalities in the heart itself, especially when chest deformity is congenital. Chest deformity also occurs as a result of congenital heart disease. Ventricular dilation and hypertrophy in children with a soft cartilaginous thorax tends to produce a bulge in the left upper chest, which is seen well in patients with a large ventricular septal defect. The developing thorax becomes fixed in its abnormal shape, and the deformity persists into adult life.

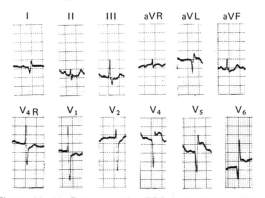

Figure 11–44. Representative ECG leads from a patient with anomalous left coronary artery originating from the aorta showing a current of injury pattern in the anterolateral left ventricular wall. (Reproduced, with permission, from Askenazi J, Nadas AS: Anomalous left coronary artery originating from the aorta. Circulation 1976;51:976.)

The heart itself may be normally situated, but the great vessels may be abnormal, as in right-sided aortic arch or absence of the left pulmonary artery, which may occur as isolated lesions or with Fallot's tetralogy. A left-sided superior vena cava may persist, either alone or with a right superior vena cava, and the inferior vena cava may enter the right atrium in an abnormal position. These lesions are seen with atrial septal defects but can also occur alone.

Dextrocardia

The heart may be situated in the right side of the chest either because of mirror image dextrocardia or because it is displaced from its normal left-sided position. Dextrocardia is usually associated with complete situs inversus involving the abdominal viscera; it is also found with other congenital heart anomalies. There may be isolated dextrocardia with a normal position of the abdominal viscera (situs solitus). In this case, associated cardiac malformations are extremely common.

The position of the atria is best determined from the ECG. If the atrial positions are reversed, the P wave is negative in leads I and aVL and positive in aVR. The position of the atria coincides with the position of the viscera, so that with few exceptions the positions of the stomach and liver give an accurate indication of the atrial position. Electrocardiography and two-dimensional echocardiography give the best indication of the position of the ventricles, and two-dimensional echo is also an effective means of determining the positions of the great vessels.

Displacement Due to Abnormalities of the Thoracic Cage

Displacement of the heart due to pectus excavatum and kyphoscoliosis may cause physical findings suggestive of heart disease. Since associated congenital heart lesions are common, the diagnosis is often difficult. Depression of the sternum may be associated with abnormalities of the position of the thoracic spine. These abnormalities narrow the anteroposterior diameter of the thorax. In this case, the heart may appear enlarged on the posteroanterior view and narrowed on the lateral view. This has been called, rather fancifully, the "pancake heart." Systolic ejection mur-

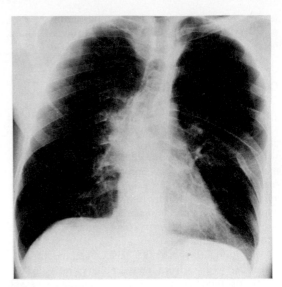

Figure 11–45. Chest x-ray of a patient with kyphoscoliosis showing rotation of the heart toward the right anterior oblique position. (Courtesy of G Gamsu.)

murs, wide splitting of the second sound, and even diastolic murmurs can occur. The ECG may show an incomplete right bundle branch block, and the large cardiac shadow on the posteroanterior view with a prominent right ventricular outflow tract may suggest atrial septal defect. In some cases, atrial septal defect is actually present. In kyphoscoliosis (Figure 11–45), the heart is often rotated, usually toward a right anterior oblique position. The outflow tract is thus abnormally prominent. The ECG shows clockwise rotation of the heart as a result of cardiac displacement, and it is often difficult to be sure that the heart is normal.

Patients with chest deformity not infrequently complain of symptoms similar to those of effort syndrome, eg, dyspnea, palpitations, sweating, fatigue, noncardiac pain, and nervousness. In the large majority of cases, there is no underlying heart disease and no specific cardiac treatment is indicated. If the chest deformity is severe, operation may be indicated for cosmetic repair of pectus excavatum. Orthopedic treatment of kyphoscoliosis should not be influenced by cardiac considerations.

REFERENCES

General

Barth CW, Roberts WC: Left main coronary originating from the right sinus of Valsalva and coursing between the aorta and pulmonary trunk. J Am Coll Cardiol 1986;7:366.

Blanche C, Chaux A: Long-term results of surgery for coronary artery fistulas. Int Surg 1990;75:238.

Cheitlin MD, DeCastro CM, McCallister HA: Sudden death as a complication of anomalous left coronary origin from the anterior sinus of Valsalva: A not-so-minor congenital anomaly. Circulation 1974;50:780.

Click RL et al: Anomalous coronary arteries: location, degree of atherosclerosis and effect on survival: A report from the Coronary Artery Surgery Study. J Am Coll Cardiol 1989;13:531.

D'Orsogna L et al: Influence of echocardiography in preoperative cardiac catheterization in congenital heart disease. Int J Cardiol 1989;24:19.

Davia JE et al: Anomalous left coronary artery origin from the right coronary sinus. Am Heart J 1984;108:165.

Donaldson RM et al: Management of cardiovascular complications in Marfan syndrome. Lancet 1980;2:1178.

Leatham A: Auscultation of the Heart and Phonocardiography, 2nd ed. Churchill Livingstone, 1975.

Lipsett J et al: Anomalous coronary arteries arising from the aorta associated with sudden death in infancy and early childhood: An autopsy series. Arch Pathol Lab Med 1991;115:770.

Marks LA, Mehta AV, Marangi D: Percutaneous transluminal balloon angioplasty of stenotic standard Blalock-Taussig shunts: effect on choice of initial palliation in cyanotic congenital heart disease. J Am Coll Cardiol 1991;18:546.

Maron BJ et al: Prospective identification by two-dimensional echocardiography of anomalous origin of the left main coronary artery from the right sinus of Valsalva. Am J Cardiol 1991;68:140.

McNamara DG, Latson LA: Long term follow-up of patients with malformations for which definitive surgical repair has been available for 25 years or more. Am J Cardiol 1982;50:560.

Morris CD, Menashe VD: 25-year mortality after surgical repair of congenital heart defect in childhood: A population-based cohort study. JAMA 1991;266:3447.

Moss AJ: What every primary physician should know about the postoperative cardiac patient. Pediatrics 1979;63:320.

Noonan JA: Association of congenital heart disease with syndromes or other defect. Pediatr Clin North Am 1978;25:797.

Nora JJ, Nora AH: Maternal transmission of congenital heart diseases: New recurrence risk figures and the questions of cytoplasmic inheritance and vulnerability to teratogens. J Am Coll Cardiol 1987;59:459.

Perloff JK et al: Adults with cyanotic congenital heart disease: Hematologic management. Ann Intern Med 1988;109:406.

Pitkin RM et al: Pregnancy and congenital heart disease. Ann Intern Med 1990;112:445.

Rao PS: Balloon valvuloplasty and angioplasty of stenotic lesions of the heart and great vessels in children. Adv Pediatr 1990;37:33.

Rigby ML, Shinebourne EA: The aetiology and epidemiology of congenital heart disease. In: Scientific Foundations of Cardiology. Sleight P, Jones JV (editors). Heinemann, 1983.

Roberts WC: Adult Congenital Heart Disease. Davis, 1986.

Roberts WC: Cardiac valvular residua and sequelae after operation for congenital heart disease. Am Heart J 1983;106:1181.

Roberts WC: Major anomalies of coronary arterial origin seen in adulthood. Am Heart J 1986;111:941.

Rudolph AM, Hoffman JIE: Pediatrics, 18th ed. Appleton & Lange, 1987.

Salloum DT et al: Anomalous coronary arteries coursing between the aorta and pulmonary trunk: Clinical indications for coronary artery bypass. Eur Heart J 1991;12:832.

Sapin P et al: Coronary artery fistula: An abnormality affecting all age groups. Medicine 1990;69:101.

Schiller NB, Snider AR: Echocardiography in congenital heart disease. Circulation 1981;63:461.

Stumper OF et al: Transesophageal echocardiography in children with congenital heart disease: An initial experience. J Am Coll Cardiol 1990;16:433.

Taussig HB: World survey of the common cardiac malformations: Developmental error or genetic variant? Am J Cardiol 1982;50:544.

Vigneswaran WT et al: Evolution of the management of anomalous left coronary artery: a new surgical approach. Ann Thorac Surg 1989;48:560.

Atrial Septal Defect

Bink-Boelkens MT et al: Arrhythmias after repair of secundum atrial septal defect: The influence of surgical modification. Am Heart J 1988;115:629.

Brandenburg RO et al: Clinical follow-up study of paroxysmal supraventricular tachyarrhythmias after operative repair of a secundum type atrial septal defect in adults. Am J Cardiol 1983;51:273.

Bricker JT et al: Dysrhythmias after repair of atrial septal defect. Texas Heart Inst J 1986;11:203.

Carabello BA et al: Normal left ventricular systolic function in adults with atrial septal defect and left heart failure. Am J Cardiol 1982;49:1868.

Cowen ME et al: The results of surgery for atrial septal defect in patients aged fifty years and over. Eur Heart J 1990;11:29.

Fiore AC et al: Surgical closure of atrial septal defect in patients older than 50 years of age. Arch Surg 1988;123:965.

Hagen PT et al: Incidence and size of patent foramen ovale during the first 10 decades of life: An autopsy study of 965 normal hearts. Mayo Clin Proc 1984;59:17.

Harjula A et al: Early and late results of surgery for atrial septal defect in patients aged over 60 years. J Cardiovasc Surg 1988;29:13.

Hurwitz RA et al: Current value of radionuclide angiocardiography for shunt quantification and management in patients with secundum atrial septal defect. Am Heart J 1982;103:421.

Hynes JK et al: Partial atrioventricular canal defect in elderly patients (aged 60 years or older). Am J Cardiol 1982;50:59.

Kitabatake A et al: Noninvasive evaluation of the ratio of pulmonary to systemic flow in atrial septal defect by duplex Doppler echocardiography. Circulation 1984;69:73.

Lipshultz SE et al: Are routine cardiac catheterization and angiography necessary before repair of ostium primum atrial septal defect? J Am Coll Cardiol 1988;11:373.

Lynch JJ et al: Prevalence of right-to-left atrial shunting

in a healthy population: Detection of Valsalva maneuver contrast echocardiography. Am J Cardiol 1984;53:1478.

Murphy JG et al: Long-term outcome after surgical repair of isolated atrial septal defect. Follow-up at 27 to 32 years. N Engl J Med 1990;323:1645.

Oakley D et al: Scimitar vein syndrome: Report of nine new cases. Am Heart J 1984;107:596.

Shub C et al: Sensitivity of two-dimensional echocardiography in the direct visualization of atrial septal defect utilizing the subcostal approach: Experience with 154 patients. J Am Coll Cardiol 1983;2:127.

Sideris EB et al: Transvenous atrial septal defect occlusion in piglets with a 'buttoned' double-disk device. Circulation 1999;81:312.

Steele PM et al: Isolated atrial septal defect with pulmonary vascular obstructive disease: Long-term follow-up and prediction of outcome after surgical correction. Circulation 1987;76:1037.

Sutton MGS, Tajik AJ, McGoon DC: Atrial septal defect in patients ages 60 years or older. Operative results and long-term postoperative follow-up. Circulation 1981;64:402.

Pulmonary Stenosis

Edwards BS et al: Morphologic changes in the pulmonary arteries after percutaneous balloon angioplasty for pulmonary arterial stenosis. Circulation 1985;71:195.

Kan JS et al: Percutaneous transluminal balloon valvuloplasty for pulmonary valve stenosis. Circulation 1984;69:554.

Kopecky SL et al: Long-term outcome of patients undergoing surgical repair of isolated pulmonary valve stenosis: Follow-up at 20-30 years. Circulation 1988;78:1150.

Lababidi Z, Wu JR: Percutaneous balloon pulmonary valvuloplasty. Am J Cardiol 1983;52:560.

Pepine CJ, Gessner IH, Feldman RL: Percutaneous balloon valvuloplasty for pulmonic valve stenosis in the adult. Am J Cardiol 1982;50:1442.

Saad AK et al: Use of a double balloon technique for percutaneous balloon pulmonary valvotomy in carditis. Br Heart J 1987;58:136.

Wren C, Oslizlok P, Bull C: Natural history of supravalvular aortic stenosis and pulmonary artery stenosis. J Am Coll Cardiol 1990;15:1625.

Fallot's Tetralogy

Barber G et al: Pulmonary atresia with ventricular septal defect: Preoperative and postoperative response to exercise. J Am Coll Cardiol 1986;7:630.

Bastos P et al: Left ventricular function after total correction of tetralogy of Fallot. Eur Heart J 1991;12:1089.

Blalock A, Taussig HB: The surgical treatment of malformations of the heart in which there is pulmonary stenosis or pulmonary atresia. JAMA 1945;128:189.

Booth DC et al: Left ventricular distensibility and passive elastic stiffness in atrial septal defect. J Am Coll Cardiol 1988;12:1231.

Calder AL et al: Progress of patients with pulmonary atresia after systemic to pulmonary arterial shunts. Ann Thorac Surg 1991;51:401.

Chandar et al: Ventricular arrhythmias in postoperative tetralogy of Fallot. Am J Cardiol 1990;65:655.

Dabizzi RP et al: Distribution and anomalies of coronary arteries in tetralogy of Fallot. Circulation 1980;61:95.

Deanfield JE et al: Ventricular arrhythmia in unrepaired and repaired tetralogy of Fallot. Br Heart J 1984;52:77.

Ferlinz J: Left ventricular function in atrial septal defect: Are interventricular interactions still too complex to permit definitive analysis? J Am Coll Cardiol 1988;12:1237.

Friedli B et al: Conduction disturbances after correction of tetralogy of Fallot: Are electrophysiologic studies of prognostic value? J Am Coll Cardiol 1988;11:162.

Garson A Jr et al: Prevention of sudden death after repair of tetralogy of Fallot: Treatment of ventricular arrhythmias. J Am Coll Cardiol 1985;6:221.

Garson A Jr, et al: Prevention of sudden death after repair of tetralogy of Fallot: Treatment of ventricular arrhythmias. J Am Coll Cardiol 1985;6:221.

Garson A Jr, Gillette PC, McNamara DG: Propranolol: The preferred palliation for tetralogy of Fallot. Am J Cardiol 1981;47:1098.

Hawkins JA et al: Early and late results in pulmonary atresia and intact ventricular septum. J Thorac Cardiovasc Surg 1990;100:492.

Hu DCK et al: Total correction of tetralogy of Fallot at 40 years and older: Long-term follow-up. J Am Coll Cardiol 1985;5:40.

In-Sook Park et al: Total correction of tetralogy of Fallot in adults: Surgical results and long-term follow-up. Texas Heart Inst J 1987;14:160.

Kirklin JK et al: Effect of transannular patching on outcome after repair of tetralogy of Fallot. Ann Thorac Surg 1989;48:783.

Kirklin JK et al: Survival, functional status, and reoperations after repair of tetralogy of Fallot with pulmonary atresia. J Thorac Cardiovasc Surg 1988;96:6.

Marie PY et al: Right ventricular overload and induced sustained ventricular tachycardia in operatively "repaired" tetralogy of Fallot. Am J Cardiol 1992;69:785.

Scott WC et al: Aneurysmal degeneration of Blalock-Taussig shunts: Identification and surgical treatment options. J Am Coll Cardiol 1984;3:1277.

Shimazaki Y et al: Pulmonary artery pressure and resistance late after repair of tetralogy of Fallot with pulmonary atresia. J Thorac Cardiovasc Surg 1990;100:425.

Walsh EP et al: Late results in patients with tetralogy of Fallot repaired during infancy. Circulation 1988;77:1062.

Ventricular Septal Defect

Blake RS et al: Conduction defects, ventricular arrhythmias, and late death after surgical closure of ventricular septal defect. Br Heart J 1982;47:305.

Chauvaud S et al: Ventricular septal defect associated with aortic valve incompetence: Results of two surgical managements. Ann Thorac Surg 1990;49:875.

Cyran SE et al: Predictors of postoperative ventricular dysfunction in infants who have undergone primary repair of ventricular septal defect. Am Heart J 1987;113:1144.

Ellis JH IV et al: Ventricular septal defect in the adult: Natural and unnatural history. Am Heart J 1987;114;115.

Hoffman JIE: Natural history of congenital heart disease: Problems of its assessment with special reference to ventricular septal defects. Circulation 1968;37:97.

Horneffer PJ et al: Long-term results of total repair of tetralogy of Fallot in childhood. Ann Thorac Surg 1990;50:179.

Jablonsky G et al: Rest and exercise ventricular function in adults with congenital ventricular septal defects. Am J Cardiol 1983;51:293.

Leung MP et al: Long-term follow-up after aortic valvuloplasty and defect closure in ventricular septal defect with aortic regurgitation. Am J Cardiol 1987;60:890.

Lock JE et al: Trans-catheter closure of ventricular septal defects. Circulation 1988;78:361.

Neutze JM et al: Assessment and follow-up of patients with ventricular septal defect and elevated pulmonary vascular resistance. Am J Cardiol 1989;63:327.

Noe DG, Guntheroth WC: Spontaneous closure of uncomplicated ventricular septal defect. Am J Cardiol 1987;60:674.

Okita Y et al: Long-term results of aortic valvuloplasty for aortic regurgitation associated with ventricular septal defect. J Thorac Cardiovasc Surg 1988;96:769.

Otterstad JE, Nitter-Hauge S, Myrthe E: Isolated ventricular septal defect in adults: Clinical and hemodynamic findings. Br Heart J 1983;50:343.

Otterstad JE, Simensen S, Erikssen J: Hemodynamic findings at rest and during supine exercise in adults with isolated uncomplicated ventricular septal defect. Circulation 1985;71:650.

Patent Ductus Arteriosus

Amy SG et al: Patent ductus arteriosus in patients more than 50 years old. Int J Cardiol 1986;11:277.

Cambier PA et al: Percutaneous closure of the small (less than 2.5 mm) patent ductus arteriosus using coil embolization. Am J Cardiol 1992;69:815.

Campbell M: Natural history of persistent ductus arteriosus. Br Heart J 1968;30:4.

Marquis RM et al: Persistence of ductus arteriosus with left to right shunt in older patients. Br Heart J 1982;48:469.

Morgan JM et al: The clinical features, management and outcome of persistence of the arterial duct presenting in adult life. Int J Cardiol 1990;27:193.

Silone ED et al: Oral prostaglandin E_2 in ductus-dependent pulmonary circulation. Circulation 1981;63:682.

Eisenmenger's Syndrome

Dawkins KD et al: Long-term results, hemodynamics, and complications after combined heart and lung transplantation. Circulation 1985;71:919.

Dexter L: Pulmonary vascular disease in acquired and congenital heart disease. Arch Intern Med 1979;139:922.

Eisenmenger V: Die angeborenen Defecte der Kammerschiedwand des Herzens. A Klin Med 1897;32 (Suppl 1).

Fremes SE et al: Single lung transplantation and closure of patent ductus arteriosus for Eisenmenger's syndrome. Toronto Lung Transplant Group. J Thorac Cardiovasc Surg 1990;100:1.

Haworth FG: Understanding pulmonary vascular disease in young children. Int J Cardiol 1987;15:101.

Henricksson P, Värendh G, Lundström NR: Haemostatic defects in cyanotic congenital heart disease. Br Heart J 1979;41:23.

Hoffman JE, Rudolph AM, Heymann MA: Pulmonary ventricular disease with congenital heart lesions: Pathologic features and causes. Circulation 1981;64:873.

Kimball KG, McIlroy MB: Pulmonary hypertension in patients with congenital heart disease. Am J Med 1966;41:883.

Perloff JK et al: Adults with cyanotic congenital heart disease: Hematologic management. Ann Intern Med 1988;109:406.

Steell G: The murmur of high pressure in the pulmonary artery. Med Chron 1888;9:182.

Warnes CA et al: Eisenmenger ventricular septal defect with prolonged survival. Am J Cardiol 1984;54:460.

Wood P: The Eisenmenger syndrome. (2 parts.) Br Med J 1958;2:701, 755.

Wood P: Pulmonary hypertension. Br Med Bull 1952;8:348.

Coarctation of the Aorta

Brewer LA III et al: Spinal cord complications following surgery for coarctation of the aorta. J Thorac Cardiovasc Surg 1972;64:368.

Carpenter MA et al: Left ventricular hyperkinesia at rest and during exercise in normotensive patients 2 to 27 years after coarctation repair. J Am Coll Cardiol 1985;6:879.

Clarkson PM et al: Results after repair of coarctation of the aorta beyond infancy: A 10 to 28 year follow-up with particular reference to late systemic hypertension. Am J Cardiol 1983;51:1481.

Cohen M et al: Coarctation of the aorta: Long-term follow-up and prediction of outcome after surgical correction. Circulation 1989;80:840.

Heikkinen L, Ala-Kulju K: Long-term results of direct aortoplasty for repair of aortic coarctation in adults. Ann Thorac Surg 1990;49:948.

Kron IL; et al: Incidence and risk of reintervention after coarctation repair. Ann Thorac Surg 1990;49:920.

Lababidi Z et al: Balloon coarctation angioplasty in an adult. Am J Cardiol 1984;54:350.

Malan JE, Benatar A, Levin SE: Long-term follow-up of coarctation of the aorta repaired by patch angioplasty. Int J Cardiol 1991;30:23.

Rao PS: Balloon angioplasty of aortic coarctation: A review. Clin Cardiol 1989;12:618.

Ebstein's Malformation

Donnelly JE, Brown JM, Radford DJ: Pregnancy outcome and Ebstein's anomaly. Br Heart J 1991;66:368.

Driscoll DJ et al: Spectrum of exercise intolerance in 45 patients with Ebstein's anomaly and observations on exercise tolerance in 11 patients after surgical repair. J Am Coll Cardiol 1988;11:831.

Ebstein W: Ueber einen sehr seltenen Fall von Insufficienz der Valvula tricuspidalis bedingt durch eine angeborene hochgradige Missbildung derselben. Arch Anat Physiol 1866;238.

Gussenhoven WJ et al: Echocardiographic criteria for Ebstein's anomaly of tricuspid valve. Br Heart J 1980;43:31.

Oh JK et al: Cardiac arrhythmias in patients with surgical

repair of Ebstein's anomaly. J Am Coll Cardiol 1985;6:1351.

Watson H: Natural history of Ebstein's anomaly of the tricuspid valve in childhood and adolescence: An international co-operative study of 505 cases. Br Heart J 1974;36:417.

Tricuspid Atresia

Cloutier A et al: Abnormal distribution of pulmonary blood flow after the Glenn shunt or Fontan procedure: Risk of development of arteriovenous fistulae. Circulation 1985;72:471.

Cowgill LD: The Fontan procedure: A historical review. Ann Thorac Surg 1991;51:1026.

Driscoll DJ et al: Five- to fifteen-year follow-up after Fontan operation. Circulation 1992;85:469.

Fontan F et al: Outcome after a 'perfect' Fontan operation. Circulation 1990;81:1520.

Fontan F et al: Repair of tricuspid atresia: Surgical considerations and results. Circulation 1974;50(Suppl 3):72.

Fontan F, Baudet E: Surgical repair of tricuspid atresia. Thorax 1971;26:240.

Girod DA et al: Long-term results after the Fontan operation for tricuspid atresia. Circulation 1987;75:605.

Kopf GS et al: Thirty-year follow-up of superior vena cava-pulmonary artery (Glenn) shunts. J Thorac Cardiovasc Surg 1990;100:662.

Patterson W et al: Tricuspid atresia in adults. Am J Cardiol 1982;49:141.

Warnes CA, Somerville J: Tricuspid atresia in adolescents and adults: Current state and late complications. Br Heart J 1986;56:535.

Zellers TM et al: Exercise tolerance and cardiorespiratory response to exercise before and after the Fontan operation. Mayo Clin Proc 1989;64:1489.

Abnormal Positions of the Heart

Bergofsky EH et al: Cardiorespiratory failure in kyphoscoliosis. Medicine 1959;38:263.

Rao PS: Dextrocardia: Systematic approach to differential diagnosis. Am Heart J 1981;102:389.

Transposition of the Great Vessels

Carvalho JS et al: Do asymptomatic school children have normal haemodynamics 6-13 years after Mustard's operation? Int J Cardiol 1990;26:259.

DiDonato RM et al: Cardiovascular response to exercise after the Mustard operation for simple and complex transposition of the great arteries with ventricular septal defect. Circulation 1989;80:1689.

Ensing GS et al: Cardiovascular response to exercise after the Mustard operation for single and complex transposition of the great vessels. Am J Cardiol 1988;62:617.

Haemmerli M, Bolens M, Friedli B: Electrophysiologi-

cal studies after the Mustard and Senning operations for complete transposition. Do they have prognostic value? Int J Cardiol 1990;27:167.

Martin BP et al: Evaluation of right and left ventricular function after anatomical correction and intra-atrial repair operation for complete transposition of the great arteries. Circulation 1990;82:808.

Musewe NN et al: Cardiopulmonary adaptation at rest and during exercise 10 years after Mustard atrial repair for transposition of the great arteries. Circulation 1988;77:1055.

Trusler GA et al: Current results of management in transposition of the great arteries, with special emphasis on patients with associated ventricular septal defects. J Am Coll Cardiol 1987;10:1061.

Turina MI et al: Late functional determination after atrial correction for transposition of the great arteries. Circulation 1989;80(Suppl I):I–162.

Wernovsky G et al: Midterm results after the arterial switch operation for transposition of the great arteries with intact ventricular septum: Clinical, hemodynamic, echocardiographic, and electrophysiologic data. Circulation 1988;77:1333.

Yamaguchi M et al: Early and midterm results of the arterial switch operation for transposition of the great arteries in Japan. J Thorac Cardiovasc Surg 1999;100:261.

Yasui H et al: Arterial switch operation for transposition of the great arteries, with special reference to left ventricular function. J Thorac Cardiovasc Surg 1989;98:601.

Corrected Transposition of the Great Arteries

Dimas AP et al: Long-term function of the morphologic right ventricle in adult patients with corrected transposition of the great arteries. Am Heart J 1989;118:526.

Lundstrom U et al: The natural and 'unnatural' history of congenitally corrected transposition. Am J Cardiol 1990;65:1222.

Congenital Aortic Stenosis

Brown JW et al: Surgical spectrum of aortic stenosis in children: A thirty-year experience with 257 children. Ann Thorac Surg 1988;45:393.

DeBoer DA et al: Late results of aortic valvotomy for congenital valvar aortic stenosis. Ann Thorac Surg 1999;50:69.

Firpo C et al: Discrete subaortic stenosis (DSS) in childhood: a congenital or acquired disease? Follow-up in 65 patients. Eur Heart J 1990;11:1033.

Shadler GF et al: Balloon dilation of congenital aortic valve stenosis. Circulation 1988;78:351.

Sharma BK et al: Supravalvular aortic stenosis: A 29-year review of surgical experience. Ann Thorac Surg 1991;51:1031.

Valvular Heart Disease; Mitral Valve Disease

12

VALVULAR HEART DISEASE

In this book we have used a clinical classification of valvular disease based on physical signs. Both mitral and aortic valve disease are dealt with under the main headings of stenosis and incompetence, with a separate description of mixed stenosis and incompetence of the mitral valve.

Etiology

Rheumatic endocarditis occurring in the course of rheumatic fever was responsible until recently for the vast majority of cases of mitral valve disease and for about half of cases of aortic valve disease. It is only in the last 35 years that this picture has changed. Improved housing conditions, reduction in the size of families—with less overcrowding—and widespread use of penicillin to treat tonsillitis and reduce the incidence of recurrences of rheumatic fever have probably been responsible for the decline in incidence of rheumatic heart disease in the Western world. Rheumatic heart disease is still an important problem in many parts of the world, however. In tropical and subtropical countries, rheumatic fever occurs earlier in life and runs a more florid course (possibly because of frequent recurrence), with more frequent and more severe cardiac muscle involvement.

Natural History

A. Chronic Valvular Lesions: Chronic valvular lesions tend to have a long course. Impairment of cardiac function may be detected when the patient is asymptomatic. There is not necessarily a direct relationship between the severity of symptoms and the degree of functional impairment of cardiac performance.

B. Acute Valvular Lesions: It has become increasingly important to distinguish the clinical features of an acute lesion—which develops over a period of minutes, days, or weeks—from the more readily recognized effects of chronic valvular lesions. Acute lesions are relatively rare (10%), and their importance depends on their severity.

MITRAL VALVE DISEASE

Except for mitral valve prolapse, rheumatic heart disease is the commonest cause of mitral valve disease. Acute clinical manifestations of rheumatic fever are detected in only about half of patients who subsequently develop mitral valve disease. The presence or absence of a history of rheumatic fever makes no difference in the course of the disease or in its clinical, hemodynamic, or pathologic findings. Congenital heart disease is rare, being encountered in less than 1% of adult cases.

Classification of Mitral Valve Disease

Mitral valve disease has been classified somewhat arbitrarily into three types: mitral stenosis, mixed mitral stenosis and incompetence, and mitral incompetence. The classification depends primarily on the physical findings rather than the history, although the history and course of the disease vary in the different lesions.

MITRAL STENOSIS

The cardinal features of mitral stenosis are shown in Figure 12–1. In mitral stenosis, rheumatic endocarditis scars the mitral valve and commonly causes fusion of the commissures and matting of the chordae tendineae, which interfere with the opening of the valve. The left atrium bears the brunt of the load, and the extent to which it dilates depends on its internal pressure and the state of the atrial myocardium. With time, calcification of the mitral valve renders it less mobile. In 10–15% of patients with tight mitral stenosis, pulmonary vascular resistance rises because the pulmonary arteriolar smooth muscle responds to the increase in pulmonary venous pressure by vasoconstriction. Severe pulmonary vascular lesions with markedly raised pulmonary vascular resistance (> 7.5 mm Hg/L/min) are virtually limited to severe mitral stenosis; lesser increases in resistance are seen

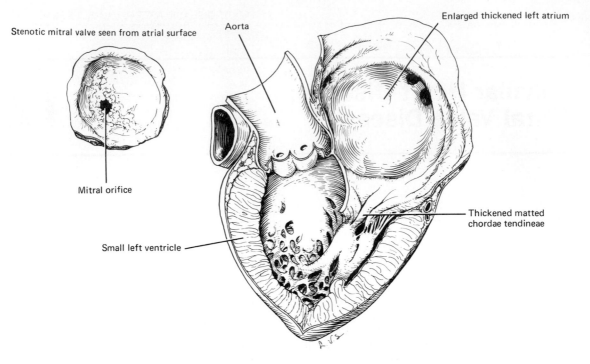

Stenotic mitral valve seen from atrial surface

Aorta

Enlarged thickened left atrium

Mitral orifice

Small left ventricle

Thickened matted chordae tendineae

Drawing of left heart in left anterior oblique view showing anatomic features of mitral stenosis.

Cardinal features: *Thickening and fusion of mitral valve cusps; raised left atrial pressure; left atrial enlargement.*

Variable factors: *Severity of obstruction; severity of rheumatic myocarditis; level of pulmonary vascular resistance.*

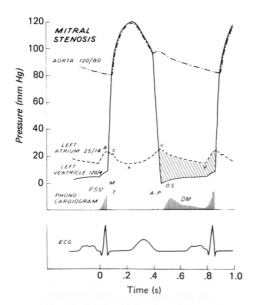

Diagram showing auscultatory and hemodynamic features of mitral stenosis. PSM, presystolic murmur; OS, opening snap; M, mitral; T, tricuspid; A, atrial; P, pulmonary; DM, diastolic murmur.

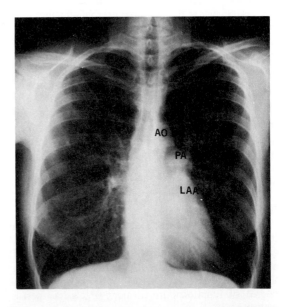

Chest x-ray of a patient with mitral stenosis showing left atrial appendage (LAA) enlargement. PA, pulmonary artery; AO, aorta.

Figure 12–1. Mitral stenosis. Structures enlarged: left atrium. Note small left ventricle. (Redrawn from the illustrations of Dr Frank H Netter, as printed in: *Heart*, Vol 5 of: *CIBA Collection of Medical Illustrations*. CIBA Pharmaceutical Company, 1969.)

in other forms of mitral disease. Increased fluid in the interstitium of the lung due to increased pulmonary capillary hydrostatic pressure compresses the small vessels and airways of the lung. This produces local hypoxia, which is in part responsible for vaso-constriction in the base of the lung. The increased vascular resistance is responsible for the decrease in pulmonary blood flow in the lung base and the redis-tribution of blood flow to the upper lobes. The condi-tion is usually reversible with relief of stenosis, in contradistinction to the pulmonary vascular disease associated with congenital lesions (see Chapter 11). A raised pulmonary vascular resistance is thus an indication—not a contraindication—for operation.

Onset of Atrial Fibrillation

In patients without pulmonary hypertension, atrial fibrillation almost always develops with the passage of time. Even if pulmonary hypertension is present, 30% of patients develop atrial fibrillation early in the course of the disease. Atrial fibrillation is most closely correlated with age, but it also depends on left atrial pressure and the severity of involvement of the left atrium in the rheumatic process.

Clinical Findings

A. Symptoms:

1. Dyspnea– The commonest presenting symp-tom (80%) in patients with mitral stenosis is shortness of breath on exertion. In women with severe lesions, this is usually noticed in early adult life (age 20–30), while the patient is still in sinus rhythm, perhaps dur-ing pregnancy. The dyspnea is due to pulmonary con-gestion that results from a rise in left atrial pressure associated with an increase in heart rate and a de-crease in left atrial emptying time. The increased stiffness of the lungs increases the work of breath-ing, and the fall in cardiac output resulting from mi-tral valve obstruction leads to an increase in heart rate that further aggravates the congestion. The onset of atrial fibrillation in a patient with significant mitral stenosis virtually always provokes dyspnea. In milder cases there may have been no dyspnea prior to the onset of arrhythmia, but in most instances the onset of atrial fibrillation exacerbates dyspnea rather than provoking it for the first time. Conversely, when a patient believed to have significant mitral stenosis develops atrial fibrillation without experiencing dysp-nea, the diagnosis is in doubt and the lesion is at most mild.

2. Paroxysmal nocturnal dyspnea– With se-vere mitral stenosis, the patient may experience sud-den, severe onset of shortness of breath after several hours of sleep. The patient awakens with a feeling of suffocation and usually must sit up or stand up to get relief. This is due to the increase in left atrial pressure brought about by the gradual increase in central blood volume brought about by recumbency with displace-ment of blood from the systemic veins to the central

veins. The dyspnea in patients with mitral stenosis may be severe enough to progress to episodes of acute pulmonary edema, especially in the presence of some additional stress.

3. Hemoptysis– Hemoptysis is the second most common presenting symptom in mitral stenosis. There may be frank pulmonary hemorrhage from rupture of a bronchial vein; frothy pink, blood-tinged sputum in pulmonary edema; or hemoptysis resulting from pul-monary infarction. Frank hemoptysis is due to open-ing of collaterals between the pulmonary veins and the bronchial veins brought about by the increased pulmonary venous pressure. The increased flow in the bronchial veins, which lie in the bronchial sub-mucosa, distends these vessels, and with rupture hemoptysis occurs.

4. Systemic embolism– Presenting symptoms due to systemic embolism are infrequent in patients with mitral stenosis. Embolism is more common after atrial fibrillation has occurred and tends to occur later in the disease in a high percentage of cases.

5. Palpitations– Palpitations are rarely the chief complaint. Any arrhythmia is likely to provoke dysp-nea, and the patient will usually complain of dyspnea rather than palpitations.

6. Symptoms in patients with raised pulmo-nary vascular resistance– Fatigue, coldness of the extremities, abdominal discomfort, and swelling of the abdomen and ankles are symptoms of right heart involvement. They suggest the presence of severe pulmonary hypertension and raised pulmonary vascu-lar resistance with right heart failure and a low car-diac output and are thus indicative of severe mitral stenosis. Symptoms of right heart failure can also occur in patients with associated organic involvement of the tricuspid valve.

7. Episodic symptoms– Confusion in diagnosis sometimes occurs when the patient's symptoms are episodic. In this case arrhythmia should be suspected, and 24-hour monitoring of the ECG is indicated.

B. Signs:
The classic signs of mitral stenosis de-velop early in the natural course of the condition and can usually be noted before symptoms develop. How-ever, the patient may have to engage in exercise in order to elicit the signs. In classic mitral stenosis, the pulse is normal or small in amplitude, and the blood pressure and systemic venous pressure are normal.

1. Palpation– The heart is not enlarged, and on palpation there is an obvious localized tapping car-diac impulse. This represents the vibrations from the loud first heart sound that originate in the cusps of the mitral valve (closing snap). There may also be a di-astolic thrill with presystolic accentuation felt at the apex and a palpable opening snap felt at the base of the heart.

2. Auscultation– On auscultation the first sound is loud, and the second sound is followed by a loud opening snap that is high-pitched and widely trans-mitted but heard best just to the right of the apex.

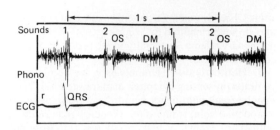

Figure 12–2. Typical phonocardiogram in mitral stenosis showing loud first sound and opening snap (OS), followed by long diastolic rumbling murmur (DM) with presystolic accentuation. (Courtesy of Roche Laboratories Division of Hoffman-La Roche, Inc.)

3. Diastolic murmur with presystolic accentuation– The characteristic finding in predominant mitral stenosis is a long, loud, rumbling mitral diastolic murmur with presystolic accentuation due to atrial systole (Figure 12–2). The murmur is often best heard in a localized area about 2.5 cm in diameter located at the apex of the heart. The patient should lie on the left side after exercise, and the physician should use the bell of the stethoscope and light pressure on the chest. The murmur may be absent in mid diastole in mild cases but still show presystolic accentuation (Figure 12–3).

There is not infrequently a mitral systolic murmur in pure mitral stenosis. The presence of a presystolic (atrial systolic) murmur excludes a diagnosis of significant mitral incompetence. Even though hemodynamically insignificant mitral incompetence is mild, it may cause a loud systolic murmur.

4. Murmurs in the presence of atrial fibrillation– When the patient develops atrial fibrillation, the presystolic murmur disappears. The heart rate becomes irregular, and after the heart rate has been slowed by digitalis therapy it becomes important to listen for the length of the diastolic murmur during the longest diastolic pauses. In patients with predominant mitral stenosis, the murmur should persist until the end of diastole even in cardiac cycles lasting 1 second. A shorter murmur suggests either mixed mitral stenosis and incompetence or decreased stroke

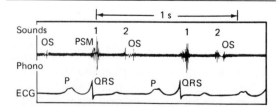

Figure 12–3. Phonocardiogram of loud first sound in mitral stenosis. Note presystolic murmur (PSM) and opening snap (OS) with no diastolic murmur following the snap. (Courtesy of Roche Laboratories Division of Hoffman-La Roche, Inc.)

volume due to a raised pulmonary vascular resistance and right heart failure.

5. Pulmonary signs– Rales at the bases of the lungs are commonly found in mitral stenosis, but their absence does not exclude the possibility of pulmonary congestion or even edema. The patient is often orthopneic because the lungs become more congested when the patient is in a supine position and the respiratory rate increases as the lungs become stiffer.

6. Signs in the presence of pulmonary hypertension– When pulmonary vascular resistance is markedly raised (> 7.5 mm Hg/L/min), the physical signs of mitral stenosis tend to be different. The patient usually has a low cardiac output and is often thin, with peripheral cyanosis, cool extremities, and a pulse of small volume. Dilated veins on the cheeks combined with peripheral cyanosis give rise to a "mitral facies" that is also seen in other patients with a chronically low cardiac output. Systemic venous pressure is likely to be raised, with a prominent *a* wave visible in the jugular pulse if sinus rhythm is present. The heart may be enlarged, with a right ventricular precordial and parasternal impulse. The auscultatory signs of mitral stenosis tend to be less florid than those in patients with low pulmonary vascular resistance because the cardiac output is lower.

In about one-third of cases, either reduction in the cardiac output or valvular calcification modifies the classic physical signs, making the diagnosis difficult. Calcification of the valve may eliminate the opening snap but should not affect the murmur. Low output may eliminate the murmur but should not affect the snap. In addition, right ventricular dilation may displace the apex of the left ventricle away from the chest wall and make the murmur difficult or impossible to hear. Calcification of the mitral valve does not always affect the physical signs, and more than half of patients with valvular calcification have an opening snap. There is often a pulmonary systolic ejection click and a short pulmonary systolic murmur in addition to a loud pulmonary valve closure sound.

a. Pulmonary incompetence– Pulmonary incompetence secondary to pulmonary hypertension may cause an immediate diastolic murmur at the base of the heart (Graham Steell murmur). This murmur is high-pitched and impossible to differentiate from the murmur of aortic valve regurgitation.

b. Tricuspid incompetence– Pansystolic murmurs are common in patients with pulmonary hypertension and are usually due to secondary tricuspid incompetence, as shown by increased systemic venous pressure, a prominent *v* wave in the neck, and increased intensity of the murmur during inspiration.

7. Signs in the presence of low output– In severely ill patients, the mitral diastolic murmur may vary in intensity because of changes in cardiac output or heart rate. The fact that one observer has heard the murmur and another has not should not be discounted, and repeated examinations may be helpful.

8. Assessment of severity from physical signs– Assessment of the severity of mitral stenosis based on physical signs is not of sufficient accuracy to be clinically valid.

C. Electrocardiographic Findings: The ECG is of little help in diagnosing or assessing the severity of predominant mitral stenosis with low pulmonary vascular resistance. A broad, notched, posteriorly oriented P wave (P mitrale) is usually all that is present. If right ventricular hypertrophy is present, pulmonary vascular resistance is almost certainly raised. The absence of right ventricular hypertrophy on the ECG does not rule out severe pulmonary hypertension, but some signs are usually present, and the progressive development of changes on the ECG is an important clue to the diagnosis of raised pulmonary vascular resistance.

D. Imaging Studies: In predominant mitral stenosis with normal pulmonary vascular resistance, the overall heart size may be normal, as shown in Figure 12–1. The left atrium is enlarged, and the left atrial appendage is usually visible on the left cardiac border. The pulmonary artery is not greatly enlarged unless pulmonary arterial pressure is over 45 mm Hg. Minor enlargement of the pulmonary artery contributes to straightening of the left cardiac border when the pulmonary artery pressure is lower. The left main bronchus may be elevated and lie more horizontally than normally. With moderate left atrial enlargement, the right border of the left atrium produces a double density on the right.

1. Pulmonary changes– The chest x-ray is useful in assessing the degree of pulmonary congestion. The most characteristic finding is the presence of Kerley's B lines, as shown in Figure 12–4. These are thickened interlobular septa that are usually seen at

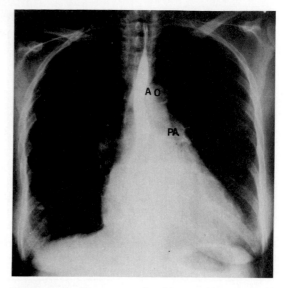

Figure 12–5. Chest x-ray of a 60-year-old woman with cardiac enlargement resulting from mitral stenosis with pulmonary hypertension. Ventricular enlargement is right-sided. (AO, aorta; PA, pulmonary artery.)

the outer edges of the lungs at the bases. The pattern of pulmonary congestion in mitral valve disease is influenced by the effects of gravity. The level of the pulmonary venous and arterial pressures is highest at the bases of the lungs.

2. Pulmonary hypertension– The response of pulmonary blood vessels to increased pressure is hypertrophy of their walls; consequently, pulmonary vascular disease is most marked at the base of the lungs. As the pulmonary arterioles thicken and develop an increased resistance to blood flow, redistribution of pulmonary blood flow occurs. As a result, the veins of the upper lobe of the lung become more prominent, and the lower lobes receive a smaller proportion of pulmonary blood flow. "Pruning" of the pulmonary arterial tree appears first at the base and later spreads to involve the entire lung. Occasionally, passive pulmonary venous congestion with intra-alveolar hemorrhage causes hemosiderosis, giving rise to a diffuse mottled pattern on the chest x-ray.

3. Ventricular enlargement– When the heart is enlarged, it is not always easy to decide on purely radiologic grounds whether the right ventricle (Figure 12–5) or the left ventricle (Figure 12–11) is enlarged.

1. Noninvasive techniques– The mitral valve is one of the structures that registers most clearly and consistently on echocardiography. The movements of the valve during systole and diastole and the effects of atrial contraction can usually be clearly discerned. Echocardiography is thus especially helpful in the diagnosis and clinical assessment of patients with mitral stenosis (Figure 12–6).

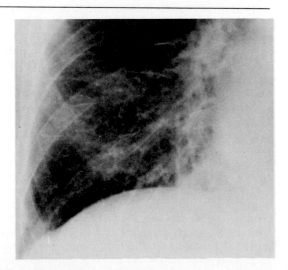

Figure 12–4. Close-up of chest x-ray of base of right lung of patient with mitral stenosis showing Kerley's B lines.

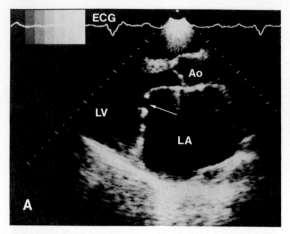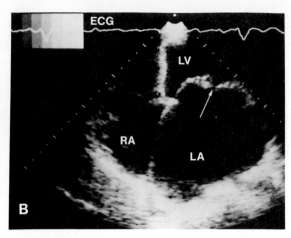

Figure 12–6. Two-dimensional echocardiographs in a patient with mitral stenosis. The arrows point to the stenosed mitral valve. **A:** Long-axis view. **B:** Four-chamber apical view. (Ao, aorta; LV, left ventricle; LA, left atrium; RA, right atrium.)

An idea of the diastolic dimensions of the mitral valve orifice can usually be obtained in short-axis views. The valve area measured by this means has been shown to correlate significantly with measurements made at cardiac catheterization.

Doppler blood velocity recordings from the mitral valve orifice can be obtained with a transducer aimed from the apex of the heart toward the mitral valve. The peak velocity of blood flow in the jet of blood passing through the valve bears a relationship to the peak pressure difference across the valve (Chapter 4). Measurement of the half-time of the fall in blood velocity in the jet at the start of diastole has been shown to provide an indirect measure of the pressure difference across the valve in patients with mitral stenosis. The value empirically expressed as $220 \div t_{1/2}$ where $t_{1/2}$ is the half-time, correlates well with hemodynamic measurements of the mitral valve gradient (Figure 12–7).

By the continuity equation, the mitral valve area can be adequately assessed:

$$MVA = \frac{A_1 \times V_1}{A_1}$$

where MVA = mitral valve area, A_1 = area of the left ventricular inflow tract, V_1 = velocity of blood flow in the inflow tract, and V_2 = velocity of blood flow at the stenotic mitral valve.

2. Invasive techniques–

a. Cardiac catheterization– Cardiac catheterization is usually not necessary to make the diagnosis of mitral stenosis or to judge its severity, because echo-Doppler techniques are quite adequate to accomplish this. When the patient is over age 40 years, when the incidence of coronary artery disease becomes significant, or if the patient has angina pectoris, catheterization is necessary to visualize the coronary arteries. If there is a question about the severity of the mitral

stenosis obtained noninvasively because of some inconsistency with the history or physical findings, cardiac catheterization should be done before surgery.

The left atrial ("wedge") pressure, the left ventricular pressure, and the cardiac output are needed for full assessment of the severity of mitral stenosis. In most laboratories, the wedge pressure is considered to be an acceptable substitute for left atrial pressure. In some centers, however, direct left atrial pressure measurements by transseptal catheterization is preferred. In patients with distorted cardiac anatomy due to marked left atrial enlargement, kyphoscoliosis, unsuspected left atrial thrombus, or left atrial tumor, transseptal catheterization is less successful and more dangerous because of the likelihood of cardiac perforation and systemic embolization.

(1) Hemodynamic measurement of severity– There is no entirely satisfactory method for measuring the hemodynamic severity of mitral stenosis, even during cardiac catheterization. The calculation of mitral valve area by means of the hydraulic formula introduced by Gorlin and Gorlin is the best available method. The three variables—cardiac output, length of diastole, and pressure difference across the valve—are included in the calculation. The normal mitral valve area is about 5 cm². A measurable gradient does not occur before the valve is reduced to about 2.5 cm², and tight mitral stenosis is said to occur at 1 cm².

(2) Technique for patients with pulmonary hypertension– In patients who have marked increases in pulmonary vascular resistance, wedge pressure measurement is critical and may occasionally prove difficult because the high pulmonary arterial pressure is associated with rapid tapering of the vessels. Pulmonary artery wedge pressures are usually measured by floating a Swan-Ganz balloon catheter out the pulmonary artery until it wedges. If a satisfac-

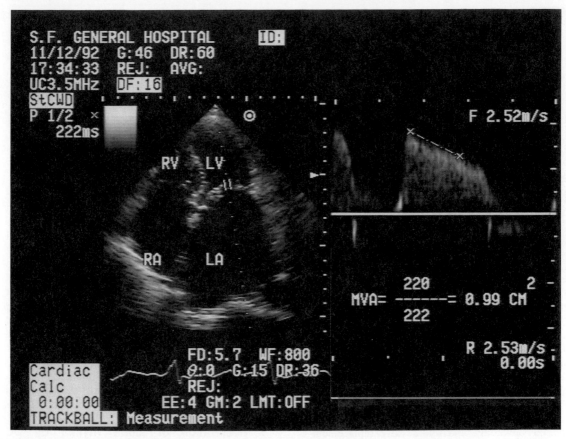

Figure 12–7. *Left:* Two-dimensional echocardiogram of patient with mitral stenosis. Area of interest is in the orifice of the mitral valve marked by two small parallel lines. *Right:* Doppler diastolic velocity profile showing calcification of mitral valve area from the Doppler half-time equation.

tory wedge pressure cannot be obtained, left atrial pressure should be obtained directly by transseptal catheterization.

b. Left ventricular angiography– Left ventricular angiography is now an important component of the overall study of patients with mitral stenosis. It is primarily used to evaluate left ventricular function and to determine the presence or absence of mitral incompetence. The multiple ectopic beats that so frequently follow the left ventricular injection of contrast material often cause mitral incompetence, even in patients with normal mitral valves. In patients with mitral stenosis, the small rigid orifice of the mitral valve may permit a small localized jet of contrast material to flow back into the left atrium. This finding does not invalidate the diagnosis of predominant mitral stenosis, however.

c. Coronary angiography– In many centers, coronary angiography is performed almost as a routine in patients with mitral valve disease who are over age 40. The yield from such investigations is low when there is no clinical evidence of coronary disease.

Differential Diagnosis

Left atrial myxoma (see Chapter 21) is the most important disorder in the differential diagnosis of mitral stenosis with or without raised pulmonary vascular resistance. The radiologic picture shown in Figure 12–8 closely resembles that of mitral stenosis, and left atrial appendage enlargement is seen. Episodic symptoms, variable heart murmurs, fever, systemic embolism, a raised sedimentation rate, and hyperglobulinemia suggest the possibility of myxoma. The lesion is 100 times less common than mitral stenosis and 100 times more common than the rare congenital lesion cor triatriatum, in which the left atrium is divided into an upper and a lower chamber by an incomplete transverse septum. Cor triatriatum may also simulate mitral stenosis. Echocardiography and angiocardiography with injection of dye into the left ventricle or pulmonary artery are helpful in diagnosis.

Course & Complications

The course of mitral stenosis is long, lasting 20 years or more in many instances. The natural history of the lesion can be altered by surgical treatment, and

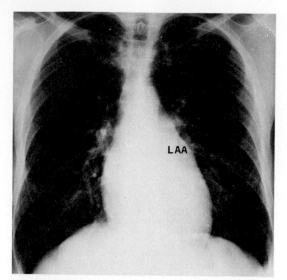

Figure 12–8. Chest x-ray in a 40-year-old man with left atrial myxoma. The left atrial appendage (LAA) is prominent.

an almost normal life expectancy may be possible with optimal treatment. If the stenosis is moderate or severe, mitral valvotomy will almost certainly be required before age 40 for the relief of dyspnea unless the level of activity is seriously curtailed by the patient. Restenosis of the valve may necessitate a second valvotomy, and mitral valve replacement is likely to be required.

The course of mitral stenosis is, however, often different in tropical, subtropical, and developing countries. Pure mitral stenosis, with minimal myocardial involvement, is less frequent, and the latent period before symptoms develop is short. Associated pulmonary hypertension is particularly prevalent on the Indian subcontinent.

A. Atrial Fibrillation: Atrial fibrillation occurs so frequently in the course of mitral stenosis that it hardly qualifies as a complication. It greatly influences the course of the lesion. The timing of onset is extremely important, and the circumstances precipitating atrial fibrillation and its clinical effects provide important diagnostic and prognostic information about the lesion. It is important to determine whether the onset of atrial fibrillation aggravated existing symptoms or heralded their appearance. If the onset of atrial fibrillation escapes notice in a patient with mitral stenosis, either the lesion is extremely mild or increased pulmonary vascular resistance is present. Atrial fibrillation markedly increases the danger of systemic embolization, especially embolic stroke. Such patients must be anticoagulated if there is no absolute contraindication.

B. Bronchitis: The congested lungs of patients with mitral disease are prone to bronchitis. This is seen more frequently in patients with mitral stenosis,

because pulmonary congestion is generally more severe than in other types of mitral valve disease.

C. Pulmonary Infarction: Pulmonary embolism and pulmonary infarction are common, especially in mitral stenosis with raised pulmonary vascular resistance. The lungs with their double arterial blood supply normally are not subject to infarction unless they are congested, and mitral stenosis is one of the commonest conditions in which pulmonary embolism is followed by pulmonary infarction.

Treatment

A. Medical Treatment:

1. Penicillin prophylaxis to prevent recurrence of rheumatic fever– Prophylactic penicillin therapy to prevent recurrence of rheumatic carditis should be considered in all young patients with mitral stenosis. The younger the patient, the stronger the indication for treatment. The upper age limit for the initiation and cessation of prophylactic penicillin therapy is not clearly defined. Most physicians do not start prophylactic therapy if the patient is older than age 30 or if there has been no evidence of activity in the previous 5 years; treatment is seldom continued past age 40. The dosage schedules are given in Chapter 17.

2. Prevention of infective endocarditis– Treatment to prevent infective endocarditis should always be recommended, especially if the valvular lesion is mild (see Chapter 16).

3. Restoration of sinus rhythm by DC countershock– Restoration of sinus rhythm in patients with atrial arrhythmia is rarely indicated before surgery in mitral stenosis. Anticoagulation is important to prevent systemic embolization and stroke. A patient with atrial fibrillation and symptoms severe enough to warrant restoration of sinus rhythm would almost certainly benefit from surgery.

B. Operative Treatment:

1. Mitral valvotomy– Surgery in mitral valve disease is seldom if ever curative. However, it is the treatment of choice. Mitral valvotomy is indicated in any patient with mitral stenosis who has significant symptoms and a mitral valve area of about 1 cm^2 or less. Mitral valvotomy is possible if the valve is flexible and there is little or no mitral regurgitation. By physical examination and echo-Doppler studies, an accurate assessment can be made about whether the patient can benefit from valvuloplasty without needing valve replacement. The operation, which is now usually performed under direct vision during cardiopulmonary bypass, is palliative; its benefits do not last indefinitely. Open mitral valvotomy improves the surgeon's ability to treat left atrial thrombus, and mitral incompetence is less likely to result. This operation also enhances the possibility of mobilizing subvalvular structures such as fused papillary muscles and matted chordae tendineae. The decision whether to proceed with mitral valvotomy or to replace the mitral valve ultimately rests with the surgeon and is often made during the operation. In some cases, during the actual valvotomy, the surgeon encounters problems that make valve replacement essential and lead to a change in plans.

Mitral valvotomy is not dangerous in patients with mitral stenosis and low pulmonary vascular resistance. The mortality rate is less than 2%, and in most centers patients with New York Heart Association class II symptoms are readily selected for operation. The principal cause of morbidity and mortality is embolism. Occasionally, massive cerebral embolism occurs with disastrous results. Mitral stenosis often occurs with little or no rheumatic myocardial involvement, and in such cases the mechanical effects of obstruction to mitral flow predominate, so that the results of surgery are good. In patients with more evidence of myocardial disease, in older patients, in those with atrial fibrillation, and in those with enlarged hearts, the benefits of valvotomy are less dramatic.

2. Catheter balloon valvuloplasty– Inflation of one or two balloon catheters positioned across the mitral valve in the manner described by Grüntzig for the treatment of arterial obstructions can be used to treat mitral stenosis. The approach is via transseptal

catheterization and involves dilating the puncture site in the atrial septum to a size (about 5 mm) that will permit the passage of the balloon catheter. A single 25-mm balloon may be used, but more often two 20-mm balloons (Figure 12–9) are required to produce sufficient dilation.

The procedure, which is technically the most difficult form of percutaneous balloon valvuloplasty, is not devoid of complications. In addition to the complications of transseptal catheterization (cardiac perforation, tamponade, and thromboembolism), the mitral valve may be damaged, and a 5-mm atrial septal defect may be created. A cardiac surgical team should be on standby alert if possible. The success rate of the procedure can be as high as 85% in experienced hands. The indications are not yet clearly defined but appear to be similar to those for mitral valvotomy—ie, young patients with "pure," "tight" mitral stenosis and clinical evidence of a flexible, noncalcified valve in sinus rhythm. Transesophageal echocardiography is needed to assess the state of the mitral valve and subvalvular area and to rule out obvious thrombus in the left atrium. The incidence of this form of mitral valve disease is now low enough outside the Third World to make it difficult for any institution to accumulate great experience with the

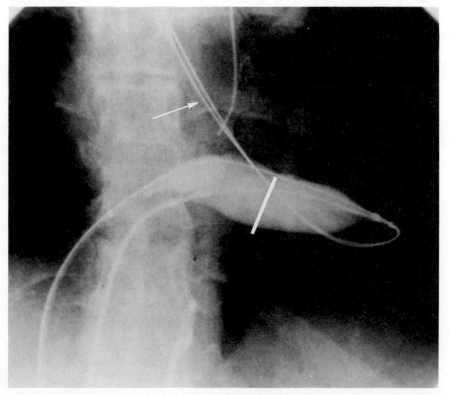

Figure 12–9. Two 20-mm balloons positioned across the mitral valve (bar) via the transseptal route. Two wires (arrow) can be seen passing via the left ventricle into the ascending aorta, with one reaching the descending aorta. (Courtesy of TA Ports.)

technique. The potential for its application is greater in the Third World. It offers a considerable advantage over open heart surgery in terms of morbidity and expense. The long-term results of this palliative procedure are not yet known. Presumably, they will be similar to the results of closed mitral valvotomy.

3. Mitral valve replacement– Mitral valve replacement is indicated in only 20–30% of cases as an initial operation in patients with mitral stenosis. If the patient is a woman of childbearing age, the use of long-term anticoagulation therapy, which is usually necessary after mitral valve replacement, is a distinct disadvantage. In patients with significant mitral regurgitation, valve replacement may occasionally be indicated as an initial operation, especially in older patients with calcified valves. Valve replacement is generally performed only when mitral valvotomy has failed to control the patient's symptoms. The mortality of mitral valve replacement is about 5%.

4. Mortality rate in patients with pulmonary hypertension– The mortality rate of surgery in patients with raised pulmonary vascular resistance is roughly related to the level of resistance. In patients with severe right heart failure, the mortality rate is 10–15%. Late deaths in heart failure (10%) and survivors with persistent pulmonary vascular disease as shown in Figure 12–10 bring the percentage of cases with unsatisfactory results to about 50%.

Prognosis

The prognosis for patients with mitral stenosis is good now that mitral valve surgery is readily available. Although the lesion cannot be cured and myocardial involvement due to rheumatic carditis is not affected by surgery, relief of dyspnea and prevention of attacks of pulmonary edema are ensured. Most patients with mitral stenosis who have had mitral valvotomy will develop symptoms again some time later, probably with the onset of atrial fibrillation in early middle age. The benefits of mitral valvotomy in patients with mitral stenosis vary and tend to be best in those who develop severe stenosis at an early age and who have no evidence of myocardial disease. Age is an important factor; if the indications for mitral valvotomy are strong and if the operation is on a young adult, the relief may last for 10–15 years, but if operation is not indicated in early adult life and is not performed until the patient is 50, the period of relief is likely to be shorter.

Raised pulmonary vascular resistance worsens the prognosis of mitral stenosis. If developing pulmonary hypertension is diagnosed early and treatment is not delayed, the prognosis is better. In older patients, however, and in patients who do not receive early treatment, the prognosis is significantly worse. Relief of mitral stenosis reverses the course of pulmonary vascular disease; the speed of reversal depends on two factors: (1) how thoroughly the mitral stenosis has been eliminated and (2) how long the original pulmonary changes have been present. Improvement may continue for up to 2 years after operation.

Long-Term Results in Operated Cases

As experience has accumulated, it has become clear that mitral valvotomy is a palliative operation and that most patients ultimately require mitral valve replacement. The long-term results of mitral valve

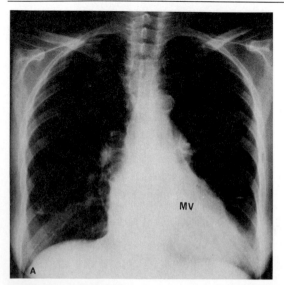
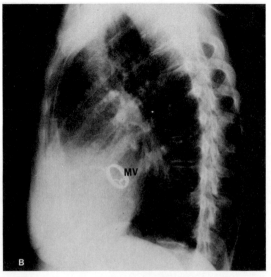

Figure 12–10. Postoperative chest x-rays of the 60-year-old woman whose preoperative x-ray is shown in Figure 12–5. Cardiac enlargement persisted after operation. The Björk-Shiley prosthetic valve (MV) is seen more clearly on the lateral view. **A,** posterior view; **B,** lateral view.

replacement are now becoming better defined as more data are available to determine the 10- to 20-year results. The 10-year survival rate after mitral valve replacement is about 50% irrespective of the type of valve used. Anticoagulation is required for all prosthetic valves and also for tissue valves if there is atrial fibrillation. Valve failure is around 10–15% over a 10-year period. No artificial valve has normal hemodynamic function, and some pressure difference is always found across the valve.

Embolism is an important complication that persists over the years and is responsible for both disability and death. It occurs at a rate of about 5% per year, but only about half of emboli cause serious problems.

MIXED MITRAL STENOSIS & INCOMPETENCE

In some cases the rheumatic involvement of the mitral valve leads to dilation and stretching of the valve tissue and subsequent scarring and retraction in addition to fusion at the commissures. In this case, stenosis is present in addition to significant leakage through the valve. After severe mitral stenosis has been treated surgically, the stenosis is less severe, but the valve is still abnormal. With time, degenerative changes, fibrosis, and calcification stiffen and immobilize the valve and produce a mixture of stenosis and incompetence. The cardinal features of this lesion (Figure 12–11) include obstruction and leakage at the mitral valve, left atrial enlargement, and left ventricular enlargement and eccentric hypertrophy. Variable features that may alter these findings are the severity of obstruction, the amount of regurgitation, and the severity of rheumatic myocardial damage.

Clinical Findings

A. Symptoms:

1. Dyspnea– Dyspnea is the commonest presenting symptom in patients with mixed mitral stenosis and incompetence. It seldom occurs while the patient is in sinus rhythm. The patient often presents with an acute episode of dyspnea associated with the development of atrial fibrillation. This onset commonly heralds the onset of other symptoms, and the patient, who may have been living a relatively normal life, becomes acutely ill with severe dyspnea and perhaps pulmonary edema. Atrial fibrillation is sometimes triggered by an intercurrent infection such as influenza or pneumonia, and a systemic or pulmonary embolism may occur simultaneously. This clinical picture is so common that it is important to consider the possibility of mitral stenosis and incompetence in any patient who suddenly becomes short of breath, especially if the heart rate is rapid and atrial fibrillation is present. The physical signs can be difficult to interpret in the acute stage when the heart rate is rapid. Episodic dyspnea may be present when there is

paroxysmal atrial arrhythmia. In such circumstances it is important to see the patient during an attack.

2. Palpitations– Palpitations are common in patients with mixed mitral stenosis and incompetence. Palpitations are generally due to atrial arrhythmia; if the heart rate is rapid, dyspnea is likely to occur because the faster the pulse, the shorter the diastolic filling period and the higher the left atrial pressure.

3. Systemic embolism– The first symptom of mixed mitral stenosis and incompetence may be due to acute systemic embolism. Sudden pain and coldness in the leg, sudden paralysis, acute loin pain due to renal infarction, flank pain due to infarction of the spleen, and infarction of the bowel due to mesenteric artery emboli sometimes occur. Embolism usually occurs in patients with atrial fibrillation, particularly when the rhythm changes, but it may happen when the patient is in sinus rhythm.

4. Pressure from a large left atrium– Symptoms due to pressure from a greatly enlarged left atrium on surrounding structures are occasionally seen. Thus, cough, hoarseness due to recurrent laryngeal nerve paralysis, and recurrent lung infection involving the left lower lobe may occur.

B. Signs: The signs in patients with mixed mitral stenosis and incompetence depend on the degree of incompetence. When incompetence is the predominant lesion, the left ventricular systolic ejection rate is more rapid than normal, and, because the forward stroke volume is normal, the peripheral pulse resembles a miniature "water-hammer" pulse. In patients with mixed mitral stenosis and incompetence it is not always easy to assess the relative importance of the stenosis, the incompetence, or the overall severity of the lesion. Many of the patients with this lesion have had mitral stenosis, and the mitral incompetence has resulted from either valvotomy or calcification and fixation of the deformed valve as well as degenerative, age-related changes and increased wear and tear.

The systemic venous pressure is not often raised unless there is associated tricuspid valve disease or right heart failure. Because pulmonary hypertension is seldom severe, the pulse is usually normal and the rhythm irregular in patients with atrial fibrillation. The heart is usually enlarged, with a hyperdynamic left ventricular impulse. The first sound may be loud and there may be an opening snap. A third heart sound may also be heard, sometimes replacing the snap rather than accompanying it. Depending on the volume of mitral diastolic blood flow, there is a pansystolic mitral murmur transmitted to the axilla and a diastolic mitral murmur of variable length (Figure 12–12). In patients with moderate mitral incompetence, the murmur may last until the end of diastole at rapid heart rates (more than 100/min).

Pulmonary congestion in mixed mitral valve disease is less marked than in mitral stenosis. Although pulmonary edema may occur at the onset of atrial fibrillation, control of the heart rate by digitalis usu-

Mitral valve seen from left atrium

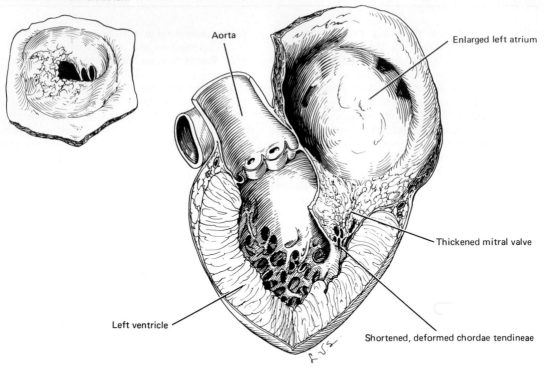

Aorta

Enlarged left atrium

Thickened mitral valve

Left ventricle

Shortened, deformed chordae tendineae

Drawing of left heart in left anterior oblique view showing anatomic features of mixed mitral stenosis and incompetence.

Cardinal features: *Obstruction and leakage at the mitral valve; left atrial enlargement; left ventricular enlargement (not hypertrophy).*

Variable factors: *Severity of obstruction; amount of leakage; severity of rheumatic myocardial damage.*

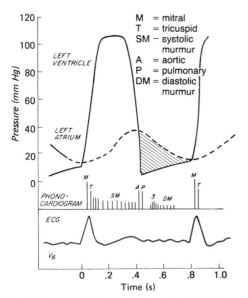

M = mitral
T = tricuspid
SM = systolic murmur
A = aortic
P = pulmonary
DM = diastolic murmur

Diagram showing auscultatory and hemodynamic features of mixed mitral stenosis and incompetence.

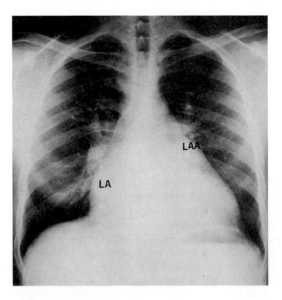

Chest x-ray showing left atrial (LA), left atrial appendage (LAA), and left ventricular enlargement in mixed mitral stenosis and incompetence.

Figure 12–11. Mitral stenosis and incompetence. Structures enlarged: left atrium, left ventricle.

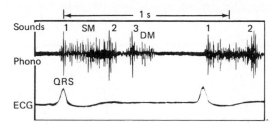

Figure 12–12. Phonocardiogram from a patient with mixed mitral stenosis and incompetence in atrial fibrillation. A pansystolic murmur (Sm) and third heart sound (3) are followed by a short diastolic murmur (DM) at a slow heart rate. (Courtesy of Roche Laboratories Division of Hoffman-La Roche, Inc.)

ally leads to rapid improvement. An increase in pulmonary vascular resistance seldom occurs and is not often severe in mixed mitral valve disease, presumably because left atrial pressure is lower than in pure stenosis.

C. Electrocardiographic Findings: The electrocardiographic findings in patients with mixed mitral stenosis and incompetence are not of diagnostic value. A broad, notched, posteriorly oriented P wave (P mitrale) is seen if the patient is in sinus rhythm. Atrial fibrillation is usually present, whereas right ventricular hypertrophy is rarely seen.

Left ventricular hypertrophy on the ECG is common but not invariable, even when mitral incompetence is more prominent than stenosis. If severe left ventricular hypertrophy is present, it is is more commonly due to systemic hypertension, aortic valve disease, or rheumatic myocardial disease than to the valve lesion.

D. Imaging Studies: Left ventricular enlargement is seen on x-ray in patients with mixed mitral stenosis and incompetence, and it is roughly proportionate to the severity of the lesion. Left atrial enlargement is seen as a double density on the right border of the heart (Figure 12–11).

Left atrial enlargement tends to be greatest in patients with mixed mitral stenosis and incompetence. In patients with giant left atrium, shown in Figure 12–13, in which the chamber assumes enormous proportions with a volume of one liter or more, mixed mitral lesions are almost always present. The left atrium forms both the right and left borders of the heart and the picture can be mistaken for that of pericardial effusion (see Chapter 18).

Enlargement of the left atrial appendage, seen on the left border of the heart, is almost invariably present.

1. Noninvasive techniques– Echocardiography is particularly helpful in assessing the lesion. Doppler echocardiography can determine the degree of stenosis, the effects and the approximate degree of incompetence, and the sizes of the left atrium and ven-

tricle. When there are no inconsistences between the history, physical findings, and noninvasive work-up and the patient is under 40 years of age without angina, surgery may be undertaken without catheterization.

2. Invasive techniques–

a. Cardiac catheterization– Right and left heart catheterization are frequently required before surgery in all patients with mixed mitral stenosis and incompetence. This is especially true when there are inconsistencies between the history, the physical examination, and the results of noninvasive investigations or when coronary arteriography is deemed necessary. Simultaneous measurements of wedge pressure, left ventricular pressure, and cardiac output are essential. The patient is frequently in atrial fibrillation, and the effects of variation in the length of diastole from beat to beat can be clearly seen in Figure 12–14. The height and configuration of wedge pressure tracings depend on the severity of the lesion, the heart rate, and the compliance of the left atrium. Equalization of the pressures in the left atrium and left ventricle usually occurs by mid diastole at slow heart rates (less than 60/min). With faster heart rates (shorter diastolic intervals), wedge pressure rises, and an end-diastolic pressure difference usually occurs. The time course of the fall in left atrial pressure following the v wave is roughly exponential, and its time constant depends on the product of the resistance to flow across the mitral valve and the compliance of the left atrium.

b. Left ventricular angiography– Left ventricular angiography is still the best available method for measuring the amount of mitral incompetence. If the left ventricular stroke volume is subtracted from the forward stroke volume (calculated by means of the Fick principle), the difference is the volume of

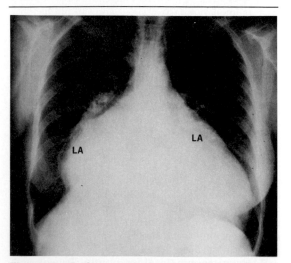

Figure 12–13. Chest x-ray of a 42-year-old woman with giant left atrium. The left atrium (LA) forms the left and right heart borders on the posteroanterior view.

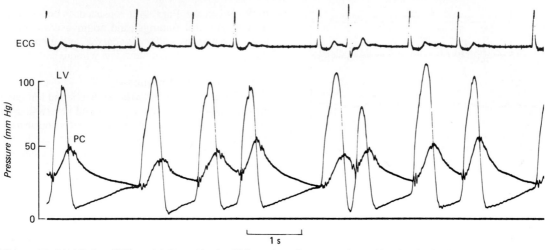

Figure 12–14. Wedge (PC) and left ventricular (LV) tracings from a patient with mixed mitral stenosis and incompetence in atrial fibrillation. The wedge pressure rises and the end-diastolic gradient increases when the heart rate increases. Lower wedge pressures are seen after a longer pause occurs between beats, and the end-diastolic gradient disappears.

blood flowing back across the mitral valve (regurgitant volumes) per beat. Echo-Doppler techniques can usually measure small or large regurgitant volumes accurately but frequently overestimate the regurgitant volume.

Differential Diagnosis

A. Atrial Septal Defect: Atrial fibrillation, cardiac enlargement, and systolic and diastolic murmurs occur in atrial septal defect, and in the middle-aged patient an erroneous history of rheumatic fever in childhood is sometimes present. With these findings, the incorrect diagnosis of rheumatic heart disease is easily made. Radiologic examination is most useful because in atrial septal defect the chest x-ray shows a large pulmonary artery, a small aorta, a big heart, a big right atrium, and a left atrium that is usually unimpressive. The ECG almost invariably shows an incomplete or complete right bundle branch block with an rsR' pattern in lead V_1. This finding should always raise the suspicion that an atrial defect exists. Cardiac catheterization is ordinarily required to establish the diagnosis with certainty, although an adequate preoperative evaluation can often be obtained with two-dimensional echocardiography and color Doppler studies.

Mitral valve disease and atrial septal defect may rarely coexist. In this condition (Lutembacher's syndrome), raised venous pressure, hepatomegaly, and peripheral edema are common, and the presence of right heart failure in a patient with mixed mitral stenosis and incompetence should always suggest an associated atrial septal defect.

B. Hypertrophic Cardiomyopathy: Patients with hypertrophic cardiomyopathy (who tend to be confused with those with mixed mitral valve disease) may have increased impedance of left ventricular inflow, with or without outflow obstruction. Hypertrophic cardiomyopathy may be present with mitral systolic and diastolic murmurs and mitral incompetence. Significant left ventricular hypertrophy is almost always seen on the ECG. Echocardiography shows narrowing of the left ventricular outflow tract and systolic anterior motion of the aortic cusp of the mitral valve.

Course & Complications

A. Atrial Fibrillation: As in pure mitral stenosis, atrial fibrillation is such a frequent occurrence that it hardly qualifies as a complication. The age at which it occurs depends to some extent on the severity of the lesion and on the rheumatic myocardial damage. In patients with severe, recurrent attacks of rheumatic carditis, atrial fibrillation may occur even in adolescence.

B. Coronary Artery Disease: In older patients, atherosclerotic coronary arterial disease may influence the clinical picture with a myocardial factor that alters prognosis.

C. Systemic Embolism: Systemic embolization is a frequent and important complication. Embolism is detected in about 20% of cases, but the true incidence is almost certainly higher when asymptomatic cases are included. Cerebral, femoral, renal, intestinal, and coronary emboli comprise most of the clinically recognized cases. Left atrial thrombi form because of stasis and account for most emboli in mixed valvular disease. The emboli resulting from left atrial thrombus clear more readily than those associated with endocarditis.

D. Infective Endocarditis: Endocarditis is a serious complication in patients with mixed mitral stenosis and incompetence. It occurs more frequently than in mitral stenosis, but not as often as in mitral incompetence. The patient is almost invariably in sinus rhythm at the time of onset (see Chapter 16).

E. Pulmonary Vascular Disease: The development of a raised pulmonary vascular resistance is much less common than in mitral stenosis, because the left atrial mean pressure is usually lower.

Treatment

A. Medical Treatment:

1. Prophylactic penicillin– Prophylactic penicillin treatment to prevent recurrence of rheumatic fever is essential when the patient is under 25 years of age; in patients over age 30, recurrences of rheumatic fever are rare, and many physicians do not prescribe rheumatic fever prophylaxis, only immediate treatment of streptococcal infection (see Chapter 17).

2. Prevention of endocarditis– Antibiotic therapy to prevent infective endocarditis should always be recommended, especially if the lesion is mild. It should be administered before the patient undergoes major dental work or minor surgical procedures (see Chapter 16).

3. Digitalization and heart rate– The immediate treatment of a patient with mixed mitral stenosis and incompetence and atrial fibrillation often consists of controlling the heart rate with digitalis because patients so commonly present with this arrhythmia. The diagnosis by auscultation of mixed mitral stenosis and incompetence can be difficult at this stage, since murmurs are more difficult to hear when the heart rate is rapid and cardiac output is low. The physician must assume that any patient presenting with rapid atrial fibrillation, dyspnea, and pulmonary congestion has mitral disease until it is proved otherwise, and full digitalization is indicated. The control of heart rate is often a serious problem, and the easier it is to achieve such control, the easier it is to manage the patient. Propranolol and verapamil have proved valuable in some cases in reducing the rate of ventricular response. A search for precipitating factors such as intercurrent chest infection, a febrile illness, anemia, or thyrotoxicosis is always indicated.

4. Restoration of sinus rhythm by DC conversion– Restoration of sinus rhythm before surgery is sometimes indicated. If the patient develops atrial fibrillation with a rapid heart rate during an intercurrent infection or in relation to some other special stress, the mitral valve lesion may be too mild to warrant surgical treatment. In this case, restoration of sinus rhythm by DC countershock (as described in Chapter 7) may be effective in maintaining sinus rhythm for several years. In general, however, the results of cardioversion are poor, not because the patient fails to obtain relief but because atrial fibrillation soon recurs. The addition of propranolol or verapamil for the control of heart rate may be useful in some patients.

5. Anticoagulant therapy– Anticoagulant ther-

apy is advised in patients with atrial fibrillation who are not treated surgically. Anticoagulation markedly reduces the incidence of embolization. Unfortunately, it does not always prevent embolism.

B. Surgical Treatment:

1. Mitral valve replacement– Mitral valve replacement is the only operation indicated for the treatment of mixed mitral stenosis and incompetence. Mechanical valves have generally proved to be the most satisfactory, especially in younger patients. In patients over 70 years of age, bioprostheses are satisfactory. Annuloplasty, valvuloplasty, and other conservative reconstructive operations on the mitral valve have proved to be less successful than valvuloplasty for mitral incompetence due to mitral valve prolapse. Since mitral valve replacement has a higher perioperative mortality rate and is associated with more late morbidity than valvotomy, surgery is generally undertaken with much greater caution than in mitral stenosis. It is important to observe the response to medical treatment in patients presenting with dyspnea at the onset of atrial fibrillation. It may be possible to postpone mitral valve replacement for several years if the arrhythmia has been precipitated by some intercurrent illness; if the heart rate was extremely rapid at the onset but has slowed significantly with digitalis therapy; and if the patient can lead a quiet life. The decision to replace the mitral valve in patients with mixed mitral stenosis and incompetence is always a serious one because the mortality rate of the operation is about 5% and improvement is seldom dramatic. Unless left ventricular function is deteriorating— as demonstrated by increasing end-systolic size of the left ventricle together with decreasing ejection fraction—the patient should be NYHA class III on therapy before mitral valve replacement is considered.

Mitral valve replacement seldom makes the heart rate easier to control, and the anticipation that surgery will help in difficult cases should not be used as an indication for operation.

2. Restoration of sinus rhythm after surgery– Restoration of sinus rhythm by DC countershock should always be considered after surgery in patients who are not in sinus rhythm. It is not indicated in patients with giant left atrium or other lesions with marked cardiac enlargement, however. Quinidine together with digitalis should always be used in an attempt to prevent recurrence of atrial fibrillation.

Prognosis

The prognosis in mixed mitral stenosis and incompetence is not greatly influenced by surgery. If myocardial function is good and the heart is not overly large, the patient can usually live a relatively normal sedentary life, and the heart rate can be controlled by digitalis. Systemic embolization is always a hazard but usually causes morbidity rather than death. Patients with extreme cardiac enlargement can nonetheless live strikingly long lives and are relatively uninfluenced by surgical treatment. Such patients develop a chronic low output state and, although seriously incapacitated by fatigue and dyspnea, manage to live a sedentary existence for 10–15 years after the lesion has become far advanced.

Long-Term Results in Operated Cases

The late results of mitral valve replacement are worse in mixed mitral valve disease than in mitral stenosis. The amount of myocardial involvement is generally greater, and the heart is larger. In addition, pulmonary hypertension is not as severe, and there is consequently less room for improvement because of regression of pulmonary vascular disease.

MITRAL INCOMPETENCE

Mitral incompetence differs from other forms of mitral valve disease in that it occurs as both an acute and a chronic lesion. The chronic lesions are further subdivided into hemodynamically insignificant and significant lesions. The hemodynamically insignificant form is present in those patients with the "click-murmur" syndrome described by Barlow, sometimes referred to as the floppy valve syndrome or mitral valve prolapse, but these terms are unsatisfactory because prolapse and "floppy valves" may cause acute mitral incompetence and imply a pathologic process that cannot be determined at the bedside.

Causes of Mitral Incompetence (Table 12–1)

The causes of mitral incompetence are diverse and are different for acute and chronic lesions.

A. Rheumatic Fever: A history of rheumatic fever is present in about 10% of cases. The lesion may be of any degree of hemodynamic severity.

B. Myxomatous Changes: Myxomatous degenerative changes in the mitral valve figure prominently in the development of mitral incompetence, and the effects of abnormal wear and tear on a slightly abnormal valve may be important in the aggravation of mitral incompetence. Stretching, tearing of the chordae tendineae, atrophy of valve tissue, and myxomatous degeneration are commonly found at operation in both acute and chronic cases. It is not clear whether the myxomatous changes are superimposed on congenital or mild rheumatic lesions or whether they occur in previously normal valves. However, it is striking that a history of a previous murmur is present in half of patients with acute mitral incompetence. This suggests that degenerative changes occur more readily in abnormal valves and that patients with the click-murmur syndrome may develop acute mitral incompetence.

C. Infective Endocarditis: Infective endocarditis

Table 12–1. Causes of mitral incompetence.

Site of Pathology	Causes
Annulus	Mitral annular calcification Dilation of left ventricle from any cause (aortic regurgitation, dilated cardiomyopathy, etc)
Valve	Rheumatic heart disease Mitral valve prolapse Infective endocarditis Trauma Congenital clefting of leaflets Connective tissue disorders (Marfan's syndrome, Ehlers-Danlos syndrome, Morquio's syndrome) Left-sided myxoma
Chordae tendineae	Idiopathic rupture Trauma Infective endocarditis
Papillary muscles	Trauma Coronary artery disease
Left ventricle, myocardium	Coronary artery disease Cardiomyopathy
Prosthetic valve	Intrinsic disruption Thrombosis and pannus formation Paraprosthetic leak

plays a particularly important role in the clinical course of mitral incompetence. It is both a causative factor and a complication. A valve that is the site of a minor, hemodynamically insignificant lesion seems to be especially prone to endocarditis, with the subsequent exacerbation of mitral incompetence in patients with click-murmur syndrome. Endocarditis is also a direct cause of mitral incompetence when highly invasive organisms become established in the bloodstream and lodge on a normal mitral valve.

D. Ischemic Heart Disease: Ischemic heart disease may be important in the development of mitral incompetence. Posteroinferior myocardial infarctions may cause ischemia or even rupture of the papillary muscle supporting the valve. Acute rupture is usually fatal, but less severe degrees of ischemia may lead to smaller numbers of ruptured chordae tendineae or produce acute mitral incompetence in the course of myocardial infarction. After myocardial infarction, temporary interference with the function of the mitral valve sufficient to cause a murmur of mitral incompetence commonly occurs. It is difficult to decide whether such lesions are hemodynamically significant.

E. Congenital Heart Disease: Clefts in the mitral and tricuspid valves are part of atrioventricular canal lesions. They are also part of the lesion in endocardial cushion defects, which are seen in association with ostium primum atrial septal defects. Isolated mitral incompetence seen in association with Marfan's syndrome, Ehlers-Danlos syndrome, or osteogenesis imperfecta is congenital in origin, and it may be that the click-murmur syndrome seen in young women is often congenital in origin. Another rare cause of mitral incompetence is coronary arteriovenous fistula.

F. Mitral Valve Ring Calcification: Calcification of the mitral valve ring is an important cause of mitral incompetence. It occurs in elderly women and produces a pathognomonic radiologic and echocardiographic picture. The condition is associated with conduction defects and is not necessarily benign.

G. Traumatic Heart Disease: Steering wheel chest injuries in automobile accidents and other forms of direct trauma to the thorax, or even the effort of attempting to lift a heavy object, may cause acute disruption of the mitral valve, usually by rupture of the chordae tendineae or even the papillary muscle. The patient may have forgotten the episode of trauma and must be questioned directly about accidents while the history is being taken.

H. Left Ventricular Dilation: Any disease causing dilation of the left ventricle can cause dilation of the mitral annulus and mitral incompetence; thus, aortic insufficiency, hypertension with heart failure, and congestive cardiomyopathy can result in mitral incompetence.

1. HEMODYNAMICALLY INSIGNIFICANT MITRAL INCOMPETENCE: CLICK-MURMUR SYNDROME (Mitral Valve Prolapse)

The cardinal features of hemodynamically insignificant mitral incompetence (Figure 12–15) include normal heart size and normal hemodynamics. A late systolic murmur with or without a late systolic click is present. The ECG and chest x-ray are usually normal, but ST and T wave changes suggestive of myocardial ischemia are not infrequently seen, and the chest x-ray may show evidence of skeletal abnormalities, with pectus excavatum, straight thoracic spine, or scoliosis.

"Click-murmur" syndrome is extremely common—the commonest form of valvular abnormality found in Western countries. If echocardiographic rather than clinical criteria are used as the basis of diagnosis, about 5% of a normal population would be found to have this lesion. Clinical examination of normal subjects with this echocardiographic abnormality reveals that while about 10% (0.5% of the normal population) have a click and 7% have a systolic murmur, the fully developed click-murmur syndrome is present in less than 2% (ie, 0.1% of the normal population).

Click-murmur syndrome is associated with the same causes as the other forms of mitral incompetence and occurs at all ages. The click and murmur may be present in infancy or may develop at any age. The incidence is highest in women in the third and fourth decades. As with other forms of mitral disease, it is logical to base the diagnostic classification on

physical findings. Echocardiography to confirm the presence of mitral valve prolapse—the commonest "cause" of the lesion—is indicated. There is no doubt that the classic physical findings can occur without mitral valve prolapse, eg, after mitral valvotomy, and also that mitral valve prolapse can occur without the physical findings in "silent" cases or with the physical signs of significant mitral incompetence.

Late systolic mitral incompetence associated with posterior displacement of the posterior cusp of the mitral valve may be due to congenital abnormality of the valve tissue (floppy valve or billowing posterior leaflet). The redundant valve tissue bulges back into the left atrium, causing incompetence late in ventricular systole, and it is this mechanism that is thought to cause the click or murmur (Figure 12–18). In later life, degenerative myxomatous changes occur in the valve, which tends to stretch, and these changes cause similar redundancy of valvular tissue. Rheumatic disease and infective endocarditis can also cause a minor late systolic mitral valve leak. Mitral incompetence is most closely related to the presence of the late systolic murmur, and a click can be present without mitral incompetence.

The hemodynamic status as evidenced by the murmur is variable, and posture, exercise, and other mechanisms that alter systemic vascular resistance may influence the murmur. Maneuvers that make the heart larger, such as lying down or squatting, make the nonejection click occur later in systole after the first sound and decrease the degree of mitral incompetence. Maneuvers that decrease the heart size, such as standing up, bring the ejection click close to the first heart sound and may increase the duration of the murmur during systole. All the pathologic processes that cause click-murmur syndrome can progress either acutely or slowly to produce hemodynamically significant mitral incompetence. Thus, mitral valve prolapse, myxomatous degeneration, and floppy valves are seen in patients in whom mitral incompetence is far from minor. The proportion of cases with progressive lesions is not yet clearly established. One study suggests that severe mitral incompetence requiring valve surgery is unusual before age 50 but increases progressively thereafter. By age 75, about 5% of men and 2% of women with mitral valve prolapse require mitral valve surgery (Wilcken, 1988).

Clinical Findings

A. Symptoms: Most patients are entirely symptom-free, and the condition is found accidentally on routine physical examination. In some cases, atypical chest pain is present, and palpitations, fatigue, and dyspnea unrelated to exertion also occur. Exercise tolerance is almost always normal. Symptoms are more common in patients who know they have the lesion, and it seems clear that cardiac neurosis (see Chapter 21) readily develops when the presence of this lesion is brought to the attention of the patient. A

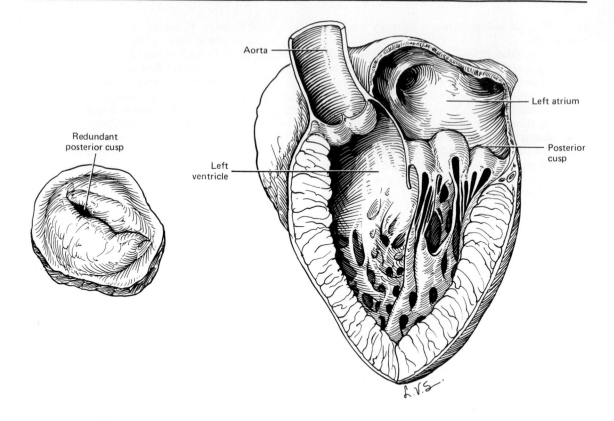

Drawing of left heart in left anterior oblique view showing anatomic features of hemodynamically insignificant mitral incompetence.

Cardinal features: *Normal heart size; redundant valve tissue.* **Variable factors:** *Clicks and murmurs.*

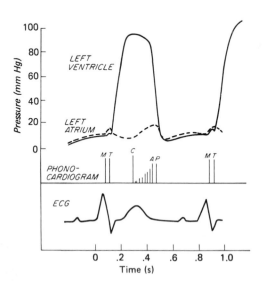

Diagram showing auscultatory and hemodynamic features of insignificant mitral incompetence. M, mitral; T, tricuspid; C, click; A, atrial; P, pulmonary.

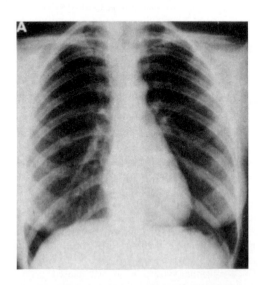

Chest x-ray in posteroanterior view of patient with click-murmur syndrome. (Reproduced, with permission, from Bontempo CP et al: Radiographic appearance of thorax in systolic click – late systolic murmur syndrome. *Am J Cardiol* 1975;**36**:27.)

Figure 12–15. Hemodynamically insignificant mitral incompetence (click-murmur syndrome). Structures enlarged: none.

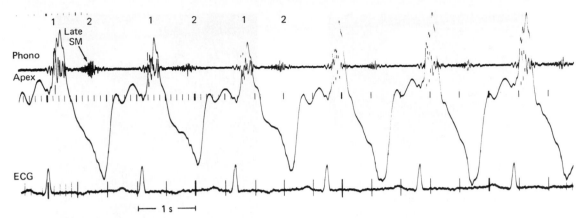

Figure 12–16. Phonocardiogram, apex cardiogram, and ECG from a patient with hemodynamically insignificant mitral incompetence. The late systolic accentuation of the murmur (late SM) can be seen.

family history of the lesion is occasionally found, and there may be a familial history of sudden death.

B. Signs: The only cardiac abnormalities are usually auscultatory in nature. Patients will often have an asthenic build and thoracic skeletal abnormalities such as pectus excavatum or kyphoscoliosis. This is the type of patient whose family is most likely to include other members with mitral valve prolapse. The characteristic sign is a late systolic murmur, as shown in Figure 12–16. It is often preceded by one or more midsystolic clicks. The murmur increases in intensity up to the second heart sound, making it difficult to time and often leading to an incorrect diagnosis of diastolic murmur. It may become pansystolic with exercise or when the patient stands up. It often has a honking quality and may on occasion be loud enough to be heard without a stethoscope. It is not uncommonly the only abnormal finding, and its timing is its most consistent feature. In some cases a click is heard without a murmur. In such patients, mitral valve prolapse without mitral incompetence is thought to be present.

C. Electrocardiographic Findings: The ECG is usually normal. An abnormal P wave (P mitrale) may be seen, and in some cases there are nonspecific ST and T wave changes in the inferior leads that suggest the possibility of myocardial ischemia.

D. Imaging Studies: The cardiac silhouette on chest x-ray is ordinarily normal. Minor left atrial enlargement is sometimes seen. The thoracic cage is not infrequently abnormal, with pectus excavatum, straight thoracic spine, or scoliosis.

1. Noninvasive techniques– Echocardiography has been primarily responsible for the apparent great increase in the frequency of diagnosis in the last 10 years. Even in patients with a click alone, echocardiographic tracings may be abnormal. Echocardiography appears to be a particularly sensitive means of detecting minor degrees of mitral valve prolapse in apparently normal subjects. Some authorities believe

that because of the saddle-like shape of the mitral annulus, the diagnosis of mitral valve prolapse should not be made on the four-chamber view alone, because portions of the valve can falsely appear to be above the annulus even in normal people. Only if the prolapse is seen in other views—especially in the parasternal long axis view—should a diagnosis of mitral valve prolapse be made. In addition to the movements of the valve itself, the size of the left atrium and ventricle can also be determined, as shown in Figure 12–17.

A negative echocardiogram does not exclude the diagnosis, and reliance on echocardiographic findings alone, in the absence of a click or murmur (or both), may result in overdiagnosis of the lesion that may do more harm than good. If stringent criteria are applied and evidence of prolapse is seen in more than one view, the condition is less likely to be overdiagnosed.

2. Invasive techniques– Since the diagnosis of chronic hemodynamically insignificant mitral incompetence is based on clinical findings and since no specific treatment is indicated, cardiac catheterization is not needed to establish the diagnosis.

Differential Diagnosis

The physical signs of click-murmur syndrome are sufficiently specific to make the diagnosis of hemodynamically insignificant mitral incompetence reasonably certain. The underlying pathology and the cause are more difficult to determine, however, and the significance of the lesion is always open to question. The presence of associated coronary artery disease may have to be ruled out by angiography in some cases.

Course & Complications

Most patients with click-murmur syndrome live normal lives. The lesion is seen in elderly persons known to have had a murmur for years. The complications that occur are thus dramatic and important but fortunately are rare.

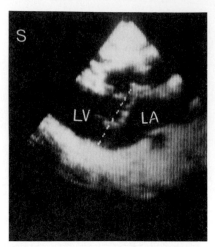 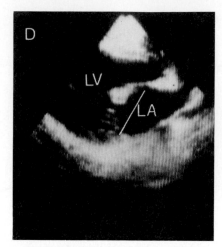

Figure 12–17. Two-dimensional echocardiograms showing systolic (S) and diastolic (D) positions of prolapsing mitral valve. The mitral valve moves backward into the left atrium during systole. (LV, left ventricle; LA, left atrium.) (Courtesy of NB Schiller.)

Several studies (Nishimura, 1985; Marks, 1989) suggest that virtually all complications occur only in those with markedly thickened, myxomatous valves as shown by echocardiography. Those with thin valves have almost no complications.

A. Infective Endocarditis: Infective endocarditis is an important complication of click-murmur syndrome. Since the hemodynamic status of the patient is virtually normal, the potential for acute valvular dis-

ruption with severe exacerbation of mitral incompetence is great.

B. Acute Disruption of the Mitral Valve: Acute mitral incompetence can develop either spontaneously or as the result of trauma in patients with click-murmur syndrome. Rupture of the chordae tendineae or stretching of a myxomatously degenerated valve is thought to be responsible for mitral valve disruption in those cases in which endocarditis is absent.

C. Coronary Artery Disease: The role of coronary artery disease in producing or exacerbating the effects of click-murmur syndrome is not clear. Hemodynamically insignificant mitral incompetence occurs in patients with coronary artery disease, especially those with minor degrees of papillary muscle dysfunction. Click-murmur syndrome occurs often enough in patients in late middle age that chance associations with coronary disease must be quite frequent.

D. Ventricular Arrhythmias and Sudden Death: Patients with click-murmur syndrome show an increased tendency to develop ventricular arrhythmias, and there is undoubtedly an increased incidence of sudden death associated with this lesion. The patient whose echocardiogram is shown in Figure 12–18 subsequently died suddenly, and since no obvious cause was found at autopsy, arrhythmia was felt to be the responsible mechanism. The incidence of sudden death is not known, but even an occurrence rate of 0.1% per year is important because the condition is so common.

E. Cerebral Ischemic Events: An association has been noted between click-murmur syndrome and transient ischemic attacks in patients under the age of 45. The most likely explanation is thought to be embolization resulting from small pieces of thrombotic material formed in association with stasis around the abnormal mitral valve.

Figure 12–18. Echocardiogram showing mitral click-murmur syndrome in a patient who subsequently died suddenly. (RV, right ventricle; S, septum; AMVL, anterior, and PMVL posterior mitral valve leaflets; MVP, mitral valve prolapse.) (Courtesy of NB Schiller.)

Treatment

Although antibiotic prophylaxis for the prevention of infective endocarditis is mandatory (see Chapter 16), click-murmur syndrome is generally so benign that no other specific treatment is needed. The patient should be followed and monitored for the development of complications. Patients with transient ischemic attacks or strokes should receive antiplatelet therapy, (eg, aspirin) or anticoagulants (or both). The possibility of sudden death from arrhythmia is always present. That it occurs only rarely is fortunate, as no form of treatment has been shown to influence the development of this complication. Treatment to prevent arrhythmia should be restricted to symptomatic patients, those with a hyperkinetic circulation or established ventricular tachycardia, and those surviving after aborted sudden death. Twenty-four-hour ambulatory electrocardiographic monitoring is indicated before the start of treatment. Patients with click-murmur syndrome in general do not lead happier lives when they are aware of the possibility of sudden death. The physician must exercise extreme care to ensure that patients with hemodynamically insignificant mitral incompetence do not become cardiac invalids. The physician should make a clear mental distinction between the patient who presents with no complaints and whose lesion is therefore discovered on routine or incidental examination and the patient who has consulted a physician because of some specific symptom thought to be related to cardiac disease.

Prognosis

The prognosis of hemodynamically insignificant mitral incompetence is not yet clear. The results of 20-year follow-up studies of patients with a late systolic murmur as the only finding indicate that infective endocarditis and acute disruption of the mitral valve due to rupture of the chordae tendineae are not infrequent sequelae. This finding correlates well with the information obtained from patients with significant mitral incompetence. A long history of a heart murmur is found in three types of patients with mitral incompetence: those with infective endocarditis, those with acute mitral valve disruption, and those with chronic hemodynamically significant mitral incompetence. It seems that many of these patients have had hemodynamically insignificant lesions that have subsequently become more severe.

2. HEMODYNAMICALLY SIGNIFICANT MITRAL INCOMPETENCE

The cardinal features of hemodynamically significant mitral incompetence (Figure 12–19) include left ventricular enlargement (hypertrophy in acute lesions), systolic backflow into the left atrium, and left atrial enlargement. The variable features that influence atrial and ventricular enlargement are the severity of the leak and the acuteness or chronicity of the process.

Pathophysiology

A. Acute Lesions: In acute mitral incompetence, the degree of pulmonary congestion is much greater than in chronic lesions. A large proportion of the force of left ventricular contraction is expended in pumping blood back across the incompetent valve into a noncompliant atrium of normal size. The volume of blood flowing forward through the aortic valve falls, reducing arterial pressure and causing reflex tachycardia and peripheral vasoconstriction, which aggravate the lesion. Pulmonary venous pressure rises, and pulmonary congestion and edema occur acutely. With marked elevation of left atrial pressure, pulmonary artery and right ventricular systolic pressures rise acutely, frequently resulting in right ventricular dilation and failure. With the sudden increase in left ventricular diastolic volume, the filling pressure of the left ventricle may increase slightly. The suddenly enlarged left ventricle in diastole within the noncompliant pericardium results in restrictive filling of the right ventricle, further elevating right ventricular diastolic pressure.

If the acute mitral incompetence is severe, the patient cannot survive without surgical treatment. With time, pulmonary vascular resistance rises, and right heart failure ultimately develops if the patient does not die in pulmonary edema. Because the left atrium is not large, normal sinus rhythm is maintained in acute mitral incompetence. In less severe cases, the hemodynamic picture gradually changes, and the left atrium dilates and becomes more compliant. The left ventricle enlarges, and as left atrial pressure falls, the resistance against which the left ventricle pumps decreases. In this way the left ventricular pressure load of acute mitral incompetence gradually changes to the volume load of chronic mitral incompetence.

1. Hemodynamic effects– The hemodynamic picture in acute mitral incompetence is shown in Figure 12–20. The findings are unique because there is pulmonary congestion with raised left atrial pressure but no left ventricular failure and no mitral stenosis. The systolic left atrial pressure is markedly raised owing to the late v wave, but the wedge pressure falls to normal levels by the end of diastole, and there is no appreciable end-diastolic pressure difference across the mitral valve. However, the average left atrial pressure is high enough to cause pulmonary edema, especially when diastole is shortened by tachycardia. Thus, the patient with acute mitral incompetence suffers from "relative" mitral stenosis and not from left ventricular failure in the initial stages.

2. Associated left ventricular disease– The hemodynamic changes mentioned above are seen in pure mechanical lesions, but the clinical picture is different in patients whose mitral incompetence is due to left ventricular disease.

Incompetent mitral valve seen
from the atrial surface

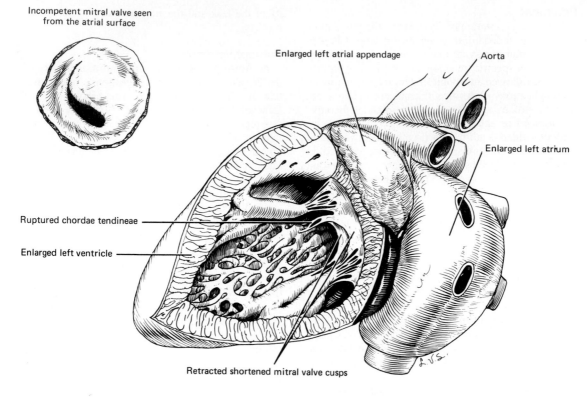

Enlarged left atrial appendage

Aorta

Enlarged left atrium

Ruptured chordae tendineae

Enlarged left ventricle

Retracted shortened mitral valve cusps

Drawing of left heart in left lateral view showing anatomic features of mitral incompetence.

Cardinal features: *Systolic backflow into left atrium; left atrial enlargement; left ventricular enlargement (hypertrophy in acute lesions).*

Variable factors: *Severity of leak; acuteness or chronicity; etiology; severity of associated left ventricular disease.*

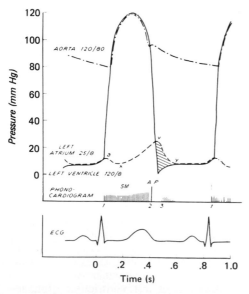

Diagram showing auscultatory and hemodynamic features of mitral incompetence. 3, third sound; SM, systolic murmur; A, atrial; P, pulmonary.

Chest x-ray of a patient with mitral incompetence showing left atrial (LA) and left ventricular (LV) enlargement.

Figure 12–19. Hemodynamically significant mitral incompetence. Structures enlarged: left atrium and left ventricle.

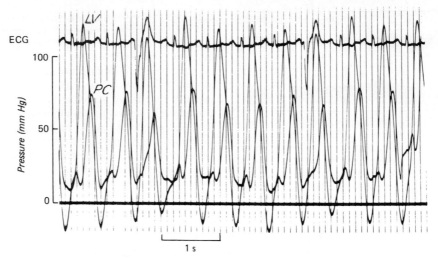

Figure 12–20. Pressure tracings in a patient with acute severe mitral incompetence showing large (70 mm Hg) *v* wave in wedge (PC) tracing and nearly normal left ventricular (LV) diastolic pressure.

The unique hemodynamic state of the patient with acute mitral incompetence is particularly susceptible to changes in systemic arterial resistance. The left ventricle pumps against two impedances in parallel during systole—aortic impedance and the impedance of the left atrium seen through the mitral valve. The magnitude of each impedance determines the overall load. An increase in left ventricular wall tension, the product of left ventricular radius and pressure, is kept to a minimum, because as the left ventricular pressure rises in systole, there is immediate ejection of blood under low pressure into the left atrium. If aortic impedance is reduced by vasodilator therapy, aortic flow will increase and mitral incompetence will decrease, lowering left atrial pressure and relieving any tendency toward pulmonary edema. This principle forms the basis for the successful use of nitroprusside and nitroglycerin in the treatment of acute mitral incompetence. If the patient survives, the acute lesions come to look more and more like those of chronic mitral incompetence, and after about a year, mitral incompetence that had an acute onset is usually indistinguishable from the chronic form of the lesion.

B. Chronic Lesions: Chronic mitral incompetence causes less hemodynamic stress than any other left-sided lesion. The left atrium bears the brunt of the load and in chronic cases dilates and becomes more compliant than normal. The mean left atrial pressure in chronic cases is thus usually less than 20 mm Hg, and left ventricular ejection against the low atrial pressure results in a pure volume overload on the left ventricle. The left ventricle dilates, and eccentric hypertrophy rapidly occurs, growing a larger ventricle around the increased volume, thus keeping the left ventricular filling pressure normal. Left ventricular stroke volume is increased. Associated left ventricular disease due to hypertension, coronary artery dis-

ease, or even possibly normal aging processes plays an important part in aggravating the hemodynamic effects of mitral incompetence.

A raised systemic vascular resistance increases the leak through the mitral valve and compromises the left ventricular output. A low output causes tachycardia and peripheral vasoconstriction, which further aggravate the lesion. Thus, age-related degenerative changes in left ventricular function may be the precipitating cause of symptoms. Left atrial dilation secondary to mitral incompetence usually leads to atrial fibrillation in middle age, but since there is no obstruction to mitral diastolic flow, patients with mitral incompetence withstand this arrhythmia better than do patients with any degree of mitral stenosis.

Clinical Findings

A. Symptoms:

1. Acute lesions– Dyspnea is the principal presenting symptom in patients with acute mitral incompetence. The onset may be acute (eg, when a cusp perforates or tears) or subacute (eg, when the mitral valve gradually shrinks and retracts after treatment of endocarditis). Dyspnea may progress to acute pulmonary edema with acute circulatory collapse, shock, and frothy pink, blood-tinged sputum. The patient may be ill at the time of onset, with a high fever and septicemia. Episodic attacks of dyspnea may occur and are associated with minor increases in cardiac output in response to the exertion of meals, washing, bowel movements, or even the excitement of visitors. Left atrial pressure is markedly dependent on the peripheral resistance in this lesion, and any increase in arterial pressure may provoke an attack of dyspnea.

2. Chronic lesions– In hemodynamically significant lesions, dyspnea is the principal presenting symptom. It is not usually as severe as in mitral ste-

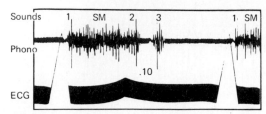

Figure 12–21. Phonocardiogram in a patient with hemodynamically significant mitral incompetence. The pansystolic murmur (SM) lasts until the second heart sound (2). The third heart sound (3) occurs 0.10 s after S_2 and lasts for about 0.05 s. Atrial fibrillation is present. (Courtesy of Roche Laboratories Division of Hoffman-La Roche, Inc.)

nosis, and the effects of an increase in heart rate are less prominent. The onset of atrial fibrillation is generally well tolerated and does not provoke the acute symptoms seen in patients who have mitral stenosis. Palpitations are more common than in other forms of mitral disease; atrial fibrillation is the commonest cause. Easy fatigability results from limited ability to increase forward effective output as left ventricular failure occurs.

B. Signs: The physical signs are depicted in Figure 12–19. The first heart sound is usually buried in the pansystolic murmur, but there is never an opening snap. The presence of an opening snap indicates that some degree of rheumatic mitral stenosis is present. With severe mitral incompetence, there is almost invariably a loud third heart sound associated with the rapid phase of left ventricular filling. It is a dull, low-pitched, thudding sound occurring about 0.10–0.18 s after the second sound (Figure 12–21). The large volume of blood crossing the mitral valve early in diastole can result in a short diastolic low-pitched flow murmur. With acute mitral incompetence, the patient is in normal sinus rhythm, and with the distended left ventricle in diastole, a fourth heart sound is frequently present.

Signs of right heart failure and raised pulmonary vascular resistance are rare except in patients with severe acute mitral incompetence resulting from acute disruption of the valve. When left ventricular failure occurs, the left ventricular diastolic pressure rises, the left atrial pressure rises, and finally the right ventricle, pumping against increased impedance, fails. This occurs extremely late in the course of chronic mitral incompetence and implies a very poor prognosis.

In patients with severe mitral incompetence, the cardiac impulse is hyperdynamic. The pulse is jerky and has been called a "small water-hammer pulse" because it resembles the pulse of aortic incompetence and has a rapid upstroke but with a small stroke volume. The size of the heart varies with the severity and acuteness of the lesion. Chronic severe lesions show large overactive hearts because of increased systolic and diastolic flows across the incompetent valve.

C. Electrocardiographic Findings: Electrocardiographic evidence of left ventricular hypertrophy eventually occurs. With sinus rhythm, left atrial abnormality is seen. In patients in whom acute mitral incompetence is not treated in the early stages, right ventricular hypertrophy may ultimately develop owing to raised pulmonary vascular resistance. Atrial arrhythmias almost inevitably develop with time in patients with mitral incompetence. Although atrial premature beats, atrial tachycardia, and atrial flutter are occasionally seen, atrial fibrillation is much more common. Atrial arrhythmia may be paroxysmal at first and become chronic later. The onset of atrial fibrillation is more closely related to the patient's age than to any other variable in mitral incompetence.

D. Imaging Studies: In patients with acute mitral incompetence, the heart is often of normal size on x-ray at the outset, and marked pulmonary congestion and edema may be the only visible signs. Starting within 1–2 weeks, however, the left atrium and ventricle enlarge and reach the proportions seen in chronic cases by the end of a year if the patient survives.

In hemodynamically significant chronic lesions, the left ventricle and left atrium are enlarged in proportion to the severity of the lesion (Figure 12–19).

The principal form of mitral incompetence in which cardiac fluoroscopy is valuable is mitral ring calcification. In this lesion, which is virtually confined to elderly women, the radiologic picture is striking (Figure 12–22). The entire calcified mitral ring

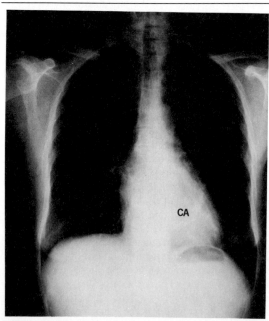

Figure 12–22. Chest x-ray of a 69-year-old woman with progressive mitral incompetence showing calcification (CA) of the mitral valve ring.

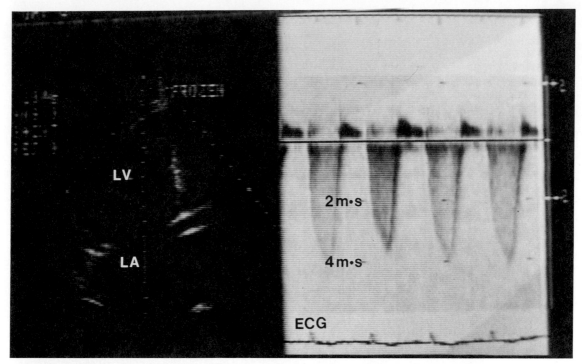

Figure 12–23. Two-chamber, two-dimensional echocardiogram **(A)** and continuous wave Doppler signal **(B)** from a patient with mitral incompetence. The peak velocity of regurgitant flow is about 4.8 m•s−1, extending to the posterior aspect of the left atrium, indicating severe incompetence. (Courtesy of NB Schiller.)

can be seen moving up and down with the heartbeat, and the lesion can be distinguished from calcification of other sites in the chest. A dense echo can be seen on echocardiography in patients with a calcified mitral annulus even when calcification is not visible on x-ray.

1. Noninvasive techniques– Mitral incompetence can be diagnosed echographically (Figure 12–23), especially in acute disruption of the mitral valve. With ruptured chordae tendineae, flailing chordae or portions of the leaflet can be seen prolapsing into the left atrium during systole. In addition to the valve itself, the size of the relevant heart chambers (left atrium and left ventricle) can be measured in the planes that are accessible to echographic investigation.

Echo-Doppler detects abnormally increased velocities of the mitral incompetence jet in the left atrium above the mitral valve. The severity of the leak can be judged by the distance from the mitral valve the jet reaches, whether it reaches the back of the left atrium or enters the pulmonary veins. The area at the mitral valve over which the jet occurs correlates roughly with the severity of the leak. With color Doppler, the turbulence caused by the increased velocity jet can detect the eccentric jet, which may be missed with continuous Doppler. In severe mitral incompetence, the jet turbulence can involve the entire left atrium

and even be seen to enter the pulmonary veins and the atrial appendage when investigated by transesophageal echocardiography. With high velocity and volume jets, the turbulent increased velocity jet can be seen to hug the left atrial wall and travel around the atrium along the walls. When this is seen, it always implies severe mitral incompetence (Figure 12–24).

With transesophageal echocardiography, the entire mitral apparatus is seen in great detail, and judgments can be made concerning the anatomic reasons for the valvular incompetence. Redundancy of the leaflets, elongation or rupture of the chordae tendineae, fibrosis and retraction or tearing of the leaflets, and dilation of the annulus can all be responsible for mitral incompetence. This information is essential in deciding whether repair of the valve is possible or whether the valve will have to be replaced (Figure 12–25).

2. Invasive techniques–

a. Acute mitral incompetence– Because noninvasive techniques can demonstrate the severity and anatomic cause of the mitral incompetence, catheterization and angiocardiography are necessary only when there is a question about the severity of the incompetence, the ventricular contractility, or the state of the coronary arteries. Right and left heart catheterization in patients with acute disruption of the mitral valve can differentiate the mechanical effects

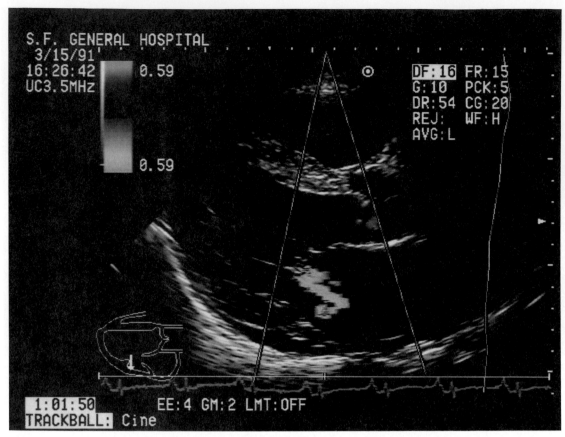

Figure 12–24. Two-dimensional color Doppler echocardiogram in the parasternal long axis view. The patient has moderate mitral regurgitation. Note jet emerging from central coaptation point of the valve. Picture taken in mid diastole.

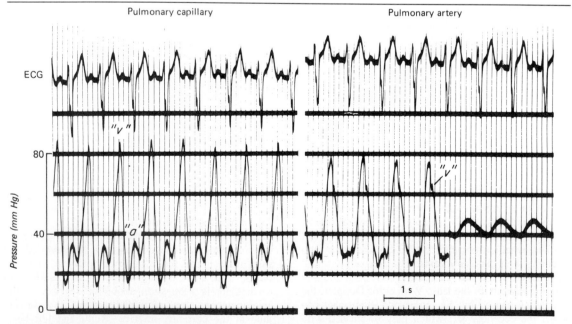

Figure 12–25. Pulmonary capillary (wedge) and pulmonary artery pressure tracings in a patient with acute mitral incompetence. The giant v wave seen in the wedge tracing is also visible in the pulmonary arterial pressure tracing.

of the lesion from those of associated myocardial or coronary disease. The hallmark of acute severe mitral incompetence is a wide pulse pressure in the wedge or left atrial tracing. The giant *v* wave, averaging over 50 mm Hg with values as high as 80 mm Hg in some cases, is quite characteristic. The *v* wave can usually also be seen in the pulmonary arterial pressure tracing as a second peak occurring in late systole which may equal or be higher than that due to right ventricular contraction (Figure 12–25). The level of the diastolic left atrial pressure is also important as a clue to the state of the myocardium. In lesions that are mainly mechanical, the left ventricular and left atrial diastolic pressures are both about 15 mm Hg, indicating that there is no left ventricular failure. Left ventricular angiography is an essential part of the study, because it shows the magnitude of mitral incompetence and demonstrates the hyperdynamic state found in pure mechanical lesions, as opposed to the sluggish ventricular contraction with mitral incompetence occurring in lesions that have poor left ventricular function. In patients who have cardiac pain and any suggestion of prior infarction, coronary angiographyis indicated. In about 15% of cases, especially in younger patients, the raised left atrial pressure resulting from acute disruption of the mitral valve may cause a marked increase in pulmonary vascular resistance.

b. Chronic mitral incompetence– In symptomatic patients with hemodynamically significant mitral incompetence, cardiac catheterization may be indicated to determine the severity of the lesion before considering surgery. If there are questions about the severity of the incompetence, the state of myocardial contractility, or the status of the coronary arteries remaining after noninvasive evaluation then catheterization is necessary. Left atrial pressure is usually only moderately raised, with a *v* wave of up to 30 mm Hg. The size of the left atrium is an important determinant of the hemodynamic findings, and in patients with a large atrium, the pressures are not usually impressive. The end-diastolic left ventricular pressure is of considerable importance. If it is raised, hypertension, active or inactive rheumatic myocarditis, or coronary disease should be suspected. The cardiac output may be abnormally low in patients with chronic mitral incompetence, especially in older persons, and the hemodynamic findings in patients with severe lesions may be unimpressive if this is the case. It is important to remember these factors when assessing the need for surgery, since valve replacement in patients even with wedge pressures of less than 20 mm Hg may have surprisingly good results.

Differential Diagnosis

Mitral incompetence must be distinguished from hypertrophic cardiomyopathy. There is a long pansystolic murmur in both conditions, and although the murmur in mitral incompetence is usually higher-pitched, has a timing that is not of the ejection type, and is transmitted to the axilla rather than centrally, the two lesions can be confused on diagnosis. Both show a third heart sound and a prominent left ventricle.

Ventricular septal defect is another condition that can be confused with mitral incompetence in both acute and chronic lesions. Again, the auscultatory findings are similar, with an overactive left ventricle, a pansystolic murmur, and third heart sound. Endocardial cushion defects with an associated ostium primum atrial defect and mitral incompetence are also difficult to differentiate from pure mitral incompetence on physical examination, and Doppler echocardiography is needed to confirm the diagnosis. In the case of acute lesions, especially in patients who have suffered a recent myocardial infarction, the distinction between acquired ventricular septal defect due to rupture of the ventricular septum and acute mitral incompetence due to papillary muscle involvement can be difficult.

Course & Complications

The course of mitral incompetence is not yet fully understood.

With increased left ventricular diastolic volume, there is dilation of the mitral annulus, which increases the regurgitant orifice and therefore the volume of regurgitation. The dilated ventricle changes the direction of chordal pull, thus decreasing the effectiveness with which the chordae prevent prolapse of the leaflet edges. Finally, the dilated annulus decreases the area of coaptation of the leaflets, which places more tension on the chordae during systole. This can cause chordal rupture, suddenly increasing the severity of mitral incompetence.

A. Systemic Embolism: Systemic embolization is an important complication. It is more common in mixed mitral stenosis and incompetence, but it also occurs in pure mitral incompetence, where it is more frequently due to infective endocarditis. Embolism is detected in about 20% of cases and almost certainly occurs more frequently without causing symptoms. The emboli resulting from left atrial thrombus clear more readily than those associated with endocarditis. Embolism is more common in patients with atrial fibrillation and is more likely to occur when the rhythm changes, either when atrial fibrillation begins or when sinus rhythm is restored.

B. Infective Endocarditis: Infective endocarditis is an important complication of mitral valvular disease in general and occurs most frequently in patients with mitral incompetence (20%). The patient is almost invariably in sinus rhythm at the onset of this complication (see also Chapter 16).

C. Coronary Artery Disease: In older patients, atherosclerotic coronary arterial disease may influence the clinical picture with a myocardial factor that alters prognosis. This is especially true of those patients with mitral incompetence, whose lesions are frequently degenerative in origin.

D. Pulmonary Vascular Disease: Pulmonary hypertension, with a raised pulmonary vascular resistance, is uncommon until late in the course except in acute mitral incompetence. The levels of left atrial pressure resulting from chronic mitral incompetence alone are usually not high enough to cause this complication.

Treatment

A. Medical Treatment: See above under Mitral Stenosis for a discussion of medical measures used in the treatment of mitral incompetence.

B. Indications for Surgical Treatment: Surgical correction is indicated for patients who despite medical management are symptomatic on ordinary activity (NYHA class III). The asymptomatic or only mildly symptomatic patient must be followed for signs of decreasing left ventricular function. The most sensitive sign of decreasing left ventricular function is an increasing end-systolic volume, especially if it occurs in a ventricle with a decreasing ejection fraction. In any case, the ejection fraction should not be allowed to fall below 55%. It is possible to follow the patient's ventricular function with noninvasive studies, echo-Doppler, or radionuclide angiography. It is unusual for a patient with severe mitral incompetence and good left ventricular systolic function to develop decreasing myocardial contractility and remain asymptomatic. One often sees patients with poor left ventricular function and severe mitral regurgitation, but in those cases the mitral incompetence is probably secondary to the dilated left ventricle caused by the poor left ventricular function. As the ability to repair the mitral valve increases and becomes more predictable, mitral valve surgery will be indicated whenever the mitral incompetence becomes hemodynamically severe.

C. Surgical Treatment:

1. Valvuloplasty in acute mitral incompetence– Acute mitral incompetence for many years is the major disorder that could be treated satisfactorily with mitral valvuloplasty. In cases in which the chordae tendineae supporting the posterior (mural) cusp of the mitral valve are torn, wedge resection of the affected part of the cusp gives excellent results. This operation has the advantage of not requiring long-term anticoagulant therapy. Over the last 20 years, techniques of mitral valve repair rather than replacement have been developed and advocated, especially by Carpentier in France and Duran in Spain. Techniques of valve repair, transferring intact chordae from the posterior to the anterior leaflet, reattaching chordae, and annular size reduction using annuloplasty rings have made it possible to repair rather than to replace valves in the majority of cases where valve disruptions have resulted in mitral incompetence.

In mitral incompetence due to rheumatic heart disease, with fibrosis and retraction of the leaflets, the chances of repairing the valve rather than replacing it are reduced. Preoperative study by transesophageal echocardiography is essential to determine the anatomic cause of the mitral incompetence and the possibility of repair.

Repair of valvular incompetence can be done with a lower mortality rate than valve replacement, and retaining the valvular-ventricular interaction by preserving the chordal attachments means that the ejection fraction does not fall after repair, as it usually does after mitral valve replacement. Valvular repair avoids all the problems seen with valvular tissue and mechanical prostheses, including a lower incidence of thromboemboli and infective endocarditis. This can be done with excellent long-term results. Deloche (1990) reported 206 consecutive patients who underwent mitral valve repair for mitral incompetence. The 15-year actuarial survival rate was 73%, and 94% were free from thromboembolism, 97% free from endocarditis, and 87% free from reoperation. Among 157 survivors 74% were in NYHA classes I and II.

These techniques of repair must be learned, and the results of repair depend on the surgeon's experience and technical ability. Because these techniques are operator-dependent, reliable repair with good results is not available in every institution performing cardiac surgery.

2. Mitral valve replacement in mitral incompetence– Until recently, mitral valve replacement was the treatment of choice in almost all cases of mitral incompetence. With mitral valve repair now possible, the indications for surgery are changing. In acute lesions, it may be difficult to decide when to operate. In patients with infective endocarditis or acute myocardial infarction, surgery should be delayed, if possible, until the acute lesion is completely healed unless the hemodynamic consequences are very severe; this is especially true in severe mitral incompetence due to ischemic heart disease. If the patient is in severe congestive heart failure, immediate afterload reduction and even intraaortic balloon pump support should be started and the patient sent to surgery immediately upon stabilization.

The lower the ejection fraction, the worse the prognosis with surgery. The operative mortality rate is high in patients with ejection fractions below 30%, and the long-term results are not good even if the patient survives. Although valve repair rather than valve replacement has a better prognosis in these patients, the ultimate long-term prognosis is bad. Since the prognosis without surgery in these patients is uniformly poor, even in these patients, if the mitral incompetence is very severe, operative repair or replacement should be offered. The hemodynamic load of acute mitral incompetence is generally not as severe as that of acute aortic incompetence, and it is usually possible to delay, particularly if systemic vasodilator therapy (afterload reduction) is employed. The timing of surgery is most critical in patients suffering from endocarditis following intravenous drug abuse or endocarditis caused by drug-resistant organisms. No satisfactory regimen has yet been established for the management of such cases, and the long-term results are poor whether valve replacement is performed early or late in the course of the disease. Patients with known associated left ventricular disease also present problems in management.

Prognosis

In patients with mitral incompetence the prognosis depends more on the cause of the valvular lesion than on its severity and acuteness.

A. Acute Mitral Incompetence: The prognosis in acute mitral incompetence is good with surgery provided that myocardial infarction or uncontrollable infective endocarditis is not the basic cause. Early diagnosis and operation performed as soon as any associated lesions have healed improve the prognosis by preventing the changes of chronic mitral incompetence.

B. Chronic Mitral Incompetence: Chronic mitral incompetence carries a good prognosis once the lesion has stabilized. The load on the left ventricle is a pure "flow" load, and left ventricular hypertrophy is by no means inevitable. Atrial fibrillation is well tolerated, and provided that systemic hypertension or coronary artery disease does not develop, valve replacement can often be put off until age 50 or later. Age-related degenerative changes in the valve and in the heart as a whole are the most important causes of progression necessitating mitral valve replacement.

Long-Term Results in Operated Cases

The late results of operation in acute mitral incompetence are better than in other forms of mitral valve disease. The results of mitral valve replacement in patients with chronic mitral incompetence resemble those in mixed mitral valve disease. The operation is palliative rather than curative, and some residual and usually progressive damage is present.

The operative mortality rate associated with mitral valve replacement in a good-risk patient is 3–5%. In patients with decreased left ventricular function or multisystem disease, it can be as high as 10–15%. After successful valve replacement, the mortality due to valve disruption, thromboembolization, infective endocarditis, and other problems is about 4% per year. With valve repair, in the best hands with properly selected patients, long-term results are excellent. Whether this will be the case as more surgeons who are less skilled attempt mitral valve repair remains to be seen.

REFERENCES

General

Barlow JB: *Perspectives on the Mitral Valve.* Davis, 1986.

Cheitlin MD: The timing of surgery in mitral and aortic valve. Curr Probl Cardiol 1987;2:69.

Cziner DG et al: Transesophageal versus transthoracic echocardiography for diagnosing mitral valve perforation. Am J Cardiol 1992;69:1495.

Law W et al: Radionuclide regurgitant index: Value and limitations. Am J Cardiol 1981;47:292.

Mann DL: Pathophysiology of valvular heart disease: Basic mechanisms. Curr Opin Cardiol 1991;6:191.

Shah PM, Bansal RC: Transesophageal echocardiography. Curr Probl Cardiol 1990;15:647.

Sheikh KH et al: The utility of transesophageal echocardiography and Doppler color flow imaging in patients undergoing cardiac valve surgery. J Am Coll Cardiol 1990;15:363.

Mitral Stenosis

Beyer RW et al: Mitral valve resistance as a hemodynamic indicator in mitral stenosis. Am J Cardiol 1992;69:775.

Block PC et al: Later (two-year) follow-up after percutaneous balloon mitral valvotomy. Am J Cardiol 1992;69:537.

Complications and Mortality of Percutaneous Balloon Mitral Commissurotomy: A report from the National Heart, Lung, Blood Institute Balloon Valvuloplasty Registry. Circulation 1992;85:2014.

Dalby AJ et al: Preoperative factors affecting the outcome of isolated mitral valve replacement. Am J Cardiol 1981;47:826.

Gordon SPF et al: Two-dimension and Doppler echocardiographic determinants of the natural history of mitral valve narrowing in patients with rheumatic mitral stenosis: Implications for follow-up. J Am Coll Cardiol 1992;19:908.

Gross RI et al: Long-term results of open radical mitral commissurotomy: Ten year follow-up study of 202 patients. Am J Cardiol 1981;47:821.

Kawanishi DT, Rahimtoola SH: Catheter balloon commissurotomy for mitral stenosis: Complications and results. J Am Coll Cardiol 1992;19:192.

Marshall R, McIlroy MB, Christie RV: The work of breathing in mitral stenosis. Clin Sci 1954;13:137.

The NHLBI Balloon Valvuloplasty Registry Participants: Multicenter experience with balloon mitral commissurotomy: NHLBI Balloon Valvuloplasty Registry Report on Immediate and 30-Day Follow-Up Results. Circulation 1992;85:448.

Ohshima M et al: Immediate effects of percutaneous transvenous mitral commissurotomy on pulmonary hemodynamics at rest and during exercise in mitral stenosis. Am J Cardiol 1992;70:641.

Rediker DE et al: Mitral balloon valvuloplasty for mitral restenosis after surgical commissurotomy. J Am Coll Cardiol 1988;11:252.

Saal AK et al: Noninvasive detection of aortic insufficiency in patients with mitral stenosis by pulsed Doppler echocardiography. J Am Coll Cardiol 1985;5: 176.

Thuillez C et al: Pulsed Doppler echocardiographic study of mitral stenosis. Circulation 1980;61:381.

Tuzcu EM et al: Immediate and long-term outcome of percutaneous mitral valvotomy in patients 65 years and older. Circulation 1992;85:963.

Wood P: An appreciation of mitral stenosis. (Two parts.) Br Med J 1954;16:1951, 1113.

Wood P et al: The effect of acetylcholine on pulmonary vascular resistance and left atrial pressure in mitral stenosis. Br Heart J 1957;19:279.

Click-Murmur Syndrome
(Mitral Valve Prolapse)

Allen H, Harris A, Leatham A: Significance and prognosis of an isolated late systolic murmur: A 9 to 22 year follow-up. Br Heart J 1974;36:525.

Barlow JB, Pocock WA: Mitral valve prolapse, the specific billowing mitral leaflet syndrome, or an insignificant nonejection systolic click. (Editorial.) Am Heart J 1979;97:277.

Bhutto ZR et al: Electrocardiographic abnormalities in mitral valve prolapse. Am J Cardiol 1992;70:265.

Boudoulas H, Wooley CF: *Mitral Valve Prolapse and the Mitral Valve Prolapse Syndrome.* Futura, 1988.

Chesler E et al: Normal catecholamine and hemodynamic responses to orthostatic tilt in subjects with mitral valve prolapse. Am J Med 1985;78:754.

Devereaux RB et al: Mitral valve prolapse: Causes, clinical manifestations, and management. Ann Intern Med 1989;111:305.

Devereaux RB et al: Relation between clinical features of mitral prolapse syndrome and echocardiography documented mitral valve prolapse. J Am Coll Cardiol 1986;8:763.

Duren DR, Becker AE, Duning AJ: Long-term follow-up of idiopathic mitral valve prolapse in 300 patients: A prospective study. J Am Coll Cardiol 1988;11:42.

Farb A et al: Comparison of cardiac findings in patients with mitral valve prolapse who die suddenly and those who have congestive heart failure from mitral regurgitation and to those with fatal noncardiac conditions. Am J Cardiol 1992;70:234.

Fontana ME et al: Mitral valve prolapse and the mitral valve prolapse syndrome. Curr Probl Cardiol 1991;16:315.

Hickey AJ, MacMahon SW, Wilcken DEL: Mitral valve prolapse and bacterial endocarditis: When is antibiotic prophylaxis necessary? Am Heart J 1985;109:131.

Jeresaty RM: Mitral valve prolapse: An update. JAMA 1985;254:793.

Kulick DL et al: Catheter balloon commissurotomy in adults. Part II: Mitral and other stenoses. Curr Probl Cardiol 1990;15:403.

Leatham A, Brigden W: Mild mitral regurgitation and the mitral prolapse fiasco. Am Heart J 1980;99:659.

Levine RA et al: Reconsideration of echocardiographic standards for mitral valve prolapse: Lack of association between leaflet displacement isolated to the apical four-chamber view and independent echocardiographic evidence of abnormality. J Am Coll Cardiol 1988;11:1010.

Marks AR et al: Identification of high-risk and low-risk subgroups of patients with mitral valve prolapse. N Engl J Med 1989;320:1031.

McMahon SW et al: Risk of infective endocarditis in mitral valve prolapse with and without precordial systolic murmurs. Am J Cardiol 1987;59:105.

Nishimura RA et al: Echocardiography documented mitral valve prolapse: Long-term follow-up of 237 patients. N Engl J Med 1985;313:1305.

Perloff JK, Child JS, Edwards JE: New guidelines for the clinical diagnosis of mitral valve prolapse. Am J Cardiol 1986;57:1124.

Pocock WA et al: Sudden death in primary mitral valve prolapse. Am Heart J 1984;107:378.

Savage DD et al: Mitral valve prolapse in the general population. 1. Epidemiologic features: The Framingham Study. 2. Clinical features: The Framingham Study. 3. Dysrhythmias: The Framingham Study. Am Heart J 1983;106:571, 577, 582.

Wilcken DEL, Hickey AJ: Lifetime risk for patients with mitral valve prolapse of developing severe valve regurgitation requiring surgery. Circulation 1988;78:10.

Wolf PA, Sila CA: Cerebral ischemia with mitral valve prolapse. Am Heart J 1987;113:1308.

Wooley CF et al: The floppy, myxomatous mitral valve, mitral valve prolapse, and mitral regurgitation. Prog Cardiovasc Dis 1991;33:397.

Mitral Incompetence

Abbasi AD et al: Detection and estimation of the degree of mitral regurgitation by range-gated pulsed Doppler echocardiography. Circulation 1980;61:143.

Carabello BA: Preservation of left ventricular function in patients with mitral regurgitation: A realistic goal for the nineties. J Am Coll Cardiol 1990;15:564.

Carabello BA: What exactly is 2+ to 3+ mitral regurgitation? J Am Coll Cardiol 1992;19:339.

Castello R et al: Quantitation of mitral regurgitation by transesophageal echocardiography with Doppler color flow mapping: Correlation with cardiac catheterization. J Am Coll Cardiol 1992;19:1516.

Cohn LH: Surgery for mitral regurgitation. JAMA 1988;260:2883.

Crawford MH et al: Determinants of survival and left ventricular performance after mitral valve replacement. Circulation 1990;81:1173.

Deloche A et al: Valve repair with Carpentier techniques. J Thorac Cardiovasc Surg 1990;99:990.

DePace NL, Nestico PF, Morganroth J: Acute severe mitral regurgitation: Pathophysiology, clinical recognition, and management. Am J Med 1985;78:293.

Freeman WK et al: Intraoperative evaluation of mitral valve regurgitation and repair by transesophageal echocardiography: Incidence and significance of systolic anterior motion. J Am Coll Cardiol 1992;20:599.

Galloway AC et al: Long-term results of mitral valve reconstruction with Carpentier techniques in 148 patients with mitral insufficiency. Circulation 1988;78(Suppl I): I–97.

Hickey AJ et al: Primary (spontaneous) chordal rupture: Relation to myxomatous valve disease and mitral valve prolapse. J Am Coll Cardiol 1985;5:1341.

Lessana A et al: Mitral valve repair: Results and the decision making process in reconstruction. Report of 275 cases. J Thorac Cardiovasc Surg 1990;99:622.

Mehta J et al: Acute haemodynamic effect of oral prazosin in severe mitral regurgitation. Br Heart J 1980;43:556.

Nestico PF et al: Mitral annular calcification: Clinical, pathophysiology, and echocardiographic review. Am Heart J 1984;107:989.

Noren GR et al: Anomalous origin of the left coronary artery from the pulmonary trunk with special reference to the occurrence of mitral insufficiency. Circulation 1964;30:171.

Oh JK: Echocardiographic evaluation of morphological and hemodynamic significance of giant left atrium: An important lesson. Circulation 1992;86:328.

Oliveira DBG et al: Chordal rupture. 2. Comparison between repair and replacement. Br Heart J 1983;50:318.

Rankin JS et al: A clinical comparison of mitral valve repair versus valve replacement in ischemic mitral regurgitation. J Thorac Cardiovasc Surg 1988;95:165.

Sarris GE et al: Restoration of left ventricular systolic performance after restoration of the mitral chordae tendineae: The importance of valvular-ventricular interaction. J Thorac Cardiovasc Surg 1988;95:969.

Sharma SK et al: Clinical, angiographic, and anatomic findings in acute severe ischemic mitral regurgitation. Am J Cardiol 1992;70:277.

Tribouilloy C et al: Assessment of severity of mitral regurgitation by measuring regurgitant jet width at it's origin with transesophageal Doppler color flow imaging. Circulation 1992;85:1248.

Wigle ED, Auger P: Sudden, severe mitral insufficiency. Can Med Assoc J 1967;96:1493.

13

Aortic Valve Disease; Multiple Valve Disease

Classification

Aortic valve disease has been classified in this text into three main categories: (1) hemodynamically insignificant aortic valve disease, (2) hemodynamically significant predominant aortic stenosis, and (3) hemodynamically significant predominant aortic incompetence.

An indirectly recorded brachial arterial diastolic blood pressure of 70 mm Hg or more is used as an arbitrary measurement below which hemodynamically significant chronic aortic incompetence is said to be present. This cutoff point is not entirely satisfactory, but it is the best single figure on which to base a classification.

Interaction of Stenosis & Incompetence

Aortic stenosis and aortic incompetence load the left ventricle in different ways. In the purest forms of stenosis, the extra left ventricular work is performed almost entirely against increased pressure, with no increase in flow. In pure incompetence there is an almost pure flow load with an increase in stroke volume, because the ventricle must eject both its normal stroke volume and the blood that returns as backflow through the valve during diastole. In chronic aortic incompetence, there is some increase in afterload because of the increased systolic pressure generated in ejecting the large stroke volume. Falling between these two extremes is a spectrum of lesions in which the ventricular load consists partly of increased pressure and partly of increased flow. Severe stenosis and severe incompetence cannot coexist. In mixed lesions, if incompetence is greater than stenosis, the stroke volume is larger and the pressure difference between the left ventricle and the aorta is exaggerated because of the large flow. If stenosis is more severe than incompetence, the narrower orifice permits less backflow during diastole, but the pressure difference during systole is large because the stenosis is relatively severe.

Left ventricular pressure is inevitably higher in patients with stenotic or predominantly stenotic lesions. Since the left ventricle tolerates pressure loads less easily than volume loads, stenotic lesions are more important than incompetent ones. Therefore, all cases with significant stenosis are included in one group (predominant aortic stenosis), and predominantly incompetent lesions form another.

Subvalvular & Supravalvular Aortic Stenosis

Among patients with predominant aortic stenosis is a small group (1% of cases) who do not have disease affecting the valves but rather congenital supravalvular or subvalvular lesions. Supravalvular aortic stenosis usually results from congenital hypoplasia of the ascending aorta, varying from a localized constriction to a long narrowed segment, whereas subvalvular stenosis is due to the presence of a fibrous ring or shelf of tissue immediately below the valve. Supravalvular stenosis occurs in a familial form in physically underdeveloped children with characteristic elfin facies and prominent ears. It also occurs in persons who appear normal, especially those with hypercalcemia in infancy. Surgical relief of the aortic obstruction is often difficult because of the diffuse hypoplasia of the aorta.

Subvalvular stenosis is also congenital and is due to ring lesions that are more amenable to surgical relief, in contrast to those of supravalvular stenosis. The clinical picture resembles that of predominant aortic stenosis, and the valve often leaks, perhaps because the subvalvular ring interferes with normal valve closure or because the valve is injured by the jet from the subvalvular obstruction. The condition is diagnosed by echocardiography or angiography. The obstructing ring is often so close to the aortic valve that withdrawal pressure tracings may fail to detect the lesion. In hypertrophic obstructive cardiomyopathy, the obstruction lies lower in the ventricle, and the clinical picture is different (see Chapter 17). A third type of subvalvular stenosis is the fibromuscular tunnel, a congenital obstruction below the valve caused by a fibromuscular thickening beneath the aortic valve, involving the interventricular septum and the anterior leaflet of the mitral valve. This tunnel is of variable length, and it is extremely difficult to relieve the obstruction surgically.

Acute & Chronic Aortic Incompetence

Aortic incompetence, like mitral incompetence, occurs in both acute and chronic forms. Acute lesions are almost always due to the effects of infective endocarditis but may occur when acute aortic dissection involves the aortic root or the aorta is torn as a result of trauma. The acute load on the left ventricle causes a clinical picture that is different from that seen in chronic lesions.

Causes of Aortic Valve Lesions

It is difficult to determine both the cause and severity of aortic valve lesions. There is often a discrepancy between the patient's symptoms and the hemodynamic severity of the lesions, and the cause often remains in doubt, even after autopsy. Both aortic stenosis and aortic incompetence may run long clinical courses lasting 20–30 years, and the physician is often confronted with patients who have hemodynamically significant lesions and yet no symptoms. Just as frequently, the patient has symptoms that are out of proportion to the hemodynamic findings. Because aortic valve lesions can run such a long clinical course, factors responsible for the progressive deterioration of the patient's clinical state are not always clear. Long-term changes may be due to valvular calcification or myocardial fibrosis.

As in mitral valve disease, rheumatic fever is an important cause of aortic valvular lesions. A history of previous rheumatic fever is present in 10% of patients with predominant stenosis and in 15% of those with predominant incompetence. Since congenital aortic valve lesions are relatively common, some patients who have been diagnosed as having had rheumatic fever in childhood actually have congenital aortic valve lesions. Among patients with a past history of rheumatic fever, 75% of those with predominant aortic stenosis are women, whereas 75% of those with pure incompetence are men. This agrees with the finding in mitral valve disease that stenosis occurs more commonly in females and incompetence in males. Aortic valve disease is more prevalent in males by a factor of 3:1 in predominant stenosis and 3:2 in predominant incompetence. These proportions vary in different series for the reason that causes vary in different geographic areas.

HEMODYNAMICALLY INSIGNIFICANT LESIONS

The cardinal features of hemodynamically insignificant aortic lesions (Figure 13–1) include normal heart size and hemodynamics and a systolic ejection murmur. The variable features are a systolic ejection click and a short aortic diastolic murmur. Auscultatory physical signs arising from the aortic valve are usually the sole abnormality. These lesions constitute 10% of cases seen in university hospital practice but make up a much larger percentage in private practice. These cases probably represent a presymptomatic phase of aortic valve disease, and some of these individuals, if followed long enough, would be seen to develop into either aortic stenosis or aortic incompe-

tence. The most important complication in such cases is infective endocarditis, with associated development or exacerbation of aortic incompetence. These lesions are seen in patients of all ages. Congenital (bicuspid valve), rheumatic, and atherosclerotic causes account for two-thirds of cases; no causative factor is identified in the others.

Clinical Features

More than half of cases are entirely asymptomatic. In the others, palpitations, fatigue, dizziness, and noncardiac dyspnea occur but without evidence of heart failure. Symptoms are more common in patients who are aware that they have a heart murmur and are unrelated to the aortic incompetence. The pulse and blood pressure are normal; a collapsing pulse or a slow-rising pulse is by definition, absent. The heart is not enlarged on clinical or x-ray examination, and no evidence of ventricular hypertrophy is detectable. (If any of these signs are present, the lesion is no longer hemodynamically insignificant.) There is always a systolic murmur at the base of the heart, preceded by an ejection click in one-third of cases and followed by a faint aortic diastolic murmur in one-third. Slight aortic dilation is occasionally seen, but valvular calcification is not necessarily present.

Cardiac catheterization is not indicated for diagnosis, but if it is performed, intracardiac pressures are normal, and there is no significant systolic pressure difference between the left ventricle and the aorta.

The role of the deposition of calcium in these slightly abnormal valves is difficult to determine, but it seems likely that valvular calcification immobilizes and narrows the valve, causing stenosis that gradually progresses but does not significantly load the left ventricle until the valve is narrowed to about one-fourth its normal area.

The other important development in such cases is infective endocarditis. Patients with hemodynamically insignificant aortic lesions are particularly prone to this complication, and the valve is likely to become acutely and severely incompetent as a result. Thus, the prevention and early recognition of endocarditis are important aspects of the management of patients with this lesion. Antibiotic prophylactic therapy preceding major dental work or minor surgery and early blood culture during febrile illnesses are mandatory. Intravenous drug abuse is particularly likely to result in infective endocarditis because contaminated needles and syringes are often used. When a rheumatic origin for the lesion is suspected, prophylactic penicillin treatment is warranted to prevent recurrences of rheumatic fever.

PREDOMINANT AORTIC STENOSIS

The cardinal features of predominant aortic stenosis (Figure 13–2) are left ventricular hypertrophy and

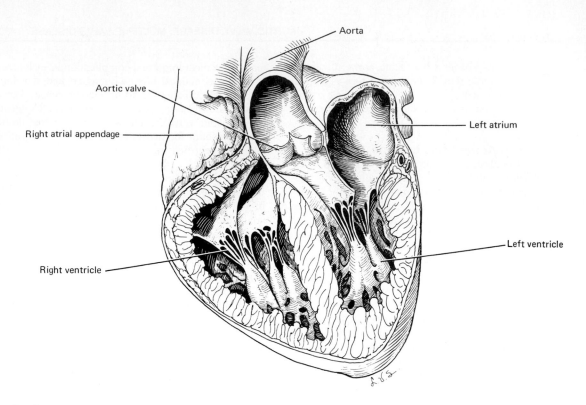

Drawing of left heart in left anterior oblique view showing anatomic features of hemodynamically insignificant aortic valve disease.

Cardinal features: *Normal heart size and hemodynamics; systolic ejection murmur.*

Variable factors: *Systolic ejection click; short aortic diastolic murmur.*

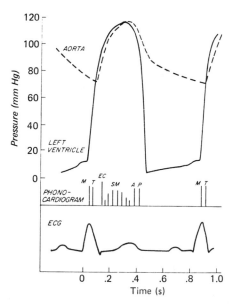

Diagram showing auscultatory and hemodynamic features of hemodynamically insignificant aortic valve disease. Note the absence of a gradient across the aortic valve. M, mitral; T, tricuspid; A, aortic; P, pulmonary valve; EC, ejection click; SM, systolic murmur.

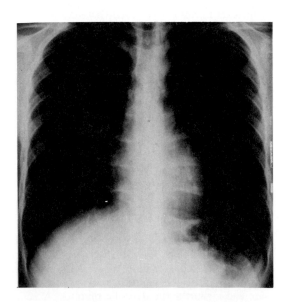

Chest x-ray showing normal heart size and shape.

Figure 13–1. Hemodynamically insignificant aortic valve disease. Structures enlarged: none.

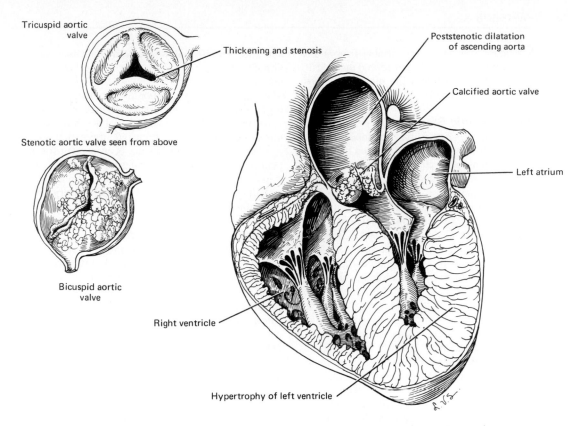

Tricuspid aortic valve

Thickening and stenosis

Stenotic aortic valve seen from above

Bicuspid aortic valve

Right ventricle

Poststenotic dilatation of ascending aorta

Calcified aortic valve

Left atrium

Hypertrophy of left ventricle

Drawing of left heart in left anterior oblique view showing anatomic features of aortic stenosis.

Cardinal features: *Left ventricular hypertrophy; systolic ejection murmur.*

Variable factors: *Severity; site of obstruction; cause; valvular calcification.*

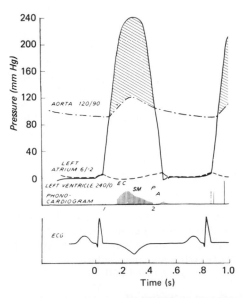

Diagram showing auscultatory and hemodynamic features of predominant aortic stenosis. EC, ejection click; SM, systolic murmur; P, pulmonary valve; A, aortic valve.

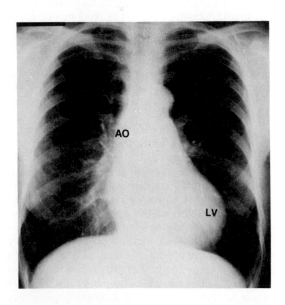

Chest x-ray of a patient with aortic stenosis showing left ventricular (LV) and aortic (AO) enlargement.

Figure 13–2. Aortic stenosis. Structures enlarged: left ventricle (thickened); poststenotic dilation of the aorta.

a systolic ejection murmur. The variable factors are the severity, which affects the hypertrophy; the side of the obstruction; the cause; and the presence or absence of valvular calcification.

Importance of Aortic Stenosis

Predominant aortic stenosis has an importance in clinical cardiology that is out of proportion to its frequency. Aortic stenosis is easily missed on clinical examination, especially if the patient is in severe left ventricular failure and the cardiac output is so low that the aortic systolic murmur is virtually inaudible. Aortic stenosis is often suspected in patients in whom there is no significant obstruction to aortic flow. In these cases, it is the presence of an aortic systolic murmur, often associated with calcification of the aortic valve on fluoroscopy, that indicates possible aortic stenosis.

Etiology

The three causes of aortic stenosis are rheumatic heart disease, congenital heart disease, and "calcific" or degenerative heart disease. The incidence of rheumatic heart disease causing aortic stenosis is decreasing in the USA. In most cases (70%), there is no clinical clue to the cause. At autopsy the valve is usually so disorganized by calcification that it is difficult to count the number of cusps. Now that aortic valve replacement has become routine, the valve is available for study at an earlier stage of the disease, and it is easier to see if there are two or three cusps. Even so, separate cusps cannot be identified in 15% of patients. Among patients with predominant aortic stenosis who undergo surgery or die of the disease, half have been found to have a bicuspid aortic valve, which indicates that the basic lesion is often congenital. Patients with bicuspid valves often have other congenital lesions, most commonly coarctation of the aorta. They are also more susceptible to the development of dissection of the aorta. Some are known to have had a murmur since early infancy, but the majority (two-thirds) have had a murmur first heard only after age 20. This latter group generally does not have congenital aortic stenosis but rather a minor congenital valvular lesion that presents as hemodynamically insignificant aortic valve disease. The congenital abnormality apparently makes the valve more than normally susceptible to wear and tear.

Severe congenital valvular aortic stenosis is rarely seen in adults and constitutes about 5% of cases. In such cases, a murmur has almost always been heard in infancy, and symptoms usually have developed in early adult life. Patients with a bicuspid valve may develop severe aortic stenosis by progressive calcification of the valve. In most cases of severe calcific aortic stenosis developing by age 60 either a bicuspid aortic valve or rheumatic heart disease is the cause. Patients with predominant aortic stenosis tend to develop valvular calcification with increasing age, and after age 40, valvular calcification is present in virtually all cases, irrespective of the cause of the lesion.

In an increasing number of patients, atherosclerotic, age-related degenerative changes in a normal valve appear to be the sole cause of aortic stenosis. In this group, the valve is tricuspid, the patient is over age 65, and a murmur has not been present for more than 5 years. There is some suggestion that aortic stenosis may develop rapidly in such patients and run a shorter course. Associated coronary artery disease is common in this group.

Progression of Aortic Stenosis

The role played by the deposition of calcium in the consequent progression of the disease seems unpredictable. Physicians must learn to recognize the signs of increasing severity of stenosis: decreasing peripheral pulse pressure, slowing and shuddering of carotid upstroke, and increasing left ventricular hypertrophy on the ECG and echocardiogram. The development of echo-Doppler techniques that reliably measure the systolic gradient across the aortic valve and, by the continuity equation, can estimate aortic valve area has been enormously important in detecting the progression of aortic stenosis. Aortic valve replacement is so much more successful in patients who have not yet developed left ventricular failure that early diagnosis and recognition of increasing severity are of the utmost importance. A special problem is the increased incidence of acquired aortic stenosis resulting from atherosclerosis in elderly persons. The disease can be extremely insidious and difficult to diagnose because there is often heart failure and a decreased stroke volume and a deep anteroposterior diameter of the chest, both of which decrease the loudness of the murmur.

That aortic stenosis runs a long presymptomatic course is evident from the finding that significant stenosis—as judged by the presence of a systolic murmur and left ventricular hypertrophy on the ECG—may be present for many years without causing any symptoms. Studies have shown that the gradient can increase at a linearized rate of 1–4 mm Hg per month. Other patients can go 10 years with no change in gradient. Even with no symptoms, progressive subendocardial fibrosis occurs when the aortic stenosis is severe, and this may be the cause of fatal ventricular arrhythmias even after valve replacement. The course of the disease after symptoms develop is rapid. Progressive left ventricular failure leads to death in 2–8 years if surgery is not performed.

Pathophysiology of Aortic Stenosis

As the aortic valve area decreases from 3 cm^2 to under 2 cm^2, sufficient obstruction to flow occurs to create a systolic gradient across the valve. The systolic murmur generated has roughly the same shape as the gradient and is powered by the stroke volume, resulting in a loud, long ejection murmur beginning as the aortic valve opens and ending as it closes. To keep the stroke volume normal, the systolic pressure developed by the left ventricle is increased, thus increasing afterload on the left ventricle. Concentric left ventricular hypertrophy occurs, thus normalizing left ventricular wall stress. With severe obstruction, the systolic ejection period is prolonged, thus decreasing the diastolic filling period, which is important in myocardial perfusion.

When the stenosis is severe, the aortic systolic pressure cannot rise as rapidly as the left ventricular pressure, thus prolonging the time to achievement of peak aortic systolic pressure. The rate of rise of the aortic systolic pressure also depends on the compliance of the aorta. Therefore, in the elderly patient with a stiff aorta, the aortic pressure rises faster for any given stroke volume and can hide the effect of severe aortic stenosis on the aortic pulse wave. When the stroke volume decreases, this leads to the classic **pulsus parvus et tardus,** the small, delayed pulse of severe aortic stenosis.

With the development of left ventricular hypertrophy, the diastolic compliance of the left ventricle is decreased, especially at end-diastole. With atrial contraction, the *a* wave can be markedly increased, causing a fourth heart sound. With left ventricular failure, the ventricle dilates and becomes stiffer, and a third heart sound is generated.

To understand the way in which severe aortic stenosis causes the three main symptoms of aortic stenosis—left ventricular failure, exertional syncope, and angina pectoris and myocardial infarction—as well as its major danger, ventricular arrhythmia and sudden death, the determinants of myocardial oxygen supply and demand must be reviewed (Table 13–1).

With aortic stenosis, there is a marked increase in myocardial oxygen demand because of increased left ventricular systolic pressure and mass. Simultaneously, because of a small decrease in aortic diastolic pressure and an increase in left ventricular filling pressure at the time of atrial systole—as well as a marked increase in coronary vascular resistance—there is a marked decrease in coronary blood flow, especially in the subendocardial region. Furthermore, because most of these patients are above the age of 50 and male, there is a significant incidence of coronary heart disease. These factors all lead to the development of intramural ischemia, angina pectoris, myocardial fibrosis, and even myocardial infarction. Ventricular arrhythmias and sudden death may also be the result of ischemia.

Exertional syncope is more complicated. The classic explanation is that there is a limitation on the ability to increase cardiac output, and, with exercise, the decreased peripheral vascular resistance in muscle and skin results in a decrease in aortic pressure and syncope. Another demonstrated reason for syncope is the development of transient, hemodynamically significant ventricular arrhythmias, both ventricular tachycardia and even bursts of ventricular fibrillation. A third explanation is the effect of the Von Bezold receptors in the left ventricle that modulate sympathetic and vagal tone, similar to these/those afferent nerves from the carotid sinus. With severe aortic stenosis, there is dissociation between the signal arising from the dropping aortic pressure and the rising left ventricular pressure. If the left ventricular signal predominates, there is inappropriate withdrawal of sympathetic tone and an increase in vagal tone, thus slowing the heart rate and vasodilating the periphery.

Finally, of unknown frequency in the causation of sudden death and even syncope is the effect of increasing ischemia on ventricular function. With ischemia, there is diastolic dysfunction, resulting in a stiffer ventricle that would interfere with ventricular filling, as well as systolic dysfunction that would decrease the force of contraction. Both of these would decrease the stroke volume, leading to a drop in aortic pressure, increasing ischemia, and setting in motion a vicious cycle leading to electromechanical dissociation.

Table 13–1. Effects of aortic valve disease on determinants of myocardial oxygen supply and demand.

Aortic Regurgitation	Aortic Stenosis	Supply	Demand	Aortic Stenosis	Aortic Regurgitation
↑↑↑	↓	Aortic diastolic pressure	Left ventricular systolic pressure	↑↑↑↑	↑↑
↓	↓	Diastolic filling period	Left ventricular diastolic volume	· · ·	↑↑↑↑
↓	↓↓↓	Coronary vascular resistance	Heart rate	· · ·	· · ·
↓↓↓↓	↓	Left ventricular diastolic pressure	Myocardial contractility	· · ·	· · ·
· · ·	· · ·	Coronary sinus and right atrial pressure	Left ventricular mass	↑↑↑↑	↑↑↑↑
			Systolic ejection period (minor)	↑↑	↑

Key:
↑ to ↑↑↑↑ = Magnitude of effect on *increasing* myocardial oxygen demand.
↓ to ↓↓↓↓ = Magnitude of effect on *decreasing* myocardial oxygen supply.

Clinical Findings

In all forms of aortic stenosis a fixed, disorganized, calcified, thickened, radiopaque mass of tissue replaces the normal flexible, thin, filmy valve structure. In congenital aortic stenosis the valve is often dome-shaped, and no cusps can be distinguished. Calcification is most closely related to age and occurs at the earliest in the late teens and 20s. The development of calcification is commonly associated with the development of an aortic systolic ejection murmur.

Aortic stenosis increases the work of the left ventricle. In cases of pure stenosis, hypertrophy first occurs at the expense of the left ventricular cavity, causing a decrease in ventricular compliance. The ventricle becomes more rounded, but overall heart size is not increased. If there is associated aortic incompetence, the left ventricle is larger, and in most cases heart size is increased by the time symptoms appear. The narrowing of the aortic valve produces turbulence, and the increased energy in the blood causes poststenotic dilation of the aorta. The calcification of the aortic valve may spread to the valve ring and thence to the anterior (aortic) cusp of the mitral valve and the mebranous part of the interventricular septum, where it may cause atrioventricular conduction defects. The coronary vessels are usually large and not atherosclerotic in younger patients with bicuspid valves, but calcific emboli may occur and cause coronary occlusion or other serious systemic embolism. Aortic stenosis developing de novo in elderly persons is more likely to be associated with coronary artery disease.

Blood is subject to extremely severe mechanical stress as it passes through the turbulent areas associated with a stenotic aortic valve. Damage to red cells in the form of excessive hemolysis may occur in patients with aortic stenosis, especially if the cells are abnormally fragile. This rare form of hemolytic anemia is also seen after aortic valve replacement.

A. Symptoms:

1. Late appearance of symptoms– Symptoms appear late in the course of aortic stenosis, and many patients with hemodynamically significant lesions have no complaints. The disease is not recognized in its earlier stages, usually because the patient does not seek medical advice. In some cases, the murmur has been present without any symptoms for so many years that the physician overlooks the possibility of aortic stenosis until it becomes severe.

The stage at which symptoms develop depends to some extent on the patient's activity level. In sedentary people the disease may be far advanced before the patient complains of symptoms. Half of patients with surgically significant aortic stenosis have had at least one episode of left ventricular failure before they undergo surgery for stenosis. In active persons, dyspnea on exertion occurs before overt left ventricular failure develops, but especially in sedentary people, an episode of paroxysmal nocturnal dyspnea may be the first symptom of disease.

The symptoms in the later stages of aortic stenosis are some of the most difficult to manage in the entire spectrum of cardiac disease. Nightly attacks of paroxysmal dyspnea, with sweating, collapse, extreme restlessness, and intractable shortness of breath, cause severe distress. Morphine and potent diuretics are the drugs of choice in the medical management of such patients, but relief of the aortic stenosis by surgery is the only treatment.

2. Dyspnea– Dyspnea on exertion is a common presenting symptom in predominant aortic stenosis. As in other forms of left ventricular overload, shortness of breath is quantitatively related to exertion and is often accompanied by a heavy, tight feeling in the chest that is discomfort rather than pain. This sensation may occasionally radiate to the arms and is characteristic of angina pectoris. Dyspnea on effort ordinarily precedes the episodes of paroxysmal nocturnal dyspnea that herald the onset of left ventricular failure.

3. Angina pectoris and myocardial infarction– Typical angina pectoris is seen as a presenting complaint in patients with significant aortic stenosis. On occasion in prolonged ischemia, discomfort results in a non-Q wave myocardial infarction. This subendocardial ischemia is due to the basis of increased demand for myocardial oxygen supply and the decreased supply of subendocardial myocardial blood flow seen in aortic stenosis. About 40% of patients with aortic stenosis and angina pectoris have coexistent coronary artery disease. In these patients, Q wave myocardial infarction can occur.

4. Syncope and presyncope– Syncope or presyncope on unaccustomed effort is the other principal symptom. It occurs in about 5% of cases, usually before the left ventricle has failed. In many patients it only occurs once, because the patient associates the syncope with overexertion and subsequently avoids lifting heavy objects, shoveling snow, running upstairs, or performing whatever activity precipitated the first attack. Loss of consciousness is usually preceded by dyspnea, which the patient disregards, perhaps because of the circumstances surrounding the overexertion. Recovery from the syncopal attack is rapid, and sudden death, which is common in aortic stenosis, seldom occurs on exertion. It is of great importance to obtain a clear history of the circumstances surrounding a syncopal episode in a patient suspected of having aortic stenosis. If syncope is provoked only by severe effort, stenosis is already severe. Syncope unrelated to excessive effort is more common than effort syncope in aortic stenosis (10%) but is not necessarily an indication that severe stenosis is present. Such syncope is often due to arrhythmia rather than an inadequate increase in cardiac output during stress. It is often confused with transient cerebral ischemic attacks due to atherosclerosis of the cerebral vessels in patients who have aortic systolic murmurs but no aortic stenosis.

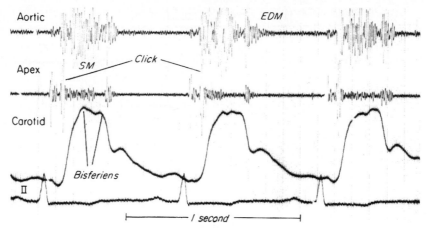

Figure 13–3. Phonocardiogram of a 36-year-old man with aortic stenosis and insufficiency. Note systolic ejection click, crescendo-decrescendo systolic murmur (SM), and short early aortic diastolic murmur (EDM). First sound faint at aortic area. Clinically, thought to be triple rhythm with presystolic gallop. The carotid pulse shows two peaks (bisferiens) whose relative heights vary.

B. Signs:

1. Pulse– The arterial pulse in patients with predominant aortic stenosis is of small amplitude if the stroke volume is decreased. The pulse is slow-rising because left ventricular ejection time through the narrowed aortic valve is prolonged. Such an arterial pulse is termed an anacrotic pulse, plateau pulse, or pulsus tardus, because the wave takes longer than normal to pass beneath the examiner's fingers. The examiner should feel the radial, brachial, femoral, and carotid pulses. The carotid pulse, being closest to the aortic valve, gives the most accurate information. The rise time is slowed and the time taken to reach peak pressure is increased in the central pulse in aortic stenosis. This sign is less reliable in older patients, in whom compliance of the arterial bed is reduced. In patients with mixed lesions in whom there is also aortic incompetence, the upstroke of the pulse is more rapid, and a double-peaked pulse (pulsus bisferiens) may be found (Figure 13–3). Pulsus bisferiens is more likely to be present in a more peripheral artery (eg, radial or brachial) and is not usually seen in the central aortic pulse. The presence of pulsus bisferiens is not of diagnostic significance.

2. Blood pressure– Blood pressure is ordinarily low, with a narrow pulse pressure, and reflects the small stroke volume in severe aortic stenosis. However, it may be normal, especially in patients with mixed lesions. Systemic hypertension, although uncommon, does not rule out surgically significant aortic stenosis. An *a* wave may be seen in the jugular venous pulse if the ventricular septum bulges to the right and impairs right ventricular filling, or if severe pulmonary hypertension develops.

3. Atrial fibrillation– The heart rate is usually regular, but about 10% of patients are in atrial fibrillation at the time of surgery. The incidence of atrial fibrillation in cases with a past history of rheumatic fever is no greater than in those with congenitally bicuspid aortic valves, but atrial fibrillation should always alert the physician to the possibility of coexisting associated mitral valve disease.

4. Left ventricular hypertrophy– The degree of left ventricular hypertrophy on physical examination—as shown by the prominence of the left ventricular heave—depends on the severity and purity of the stenosis. If the chest wall is thin, a left ventricular heave is readily seen and felt, but in many patients it is necessary to rely on the ECG or echocardiogram for evidence of left ventricular hypertrophy. The degree of left ventricular enlargement on physical examination depends largely on the degree of aortic incompetence accompanying the aortic stenosis. The examining hand readily perceives the dynamic quality of the ventricular impulse, which primarily reflects left ventricular stroke volume. The degree of left ventricular enlargement is better detected on the chest x-ray than on physical examination, especially when left ventricular failure has reduced the stroke volume.

Some degree of aortic incompetence is usually present. The greater the incompetence, the larger the heart. Predominant aortic stenosis varies from cases with no incompetence to those with an aortic leak sufficient to give a normal or slightly widened pulse pressure and a slightly hyperdynamic left ventricular impulse.

5. Heart sounds– Depending on the anatomy of the valve and the degree of calcification, an aortic valve closure sound may or may not be present. If A_2 is audible, paradoxic (reversed) splitting of the second heart sound may be heard if severe stenosis or left bundle branch block is present (Figure 13–4). Third and fourth heart sounds are commonly heard. The characteristic murmur of aortic stenosis is harsh,

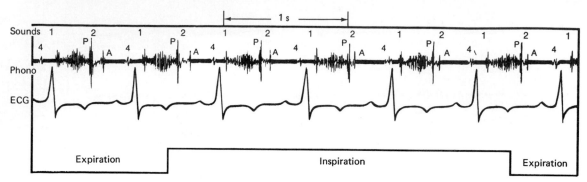

Figure 13–4. Phonocardiogram and ECG in aortic stenosis. The phonocardiogram shows ejection murmur, presystolic gallop (4), soft late A_2, and paradoxic splitting of the second heart sound (2). (Courtesy of Roche Laboratories Division of Hoffman-La Roche, Inc.)

similar to the sound made when "clearing the throat," and its timing is ejection in nature, starting after isovolumetric contraction has occurred, ie, 0.06 s or more after the first heart sound (Figure 13–2). It is usually associated with a systolic thrill at the base. It is preceded by an ejection click (Figure 13–3) when the aortic valve is more flexible and ventricular ejection more rapid. The murmur may be heard at the base or the apex of the heart. It is often heard well in the neck, but this does not mean it is aortic in origin, since pulmonary systolic murmurs and bruits of carotid artery stenosis are also well heard there. The murmur starts after the first heart sound and stops before the second heart sound. It is louder after a long pause following an ectopic beat, and it varies with cardiac filling in atrial fibrillation. This finding differentiates the ejection murmur of aortic stenosis from the regurgitant murmur of mitral incompetence. It may be audible only at the apex of the heart and can be easily missed if the patient is in severe left ventricular failure. A faint aortic diastolic murmur along the left sternal edge is usually present, but its loudness does not necessarily correspond to the severity of associated aortic incompetence, which is judged instead by the character of the pulse, the size of the heart, and the dynamic qualities of the left ventricular impulse.

Rales at the bases of the lungs are heard in patients with left ventricular failure, and signs of right ventricular failure with raised jugular venous pressure, hepatomegaly, and peripheral edema are extremely late manifestations of the disease. They are generally due to the development of a raised pulmonary vascular resistance (> 3.5 mm Hg/L/min), which occurs in about 10% of cases and is seen only in the preterminal stage of the disease.

C. Electrocardiographic Findings: Electrocardiographic evidence of left ventricular hypertrophy is characteristically severe in predominant aortic stenosis. In about 10% of cases, left or right bundle branch block or even complete block is found. Left bundle branch block interferes with the electrocardiographic recognition of left ventricular hypertrophy, but right bundle branch block does not. Significant aortic stenosis may be present in patients in whom the ECG shows little or no evidence of left ventricular hypertrophy (Figure 13–5). Moderately severe or gross evidence of left ventricular hypertrophy on the ECG is seen in about 75% of cases. Changes due to associated myocardial ischemia or myocardial infarction may be present, making electrocardiographic interpretation difficult. Patients with severe aortic stenosis who have ventricular failure and a low cardiac output have either a soft murmur or none at all. Such patients almost invariably have electrocardiographic left ventricular hypertrophy, however. When a patient—especially an elderly one—is seen with left ventricular failure and left ventricular hypertrophy, aortic stenosis must be ruled out even if no murmur is audible.

D. Imaging Studies: The chest x-ray shows a rounded shadow forming the left border of the heart; this represents the hypertrophied left ventricle. The overall heart shadow is enlarged in patients with left ventricular failure and in those with significant aortic incompetence, but not necessarily in those with early stenotic lesions in whom the left ventricle hypertrophies at the expense on the left ventricular cavity. The progression of the lesion over 10 years is shown in Figure 13–6. Poststenotic dilation confined to the origin of the ascending aorta is the rule. It is best seen on the left anterior oblique view. Calcification of the aortic valve, although often visible on the x-ray, should be sought at fluoroscopy. The characteristic dense shadow of the calcified aortic valve lies surprisingly low in the cardiac silhouette, moves up and down with the heartbeat, and lies more medially and less posteriorly than a calcified mitral valve. The presence of calcium in the aortic valve can readily be detected during cardiac catheterization when the catheter comes up against the aortic valve. Signs of pulmonary congestion and slight left atrial enlargement

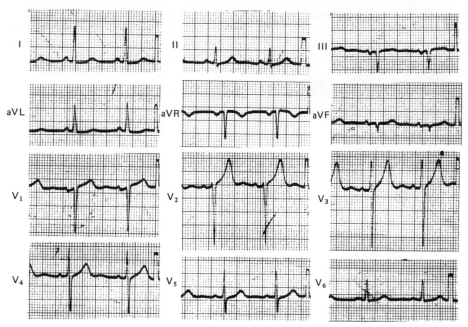

Figure 13–5. ECG of a 77-year-old woman with severe aortic stenosis. Left ventricular pressure 260/5 mm Hg; aortic pressure 130/67 mm Hg. There is little evidence on the ECG of left ventricular hypertrophy.

are common, but prominence of the pulmonary artery is only seen in a few patients presenting late in the course of the disease.

1. Noninvasive techniques– Doppler echocardiography is most helpful in diagnosing the presence and estimating the severity of aortic stenosis. Doppler blood velocity measurements provide a relatively ac-

curate means of establishing severity. The peak velocity in the jet of blood passing through a stenotic valve depends on the severity of the obstruction. An indication of the pressure difference can be obtained by applying a simplified form of the Bernoulli equation (see Chapter 4). The values for the pressure gradient across the aortic valve calculated from continuous

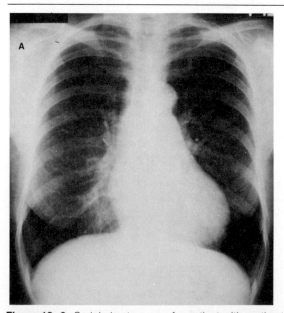
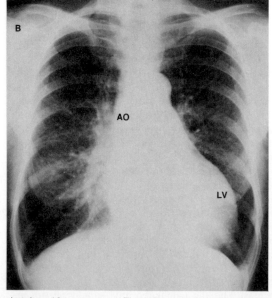

Figure 13–6. Serial chest x-rays of a patient with aortic stenosis taken 10 years apart. The left ventricle (LV) and aorta (AO) are prominent in both x-rays. The heart is larger and the right hilar vessels more prominent in the film shown at right, which was taken after the development of symptoms. Pressure tracings from this patient are shown in Figure 13–9.

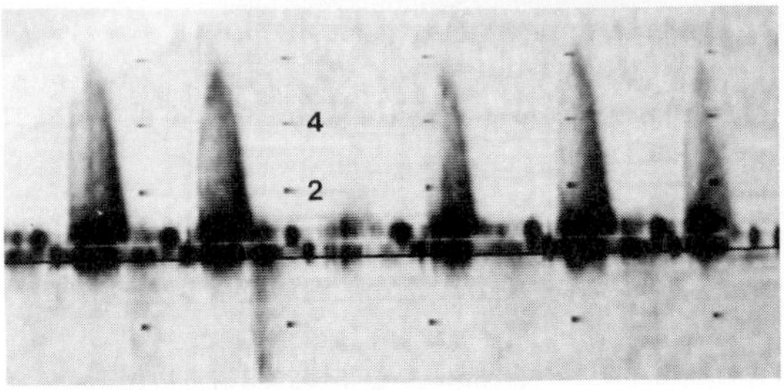

Figure 13–7. Continuous wave Doppler signal in aortic stenosis. The peak velocity recorded by continuous wave Doppler is 5.5 cm•s⁻¹. By the Bernoulli principle, this represents a peak pressure difference of 120 mm Hg. (Courtesy of NB Schiller.)

wave Doppler measurements have been shown to correlate well with measurements made at cardiac catheterization. A Doppler tracing from a patient with severe aortic stenosis is shown in Figure 13–7.

Color Doppler is helpful in demonstrating an eccentric jet that is difficult to access through the available echo "windows." In older patients, the anteroposterior diameter of the chest wall increases, and with aortic arteriosclerosis the root and ascending aorta assume a more horizontal orientation. The jet of aortic stenosis can be oriented in a direction where it cannot be accessed at an angle that will provide an accurate assessment of maximal jet velocity. Color Doppler helps to identify the location of the jet and thus provides the best estimate of maximum gradient.

The gradient of most significance is the mean gradient. This measurement correlates very well with the mean gradient obtained at catheterization. By the continuity equation, an estimate of aortic valve area can be obtained that also correlates well with that obtained by catheterization.

2. Invasive techniques–

a. Right and left heart catheterization– Catheterization can provide an accurate measurement of the systolic gradient as well as the systolic blood flow across the aortic valve. However, with the development of echo-Doppler techniques to obtain similar information, it is no longer essential in many cases to catheterize the patient to evaluate the severity of aortic stenosis. This is especially true when the gradient is either small or large in patients not in heart failure, since even large variations in cardiac output would not change the grade of severity. However, in patients with heart failure or for other reasons when the cardiac output may be decreased, the gradient may be low in spite of severe aortic stenosis. If the low gradient is caused by the low cardiac output, dobutamine infusion can raise the cardiac output. If the patient has severe aortic stenosis, the systolic gradient should increase and the calculated area should remain unchanged. If the low cardiac output is due to poor left ventricular function, the cardiac output will rise but

the gradient will not change, since the valve will open farther and the calculated valve area will increase. Whenever there is a discrepancy between the clinical findings and the noninvasive findings, the patient should have the advantage of cardiac catheterization before a decision for or against surgery is made.

Right heart catheterization may show a large right atrial *a* wave, raised pulmonary arterial pressure, and even moderately raised pulmonary vascular resistance in patients with severe lesions who are seen late in the course of the disease. In most cases, the right-sided pressures are normal, and the left atrial (wedge) pressure shows a large left atrial *a* wave due to increased force of left atrial contraction against a poorly compliant left ventricle. Left heart catheterization is most commonly performed using the retrograde aortic route.

Retrograde percutaneous femoral arterial catheterization is not always successful. Transseptal catheterization passing a catheter across the mitral valve into the left ventricle and simultaneous retrograde aortic catheterization are preferred in some centers, and this approach succeeds in about 85% of cases. It is important to measure left ventricular pressure, aortic pressure, and cardiac output simultaneously. An example of left ventricular and aortic pressure tracings in a patient with severe aortic stenosis is shown in Figure 13–8. Calculation of the valve area by the Gorlin formula provides the most valuable index of severity. As in mitral disease, the presence of incompetence invalidates the measurement of valve area, but the Gorlin formula can provide a minimal value for valve area if it is assumed that incompetence is absent.

If it proves difficult to pass a catheter across the aortic valve, supravalvular angiography may be helpful in indicating the position of the aortic valve orifice, but the angiographic findings cannot be used as an indication of the severity of stenosis. In retrograde studies, the severity of aortic stenosis does not correlate directly with the ease with which a catheter can be passed across a stenotic valve. The degree of aortic dilation and the position of the valve are more important factors in determining success of the procedure.

b. Left ventricular puncture– Another method of measuring the gradient across the aortic valve is by transthoracic needle puncture through the apex of the heart into the left ventricle. A catheter can be introduced over a guide wire so that both pressure measurements and left ventricular angiocardiography can be done. This is the only way access to the left ventricle can be obtained in a patient with both an aortic and a mitral mechanical valve. Retrograde passage of a catheter can be safely accomplished across a tissue valve, but it is unwise to pass catheters across mechanical valves because of the danger of dislodging a leaflet or poppet. The procedure is performed with a 20-gauge lumbar puncture needle under fluoroscopic control, using 50–100 mg of intravenous meperidine as an analgesic. The procedure is surprisingly well

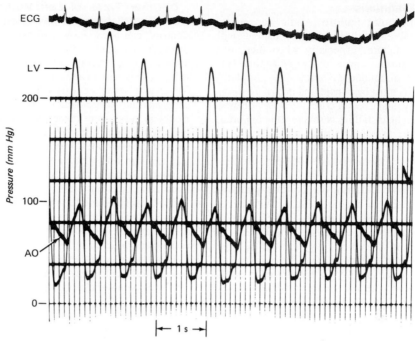

Figure 13–8. Simultaneous left ventricular (LV 270–240/40) and aortic (AO 100/60) pressure tracings in the patient whose chest x-rays are shown in Figure 13–6. Pulsus alternans is present and is more prominent on the left ventricular tracing.

tolerated and usually painless. Satisfactory tracings are obtained in about 85% of cases, and since the left ventricle is almost invariably hypertrophied, the dangers of hemorrhage and tamponade are minimal. A small pneumothorax is the most frequent complication and occurs in about 10% of cases. The patient's status must be monitored for several hours after the procedure in order to detect any early evidence of complications.

c. Selective coronary angiography– Some cardiologists advocate coronary arteriography in all patients with aortic stenosis. In general, however, the state of the coronary vessels alters the prognosis of aortic stenosis but not the treatment or the decision to operate, which depend on the severity of the obstruction. Because coronary arteriography increases the morbidity and mortality rates of an already difficult investigation, it is not advised in younger patients with severe or moderately severe aortic stenosis. In cases in which the hemodynamic severity of the stenosis does not definitely warrant surgery, coronary angiography can help the cardiologist decide whether or not to operate. Coronary angiography is usually done in patients over age 40 even if there are no symptoms of angina pectoris because the incidence of significant coronary artery disease increases at this age. Coronary angiography is definitely indicated in patients with angina pectoris or those who have had a myocardial infarction.

Increasing numbers of patients are being found to have both aortic stenosis and coronary artery disease. This probably reflects the increasing late development of aortic stenosis in older patients who already have coronary lesions. Now that aortocoronary bypass has come to be a commonplace operation with a low mortality rate, a larger number of patients are being treated by combined aortic valve replacement and aortocoronary bypass. There is still some difference of opinion about the indications for coronary bypass surgery in patients with aortic stenosis without angina pectoris in whom coronary lesions are found at angiography. There are studies showing no difference in mortality rate between patients with aortic valve replacement without significant coronary artery disease and those with aortic valve replacement and coronary bypass surgery of significant lesions. Presumably, some late deaths would have occurred in the patients with coronary lesions had they not been bypassed. There has been no study in which patients with severe aortic stenosis and coronary artery disease have been randomized to receive coronary bypass surgery plus aortic valve replacement or to have aortic valve replacement alone. Most surgeons elect to bypass significant lesions, especially those in the left anterior descending coronary artery. If a left main coronary lesion is present or the aortic valve disease is mild and angina is present, bypass surgery is indicated—but the value of "prophylactic" bypass surgery in patients with aortic valve disease without angina is not yet established.

Differential Diagnosis

A. Left Ventricular Failure: Aortic stenosis enters into the differential diagnosis of all patients with left ventricular failure, especially when there is a basal systolic murmur and a history of angina, syncope, dizziness, or conduction defect. The possibility of aortic stenosis must be considered in hypertension, cardiomyopathy, and even in coronary artery disease, especially when heart failure is severe. It is important to recognize the systolic murmur and rule out the possibility of aortic stenosis by all available means, including cardiac catheterization if echo-Doppler studies are inconclusive.

B. Hypertrophic Obstructive Cardiomyopathy: Aortic stenosis should not be confused with hypertrophic obstructive cardiomyopathy. In the latter condition (see Chapter 17), the pulse is jerky and the upstroke rapid and often bifid, in contrast to the slow-rising pulse of aortic stenosis. If there is associated aortic incompetence modifying the upstroke of the pulse in a patient with predominant aortic stenosis, there will be an aortic diastolic murmur, which virtually rules out obstructive cardiomyopathy. Compared with valvular aortic stenosis, the murmur of obstructive cardiomyopathy is longer, harsher, and usually heard best to the left of the sternum. The variation occurring in the murmur when diagnostic measures are used to influence the extent of outflow tract narrowing is helpful in establishing the diagnosis of obstructive cardiomyopathy. Echocardiography is particularly helpful in differential diagnosis because it shows systolic anterior motion of the mitral valve in hypertrophic cardiomyopathy and aortic valve thickening in aortic stenosis.

C. Other Lesions: The physical signs in mitral incompetence and ventricular septal defect are seldom confused with those of predominant aortic stenosis. In these disorders, the murmur is pansystolic, and the carotid upstroke is rapid. When the patient has both aortic stenosis and mitral incompetence, it is difficult to distinguish between them, and clinical assessment of the relative severity of the two lesions is usually impossible. In some cases of aortic valve disease, especially when the valve is calcified, there is a characteristic high-pitched "seagull cry" murmur.

Coarctation of the aorta is another lesion that may occasionally coexist with aortic stenosis and be confused with it. The murmur of coarctation occurs later in systole and reaches its peak about the time of the second heart sound. There is characteristically a prominent carotid arterial pulsation as well as absent or diminished femoral pulses and delay between the peaks of the brachial and femoral pulses, with hypertension in the arms (Chapter 11). Although coarctation of the aorta is commonly associated with bicuspid aortic valve, the coarctation is likely to cause problems long before the abnormal valve gives rise to difficulties that are associated with the development of aortic stenosis.

D. Other Types of Left Ventricular Outflow Tract Obstruction: As mentioned earlier, "aortic stenosis" can occur above and below the valve. With supravalvular stenosis there is a web or hourglass or a long hypoplastic segment of the aorta above the valve. The murmur can be indistinguishable from that of valvular aortic stenosis. Clues to the diagnosis of supravalvular aortic stenosis are that aortic insufficiency is not seen in this type of aortic stenosis; that because the jet is directed into the innominate artery, the systolic pressure is higher in the right arm than the left; and that with supravalvular aortic stenosis, poststenotic dilation of the ascending aorta is absent and there is no ejection click.

Clues to subvalvular aortic stenosis are the presence in discrete membranous subaortic stenosis of aortic insufficiency in 85% of cases as well as the lack of an ejection click.

Echo-Doppler studies can definitively diagnose the type of left ventricular outflow tract obstruction and should be done in every patient with suspected aortic stenosis.

Complications

A. Sudden Death: Patients with predominant aortic stenosis have an increased incidence of sudden death. The exact incidence is unknown but is probably underestimated. Of all patients with aortic stenosis who die, about 25% die suddenly. Before surgery, sudden death is most unusual as the first symptom of aortic stenosis and is usually seen in the patient who already has other symptoms. Sudden death is clearly not confined to patients with severe stenosis, since it is the most common cause of late death following aortic valve replacement. This finding suggests that residual myocardial fibrosis may cause arrhythmias or that valve malfunction may occur acutely. The general consensus is that arrhythmia is responsible for most cases of sudden death in aortic stenosis. In aortic stenosis, the effects of a sudden fall in arterial pressure resulting from arrhythmia are probably greater than normal for both mechanical and reflex reasons. In some cases, a vicious circle occurs when myocardial ischemia depresses left ventricular function, which leads to a fall in aortic pressure, which impairs coronary perfusion and causes further ischemia. In terms of mechanics, cardiac output takes longer to return to normal after an arrhythmia has developed. In terms of reflexes, the central nervous system tends to receive contradictory information from the carotid and aortic baroreceptors on the one hand and the left ventricular stretch receptors (von Bezold receptors) on the other, because left ventricular pressure is high and aortic pressure is relatively low.

B. Left Ventricular Failure: Left ventricular failure is an almost inevitable consequence of aortic stenosis and occurs relatively late. It is the strongest possible indication for surgical treatment because it is consistently relieved by surgery. Medical measures for its control should be regarded as part of the preoperative preparation and not as a substitute for surgery.

C. Conduction Defects: Complete atrioventricular block occasionally complicates aortic stenosis, and its association with slow heart rates and large stroke volumes makes clinical assessment of the lesion difficult. The hemodynamic signs of aortic stenosis seem more severe when the heart rate is slow. The heart is larger, the systolic murmur and thrill are more impressive, and the pressure difference between the left ventricle and the aorta is greater. Usually, however, all that is necessary to assess the stenosis is a calculation of the aortic valve area by means of the Gorlin formula, since the heart rate does not influence the calculated valve area.

D. Infective Endocarditis: Infective endocarditis is an important but rare complication of aortic stenosis. It occurs in about 2% of cases and is less common than in mitral or aortic incompetence.

E. Embolization: Occasionally, small flecks of calcification from the aortic valve can break off and embolize. If they lodge in small vessels supplying organs sensitive to ischemia, symptoms can occur. Stroke and sudden visual impairment, with calcified emboli seen in the retinal artery, have been reported.

Treatment

A. Medical Treatment: It is important that the treatment for left ventricular failure in aortic stenosis not be restricted to medical means. Intervention is the first and not the last resort. Digitalis, diuretics, and salt restriction are effective in left ventricular failure caused by aortic stenosis, and they should be used preoperatively. Treatment in severe aortic stenosis is a matter of some urgency.

B. Operative Treatment:

1. Aortic valve replacement– Replacement of the aortic valve is required in all symptomatic patients with moderate or severe stenosis (pressure difference 50 mm Hg or more or aortic valve area 0.8 cm² or less). Age is no bar to surgery, and the discomfort of intractable left ventricular failure should be avoided if at all possible. In young patients (under age 30) with uncalcified, severely stenotic valves, even if asymptomatic, palliative open aortic valvotomy is justified to avoid as long as possible the long-term hazards of valve replacement. The physician should remember that after valvotomy a second operation to replace the aortic valve will almost certainly be necessary in a decade or two.

The problem of when to replace the aortic valve in the asymptomatic patient with severe aortic stenosis is still controversial. If the incidence of sudden death as the first symptom is greater than the operative mortality rate, it is obvious that surgery would be beneficial. Several noncontrolled retrospective studies (Kelly, 1988; Pellika, 1990) have shown that sudden death as the first event in the totally asymptomatic patient with severe aortic stenosis is very unusual. The recommendation emerging from these studies has been to wait for symptoms to appear before offering aortic valve replacement. In the author's opinion, the problem with this advice is that symptoms are subjective, and the difference between two patients with the same degree of severe aortic stenosis may be that one patient experiences the sensation of angina or dyspnea on climbing stairs and the other does not, or does not report it to the physician. It is reasonable to wait for symptoms in elderly patients (eg, over age 70–75 years) before recommending surgery. In younger patients, there is evidence that progressive intramural fibrosis is an early consequence of severe aortic stenosis (Cheitlin, 1978) and that irreversible changes in the left ventricle may be taking place that will influence the course of the patient even after valve replacement and may limit the benefits of later surgery. For this reason, this author recommends valve replacement to patients under age 70 years when severe aortic stenosis (valve area ≤ 0.75 cm²) is diagnosed even if they are asymptomatic.

Attempts have been made to debride the calcific aortic valve ever since the introduction of open heart surgery. Creation of severe aortic valve incompetence and rapid recalcification and stenosis have made this approach untenable. Recently, intraoperative debridement of the calcified valve using ultrasound was advocated but met the same fate as simple debridement and is no longer used.

The choice of artificial valve rests with the surgeon. Homograft, heterograft, ball, flap, and disk valves have been used (Figure 13–9). The Starr-Edwards ball and cage valve was the first successful aortic valve and is still probably the most widely used around the world. The low-profile bileaflet St. Jude valve has a longer effective orifice and is

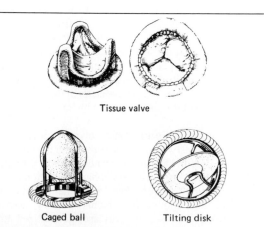

Tissue valve

Caged ball   Tilting disk

Figure 13–9. Examples of artificial heart valves. (Reproduced, with permission, from Way LW [editor]: *Current Surgical diagnosis & Treatment,* 8th ed. Appleton & Lange, 1988.)

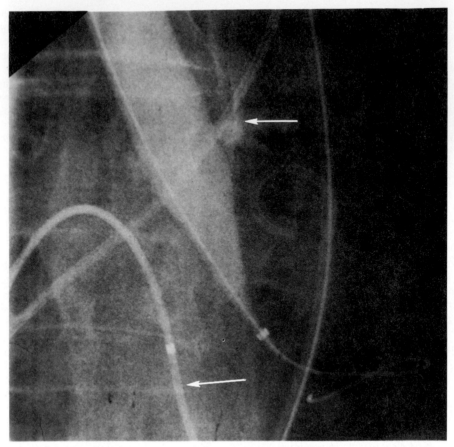

Figure 13–10. Balloon catheter positioned across a calcified stenotic aortic valve. The guide wire is coiled in the left ventricle. The upper arrow points to calcium in the aortic valve. The lower arrow indicates a pacing catheter in the right ventricle. (Courtesy of TA Ports.)

at present—now that the Björk-Shiley valve is no longer available—the most commonly used valve in the United States. It is generally thought that homograft and heterograft tissue valves do not require postoperative anticoagulant therapy indefinitely, as opposed to all types of prosthetic valves, in which lifetime anticoagulation is needed. The mortality rate of aortic valve replacement depends on the stage of the disease at the time of surgery; the average is about 5%. The mortality rate is greatest in patients with marked left ventricular hypertrophy or severe heart failure.

2. Catheter balloon aortic valvuloplasty– Balloon valvuloplasty has been advocated increasingly as palliative treatment of aortic stenosis at the extremes of life. In young persons with congenital lesions, it is often important to defer valve replacement until early adult life. In symptomatic patients over 80, associated coronary disease, lung disease, generalized atherosclerosis, or general debility may make balloon valvuloplasty the treatment of choice.

a. Technique– A 25-mm balloon catheter is passed percutaneously via a large (No. 12F) sheath in the femoral artery and positioned across the aortic valve as shown in Figure 13–10. Dilation of the balloon to a pressure of 6–8 atm for up to 30 seconds is surprisingly well tolerated. The mechanism for the hemodynamic improvement is usually fracture of calcified nodules or separation of fused commissures. A second balloon may sometimes be needed to maximize dilation. It is passed from the opposite groin.

b. Results of treatment– Even a minor increase in the valve area effectively relieves intractable symptoms of left ventricular failure in elderly patients. However, the procedure is palliative, and even short-term follow-up studies indicate that restenosis is frequent, as is the high incidence of late demise. The procedure can be repeated with success in some patients but is not a substitute for valve replacement in the patient who has a reasonable chance of surviving surgery.

Passing the balloon catheter across the stenosed valve can be difficult, and the multiple large catheters and sheaths that are used may lead to arterial complications with hemorrhage, aortoiliac perforations, and thrombosis. Calcified emboli, leaflet rupture, and serious aortic incompetence do not appear to be frequent complications.

Balloon valvuloplasty in the adult is probably indicated only in the very symptomatic elderly patient with multisystem disease who is not a candidate for valve surgery.

3. Surgical treatment of nonvalvular lesions– Supravalvular aortic stenosis is more difficult to treat than valvular stenosis because the ascending aorta is often hypoplastic. Congenital subvalvular ring stenosis can be excised, bringing dramatic relief. Valve replacement is not needed.

Operation for correction of a fibromuscular tunnel is more difficult. Attempts to remove the fibroelastic material directly are in general inadequate. At present, the Konno procedure is advocated, where the left ventricular outflow tract is approached through the right ventricle and by opening the ventricular septum. An adequate outflow tract is established, and the aortic valve ring is opened, usually with insertion of a mechanical valve. The septum is then patched closed, as is the right ventricle.

4. Results of treatment– Like the mortality rate, the results of surgical treatment vary depending on when operation is performed and whether coronary artery disease or other valve lesions are present. If the left ventricle is markedly dilated as a result of longstanding left ventricular failure, results will be worse than in early cases with hearts of normal size. Ideally, patients should be closely followed and operation recommended at the first sign of significant symptoms. In practice, however, diagnosis is made late in the course of the disease in about half of cases, usually because the patient does not seek help, and sometimes because the correct diagnosis is missed.

In young patients, because of the progressive intramural fibrosis that occurs in severe aortic stenosis, valvotomy is indicated even in asymptomatic patients. For the same reason, the author believes that asymptomatic patients with a reasonable expectation of long survival after surgery should be offered valve replacement when the aortic stenosis is severe, with a calculated valve area of 0.75 cm^2 or less. In older patients (above age 75 or 80), there is no evidence that the asymptomatic patient will benefit from operation. In this age group, it is the majority opinion that patients should be offered surgery only if and when symptoms develop. Since aortic stenosis is a reversible afterload burden on the left ventricle, if the valve is replaced there is no stage of poor left ventricular function that contraindicates surgery. Many of these patients with low ejection fractions preoperatively will have normal or near-normal ejection fractions after valve replacement.

Prognosis

Without surgery, the prognosis in aortic stenosis after the development of signs and symptoms of heart failure is poor. With treatment of heart failure, the patient may live for up to 5 years, but distressing episodes of recurrent left ventricular failure with pulmonary edema make the average survival time shorter.

Long-Term Results in Operated Cases

Aortic valve replacement for predominant aortic stenosis is the most satisfactory of all valve replacement operations. The degree of disability in the survivors is much less than in unoperated patients, and left ventricular failure is almost inevitably relieved. Approximately 75% of those who survive to leave hospital are still alive 5 years later, and after 10 years 50% are still living.

PREDOMINANT AORTIC INCOMPETENCE

The cardinal features of hemodynamically significant predominant aortic incompetence (Figure 13–11) include a large hypertrophied left ventricle, a large aorta, increased stroke volume, and wide pulse pressure. Variable factors include the severity of the process, the nature of the lesion (acute or chronic), and the cause.

Hemodynamically significant aortic incompetence creates an important extra load on the left ventricle. The blood that flows back across the aortic valve during diastole must be ejected during systole, and the consequent large stroke volume increases the work of the heart. The extra work is mainly "flow" work rather than "pressure" work, but peak systolic pressure tends to be raised and aortic diastolic pressure lowered because of rapid runoff of aortic blood into the peripheral arterial bed and back into the left ventricle. The arbitrary basis on which aortic incompetence is classified as hemodynamically significant here is the level of diastolic pressure. As stated at the beginning of the chapter, a value of less than 70 mm Hg constitutes the arbitrary dividing line, and patients with aortic incompetence and arterial diastolic pressures higher than that are considered to have hemodynamically insignificant aortic incompetence. The selection of this diastolic pressure as a criterion for hemodynamically significant aortic incompetence would misclassify those patients with essential hypertension who develop severe aortic regurgitation but whose aortic diastolic pressure might still be above 70 mm Hg.

Pathophysiology of Aortic Incompetence

A. Acute Aortic Incompetence: With sudden severe incompetence of the aortic valve, there is rapid runoff from the aorta, both to the periphery and back into the left ventricle. With sudden increase in left ventricular volume, the left ventricular muscle re-

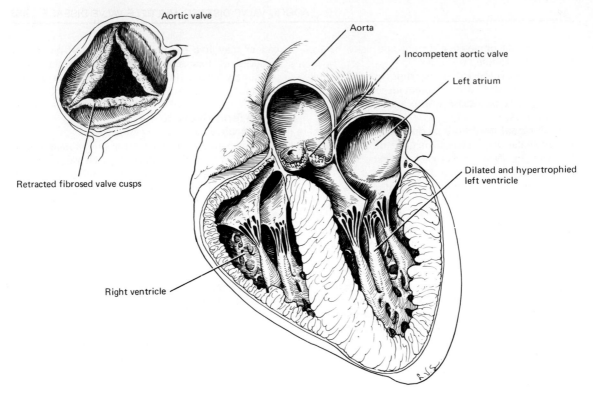

Drawing of left heart in left anterior oblique view showing anatomic features of aortic incompetence.

Cardinal features: *Large hypertrophied left ventricle; large aorta; increased stroke volume; wide pulse pressure.*

Variable factors: *Severity; acuteness or chronicity; cause.*

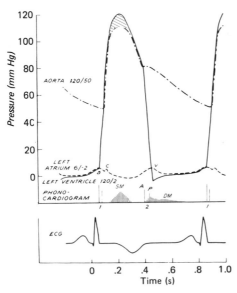

Diagram showing auscultatory and hemodynamic features of predominant aortic incompetence. SM, systolic murmur; A, aortic valve; P, pulmonary valve; DM, diastolic murmur.

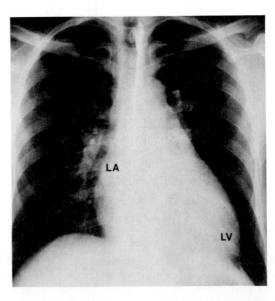

Chest x-ray of a patient with aortic incompetence and no signs of left heart failure. The long shadow of the enlarged left ventricle (LV) and slight left atrial (LA) enlargement can be seen.

Figure 13–11. Aortic incompetence. Structures enlarged: left ventricle, aorta.

sists, as does the noncompliant normal pericardium. As a result, the intrapericardial pressure rises, and to maintain a normal transmural pressure to fill the heart normally in diastole, the left ventricular filling pressure also rises sharply. This results in left atrial and pulmonary capillary pressure elevations and pulmonary congestion. As was the case with sudden mitral incompetence, the sudden increase in left atrial pressure causes an abrupt rise in afterload in the left ventricle and may cause it to fail. Also with the increase in size of the left ventricle inside a noncompliant pericardium, left ventricular filling may be interfered with, further causing a rise in right ventricular and right atrial diastolic pressure. Because the forward stroke volume may be limited, there may be peripheral vasoconstriction, and because the aortic diastolic pressure cannot fall below the elevated left ventricular diastolic pressure, the aortic diastolic pressure may fall only moderately. Thus, many of the peripheral signs of aortic incompetence may be absent. Still, the aortic pressure falls rapidly, acting like the left ventricle, so the cardiac pulse has the collapsing quality that indicates severe aortic incompetence.

With limited forward stroke volume, there is frequently sinus tachycardia, which, by limiting the diastolic filling period, reduces the minute regurgitant volume.

Because of the high filling pressure in the left ventricle and the low aortic diastolic pressure, there is markedly reduced coronary blood flow, especially to the compressed subendocardium in diastole. At the same time, with a sudden increase in left ventricular volume and tachycardia, there is increased myocardial oxygen demand. This leads to myocardial ischemia, angina, and infarction, further myocardial dysfunction, arrhythmias, and sudden death.

B. Chronic Aortic Incompetence: If the diastolic regurgitant volume increases gradually, the dilated left ventricle undergoes eccentric hypertrophy, and a large left ventricle develops that is capable of ejecting large stroke volumes sufficient to accommodate the regurgitant volume and yet keep the forward stroke volume normal. Because the ventricle has enlarged around the larger diastolic volume, the filling pressure remains normally low. The large stroke volume results in increased left ventricular and aortic systolic pressures, thus increasing the afterload on the left ventricle. The diastolic pressure drops rapidly because of the runoff back into the left ventricle. Since the left ventricular diastolic pressure is low in chronic aortic incompetence the aortic diastolic pressure drops to low levels and the pulse pressure is wide. This wide pulse pressure accounts for many of the peripheral signs of chronic aortic incompetence. The wide pulse pressure also stimulates the baroreceptor reflex, causing vasodilation, which further widens the pulse pressure.

The effect of aortic incompetence on the myocardial oxygen supply and demand relationship is shown in Table 13–1. It is apparent that—for slightly different reasons—aortic incompetence can lead to symptoms seen also with aortic stenosis. In addition, by virtue of the Venturi effect of the diastolic rush of blood past the coronary ostia, aortic incompetence can cause a decrease in pressure at the ostium which further decreases coronary blood flow.

Acute Lesions

Aortic incompetence occurs both as an acute lesion (20% of cases) and a single chronic lesion (80% of cases). Acute aortic incompetence occurs when valve lesions develop either instantaneously—when a cusp perforates or tears—or over a few days or weeks—when valve tissue is gradually eroded by infection, or when fibrosis, associated with healing of an infection, scars and contracts the valve. Because of the increased afterload in acute aortic incompetence and its more profound effect on myocardial blood flow, acute aortic incompetence imposes a more serious load on the left ventricle than acute mitral incompetence, and the chances that the patient's hemodynamic status will stabilize without surgical treatment are small. If the damage is less severe or less acute, the possibility for survival is better; and if the patient survives, the clinical picture in acute aortic incompetence by the end of about one year resembles that in chronic lesions.

Chronic Lesions

Chronic aortic incompetence results in marked peripheral vasodilation, which is attributable in part to reflex baroreceptor effects. The wide aortic and carotid pulse pressures cause reflex vasodilation and relative bradycardia. With exercise, the cardiac output increases, there is peripheral vasodilation of the muscular capillaries, and a further fall in systemic vascular resistance occurs. With tachycardia, the diastolic filling period is shortened, thus decreasing the number of times per minute when regurgitation can occur. As a result, the proportion of the left ventricular stroke volume returning to the left ventricle during diastole falls, and the hemodynamic status becomes close to that seen in normal subjects. In contrast, anything that increases the systemic vascular resistance, such as isometric exercise, exposure to cold, sympathetic nervous system stimulation, mental stress, or cardiac failure, tends to increase the volume of blood returning to the ventricle during diastole and makes the load on the heart more a "pressure" load and less a "flow" load.

Left Ventricular Hypertrophy & Dilation

Aortic incompetence leads to left ventricular dilation, which constitutes an important stimulus to eccentric hypertrophy of the left ventricular muscle. Hypertrophy involves an increase in the size of muscle cells and an increase in the connective tissue elements of the heart. In time, long-standing hypertrophy almost inevitably leads to myocardial fibrosis and becomes irreversible, so that heart muscle cells do not return to normal when the stimulus causing the hypertrophy is removed. With time, the left ventricle fails; the reasons are not fully understood, but myocardial fibrosis and age-related changes in ventricular muscle may play a role. This occurs relatively late in the course of chronic lesions. The development of ventricular failure is influenced by the severity of the incompetence and the state of the myocardium. It is also possible that the patient's activity level may play a part; earlier failure may develop in patients with more strenuous occupations. When it occurs, left ventricular failure is often acute and severe because reflex vasoconstriction takes the place of the normal vasodilation seen in chronic lesions, further aggravating ventricular failure by increasing systemic vascular resistance and hence the amount of incompetence. The most striking clinical manifestations of left ventricular failure are an increase in arterial diastolic pressure and the change from vasodilation to vasoconstriction that often accompanies failure and tends to obscure peripheral signs of aortic incompetence.

Causes of Aortic Incompetence (Table 13–2)

A. Acute Lesions: The most important cause of acute aortic incompetence is infective endocarditis. Patients who initially have normal aortic valves may contract infective endocarditis when they are debilitated because of immunosuppressive therapy, chronic illness, or intravenous drug abuse or when the infecting organism is highly invasive; in these cases, organisms of minimal pathogenicity may be the infective agent. Infective endocarditis also affects valves that are already diseased as a result of rheumatic or congenital involvement. The milder the original valve disease, the greater the potential for acute hemodynamic deterioration.

Another and rarer cause of acute aortic incompetence is aortic dissection. In this condition, a tear in the aortic intima extends to the neighborhood of a cusp of the aortic valve and causes the valve lesion. Marfan's syndrome and hypertension are the main causes of aortic dissection. Lesions from blunt trauma or penetrating wounds may cause aortic incompetence.

B. Chronic Lesions: Chronic aortic incompetence has several causes and occurs at all ages. It is more common in males by a factor of 3:2 and appears in our experience to be the commonest valvular lesion in black males. Rheumatic fever is still an important cause of aortic incompetence, though the incidence in the United States has decreased markedly. In the past, there was a history of rheumatic fever in about 25% of cases of chronic aortic regurgitation. If it is assumed that in 50% of cases rheumatic fever is subclinical, it follows that about half of cases of chronic

Table 13–2. Causes of aortic incompetence.

Onset	Causes
Acute	Infective endocarditis Rupture of myxomatous leaflet Traumatic rupture Dissection of the aorta Detachment of prosthetic aortic valve

Chronic	Disease of aortic valve and aortic root
	Rheumatic heart disease
	Aortitis
	   Takayasu's disease
	   Granulomatous aortitis
	   Temporal arteritis
	   Reiter's syndrome
	Aortic aneurysm
	   Marfan's disease
	   Aortic root disease
	   Aortic medial necrosis
	   Dissection of the aorta
	   Arteriosclerosis of the aorta
	Connective tissue disease
	   Ehlers-Danlos syndrome
	   Pseudoxanthoma elasticum
	   Morquio's syndrome
	Congenital valve lesions
	   Bicuspid aortic valve
	   Sinus of Valsalva aneurysm
	   Interventricular septal defect with aortic incompetence
	   Quadricuspid valve
	   Valvular aortic stenosis
	   Discrete membranous subvalvular aortic stenosis
	Trauma
	Other collagen diseases
	   Disseminated lupus erythematosus
	   Rheumatoid arthritis
	   Rheumatoid spondylitis

aortic incompetence were of rheumatic origin. This is certainly no longer the case.

Syphilis is a decreasing common cause of aortic incompetence. The average age of these patients is over 60 years, and associated atherosclerosis is almost always present.

Cases in which a congenital cause is confirmed are increasing as a result of echocardiographic diagnosis. The bicuspid aortic valve is present in 1–2% of the population and so is probably the commonest cause of all cases of aortic incompetence. A congenital cause should be suspected when associated lesions such as ventricular septal defect, Fallot's tetralogy, patent ductus arteriosus, or coarctation of the aorta are seen; when noncardiac congenital lesions such as Marfan's syndrome are present; or when the murmur is heard in infancy.

Ankylosing spondylitis and Reiter's syndrome are rare causes of aortic incompetence (5% of cases) in which the atrioventricular conduction system may be involved. The characteristic hip or sacroiliac joint involvement of ankylosing spondylitis may precede or follow the valve lesion and is sometimes only detected on x-ray examination.

Hypertension and atherosclerosis are rarely (3% of cases) the cause of hemodynamically significant aortic incompetence. More commonly these conditions produce an aortic diastolic murmur, with only slight widening of the aortic pulse pressure and no lowering of the aortic diastolic pressure.

Clinical Findings

A. Symptoms:

1. Acute lesions– Dyspnea is the commonest presenting cardiac symptom in acute lesions (50% of cases). Since infective endocarditis is by far the commonest cause, the patient usually is febrile and may be acutely ill with septicemia at the time that the aortic valve lesion develops. In other cases, the onset is slower and subacute: the aortic lesion appears or worsens as endocarditis heals, and the valve shrinks as it fibroses weeks or months after the endocarditis has responded to antibiotic therapy. In other patients with infective endocarditis, systemic embolism may be the presenting symptom, with a cerebrovascular accident, an acute coronary occlusion, or a cold, painful leg as the first sign of acute aortic incompetence. Acute aortic incompetence occurring in association with chest pain suggests the possibility of acute aortic dissection involving the noncoronary or right coronary cusp of the aortic valve. This uncommon lesion is not always painful. If the right coronary artery is involved, the patient may present with an inferior wall myocardial infarction. If the left coronary is occluded, the patient almost inevitably dies.

The dyspnea of acute aortic incompetence is often paroxysmal and associated with orthopnea and cough, with frothy pink sputum resulting from acute pulmonary edema. Chest pain may occur because of acute myocardial ischemia and peripheral circulatory collapse. Symptoms of shock, with anxiety, confusion, and mental obtundation, are occasionally seen. Sudden death due to ischemia, arrhythmia, or electromechanical dissociation is common.

2. Chronic lesions–

a. Symptoms unrelated to severity– There are two varieties of symptoms in chronic aortic incompetence, those due to the patient's awareness of increased force of the heartbeat and those due to left ventricular disease and heart failure. One-third of patients with hemodynamically significant aortic incompetence complain of palpitations, which on questioning turn out to be associated with sensations arising from forceful left ventricular contraction, producing a large stroke volume. The patient often notices the symptoms when lying in bed at night. These sensations sometimes provoke the symptoms of anxiety seen in cardiac neurosis, with stabbing inframammary pain, fatigue, and dyspnea with sighing respirations. The patient may have ventricular premature beats that further accentuate the symptoms. These symptoms usually occur in early adult life and can be present for 20 years or more without significant progression of the valvular lesion. More frequently (two-thirds of cases), the patient has no symptoms and is able to lead a surprisingly normal, active life in spite of a hemodynamically serious lesion. It is important to recognize certain symptoms as "functional" in patients with aortic incompetence and not interpret them as a necessary indication for surgery. Ventricular arrhythmia is probably the most important cause of symptoms at this stage, since it is thought that it may precede ventricular tachycardia or fibrillation, and these developments may account for the sudden death that is rarer in chronic aortic incompetence than in stenosis but that nevertheless occurs. The onset of syncope is particularly worrisome, since it may be due to malignant ventricular arrhythmias. The presence of symptoms in a patient with aortic incompetence is always an indication for thorough investigation; but if the valvular lesion is well tolerated, the patient (especially if young) should usually simply be closely followed, and the physician should watch for the development of serious symptoms.

b. Symptoms of left ventricular failure– When aortic incompetence is the sole lesion, serious symptoms due to left ventricular failure occur late in the course of the disease. Dyspnea is by far the commonest symptom (75% of cases) and may be associated with a feeling of heaviness in the chest and substernal discomfort. Left ventricular failure due solely to chronic aortic incompetence usually occurs after age 40, and patients who lead sedentary lives may not be aware of the insidious progression of pulmonary congestion because they have never exerted themselves sufficiently. In these patients, an acute episode of paroxysmal nocturnal dyspnea or frank pulmonary edema may be the presenting event.

Chest pain is the next most common symptom in aortic incompetence. It is particularly common in patients with syphilitic lesions and in older persons with associated coronary arterial disease. Anginal pain may be present at rest or during exercise; in general, it is due to increased metabolic demands of the hypertrophied myocardium coupled with decreased diastolic perfusion of the coronary bed, rather than to decreased supply resulting from obstructive atherosclerotic lesions in major coronary vessels. Syncope and dizziness are less common than in patients with predominantly stenotic lesions, and syncope during unaccustomed effort (the type seen in aortic stenosis) does not occur.

c. Development of left ventricular failure– The late symptoms in aortic incompetence carry a poor prognosis. This is in part due to reflex factors that cause a vicious circle. When forward effective cardiac output falls as the left ventricle fails, the normal peripheral vasodilation seen in aortic incompetence is replaced by vasoconstriction. This peripheral vasoconstriction increases the work of the left ventricle, increases aortic incompetence, and aggravates left ventricular failure. The relatively high arterial diastolic pressure that results may mislead the physician into thinking that significant aortic incompetence is not present. Left ventricular failure is thus especially sudden in aortic incompetence and is often provoked by factors involving autonomic nervous system control of blood pressure and blood volume, such as excitement, excessive sodium intake, recumbency, overexertion, excessive mental stress, and violent dreams, all of which cause a rise in systemic arterial pressure. The patient's occupation may also influence the occurrence of left ventricular failure. Patients with strenuous jobs involving heavy manual labor may develop larger hearts corresponding to a given level of severity in the lesion and hence develop left ventricular failure earlier than patients who avoid excessive exertion. The role of mental stress may also be important in patients with this lesion, because it is increased systemic arterial pressure and increased peripheral resistance that tend to aggravate incompetence more than any increase in cardiac output.

d. Sweating– Patients with predominant aortic incompetence have a tendency to sweat more, which may be due to increased sympathetic tone or increased perfusion of the skin associated with low peripheral resistance.

B. Signs: The rapid runoff of blood from the aorta during diastole dominates the physical signs of hemodynamically significant aortic incompetence.

1. Peripheral circulation– Prominent carotid pulsations in the neck, throbbing peripheral arteries, and a prominent left ventricular impulse that moves the whole left side of the chest produce easily visible evidence of the large left ventricular stroke volume and increased rate of systolic ejection seen in this lesion. These peripheral circulatory signs are seen in both acute and chronic lesions and are present in all patients except those in severe left ventricular failure. The rapid aortic runoff is due to increased blood flow back into the left ventricle and into the dilated peripheral arterial bed. It is important to remember that rapid runoff from the aorta into cardiac chambers or blood vessels other than the left ventricle is an equally potent cause of the peripheral signs ordinarily associated with aortic incompetence. Large patent ductus arteriosus, aortopulmonary window, rupture of an aneurysm of the aortic sinus (sinus of Valsalva) with consequent left-to-right shunt, or a major systemic arteriovenous fistula may produce similar physical signs.

Systemic arterial pressure is the most readily measured indication of the severity of the peripheral signs of rapid aortic runoff. There is a wide pulse pressure, with high systolic and low diastolic pressure. Arteria pressure measured indirectly with a blood pressure cuff is not always accurate, and a diastolic pressure reading of zero—ie, an audible sound over the artery with no cuff in position—is never correct although it is often seen in patients with aortic incompetence. The point at which the Korotkoff sounds become muf-

fled gives a better indication of the level of diastolic arterial pressure in aortic incompetence. The wide pulse pressure gives rise to the typical collapsing pulse in which the pulse wave rises rapidly to a peak and falls away quickly.

2. Secondary signs– Secondary physical signs due to rapid aortic runoff are numerous and usually have eponymic designations. Head movement in time with the heartbeat is called de Musset's sign after the French poet Alfred de Musset, in whom it was noticed by his brother, who was a physician. Quincke's pulse denotes capillary pulsation in the extremities; Duroziez's sign refers to systolic and diastolic murmurs over the compressed femoral artery; and Hill's sign denotes increased blood pressure in the legs above that measured in the arms. Corrigan's pulse refers to the collapsing pulse, which is also called a "water-hammer" pulse after a 19th century children's toy of that name. Pulsations in the digital and ulnar arteries are readily felt, and the hands and feet are warm and sweaty.

In chronic aortic incompetence, the left ventricular impulse is heaving and hyperdynamic, and the apex beat is displaced downward and to the left. These physical signs depend largely on the size of the heart and are less obvious in acute aortic incompetence in which left ventricular dilation and hypertrophy has not yet developed.

3. Auscultatory findings– The characteristic physical sign on auscultation is a high-pitched, blowing diastolic murmur beginning immediately after the second sound at the start of diastole (Figure 13–11). It is called an "immediate" diastolic murmur to distinguish it from the "delayed" diastolic murmur of mitral stenosis, which does not start until left ventricular pressure has fallen below the level of left atrial pressure, ie, about 0.1 s after the start of diastole. The diastolic murmur of aortic incompetence lasts until backflow through the valve stops; the length of the murmur thus depends on the severity of the lesion and the compliance of the left ventricle. In severe cases, the murmur lasts throughout diastole and may be associated with a third heart sound (Figure 13–12).

The pitch and loudness of the murmur depends on the diastolic pressure gradient and volume of blood regurgitation. The smaller the regurgitant orifice, the higher the gradient, and the smaller the regurgitated volume, the higher the pitch and the softer the murmur. Doppler echocardiography can demonstrate minimal aortic regurgitation with frequencies so high that there is no audible diastolic murmur. The larger the regurgitant orifice, the lower the gradient, and the greater the volume of blood regurgitated, the lower the pitch and the louder the murmur.

The inevitable increase in left ventricular stroke volume ordinarily causes a systolic murmur that is of no value in diagnosis or in the differentiation of aortic incompetence from predominant aortic stenosis. The site at which the immediate diastolic murmur of aortic

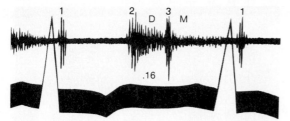

Figure 13–12. Phonocardiogram of a patient with aortic incompetence. A third sound is buried in the murmur (DM) that follows immediately after the second sound (2). (Courtesy of Roche Laboratories Division of Hoffman-La Roche, Inc.)

incompetence is heard best depends on the degree of aortic dilation and the direction of the regurgitant jet. If the aorta is large, as in syphilitic lesions, the murmur is heard best to the right of the sternum. If the aorta is small, as in rheumatic lesions, the murmur is heard best to the left of the sternum. The murmur of aortic incompetence is sometimes only heard in the lower intercostal spaces (fourth or fifth) beside the sternum and is usually not heard well at the apex. When aortic incompetence is severe, an additional separate low-frequency apical diastolic murmur is heard. This murmur, which is called an Austin Flint murmur (Figure 13–13), is middiastolic or presystolic. The pathogenesis of the murmur is uncertain. It

seems to be related to the interaction between the regurgitant jet and the left ventricular wall. Atrial contraction can influence the pattern of flow in this region and cause presystolic accentuation of the murmur, which is only heard in patients with severe aortic incompetence. Thus, the differential diagnosis is not between mitral stenosis and aortic incompetence, but between aortic incompetence and aortic incompetence plus mitral stenosis.

The murmurs of aortic incompetence may be similar in both the acute and the chronic form. In some patients with acute lesions, the murmurs may be of lower frequency; they may be shorter or even absent in patients with high diastolic left ventricular pressure and tachycardia.

4. Differences between acute and chronic lesions– Physical signs due to the hemodynamic effects of aortic incompetence may be strikingly different in acute and chronic lesions. For example, left ventricular dilation and hypertrophy and aortic dilation are not seen at the onset of acute aortic incompetence, whereas peripheral circulatory collapse, sweating, marked tachycardia, and signs of shock, with tachypnea, basal rales, and other signs of acute severe incompetence arc not seen in patients with chronic lesions, except in severe left ventricular failure. The aortic diastolic murmur and the pulse pressure are the two signs that should be monitored continuously in patients with infective endocarditis who are at risk of developing aortic incompetence.

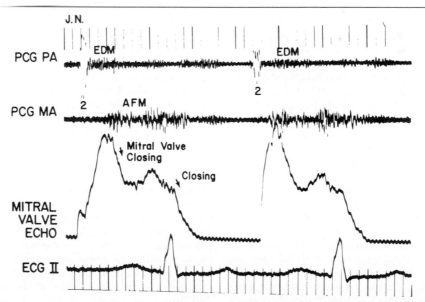

Figure 13–13. Phonocardiogram (PCG), echocardiogram, and ECG of a patient with a two-component Austin Flint murmur (AFM). The murmur has its onset in mid diastole as the early diastolic aortic murmur (EDM) is diminishing, and it occurs while the mitral valve is closing. The second component of the murmur occurs coincidentally with atrial systole. At the time of this murmur, the mitral valve opens incompletely. The mitral valve echocardiogram shows the position of the anterior cusp. The rapid backward motion associated with mitral valve closure is interrupted by atrial systole. (PA, pulmonary area; MA, mitral area.) (Reproduced, with permission of the American Heart Association, Inc., from Fortuin NJ, Craige E: On the mechanism of Austin Flint murmur. Circulation 1972;45:558.)

C. Electrocardiographic Findings: Electrocardiographic evidence of left ventricular hypertrophy is always present in patients with chronic hemodynamically significant aortic incompetence unless left bundle branch block or complete atrioventricular block obscures the changes. The degree of left ventricular hypertrophy—as judged by the height of the R wave in the left-sided chest leads, the depth of the S wave in the right-sided leads, and the associated ST–T changes—is moderate or considerable in more than half of patients. In about 10% of patients, right or, more commonly, left bundle branch block or even complete atrioventricular block is present. Atrial fibrillation is less common than in any other isolated left-sided lesion (5% of patients), perhaps because left ventricular failure is seldom chronic, and unrecognized mitral valve disease occurs less frequently. In acute aortic incompetence, left ventricular hypertrophy may be absent when the patient is first seen and may develop over a period of months. In other patients in whom aortic incompetence is present before infective endocarditis develops, left ventricular hypertrophy may become progressively more severe.

D. Imaging Studies: The cardiac silhouette in severe aortic incompetence shows evidence of dilation of the left ventricle, as shown in Figure 13–11. The long wide curve of the left lateral wall of the heart on the posteroanterior view extends below the diaphragm; on the left anterior oblique view, the posterior sweep of the left ventricle overlies the dorsal spine and extends posterior to the inferior vena caval shadow. The physician must exercise care in interpreting x-ray evidence of left ventricular enlargement, since the left and right ventricles can on occasion be confused with one another. Electrocardiographic and echocardiographic confirmation is always helpful and is required before the physician concludes that x-ray findings are due to the enlargement of a particular ventricle. Aortic dilation, as shown in Figure 13–14, is an important finding in patients with nonrheumatic aortic incompetence. Although calcification of the aortic valve is rare (< 10% of cases), linear "eggshell" calcification of the ascending aorta (Figure 20–2) is diagnostic of aortitis and almost pathognomonic of a syphilitic lesion. Calcification of the arch and descending portions of the aorta is not important as a diagnostic sign and is commonly seen in older, atherosclerotic patients.

In acute aortic incompetence, left ventricular enlargement on the chest x-ray may be absent when the patient is first seen. If the patient survives, the left ventricle enlarges at about the same rate as the electrocardiographic changes of hypertrophy develop (3 weeks to 6 months). There is x-ray evidence of pulmonary congestion with acute lesions. It is important to distinguish these changes from those seen in pulmonary infarction or pneumonia. The lesions are almost always bilateral but not always symmetric, and the characteristic "bat's wing" distribution of sub-

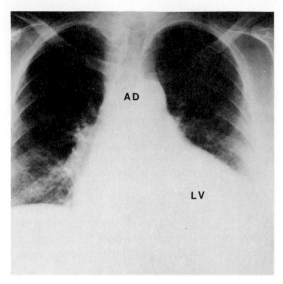

Figure 13–14. Chest x-ray of a patient with severe aortic incompetence and left heart failure. The large left ventricle (LV) and aortic dilation (AD) are clearly seen.

acute pulmonary edema with shadows extending out from the roots of the lungs is often seen.

1. Noninvasive techniques– Echocardiography is valuable in detecting diastolic fluttering of the aortic leaflet of the mitral valve during diastole (Figure 13–15) and aortic valve prolapse or vegetations on the aortic valve. In severe, acute cases of aortic incompetence, the mitral valve closes early in diastole as the diastolic rush of blood from the aorta enters the ventricle. This echocardiographic sign has been used as an indication of severity; it is probably valid in patients with tachycardia.

Doppler blood velocity measurements have been used to assess the severity of aortic incompetence. Ascending aortic blood flow is normally confined to systole, and diastolic flow is an indication of abnormal runoff via a low resistance pathway. In aortic incompetence, the flow takes place both forward, into the dilated peripheral bed; and backward, into the left ventricle. Semiquantitative estimates of the magnitude of backflow can be made using Doppler techniques to measure blood velocity in the ascending aorta. The results correlate well with other estimates of the regurgitant flow. Color Doppler studies can be used to outline the extent of regurgitant flow into the left ventricle—the broader the base of the regurgitant jet, the greater the severity of the lesion (Figure 13–16).

Radionuclear measurement of the left ventricular ejection fraction and end-systolic and diastolic left ventricular volumes is proving valuable in following the course of patients with aortic incompetence. The technique can be applied during exercise, and the exercise does not have to be maximal to bring out

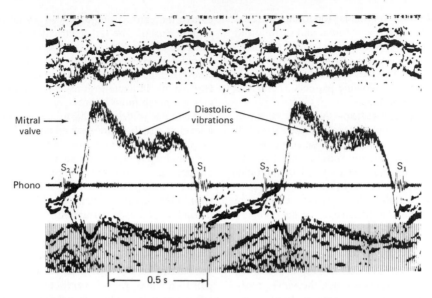

Figure 13–15. Echocardiogram showing diastolic vibration of mitral valve leaflet in a patient with aortic incompetence.

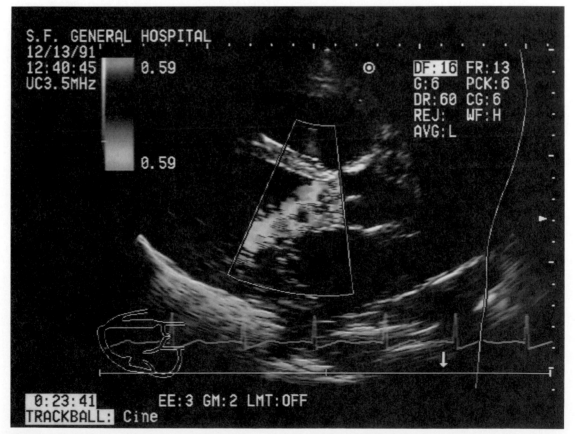

Figure 13–16. Color Doppler. Four-chamber view of a patient with aortic regurgitation. The entire left ventricular outflow tract is filled with the mosaic color of the regurgitant jet. White arrow on ECG shows that the picture was taken in late diastole.

the impairment in left ventricular function. On serial studies, an increasing left ventricular and systolic and end-diastolic volume with a decreasing ejection fraction implies decreasing myocardial function. The ease with which serial studies can be done makes this an attractive means of following patients.

2. Invasive techniques—

a. Cardiac catheterization— As with other valvular lesions, the noninvasive techniques described above are usually sufficient to diagnose aortic incompetence, estimate the severity of the regurgitant volume, and assess the function of the left ventricle. Catheterization is not necessary if the clinical picture and the noninvasive data are consistent with severe aortic incompetence and if the status of the coronary arterial system does not need to be visualized. If there is inconsistency between the noninvasive data and the clinical picture, cardiac catheterization and retrograde aortography are essential. If there is doubt that the runoff from the aorta is through the valve, retrograde aortography is likewise essential. In this way, an unsuspected sinus of Valsalva aneurysm ruptured into the outflow tract of the right ventricle or the rarer aortic-left ventricular tunnel can be distinguished from aortic incompetence.

Since left ventricular failure occurs so late in the course of aortic incompetence, most patients with chronic lesions show normal right heart pressures when they are first studied. In older patients with clinical evidence of left heart failure, raised wedge and left ventricular diastolic pressures are found, although the cardiac output is usually normal or even slightly raised. The left ventricular and wedge pressures are usually lower than expected, and pulmonary vascular resistance is rarely increased (< 10% of cases); the increase is at most moderate (3.5–7.5 mm Hg/L/min). In acute lesions, the hemodynamic findings are much more impressive, and the wedge pressure and left ventricular diastolic pressure are often at a level at which pulmonary edema is likely to occur (> 35 mm Hg). The pressure in the left ventricle may rise rapidly during diastole to high levels, resembling the pressure curves seen in constrictive pericarditis, and a reversed gradient across the mitral valve may be seen in severe cases (Figure 13–17). The characteristic finding of a wide aortic pulse pressure is present in all chronic aortic incompetence patients except those in severe left ventricular failure. The aortic pulse pressure is usually less than that in a peripheral artery, and that in turn is less than the indirectly recorded pulse pressure. As left ventricular failure develops, left ventricular diastolic pressure rises, establishing a lower limit to the aortic pressure of about 40 mm Hg. The level of left ventricular diastolic pressure varies with the compliance of the left ventricle. This is greater in large dilated ventricles in chronic lesions. The highest ventricular diastolic pressures are seen in patients with acute lesions and small hearts. In such patients, values of 60 mm Hg can occur, as seen in Figure 13–18, and the pulse pressure may not be markedly widened.

b. Angiography— Supravalvular aortography is

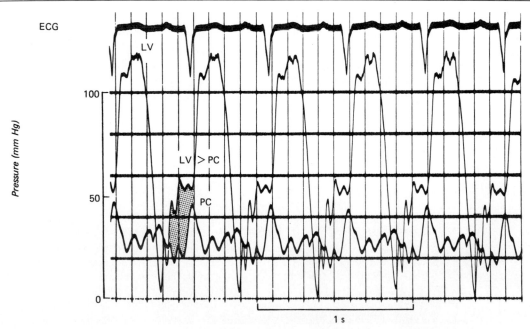

Figure 13–17. Left ventricular (LV) and wedge (PC, pulmonary capillary) pressure tracings in a patient with acute severe aortic incompetence. During the crosshatched period of diastole, the left ventricular pressure exceeds the pulmonary capillary pressure; this constitutes the reverse mitral gradient.

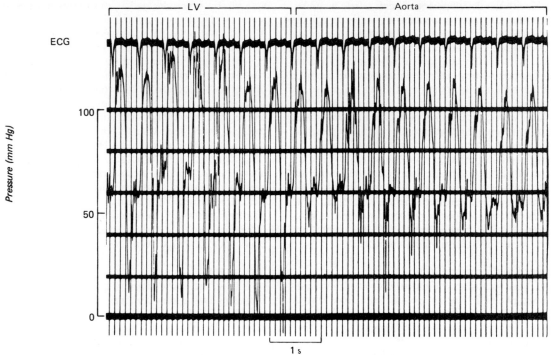

Figure 13–18. Withdrawal pressure tracing from left ventricle (LV) to aorta in a patient with acute severe aortic incompetence showing equalization of end-diastolic pressure at 60 mm Hg.

important in assessing aortic incompetence. The rapidity and density with which the left ventricle opacifies is roughly proportionate to the severity of the leak. Angiocardiography establishes the valvular nature of the lesion and provides opacification of the left ventricle sufficient to assess left ventricular function without a catheter in the chamber. Angiography also makes it possible to detect or rule out associated mitral incompetence with greater certainty because ectopic beats (which often produce spurious mitral incompetence) occur less frequently, and positioning of the catheter to avoid interfering with the action of the mitral valve apparatus is not a problem. The end-diastolic volume of the left ventricle is increased in aortic incompetence, often with a normal end-diastolic pressure, indicating increased compliance of the ventricle. The total stroke volume is always greater than normal, and the ejection fraction is reasonably well maintained until left ventricular failure occurs. If the left ventricular stroke volume is measured independently from the effective forward stroke volume, it is possible to calculate the volume of blood flowing back across the aortic valve during diastole. This is usually expressed as a proportion of the total stroke volume or "regurgitant fraction." A value of 50% or more is found in patients with severe lesions and indicates that half the stroke volume returns to the ventricle during diastole. Coronary arteriography is frequently performed as a routine procedure in pa-

tients with aortic incompetence, but as in aortic stenosis, the state of the coronary arteries should not influence the decision to operate, which depends instead on the hemodynamic severity of the aortic valve lesion.

Differential Diagnosis

A. Pulmonary Incompetence: The murmur of aortic incompetence can be readily confused with the murmur of pulmonary incompetence in patients with severe pulmonary hypertension. Pulmonary incompetence rarely occurs in patients who do not have moderate or severe pulmonary hypertension. In patients with pulmonary hypertension, the hypertrophied right ventricle relaxes at about the same time as the left ventricle, causing the characteristic immediate, high-pitched diastolic murmur that is indistinguishable from that of aortic incompetence.

In patients with low pulmonary arterial pressure, the murmur of pulmonary incompetence is different and is therefore not likely to be confused with an aortic murmur. When pulmonary arterial pressure is low, the right ventricle relaxes more slowly and the murmur starts later and is pitched lower.

B. Sinus of Valsalva Aneurysm: Aneurysm of the sinus of Valsalva is a congenital abnormality that generally does not cause a problem until it ruptures, into either the right atrium or the right ventricle. Rupture produces a clinical picture that is readily confused with the development of acute aortic incompetence. Rupture may be spontaneous and occur acutely or subacutely; it also occurs in the course of infective endocarditis. The presenting symptom is usually dyspnea, with paroxysmal nocturnal dyspnea, and the most important physical sign is the development of a murmur that may be almost continuous and is usually both systolic and diastolic. There are signs of rapid runoff, with a collapsing pulse, and a wide pulse pressure resembling that seen in aortic incompetence.

C. Rapid Aortic Runoff in Other Conditions: Other disorders can cause the characteristic physical signs of rapid runoff of blood from the aorta into some low-pressure area or into other areas in the circulation. There disorders include patent ductus arteriosus, aortopulmonary window, systemic arteriovenous fistula, truncus arteriosus, and ventricular septal defect with aortic incompetence.

Course & Complications

A. Left Ventricular Failure: Left ventricular failure occurs late in the course of uncomplicated chronic aortic incompetence and should be thought of as part of the disease rather than a complication. The part played by myocardial fibrosis in causing left heart failure is difficult to determine. Myocardial hypertrophy results in an increase in connective tissue elements of the heart as well as an increase in the size of the individual muscle cells. The role of current or previous rheumatic myocarditis in the development of left ventricular failure is a matter of continuing controversy but is probably of minimal importance.

Severe coronary arterial disease is not usually present in patients with hemodynamically significant aortic incompetence who present in a hospital, presumably because the patient population in which severe aortic incompetence is seen is relatively young. In syphilitic aortic incompetence, coronary ostial stenosis is an important associated finding that may cause progressively more severe angina.

Left ventricular failure is difficult to predict in aortic incompetence, and the premonitory symptoms of increasing dyspnea with decreasing effort over several months or years are not always seen. The onset of left ventricular failure is more abrupt in aortic incompetence than in any other form of chronic left ventricular disease, probably because the change is so abrupt from marked peripheral vasodilation to severe vasoconstriction associated with a falling cardiac output.

B. Infective Endocarditis: Infective endocarditis is the most important complication of aortic incompetence. Therapeutic advances, increased use of intravenous medication, the increased incidence of intravenous drug abuse, and the use of immunosuppressive drugs have since increased both the variety of organisms and the range of pathogenicity. Infective endocarditis is a greater hazard at the aortic valve than at any other site and is most dangerous when aortic incompetence is mild. The reason that endocarditis involving the aortic valve carries such a poor prognosis is that the valve is of crucial hemodynamic importance and is situated close to the main coronary vessels and conduction system. Ulcerative lesions of the cusps and the aortic root can cause acute, subacute, or chronic exacerbation of aortic incompetence, with or without perforation into adjacent cardiac chambers. (See Chapter 16 for details of treatment of infective endocarditis.)

C. Conduction Defects: Atrioventricular conduction defects are an occasional complication, especially in patients with ankylosing spondylitis or Reiter's syndrome. In patients with marked left ventricular hypertrophy and dilation, left bundle branch block may occur, and all varieties of atrioventricular conduction delay are seen.

Treatment

With severe aortic incompetence, afterload reduction using hydralazine has been shown to acutely and chronically reduce the regurgitant volume, decrease end-systolic and end-diastolic left ventricular volumes, and increase ejection fraction (Greenberg, 1988). Other afterload-reducing agents such as the angiotensin-converting enzyme inhibitors are probably similarly effective. Certainly, preload and afterload reduction can be lifesaving in acute aortic incompetence, and nitroprusside has been used in this role. Whether chronic afterload reduction can postpone the time of onset of congestive heart failure or the need for aortic valve replacement is not known. In the patient who is not yet a candidate for aortic valve replacement, we use an angiotensin-converting enzyme inhibitor for afterload reduction. However, this should never be a substitute for aortic valve replacement in a patient with severe aortic incompetence who is a surgical candidate.

Aortic valve replacement is the only effective treatment for aortic incompetence. However, this lesion is the one with the most problematic indications for surgery. At present, only with dissection of the aorta and aortic incompetence is there a good chance of successfully resuspending the aortic valve. In several centers, techniques are being developed to repair the valve and decrease aortic incompetence. The long-term results of repair are still not known, and at present repair of the valve must still be considered experimental. Both the timing of surgery and the choice of prosthetic valve are still controversial. Since aortic valve replacement has become widely available, surgical treatment of chronic aortic incompetence has been instituted at progressively earlier stages of the disease. The chief difficulty is that if surgery is delayed until heart failure is obvious, the results of operation are poor because the large, hypertrophied, dilated, and often fibrotic heart does not recover normal function because irreversible myocardial fibrosis has irrevocably compromised left ventricular function.

The dilemma is that heart failure develops late in the course of the disease, and its onset cannot be predicted with sufficient accuracy to enable the surgeon to make a rational decision about surgical treatment. If the long-term durability of prosthetic valves were good and the surgical mortality rate were negligible, earlier valve replacement could be recommended. However, the long-term durability of prosthetic valves is not yet known, and as yet neither the mortality nor the morbidity rates of aortic valve replacement—nor the long-term complication rates associated with artificial valves or homografts— are low enough to warrant prophylactic valve replacement.

If surgery is performed, an additional difficulty lies in anchoring the valve securely. In endocarditis, there is the danger of extension of the infection into the aortic ring, with paravalvular abscess, resulting in friable tissue and the danger of residual infection in the area of the anchoring sutures. There is often associated disease of the aortic wall that makes sutures more likely to tear out and necessitate a second open heart operation. Severe morbidity or even death may then result.

A 20-year-old asymptomatic patient with uncomplicated hemodynamically significant aortic incompetence can probably expect an average of about 20 years of life free from symptoms. Some more precise indications for surgery, such as massive cardiac enlargement, an arbitrary age (eg, 40 years), or the hemodynamic response to some stress such as exercise or angiotensin infusion, might be more logical than the present situation in which some "excuse" is generally required before surgery is recommended in an asymptomatic patients. When significant dyspnea, angina, syncope, or left heart failure develop, surgery is mandatory. Medical treatment of left ventricular failure should only be a prelude to operation.

Exercise testing is less helpful than might be expected, because the patient with aortic incompetence generally tolerates exercise well. Signs of increasing left ventricular hypertrophy on the ECG and chest x-ray are not too helpful, since both have been documented 20–30 years before left ventricular failure occurred. At present, it is believed that the best means of following patients with hemodynamically significant aortic incompetence for decreasing myocardial contractility is to measure the left ventricular volumes in diastole and systole. As myocardial contractility decreases, there is a progressive increase in end-systolic and end-diastolic volume and a concomitant decrease in ejection fraction. Since afterload is increased in aortic incompetence, some decrease in ejection fraction is attributable to afterload, which will be reversed after valve replacement. Consequently, one should follow the ventricular volumes and ejection fraction at yearly intervals noninvasively with echo-Doppler or radionuclide angiography. If there is progressive change indicating decreased contractility or if there are progressive symptoms, valve replacement is indicated.

In the authors' experience, exercise stress testing and measurement of ejection fraction are not useful in deciding on the timing of surgery. A decrease instead of the normal rise in ejection fraction with exercise means that cardiac reserve is limited and that the onset of symptoms is near. However, in an asymptomatic patient with normal resting systolic function, a drop in ejection fraction with exercise by itself would not be an indication for surgery.

In patients with acute or acutely exacerbated lesions, surgery is almost always needed, and acute and progressive hemodynamic deterioration may force operation. Patients with infective endocarditis, especially those with acute fulminant lesions, should be treated at a center where emergency cardiac surgery is available, because the need for operation may arise at any time in the course of the disease. The course of infective endocarditis is so unpredictable and varies so widely with the type of causative organism, the prior state of the valve, and the general health of the patient that it is impossible to set up any rational guidelines for the management of patients with this lesion. Medical treatment alone is unlikely to stabilize the hemodynamic status of patients with aortic incompetence occurring de novo. In these patients, aortic valve replacement is almost inevitable, and the principal question is the timing of surgery.

When endocarditis is present, appropriate antimicrobial treatment should be started; when an adequate serum concentration of antibiotic has been achieved, valve replacement should be undertaken. Waiting for adequate control of the infection has been tried in the past, but deterioration can occur so rapidly that the patient may die before the operation can be performed. Present evidence suggests that if bactericidal levels of the appropriate antibiotics have been maintained for 12–24 hours, valve replacement can be done with minimal chance of reinfection.

Serious problems arise in patients who are addicted to heroin and in whom fungi or saprophytic organisms such as Pseudomonas or Serratia marcescens are present. In such cases, valve replacement offers the only hope of cure. The reinfection rate is extremely high, and the prognosis is dismal. There is little doubt that satisfactory results can be obtained in no more than 50% of patients. The patient must be closely followed for over one year because hemodynamic deterioration following infective endocarditis may occur late in the disease, when healing causes retraction and fibrosis of the damaged valvular tissue.

As it does in aortic stenosis, the choice of artificial valve rests with the surgeon. Heterograft or other tissue aortic valves have the advantage of not requiring long-term anticoagulation, but this factor must be balanced against their tendency to stiffen, calcify, and leak with time. The mortality rate of surgery depends on the clinical status of the patient and the experience of the surgeon and averages 2–5% in chronic cases.

The mortality rate is two to three times higher in second operations, mainly because the patient's clinical condition is almost inevitably worse. In patients with infective endocarditis, it is clearly advantageous to wait until the infection has been controlled, if possible. It has been shown, however, that it is possible to operate in the presence of infection without significantly compromising the results if appropriate amounts of the proper antibiotics are administered. Thus, the patient's hemodynamic state clearly takes precedence over optimal management of the infection.

Prognosis

Aortic incompetence has a better prognosis than aortic stenosis, since the load on the ventricle is better tolerated, primarily because it is a "volume" load. In acute lesions, aortic incompetence carries a worse prognosis than mitral incompetence because the load on the ventricle is greater and there is an increased possibility of myocardial ischemia; because a severe systemic infection is often present when the lesion develops; and because fistula formation and conduction defects are more likely to occur.

The prognosis of left ventricular failure in aortic incompetence is poor because it occurs at such a late stage in the disease. In milder lesions, the threat of endocarditis is the most important and least predictable factor in prognosis.

Long-Term Results in Operated Cases

If valve replacement is delayed until the heart is very large and there is evidence of left ventricular failure, the late results of valve replacement in patients with aortic incompetence are the least satisfactory of all valve replacement surgery. Most patients who come to surgery with chronic lesions at this stage have large, fibrotic left ventricles which, though their function improves, never return to normal size or recover a normal ejection fraction.

At present, with the indications for surgery set forth above, the results of surgery are good, with an operative mortality rate in the range of 3–5% and a 5-year survival rate of 90%.

Patients with acute lesions almost all have infective endocarditis; in some of these patients, the valve may be dislodged because of ulcerative lesions in the area in which it is anchored. If sutures tear out from an area where inflammatory changes have weakened the tissues, the valve ring may become unseated and move with each heartbeat. This tends to tear out more sutures and is an urgent indication for reoperation.

MULTIPLE VALVE INVOLVEMENT

Combined Mitral & Aortic Valve Disease

Involvement of both aortic and mitral valves is almost pathognomonic of rheumatic heart disease, and patients with lesions of both valves have a higher incidence of a history of rheumatic infection in childhood (70%) than any other group of patients with valve disease. When both aortic and mitral valves are involved, the variability of the clinical picture greatly increases. The importance of the lesion at each valve can vary; the nature of each lesion (stenosis, incompetence, or mixture of the two) is diverse; and it is possible that rheumatic myocardial involvement plays a more important part in the clinical course because the rheumatic infection is more severe and more often recurrent in these cases. It can be seen from the classification of mitral and aortic disease in this text that 20 or more subclassifications of different mixed valvular diseases can be described. It is beyond the scope of this text to do more than point out some of the more obvious relationships between aortic and mitral disease and to make a few general comments about the clinical picture.

Combined mitral and aortic valve disease constitutes about 10% of cases of valvular disease. Such patients have hemodynamically significant disease of each valve. Predominant aortic and predominant mitral disease are about equal in frequency in combined lesions. Mitral stenosis decreases the apparent severity of aortic disease, particularly in aortic incompetence, and the combination of mitral stenosis and aortic incompetence is surprisingly well tolerated. After mitral stenosis has been relieved by valvotomy, aortic incompetence often appears to be more severe, and the presence by ECG or echocardiogram of left ventricular hypertrophy owing to aortic incompetence in a patient with predominant mitral stenosis is sufficient warning to warrant serious consideration of aortic valve replacement at the time of mitral valve surgery.

Mitral stenosis and aortic stenosis tend to mask one another, so that one or the other appears to be the dominant lesion clinically. The significance of the less dominant lesion is often underestimated. Severe aortic incompetence, because of rapid diastolic filling of the left ventricle, tends to mask the presence of severe mitral stenosis. Even at catheterization, the gradient across the mitral valve may be underestimated unless the patient is exercised. This shortens the diastolic filling period, raises the mitral diastolic gradient, and allows for a more accurate assessment of the severity of mitral stenosis.

When aortic valve disease is the major lesion, significant mitral incompetence is more serious than mitral stenosis. In either aortic stenosis or aortic incompetence, mitral incompetence is aggravated, and extreme cardiac enlargement and early heart failure are common.

Among the characteristic clinical pictures of combined valvular disease that should be mentioned is the combination of aortic stenosis with insignificant or mild mitral incompetence. This lesion gives rise to a characteristic high-pitched "seagull cry" murmur. In some cases, extension of aortic calcification into the aortic cusp of the mitral valve can be demonstrated. Combined mitral and aortic valve prolapse due to myxomatous degeneration can also occur, and infective endocarditis may also affect more than one valve.

Clinical Course of Combined Lesions

Patients with combined mitral and aortic valve lesions tend to be symptomatic at an earlier age than patients with single valve lesions. The heart is usually larger, and atrial fibrillation tends to develop at an earlier age. The disease of each valve is less advanced in combined lesions because the valvular lesions are additive.

Physical signs are more difficult to interpret in mixed lesions, and it is not always easy to distinguish the delayed diastolic or presystolic murmur of severe aortic incompetence (Austin Flint murmur) from the murmur of associated mitral stenosis. Similarly, an immediate basal diastolic murmur of pulmonary incompetence (Graham Steell murmur) in mitral stenosis with raised pulmonary vascular resistance can be confused with the murmur of associated aortic incompetence. In patients with predominant aortic valve disease, the distinction between functional and organic mitral incompetence is often difficult. In the presence of left heart failure, a systolic murmur of mitral incompetence is often found, but it may be difficult to distinguish from the aortic systolic murmur; in mixed mitral stenosis and incompetence, the organic nature of the systolic murmur can be more readily recognized. The development of echo-Doppler techniques has contributed greatly to the proper identification of combined lesions and to the assessment of their individual hemodynamic significance.

In combined aortic and mitral valve disease, either valve lesion may become acutely worse in the course of infective endocarditis. The presence of a chronic lesion of one valve exaggerates the effects of an acute lesion of the other valve. Infective endocarditis and systemic embolism are as common in combined aortic and mitral valve disease as they are in aortic or mitral incompetence alone.

Double Valve Replacement

Surgical replacement of both valves, or aortic valve replacement with mitral valvotomy, generally leads to less satisfactory results than single valve replacement. This is probably because more extensive myocardial disease may be present in patients with combined lesions. It may also be associated with increased myocardial damage referable to the longer pump times needed to repair multiple valve lesions. Simultaneous valve replacement is preferable to serial valve replacement, since the second cardiotomy is always more difficult than the first. The surgeon should have as much information as possible on which to base the decision whether to replace one valve or two, and full preoperative hemodynamic studies are mandatory. Long-term survival after double valve replacement is similar to that after single valve replacement. This may be because valve lesions are additive, and double valve replacement is therefore usually undertaken at an earlier stage of development of each individual valve lesion. A recent study of multiple valve operations with long-term follow-up in 513 patients reported a 12.5% overall hospital mortality rate and excellent improvement in functional capacity from 95% preoperative NYHA III and IV to 80% postoperative NYHA I and II. The 5-year rate of freedom from late combined valve-related morbidity and death was 72% (Galloway, 1992).

The management of patients with combined aortic and mitral valve lesions always presents problems because the cases are naturally more complex and different, and sufficient experience of treatment regimens is generally lacking.

Combined Mitral & Tricuspid Valve Disease

Functional tricuspid incompetence has already been mentioned as a common complication of mitral stenosis with raised pulmonary vascular resistance (Chapter 12). At surgery, if tricuspid regurgitation is significant, tricuspid ring annuloplasty is successful in eliminating or at least reducing the severity of the defect. It is rare that an artificial or biologic prosthetic valve is needed. In about 2% of patients with mitral valve disease, organic tricuspid valve disease is present and causes right heart failure. The mitral valve lesion is almost always mixed mitral stenosis and incompetence, and pulmonary vascular resistance is not greatly raised (average 2 mm Hg/L/min). An important clue to the presence of tricuspid valve disease is the increase in murmur that occurs with inspiration. This can be heard in about half of cases. Markedly raised systemic venous pressure (average 24 mm Hg), frequently with a large jugular venous *v* wave, is the most striking clinical feature, and cardiac enlargement is usually massive. But not as great as in giant left atrium. Low cardiac output and atrial fibrillation are almost inevitable, and the lesions tend to run a chronic course in which valve replacement provides less benefit than in disease of the mitral valve alone. Tricuspid stenosis is characterized by a rumbling diastolic murmur along the left sternal border similar to the diastolic murmur of mitral stenosis but heard at the apex. The murmur of tricuspid stenosis increases with inspiration. There may be a tricuspid opening snap. An additional clue is the presence of a large jugular venous *a* wave as the atrium contracts against the stenotic valve. Isolated rheumatic tricuspid valve disease without mitral valve involvement can theoretically occur, but it is rare enough to be of negligible importance.

Triple-Valve Disease

The remarks that have been made about double-valve disease are even more applicable to triple-valve disease, in which aortic, mitral, and tricuspid valves are involved. Since the lesions are additive, the results of surgery are never as satisfactory as in disease affecting a single valve. All artificial valves currently available are functionally inferior to a normal valve. The presence of three such valves in series in the heart is likely to cause a significant load on the myocardium and tends to make the prognosis worse and decrease the degree of functional improvement that the patient experiences after surgery.

CARCINOID VALVULAR HEART DISEASE

Carcinoid tumors that arise from the chromaffin tissue in the gastrointestinal tract—usually in the ileum—produce vasoactive substances such as serotonin, bradykinin, and tryptophan. These vasoactive substances cause endothelial damage to the right side of the heart, resulting in fibrosis and thickening of the heart valves. Tricuspid incompetence and, less frequently, pulmonary stenosis are the end results of the damage, which also affects the endocardium of the right atrium and ventricle. The primary tumors can be small, and hepatic metastases are almost invariably present in patients with cardiac involvement.

Clinical Findings

A. Symptoms: Patients with carcinoid syndrome complain of episodes of facial and upper trunk flushing in response to alcohol ingestion, eating, and emotional reactions. The release of vasoactive substances into the bloodstream is thought to be responsible. Abdominal pain, diarrhea, and renal and hepatic failure are also seen. Dyspnea is uncommon.

B. Signs: Hepatic enlargement and a peculiar violaceous color of the face and neck are often seen, and abdominal distention and ascites occur. The cardiac signs are not present in all cases. A systolic murmur of tricuspid incompetence is the commonest finding. It is louder on inspiration and often associated with *a* and *v* waves in the jugular venous pulse. A systolic ejection murmur due to pulmonary stenosis is less common, and diastolic murmurs are a late manifestation. Frank right heart failure with edema appears late

in the disease and may be difficult to assess in the presence of severe hepatic involvement.

C. Electrocardiographic Findings: P wave abnormalities are usually all that are seen, and right ventricular hypertrophy is rare.

D. Imaging Studies: Dilation of the right heart seen on x-ray occurs late in the disease. Echocardiography is helpful in detecting valve lesions. Doppler techniques can detect and help quantify the degree of tricuspid regurgitation or pulmonary valve stenosis. Cardiac catheterization is seldom indicated, because the cardiac involvement is usually not severe. Liver scans may reveal defects from metastases.

E. Laboratory Findings: The diagnosis of carcinoid tumor is established by finding 5-hydroxyindoleacetic acid in the urine. It is a metabolic product of serotonin. A value of more than 25 ng/24 h is considered diagnostic and usually implies hepatic metastases. An amount exceeding 200 ng/24 h is usually found in patients with cardiac involvement. A variety of foods (bananas, apples) and drugs (phenothiazines) may cause false-positive reactions.

Biopsy of the liver or the primary tumor shows the characteristic histologic findings.

Differential Diagnosis

Isolated tricuspid incompetence is rare in rheumatic heart disease. Infective endocarditis involving the tricuspid valve, restrictive right-sided cardiomyopathy, and tumor involving the right atrium are the most important differential diagnostic problems.

Course & Complications

The tumor grows slowly in most cases, although it metastasizes early. The cardiac manifestations rarely cause serious problems but can progress to the stage at which valve replacement must be considered. Atrial fibrillation may occur in severe cases. In some patients the vasoactive substances are not inactivated in the lungs, and left-sided lesions have been reported.

Treatment

Resection of the primary tumor is the most helpful procedure. Chemotherapy with cytotoxic drugs (eg, cyclophosphamide) is used to treat hepatic metastases. Various serotonin antagonists (eg, methysergide) have been used to treat the flushing attacks, with generally disappointing results. Phenothiazines have been useful in some cases. Digitalis and diuretics are used for the treatment of right heart failure, and tricuspid or pulmonary valve replacement is seldom needed.

Prognosis

The disease is more slowly progressive than might be expected, and survival for 5–10 years after the initial symptoms develop is not uncommon. The cardiac involvement seldom influences the prognosis, which depends on the hepatic metastases.

IATROGENICALLY MODIFIED VALVULAR HEART DISEASE

1. MITRAL VALVOTOMY

Mitral commissurotomy is an important iatrogenic factor modifying the course of valvular heart disease. Even relatively ineffective closed mitral valvotomy is capable of influencing the clinical course of mitral stenosis. The operation is palliative rather than curative, and in 2–15 years after valvotomy the patient is likely to experience a recurrence of dyspnea. With open mitral valvuloplasty, there is a good long-term prognosis, ie, a period of 10–20 years without symptoms and no need for reoperation. If the patient can be returned to normal sinus rhythm and remains in sinus rhythm, the incidence of emboli also is decreased. In some cases (about 20%), a second valvotomy is performed, but in most cases mitral valve replacement is necessary at the second operation.

Clinical Findings

A. Symptoms: In patients who have had a previous mitral valvotomy, symptoms are difficult to assess. Dyspnea is the commonest symptom, and, as in all patients with mitral valve disease, the relation between the onset of atrial fibrillation and the onset of dyspnea is of prime importance. A clinical picture resembling that of mixed mitral valve disease is common. Patients who have gained relief through mitral valvotomy are likely to experience a significant increase in dyspnea when atrial fibrillation occurs. There is often a relationship between the length of the asymptomatic interval following valvotomy and the age of the patient. A woman who has had a mitral valvotomy in her 20s is likely to have 15 symptom-free years before atrial fibrillation develops, whereas a 35-year-old woman is likely to develop atrial fibrillation within about 5 years of operation.

B. Signs: The physical signs in iatrogenically modified cases usually reflect the preoperative findings. A loud opening snap and loud first heart sound are often present, and the timing of the opening snap reflects the preoperative and not the postoperative status of the patient. In such cases, the length of the diastolic murmur measured at the bedside becomes the best indicator of the severity of stenosis. A systolic murmur may appear after surgery, but, as is the case in patients who have not undergone operation, its significance is open to question, and other clinical evidence of mitral incompetence must always be sought.

C. Electrocardiographic Findings: In a few cases, regression of the changes of right ventricular hypertrophy is seen, but in most patients the ECG shows little change from the preoperative tracing. Sooner or later, atrial fibrillation will almost certainly develop.

D. Imaging Studies: The absence of the left atrial appendage as a bulge on the left heart border on x-ray is a characteristic finding in patients who have undergone operation (Figure 13–19). If the pulmonary artery was enlarged before operation, it seldom returns to normal size, and the same is true of the left atrium. Changes in the degree of pulmonary congestion are perhaps the best indicators of the success of surgical treatment.

Exercise testing and echocardiography are helpful noninvasive techniques used in screening patients to decide whether they should undergo catheterization again. However, Doppler echocardiographic findings tend to be influenced by the preoperative status of the valve. Doppler studies are helpful in estimating the severity of any residual mitral valve gradient. By the continuity equation, mitral valve area can be estimated. Cardiac catheterization, with measurement of the wedge pressure, left ventricular pressure, and cardiac output, provides the best objective evidence of the patients' postoperative status. It is thus highly advantageous to have a preoperative study available for comparison. The decision to perform a second operation is important, since the chances are high (80%) that valve replacement will be needed at that time.

Treatment

Almost all patients who have had mitral valvotomy ultimately require valve replacement. Temporizing with a second valvotomy is generally attempted when the valve is flexible and shows little or no calcification.

2. PATIENTS WITH ARTIFICIAL VALVES

Patients who have had mitral or aortic valve replacement are becoming more common in everyday medical practice. In the past, the largest number of such patients have Starr-Edwards ball and cage prostheses. Other forms of plastic and metal valves, such as the Björk-Shiley disk valve (now withdrawn because of strut fracture), the St. Jude bileaflet valve, and homograft or heterograft (Hancock and Carpenter-Edwards) tissue valves are also used.

The clinical picture in patients who have had valve replacement varies greatly and depends on the type of valve used, the nature of the original lesion, the stage at which operation was performed, and the success of the operation. Few patients are free of symptoms; the problems encountered are most commonly related to thrombosis, embolism, valve dehiscence, leakage or

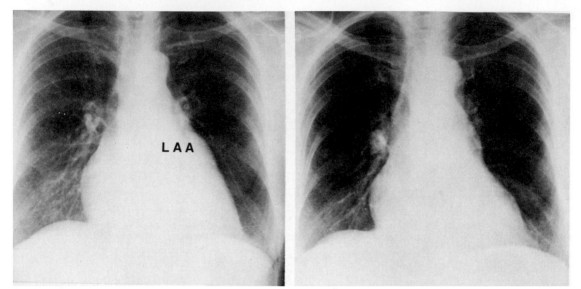

Figure 13–19. Preoperative and postoperative chest x-rays of a patient with mitral stenosis. The left atrial appendage (LAA) has been resected.

obstruction of the valve, infective endocarditis, hemolysis, and hemorrhage from excessive anticoagulant therapy.

A late form of iatrogenically modified mitral valve disease occurs after mitral valve replacement. Pulmonary vascular disease is occasionally partially irreversible, and when its development is arrested, cardiac function often continues to deteriorate as degenerative age-related changes occur. Patients with raised pulmonary vascular resistance often develop chronic severe right heart failure that responds poorly to treatment. In such cases, left ventricular failure may also be present, as shown by a rise in end-diastolic left ventricular pressure. Patients with such lesions are usually subjected to investigation in the hope of finding some surgically treatable lesion, but in practice they are usually exhibiting the long-term effects of rheumatic carditis, poor preservation of myocardium at surgery, or excessive delay of operation.

Clinical Findings

A. Symptoms: Many patients with artificial valves have residual shortness of breath on exertion. Most have at least a small pressure gradient across the valve at rest that becomes larger when the cardiac output and heart rate increase during exercise. The patient may also complain of the loud noise made by the artificial valve as it opens and closes with each heartbeat, but most patients become accustomed to the sensation within a few weeks after operation. This is less common in valves other than Starr-Edwards.

B. Signs: The physical signs arising from an artificial valve depend on the nature and type of valve used. Tissue valves do not give rise to the loud open-

ing and closing clicks heard with metal and plastic prostheses. However, they do tend to leak with the passage of time as the tissue stiffens and calcifies or tears. Thus, mitral systolic and aortic diastolic murmurs are not uncommon. The opening and closing clicks of plastic and metal valves are characteristic for each individual brand of valve. In general, there is a loud opening click at the start of systole and a loud closing click at the end of systole. The clicks are usually louder than the normal heart sounds and interfere with auscultation of natural valves. Diastolic murmurs are abnormal in patients with tissue valves—the longer the murmur, the greater its significance. Systolic and diastolic murmurs are difficult to interpret in patients with artificial valves, and more importance should be given to changes in the auscultatory findings than to the findings themselves.

C. Electrocardiographic Findings: There are no characteristic electrocardiographic changes in patients with artificial heart valves.

D. Imaging Studies: Artificial heart valves composed of metal are clearly seen on chest x-rays, and each has a characteristic shape. The opaque plastic ball can usually be seen moving up and down with the heartbeat on cinefluoroscopy. The position of the artificial valve varies considerably from case to case, and a change in the position of the valve or in its movement during the cardiac cycle is important evidence of valvular dysfunction. Tissue valves may calcify with time and become visible on the chest x-ray.

1. Noninvasive techniques– Because plastic and metal valves reflect ultrasound well, they are readily detected by echocardiography. However, it is difficult to determine valve function by this means of study. Doppler techniques offer a better indication of valve function. Transesophageal echocardiography has been a major advance in the evaluation of patients with prosthetic valves. Transthoracic echocardiography results in a high degree of reflectance and of echoes off the metal of the valve, and so there is difficulty imaging behind the metal valve in the left atrium. With transesophageal echocardiography, the echoes come from the esophagus, directed anteriorly imaging the left atrium, the prosthetic valve, and the aortic valve wall. The mitral valve, the aortic ring, the outflow tract of the left ventricle, and the mitral prosthetic valve are all well visualized. Because there are sufficient echoes posterior to the prosthetic valve, detection of valvular and paravalvular insufficiency and thrombus is far better than with transthoracic echocardiography.

2. Invasive techniques– Cardiac catheterization and angiography are usually needed to decide whether prosthetic valve malfunction is severe enough to warrant reoperation. Most physicians carefully avoid passing a catheter through a prosthetic valve for fear of causing damage or dislodging a leaflet. When catheters have been inadvertently passed through artificial valves, little ill effect has been noticed. The most important information sought in studies of patients with artificial valves is the pressure difference across the valve and the flow through it. Angiography is commonly used to test for valvular incompetence.

Particular problems arise in the investigation of patients with combined mitral and aortic valve replacement. Retrograde catheterization of the left ventricle with passage of a catheter across the artificial aortic valve is not recommended. In addition to the possibility of damage to the valve, the fact that leakage of the valve caused by the presence of the catheter may disturb the hemodynamic pattern contraindicates this approach. The only alternative is direct left ventricular puncture. If angiography is essential, a short angiocatheter may be used, placed percutaneously in the left ventricle. This is now rarely needed with transesophageal echocardiography.

Differential Diagnosis

The principal problem in differential diagnosis is distinguishing artificial valve malfunction from disease of another valve.

Long-Term Results
& Complications

The long-term results of valve replacement depend to a considerable extent on the type of valve used—prosthetic versus homograft and xenograft. Data for Starr-Edwards ball and cage valves are now available for 20 years, while the commonest other prosthetic valve—the Björk-Shiley disk valve—has been in use for about 15 years and the St. Jude valve for 5–10 years. The several other types of prosthetic valves that have been introduced have either been abandoned or not used widely enough to generate adequate follow-up data. Data for tissue valves are also available for almost 30 years, but only in small numbers of patients with aortic homografts. The results with porcine xenografts (Hancock and Carpenter-Edwards valves) now cover about 20 years and those for the Ionescu-Shiley valve made of glutaraldehyde-treated pericardial tissue a slightly shorter time.

A. Prosthetic Valves: The principal problem with prosthetic valves has always been thromboembolism. Anticoagulation with coumarin anticoagulants is essential, and in spite of this therapy the incidence of thromboembolism is about 4% per patient year in mitral valve replacement and 1–2% in aortic valve replacement. About half of the emboli are serious—ie, cause a stroke, hematuria, or a painful cold limb. The incidence of embolism has tended to remain constant over the years of follow-up, and sudden cessation of anticoagulation is particularly likely to result in a "rebound" hypercoagulable state. The durability of the Starr-Edwards valve is well established now that problems related to ball variance have been dealt with. The Björk-Shiley valve provided a slightly larger area for flow and had similar thrombogenic characteristics. It has now been withdrawn because of the frequency of fractures of the downstream struts, particularly with the largest valves.

Valve failure does occur with prosthetic valves, which may stick either in the open or the closed position, especially when thrombus or pannus grows into the valve. This form of valve failure is more likely in the mitral than in the aortic position and can occur abruptly without warning. Both survival and maintenance of adequate valve function are more likely in the aortic than in the mitral position, probably because there is less stasis in the neighborhood of the aortic valve.

B. Tissue Valves: The principal advantage of a tissue valve is that anticoagulation is not required, except in patients in atrial fibrillation after mitral valve replacement and for the first few months after insertion. Thromboembolism still occurs, but less commonly than with prosthetic valves. Tissue valves are preferable, therefore, in people in whom anticoagulation is undesirable or difficult, such as in women who want to become pregnant, in which case coumarin anticoagulation is contraindicated. The tendency for tissue valves to stiffen, calcify, leak, and cause obstruction to flow detracts from their overall durability. This tendency was most marked in formaldehyde-treated freeze-dried aortic homografts. While the results with glutaraldehyde-treated porcine xenograft (Hancock) valves were encouraging after 4 years of follow-up, longer-term studies have shown that late failure between 5 and 10 years is an important problem. One advantage of tissue valves is that their failure occurs relatively slowly, and an increase in symptoms, with changes in the physical signs and often calcification of the valve, makes it possible to recognize the problem and replace the valve. Aortic valve homografts are more technically demanding to place, and availability is limited. However, 20 years of follow-up showed a 67% freedom from valve-related deaths. There was only one thromboembolic episode in 555 patients, and none in patients receiving anticoagulants. These results are superior to those achieved with any other tissue or mechanical valve (Matsuki, 1988). Calcification and valve failure occur rapidly in patients in whom calcium and phosphorus metabolism is active. Therefore, tissue valves should not be used in children or in patients with chronic renal failure. Since valve failure and therefore reoperation after 10–15 years are inevitable, tissue valves should not be used in most young patients but should be reserved for elderly patients, for whom the advantage of not needing anticoagulation makes them most desirable.

C. Infective Endocarditis: Infective endocarditis involving an artificial valve is an unusual but dangerous complication, occurring at a rate of about 0.5–1% per patient year with all types of valve (see Chapter 16). The later the infection occurs after surgery, the better the chance of cure with antibiotic therapy. Endocarditis involving tissue valves may be curable without replacing the valve, but if the infection occurs on a prosthetic valve, a second operation is almost inevitable except in patients with endocarditis caused by very sensitive pathogens. The mortality rate of endocarditis on an artificial valve approaches 30–50%, and since the complication is so serious, antibiotic coverage for major dental work and other minor surgical procedures is highly important.

D. Hemolysis: Hemolysis due to trauma to red cells is virtually confined to patients with prosthetic valves. An elevated serum LDH concentration is seen in most patients with prosthetic valves. It is seldom a serious problem but is more likely to occur after multiple valve replacement. Perivalvular leak is likely to aggravate hemolysis, which should be suspected in any patient with anemia.

E. Hemorrhage From Anticoagulant Therapy: Long-term anticoagulation with warfarin is not without its complications, especially in older patients. Hemorrhage, particularly from the gut, requires thorough investigation, looking for peptic ulceration, carcinoma of the colon, and other noncardiac lesions. Similarly, hematuria and hemoptysis and in fact hemorrhage from any site require full investigation before the conclusion that the anticoagulant therapy is responsible can be justified. It is inadvisable to stop anticoagulant therapy suddenly or completely, but reduction in the dose of anticoagulant, with close monitoring of the prothrombin level, is essential. With realization that the change from human brain to rabbit brain thromboplastin was the reason for excessive anticoagulation and the introduction of International Normalized Ratio (INR) reporting of prothrombin times, there has been a reduction in the incidence of serious bleeding in anticoagulated patients. At present, with prosthetic valves, maintenance of a prothrombin time of 3–4 INR is recommended. Anticoagulant therapy with warfarin may have to be stopped and therapy with heparin started about 6 hours before noncardiac surgery. Warfarin may then be resumed as soon after surgery as the postoperative threat of hemorrhage permits. In the patient with a prosthetic valve who becomes pregnant, warfarin is contraindicated—especially in the first and third trimesters—because of its effects on the fetus. Therefore, when pregnancy is recognized, the patient must be maintained on depot subcutaneous heparin injections every 12 hours throughout pregnancy, since heparin does not cross the placental barrier.

F. Thromboembolism: Thrombosis around the artificial valve, with consequent stenosis and systemic embolism, is the commonest complication of artificial valves. Anticoagulant therapy is needed in all types of valves except tissue valves. When thrombus forms around a prosthetic valve, it may disturb valve function and interfere with both the opening and the closing of the valve. In some cases, especially early after operation, valve displacement due to tearing out of the sutures anchoring the valve leads to paravalvular leak. In other cases the valve mechanism itself may fail and cause leakage. Sudden death is still an important complication of valve replacement. The mechanism is not always clear, but escape of a worn ball from the cage mechanism has been reported. In other cases, the valve mechanism sticks shut. Most cases of sudden death are probably related to malignant ventricular arrhythmias, presumably caused by fibrosis in the ventricle.

Treatment

A second valve replacement is the only effective therapy for artificial valve malfunction. Both the patient and the physician are naturally reluctant to take this major step, and clear evidence of malfunction is required before a second artificial valve is inserted. In some cases, one of the natural valves proves to be the cause of the problem and needs replacement.

Prognosis

The long-term prognosis of patients with artificial valves is not yet established. In the age group in which valve replacement usually occurs, the late linear mortality rate is about 3% per year, with a significant incidence of 3% per year of late morbidity from thromboembolism, infection, valve disruption, and other frequently valve-related events.

REFERENCES

General

Cheitlin MD et al: Task Force II: Acquired valvular heart disease. J Am Coll Cardiol 1985;6:1209.

Cohn LH: Valvular surgery. Curr Opin Cardiol 1991;6:235.

Cosh JA, Lever JY: The aortic valve. Cardiovasc Rev Rep 1985;6:743.

Mann DL: Pathophysiology of valvular heart disease: Basic mechanisms. Curr Opin Cardiol 1991;6:191.

Morrison GW et al: Incidence of coronary artery disease in patients with valvular heart disease. Br Heart J 1980;44:630.

Mullany CJ et al: Coronary artery disease and its management: Influence on survival in patients undergoing aortic valve replacement. J Am Coll Cardiol 1987;10:66.

Rahimtoola SH: Perspective of valvular heart disease: An update. J Am Coll Cardiol 1989;14:1.

Shah PM et al: Echocardiography in valvular heart disease. Curr Opin Cardiol 1990;5:157.

Terdjman M et al: Aneurysms of sinus of Valsalva: Two-dimensional echocardiographic diagnosis and recognition of rupture into right heart cavities. J Am Coll Cardiol 1984;3:1227.

Thompson R, Ross I, Elmes R: Quantification of valvular regurgitation by cardiac gated pool imaging. Br Heart J 1981;46:629.

Aortic Stenosis

Cheitlin MD et al: The distribution of fibrosis in left ventricle in congenital aortic stenosis and coarctation of the aorta. Circulation 1978(Suppl II)58:243.

Cheitlin MD et al: Rate of progression of severity of valvular aortic stenosis in the adult. Am Heart J 1988;61:123.

Come PC et al: Prediction of severity of aortic stenosis: Accuracy of multiple noninvasive parameters. Am J Med 1988;85:29.

Currie PJ et al: Continuous-wave Doppler echocardiographic assessment of severity of calcific aortic stenosis: A simultaneous Doppler-catheter correlative study in 100 adult patients. Circulation 1985;71:1162.

Exadactylos N, Ugrue DD, Oakley CM: Prevalence of coronary artery disease in patients with isolated aortic valve stenosis. Br Heart J 1984;51:121.

Horstkotte D, Loogan F: The natural history of aortic valve stenosis. Eur Heart J 1988;9(Suppl):57.

Hsieh K et al: Long-term follow-up of valvotomy before 1968 for congenital aortic stenosis. Am J Cardiol 1986;58:338.

Kelly TA et al: Comparison of outcome of asymptomatic to symptomatic patients older than 20 years of age with valvular aortic stenosis. Am J Cardiol 1988;61:123.

McKay RG et al: Balloon dilatation of calcific aortic stenosis in elderly patients: Postmortem, intraoperative, and percutaneous valvuloplasty studies. Circulation 1986;74:119.

McKenney PA et al: Echocardiographic frequency and severity of aortic regurgitation after ultrasonic aortic valve debridement for aortic stenosis in persons aged greater than 65 years. Am J Cardiol 1992;70:125.

Monrad ES et al: Time course of regression of left ventricular hypertrophy after aortic valve replacement. Circulation 1988;77:1345.

Murphy ES et al: Severe aortic stenosis in patients 60 years of age and older: Left ventricular function and 10 year survival after valve replacement. Circulation 1981;64(Suppl 2):184.

Nair CK et al: Cardiac conduction defects in patients older than 60 years with aortic stenosis with and without mitral anular calcium. Am J Cardiol 1984;54:169.

Nishimura RA et al: Doppler echocardiographic observations during percutaneous aortic balloon valvuloplasty. J Am Coll Cardiol 1988;11:1219.

Reis RL et al: Congenital fixed subvalvular aortic stenosis. Circulation 1971;43(Suppl 1):11.

Roger VL et al: Progression of aortic stenosis in adults: New appraisal using Doppler echocardiography. Am Heart J 1990;119:331.

Safian RD et al: Balloon aortic valvuloplasty in 170 consecutive patients N Engl J Med 1988;319:125.

Villan B et al: Effect of aortic valve stenosis (pressure overload) and regurgitation (volume overload) on left ventricular systolic and diastolic function. Am J Cardiol 1992;69:927.

Wagner S, Selzer A: Patterns of progression of aortic stenosis: A longitudinal hemodynamic study. Circulation 1982;65:709.

Wood P: Aortic stenosis. Am J Cardiol 1981:553.

Cribier A, Letac B: Percutaneous balloon aortic valvuloplasty in adults with calcific aortic stenosis. Curr Opin Cardiol 1991;6:212.

Pellikka PA et al: The natural history of adults with asymptomatic, hemodynamically significant aortic stenosis. J Am Coll Cardiol 1990;15:1012.

Roger FL et al: Progression of aortic stenosis in adults: New appraisal using Doppler echocardiography. Am Heart J 1990;119:331.

Aortic Incompetence

Bonow RO et al: The natural history of asymptomatic patients with aortic regurgitation and normal left ventricular function. Circulation 1983;68:509.

Bouchard A et al: Value of color Doppler estimation of regurgitated volume in patients with chronic aortic insufficiency. Am Heart J 1989;117:1099.

David TE et al: Heart valve operation in patients with acute infective endocarditis. Ann Thorac Surg 1990;49:701.

Dumesnil JG: Beneficial long-term effects of hydralazine in aortic regurgitation. Ann Intern Med 1990;150:757.

Fioretti P et al: Postoperative regression of left ventricular dimensions in aortic insufficiency: A long-term echocardiographic study. J Am Coll Cardiol 1985;5:856.

Greenberg B et al: Long-term vasodilator therapy of chronic aortic insufficiency. Circulation 1988;78:92.

Huxley RL et al: Early detection of left ventricular dysfunction in chronic aortic regurgitation as assessed by contrast angiography, echocardiography, and rest and exercise scintigraphy. Am J Cardiol 1983;51:1542.

Karalis DG: Transesophageal echocardiographic recog-

nition of subaortic complications in aortic valve endocarditis: Clinical and surgical implications. Circulation 1992;86:353.

Landzberg JS et al: Etiology of the Austin Flint murmur.
J Am Coll Cardiol 1992;20:408.

Massie BM et al: Ejection fraction response to supine
exercise in asymptomatic aortic regurgitation: Relation to simultaneous hemodynamic measurements. J
Am Coll Cardiol 1985;5:847.

Rahimtoola SH: Vasodilator therapy in chronic severe
aortic regurgitation. (Editorial.) J Am Coll Cardiol
1990;16:430.

Roberts WC, Day PJ: Electrocardiographic observations
in clinically isolated, pure, chronic, severe aortic regurgitation: Analysis of 30 necropsy patients aged 19
to 65 years. Am J Cardiol 1985;55:431.

Roman MJ et al: Reversal of left ventricular dilatation,
hypertrophy, and dysfunction by valve replacement in
aortic regurgitation. Am Heart J 1989;118:553.

Russell RO Jr: Timing of aortic valve replacement in
chronic aortic valve regurgitation. (Editorial.) J Am
Coll Cardiol 1988;11:930.

Shen WF et al: Evaluation of relationship between myocardial contractile state and left ventricular function in
patients with aortic regurgitation. Circulation 1985;71:
31.

Scognamiglio R et al: Long-term nifedipine therapy in
asymptomatic patients with chronic severe aortic regurgitation. J Am Coll Cardiol 1990;16:424.

Prosthetic Valves

Galloway AC et al: Ten-year experience with aortic valve
replacement in 482 patients 70 years of age or older:
Operative risk and long-term results. Ann Thorac
Surg 1990;49:84.

Grunkemeier GL, Rahimtoola SH: Artificial heart
valves. Annu Rev Med 1990;41:251.

Jameson WRE et al: The Carpentier-Edwards standard
porcine bioprosthesis. J Thorac Cardiovasc Surg
1990;99:543.

Jones EL et al: Ten-year experience with the porcine
bioprosthetic valve: Interrelationship of valve survival
and patient survival in 1,050 valve replacements. Ann
Thorac Surg 1990;49:370.

Matsuki O et al: Long-term performance of 555 aortic
homografts in the aortic position. Ann Thorac Surg
1988;46:187.

Nair CK et al: Ten-year results with the St Jude Medical
Prosthesis. Am J Cardiol 1990;65:217.

Nellessen U et al: Transesophageal two-dimensional
echocardiography and color Doppler flow velocity
mapping in the evaluation of cardiac valve prosthesis.
Circulation 1988;78:848.

Multiple Valve Disease

Galloway AC et al: Multiple valve operation for advanced valvular heart disease: Results and risk factors
in 513 patients. J Am Coll Cardiol 1992;19:725.

Gash AK et al: Left ventricular performance in patients
with coexistent mitral stenosis and aortic insufficiency. J Am Coll Cardiol 1984;3:703.

Gersh BJ et al: Results of triple valve replacement in
91 patients: Perioperative mortality and long-term
follow-up. Circulation 1985;72:130.

Herrera CJ et al: Value and limitations of transesophageal

echocardiography in evaluating prosthetic or bioprosthetic valve dysfunction. Am J Cardiol 1992;69:
697.

McGrath LB: Tricuspid valve operations in 530 patients:
Twenty-five year assessment of early and late phase
events. J Thorac Cardiovasc Surg 1990;99:124.

McGrath LB et al: Tricuspid valve operations in 530
patients: Twenty-five-year assessment of early and
late phase events. J Thorac Cardiovasc Surg 1990;49:
124.

Wong M et al: The value of Doppler echocardiography in
the treatment of tricuspid regurgitation in patients
with mitral valve replacement: Perspective and two-
year postoperative findings. J Thorac Cardiovasc Surg
1990;99:1003.

Carcinoid Valve Disease

Himelman RB, Schiller NB: Clinical and echocardiographic comparison of patients with the carcinoid
syndrome with and without carcinoid heart disease.
Am J Cardiol 1989;63:347.

Lundin L et al: Carcinoid heart disease: Relationship
of circulating vasoactive substances to ultrasound-
detectable cardiac abnormalities. Circulation 1988;77:
264.

Reid CL et al: Echocardiographic features of carcinoid
heart disease. Am Heart J 1984;107:801.

Artificial Valves

Blackstone EH, Kirklin JW: Death and other time-
related events after valve replacement. Circulation
1985;72:753.

Calderwood SB et al: Risk factors for the development of
prosthetic valve endocarditis. Circulation 1985;72:31.

Cohn LH et al: Five to eight-year follow-up of patients
undergoing porcine heart-valve replacement. N Engl J
Med 1981;304:258.

Cunha CLP et al: Echophonocardiographic findings in
patients with prosthetic heart valve malfunction.
Mayo Clin Proc 1980;55:231.

Forman R, Firth BG, Barnard MS: Prognostic significance of preoperative left ventricular ejection fraction
and valve lesion in patients with aortic valve replacement. Am J Cardiol 1980;45:1120.

Gersh BJ et al: Results of triple valve replacement in
91 patients: Perioperative mortality and long-term
follow-up. Circulation 1985;72:130.

Ivert TSA et al: Prosthetic valve endocarditis. Circulation 1984;69:223.

Jaffe WM et al: Infective endocarditis, 1983–1988:
Echocardiographic findings as factors influencing
mortality. J Am Coll Cardiol 1990;15:1227.

Kotler MN et al: Noninvasive evaluation of normal and
abnormal prosthetic valve function. J Am Coll Cardiol 1983;2:151.

Lakier JB et al: Porcine xenograft valves; Long-term
(60–80 month) follow-up. Circulation 1980;62:513.

Lytle BW et al: Replacement of aortic valve combined
with myocardial revascularization: Determinants of
early and late risk for 500 patients, 1967–1981. Circulation 1983;68:1149.

McClung JA et al: Prosthetic heart valves: A review.
Prog Cardiovasc Dis 1983;26:237.

McGoon MD et al: Aortic and mitral valve incompetence: Long-term follow-up (10 to 19 years) of pa-

tients treated with the Starr-Edwards prosthesis. Circulation 1984;3:930.

Mehlman DJ: A guide to the radiographic identification of prosthetic heart valves: An addendum. Circulation 1984;69:102.

Penta A et al: Patient status 10 or more years after "fresh" homograft replacement of the aortic valve. Circulation 1984;70(Suppl 1):182.

Santinga JT et al: Factors relating to late sudden death in patients having aortic valve replacement. Ann Thorac Surg 1980;29:249.

Saour JN et al: Trial of different intensities of anticoagulation in patients with prosthetic heart valves. N Engl J Med 1990;322:428.

Sareli P et al: Maternal and fetal sequelae and anticoagulation during pregnancy in patients with mechanical heart valves prostheses. Am J Cardiol 1989;63:1462.

Siemienczuk D et al: Chronic aortic insufficiency: Factors associated with progression to aortic valve replacement. Ann Intern Med 1989;110:587.

Starr A: The Starr-Edwards valve. J Am Coll Cardiol 1985;6:899.

14

Conduction Defects

ELECTROPHYSIOLOGY

Our understanding of disorders of the formation (initiation) and conduction (transmission) of the electrical impulse of the heart is based on the descriptions of electrophysiologic events in Chapter 1. In this and the next chapter (Cardiac Arrhythmias), we describe disturbances in the electrical activity of the heart manifested by electrocardiographic changes and by symptoms and signs of heart disease. See Chapter 7 for further discussion of pacemakers.

The Cell Membrane Basis for Excitability & Repolarization (Adapted from Fitzgerald, 1991)

The myocardial cell in the resting state has an electrical potential across the cell membrane of approximately −90 mV compared with the extracellular space. Excitation of myocardial cells generates an action potential in response to an adequate (threshold) stimulus (Fozzard, 1977).

The electrical potential that exists for cell membranes is generated by a fundamental property of the membrane, ie, the capacity to restrict movements of ions between the extracellular and intracellular spaces. This regulation of ionic movements is accomplished through "ion channels"—protein channels within the phospholipid bilayer of the cell membrane. The energy driving ionic movement is generated by electrical voltage and ion concentration gradients and is modulated by messengers that allow selective transport of ions. In this way, ionic gradients across the cell membrane are maintained, and ionic movement across the membrane form the basis for excitation and recovery or repolarization. Natural mediators such as catecholamines, autonomic stimulation, and antiarrhythmic drugs work via changes in ion movements through these channels.

The intracellular cytosol contains large organic molecules, mainly structural proteins that have a negative charge (anions) and which cannot cross the cell membrane. This negative charge is counterbalanced by positively charged ions (cations) and thus maintain electrical neutrality within the cell. The main cations in the intracellular space are K^+ and in the extracellular space Na^+.

The resting cell membrane has a very low conductance for Na^+, and any leak of Na^+ into the cell activates an energy-consuming Na^+-K^+ "ion pump" in the cell membrane that exchanges three Na^+ for two K^+. This pump keeps the intracellular K^+ high and the Na^+ low, maintaining an osmotic balance between the inside and outside environments. This also creates a large K^+ concentration gradient across the cell membrane, and K^+ is distributed through concentration gradient and electrical forces in such a way that electrochemical equilibrium is maintained and the electrical potential difference across the cell membrane is about −90 mV.

If an appropriate stimulus reduces the negativity of the membrane to threshold level, activation of ion channels produces rapid depolarization, later followed by a slower reconstitution of the resting membrane potential called **repolarization.**

In cardiac muscle there are two types of depolarization, one considerably faster than the other. The fast channel is found in the cell membrane of the atrial cells, the His-Purkinje system, and the ventricular cells, which have a transmembrane resting potential of −80 mV to −90 mV. An appropriate stimulus depolarizes the cell membrane to the threshold of the Na^+ channel (−60 mV). The Na^+ channels open, and a rapid influx of Na^+ occurs powered by the Na^+ concentration gradient. This phase 0 of the action potential (Figure 1–17) has a maximum velocity of 100–150 V/s, and in 1–5 ms the transmembrane potential goes from −90 mV to +30 mV.

As the membrane potential becomes more positive, Na^+ conductance decreases, Ca^{2+} channels open, and a slower Ca^{2+} current enters the cell. Inactivation of the Na^+ current and perhaps a small outward current causes a short period of repolarization (phase 1), bringing the membrane potential from +30 mV toward 0 mV.

Phase 2 of the action potential is due to a decrease in K^+ conductance out of the cell and incomplete inactivation of the inward Ca^{2+} current, resulting in an equilibrium phase near zero potential lasting 100 ms. Later, K^+ channels open, causing outward flow of K^+ impelled by the concentration gradient, which results in repolarization (phase 3), bringing the resting membrane potential back to −90 mV (phase 4). Thereafter, there is restoration of the resting membrane ionic distribution with Na^+ pumped out of the cell in exchange for K^+.

These "slow" action potentials are found in sinoatrial and atrioventricular nodes. The resting membrane potential in these cells is −50 mV to −70 mV.

The upstroke of the action potential is mediated by the slow inward Ca^{2+} current with a threshold of –50 mV to –40 mV and an upstroke velocity of 1–15 V/s. Phase 1 is absent, and phase 2 is abbreviated. Phase 4 consists of a spontaneous diastolic depolarization, producing the property of automaticity.

Voltage clamp experiments have demonstrated several K^+ currents. In sinus nodal tissue, there is a time- and voltage-dependent outward K^+ current activated on depolarization beyond –50 mV, which is important for repolarization of the action potential. A gradual decay in this current leads to intracellular accumulation of K^+ in the cell. There are also two separate components to the slow inward Ca^{2+} current, one flowing through L-type channels and activated at –40 mV, probably responsible for the action potential upstroke of the nodal cells. A second, lower threshold Ca^{2+} current, activated at –50 mV, is identified in atrial and ventricular cells. These channels are identified by being blocked by different chemicals, eg, L-type channels are blocked by nifedipine, whereas both Ca^{2+} channels are blocked by cadmium.

There is an inward current, identified when the sinoatrial cells are hyperpolarized from –100 mV to –90 mV. This is a nonspecific channel, carrying either Na^+ or K^+ augmented by catecholamines, which may be important in the sinoatrial node when there is increased adrenergic tone. There is a potential background inward current leak, possibly of Na^+, which tends to raise the resting membrane potential toward threshold. Whether this occurs through specific ion channels, via an electrogenic ion pump, or through the lipid part of the membrane is not known, nor is it known what role this current plays in pacemaker activity.

The pacemaker current therefore probably results via interaction of several ionic currents through several channels. It results from a slow decay in outward K^+ conductance in diastole, causing a rise in membrane potential. At less negative membrane potentials, other ion channels are activated, further raising the membrane potential to threshold.

Electrical Properties of Cardiac Cells

Understanding disorders of conduction and cardiac rhythm requires knowledge of the inherent properties of cardiac tissue—automaticity, excitability and refractoriness, conductivity, and the capacity for re-entry.

The sinoatrial node (sinus node) is a small group of cells situated at the junction of the superior vena cava and the right atrium that initiates the cardiac impulse and results in normal sinus rhythm (see Figure 1–16). Spread of the impulse as it passes through the heart is represented on the ECG as the P wave, QRS complex, ST segment, and T wave. Normally, the heart rate is determined by the rate of diastolic depolariza-

tion of the sinoatrial nodal cells, as shown by the degree of the phase 4 slope (see Figures 1–18 and 1–19). The sinoatrial node is under the influence of the autonomic nervous system; stimulation of the vagus nerve, either spontaneously, by reflex, or by drugs, slows the heart rate, decreasing the slope of phase 4. Sympathetic cardiac stimulation by drugs or via the central nervous system directly or reflexly increases the heart rate and increases the slope of phase 4.

A. Automaticity: All cardiac cells possess the capacity to beat spontaneously. Certain cells of the specialized conduction system are able to initiate an action potential that sequentially activates the entire heart; this capability is known as automaticity. Automaticity is most marked in the sinoatrial nodal cells, as shown by the steepest phase 4 slope of any of the specialized cardiac cells, and these cells normally serve as the pacemaker of the heart. The more distal the cell from the sinoatrial node, the more gradual the slope of phase 4 (ie, the slope is more gradual in cells at the atrioventricular junction and most gradual in cells in the Purkinje fibers). If any of the more proximal pacemaker cells fail, a more distal latent cell may become the pacemaker, preventing cardiac standstill and producing **escape rhythms.** The rate of automatic discharge is slower in the more distal pacemakers. Cells in the junctional tissues near the atrioventricular node in the bundle of His or in the Purkinje system commonly take over when the sinoatrial node pacemakers fail for any reason.

Automaticity in any cardiac cell may be increased by disease, drugs, or overactivity of the sympathetic nervous system, and latent cells may assume the role of pacemaker when not needed. When secondary pacemakers take over because of failure of the primary pacemakers, they are like junior officers taking command of the ship when the captain collapses. When subsidiary pacemakers take over because of increased automaticity, they are like mutineers, because the primary pacemakers are still functioning. Although increased automaticity does occur, the role of latent pacemakers is basically to provide a backup mechanism in the event that the more proximal cells fail to "fire."

B. Excitability and Refractoriness: The ability of a cell to respond to a stimulus and initiate an action potential is called excitability. The term also denotes the ability of a cell to respond to a propagated impulse from a neighboring cell. The action potential itself serves as a stimulus to excite neighboring cells, and in this way, in a sequential and orderly manner, the heart is depolarized.

Refractoriness is the property by which cardiac cells fail to respond to an oncoming stimulus because repolarization is incomplete and the voltage of the interior of the cell has not become sufficiently negative to initiate or propagate an action potential. It is related to excitability in that the cell is totally unexcitable when the voltage is less negative than threshold and no stimulus, no matter how strong, can evoke a propagated response. This is the absolute refractory period. As the voltage of the cell becomes more negative at the end of phase 3, the resting membrane potential may not have reached its normal value of -90 mV but may be sufficiently negative that a powerful stimulus can evoke a response even though it may not be strong enough to be fully propagated and may depolarize only a few neighboring cells. Shortly after this relative refractory period and before the normal resting maximum diastolic pressure potential has been reached, there is a short "supernormal" phase corresponding to the downstroke of the T wave, during which time a smaller than usual current can induce a propagated response. The supernormal (vulnerable) phase is responsible for the so-called **R on T phenomenon,** in which a ventricular premature beat falling on the descending limb of the T wave may induce repetitive ventricular ectopic discharges, including ventricular fibrillation.

The refractory period varies in different parts of the heart, being shortest in the atrium and longest in the Purkinje system and in the atrioventricular node. This variability of recovery of excitability, or refractoriness, is exaggerated in portions of the ventricle or conduction system in diseases such as ischemic heart disease. Altered, uneven recovery of excitability in ischemic cells may be responsible for the frequency of ventricular arrhythmias in coronary heart disease. Recovery of refractoriness, excitability, and conduction velocity varies from one cell to another and from one tissue region to another. This variability affects repolarization, heart rate, and duration of the action potential and can thus initiate reentry arrhythmias (Han, 1971). Drugs rather than disease may exaggerate these changes; digitalis, for example, shortens the action potential, whereas quinidine prolongs it. Hypokalemia lengthens and hyperkalemia shortens the action potential.

C. Conductivity: Conduction of an electrical impulse from one cell to another is a fundamental property of cardiac tissue and results from the spread of electrical activity from one specialized cell to another and finally to myocardial cells. The velocity of conduction varies in different tissues of the heart and is 100 times more rapid in the Purkinje system than in the atrioventricular node. It is about 20–30 mm/s in the atrioventricular node, 3000–5000 mm/s in the Purkinje system, and about 500–600 mm/s in the ventricle. Slow conduction through the atrioventricular node prolongs the absolute refractory period in nodal cells and prevents rapid atrial impulses from activating the ventricles at the same rapid rate as the atria. In normal adults, this prevents them from beating so rapidly that they cannot maintain a normal cardiac output. Infants do not have the same conduction delay in the atrioventricular node and can have

atrial arrhythmias with ventricular rates as high as 300/min.

The **velocity of conduction** is related to the magnitude of the resting membrane potential when the action potential begins. The velocity is slower, and there is a decreased rate of rise of phase 0, when the resting membrane potential is less negative. The velocity of the conduction is also related to the heart rate. Decrease in the slope and amplitude of phase 4 depolarization increases the time between successive action potentials and the velocity of conduction in the subsequent beat. When the velocity of conduction is slowed sufficiently as a result of decreased maximum resting membrane potential, conduction may be sufficiently impaired so that it decreases as the depolarization wave spreads distally, with the result that the impulse may not be propagated throughout the entire conduction system. The ability of the excitation wave to propagate may progressively deteriorate. The term **decremental conduction** denotes the progressive decrease in conduction that results from alterations in the characteristics of the action potential owing to cellular abnormalities in the conduction pathway until ultimately a propagated impulse cannot be sustained. Decremental conduction may leave in its wake cells that have been incompletely repolarized and therefore have become refractory to an oncoming antegrade stimulus. This may not be obvious on the ECG and is one form of **concealed conduction,** which may also result when premature beats partially penetrate but do not pass through the atrioventricular node to the remainder of the conduction system. Such failure to conduct completely is called concealed conduction regardless of whether the spread is antegrade from the atria or retrograde from the ventricles. Concealed conduction may cause conduction delay or block anywhere along the normal pathway. Failure or delay in conduction may not be uniform—ie, it may be more manifest in one fiber than in a neighboring one. It may thus be important in setting up a reentry circuit, causing premature beats or tachycardia.

Failure of conduction is usually due to pathologic processes such as fibrosis, ischemia, hypoxia, acidosis, hyperkalemia, or drugs, any of which decreases the maximum resting membrane potential or shortens repolarization, allowing the resting membrane potential during diastole to be closer to the threshold potential. This decreases the velocity of the upstroke of phase 0 of depolarization, thereby decreasing the velocity of conduction.

D. Reentry: Reentry is not a property of cardiac cells per se but is thought to be the mechanism by which arrhythmias can develop in any portion of the heart through disturbances in the fundamental properties noted above. An automatic cell, by increasing the slope of phase 4 depolarization and increasing its automaticity, can become the pacemaker of the heart, producing either a premature beat or tachycardia.

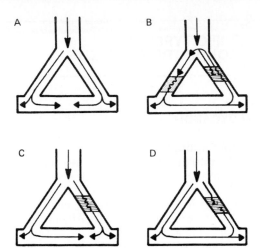

Figure 14–1. Schematic diagram of reentrant pathway and means for its modification. **A:** Normal propagation through the distal conducting system to the ventricle. Conduction proceeds with equal velocity through both limbs of a terminal Purkinje fiber bundle and then activates the myocardium. **B:** Shaded area on right indicates diseased tissue, including partially depolarized Purkinje fibers. Antegrade activation through the site is blocked. Activation is slowed (shaded area on left) but proceeds normally through the other limb to the myocardium and then activates the depressed segment (which is no longer refractory) in a retrograde direction. This impulse succeeds in propagating slowly through the depressed segment and reenters the proximal conducting system. **C:** If physiologic changes occur or appropriate pharmacologic agents are administered (see text), conduction may improve through the depressed segment and result in reestablishment of antegrade activation and abolition of reentry. **D:** If changes occur (or are induced) that result in block of retrograde activation as well as antegrade activation, then bidirectional conduction block occurs. This condition, too, would suppress a reentrant arrhythmia. (Modified and reproduced, with permission, from Rosen MR et al: Electrophysiology and pharmacology of cardiac arrhythmias. 5. Cardiac antiarrhythmic effects of lidocaine. Am Heart J 1975;89:526.)

Similarly, through operation of a reentry mechanism, a premature beat can be propagated by a circuitous route through an area of the heart and permit continuous repetitive depolarization and tachycardia.

Figure 14–1 shows in schematic fashion a reentrant pathway and how it can be modified.

1. Requirements for reentry– Normally, the cardiac impulse propagates evenly through the distal conducting system to the ventricles, with equal velocity in each of the closely related cardiac fibers (for purposes of illustration called "limbs" of a terminal Purkinje fiber bundle, as illustrated in Figure 14–1). Use of the term "limb" is not meant to imply that every area of the Purkinje system has only two fibers. Reentry requires that one portion of the myocardial fiber in a bundle of fibers be blocked in one direction (usually antegrade), because that limb is partially depolarized and cannot conduct properly (unidirectional block). Reentry also requires that antegrade activation through the other limb of the distal Purkinje fiber be slowed but spread in the normal direction to the ventricle. It then returns to the point of origin in a retrograde manner and activates the initially blocked limb or fiber. The impulse proceeds slowly in retrograde fashion through the segment that had antegrade block until it reaches the proximal conducting fiber, which by this time has recovered its excitability and is no longer refractory as a result of excitation; this allows a retrograde impulse from the originally blocked segment to reenter the normal segment or limb, setting up a reentry circuit that may then become repetitive.

Reentry requires, then, both impaired conduction (in one limb) and unidirectional block (in the other). Decremental conduction (as discussed above) may slow conduction in one fiber or produce antegrade unidirectional block in another fiber and so foster reentry. Parts C and D of Figure 14–1 show how the reentry rhythm can be terminated, either by improving conduction in the depressed segment and thus allowing the initial impulse to spread equally through both limbs of the fibers, or by increasing the retrograde block in the blocked segment so that the original impulse cannot be conducted to the proximal site.

A new stimulus, either from an atrial premature beat or from retrograde excitation of the atria by ventricular premature beats, is the usual mechanism for initiating paroxysmal atrial tachycardia, with the reentry circuit involving the atrioventricular node. A repetitive reentry circuit can be interrupted by drugs such as digitalis or verapamil if the reentry circuit involves the atrioventricular node. These drugs increase atrioventricular nodal block, prolonging conduction in the atrioventricular node and making it refractory to any new impulse that reaches the atrioventricular node as part of the reentry circuit. Return (echo) beats find the atrioventricular node unexcitable, so that it cannot continue to propagate the reentry circuit impulse.

2. Occurrence and causes of reentry– A reentry circuit can occur anywhere in the heart. In paroxysmal atrial tachycardia, it usually includes the atrioventricular node. Atrial flutter is thought to result from a reentry pathway in the atria. In the ventricle, a reentry circuit may occur in a diseased portion of the tissue. If there is an "excitable gap" between the head and the tail of the reentry pathway (circus movement), there may be a continuous excitation wave that sets up a paroxysm of arrhythmia. Unidirectional block in one segment may be induced by ischemia, hypoxia, acidosis, potassium leak from necrotic cells, or (experimentally) by cooling. As a result of the relative automaticity of one group of cells, currents may be set up that stimulate neighboring cells and may lead to a propagated paroxysmal arrhythmia either via the reentry mechanism or via a direct ectopic rhythm (automaticity). Pathologic states such as ischemia do not affect all fibers uniformly; the resulting irregular return of cells to their maximum resting diastolic potential and with varying conduction velocity may lead to arrhythmias. Ventricular arrhythmias may be due to propagation from an ectopic site that has assumed greater automaticity because of early recovery of excitability; in other cases, reentry may be the mechanism. Recovery of excitability and altered refractory periods are common, especially in the border zone between necrotic and surviving cells that behave as chronically ischemic cells. This may explain the high incidence of arrhythmias after healed myocardial infarction and why unexpected ventricular fibrillation and sudden death may occur.

E. Triggered Activity: The term "triggered activity" denotes oscillatory changes in membrane voltage potentials set off by a propagated depolarization. When this oscillation in membrane potential occurs early, before completion of repolarization, it is called early afterdepolarization (EAD); when it occurs after repolarization, it is called delayed afterdepolarization (DAD) (Cranefield, 1988). These afterdepolarizations, when increased in magnitude, are a mechanism for the production of arrhythmias.

The amplitude of the oscillations early after depolarization is increased by a slow heart rate. Since the oscillations occur on the downslope of the T wave in the scalar ECG, they tend to prolong the QT interval. The arrhythmias produced by EAD can be precipitated by a slow heart rate.

Early afterdepolarizations result from a reduced repolarization current compared with the depolarization current, which is caused by a reduced outward current, increased inward current, or both. EAD can be abolished by a variety of drugs blocking Ca^{2+} inward current and Na^+ channel blockers as well as by an increased heart rate. This, plus the fact that a variety of antiarrhythmic drugs such as quinidine, calcium current agonists, and catecholamines can induce EAD, implicate L-type Ca^{2+} channels and a diversity of other channels and currents have been implicated in the genesis of these EADs. Early afterdepolarizations are implicated in the genesis of arrhythmias seen in torsade de pointes and the prolonged QT interval arrhythmias (Jackman, 1988; January, 1990). The amplitude of delayed afterdepolarization (DAD) is increased with fast heart rates, and these DADs have been implicated as the cause of premature ventricular beats and ventricular tachycardia seen in digitalis toxicity as well as acute myocardial infarction (Rosen, 1988). Accelerated junctional escape may be due to DAD. One possibility is that DADs are the result of release of calcium into the cytosol, perhaps from the sarcoplasmic reticulum. This triggers a transient inward Na^+ current, causing the DADs.

SPECIFIC TYPES OF CONDUCTION DEFECTS

BRADYCARDIA

Clinical Findings

A. Symptoms and Signs: The assessment of sinus bradycardia is difficult, since the definition itself is by no means uniform. Many authorities state that any regular sinus rate less than 60/min constitutes sinus bradycardia. Others use lower figures, such as 55/min or 50/min. The age of the patient plays a role, because slower heart rates (< 55/min) are more prevalent in healthy young individuals, especially athletes; are usually attributed to high vagal tone; are rarely associated with symptoms; and require no special investigative studies or treatment. Equivalent slow rates or more marked bradycardia (< 45/min) may produce symptoms in older individuals, because with the development of coronary artery disease and impaired left ventricular function, stroke volume may not be able to increase to compensate for the slow heart rate and there may be a fall in cardiac output. Sinus bradycardia at any age is fairly common unless one defines it as a rate less than 40/min.

The sinoatrial node is controlled by both cholinergic and adrenergic autonomic nervous impulses reflexly stimulated from any part of the body. Noncardiac causes of sinus bradycardia involving this system must be evaluated in light of the function of the sinoatrial node as the common end pathway for many efferent impulses from the central nervous system.

Pathologically, there may be various infiltrative and inflammatory changes in the tissue framework of the sinoatrial node as well as lesions involving the sinoatrial nodal artery. With aging, there is a loss of pacemaker cells in the sinoatrial node as the probable cause of resting sinus bradycardia so commonly seen in the elderly.

The clinical significance of sinus bradycardia or sinoatrial nodal or atrial dysfunction depends on whether atrioventricular junctional escape pacemakers or His bundle escape pacemakers take over the rhythm of the heart at rates that are only slightly slower than the normal sinus rate. If there is concomitant involvement of both sinoatrial and atrioventricular nodal areas, so that bundle branch or ventricular pacemakers are required, the prognosis for life is worse because these lower pacemakers are slower and less reliable, and artificial pacemakers are often indicated. The role of drugs—especially beta-adrenergic blocking agents, opioids, phenothiazines and other tranquilizers—must always be considered in sinus bradycardia. The decreased phase 4 depolarization slope that occurs in hypothyroidism and other metabolic disturbances should also be considered in the analysis of sinus bradycardia.

B. Myocardial Infarction and Bradycardia: The artery to the sinoatrial node arises in most people from the right coronary artery, but in about one-third of individuals it arises from a branch of the left circumflex artery; sinus bradycardia, therefore, is usually found in patients with acute inferior myocardial infarction resulting from occlusion of the right coronary artery. Bradycardia is often transient or reversible, owing to ischemia of the sinoatrial node and increased vagal tone, and can be reversed with time or with atropine. The slow heart rate is significant for two reasons: (1) By decreasing cardiac output and blood pressure, bradycardia may interfere with coronary perfusion and thus extend the infarction; and (2) a slow ventricular rate with variable conduction delay and repolarization may allow ectopic impulses to take over the rhythm of the heart in the ischemic or damaged ventricular muscle supplied by the right coronary artery.

C. His Bundle Recordings: His bundle recordings (Figure 14–2) have shown that the PR interval includes the spread of the impulse from the sinoatrial node through the atria and the bundle of His as well as the first part of its two main branches. The current from the His bundle is of sufficiently small magnitude that the surface ECG does not pick up its individual potentials. It can be recorded by bipolar electrode catheter placed across the tricuspid valve near the His bundle and can be seen to occur during the PR interval of the surface ECG. The activity and timing of the conduction system between the sinoatrial node and the ventricles can then be determined. His bundle recordings have enhanced our understanding of the pathophysiology of atrioventricular conduction defects, especially the diagnostic, prognostic, and therapeutic significance of pacemaker activity above, in, and below the atrioventricular node.

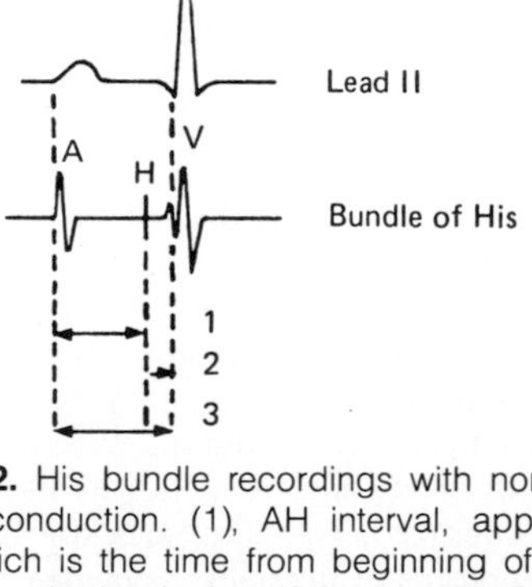

Electrophysiologic methods of determining sinoatrial node activity, such as sinoatrial node recovery time, are useful but have significant limitations. The recovery time can be determined by noting the time taken for a sinus beat to occur when rapid atrial pacing is stopped. Sinoatrial node recovery time is variable in the same patient at different times, and there is a considerable overlap between normal and abnormal patients (Table 14–1).

Differential Diagnosis

Because there is evidence that sinus bradycardia may not be as benign as once thought and because varying degrees of sinoatrial node and atrial dysfunction as well as atrioventricular conduction defects may develop over a period of years, ambulatory 24-hour electrocardiographic recordings should be obtained on symptomatic older patients (over age 50) with dizziness, light-headedness, or syncope to rule out transient unrecognized atrial arrhythmias or conduction defects. This is most important if there is concomitant evidence of intraventricular conduction defects such as right or left bundle branch block or bifascicular block (usually right bundle branch block and left anterior hemiblock). (See Atrioventricular Conduction Defects, below.) If the patient is without symptoms and has only modest bradycardia (eg, < 50/min) and has normal exercise tolerance, further investigation is not indicated, but the patient should be seen once a year and told to report any unusual symptoms such as near-syncope, dizziness, or awareness of cardiac arrhythmias (Table 14–2).

Treatment

See Bradycardia-Tachycardia Syndrome, below.

TACHYCARDIA

Sinus tachycardia (> 100 beats/min) can occur in any condition that increases the slope of phase 4 depolarization of the sinoatrial nodal cells, which therefore reach "threshold" sooner and thus result in rapid heart rates. This occurs in exercise, anemia, fever, emotional stress, thyrotoxicosis, following administration of adrenergic drugs such as epinephrine, or following any stimuli that increase adrenergic activity, which increases the release of norepinephrine. Beta-adrenergic blocking agents slow the heart rate at rest and during exercise by interfering with the adrenergic activity in the sinoatrial node. Cholinergic or vagal stimuli slow the sinus rate; the effects can be reversed by atropine.

When sinus tachycardia occurs in acute myocardial

Figure 14–2. His bundle recordings with normal atrioventricular conduction. (1), AH interval, approximately 120 ms, which is the time from beginning of atrial depolarization to the beginning of the bundle of His spike. (2), HV interval, approximately 50 ms (upper limits of normal are 55–60 ms), which represents the time from the bundle of His spike to the beginning of ventricular depolarization. (3), AV time, which is the PR interval. (Reproduced, with permission, from Goldman MJ: *Principles of Clinical Electrocardiography*, 12th ed. Lange, 1986.)

Table 14–1. Clinical test for evaluation of sinoatrial node function.[1,2]

Test	Criteria of Abnormal Response	Comments
Atropine (0.04 mg/kg IV)	<50% increase in sinus rate	Relatively easy, safe test; helpful only if positive.
Isoproterenol (3 µg/min IV)	<25% increase in sinus rate	Helpful if positive; may be dangerous in ventricular arrhythmia and ischemic heart disease.
Sinoatrial node recovery time (SNRT)	$SNRT_c > 450$ ms $SNRT_c = SNRT - BCL$ or $SNRT > 140\%$ BCL	Highly specific, moderately sensitive; invasive procedure.
Sinoatrial conduction time (SACT)	SACT > 120 ms	Moderately specific, highly sensitive; invasive procedure.
Ambulatory electrocardiographic monitoring	Sinus bradycardia, sinus arrest, sinoatrial block, bradytachyarrhythmias	Excellent test; can correlate symptoms with arrhythmias.
Treadmill testing	<90% of predicted maximum heart rate for age and sex; development of exercise-induced sinus bradycardia	Difficult to assess in the elderly and debilitated patients.
Intrinsic heart rate	>10% decrease in age-predicted rate; IHR = 117.2 beats/min (0.53 × age)	Wide experience unavailable.

[1] Reproduced, with permission, from Talano JV et al: Sinoatrial node dysfunction: An overview with emphasis on autonomic and pharmacologic consideration. Am J Med 1978;64:773
[2] $SNRT_c$, sinoatrial node recovery time corrected; SNRT, observed sinoatrial node recovery time; BCL, basic cycle length; IHR, intrinsic heart rate; SACT, sinoatrial conduction time.

Table 14–2. Ambulatory 24-hour monitoring findings in 95 patients with dizziness or syncope.[1,2]

Clinical Findings	Number of Patients
No abnormalities detected	22
Findings definitely correlating with symptoms	46
Paroxysmal atrial fibrillation	6
Paroxysmal atrial flutter	1
Paroxysmal atrial tachycardia	11
Ventricular tachycardia	10
Sinus bradycardia	3
Sinotrial block of standstill	5
Atrioventricular block, second-degree	4
Atrioventricular block, third-degree	3
Defective pacemaker	5
Findings possibly related to symptoms	42
Frequent premature atrial contractions	11[3]
Frequent premature ventricular contractions	31[4]
Findings not related to symptoms	17
Sinus tachycrdia (≥ 120 beats/min)	8
Sinus bradycardia (≤ 50 beats/min)	1
Intermittent bundle branch block	3
Atrioventricular block, first-degree	5

[1] Reproduced, with permission, from Van Durme JP: Tachyarrhythmias and transient cerebral ischemic attacks. Am Heart J 1975;89:538.
[2] Patients who presented different types of arrhythmia or conduction defect were listed under each separate item.
[3] Five patients developed paroxysmal atrial tachycardia; 2 patients developed atrial fibrillation.
[4] Ten patients developed ventricular tachycardia.

infarction, it increases the work of the heart and may extend the size of the myocardial infarction. Sinus tachycardia in acute myocardial infarction is frequently associated with impaired left ventricular function and a decreased stroke volume. It is a bad prognostic sign. If the patient has an obstructive lesion such as mitral stenosis, tachycardia decreases the duration of ventricular filling and causes an increase in the pulmonary artery wedge pressure that induces pulmonary venous congestion and dyspnea.

BRADYCARDIA-TACHYCARDIA SYNDROME
(Sick Sinus Syndrome)

The bradycardia-tachycardia syndrome, consisting of alternating bradycardia due to sinus arrest, sinus bradycardia, or sinoatrial exit block combined with tachycardia from paroxysmal atrial or junctional arrhythmias, may produce symptoms referable to either slow or fast heart rates (Sutton, 1986). It is being reported with increasing frequency as its importance becomes recognized. The term "sick sinus syndrome" denotes symptoms of dizziness, syncope, and bradycardia due to the slow rate resulting from failure of impulse formation in the sinoatrial node or its conduction to the atrioventricular node. The term "bradycardia-tachycardia syndrome" is preferred by some cardiologists because patients characteristically have paroxysmal atrial or junctional tachyarrhythmias in addition to the slow heart rates; this is because the pathologic process, usually fibrosis, is not confined to the sinoatrial node but may involve parts of the atrium, the atrioventricular node, the bundle of His, and the His-Purkinje system. Recent pathologic investigations have shown that this fibrotic process is much more common than was once thought. The mechanism of bradycardia-tachycardia syndrome can therefore be sinus bradycardia, sinus node arrest, sinoatrial conduction defect, or disease of the atrioventricular node, with escape mechanisms in junctional pacemakers. Atrial arrhythmias can result.

In addition to the pathologic finding of nonspecific fibrotic degenerative disease of the conduction system, the bradycardiac syndromes may be associated with the more common diseases such as coronary disease, hypertension, aortic and mitral valve disease, and primary cardiomyopathy, but these conditions may be only incidental.

Clinical Findings

A. Symptoms and Signs: Characteristic findings of bradycardia-tachycardia syndrome are intermittent symptoms referable to a slow heart rate or to rapid supraventricular arrhythmias (paroxysmal atrial or junctional tachycardia, atrial flutter, or atrial fibrillation).

In some patients, the fast and slow rates may alternate. On one occasion the patient may have paroxysmal arrhythmia with palpitations and impaired cerebral, coronary, and extremity flow from rapid ventricular rates; on another occasion, the slow heart rate caused by dysfunction of the sinoatrial node or transmission from the sinoatrial to the atrioventricular node may result in inadequate perfusion of the brain, with dizziness, impaired cerebral function, and either presyncope or syncope. Impairment of coronary flow may result in angina pectoris or symptoms of cardiac failure or general weakness. In patients who present with paroxysmal atrial arrhythmias, the disorder of the sinoatrial node or sinoatrial conduction dysfunction may only be recognized by the presence of sinus bradycardia between attacks or by noting that when the tachycardia is terminated (either with drugs or with cardioversion), the sinoatrial node shows a period of standstill and slow return to normal function. Five to 10 percent of cases of cardiovascular syncope were found by Easley (1971) to occur in this manner. A history of syncope that immediately follows the cessation of tachycardia suggests the diagnosis.

In a prospective study (Rokseth, 1974), sinoatrial or sinus node disease occurred in about one-third of all clinical conduction defects. Many patients were seen by a neurologist because the symptoms were vague and misinterpreted. Sixty percent of patients had atrial arrhythmias, and the incidence was higher if long-term ambulatory monitoring of the ECG was used.

Sinus bradycardia, especially in older individuals, should be looked on with suspicion and not dismissed

Table 14–3. Incidence of sinus abnormalities and atrioventricular block in patient population.[1]

	Number of Cases[2]	Percentage of Total Cases
Sinus		
Bradycardia	129	7.7
Tachycardia	429	25.6
Pause, arrest, or sinoatrial block	63	3.8
Atrioventricular block		
First-degree	32	1.9
Second-degree	39	2.3
Third-degree (complete)	10	0.6

[1] Reproduced, with permission, from Bleifer SB et al: Diagnosis of occult arrhythmias by Holter electrocardiography. Prog Cardiovasc Dis 1974; 16:569.
[2] The numbers and percentages are not mutually exclusive, since a patient may demonstrate more than one abnormality.

as a sensitive carotid sinus or "vagotonia." Patients with marked sinus bradycardia or with symptoms that could be related to a slow heart rate should have ambulatory monitoring of the ECG for 12–24 hours or more (Table 14–3). Some patients with sinus nodal dysfunction manifest only chronotropic incompetence in that they cannot raise their heart rate appropriately with exercise. Another danger of sick sinus syndrome is the development of atrial fibrillation, which can predispose the patient to systemic embolization. Episodes of short or long paroxysmal atrial tachycardia, atrial fibrillation, or atrial flutter may not have been suspected on the basis of the clinical history. His bundle recordings of atrial and His bundle depolarizations may show a variety of conduction disturbances between the sinoatrial node and other parts of the specialized conduction system (not solely the atrioventricular node) in a reentry circuit, as is usual in paroxysmal atrial tachycardia.

B. Electrophysiologic and Special Studies, Including His Bundle Studies: Electrophysiologic methods of determining sinoatrial node activity, such as sinoatrial node recovery time, are useful but have significant limitations. The recovery time can be determined by noting the recovery time for a sinus beat when rapid atrial pacing is stopped. Sinoatrial node recovery time is variable in the same patient at different times, and there is a considerable overlap between normal and abnormal patients (Table 14–1).

In addition to continuous monitoring of the ECG over a period of hours, either while the patient is ambulatory or in the coronary care unit, other studies may be helpful in making the diagnosis. The response of the sinus rate to exercise or atropine, His bundle recordings, atrial pacing, atrial extrastimulus testing, and overdrive suppression of the sinoatrial node may reveal dysfunction of the sinoatrial node or its connections to the atrioventricular node. Examples of such dysfunction are delayed recovery of the sinoatrial node following rapid atrial pacing (sinoatrial node recovery time) and prolonged sinoatrial conduction time after atrial extrastimulus testing with progressively increasing prematurity. These studies are still investigational, and their role in diagnosis is uncertain. If the prolonged pauses during atrial pacing studies reproduce the spontaneous symptoms of the patient, the role of bradycardia can be considered established, and placement of a right atrial (AAI) pacemaker may relieve the symptoms. The atrial arrhythmias are often due to chance reexcitation of already repolarized fibers; differences in the rate of repolarization result from variable refractory periods that are prevalent when the heart rate is slow. Han (1966) has shown that vagal stimulation decreases the refractory period unevenly in different parts of the atrium, which might lead to reentry atrial arrhythmias.

If the patient with sinus bradycardia is asymptomatic and yet has both bifascicular block and a prolonged PR interval on the ECG, suggesting trifascicular block, the hazard of complete atrioventricular block is sufficient to make one follow the patient closely and proceed with His bundle and other specialized studies if symptoms appear.

C. Precautions Before Undertaking Special Investigations in Chronic Sinoatrial Disease: Before resorting to invasive techniques such as atrial pacing and His bundle recordings, one should (as indicated earlier) rule out paroxysmal arrhythmias (both atrial and ventricular), drug effects (especially beta-blockers, sympathetic blocking agents, and calcium channel-blocking agents), hypothyroidism, anemia due to blood loss or hematologic disorders, postural hypotension, transient ischemic attacks, what in early days was called "swooning" (vasovagal attacks), and the vague dizziness and confusion of cerebrovascular disease without focal neurologic signs. The differential diagnosis of nonspecific dizziness and weakness in elderly people includes many noncardiac conditions. This problem is discussed in more detail in Chapter 2. Twenty-four-hour monitoring of the ECG is indicated in all such patients to exclude a tachy- or bradyarrhythmia that is amenable to treatment. The variety of abnormalities detected is illustrated in Table 14–2.

Myocardial ischemia induced by effort may be associated with hypotension and cerebral symptoms. Electrocardiographic monitoring may identify these patients. The specialized studies discussed below require equipment that is available only in larger centers. Simple noninvasive tests (eg, exercise tests or 24-hour monitoring of the ECG) (see Chapter 5) should be performed in symptomatic patients before referral to a major center for invasive studies.

Before accepting ambulatory electrocardiographic evidence of sinoatrial nodal block or pause that did not reproduce the patient's symptoms as a cause of unexplained syncope, serious consideration should be given to electrophysiologic study. Syncope as a result of sick sinus syndrome is unusual. Electrophysiologic study of 141 consecutive patients with unexplained syncope found none with sinus node dysfunction as the cause. Twenty percent of the patients had bradyarrhythmia as the cause, about half with atrioventricular nodal disease and half with infra-His bundle disease. In 13%, ventricular tachyarrhythmias were the cause of syncope (Bachinsky, 1992).

D. Atropine Test: Atropine sulfate, 0.5 mg intravenously, usually increases the heart rate in normal individuals to over 100/min. In a group of patients with bradycardia-tachycardia syndrome, Rosen (1971) found that no patient developed a heart rate greater than 90/min after administration of 1 mg of atropine intravenously.

Although atropine can be used as a test of the ability of the sinoatrial node to increase its rate of discharge, there are occasions when atropine produces tachycardia and may induce angina pectoris or an arrhythmia, especially in the presence of coronary heart disease. Small doses (eg, 0.25 mg or 0.5 mg intravenously) should be given first, therefore, and the effect on heart rate noted before larger doses are used. Slow heart rates with varying rates of recovery of excitability in different parts of the atrium can lead to reentry atrial premature beats and perhaps atrial tachycardia or fibrillation.

Differential Diagnosis

The differential diagnosis of sick sinus syndrome includes all conditions causing bradycardia and atrial tachyarrhythmias. In addition, because the symptoms are often vague and nonspecific, one must consider psychophysiologic reactions, transient ischemic attacks due to cerebrovascular disease, vasovagal fainting, and all conditions in which elderly individuals may have transient cerebral symptoms other than sinus node, sinoatrial, or atrioventricular conduction disturbances. Cerebral symptoms are nonspecific when due to conduction defects and may result from abnormalities anywhere in the transmission system from the sinoatrial node to the Purkinje system. Special studies are needed to identify the site of delay in conduction.

If vague symptoms suggesting cerebral or cardiac ischemia appear with exercise and the sinus rate is slow (usually < 45/min), one should exercise the patient to determine if the atrial rate can be increased appropriately. If the cardiac rate does not increase following moderate exercise to more than 110/min or if symptoms suggest decreased perfusion of the brain or heart, one can suspect chronotropic incompetence as a result of sinus node dysfunction and proceed to electrophysiologic testing.

Treatment

A. Drug Treatment: If the patient is asymptomatic, no treatment is indicated. If, in addition to the sinus bradycardia, the patient has symptoms of cerebral insufficiency suggesting sinoatrial syncope, an AAI or DDD pacemaker should be considered.

The physician should make certain that the symptoms and slow heart rate are not due to use of phenothiazines, quinidine, or beta-adrenergic blocking drugs given to prevent atrial arrhythmias. Digitalis given in large doses to prevent or treat paroxysmal atrial fibrillation may cause or prolong the period of sinus arrest. Combining several medications such as digoxin and verapamil or diltiazem, each of which suppress sinoatrial nodal activity, can precipitate sinoatrial nodal block, long pauses, or atrioventricular nodal block and syncope. Withdrawal of these medications is an important first step before use of a pacemaker is considered.

B. Pacemaker Implantation: (See Chapter 7 and below.) The most effective method of therapy in symptomatic patients is insertion of a pacemaker to maintain an adequate heart rate and prevent syncopal attacks. There is increasing evidence that it is important to pace the atrium in order to prevent the development of atrial fibrillation (Ryden, 1988; Camm, 1990; Santini, 1990). The type of pacemaker employed depends upon the atrial rhythm and the extent of conduction system disease, which may be present in one-third of patients with sick sinus syndrome (Santini, 1990), especially in older patients.. The appropriate pacemaker should increase the ventricular rate in response to exercise and ensure proper timing between atrial and ventricular contraction. Since patients with sinus nodal dysfunction can have a high incidence of chronotropic incompetence, rate-responsive AAIR or DDDR has been advocated (Rosenqvist, 1990). If atrial arrhythmias are present, the DDD pacemaker can be reprogrammed to VVI mode. The physician can then use antiarrhythmic drugs to prevent atrial tachyarrhythmias without being concerned about their cardiac depressant effects. With the improvement in cardiac function that follows restoration of a normal heart rate by the introduction of a demand pacemaker, the atrial arrhythmias may not recur. Sinoatrial node dysfunction with bradycardia-tachycardia syndrome is the indication for implantation of about one-third of all demand pacemakers for cardiac syncope. If these patients have abnormalities below the His conduction system, a DDD pacemaker is needed.

Before use of a pacemaker is considered, it must be established that the symptoms are caused by a conduction defect, either sinoatrial node abnormality or alternating bradycardia and tachycardia. The presence of sinus bradycardia alone, while requiring careful follow-up, is not an indication for pacemaker therapy. Patients with vague symptoms such as dizziness, fatigue, or even syncope do not require a pacemaker unless it is established that the symptoms are due to a conduction defect. Sudden death is rare in sinoatrial node disease, in contrast to atrioventricular block,

and pacemaker therapy is used for relief of symptoms. The indications for pacemaker insertion are controversial, and many physicians believe this option is elected too frequently in sinus node disease.

Although patients with sinoatrial disease are an average of 10 years younger than those with atrioventricular conduction disease and generally have a more benign prognosis than those with atrioventricular block, major Stokes-Adams attacks may occur. A pacemaker should be inserted when it has been established that presyncope or syncope is due to sinoatrial disease. Practice guidelines for the use of pacemakers in sick sinus syndrome have been published by a task force of the American College of Cardiology/ American Heart Association (Dreifus, 1991).

The slow progression of bradycardia-tachycardia syndrome to complete atrioventricular block makes it difficult sometimes to decide whether to be conservative or aggressive in treatment. In general, as long as the patient is asymptomatic, nothing is necessary except to carefully note the response to noninvasive procedures such as exercise, posture, Valsalva's maneuver, squatting, or atropine. If the cause has been identified as coronary heart disease, if the progress of the disease seems rapid, or if the patient develops symptoms due to both bradycardia and tachycardia, definitive pacemaker and antiarrhythmic therapy should be initiated. Before a permanent transvenous pacemaker is introduced—especially if there is doubt about the relationship between the cerebral symptoms and bradycardia—a temporary pacemaker should be tried, and the effect of increased heart rate on the cerebral symptoms should be noted.

Pacemakers are not innocuous and should be used only on adequate indications, but it is just as wrong not to use pacemakers when they are clearly indicated as to recommend their introduction unnecessarily. Permanent pacing may not necessarily result in improved survival time (Rasmussen, 1981). The results of transvenous pacing in patients with bradycardia-tachycardia syndrome have been uniformly good with respect to relief of symptoms from slow heart rates, but additional drugs are often necessary to control the paroxysmal arrhythmia.

Prognosis

Because the most common pathologic process is fibrosis of the conduction system, which is usually slowly progressive, the physician should follow the patient even if there are no symptoms in order to note the development of symptoms, arrhythmias, or atrioventricular conduction defects that may presage the onset of Stokes-Adams attacks. Atypical symptoms may not be interpreted correctly, and sinoatrial disease may be found only if special studies such as 24-hour monitoring of the ECG are periodically undertaken. Unexplained cerebral symptoms are most important to note in patients with bradycardia. Unexplained atrial fibrillation, especially when associated with bradycardia occurring between paroxysmal attacks, should also alert the physician to the possibility of the condition and its long-term guarded prognosis.

ATRIOVENTRICULAR CONDUCTION DEFECTS

Atrioventricular conduction defects may occur anywhere from the atrioventricular node to both bundle branches. His bundle recordings have demonstrated single and multiple blocks, which may be localized in the atrioventricular node, the bundle of His, or anywhere in the conduction system distal to the bundle of His. Atrioventricular defects may be acute, transient, and reversible or may be chronic. Examples of acute defects are those associated with acute myocardial ischemia or infarction (discussed in detail below because of its importance) and those associated with acute myocarditis, rheumatic fever, heart block following surgery, drug toxicity, and hyperkalemia (discussed in other chapters). See Table 14–4.

Chronic atrioventricular defects may be intermittent or permanent and are usually due to structural defects in the conduction system that occur during the course of chronic disease. The most common causes of chronic defects are coronary heart disease, dilated cardiomyopathy, fibrosis of the conduction system (Lev's disease or Lenegre's disease), and myocardial infiltrative diseases (Table 14–4). In coronary heart disease, the conduction defect may be acute, as in acute myocardial ischemia or infarction, or chronic, as in chronic coronary heart disease following myocardial infarction.

Atrioventricular defects, whether acute or chronic, are important because they may lead to advanced heart block, syncope, or Stokes-Adams attacks with

Table 14–4. Causes of atrioventricular block.

1. Degenerative disease of conduction system (Lev's disease, Lenegre's disease).
2. Myocardial infarction or ischemia without infarction.
3. Dilated cardiomyopathy.
4. Drug toxicity due to digitalis, quinidine, phenothiazines, tricyclic antidepressants.
5. Valvular heart disease (especially aortic stenosis and aortic insufficiency).
6. Connective tissue and myocardial disorders (eg, sarcoidosis, scleroderma, amyloidosis, systemic lupus erythematosus, thyroid disease).
7. Surgical heart block.
8. Hyperkalemia and following use of antiarrhythmic drugs.
9. Cardiac tumors (usually secondary but sometimes primary).
10. Chagas' disease of the heart; rarely, syphilitic gumma.
11. Lyme disease.
12. Congenital.
13. Acute rheumatic fever.
14. Atrioventricular ring infection in infective endocarditis.
15. Trauma.

ventricular standstill or ventricular fibrillation. Insertion of a pacemaker may be required if advanced or complete heart block occurs.

Atrioventricular conduction defects vary from **partial (first-degree) block** to **second-degree block** to **complete (third-degree) block** (Figures 14–3 to 14–6). Partial atrioventricular block consists of prolongation of the PR interval to 0.21 s or more at normal heart rates and represents a delay in conduction of the cardiac impulse from the sinoatrial node to the ventricles, recognized only on ECG. In second-degree block, not every sinus impulse reaches the ventricles, with the result that failure of ventricular contraction occurs and is apparent by the absence (dropping) of a beat. Failure of conduction on the part of the ventricles allows the conduction system to recover, so that a subsequent beat is transmitted to the ventricles. The basic definition and classification of second-degree block (Mobitz type I and Mobitz type II; see below) have been clarified by His bundle recordings and electrical stimulation of the heart. In complete (third-degree) atrioventricular block, the lesion is in the atrioventricular node or distal to the His bundle. It is often part of a generalized pathologic process (Table 14–4) and associated with bilateral bundle branch block, but it may occur without any conduction defect in either the right or the left bundle branches.

1. ACUTE ATRIOVENTRICULAR CONDUCTION DEFECTS

Myocardial Infarction & Acute Conduction Defects*

Continuous electrocardiographic monitoring of patients in coronary care units has shown that atrioventricular conduction defects are common in acute myocardial infarction. Overall, complete atrioventricular block occurs in 6–10% of cases, depending on the sample of patients, and, especially in anterior wall infarction, is associated with a high mortality rate not necessarily as a result of the heart block itself. Atrioventricular block, especially in the presence of anterior myocardial infarction, implies a large infarct with considerable myocardial damage in the area of the septum and consequent cardiac failure or cardiogenic shock.

A. Inferior Infarcts: When atrioventricular conduction defects occur in inferior infarction, the damage to the conduction tissue is usually reversible and transient. It is due to temporary ischemia or edema of the atrioventricular node caused by occlusion of the atrioventricular nodal artery—a branch of the right coronary artery in 90% of patients—and is characterized by progression through all degrees of atrioventricular block to complete atrioventricular block, though Stokes-Adams attacks are uncommon. The

---

*See also Chapter 8.

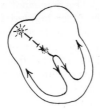
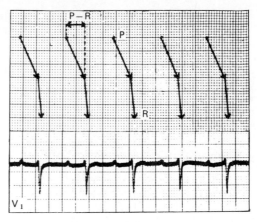

Figure 14–3. First-degree atrioventricular block. The PR interval is prolonged to 0.28 s. (Reproduced, with permission, from Goldman MJ: *Principles of Clinical Electrocardiography,* 12th ed. Lange, 1986.)

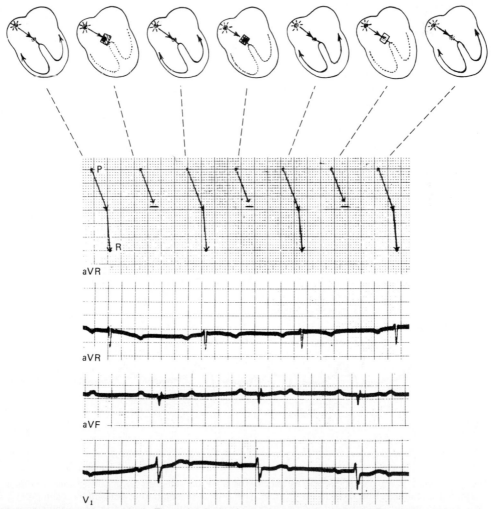

Figure 14–4. 2:1 atrioventricular block. The atrial rhythm is regular at a rate of 82/min. Every other atrial beat produces ventricular stimulation. (Reproduced, with permission, from Goldman MJ: *Principles of Clinical Electrocardiography,* 12th ed. Lange, 1986.)

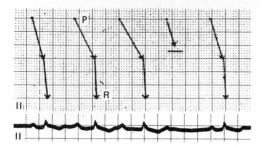

Figure 14–5. Second-degree atrioventricular block of Wenckebach type (Mobitz type I). The atrial rhythm is regular. In lead II, the first PR interval = 0.18 s, the second = 0.28 s, and the third = 0.36 s. The fourth atrial beat fails to activate the ventricle. (Reproduced, with permission, from Goldman MJ: *Principles of Clinical Electrocardiography*, 12th ed. Lange, 1986.)

QRS complex is almost always normal in width. With complete atrioventricular block, there is escape of a junctional pacemaker, resulting in a heart rate greater than 50/min. His bundle recordings indicate that the atrioventricular block is usually in the atrioventricular node and rarely involves the bundle of His or its branches, and the prognosis is correspondingly better than when the block is infranodal. Cardiac pacemakers are less often required than in anterior infarction and in many centers are not used at all unless the patient has episodes of syncope or fall in blood pressure or cardiac output, especially if the junctional pacemaker is satisfactory (> 50 beats per minute). The conduction defect usually lasts for a few days— rarely as long as a week—and the prognosis is good

for the acute episode. The frequency of transient complete atrioventricular block in inferior infarctions is at least twice that in anterior infarctions.

B. Anterior Infarcts: In anterior myocardial infarction with conduction defects, there is usually widespread necrosis of the septum involving the bundle of His and its branches, usually preceded by the sudden onset of unifascicular or bifascicular block— most often right bundle branch block or left anterior hemiblock. The sequential change to and from bundle branch block to left anterior hemiblock (fascicular block) and complete atrioventricular block as well as various arrhythmias may be rapid and take place over minutes to an hour. His bundle recordings show that the conduction defect is below the atrioventricular node; the QRS duration is usually widened; the interval between the bundle of His spike and the beginning of the QRS complex (the HV interval) is prolonged; the escape heart rate is usually less than 40 beats/min; and the escape pacemaker is in the bundle branches or lower in the Purkinje system. Stokes-Adams attacks and sudden death are an ever-present danger. Insertion of a prophylactic demand ventricular pacemaker is indicated when certain manifestations of ventricular conduction defect such as trifascicular bundle branch block (first-degree atrioventricular block with right bundle branch block with left anterior or posterior hemiblock, or with left bundle branch block) or Mobitz type II second-degree atrioventricular block develops during the course of acute anterior infarction, because complete atrioventricular block and Stokes-Adams attacks may appear rapidly (Fitzpatrick, 1992). The mortality rate is high when atrioventricular conduction defects develop for the first

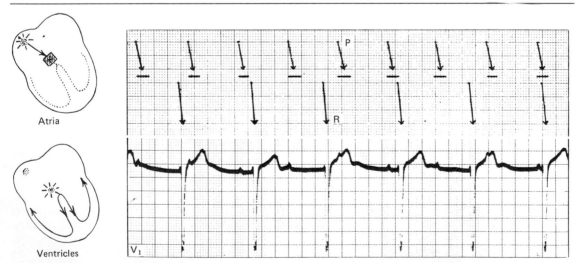

Figure 14–6. Diagram of complete atrioventricular block. The atria are activated by impulses arising normally in the sinoatrial node. In this example, the atrial rate = 72/min. The atrial impulses do not activate the ventricles. A second cardiac pacemaker is located near the atrioventricular node and stimulates the ventricles. The ventricular rate = 54/min. The atrial and ventricular rhythms are independent of each other. (Reproduced, with permission, from Goldman MJ: *Principles of Clinical Electrocardiography*, 12th ed. Lange, 1986.)

time in anterior infarction, because the necrosis is extensive and left ventricular function is severely impaired, with decreased cardiac output, raised left ventricular filling pressure, decreased ejection fraction, and a low stroke work index. There may be pump failure and even an abrupt development of ventricular aneurysm, septal perforation, or mitral insufficiency. The mortality rate is high even if a pacemaker is introduced, because cardiac function is sufficiently impaired by the widespread necrosis so that even if Stokes-Adams attacks are prevented, the patient may die of "pump failure," cardiogenic shock, or ventricular fibrillation. The complication rate of temporary pacing in acute myocardial infarction can be high. In one study (Jowett, 1989) of 162 patients, the complication rate was 19.8%, with four deaths related to the procedure. The mortality rate in the patients with anterior myocardial infarction was 74%, and it is not obvious that the pacemaker was always necessary. If the patient survives the episode of complete atrioventricular block with Stokes-Adams attacks in anterior infarction, it may be wise to replace the temporary ventricular pacemaker with a permanent one because there are some (though few) data indicating that these patients have a high incidence of sudden death within the ensuing 1–2 years if they are not paced (Dreifus, 1991).

2. CHRONIC ATRIOVENTRICULAR CONDUCTION DEFECTS

Clinical Findings

A. Partial (First-Degree) Atrioventricular Block: Clinically, patients with partial atrioventricular block (PR interval prolonged to 0.21 s or more at normal heart rates) alone are usually asymptomatic, and the diagnosis is made on routine electrocardiography. It may be suspected clinically if there is a very soft first heart sound, because of the inverse relationship between the PR interval and the loudness of the first sound. With long PR intervals, the mitral valve leaflets have become nearly apposed prior to ventricular systole; when they finally close completely with ventricular systole, tension at closure of the valve is associated with minimal sound. Conversely, a loud first heart sound indicates that the mitral valve leaflets were still deep in the ventricle just before ventricular systole, making first-degree atrioventricular block unlikely. This is correlated with a normal or short PR interval.

Although there is conduction delay between the atria and the ventricles in partial atrioventricular block, each atrial impulse is transmitted regularly to the ventricles. Conduction is delayed following an early premature beat, and partial atrioventricular block may be seen only in one or two beats following the long pause after an early premature beat. The refractory periods of the atrioventricular node and of

the ventricular myocardium are inversely proportionate to the preceding cycle length. Partial atrioventricular block that occurs unexpectedly in one or two beats should suggest an atrial premature beat (often nonconducted) or a His bundle premature beat that may not be easily visible on the ECG; this has been termed **concealed conduction** by Langendorf (1948) and refers to incomplete penetration of the atrioventricular node by the atrial premature beats, which are not discernible on the routine ECG but which can be seen in His bundle recordings. The next sinus beat finds the atrioventricular node partially refractory, which results in prolongation of the PR interval. An abrupt, transient, prolonged PR interval may thus justify the inference that conduction has been delayed by an event such as an atrial premature beat that is not visible by conventional means. The finding has no more significance than the atrial premature beat itself.

1. His bundle recordings– The PR interval has been shown by His bundle recordings to consist of the **AH interval** (65–156 ms), representing the spread of the impulse from the low atrial region to the bundle of His, and the **HV interval** (35–55 ms), representing the spread of the impulse from the bundle of His to the beginning of the QRS complex. Electrophysiologic studies have shown that when the prolongation of the PR interval is due to prolongation of the AH interval, the disease process is in the atrioventricular node; when the HV interval is prolonged, the pathologic processes are distal to the His bundle. The AH interval is prolonged by drugs such as digitalis and by acute myocarditis, thyrotoxicosis, acute inferior infarction, and rapid atrial pacing. In general, a prolonged AH interval (proximal block) is of more favorable prognostic significance than a prolonged HV interval (distal block).

When the AH interval is normal but the HV interval is prolonged (especially to more than 70 ms), the conduction delay is distal to the His bundle or its branches. This infranodal delay is more serious because it indicates disease of the ventricular conduction system, with a higher prevalence of chronic myocardial disease, and an adverse clinical course that may lead to sudden death. However, deaths (including sudden deaths) are usually the result of underlying cardiac disease and infrequently due to the development of heart block and Stokes-Adams attacks (Dhingra, 1981; McAnulty, 1984; Scheinman, 1982). The incidence of sudden death was no different in patients with a prolonged HV interval who were not paced from the incidence in those who were (Morady, 1984; McAnulty, 1984). It is apparent from multiple studies that the rate of progression of bifascicular and even trifascicular block to complete heart block is low. Furthermore, no single clinical or electrocardiographic variable identifies patients at risk of sudden death from future bradyarrhythmias. Pacemakers are not advised unless the HV interval exceeds 100 ms, and even this is controversial. Neurologic symptoms due to paroxysmal complete atrioventricular block require a pacemaker.

2. Trifascicular block with prolonged PR and HV intervals and bundle branch block– Trifascicular block implies conduction abnormalities involving all three fascicles of the bundle branches. On electrophysiologic study, it is demonstrated by an HV interval greater than 70 ms in the presence of left or right bundle branch block. On the surface ECG, trifascicular block can be suspected when there is (1) first-degree atrioventricular block and right or left bundle branch block (or both) or (2) right bundle branch block and either left anterior or left posterior hemiblock. If symptoms related to atrioventricular block develop, a permanent pacemaker should be inserted to relieve symptoms; however, this has not been shown to prolong life (Morady, 1984; Scheinman, 1982). Patients with prolonged HV intervals are more apt to have a greater incidence of coronary disease, ventricular arrhythmias, and cardiac failure; the high mortality rate is usually due to these causes. If the atrioventricular block is associated with a prolonged AH interval only, one can conclude that although heart disease is present, the risk of complete atrioventricular block is minimal.

B. Second-Degree Atrioventricular Block: In second-degree atrioventricular conduction delay, not every sinus impulse reaches the ventricles, with the result that failure of ventricular contraction occurs and is apparent on auscultation at the bedside by the absence (dropping) of the beat. The failure of conduction on the part of the ventricles allows the conduction system to recover, so that a subsequent beat is transmitted to the ventricles (Figures 14–5 and 14–7).

Second-degree atrioventricular block may be of two forms (Figure 14–7): (1) partial progressive atrioventricular block (also called **Wenckebach** or **Mobitz type I**), in which the PR interval progressively increases, culminating in a dropped beat; and (2) infra-His block (also called Mobitz type II), in which there may be a sudden dropped beat without change in PR interval, or there may be a 3:1 or 4:1 block, in which every third or fourth beat is dropped but the PR interval is not progressively prolonged in the beat prior to the dropped beat. The classification of Mobitz type I and Mobitz type II is only partially helpful, because some patients demonstrate both types of block in the same lead and because the site of the conduction delay in 2:1 block cannot be predicted reliably. Although in many patients with 2:1 block the block is distal to the bundle of His, it may be in the atrioventricular node. The width of the QRS complex in the conducted beats is helpful in locating the block—narrow if the block is in the atrioventricular node and wide if below it. Multiple blocks may also be present.

Clinical correlation and electrophysiologic studies have shown that Mobitz type I, or partial progressive atrioventricular block, is usually due to conduction delay in the atrioventricular node and associated with a QRS complex of normal width and a heart rate of more than 50 beats/min; it rarely produces Stokes-Adams attacks. This is in contrast to Mobitz type II, which has been shown by His bundle recordings to be

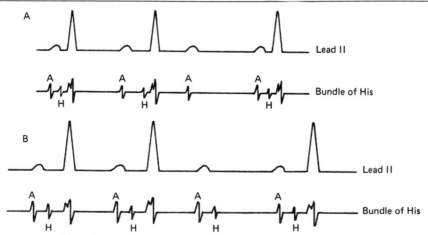

Figure 14–7. Diagrammatic illustrations of bundle of His recordings in second-degree atrioventricular block. **A:** Mobitz type I (Wenckebach) block: The first complex has a normal PR interval with normal AH and HV intervals. The second complex has a prolonged PR interval owing to lengthening of the AH interval. The third P wave is not conducted and is not followed by a bundle of His spike. This indicates that the site of the block is proximal to the His bundle in the atrioventricular node. **B:** Mobitz type II block: The first two beats are sinus-conducted, with a prolonged PR interval due to lengthening of the HV interval. The third P wave is not conducted and is followed by a His spike. This indicates that the block is distal to the His bundle. The PR interval is constant for the conducted beats, and the QRS interval is prolonged. (Reproduced, with permission, from Goldman MJ: *Principles of Clinical Electrocardiography,* 12th ed. Lange, 1986.)

due in most cases to conduction delay within or distal to the bundle of His but definitely distal to the atrioventricular node; this form is usually associated with a wide QRS complex, is more apt to progress to complete atrioventricular block with Stokes-Adams attacks, and is associated with a prolonged HV interval in about half of cases. It seems paradoxic that 2:1 atrioventricular block may be associated with a normal HV interval in the conducted beat, but this occurs because of variable conduction delay in different parts of the system. A similar situation obtains in complete atrioventricular block without a phase of partial or complete atrioventricular block. A balanced discussion of second-degree atrioventricular block is that of Zipes (1979).

1. Wenckebach pauses– In partial progressive atrioventricular block (Wenckebach type), the increment in the PR interval between the first and second conducted beats is usually greater than in subsequent conducted beats, with the PR intervals becoming longer and the RR shorter with each beat. The pauses may vary, so that the rhythm can be 2:1, 4:3, 5:4, etc. Although in Mobitz type II the second-degree block is usually associated with a 2:1 rhythm, there may be other intervals such as 3:1 or 4:1. As implied above, His bundle recordings are needed in 2:1 block to see whether the HV interval is prolonged and whether the block is proximal or distal to the His bundle.

2. Dropped beats– Patients are usually unaware of the dropped beat, and the diagnosis is often made incidentally from a routine ECG or during continuous monitoring of the ECG. Dropped beats must be differentiated from premature beats by noting that there is no heart sound at the apex. Premature beats, even when quite premature, usually cause tensing of the mitral valve and a first heart sound heard faintly at the apex (unless they are blocked supraventricular premature beats). If the contraction is not sufficient to open the aortic valve, no pulse may be felt.

3. His bundle recordings– The division of the PR interval into the AH interval and the HV interval (see above) by His bundle recordings has led to an attempt to classify second-degree atrioventricular block according to duration of the HV interval (nodal if the HV interval is normal; infranodal if it is prolonged). Measurement of the HV interval is imprecise, and the interval may be either normal or abnormal, with either a normal or abnormal PR interval or with evidence of infranodal ventricular conduction defect such as left or right bundle branch block or hemiblock (see below).

C. Complete (Third-Degree) Atrioventricular Block: Block usually progresses from first- to second- to third-degree (Figure 14–8), but complete block may occur without preceding partial block, or the PR interval may be normal immediately after a period of complete block. Runs of ventricular tachycardia or fibrillation may interrupt complete atrioventricular block, may be precipitated by exercise, and may be the mechanism for a Stokes-Adams attack (Figure 14–9). The site of the complete atrioventricular block is often suggested by the width of the QRS complex and the ventricular rate. In atrioventricular nodal complete block, the width is usually normal, and the escape pacemaker has a rate of more than 50/min (Narula, 1971). When the block is distal to the His bundle, the QRS complex is usually widened and the ventricular rate slower. Because of the block, there is dissociation between the atrial and ventricular contractions, but atrioventricular dissociation is not synonymous with atrioventricular block. Atrioventricular dissociation is always present in complete atrioventricular block but may also be present in its absence, as in nonparoxysmal junctional tachycardia or ventricular tachycardia. In these situations, the junctional or ventricular pacemaker rate is faster than the sinus rate and does not permit the latter to activate the ventricles.

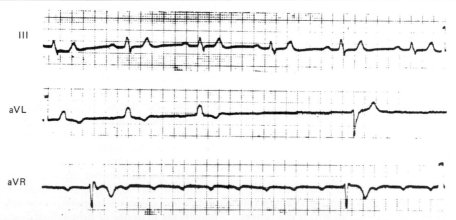

Figure 14–8. Transition from 2:1 atrioventricular block to complete block with ventricular escape following a period of ventricular standstill in a 53-year-old man.

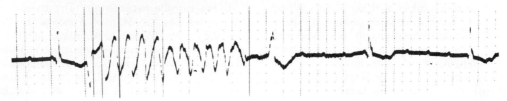

Figure 14–9. Complete atrioventricular block with run of ventricular tachycardia in a 55-year-old woman with atrial flutter.

1. "Escape" pacemakers– In complete atrioventricular block, survival of the patient depends upon activation of pacemakers distal to the block, which are called "escape" pacemakers. When the block is in the atrioventricular node, the pacemaker may be in the junctional tissue or proximal bundle of His, which has an inherently faster rate of spontaneous phase 4 depolarization than do pacemakers lower in the Purkinje system. When the atrioventricular block is distal to the bundle of His, the "escape" pacemaker may be in one of the bundle branches or in the ventricles. These are less reliable and may fail temporarily, leading to cessation of ventricular activity, with Stokes-Adams attacks.

2. Stokes-Adams attacks– Stokes-Adams attacks are manifested by cerebral symptoms due to cerebral ischemia from ventricular asystole in complete atrioventricular block or ventricular conduction defects. Ventricular asystole may follow a period of ventricular fibrillation; therefore, a patient seen late may be thought to have primary ventricular asystole when in fact it was preceded by ventricular fibrillation. In almost all cases of cardiac arrest observed at onset, the mechanism is ventricular fibrillation with or without preceding ventricular tachycardia, followed by asystole. The latter obviously can occur de novo. The cerebral symptoms reflect a continuum from momentary transient giddiness to loss of consciousness, convulsions, and sudden death, depending upon the duration of interruption of the cardiac output. The momentary lapse of consciousness resembles a petit mal episode and may last only a few seconds. The attacks are abrupt and unpredictable, can occur without warning many times a day or at intervals of days to years, are variable in severity (duration of syncope), and occur in recumbency as well as in the erect position. The patient falls to the ground without warning and becomes pale and pulseless but rapidly recovers when the ventricles resume beating. There is usually a postischemic flush, and the reactive hyperemia is often so obvious that both the patient and witnesses can describe it. As soon as the ventricles resume beating, the patient feels well and can resume activity. This is in sharp contrast to epilepsy or vasovagal fainting, in which the patient has premonitory symptoms and feels weak and nauseated both before and after. Absence of premonitory symptoms, pallor during and hyperemia after the attack, and rapid recovery are characteristic of Stokes-Adams attacks.

3. Symptoms other than syncope– Depending upon the heart rate and the underlying condition of the ventricle, the patient may be totally asymptomatic despite the presence of complete atrioventricular block or may complain of fatigue and weakness because a normal cardiac output cannot be maintained at the slow rate, especially with physical activity. Any manifestations of cardiac failure or cerebral symptoms due to impaired cerebral perfusion may then develop. A ventricular rate of more than 40/min is usually necessary for the patient to be free of symptoms. There may be episodes of transient lightheadedness rather than typical Stokes-Adams attacks if the duration of ventricular standstill is short. If ventricular fibrillation occurs, defibrillation is necessary. Asystole lasting 2–3 minutes is usually fatal if not treated.

4. Signs– The physical signs of complete atrioventricular block are due to the slow ventricular rate, the long period of variable diastolic ventricular filling, the large stroke volume resulting from the slow heart rate, and the presence of independent atrial and ventricular contractions. The slow ventricular rate increases only slightly (approximately 5 beats/min) with exercise or following a sympathomimetic drug and is associated with a wide pulse pressure and raised systolic pressure if ventricular function is normal. The large stroke volume produces a variable pulmonary systolic ejection murmur and third heart sound. The most important signs are those related to independent atrial and ventricular contractions with evidence of atrioventricular dissociation. Depending upon the timing of the contractions of the atrium and ventricles, the first sound varies in intensity, so that there may be intermittent loud first sounds as well as atrial sounds. There may be intermittent **"cannon" *a* waves** when the right atrium contracts against a closed tricuspid valve.

5. His bundle recordings– Patients with slow ventricular rates and symptoms should have 24-hour ambulatory electrocardiographic monitoring to determine if the episodes of near-syncope or syncope are associated with the development of complete atrioventricular block. Light-headedness and dizziness are common symptoms in older people, and it must be definitely established that the symptom is due to complete block before the decision is made to insert a pacemaker. Even with other evidence of conduction delay in the bundle branches with bilateral bundle branch block or a prolonged HV interval by His bundle recording, dizziness and weakness may be due to other atrial or ventricular arrhythmias, postural hypotension, anemia, diffuse cerebral arteriosclerosis, or general debility and not to complete block. This is especially important in patients with bilateral bundle branch block with or without a prolonged PR interval who have syncope or near syncope. His bundle recordings have shown that whether or not the PR interval or HV interval is prolonged, one cannot automatically assume that episodes of syncope or near syncope are due to intermittent complete atrioventricular block. The longer the HV interval, the more likely that episodic syncope is due to the development of complete atrioventricular block, but this is not invariable.

In a study of 141 consecutive patients with syncope of unknown cause undergoing electrophysiologic studies, six clinical predictors of the results of the electrophysiologic study were found (Bachinsky, 1992). Organic heart disease, premature ventricular beats, and nonsustained ventricular tachycardia by ambulatory electrocardiography predicted serious ventricular tachyarrhythmias at electrophysiologic study with a sensitivity of 100%. Sinus bradycardia, first-degree atrioventricular block, and bundle branch block were predictive of bradyarrhythmias as the cause of syncope, with a sensitivity of 79%.

Treatment

A. Partial (First-Degree) Atrioventricular Block:
Treatment involves serial observation with ECGs if the conduction defect is chronic. Attempts should be made to eliminate the cause if block is due to use of digitalis or other antiarrhythmic agents, beta-blocking agents, quinidine, or procainamide; to hyperkalemia; or to myocarditis. A decrease in the PR interval following exercise is an encouraging sign, indicating that the conduction defect is benign and in the atrioventricular node. In the absence of clinical cardiac disease, first-degree atrioventricular block is a benign condition (Mymin, 1986). If the patient is symptomatic, with episodic dizziness or syncope suggesting intermittent Stokes-Adams attacks, 24-hour continuous ambulatory electrocardiographic monitoring is indicated to determine if symptoms are due to complete atrioventricular block or another cause (eg, ventricular arrhythmias) not related to bradyarrhythmia.

Patients with first-degree atrioventricular block who have cerebral symptoms proved to be due to bradyarrhythmia are generally advised to undergo insertion of a pacemaker (see below), especially if ambulatory monitoring reveals episodes of more advanced block associated with symptoms. If symp-tomatic patients are shown by His bundle recordings to have a prolonged AH interval and a normal HV interval, the conduction defect is atrioventricular nodal or supranodal, and the risk of development of complete atrioventricular block is minimal even in the presence of known heart disease. Insertion of a pacemaker in patients with a prolonged HV interval is indicated only if the patient has neurologic symptoms or if episodes of syncope are known to be due to high-grade atrioventricular block.

B. Second-Degree Atrioventricular Block:
If second-degree block is in the atrioventricular node (Mobitz type I), even with inferior myocardial infarction, clinical observation is usually sufficient, because progression to *complete* symptomatic atrioventricular block and Stokes-Adams attacks is uncommon (Dreifus, 1991). In patients with inferior myocardial infarction and complete atrioventricular block, it is still not clear whether a temporary pacemaker should be introduced. We believe it is acceptable to insert a pacemaker in such patients with inferior infarction who develop complete atrioventricular block from second-degree block in the atrioventricular node, especially if it occurs early or if symptoms develop that suggest Stokes-Adams attacks. The likelihood of Stokes-Adams attacks is less in these patients than it is in those with complete atrioventricular block distal to the atrioventricular node, but attacks do occur. Atropine, 0.3–0.5 mg intravenously, may decrease the degree of atrioventricular block and perhaps avoid the need for insertion of a temporary pacemaker. With the development of a reliable external pacemaker, the electrode patches are frequently placed in preparation for use of the external pacemaker if the junctional pacemaker slows to the point of hemodynamic compromise or fails entirely.

In chronic atrioventricular block distal to the atrioventricular node (Mobitz type II), there is controversy about the necessity for placing a permanent pacemaker if the patient is asymptomatic, though at present the authors believe doing so is justified since with Mobitz II block sudden failure of the distal pacemaker is not uncommon (Dreifus, 1991). However, if the patient has symptoms suggesting episodic syncope or its equivalent or if the block develops acutely in the setting of acute anterior infarction with acute development of bifascicular block, a temporary demand pacemaker is immediately indicated. It is important to determine whether the bifascicular block preceded the acute infarction; if it did, the prognosis is better and a pacemaker need not be inserted. The decision about what course of action to take will also depend upon the age of the patient, the degree of hemodynamic impairment, and the degree of associated atherosclerosis.

C. Complete (Third-Degree) Atrioventricular Block:
Drugs are not used chronically today in complete atrioventricular block because of the almost universal availability of pacemakers. During the interval

between recognition of a Stokes-Adams attack and introduction of a temporary or permanent pacemaker, it is wise for the patient to be in the hospital with continuous electrocardiographic monitoring and an intravenous infusion of isoproterenol available. In this situation, placement of the electrode patches for the external pacemaker to standby is appropriate.

The treatment of asymptomatic complete atrioventricular block discovered accidentally is a matter of dispute. The prognosis is worse when a pacemaker is not used, because patients with complete block, especially if over age 60, may develop Stokes-Adams attacks, ventricular arrhythmias, or cardiac or cerebral perfusion abnormalities. For this reason, most authorities would recommend a permanent pacemaker in spite of the controversy.

In the past, it was thought that congenital complete atrioventricular block had a favorable prognosis if patients were asymptomatic. However, in long-term follow-up, 35 patients, most less than age 20 years when first seen, developed symptoms, presumably due to atrioventricular block, and two-thirds required pacemaker insertion. Symptoms were often absent for many years. The prognosis was worse in patients who developed symptoms in infancy, but most patients required pacemakers before age 50 (Reid, 1982).

If the patient has had a single unequivocal Stokes-Adams attack, a pacemaker should be introduced because recurrent attacks are the rule, and any individual episode may be fatal. When atrioventricular block is varying from 2:1 to complete, a pacemaker should be inserted because during the transition there may be ventricular asystole with Stokes-Adams attacks and the patient is at greater risk of ventricular fibrillation. In patients with permanent or intermittent complete atrioventricular block, pacemakers can dramatically improve cardiac failure, relieve cerebral symptoms with syncope or near-syncope, and improve survival. The pacemaker should be set at 70–80 beats/min; the programmable pacemakers permit variation of rate, depending upon the response of the patient.

If the relevance of the symptoms to the cardiac rhythm is uncertain in patients with bradyarrhythmias who suffer symptoms of heart failure or low cardiac output with dizziness or fainting, a temporary pacemaker can be inserted to see what effect it has on the symptoms. If the patient has documented complete atrioventricular block with Stokes-Adams attacks, a temporary pacemaker is not required, and a permanent pacemaker should be inserted promptly. The mortality rate in a group of patients paced for atrioventricular block compared with that expected in the population at large was 1.7:1 in one study (Ginks, 1979). The mortality rate was higher in the first year of pacing than subsequently. The most important factor influencing prognosis was a history of myocardial infarction. Late sudden death occurred in one-fourth of patients, probably due to ventricular tachyarrhythmia.

D. Unexplained Syncope: Syncope is a common clinical problem with many causes. The commonest reason for syncope is vasovagal reflex bradycardia or vasodilation, resulting in hypotension. On noninvasive workup, the cause of the syncope is apparent about half the time. In the rest of the patients, the syncope is of unknown cause. In the presence of clinical heart disease—either coronary disease or cardiomyopathy—the incidence of ventricular tachyarrhythmias as the cause of the syncope is high, and these patients deserve electrophysiologic study. If a monomorphic ventricular tachycardia can be induced, the patient should have an antiarrhythmic drug selected by virtue of its ability to prevent the induction of arrhythmia by electrophysiologic stimulation (Fogoros, 1992). Electrophysiologic studies in patients with unexplained syncope have shown that about one-third have ventricular arrhythmias, a smaller percentage conduction defects, and approximately half an unknown cause. Appropriate therapy can be instituted in one-fourth to one-third of these patients, and about half have no further episodes of syncope even in the absence of definitive treatment (Hess, 1982; Manolini, 1990).

PACEMAKERS

The modern implantable pacemaker is a complex miniaturized electronic device capable of sensing electrical activity in the atrium, the ventricle, or both. If it senses no electrical activity within a preprogrammed period, it can electrically stimulate the appropriate chamber. It can also sense depolarization and trigger a further impulse. Most pacemakers allow electronic reprogramming of multiple parameters such as heart rate, impulse amplitude and duration, sensitivity, and refractory period, as well as delay intervals; the preprogrammed values can be printed out on demand. The five-letter international code for the characteristics of pacemakers is described in Table 7–1.

The pacemaker's programmability and reprogrammability after implantation allow the clinician to tailor the pacemaker to the patient, maximize battery life, and reduce the frequency of pacemaker replacement. Reprogramming sensitivity can diminish excessive pacemaker firing caused by extraneous electrical signals. Changes in refractory period can avoid erroneous sensing of T waves. Increases in output can compensate for increasing threshold. However, programmable features are underutilized; most pacemakers are never reprogrammed after insertion.

VVI & DDD Pacemakers

The indications for using a specific type of pacemaker are determined by the manifestations of the disease as well as by certain patient characteristics. The VVI pacemaker, for example, is a ventricular standby pacemaker that will prevent the ventricular response from dropping below a predetermined rate but will not respond to exercise or other physiologic demands by an appropriate increase in heart rate. The DDD (or double-chamber) pacemaker will respond to increases in atrial rate with appropriate increases in ventricular rate, thus increasing cardiac output for increased physiologic demands. This is the best pacemaker for young patients, who can be expected to benefit from such a feature.

Another problem with the VVI pacemaker is that it can produce a retrograde depolarization of the atrium and result in an atrial contraction after ventricular contraction, causing a "cannon" *a* wave in the jugular pulse; there is also loss of the appropriate atrial "kick" just before ventricular systole, which in some patients causes a drop in stroke volume and systolic blood pressure. Together, these physiologic effects result in "pacemaker syndrome"—a feeling of fullness in the neck and head and faintness. The DDD pacemaker can avoid this problem but, if improperly programmed, can produce retrograde conduction of ventricular depolarization back to the atrium, resulting in a reentrant supraventricular "pacemaker tachycardia." Patients without an effective atrial rhythm, such as those with atrial tachyarrhythmias, atrial flutter, or atrial fibrillation, which can be either chronic or intermittent, are not candidates for pacemakers in the DDD mode.

The VVI pacemaker is still commonly used, but DDD pacemakers can be programmed to function as any type of pacemaker and are therefore being used with increasing frequency. In 1989, a survey found that 32% of first-time pacemaker implants that year in the USA were dual-chamber pacemakers (Bernstein, 1989). If the DDD pacemaker did not require an extra atrial lead, increased expense, and more complex follow-up studies, it would be used exclusively in patients without atrial arrhythmias.

Indications for Pacemaker Implantation

In general, pacemakers should be reserved for patients who are symptomatic, either with hemodynamic instability or symptoms of low cardiac output and cerebral dysfunction proved to be due to a bradyarrhythmia or a tachyarrhythmia that will benefit from the use of a pacemaker—ie, they should be reserved for patients with arrhythmia-dependent symptoms. Table 14–5 summarizes the indications for pacemaker implantation.

A DDD (double-chamber) pacemaker is recommended if the patient has a competent atrial rhythm and (1) is young and likely to benefit from the physiologic pacemaker, which allows increase in ventricular rate appropriate to increased demand with exer-

Table 14–5. Indications for pacemaker implantation.[1]

1. Acquired complete atrioventricular heart block—symptomatic or asymptomatic, permanent or transient.
2. Congenital complete heart block with symptoms due to bradyarrhythmia.
3. Mobitz type II second-degree atrioventricular block.
4. Mobitz type I second-degree atrioventricular block, chronic in duration with symptoms of hemodynamic instability due to the block.
5. Sinus bradycardia with rate under 40/min and hemodynamic instability, seizures, syncope or dizziness, mental confusion, or congestive heart failure that improves on temporary pacing. Correlation between symptoms and bradycardia must be documented.
6. Sinus bradycardia causing symptoms as in 5, above, but due to the use of a drug that cannot be avoided, eg, beta-blockers in patients with angina pectoris, antiarrhythmic drugs, or any hypertensive drugs resulting in sympathetic and symptomatic bradyarrhythmias.
7. Sinoatrial node dysfunction with symptoms of hemodynamic instability, presyncope, or syncope due to bradyarrhythmia.
8. Sinus bradycardia with bradycardia-dependent ventricular or supraventricular tachyarrhythmias.
9. Carotid sinus syncope in which dizziness or syncope is due to the chronotropic depression with ventricular arrhythmias and not to the vasopressor component.
10. Transient complete heart block or Mobitz type II second degree atrioventricular block in patients with bi- or triventricular block, prophyllactically following recovery from acute myocardial infarction.
11. Ventricular tachycardia controlled by overdrive ventricular pacing.

[1] Modified and reproduced, with permission, from *Medicare Coverage Issues Manual.* US Department of Health & Human Services, 1988; and Harthrone JW: Cardiac pacemakers. Curr Probl Cardiol 1987;12:649.

cise; (2) has symptoms of "pacemaker syndrome" with VVI pacing or the systolic blood pressure drops on VVI pacemaking; or (3) atrial contraction is necessary for optimal ventricular function.

Pacemakers have now been designed to increase ventricular rate in response to physiologic signals of increased demand for cardiac output other than the increased sinus rate (so-called rate-modulated pacemakers), including increased muscular activity (through a piezoelectric crystal), increased respiratory rate, increased temperature of the venous blood, and alterations of the exercise QT interval. These pacemakers could be used in patients who are chronotropically incompetent, ie, who have atrial arrhythmias, such as atrial flutter or fibrillation.

The dual-chamber pacemaker in the DDD mode, especially with rate modulation (DDDR mode), returns the patient with complete heart block and a normally functioning left ventricle to a near-normal physiologic state. Compared with the VVI pacemaker, the cardiac output in response to activity is more nearly normal, in part because an optimal atrioventricular interval for maximizing stroke volume can be programmed. With exercise, the normal increase in heart rate allows for a normal increase in cardiac output. Studies on the chronic effects of different pacing modes have indicated that dual-chamber pacing may reduce the heart size and have a long-term beneficial effect on exercise capacity. Estimates are that in 60–80% of patients who need pacemakers, dual-chamber DDD pacemakers are indicated (Buckingham, 1992).

The patient with an implanted pacemaker must have a log kept and updated at all visits of all changes made in any of the parameters, such as rate, refractory period, and delay times. Following patients with DDD pacemakers requires information about which pacemaker was implanted and its particular characteristics. Experience in this area is essential. The inexperienced physician can misinterpret a normal function of these programmable pacemakers as evidence of malfunction, leading to inappropriate replacement (Furman, 1990).

There is evidence that pacemakers have in some cases been implanted for insufficient reasons. In view of this problem, the indications for pacemaker implantation should be unequivocally established and documented in the patient's record.

Proper Functioning of Pacemakers (See also Chapter 7.)

After being provided with a pacemaker, the patient should be closely observed to confirm its proper functioning, especially during the first month. Recurrence of symptoms suggests that positioning of the electrode catheter has been faulty or that the catheter has moved, and 24-hour ambulatory electrocardiographic monitoring should be employed to correlate symptoms with the possibility of such faulty pacing. The rate of the pacemaker and its functioning should be checked periodically—weekly for the first month, monthly for 3 months, then once a year, then more frequently as battery failure is anticipated. The patient or a family member should be taught to count the pulse rate, understand the significance of changes in rate, and immediately report such changes to the physician.

VENTRICULAR CONDUCTION DEFECTS & BUNDLE BRANCH BLOCK

Bundle branch block is an electrocardiographic finding, usually an unexpected one. It is uncommon before age 60 and increases in frequency with age. Most patients with bundle branch block have associated cardiovascular disease or develop it within a few years; approximately 20% have no obvious abnormality of the heart. Bundle branch block is diagnosed when the QRS complex equals or exceeds 0.12 s, with late delay in the right precordial leads in right bundle branch block and in the left ventricular leads

in left bundle branch block, combined with depressed ST and asymmetrically inverted T waves opposite to the direction of the QRS delay in the leads with late delay in the QRS complex. The block may be intermittent (Figure 14–10) or may develop over a period of years.

The term "bundle branch block" implies that the branch is in fact blocked, whereas anatomically and functionally there is merely a delay in conduction in the bundle branches. The term "conduction delay" rather than "block" is therefore preferable, and the degree of the delay can be expressed as minor, incomplete, or complete.

When a right or left bundle branch block occurs in the presence of associated cardiac disease, its significance depends on the nature of the cardiac disease, associated defects in the fascicles of the left bundle, a prolonged PR interval, and symptoms suggesting intermittent, more advanced heart block.

Examination over a period of months or years or monitoring of the ECG for 24 hours in patients with either right or left bundle branch block may reveal paroxysmal atrioventricular block, indicating that the ventricular conduction defects precede and may be the earliest precursors of complete atrioventricular block. Twenty-four-hour electrocardiographic monitoring and careful clinical observation are indicated in patients with isolated bundle branch block who have symptoms suggesting bradyarrhythmia.

Left Bundle Branch Block

Left bundle branch block is most frequently found in individuals with clinical evidence of heart disease. It is extremely rare as a congenital abnormality. In the absence of other evidence of heart disease, it can be associated with many years of normal life (Rotman, 1975). Latent coronary disease may be the cause (Fisch, 1980). In the absence of any evident heart disease, it is probably due to discrete abnormality of the conduction system (Lenègre's disease) or calcification of valve rings (Lev's disease).

The left bundle is not a discrete entity, as is the right bundle, and the division into left anterior and left posterior divisions is purely arbitrary. Left bundle branch block obscures the electrocardiographic diagnosis of acute myocardial infarction (Figure 14–11); radioisotopic methods (see Chapter 8) may be useful in diagnosis under these circumstances. Abnormal thallium-201 scintigrams have been described in left bundle branch block in the absence of coronary artery disease. This is believed to be due to a combination of hemodynamic effects contributing to reduced coronary filling of the septum in diastole (Larcos, 1991). The diagnostic accuracy may be improved if single-photon emission computed tomography (SPECT) is used, and the presence of coronary disease in a patient with left bundle branch block can be predicted best when an apical defect is present, not just a septal or anterior defect (Matzer, 1991).

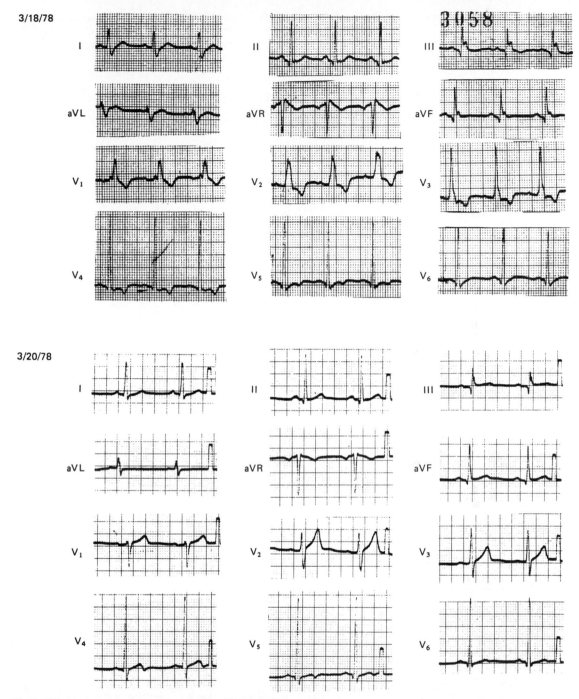

Figure 14–10. Intermittent right bundle branch block (top tracing) in a 63-year-old man with postoperative esophagitis. Two days later, conduction was normal (bottom tracing).

Myocardial ischemia can also be masked by a pacemaker rhythm and may become apparent when the pacemaker is turned off. The abnormal depolarization caused by a pacemaker is associated with an abnormal repolarization. When the pacemaker is turned off, the abnormal repolarization may persist, causing abnormal T waves that do not necessarily imply myocardial ischemia. Care must be taken to exclude nonspecific T wave changes.

If the patient with left bundle branch block requires general anesthesia for noncardiac surgery, a temporary pacemaker need not be inserted, since this has

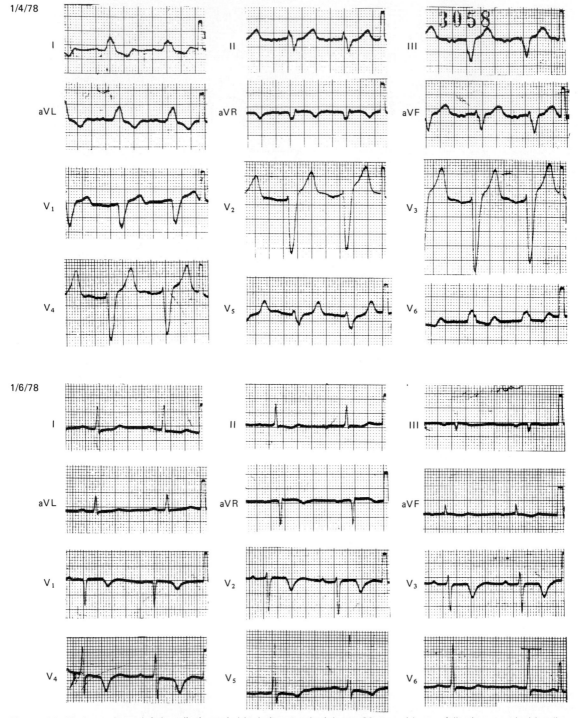

Figure 14–11. Intermittent left bundle branch block (top tracing) in an 80-year-old man following gastric bleeding. Second tracing 2 days later (bottom tracing) reveals apparent acute myocardial ischemia, but repolarization changes after left bundle branch block occur in the absence of any known heart disease.

not been associated with the precipitation of high degrees of atrioventricular block. Transient complete heart block occurred in only one of 52 patients with chronic right bundle branch block and left axis deviation (bifascicular block) who required noncardiac surgery (Pastore, 1978). However, if a right-sided cardiac catheter is to be inserted in a patient with preexisting left bundle branch block, a temporary pacemaker should be placed, because the catheter could cause right bundle branch injury and precipitate complete heart block.

Right Bundle Branch Block

Right bundle branch block, especially incomplete block, occurs in many normal individuals and may be congenital. If one includes as showing right ventricular conduction defects those ECGs with an r′ in the right precordial leads, the percentage in the general population may be as high as 10%. Transient right bundle branch block (complete or incomplete) may follow the development of acute right ventricular dilation in acute pulmonary embolism. Pulmonary hypertension develops transiently, causing right ventricular dilation and an electrocardiographic pattern of right ventricular conduction defect.

Right bundle branch block is more common in acute myocardial infarction than is left bundle branch block and may be rapidly followed by complete atrioventricular block, especially if the patient has associated left anterior hemiblock. The right bundle is supplied anatomically by the first septal perforator branch of the left anterior descending artery. Right bundle branch block, therefore, is common when necrosis of the proximal portion of the septum occurs as a result of occlusion of the proximal left anterior descending artery. His bundle recordings have shown that whether the PR interval is normal or prolonged, HV prolongation may be present in chronic right or chronic left bundle branch block, indicating extension of the conduction defect to the more distal branches of the bundles. This is more common in left block than in right block.

Isolated right bundle branch block has been subdivided into proximal block and distal block, with different prognoses. Patients with distal delay have episodes of syncope or near-syncope, which are rare in proximal block. The distinction can be made by noting whether the delay in pulmonary valve opening is mainly between mitral and tricuspid valve closure (proximal block) or between tricuspid valve closure and pulmonary valve opening (distal block) (Dancy, 1982).

Bilateral Bundle Branch Block

In bilateral bundle branch block (right bundle branch block and left anterior hemiblock, right bundle branch block and left posterior hemiblock, or right or left bundle branch block with prolonged PR interval or alternating right and left bundle branch

block), the heart presumably depends on the remaining fascicle for conduction of the atrial impulse to the ventricle (Fisch, 1980). The incidence of complete atrioventricular block is probably about 1% per year in unselected asymptomatic patients found or known to have bifascicular block (Figure 14–12).

The presence of an atrioventricular conduction defect, whether it be a prolonged HV interval or second-degree block, does not necessarily mean that Stokes-Adams attacks are likely or that a pacemaker is necessary. *Further prospective studies and clinical judgment are required before pacemaker implantation can be justified solely on the basis of the ECG or HIS bundle findings in the absence of symptoms shown to be due to bradyarrhythmias* (Dreifus, 1991).

Unifascicular & Bifascicular Block

The main left bundle branch of the bundle of His usually divides into two main branches, the left anterior superior and the left posterior fascicles. Anatomically, the division is often much more complex, but for clinical purposes it is sufficient to assume only the two divisions. A third "septal" fascicle is postulated to supply the septum. Left anterior fascicular block is diagnosed when the frontal plane QRS axis is to the left and superior, between −45 and −90 degrees. There is an r wave and a prominent S wave in leads II and III. There are also q waves in leads I and aVL. The differentiation from an old inferior myocardial infarction is not always easy. Left posterior hemiblock is diagnosed when there is right axis deviation greater than 120 degrees, provided right ventricular hypertrophy or old lateral myocardial infarction (both of which may cause right axis deviation) can be excluded. In the presence of right bundle branch block, left anterior and left posterior hemiblock can be diagnosed if the initial 0.04–0.06 s of the QRS are markedly leftward or rightward, respectively.

Left anterior hemiblock is much more common than left posterior hemiblock. Although the incidence of chronic asymptomatic left anterior hemiblock increases with age, it is not a sensitive indicator of clinical cardiac disease (Corne, 1978). The prevalence of left anterior hemiblock in 16,000 life insurance applicants was only 2.5%.

The causes of bifascicular block are chiefly those of ventricular conduction defects anywhere: hypertensive or coronary heart disease, fibrosis of the conduction system, and primary myocardial disease. Bifascicular block is more common in men. The average age of patients when first seen is about 60 years. Coronary disease, arrhythmias on ambulatory electrocardiographic monitoring, and congestive heart failure are more common when the HV interval is prolonged (Dhingra, 1981).

In bifascicular block with right bundle branch block and left anterior or left posterior hemiblock, it is assumed that two of the three fascicles that are extensions from the bundle of His are involved, and

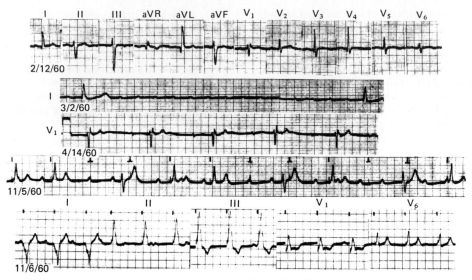

Figure 14–12. Five successive ECGs of a 58-year-old man suffering from Stokes-Adams attacks. First tracing, February 12, 1960. Regular sinus rhythm 66/min, practically normal PR interval measuring 0.20 s, atypical right bundle branch block with QRS axis –60 degrees, and left anterior hemiblock (bifascicular block), T axis +20 degrees, QRS duration = 0.12 s, rSr' pattern in V₁ (r' delay = 0.08 s), qr or QR pattern in aVR and aVL; measured in aVL, the left ventricular activation time would be delayed to 0.09 s. The third tracing, recorded on April 14, 1960, showed a complete atrioventricular block (76/36), with a right ventricular delay (identical in pattern with what is seen in sinus rhythm); a ventricular pause of 7 seconds is seen in the record of March 2. The last two tracings, recorded after electrical stimulation, showed in one an intermittent response and in the other a regular response. (Reproduced, with permission, from Lenègre J: Etiology and pathology of bilateral bundle branch block in relation to complete heart block. Prog Cardiovasc Dis 1964;6:409.)

survival depends on adequate functioning of the remaining third fascicle. Careful follow-up (including ambulatory electrocardiographic monitoring) is sufficient in asymptomatic bifascicular block unless the patient develops cerebral symptoms thought (or found by ambulatory monitoring) to be due to atrioventricular block. If the symptoms strongly suggest Stokes-Adams attacks and the diagnosis is documented by continuous monitoring of the ECG, a pacemaker is recommended (Scheinman, 1982).

Although patients with bifascicular block may die suddenly, only 5% in one study had developed documented complete atrioventricular block over a period of years. Many patients with bifascicular block have a history of angina, bundle branch block, or ventricular arrhythmias, and sudden death can occur without complete atrioventricular block. Although sudden death is a major cause of death in these patients, most deaths are due to ventricular arrhythmias or cardiac failure and not to atrioventricular block. Prophylactic pacing is therefore not recommended unless patients with dizziness or syncope have documented bradyarrhythmias associated with their symptoms. In these chronically ill patients, dizziness and syncope may be due to many causes, including drugs, conduction defects, bleeding, postural hypotension, paroxysmal arrhythmias, aortic stenosis, cardiomyopathy, and vasovagal fainting, among others. Table 14–6 tabulates

the causes of syncope in patients with chronic bifascicular block and demonstrates the rarity with which atrioventricular or sinoatrial block occurs in these patients.

Because of the hazard of abrupt onset of complete

Table 14–6. Causes of syncope in 30 of 186 patients with chronic bifascicular block.[1,2]

Cause	RBBB and LAH (124)[3]	RBBB and LPH (24)[3]	LBBB (38)[3]
Second- or third-degree atrioventricular block	3	1	1
Sinoatrial block		1	
Orthostatic hypotension	2		
Seizure disorders	3		
Gastrointestinal bleeding			1
Ventricular arrhythmia	5	1	3
Unknown	8		
TOTAL	21	3	6

[1] Reproduced, with permission, from Dhingra RC et al: Evaluation and management of conduction disease. Cardiovascular Med 1978;3:493.
[2] RBBB, LBBB, right and left bundle branch block; LAH, LPH, left anterior and posterior hemiblock.
[3] Number of patients in subgroup.

atrioventricular block and syncope, a conservative course of action is *not* advised in acute anterior myocardial infarction—a pacemaker should be promptly introduced when left anterior hemiblock with right bundle branch block (bifascicular block) develops.

Bifascicular block with right bundle branch block and left posterior hemiblock is often overdiagnosed because right axis deviation exceeding 110 degrees can be found in normal thin individuals or those with right ventricular hypertrophy. A marked superior axis, even to the right, can occur with some varieties of anterolateral myocardial infarction. Left posterior hemiblock is an uncommon condition.

Intermittent or Rate-Dependent Conduction Defects

Conduction defects are not static, and electrocardiographic abnormalities may be present on one occasion and absent at other times (Figure 14–12). Atrioventricular block, bundle branch block, and bifascicular block may vary with the heart rate and be either bradycardia- or tachycardia-dependent. The mechanism of tachycardia-dependent bundle branch block is probably related to abnormal prolongation of refractoriness with an increased heart rate (Chiale, 1990).

VENTRICULAR PREEXCITATION (Accelerated Conduction Syndrome; Wolff-Parkinson-White Syndrome)

Ventricular preexcitation is usually congenital. The most common variety of preexcitation, the Wolff-Parkinson-White syndrome, is characterized by excitation of the ventricles earlier than would be expected from the normal activation sequence from the sinoatrial node, the atrioventricular node, and the Purkinje system. The ventricle is preexcited usually by an accessory pathway (the bundle of Kent) that bypasses the atrioventricular node. Additional bypass tracts have been described. Preexcitation in Wolff-Parkinson-White syndrome can be seen in the ECG: the PR interval is short (< 0.12 s), and the QRS interval is widened because of an initial slurred portion, the delta wave. A variant of preexcitation in which there is accelerated conduction through a portion of the atrioventricular node, such that the QRS interval is normal but the PR interval is short, is known as the Lown-Ganong-Levine syndrome. This syndrome may also be caused by an atrio-His muscular pathway.

Preexcitation may occur by a number of accessory pathways (Figure 14–13). Early activation of the ventricle occurs along a complex system of accessory pathways, as shown by epicardial mapping and surgical interruption of the pathways (Gallagher: Epicardial mapping, 1978). The lateral accessory pathway (bundle of Kent) enters a portion of the ventricular

myocardium from the atrium. Mahaim fibers may pass from the bundle of His to the ventricular myocardium, and pathways may spread from the internodal atrial tracks to the ventricular myocardium, bypassing the upper part of the atrioventricular node via the James fibers. The precise anatomy of the bypass track can only be determined by epicardial mapping. The orientation of the delta wave gives a clue to the location of the accessory pathways, which may be anterior, posterior, septal, lateral, or a combination of these sites (Figure 14–13; Table 14–7).

Preexcitation may be constant or intermittent, the latter often brought on by a change in atrial rate. Because the ventricle is activated both via the accessory pathway and via the normal atrioventricular nodal pathway, fusion ventricular beats may occur. The syndrome occurs in 0.5–2% of the population, and paroxysmal atrial arrhythmias occur in half of affected individuals. Table 14–8 summarizes the effect of drugs.

1. LOWN-GANONG-LEVINE SYNDROME

The Lown-Ganong-Levine syndrome (Lown, 1952) is characterized on the ECG by a short PR interval and normal QRS interval without a delta wave. It is thought to represent a variety of short-circuiting of the upper part of the atrioventricular node (via James fibers) and is also associated with increased frequency of paroxysmal atrial arrhythmias. The arrhythmias observed in Lown-Ganong-Levine syndrome include mostly atrial and ventricular premature beats; however, paroxysmal supraventricular tachycardia as well as ventricular tachycardia may occur (Benditt, 1978). Concealed accessory pathways for retrograde conduction occur in some patients with paroxysmal tachycardia, and individual electrophysiologic evaluation is necessary. The explanation for the reentrant paroxysmal tachycardia in Lown-Ganong-Levine syndrome may be that the patient possesses essentially normal dual atrioventricular pathways but one conducts faster than the other (Josephson, 1977). Aberrancy occurs because the ventricular complex resulting from the atrial premature beat occurs during the relative refractory period of the preceding depolarization before repolarization is complete. Ventricular depolarization following the atrial premature beat begins, therefore, at a less negative maximum resting potential and alters phase 0 of the action potential.

If such a patient has supraventricular tachycardia and the dual pathway occurs within the atrioventricular node, catheter ablation would result in complete heart block. In junctional supraventricular tachycardia and supraventricular tachycardias associated with Wolff-Parkinson-White syndrome, the two pathways are usually anatomically separate and can be individually ablated. Therefore, if the supraventricular

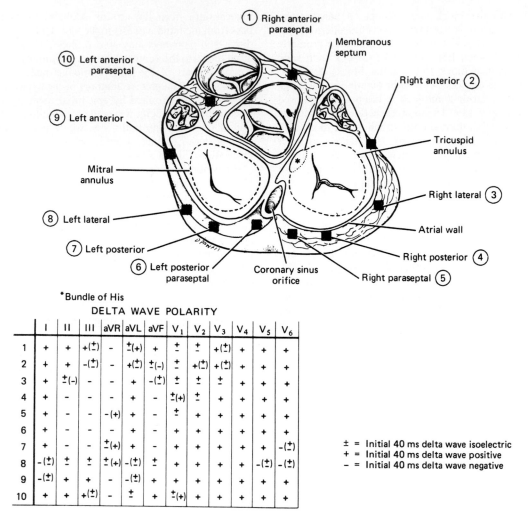

Figure 14–13. Polarity of the delta wave in different leads in various types of preexcitation. (Reproduced, with permission, from Gallagher JJ et al: The preexcitation syndromes. Prog Cardiovasc Dis 1978;20:285.)

Table 14–7. Summary of electrocardiographic findings for localizing an accessory atrioventricular pathway.[1]

Region of Bypass Tract	Leads With Negative Delta Wave	QRS Axis in Frontal Plane (degrees)	Precordial Lead With R > S
Left lateral	I or aVL (or both)	Normal	V_{1-3}
Left posterior	III and aVF	−75 to +75	V_1
Posteroseptal	III and aVF	0 to −90	V_{2-4}
Right free ventricular wall	aVR	Normal	V_{3-5}
Anteroseptal	V_1 and V_2	Normal	V_3 and V_5

[1] Adapted, with permission, from Lindsay BD, Crossen KJ, Cain ME: Concordance of distinguishing electrocardiographic features during sinus rhythm with the location of accessory pathways in the Wolff-Parkinson-White syndrome. Am J Cardiol 1987;59:1093.

Table 14–8. Effect of drugs in Wolff-Parkinson-White syndrome.[1,2]

| Drug | Duration of Effective Refractory Period | | | | | Shortest RR Interval Between 2 Preexcited Beats During Atrial Fibrillation |
	Atrium	Atrio-ventricular Node	His-Purkinje	Ventricle	Accessory Pathway	
Digitalis	±	+	0	±	−	−
Quinidine	+	−	+	+	+	+
Procainamide	+	−	+	+	+	+
Lidocaine	±	±	−	+	+	+
Disopyramide	+	−	±	+	+	?
Amiodarone	+	+	+	+	+	+
Ajmaline (IV)[3]	+	0	+	+	+	+
Propranolol	0	+	0	0	0	0
Phenytoin	±	−	−	±	±	?
Verapamil	±	+	0	±	±	?

[1] Modified and reproduced, with permission, from Gallagher JJ et al: The preexcitation syndromes. Prog Cardiovasc Dis 1978; 20:285.
[2] +, prolonged; −, shortened; 0, no change; ±, variable; ?, unknown.
[3] Investigational.

tachycardia with Lown-Ganong-Levine syndrome cannot be managed medically, the only alternative is to attempt to injure the atrioventricular node in hope of then being able to control the arrhythmia medically or ablate the atrioventricular node and place a dual-chamber pacemaker. This may be because a dual pathway in the atrioventricular node rather than an accessory bypass track may be responsible for the preexcitation.

2. WOLFF-PARKINSON-WHITE SYNDROME

Preexcitation due to Wolff-Parkinson-White syndrome (Wolff, 1930) has been classified according to the location of the accessory bypass, but the classification is incomplete because a variety of subtypes have recently been discovered by electrophysiologic study. Conventionally, type A preexcitation is from the left accessory bypass, producing an electrocardiographic pattern in V_1 resembling right ventricular hypertrophy or right bundle branch block. Type B preexcitation results from early activation via the right lateral accessory pathway, producing an electrocardiographic change similar to that of left bundle branch block (Figure 14–14). Subgroups can be identified by special electrophysiologic techniques that by epicardial mapping may identify patients who may be helped by ablation of the accessory or anomalous pathways.

The electrocardiographic classification originally proposed by Rosenbaum (1945) has been extended by the work of Gallagher (Preexcitation syndromes, 1978), with special reference to the polarity of the delta wave, resulting in probable identification of ten different anatomic locations of accessory pathways

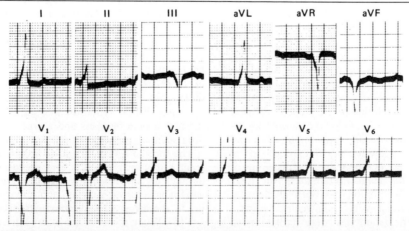

Figure 14–14. Wolff-Parkinson-White syndrome in a 26-year-old woman. The superior orientation of the delta vector (type B) produces QS complexes in aVF that simulate inferior infarction. Note the short PR and the slurred initial upstroke of the QRS (the delta wave), producing a wide QRS complex in leads I, aVL, V_5, and V_6.

(Figure 14–13). Orientation of the delta wave may simulate anterior or inferior myocardial infarction and right or left ventricular hypertrophy.

The spatial orientation of the delta vector in patients with Wolff-Parkinson-White syndrome gives some indication of the location of the accessory pathway, but electrophysiologic studies are required for precise localization. Some pathways are difficult to identify, but some can be inferred. The polarity of the delta wave in various types of epicardial preexcitation is illustrated in Figure 14–13. Epicardial mapping to determine the site of the accessory pathways should be performed only if the patient has atrial arrhythmias or syncopal attacks and catheter ablation is contemplated. On the other hand, His bundle recordings with programmed electrical stimulation are desirable in almost all cases of Wolff-Parkinson-White syndrome with atrial tachyarrhythmias to determine the refractory period of the accessory pathway. If the refractory period is short, drugs such as digitalis, which shorten it further, are hazardous, especially if the patient has atrial fibrillation (Table 14–8).

The effective refractory period of the accessory pathway ranges from 200 ms to as long as 900 ms, with most of the periods between 200 and 400 ms (Gallagher, 1976; Della Bella, 1991). This wide range must be appreciated, as must the significance of the short refractory periods, which may result in rapid ventricular responses to atrial fibrillation.

Clinical Findings

A. Symptoms and Signs: The diagnosis is made electrocardiographically even in patients who do not have a history of paroxysmal arrhythmia. During the arrhythmia it may be difficult to see the characteristic pattern, especially if there is a rapid atrial rate. The typical findings include a short PR interval, a wide QRS complex, and a slurred delta wave at the onset of the QRS, representing ventricular preexcitation via the bypass through the accessory pathway. The total PR interval plus the QRS interval is essentially normal. The delta wave is usually short—about 0.05 s— and the PR interval in rare cases may be essentially normal. About half of patients have no symptoms; the remainder have episodes of paroxysmal atrial arrhythmia, both reciprocating tachycardia and atrial fibrillation, which in some cases may only be noted by 12- to 24-hour ambulatory electrocardiographic monitoring (Arai, 1990). Palpitations due to arrhythmia are the presenting symptom in many patients; they may last a few seconds and produce trivial or no concern or may last hours and be disabling. It was once thought that death was rare during an attack of arrhythmia. This opinion has been challenged, possibly because of the very rapid ventricular rates that may occur if the patient has atrial fibrillation and because of the adverse effect of digitalis in such circumstances, with occasional deterioration to ventricular fibrillation and death. Digitalis increases con-

duction through the accessory pathway and does not slow the ventricular rate.

Although there are well-documented sudden deaths related to the development of atrial fibrillation and rapid antidromic conduction down the bypass tract at a rate high enough to precipitate ventricular tachycardia, this is still rare considering all the patients at risk with Wolff-Parkinson-White syndrome. The reported patients who have died suddenly have all been symptomatic and all on digitalis, which can facilitate conduction down the bypass tract. In asymptomatic patients with Wolff-Parkinson-White syndrome, the incidence of sudden death is very rare, and there is certainly no reason to order an electrophysiologic study. In a study of nearly 4000 Royal Canadian Air Force men followed for 40 years, there were 19 with Wolff-Parkinson-White syndrome. There was no excess morbidity or mortality compared with those without the syndrome or even in those with the syndrome who had symptomatic arrhythmias (Krahn, 1992). This is consistent with the benign natural history of Wolff-Parkinson-White syndrome in asymptomatic men reported from the United States Air Force (Hiss, 1962).

Approximately one-third of patients with Wolff-Parkinson-White syndrome develop atrial fibrillation at some time. The duration of the refractory period of the accessory pathway is of considerable therapeutic importance in these patients (Della Bella, 1991); if it shortens at rapid atrial rates, the frequent impulses from the atrium in atrial fibrillation may spread directly to the ventricle via the accessory pathway, causing rapid ventricular rates and collapse. Ventricular fibrillation may follow. Patients in whom the accessory pathway has a short refractory period usually have a rapid ventricular response if atrial fibrillation occurs. If the ventricular rate cannot be determined during an attack of atrial fibrillation, atrial fibrillation can be induced in an electrophysiologic study by rapid atrial stimulation to determine the ventricular rate. If the ventricular rate is rapid, with an R–R interval of 220 ms or faster, indicating direct transmission of rapid atrial impulses to the ventricle via the accessory pathway, drugs such as digitalis and verapamil that shorten the effective refractory period of the accessory pathway should not be used. These drugs can be avoided in patients with Wolff-Parkinson-White syndrome and atrial fibrillation by the use of beta-blockers and a type I antiarrhythmic drug such as quinidine or procainamide.

The mechanism of the atrial arrhythmia is that of reentry, in which impulses from the atria usually pass through the normal atrioventricular conduction system to the ventricle and then return in retrograde fashion to the atria via the anomalous pathway (Figure 14–15). When the atria, the atrioventricular junction, and the atrioventricular node are no longer refractory, the retrograde impulse may reexcite portions of the specialized normal atrioventricular pathway that con-

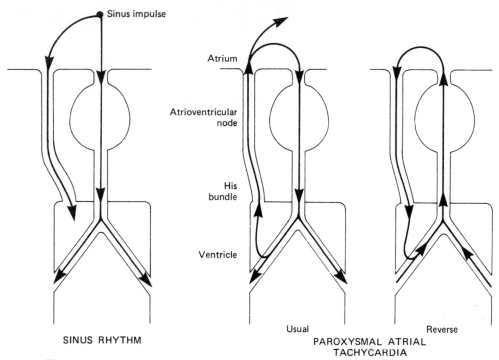

Sinus impulse

Atrium

Atrioventricular node

His bundle

Ventricle

SINUS RHYTHM

Usual   Reverse
PAROXYSMAL ATRIAL
TACHYCARDIA

Figure 14–15. Diagram of the normal conduction system and the accessory atrioventricular connection showing the conduction sequence during sinus rhythm in the left-hand panel and during tachycardia in the two right-hand panels. (Arrows show the direction of the reverse of the conduction sequence during tachycardia if the impulse spreads from the atrium via the bypass accessory pathway and returns through the atrioventricular node in retrograde fashion.) (Modified and reproduced, with permission, from Spurrell RAJ, Krikler DM, Sowton E: Problems concerning assessment of anatomical site of accessory pathway in Wolff-Parkinson-White syndrome. Br Heart J 1975;37:127.)

duct to the ventricles and so set up a self-perpetuating circuit and normalize the QRS. Recent electrophysiologic studies have shown that the circuit is antegrade through the normal atrioventricular pathway (orthodromic) and retrograde through the anomalous bypass pathway because the refractory period of the latter is usually (not always) shorter. Less commonly, the reverse pathway may be the mechanism of the reentry tachycardia. The impulse is retrograde via the atrioventricular node and antegrade through the accessory pathway (antidromic) (Figure 14–15), and the pattern thus simulates ventricular tachycardia because of the aberrant QRS complexes. In about 10% of cases, there are multiple accessory pathways (Wellens, 1990; Arai, 1990).

B. His Bundle and Intracardiac Recordings: His bundle recordings and epicardial mapping have further delineated the mechanisms of Wolff-Parkinson-White syndrome.

The relationship of the His bundle spike to the delta wave is a function of the HV interval. The HQ or the HV interval is less than normal (usually 30–50 ms) when Wolff-Parkinson-White syndrome is present. When conduction from the atrioventricular node is prolonged, the H spike may either follow the delta wave or be "lost" in the QRS complex because excita-

tion of the ventricles precedes that of the His bundle, presumably by bypass tracks.

Wellens (1974) found an almost linear relationship between the shortest RR interval (the most rapid ventricular response) during atrial fibrillation and the effective refractory period of the accessory pathway. When the effective refractory period was 200 ms, the RR interval was 200 ms. When the effective refractory period was 300 ms, the shortest RR interval during atrial fibrillation was 300 ms. This was true in each patient in a series of 16 patients in whom consecutive RR intervals were measured. The duration of the refractory period following administration of various antiarrhythmic agents has been studied (see also Table 14–8 and below). All of the common antiarrhythmic agents either increased the refractory period of the accessory pathway or had no effect—with the exception of digitalis, which decreased it. Procainamide and quinidine increased the HV interval, but digitalis, phenytoin, atropine, propranolol, lidocaine, and verapamil had no effect. The drugs had contrasting effects on the refractory period of the atrioventricular node. Digitalis, propranolol, and verapamil prolonged it; quinidine had a variable effect, decreasing it in some and increasing it in others; and atropine and lidocaine decreased it. Procainamide may

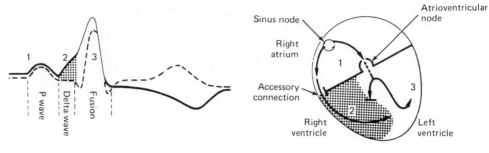

Electrocardiogram
1. Normal P waves with shortened PR interval.

Epicardial mapping
1. Antegrade conduction from the sinus node to the atrioventricular node.

2. Premature activation of the ventricle from the accessory pathway, which forms the delta wave.

3. Late fusion of both ventricular depolarizations.

Figure 14–16. Basis of the ECG in Wolff-Parkinson-White syndrome. (Reproduced, with permission, from Boineau JP et al: Epicardial mapping in Wolff-Parkinson-White syndrome. Arch Intern Med 1975;135:422.)

increase the refractory period of the accessory pathways from 275 ms to 400 ms and is therefore a safe drug to use in Wolff-Parkinson-White syndrome (Boahene, 1990).

C. Epicardial Mapping: Epicardial mapping reveals the basis of the ECG in Wolff-Parkinson-White syndrome and identifies the accessory pathways by noting the activation of the ventricles that coincides with the delta wave. As shown in Figure 14–16, the delta wave coincides with the antegrade activation of the right ventricle at the time of the delta wave. The latter part of the QRS is a fusion wave that results from activation of the ventricle from both the accessory pathway and the normal pathway. When the ventricle is activated early but the QRS complex is normal in duration, the connection between the atria and the His bundle is by way of the James fibers, bypassing the upper part of the atrioventricular node. This is probably the mechanism of the Lown-Ganong-Levine syndrome.

The technique of epicardial mapping is described in detail by Gallagher et al (Epicardial mapping, 1978) (see also Figure 14–16). Details of the procedure are given, and the authors describe their efforts to define both the atrial and ventricular insertions of the accessory pathways by both retrograde and antegrade mapping. The timing of the arrival of the excitation wave in various parts of the ventricle defines the site of the accessory pathway and is best predicted by the delta vectors, as in Figure 14–13.

Treatment

Asymptomatic patients in whom the condition is discovered by chance during a routine ECG should be informed of the nature and significance of the syndrome.

The effects of various drugs on the refractory period of the accessory pathway, the atrioventricular node, and the HV interval of atrioventricular conduc-

tion have already been discussed and summarized in Table 14–8. Verapamil shortens the effective refractory period of the accessory pathway and should be avoided. Amiodarone prolongs the effective refractory period of both the atrium and the ventricle, preventing the initiation of reentry tachycardia as well as prolonging the refractory period of the accessory pathway. Procainamide and quinidine have less toxicity and may be tried before amiodarone, though the last is most effective.

There is no indication for electrophysiologic studies or "prophylactic" antiarrhythmic drugs. Until recently, surgical or catheter ablation was reserved for patients with paroxysmal supraventricular tachycardias that were uncontrolled on medical management. This was justified when the method of ablation was with electrical energy, which created a relatively large volume of myocardial necrosis. With the development of radiofrequency catheter ablation, the lesions created are small, and with modern mapping techniques the rate of successful ablations of bypass tracts in all locations is over 90%. In one study, the accessory pathway was successfully eliminated in 99% of 166 patients (Jackman, 1991). There is a growing consensus that in patients with paroxysmal supraventricular tachycardia, rather than lifelong medical management, radiofrequency catheter ablation is the treatment of choice (Prystowsky, 1990; Arai, 1990). There appears to be no role at present for surgical ablation of bypass tracts.

In patients with syncope or atrial fibrillation, an electrophysiologic study to induce atrial fibrillation and measure the shortest RR interval is recommended. Patients who can conduct rapidly with the ventricle over the bypass tract are the ones at risk of ventricular fibrillation, and ablation of the bypass tract is indicated.

A. Hazard of Digitalis When Atrial Fibrillation Occurs in Wolff-Parkinson-White Syndrome: If the atrial arrhythmia is fibrillation, digitalis should *not* be used, because it increases the block in the atrioventricular node while decreasing the refractory period of the accessory pathway, permitting favored passage of the cardiac impulse via the accessory pathway. The rapid atrial impulses may then be transmitted without the protective blocking action of the atrioventricular node directly to the ventricle, and rapid ventricular rates of atrial fibrillation, ventricular tachycardia, or even ventricular fibrillation may ensue. Patients with RR intervals of 220 ms or less during spontaneous atrial fibrillation may develop ventricular fibrillation following administration of digitalis. Digitalis could be directly related to the onset of ventricular fibrillation in slightly less than half of patients who had atrial fibrillation with a short refractory period of the accessory pathway (Sellers, 1977). Sudden death in patients with Wolff-Parkinson-White syndrome may be due to rapid conduction across an accessory pathway with a short refractory period. The cycle length of the anomalous pathway is not shortened by digitalis in all patients; the ventricular rate during spontaneous or induced atrial fibrillation may be a more direct measure of the likelihood of ventricular fibrillation if digitalis is given.

The frequency of atrial fibrillation becomes greater with age; it is uncommon in children. In 140 patients with Wolff-Parkinson-White syndrome who had their initial episode of supraventricular tachycardia before 18 years of age, the waxing and waning of paroxysmal tachycardia was studied. In those with paroxysmal tachycardia before age 2 months, paroxysms persisted in only 7%. In one-third, the paroxysms disappeared and reappeared at 8 years of age. Among patients whose tachycardia was present after age 5 years, persistence was reported in 78% (Perry, 1990; Guiraudon, 1986).

B. Management of Atrial Arrhythmia in Wolff-Parkinson-White Syndrome : Most cases of paroxysmal atrial tachycardia can be treated in the usual fashion, ie, with interruption of the reentry circuit. This can be achieved by increasing the block in the atrioventricular node by maneuvers such as carotid sinus massage, drugs that stimulate the vagus nerve—or digitalis if the rhythm is paroxysmal atrial tachycardia and not atrial fibrillation—or catheter ablation of the aberrant pathway (see Chapter 15). Drugs that *increase* the block in the accessory pathway—procainamide and quinidine—are the most effective. Propranolol has little effect on the accessory pathway but a selective blocking effect on the atrioventricular node. About 20% of patients who have paroxysmal atrial tachycardia in the absence of obvious evidence of Wolff-Parkinson-White syndrome on the ECG have a retrograde accessory pathway, so-called **concealed Wolff-Parkinson-White syndrome**. There are no clear diagnostic criteria on the surface ECG by which those with a concealed accessory atrioventricular pathway can be identified. It may be suspected if

paroxysmal atrial tachycardia occurs without an antecedent atrial premature beat, especially if paroxysmal atrial tachycardia occurs after shortening of the preceding cycle length (Sung, 1977).

Encainide and amiodarone have suppressed arrhythmias in patients with preexcitation who did not respond to conventional drugs. These newer drugs increase the refractoriness of the accessory pathway (Prystowsky, 1984).

1. Atrial pacing– Atrial pacing has been used therapeutically with the hope that a random beat might by chance excite a portion of the reentry pathway, making it refractory to the oncoming circuit wave. There is a risk that atrial pacing may increase the ventricular rate.

2. Emergency treatment– DC shock (cardioversion) or intravenous procainamide should be considered in emergency situations. It is unwise to use beta-blockers and verapamil, because although they do not decrease the refractory period of the accessory pathway per se, they decrease it *relative* to that of the atrioventricular node. The refractory period of the atrioventricular node is prolonged by propranolol and verapamil.

3. Catheter ablation– Until recently, surgical ablation—at times using cryosurgical ablation at surgery, was the favored approach for elimination of bypass tracts. Although this technique was highly successful (Prystowsky, 1990), it requires thoracotomy and frequently an extensive incision in the atrioventricular groove, with extensive associated damage. There was also the danger of injury to the coronary arteries, and even an occasional fatality. With the development of catheter ablation techniques, the frequency with which surgery is done has decreased, and with the success of radiofrequency catheter ablation, surgery will be done very rarely and only in patients where elimination of the bypass tract is necessary and where catheter ablation has failed.

IDIOPATHIC LONG QT SYNDROME

Idiopathic long QT syndrome is an uncommon condition first described in deaf siblings (Jervell and Lange-Nielsen syndrome), though deafness is not always present. The syndrome is characterized by recurrent syncope, a long QT interval (usually 0.5–0.7 s, sometimes intermittent), ventricular arrhythmias (torsade de pointes), and sudden and unexpected death (Moss, 1991). Patients with the disease demonstrate neural degeneration of the conduction system. The syndrome may be acquired, resulting from electrolyte imbalance, neurologic disorders, or toxicity to cardiac drugs (eg, quinidine or other antiarrhythmic drugs) or psychotropic drugs. The role of these various causes in producing sudden death is unclear (Jackman, 1988).

The sympathetic nervous system (especially the

left stellate ganglion) and autonomic imbalance play a role in the pathogenesis of the syndrome (Neural mechanisms..., 1991). Acute arrhythmic episodes are treated by local anesthetic block of the left stellate ganglion, and recurrent episodes are treated by resection of this ganglion as well as of the first three or four thoracic ganglia (Schwartz, 1991). Before resection of the left stellate ganglion is considered, patients should be treated with propranolol or other beta-adrenergic blocking drugs or with phenytoin, which has proved beneficial in some patients.

Antiarrhythmic drugs, especially type Ia and type Ic drugs such as quinidine, procainamide, encainide, and flecainide, are associated with torsade de pointes, ventricular tachycardia, and prolongation of the QT interval. This proarrhythmic effect of antiarrhythmic, psychotropic, and other drugs such as antihistamines must be differentiated from the congenital long QT syndromes.

REFERENCES

Electrophysiology

Castellanos A Jr, Castillo CA, Agha AS: Symposium on electrophysiological correlates of clinical arrhythmias: 3. Contribution of His bundle recordings to the understanding of clinical arrhythmias. Am J Cardiol 1971;28:499.

Cranefield PF, Aronson RS: *Cardiac Arrhythmias: The Role of Triggered Activity and Other Mechanisms.* Futura, 1988.

Fisch C: Concealed conduction. Cardiol Clin 1983;1:63.

Fitzgerald D et al: Anatomy of cardiac conduction studies: Basic concepts in cardiac electrophysiology. In: *Cardiac Arrhythmias: A Practical Approach.* Naccarelli GV (editor): Futura, 1991.

Fozzard HA: Cardiac muscle: Excitability and passive electrical properties. Prog Cardiovasc Dis 1977;19:343.

Fozzard HA, DasGupta DS: Electrophysiology and the electrocardiogram. Mod Concepts Cardiovasc Dis 1975;44:29.

Han J: The concepts of re-entrant activity responsible for ectopic rhythm. Am J Cardiol 1971;28:253.

Jackman WM et al: The long QT syndrome: A critical review, new clinical observations, and a unifying hypothesis. Prog Cardiovasc Dis 1988;31:115.

January CT, Makielski JC: Triggered arrhythmias: New insights into basic mechanisms. Curr Opin Cardiol 1990;5:65.

Josephson ME, Seides SF: *Clinical Cardiac Electrophysiology: Techniques and Interpretations*, Lea & Febiger, 1979.

Langendorf R: Concealed A-V conduction: The effect of blocked impulses on the formation and conduction of subsequent impulses. Am Heart J 1948;35:542.

Massing GK, James TN: Anatomical configuration of the His bundle and bundle branches in the human heart. Circulation 1976;53:609.

Narula OS (editor): *His Bundle Electrocardiography and Clinical Electrophysiology.* Davis, 1975.

Rosen MR, Wit AL: Triggered activity. Prog Cardiol 1988;1/1:39.

Scheinman MM, Morady F: Invasive cardiac electrophysiologic testing: The current state of the art. (Editorial.) Circulation 1983;67:1169.

Wellens HJJ: Contribution of cardiac pacing to our understanding of the Wolff-Parkinson-White syndrome. Br Heart J 1975;37:231.

Pathology & Causes

Fraser GR, Froggatt P, James TN: Congenital deafness associated with electrocardiographic abnormalities, fainting attacks and sudden death: A recessive syndrome. Q J Med 1964;33:361.

Frink RJ, James TN: Normal blood supply to the human His bundle and proximal bundle branches. Circulation 1973;47:8.

Hudson REB: Surgical pathology of the conducting system of the heart. Br Heart J 1967;29:646.

James TN et al: De subitaneis mortibus. 30. Observations on the pathophysiology of the long QT syndromes with special reference to the neuropathology of the heart. Circulation 1978;57:1221.

Lev M: The pathology of atrioventricular block. Cardiovasc Clin 1972;4:159.

Bradycardiac Syndromes

Alpert MA, Flaker GC: Arrhythmias associated with sinus node dysfunction: Pathogenesis, recognition, and management. JAMA 1983;250:2160.

Alpert MA et al: Comparative survival following permanent ventricular and dual-chamber pacing for patients with chronic symptomatic sinus node dysfunction with and without congestive heart failure. Am Heart J 1987;113:958.

Bachinsky WB et al: Usefulness of clinical characteristics in predicting the outcome of electrophysiologic studies in unexplained syncope. Am J Cardiol 1992;69:1044.

Bleifer SB et al: Diagnosis of occult arrhythmias by Holter electrocardiography. Prog Cardiovasc Dis 1974;16:569.

Camm J, Katritsis D: Ventricular pacing for sick sinus syndrome: A risky business? PACE 1990;13:695.

Dreifus LS et al: Guidelines for implantation of cardiac pacemakers and antiarrhythmic devices. J Am Coll Cardiol 1991;18:1.

Easley RM Jr, Goldstein S: Sino-atrial syncope. Am J Med 1971;50:166.

Gillette PC: Recent advances in mechanisms, evaluation, and pacemaker treatment of chronic bradydysrhythmias in children. Am Heart J 1982;102:920.

Han J et al: Temporal dispersion of recovery of excitability in atrium and ventricle as a function of heart rate. Am Heart J 1966;71:481.

Kang PS et al: Role of autonomic regulatory mechanisms

in sinoatrial conduction and sinus node automaticity in sick sinus syndrome. Circulation 1981;64:832.

Miura DS, Keefe DL, Dangman K: Sinus-node dysfunction: Invasive and noninvasive evaluation. Cardiovasc Rev Rep 1987;8:64.

Rasmussen K: Chronic sinus node disease: Natural course and indications for pacing. Am Heart J 1981;2:455.

Rokseth R, Hatle L: Prospective study on the occurrence and management of chronic sinoatrial disease, with follow-up. Br Heart J 1974;36:582.

Rosen KM et al: Cardiac conduction in patients with symptomatic sinus node disease. Circulation 1971;43:836.

Rosenqvist M et al: Atrial rate responsive pacing in sinus node disease. Eur Heart J 1990;11:537.

Ryden L: Atrial inhibited pacing: An underused mode of cardiac stimulation. PACE 1988;11:1375.

Santini M et al: Relation of prognosis in sick sinus syndrome to age, conduction defects, and modes of permanent cardiac pacing. Am J Cardiol 1990;65:729.

Sutton R, Kenny R: The natural history of sick sinus syndrome. PACE 1986;9:1110.

Tresch DD, Fleg JL: Unexplained sinus bradycardia: Clinical significance and long-term prognosis in apparently healthy persons older than 40 years. Am J Cardiol 1986;58:1009.

Atrioventricular Conduction Defects

Barold SS, Coumel P: Mechanisms of atrioventricular junctional tachycardia: Role of reentry and concealed accessory bypass tracts. Am J Cardiol 1977;39:97.

Bernstein AD, Parssonnet V: Survey of cardiac pacing in the United States in 1989. Am J Cardiol 1992;69:331.

Bhatia S, Goldschlager N: Office evaluation of the pacemaker patient: Detection of normal and abnormal pacemaker function. JAMA 1985;254:1346.

Buckingham TA et al: Pacemaker hemodynamics: Clinical implications. Prog Cardiovasc Dis 1992;34:347.

Dewey RC, Capeless MA, Levy AM: Use of ambulatory electrocardiographic monitoring to identify high-risk patients with congenital complete heart block. N Engl J Med 1987;316:835.

Dhingra RC et al: Significance of the HV interval in 517 patients with chronic bifascicular block. Circulation 1981;64:1265.

Fitzpatrick A, Sutton R: A guide to temporary pacing. Br Med J 1992;304:365.

Fogoros RN et al: Long-term outcome of survivors of cardiac arrest whose therapy is guided by electrophysiologic study. J Am Coll Cardiol 1992;19:780.

Furman S, Gross J: Dual chamber pacing and pacemakers. Curr Probl Cardiol 1990;15:123.

Ginks W, Leatham A, Siddons H: Prognosis of patients paced for chronic atrioventricular block. Br Heart J 1979;41:633.

Harthorne JW: Cardiac pacemakers. Curr Probl Cardiol 1987;12:651.

Hess DS, Morady F, Scheinman MM: Electrophysiologic testing in the evaluation of patients with syncope of undetermined origin. Am J Cardiol 1982;50:1309.

Kastor JA: Atrioventricular block. (Two parts.) N Engl J Med 1975;292:462, 572.

Jowett NI et al: Temporary transvenous cardiac pacing: 6 years experience in one coronary care unit. Postgrad Med J 1989;65:211.

Lagergren H et al: Three hundred and five cases of permanent intravenous pacemaker treatment for Adams-Stokes syndrome. Surgery 1966;59:494.

Langendorf R: Concealed A-V conduction: The effect of blocked impulses on the formation and conduction of subsequent impulses. Am Heart J 1948;35:542.

Langendorf R, Cohen H, Gozo EG Jr: Observations on second degree atrioventricular block, including new criteria for the differential diagnosis between type I and type II block. Am J Cardiol 1972;29:111.

Lie KI et al: Mechanism and significance of widened QRS complexes during complete atrioventricular block in acute inferior myocardial infarction. Am J Cardiol 1974;33:833.

Luceri RM et al: The arrhythmias of dual-chamber cardiac pacemakers and their management. Ann Intern Med 1983;99:354.

Manolis AS et al: Syncope: Current diagnostic evaluation and management. Ann Intern Med 1990;112:850.

McAlister HF et al: Lyme carditis: An important cause of reversible heart block. Ann Intern Med 1989;110:338.

McAnulty JH, Rahimtoola SH: Bundle branch block. Prog Cardiovasc Dis 1984;26:333.

Morady F, Peters RW, Scheinman MM: Bradyarrhythmias and bundle branch block. In: *Cardiac Emergencies.* Scheinman MM (editor). Saunders, 1984.

Mymin D et al: The natural history of primary first-degree atrioventricular heart block. N Engl J Med 1986;315:1183.

Narula OS et al: Atrioventricular block: Localization and classification by His bundle recordings. Am J Med 1971;50:146.

Parssonnet V, Bernstein AD: Pacing in perspective: Concepts and controversies. Circulation 1986;73:1087.

Puech P: Atrioventricular block: The value of intracardiac recordings. In: *Cardiac Arrhythmias: The Modern Electrophysiological Approach.* Krikler DM, Goodwin JF (editors). Saunders, 1975.

Reid JM, Coleman EN, Doig W: Complete congenital heart block. Br Heart J 1982;48:236.

Rowland E, Evans T, Krikler D: Effect of nifedipine on atrioventricular conduction as compared with verapamil: Intracardiac electrophysiological study. Br Heart J 1979;42:124.

Scarpelli FM, Rudolph AM: The hemodynamics of congenital complete heart block. Prog Cardiovasc Dis 1964;6:327.

Scheinman MM et al: Value of the H-Q interval in patients with bundle branch block and the role of prophylactic permanent pacing. Am J Cardiol 1982;50:1316.

Watanabe Y, Dreifus LS: Factors controlling impulse transmission with special reference to A-V conduction. Am Heart J 1975;89:790.

Zipes DP: Second-degree atrioventricular block. Circulation 1979;60:465.

Ventricular Conduction Defects & Bundle Branch Block

Brohet CR et al: Vectorcardiographic diagnosis of right ventricular hypertrophy in the presence of right bundle branch block in young subjects. Am J Cardiol 1978;42:602.

Brooks N, Leech G, Leatham A: Complete right bundle-branch block: Echophonocardiographic study of first heart sound and right ventricular contraction times. Br Heart J 1979;41:637.

Castellanos A Jr, Lemberg L: Diagnosis of isolated and combined block in the bundle branches and the divisions of the left branch. Circulation 1971;43:971.

Chiale PA et al: Contrasting effects of verapamil and procainamide on rate-dependent bundle branch block: Pharmacologic evidence for the role of depressed sodium channel responses. J Am Coll Cardiol 1990;15:633.

Chilson DA et al: Functional bundle branch block: Discordant response of right and left bundle branches to changes in heart rate. Am J Cardiol 1984;54:313.

Corne RA, Beamish RE, Rollwagen RL: Significance of left anterior hemiblock. Br Heart J 1978;40:552.

Dancy M, Leech G, Leatham A: Significance of complete right bundle-branch block when an isolated finding. Br Heart J 1982;48:217.

Demoulin JC, Kulbertus HE: Histopathologic correlates of left posterior fascicular block. Am J Cardiol 1979;44:1083.

Dhingra RC et al: Significance of the HV interval in 517 patients with chronic bifascicular block. Circulation 1981;64:1265.

Dunn M: Left bundle branch block: Variations on a theme. (Editorial.) J Am Coll Cardiol 1987;10:81.

Fisch GR, Zipes DP, Fisch C: Bundle branch block and sudden death. Prog Cardiovasc Dis 1980;23:187.

Fleg JL: Asymptomatic right bundle branch block: Prognosis. Prim Cardiol 1985;11:55.

Freedman RA et al: Bundle branch block in patients with chronic coronary artery disease: Angiographic correlates and prognostic significance. J Am Coll Cardiol 1987;10:73.

Havelda CJ et al: The pathologic correlates of the electrocardiogram: Complete left bundle branch block. Circulation 1982;65:445.

Hindman MC et al: The clinical significance of bundle branch block complicating acute myocardial infarction. (2 parts.) Circulation 1978;58:679, 689.

Kafka H, Burggraf GW, Milliken JA: Electrocardiographic diagnosis of left ventricular hypertrophy in the presence of left bundle branch block: An echocardiographic study. Am J Cardiol 1985;55:103.

Kunkel F, Rowland M, Scheinman MM: The electrophysiologic effects of lidocaine in patients with intraventricular conduction defects. Circulation 1974;49:894.

Larcos G et al: Diagnostic accuracy of exercise thallium-201 single-photon emission computed tomography in patients with left bundle branch block. Am J Cardiol 1991;68:756.

Liao YL et al: Characteristics and prognosis incomplete right bundle branch block: An epidemiologic study. J Am Coll Cardiol 1986;7:492.

Luy G, Bahl OP, Massie E: Intermittent left bundle branch block. Am Heart J 1973;8:332.

Matzer L et al: A new approach to the assessment of tomographic thallium-201 scintigraphy in patients with left bundle branch block. J Am Coll Cardiol 1991;17:1309.

Pastore JO et al: The risk of advanced heart block in surgical patients with right bundle branch block and left axis deviation. Circulation 1978;57:677.

Rosenbaum MB et al: The differential electrocardiographic manifestations of hemiblocks, bilateral bundle branch block and trifascicular blocks. In: Advances in Electrocardiography. Schlant RC, Hurst JW (editors). Grune & Stratton, 1972.

Rotman M, Triebwasser JH: A clinical and follow-up study of right and left bundle branch block. Circulation 1975;51:477.

Scheinman MM, Morady F: Invasive cardiac electrophysiologic testing: The current state of the art. (Editorial.) Circulation 1983;67:1169.

Scheinman MM et al: Value of the H–Q interval in patients with bundle branch block and the role of prophylactic permanent pacing. Am J Cardiol 1982;50:1316.

Sung RJ et al: Clinical and electrophysiologic observations in patients with concealed accessory atrioventricular bypass tracts. Am J Cardiol 1977;40:839.

Warner RA et al: Improved electrocardiographic criteria for the diagnosis of left anterior hemiblock. Am J Cardiol 1983;51:723.

Ventricular Preexcitation Syndromes

Arai A, Kron J: Current management of the Wolff-Parkinson-White syndrome. West J Med 1990;152:383.

Benditt DG et al: Characteristics of atrioventricular conduction and the spectrum of arrhythmias in Lown-Ganong-Levine syndrome. Circulation 1978;57:454.

Boahene KA et al: Termination of acute atrial fibrillation in the Wolff-Parkinson-White syndrome by procainamide and propafenone: Importance of atrial fibrillation cycle length. J Am Coll Cardiol 1990;16:1408.

Boineau JP: Mapping: Cardiac activation and repolarization. Circulation 1981;64:208.

Della Bella P et al: Atrial fibrillation in patients with an accessory pathway: Importance of the conduction properties of the accessory pathway. J Am Coll Cardiol 1991;17:1352.

Fischell TA et al: Long-term follow-up after surgical correction of Wolff-Parkinson-White syndrome. J Am Coll Cardiol 1987;9:283.

Gallagher JJ et al: Epicardial mapping in the Wolff-Parkinson-White syndrome. Circulation 1978a;57:854.

Gallagher JJ et al: The preexcitation syndromes. Prog Cardiovasc Dis 1978b;20:285.

Gallagher JJ et al: Techniques of intraoperative electrophysiologic mapping. Am J Cardiol 1982;49:221.

Gallagher JJ et al: The Wolff-Parkinson-White syndrome and the preexcitation dysrhythmias: Medical and surgical management. Med Clin North Am 1976;60:101.

Guiraudon GM et al: Surgery for Wolff-Parkinson-White syndrome: Further experience with an epicardial approach. Circulation 1986;74:525.

Hiss RE, Lamb LE: Electrocardiographic findings in 122,043 individuals. Circulation 1962;25:947.

Harper RW et al: Effects of verapamil on the electrophysiologic properties of the accessory pathway in patients with the Wolff-Parkinson-White syndrome. Am J Cardiol 1982;50:1323.

Jackman WB et al: Catheter ablation of accessory atrioventricular pathways (Wolff-Parkinson-White syndrome). N Engl J Med 1991;324:1605.

Josephson ME, Kastor JA: Supraventricular tachycardia in Lown-Ganong-Levine syndrome: Atrionodal versus intranodal reentry. Am J Cardiol 1977;40:521.

Krahn AD et al: The natural history of electrocardiographic preexcitation in men. Ann Intern Med 1992;116:456.

Leitch JW et al: Prognostic value of electrophysiology testing in arrhythmic patients with Wolff-Parkinson-White patterns. Circulation 1990;82:1718.

Lindsay BD, Crossen KJ, Cain ME: Concordance of distinguishing electrocardiographic features during sinus rhythm with the location of accessory pathways in the Wolff-Parkinson-White syndrome. Am J Cardiol 1987;59:1093.

Lown B, Ganong WF, Levine SA: The syndrome of short P-R interval, normal QRS complex, and paroxysmal rapid heart action. Circulation 1952;5:693.

Mandel WJ, Danzig R, Hayakawa H: Lown-Ganong-Levine syndrome: A study using His bundle electrograms. Circulation 1971;44:696.

Milstein S, Sharma AD, Klein GJ: Electrophysiologic profile of asymptomatic Wolff-Parkinson-White pattern. Am J Cardiol 1986;57:1097.

Morady F et al: Electrophysiologic testing in the management of patients with the Wolff-Parkinson-White syndrome and atrial fibrillation. Am J Cardiol 1983;51:1623.

Perry JC, Garson A Jr: Supraventricular tachycardia due to Wolff-Parkinson-White syndrome in children: Early disappearance and late recurrence. J Am Coll Cardiol 1990;16:1215.

Prystowsky EN et al: Clinical efficacy and electrophysiologic effects of encainide in patients with Wolff-Parkinson-White syndrome. Circulation 1984;69:278.

Prytstowsky EN et al: Nonpharmacologic treatment of the Wolff-Parkinson-White syndrome and other supraventricular tachycardias. Annu Rev Med 1990;41:239.

Reddy GV, Schamroth L: The localization of bypass tracts in the Wolff-Parkinson-White syndrome from the surface electrocardiogram. Am Heart J 1987;113:984.

Rosenbaum FF et al: The potential variations of the thorax and the esophagus in anomalous atrioventricular excitation (Wolff-Parkinson-White syndrome). Am Heart J 1945;29:281.

Sellers TD, Bashore TM, Gallagher JJ: Digitalis in the preexcitation syndrome: Analysis during atrial fibrillation. Circulation 1977;56:260.

Sung RJ et al: Clinical and electrophysiologic observations in patients with concealed accessory atrioventricular bypass tracts. Am J Cardiol 1977;40:839.

Waldo AL et al: Appropriate electrophysiologic study and treatment of patients with the Wolff-Parkinson-White Syndrome. J Am Coll Cardiol 1988;11:1124.

Waspe LE et al: Susceptibility to atrial fibrillation and ventricular tachyarrhythmia in the Wolff-Parkinson-White syndrome: Role of the accessory pathway. Am Heart J 1986;112:1141.

Wellens HJ, Brugada P, Penn OC: The management of preexcitation syndromes. JAMA 1987;257:2325.

Wellens HJJ, Durrer D: Wolff-Parkinson-White syndrome and atrial fibrillation: Relation between refractory period of accessory pathway and ventricular rate during atrial fibrillation. Am J Cardiol 1974;34:777.

Wellens HJJ et al: The electrocardiogram in patients with multiple accessory atrioventricular pathways. J Am Coll Cardiol 1990;16:745.

Wolff L, Parkinson J, White PD: Bundle branch block with short P-R interval in healthy young people prone to paroxysmal tachycardia. Am Heart J 1930;5:685.

Idiopathic Long QT Syndrome

Crampton R: Preeminence of the left stellate ganglion in the long Q-T syndrome: Circulation 1979;59:769.

Eldar M et al: Permanent cardiac pacing in patients with the long QT syndrome. J Am Coll Cardiol 1987;10:600.

Gallagher JJ et al: Catheter technique for closed-chest ablation of the atrioventricular conduction system: A therapeutic alternative for the treatment of refractory supraventricular tachycardia. N Engl J Med 1982;306:194.

Jackman WM et al: Ventricular tachyarrhythmias in the long QT syndromes. Med Clin North Am 1984;68:1079.

Jackman WM et al: The long QT syndromes: A critical review, new clinical observations and a unifying hypothesis. Prog Cardiovasc Dis 1988;31:115.

James TN et al: De subitaneis mortibus. 30. Observations on the pathophysiology of the long QT syndromes with special reference to the neuropathology of the heart. Circulation 1978;57:1221.

Moss AJ et al: The long QT syndrome: Prospective longitudinal study of 328 failures. Circulation 1991;84:1136.

Moss AJ: Prolonged QT-interval syndromes. JAMA 1986;256:2985.

Neural mechanisms in sudden cardiac death: Insights from long QT syndrome. (Editorial.) Lancet 1991;338:1181.

Roden DM, Woosley RL, Primm RK: Incidence and clinical features of the quinidine-associated long QT syndrome: Implications for patient care. Am Heart J 1986;111:1088.

Rubin SA et al: Usefulness of Valsalva manoeuvre and cold pressor test for evaluation of arrhythmias in long QT syndrome. Br Heart J 1979;42:490.

Schwartz PJ et al: Therapy of the congenital long QT syndrome. Circulation 1991;84:503.

Surawicz B, Knoebel SB: Long QT: Good, bad or indifferent? J Am Coll Cardiol 1984;4:398.

15   Cardiac Arrhythmias

Cardiac arrhythmias can occur in a wide variety of circumstances in patients with no evidence of heart disease or in those with heart disease due to any cause. For purposes of description, we have divided disturbances of rhythm into (1) supraventricular (atrial or junctional) arrhythmias and (2) ventricular arrhythmias. The electrophysiologic principles applicable to the study of cardiac arrhythmias are included with the discussion of that subject in Chapter 14.

The usual history of cardiac arrhythmia is of a sudden onset of palpitations that the patient may describe as regular or irregular, though it may not always be possible to characterize them one way or the other. It may help if the physician taps out various rhythms and rates and asks, "Is it like this? Or like this?" etc. The patient may complain not of palpitations but rather of the consequences of the arrhythmia, such as weakness, chest pain, dizziness, dyspnea, and confusion. Some patients have no symptoms with arrhythmia. In some patients, sudden cardiac arrest with rapid ventricular tachycardia or fibrillation is the first manifestation of an arrhythmia.

If the arrhythmia occurs in an older patient with coronary heart disease, severe symptoms of near-syncope, chest pain, palpitations, dyspnea, and disturbed left ventricular function with low cardiac output may develop.

In arrhythmias of longer duration, there may be progressive deterioration of cardiac function, with impaired perfusion of vital organs resulting from decreased cardiac output. With persistent tachycardia, left ventricular systolic dysfunction may occur. The patient may develop the clinical picture of dilated cardiomyopathy with severe congestive heart failure. The patient may then develop symptoms resulting from inadequate perfusion of the brain, heart, kidneys, skin, and extremities. The fact that the patient tolerates the arrhythmia at the outset does not guarantee that circulatory embarrassment will not develop with time. This is especially true in patients in the coronary care unit, in whom cardiac failure may develop gradually.

Palpitations may be due to increased forcefulness of the heartbeat as well as to arrhythmia or due to one or the other at different times. An "event recorder" or continuous ambulatory electrocardiographic monitoring to determine the rhythm is often necessary. Some arrhythmias last seconds or minutes, while others, such as atrial fibrillation, last hours, days, or indefinitely.

The diagnosis may be simple after a routine ECG, or it may be complex, requiring extensive studies with carotid sinus massage, Valsalva's maneuver, rapid atrial pacing, His bundle studies with intracardiac recording and stimulation, and, in selected cases, echocardiography, coronary arteriography, and left ventricular cineangiograms. It may be necessary to determine the relationship of the QRS complex and the P wave to the His bundle deflection, the effect of posture and drugs, and the adequacy of the baroreceptor reflexes in order to identify the type of arrhythmia and determine whether it is ventricular or supraventricular. The examiner should obtain a history of previous episodes, the circumstances under which the arrhythmia occurs, an indication of the patient's tolerance of them, their frequency and duration, the extent of circulatory impairment, and the response to treatment, if any.

It is important to estimate the severity of the arrhythmia (ie, the impact on left ventricular function, blood pressure, cerebral and coronary perfusion, and renal function). The importance of the heart rate, the duration of the arrhythmia, and the presence of underlying heart disease must be emphasized. The arrhythmia may be trivial or urgent, depending on the cause, the effect on the circulation, and the age of the patient.

The consequences of a cardiac arrhythmia depend upon its effect on cardiac hemodynamics; on cerebral, coronary, and renal perfusion; on blood pressure, left ventricular function, and cardiac rate (rapid or slow); on the duration of the arrhythmia; and on the presence or absence of underlying heart disease. If the arrhythmia occurs in a young person with no underlying heart disease and the increase in ventricular rate is only modest (< 160/min), hemodynamic function is rarely impaired, and perfusion of vital organs (brain, heart, and kidneys) and extremities is adequate.

Whether the disturbance in rhythm is regular or irregular has an important influence on the patient's tolerance; an irregular rhythm such as atrial fibrillation is less well tolerated than paroxysmal atrial tachycardia at a similar rate. Incomplete ventricular filling in the absence of atrial systole can significantly reduce cardiac output in a cardiac arrhythmia.

SUPRAVENTRICULAR (ATRIAL OR JUNCTIONAL) ARRHYTHMIAS

SUPRAVENTRICULAR PREMATURE BEATS
(Atrial Extrasystoles, Atrial Premature Beats)

Premature beats are important only if they interfere with hemodynamic function of the left ventricle, impair cardiac output, and decrease perfusion to vital organs, or if they are precursors of more serious arrhythmia. Supraventricular premature beats are rarely important in this sense.

Supraventricular premature beats are more apt to occur if there is atrial or conduction system disease such as left atrial enlargement in mitral stenosis. Beats occurring in these conditions may presage the development of atrial fibrillation. When atrial fibrillation is converted to sinus rhythm, reappearance of atrial premature beats often indicates that atrial fibrillation will soon recur.

In community prospective studies, supraventricular beats are not related to sudden death, as are ventricular premature beats in coronary disease.

Clinical Findings

A. Symptoms: Atrial premature beats are conducted in antegrade or retrograde manner; they commonly depolarize the sinoatrial node, and for that reason there may be a pause following the premature beat that is longer or shorter than the pause between two normally conducted sinus beats. Except in hypertrophic cardiomyopathy, in which the stroke output following a pause is usually weaker than normal, the ventricular beat following the pause is usually stronger, ejecting an increased stroke volume, and the patient may have a variety of symptoms referable to awareness of the strength of this beat. When supraventricular beats are frequent or occur in runs, such beats may decrease the cardiac output and impair perfusion to the essential organs, causing mental confusion, dyspnea, angina, palpitations, or weakness.

Supraventricular premature beats are common in healthy individuals and increase in frequency with age. They are not by themselves an indication of cardiac disease, and antiarrhythmic drug therapy is not indicated in the absence of symptoms.

B. Signs: Supraventricular premature beats, like ventricular premature beats, may be recognized at the bedside when an extra beat is detected that disturbs the dominant rhythm. The origin of the extra beat, whether supraventricular or ventricular, is difficult to distinguish on auscultation. If the premature beat ret-

rogradely penetrates the sinus node and discharges it, the next normal sinus beat is delayed, but the pause is not "compensatory" and the basic rhythm is altered. Unless the premature beats occur near the junction of the atria and the atrioventricular node (junctional premature beats), cannon waves do not occur (see Chapter 3). Cannon waves may occur if the atria contract when the tricuspid valve is closed, since both atria and ventricles contract within a short interval.

The pause that follows the premature beat may allow the physician to diagnose the underlying cardiac condition, and it is useful to listen carefully to the postpause beat. In aortic stenosis, for example, the murmur may be louder as a result of the more forceful ventricular contraction following the pause. In mitral incompetence, the murmur is not louder. In hypertrophic cardiomyopathy, the long pause with increased left ventricular volume may reduce the left ventricular outflow obstruction (see Chapter 17), and the systolic murmur will become softer. However, because of increased contractility in the postextrasystolic beat, the murmur may become louder. When long pauses are felt in the radial or carotid arteries, the possibility of a "dropped" beat due to atrioventricular block must be considered. Valve tensing sounds due to early premature beats can be heard (unless they are nonconducted atrial premature beats), whereas "dropped" beats cannot.

1. Electrocardiography– Supraventricular premature beats are best recognized on the ECG, especially after careful inspection of a long strip (Figure 15–1). The usual pattern is that of P waves having a contour different from that of regular sinus P waves. These P waves are premature and may be associated with an aberrant QRS complex that usually has a right bundle branch block configuration. They may be nonconducted if they occur early and may be missed unless careful inspection of the T wave preceding a pause shows that it is slurred or notched or otherwise different from other T waves in the lead, thus indicating that a premature P wave is buried in the T wave complex.

The ectopic (premature) P wave has been called P′ and should be carefully sought if the RR interval or the dominant rhythm is disturbed or if the PR interval in the succeeding beat is prolonged because of concealed conduction in the atrioventricular node. P′ complexes may often explain the cause of bradycardia. When atrial premature beats occur in bigeminy, ie, in every other beat, the patient may be thought to have 2:1 block or sinus bradycardia when in fact the rhythm is that of atrial premature beats, which are clinically less significant.

2. Concealed atrial premature beats– Occasionally, the premature beat or P′ beat may be isoelectric to the lead examined and thus not obvious and only suspected or recognized by its effects on the subsequent PR interval or by the pause that follows

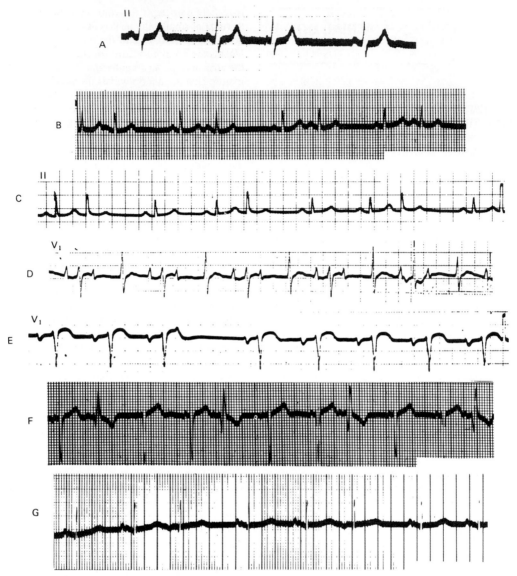

Figure 15–1. Atrial premature beats. **A:** Atrial premature beats, lead II. **B:** Atrial bigeminal rhythm, lead II. **C:** Atrial premature beats with slight aberrant conduction and subtle changes when P is superimposed on T waves, lead II. **D:** Normal sinus rhythm with atrial bigeminy that represents either nonconducted premature beats followed by junctional escape beats with aberrant intraventricular conduction or atrial premature beats with prolonged PR interval, lead V_1. **E:** Nonconducted atrial premature beat after third QRS complex, lead V_1. **F:** Atrial premature beats with aberrant conduction of right bundle branch block pattern, lead V_1. **G:** Atrial or junctional premature beats, lead II.

the so-called concealed premature beat. Atrial premature beats may be "concealed" when they partially penetrate the atrioventricular node and do not spread to the ventricles, but they nonetheless influence the refractory period of the atrioventricular node and so alter the succeeding PR interval. Supraventricular beats may not be recognized despite careful inspection but may be found and proved by His bundle recording that reveals a premature atrial or His bundle

spike. If the presence of a premature beat that is not obvious on the ordinary ECG is strongly suspected, the ECG can be recorded at double standardization, or different leads that tend to exaggerate the size of the P′ wave may be employed.

Other means of amplifying the size of the supraventricular depolarizations include the bipolar Lewis lead (right arm electrode in the second intercostal space to the right of the sternum two interspaces above lead V_1 and left arm electrode in the fourth intercostal space to the right of the sternum, the normal position for lead V_1, and both recorded on lead I), esophageal leads (electrode directly posterior to the left atrium), and right atrial electrode catheters that display large P′ as well as P waves. The P′ or ectopic atrial depolarization usually has a polarity different from the normal sinus P wave and may be inverted in leads II, III, and aVF and upright in aVR. These are low atrial or junctional.

3. Initiation of paroxysmal tachycardia– If the atrial premature beats occur at a critical time after the previous QRS complex (so-called **critical coupling interval**) and if conduction delay through a portion of the conduction system—usually the atrioventricular node or a bypass tract—is present, a reentry circuit may be established, and the premature atrial beat may initiate supraventricular tachycardia. Programmed electrical stimulation has shown that atrial premature beats with a progressively shorter coupling interval combined with delay in conduction through the atrioventricular node are the causal mechanism in most cases of supraventricular tachycardia, though such tachycardias may be due to increased automaticity, such as occurs in coronary disease or following digitalis.

Treatment

Atrial premature beats rarely require drug treatment unless they are frequent, multiform, chaotic, or associated with hemodynamic changes. (See Treatment of Supraventricular Tachycardia.)

SUPRAVENTRICULAR TACHYCARDIA

Classification

A number of mechanisms for supraventricular tachycardia have now been clarified. The mechanisms involve reentry and automaticity (Chapter 14) (Figure 15–2). There are four types.

A. Reentrant Atrial Tachycardia: Reentry is seen in a number of atrial tachycardias, including atrial fibrillation, atrial flutter, and intra-atrial tachycardia. The pathway is entirely in the atrium, and the atrioventricular node is not involved in the circuit. The classic reentrant atrial tachycardia is atrial flutter, where the circuit involves macroreentry in the pathway around the orifices of the venae cavae and the tricuspid ring, which act as barriers to conduction. Atrial flutter is characterized by an atrial vector parallel to lead II, producing a very regular saw-toothed atrial pattern on the surface ECG with a rate of 250–340 beats/min.

Intra-atrial reentrant tachycardia is similar to atrial flutter, involving a slower, less predictable pathway in the atrium. There is a higher prevalence of structural myocardial disease and the pathway is slower, producing a longer cycle length and slower atrial rate.

B. Atrioventricular Nodal Reentrant Tachycardia: This is the commonest form of supraventricular tachycardia, comprising about 50–60% of cases. The pathway involves the atrioventricular node and probably a small rim of paranodal atrial myocardium. Electrophysiologically, this rhythm depends on the circuit, involving a slow α and fast β pathway. Although both pathways could be intranodal, there is increasing evidence by radiofrequency catheter ablation that the fast and slow pathways are anatomically separated, with the slow pathway in the posterior node near the coronary sinus ostium and the fast pathway in the anterior nodal region. Typically, the arrhythmia is initiated after an atrial extrasystole, where the impulse is blocked in the fast pathway and antegrade conduction into the ventricle occurs through the slow pathway. The fast pathway acts as the retrograde limb of the reentry circuit, and the typical "slow-fast" tachycardia is seen. Since retrograde conduction to the atrium occurs rapidly, the retrograde P wave is buried in the QRS and is not seen. Less commonly, the conduction to the retrograde limb is relatively slow, and the retrograde P wave is seen after the QRS, the "fast-slow" versus "long R–P′" tachycardia (Figure 15–2).

C. Atrioventricular Reciprocating Tachycardia or Atrioventricular Reentrant Tachycardia Utilizing a Concealed Bypass Tract: In this reentrant rhythm, antegrade conduction into the ventricle is through the atrioventricular node, and the circuit involves ventricular myocardium and retrograde conduction to the atrium or macroreentry over a "concealed" bypass tract or bundle of Kent. The bypass tract is "concealed," since antegrade conduction does not occur over this tract, only retrograde conduction. At other times or in other patients, the bypass tract conducts antegrade and the reentry occurs retrograde over the atrioventricular node. Typically, the conduction is "orthodromic" or down the atrioventricular node and retrograde through the "concealed" bypass tract. Less commonly, the sequence is down the bypass tract, with reentry occurring through the atrioventricular node, and the reciprocating tachycardia is called "antidromic."

In the usual orthodromic tachycardia, since the reciprocating pathway is over ventricular muscle to the bypass tract. the R–P′ interval is long, and the retrograde P wave occurs late after the QRS. In patients with a posteroseptal bypass tract, there can be decremental conduction in the tract, forming the substrate for an incessant long R–P′ tachycardia termed the permanent form of junctional reciprocating tachycardia.

Reciprocating tachycardias comprise 30–40% of supraventricular tachycardias.

D. Automatic Tachycardias: There are uncommon tachycardias with enhanced automaticity or trig-

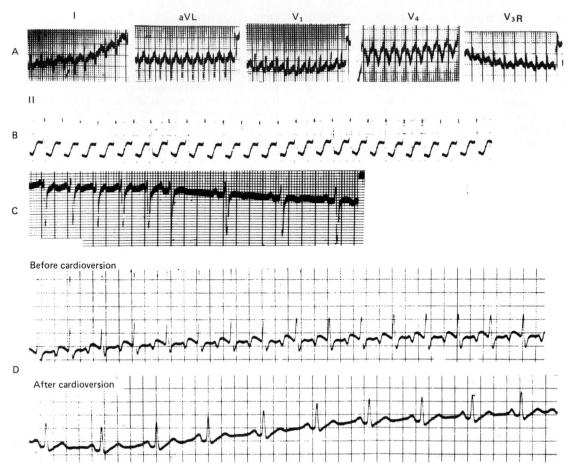

Figure 15–2. Supraventricular tachycardia. **A:** Supraventricular tachycardia in 3-week-old girl with a heart rate of 300/min. **B:** Probable myocardial ischemia during supraventricular tachycardia at a rate of 220/min. **C:** Supraventricular tachycardia with spontaneous subsidence in a 57-year-old woman. **D:** Paroxysmal supraventricular tachycardia with 1:1 conduction. Change in height of R waves indicates altered ventricular conduction converted by cardioversion in a 36-year-old woman to 2:1 conduction.

gered activity as the underlying electrophysiologic mechanism. They comprise about 10% of the supraventricular tachycardias and can be intermittent, repetitive, or incessant. They are characterized by a graded increase in rate for several beats (a "warm-up" period) at their onset before they become regular. The P wave morphology depends on the point of origin in the atrium or intra-atrial septum. If the origin is near the sinoatrial node, P wave morphology is normal and the rhythm looks like sinus tachycardia.

Atrial phase 4 depolarization or enhanced automaticity can occur in a number of disease states, in metabolic or electrolyte derangements, or with a number of drugs. It is therefore seen with uremia, hypokalemia, alcohol intoxication, and catecholamine drugs. Triggered activity is seen with digitalis and enhanced by sympathetic tone and hypokalemia. Because this rhythm is not dependent on a reentrant pathway, it cannot be terminated by overdrive pacing.

Multifocal atrial tachycardia is seen most often in

patients with chronic pulmonary disease and is not electrophysiologically well understood. It is characterized by a rate greater than 100/min and three or more distinct P wave morphologies. It is therefore probably an arrhythmia generated by multiple foci of abnormal atrial impulse generators, perhaps due to triggered automaticity. For this reason, since triggered activity is attributed to early afterdepolarization mediated by calcium and perhaps potassium currents, calcium channel blocking agents have been effective in this arrhythmia.

Mechanism of
Supraventricular Tachycardia

The mechanism of paroxysmal supraventricular tachycardia is reentry in about 75% of cases. The remainder of cases are due to increased automaticity or, in a small percentage of cases, to triggered activity as a result of increased afterpotentials (see Reentry). The mechanism by which the supraventricular tachycardias occur has therapeutic implications. Reentrant atrial tachycardias and atrioventricular nodal reentrant tachycardias, because they depend on a reentrant pathway, can be interrupted by depolarizing the pathway at a time that interrupts the circus depolarization. These rhythms can be interrupted permanently by ablating a section of the pathway. With automatic atrial tachycardias, interruption by pacing is not possible, and ablating those foci is much more difficult.

Supraventricular tachycardia is due to the same causes as premature beats. It often occurs in individuals with no evident heart disease. It may result from disease of the atria or bundle of His, as in atrial septal defect, mitral stenosis, or coronary disease involving the artery to the sinoatrial or atrioventricular node. The latter is usually confined to acute myocardial infarction, and paroxysmal supraventricular tachycardia is infrequent in patients with chronic coronary heart disease. Tobacco, coffee, stimulant drugs, and, most importantly, alcohol have been invoked as causal factors.

1. PAROXYSMAL SUPRAVENTRICULAR TACHYCARDIA

Although the electrophysiologic mechanisms of the various supraventricular tachycardias differ, the clinical features may be indistinguishable. The diagnosis of the type of supraventricular tachycardia may be suspected by careful examination of the scalar ECG. At other times, only electrophysiologic studies can elucidate the mechanism.

Paroxysmal supraventricular tachycardia results in a sudden increase in heart rate to 150–250/min, although rates of 300/min have been observed in infants, probably because atrioventricular conduction is accelerated in infants and the refractory period of the atrioventricular node is shorter. Young adults may have ventricular rates of 300/min for short periods at the onset that may result in syncope.

Many normal individuals have rapid heart rates with paroxysmal supraventricular tachycardia but do not develop "ischemic" ST segments during the attack or after it, or if they do, the ST changes may last only minutes to hours. Since patients rarely die during an attack, pathologic confirmation is not available. Some patients who develop "ischemic" ST segments during paroxysmal atrial tachycardia but who do not have angina on effort when they are in sinus rhythm may over a period of a few years develop angina pectoris, suggesting that subclinical coronary disease was unmasked by the rapid rate of the paroxysmal atrial tachycardia. The amount of ischemia or cellular damage that results from rapid rates with paroxysmal atrial tachycardia must be small, because few of these patients develop serum enzyme abnormalities or clinical manifestations suggesting non-Q wave infarction. Nevertheless, it is common to find ischemic ST segment changes during paroxysmal supraventricular tachycardia in patients who have no symptoms and sho do not have agina pectoris between attacks.

Clinical Findings

A. Symptoms: Typically, paroxysmal supraventricular tachycardia starts and ends abruptly, and usually the patient can recognize this. Palpitations may be the only symptom, but if there is underlying heart disease, the patient may complain of weakness, dizziness, anginal pain, or dyspnea. Central nervous system disturbances, when they occur, are usually diffuse and not focal, as is apt to be the case in cerebral ischemic attacks due to internal carotid artery disease. Angina pectoris may appear with the onset of tachycardia even if the patient has had no history of angina. The patient may be unaware of the rapid heart rate and complain only of angina. It is important to consider the onset of arrhythmias as a cause of the angina pectoris that appears at rest or during the night and is unrelated to exercise. The presence of underlying coronary disease is suggested not only by the appearance of angina during tachycardia but also by the appearance of typical ischemic ST segments on the ECG during the attack of rapid heart action. Infants may develop heart failure, especially if the heart rate exceeds 300/min; this is often the presenting manifestation of supraventricular tachycardia.

B. Signs:

1. Urine– In paroxysmal supraventricular tachycardia, the patient may pass a large quantity of urine within a few minutes of onset, a phenomenon that is thought to be due to release of atrial natriuretic factor induced by volume or stretch changes in the atria.

2. Degree of atrioventricular conduction– Conduction is almost always 1:1, and there is no clinical evidence of atrial and ventricular asynchrony, so there is nothing abnormal to be heard at the bedside other than the rapid heart rate. The first sound does not vary in intensity, and no cannon waves can be seen in the jugular venous pulse. The major exception occurs when the atrial tachycardia is due to digitalis toxicity, in which instance, because digitalis also decreases conduction through the atrioventricular node, 2:1 block is frequent and may be overlooked when the atrial rate is about 150/min and the ventricular rate about 75/min. Because the ventricular rate is normal, the patient has no palpitations or other symptoms, and were it not for the evidence on the ECG of rapid atrial rates with 2:1 ventricular response, digitalis toxicity could be overlooked. Figure 15–3 shows ECGs in coronary heart disease before and after treatment. Although digitalis is the usual cause of atrial tachycardia with 2:1 conduction, there are well-documented instances in which the patient with this disorder has not received digitalis; the physician is thus not warranted in diagnosing digitalis toxicity on the basis of the arrhythmia alone.

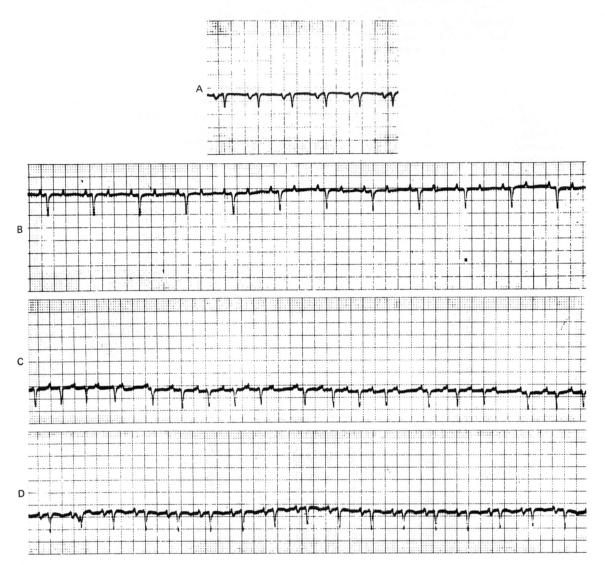

Figure 15–3. Atrial tachycardia before, during, and after treatment in a man age 52 weighing 60 kg, with coronary heart disease. **A:** 5:00 PM 7/22/55. Coronary heart disease before treatment with digoxin and a mercurial diuretic (Mercuhydrin, 2 mL intramuscularly). Note sinus rhythm. **B:** Atrial tachycardia with an atrial rate of 150/min and a ventricular rate of 75/min with 2:1 block after digoxin, 2.5 mg, and Mercuhydrin, 1 mL intramuscularly in 24 hours, with weight loss of 3.6 kg not recognized. On second day, a further dose of 1 m digoxin and 1 mL Mercuhydrin was given, with weight loss of 5.9 kg in 48 hours. **C:** 9:00 PM 7/25/55, 4 hours after administration of 11 meq potassium orally. Atrial tachycardia (rate 125/min) with Wenckebach phenomenon is now present. **D:** 11:45 PM 7/25/55, 1 hour and 45 minutes after a second dose of 11 meq potassium. Sinus tachycardia is now present. (All strips are lead V_1)

Digitalis toxicity is less commonly manifested by atrial tachycardia with 1:1 conduction or by varying degrees of atrioventricular block with or without atrial tachycardia or atrial fibrillation. Digitalis may not only cause atrial tachycardia with 2:1 conduction but may also produce partial progressive atrioventricular block with Wenckebach phenomenon, as shown in Figure 15–3C.

3. Jugular venous pulse– It is helpful to study the jugular venous pulse carefully in these instances;

rapid a waves at twice the rate of the ventricular response may lead to the correct diagnosis. The same is true in atrial flutter (see below), when the conduction from the atria to the ventricles is 4:1 and the ventricular rate at 75/min does not make one suspect that the atria are beating at a more rapid rate. The ECG can usually define the atrial rate unless the atrial waves are isoelectric.

4. Concealed accessory pathways– As many as 20% of patients with supraventricular tachycardia may have a concealed retrograde accessory pathway. These patients may have had a definite delta wave in childhood that disappeared in later life; electrophysiologic studies demonstrate the anomalous pathway. In atrioventricular nodal reciprocating tachycardia utilizing a concealed bypass tract, the retrograde P wave occurs late, after the QRS. The differentiation of this variety of reentry from atrioventricular nodal tachycardia may be difficult without special studies. In centers that do frequent electrophysiologic examinations of such patients, surgical ablation of the anomalous pathway has been recommended as primary therapy, since there is a high degree of success in permanently eliminating the arrhythmia and thus obviating the need for chronic antiarrhythmic therapy.

Differential Diagnosis

Atrial flutter is an atrial arrhythmia thought to be due to a circus movement, arising low in the atria, with atrial rates varying from 150/min to 350/min; at the lower range, atrial flutter may be difficult to distinguish from atrial tachycardia, just as atrial tachycardia with a rapid atrial rate may be difficult to distinguish from atrial flutter. One must then rely upon probabilities. In the usual case of supraventricular tachycardia, the atrial rate is less than 200/min, and in most cases of atrial flutter, the atrial rates are approximately 300/min. Atrial or supraventricular tachycardia usually occurs in younger individuals, often those with no heart disease or with heart disease that obviously involves the atria; it can then be inferred that the rapid supraventricular rhythm is more likely to be supraventricular tachycardia than atrial flutter. In contrast, atrial flutter, like atrial fibrillation, is more apt to occur in older individuals with obvious heart disease such as coronary heart disease or mitral stenosis. A conduction block from atria to ventricles of 4:1—or variable conduction such as alternating 2:1, 3:1, 4:1—occurs in atrial flutter but is uncommon in supraventricular tachycardia.

Treatment

See p 480.

2. NONPAROXYSMAL JUNCTIONAL (SUPRAVENTRICULAR) TACHYCARDIA

When sinoatrial nodal function is depressed, supraventricular tachycardia may occur, usually with a rate less than 130/min. This may occur during digitalis therapy, in acute myocardial infarction, and often after open heart surgery. The cause is obscure. It may be that secondary junctional pacemakers "escape" as a result of depressed sinoatrial node function or that the automaticity of the junctional tissues is enhanced by metabolic abnormalities secondary to hypoxia, ischemia, and associated digitalis therapy.

This condition is called nonparoxysmal junctional tachycardia and is usually associated with a narrow QRS complex. The junctional pacemaker may activate the atria retrogradely or may beat independently of the atria and result in atrioventricular dissociation.

When the mechanism is not "escape" but enhanced automaticity, it is postulated that the released metabolites or potassium from the ischemic and hypoxic myocardial cells may increase the slope of phase 4 diastolic depolarization of the action potential of the involved cells, further increasing automaticity of the junctional tissues.

In some instances, both the sinoatrial node and the junctional area "fire" independently, and atrioventricular dissociation occurs. This can be recognized on the ECG by noting intermittent capture of the ventricles by a sinus impulse that fortuitously reaches the ventricle when it has recovered excitability following depolarization from the junctional beat. Pick (1957) described nonparoxysmal junctional tachycardia and noted that the ventricular rate was slower than with ordinary supraventricular tachycardia. In contrast to the sudden onset and sudden offset that characterize paroxysmal supraventricular tachycardia, nonparoxysmal junctional tachycardia has a gradual onset and offset and is often seen transiently in the first few days after acute myocardial infarction. Although the QRS interval is often narrow, it may be wide and slurred if there is aberrant conduction to the ventricles.

Clinical Findings

A. Symptoms: The symptoms in nonparoxysmal junctional tachycardia depend upon the ventricular rate and hemodynamic effects. Symptoms may be absent because the ventricular rate is usually between 80/min and 120/min, or there may be palpitations, dyspnea, or fatigue. The diagnosis is often not suspected at the bedside but made on the basis of the clinical setting and the ECG.

B. Signs: The signs are similar to those of paroxysmal supraventricular tachycardia, but there may be signs of atrioventricular dissociation (see above).

Differential Diagnosis

Nonparoxysmal junctional tachycardia with aberrancy must be differentiated from accelerated idioventricular rhythm during acute myocardial infarction, which usually has more abnormal ventricular complexes. Differentiation is often not possible with conventional ECGs, and His bundle recordings are necessary to make a definitive diagnosis. Clinically, this is rarely necessary. The ventricular origin is also more probable when the clinical situation abruptly worsens or when the signs of ventricular tachycardia (see Clinical Differentiation, below) can be elicited. If fusion beats of gradual onset and offset occur preceding and following the run of tachycardia, the rhythm is ventricular in origin.

Lead II

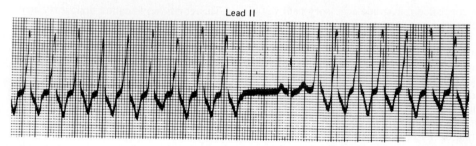

Figure 15–4. Tachycardia (ventricular or junctional?) interrupted by single normal beat in a 43-year-old man.

The regularity of the heart rate in nonparoxysmal junctional tachycardia may differentiate this rhythm from sinus tachycardia. In sinus tachycardia, the rate is rapid, essentially regular at short intervals, and almost always less than 180/min. It may be slightly irregular and vary with simple maneuvers such as posture, mild exercise, respiration, breath-holding, or carotid sinus pressure. If the heart rate is counted for a full minute, especially after changes in position and other maneuvers just mentioned, it will be shown to be slightly irregular and variable in sinus tachycardia. In paroxysmal supraventricular tachycardia, however, the heart rate is not influenced by these procedures unless the attack is terminated abruptly.

If the surface ECG shows a sinus tachycardia that abruptly stops with a slower sinus rate succeeding it, the diagnosis of sinus node reentry tachycardia can be made.

Sinus tachycardia results from a number of factors, eg, fever, infection, anemia, anxiety, leukemia, thyrotoxicosis, or connective tissue disorders.

A. Differentiation of Ventricular and Supraventricular Tachycardia on the ECG: (Figure 15–4.) If the QRS complex is narrow and preceded by P waves, the rhythm is supraventricular.

When P waves cannot be seen and when QRS complexes are wide (eg, duration ≥ 0.12 s), the differentiation between ventricular tachycardia and supraventricular tachycardia with aberrant conduction is often difficult (Table 15–1). The key to the differentiation is identification of the P waves and their relationship to the ventricular complex. In ventricular tachycardia, atrioventricular dissociation occurs, and the ventricles are usually beating at a faster rate than the atria. However, in rare cases there may be retrograde conduction to the atria, with retrograde 1:1 conduction and one P wave for every QRS complex. In paroxysmal supraventricular tachycardia, the atria and ventricles beat at the same rate.

Careful inspection of the T waves and QRS complexes for the possible presence of "buried" P waves is important in determining the atrial rate and deciding if there are two independent pacemakers. Multiple conventional or Lewis leads, esophageal leads, right atrial electrode catheter electrograms, or His

bundle recordings may be required to amplify the P waves or to relate them to the QRS complexes (Figures 15–5 and 15–6).

When the QRS complex is wide, supraventricular tachycardia is probable when (1) the pattern in lead V_1 is that of right bundle branch block with an rSr′ or rsR′ pattern because of a prolonged refractory period in the right bundle or (2) the QRS configuration in the first few beats of tachycardia is similar to the pattern of supraventricular premature beats that may have been present previously. However, the rSr′ pattern in lead V_1 could still represent junctional tachycardia with aberrancy rather than paroxysmal supraventricular tachycardia.

Ventricular tachycardia is the more likely diagnosis (1) if the QRS pattern is like that in left bundle branch block or has a QR pattern in lead V_1, or (2) if the QRS configuration in the current tachycardia is similar to that of the ventricular premature beats on a previous ECG.

Using His bundle recordings to establish the site of origin of the tachycardia, Wellens (1985) found that the diagnosis of a ventricular origin was favored (but not established) by (1) QRS duration exceeding 0.14 s; (2) left axis deviation greater than −30 degrees; (3) atrioventricular dissociation during tachycardia; (4) capture or fusion beats (infrequent); (5) monophasic (R) or biphasic (qR, QR, or RS) complexes in V_1; and (6) an rS or QS complex in lead V_6. The diagnosis of a supraventricular origin was favored by

Table 15–1. Criteria of Puech (1970) and Waxman (1977) for the diagnosis of ventricular tachycardia.

- QRS complexes exceeding 0.12 s not associated with preexisting bundle branch block.
- Atrioventricular dissociation or ventriculoatrial block present.
- Irregular fusion and normal capture beats.
- Normalization of the QRS complexes by ventricular capture during tachycardia with wide QRS complex.
- Failure to produce aberration by rapid atrial pacing at a rate greater than the underlying tachycardia.
- Absence of a His bundle potential preceding ventricular activation during tachycardia, whereas during sinus rhythm such a potential precedes the QRS complex.

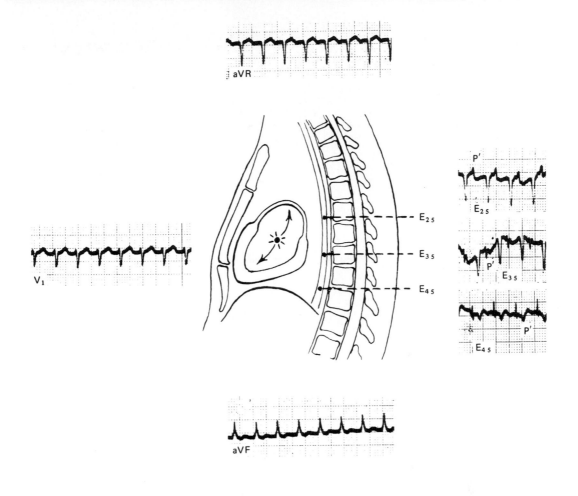

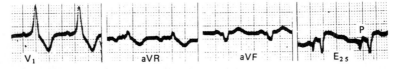

Figure 15–5. Supraventricular reentry atrioventricular nodal tachycardia, diagnosed with the aid of esophageal leads that amplify the P waves. The bottom strip was taken after reversion to sinus rhythm and demonstrates a typical Wolff-Parkinson-White syndrome conduction (type A). (Reproduced, with permission, from Goldman MJ: *Principles of Clinical Electrocardiography,* 12th ed. Lange, 1986.)

the following: (1) a triphasic QRS complex, especially if there was initial negativity in leads I and V_6; (2) ventricular rates exceeding 170/min; (3) QRS duration greater than 0.12 s but less than or equal to 0.14 s; and (4) the presence of preexcitation syndrome.

With wide QRS complexes, the diagnosis of ventricular tachycardia can also be made on the basis of the following criteria: (1) The QRS complexes during the tachycardia are 120 ms or more in duration and totally different from the complexes during supraventricular rhythm. (2) Atrioventricular dissociation or ventriculoatrial block is present. (3) Intermittent fusion and normal capture beats occur. (4) Atrial pacing to rates in excess of the tachycardia does not produce aberration. (5) No His bundle potential precedes ventricular activation during the tachycardia; His bundle potential precedes each QRS complex with a normal HV interval when sinus rhythm is restored (Puech, 1970; Akhtar, 1988; Tchou, 1988).

B. Clinical Differentiation: Clinical bedside evaluation may provide evidence of atrial and ventricular asynchrony, eg, varying intensity of the first heart sound and cannon waves in the jugular venous pulse.

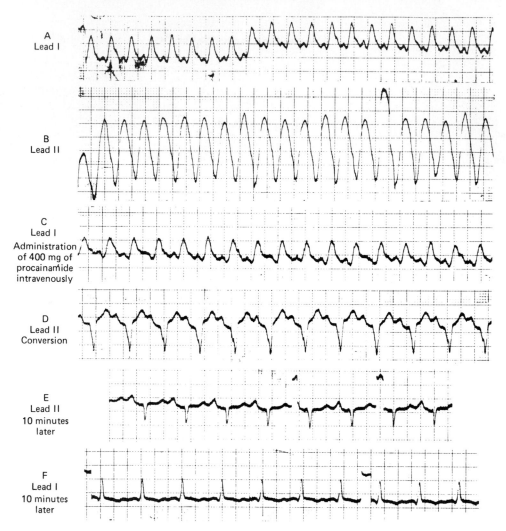

Figure 15–6. Paroxysmal supraventricular tachycardia 7 days after aortoiliac thromboendarterectomy. Sudden tachycardia after bowel movement. **A** and **B:** Before treatment. The pattern resembles ventricular tachycardia because of the wide QRS complexes, but a P wave is seen before each QRS complex in **A,** indicating that the rhythm is atrial tachycardia with aberrant conduction. **C:** Ventricular slowing following administration of 400 mg of procainamide intravenously (2 hours after 1 g quinidine gluconate intramuscularly over a 4-hour period with a quinidine blood level of 3.1 mg/mL). **D:** Sinus rhythm with intraventricular block at time of conversion. **E** and **F:** 10 minutes later, showing normal intraventricular conduction.

Cannon waves are large abrupt *a* waves in the jugular venous pulse ("venous Corrigan waves") occurring as the atria contract when the tricuspid valve is closed.

C. Value of Underlying Condition in Differentiation: The age of the patient and the setting in which the tachycardia occurs are helpful in diagnosis. Ventricular tachycardia is more likely if the patient has acute myocardial infarction, coronary heart disease, or other disease of the left ventricle, such as hypertrophic cardiomyopathy, aortic stenosis, or hypertensive disease. As noted previously, if the patient is young and free of heart disease and the precipitating factor was an acute emotional event, supra-

ventricular tachycardia is the more likely diagnosis. It must be emphasized again, however, that none of these criteria are absolute and that all indicate only the probable site of origin of the tachycardia. About 5–10% of patients with ventricular tachycardia have no known or obvious heart disease, whereas supraventricular tachycardia may occur in patients with known heart disease even if the patient is young. If it is essential to make the differentiation in order to determine therapy, His bundle recordings are helpful by demonstrating the presence of a His bundle spike preceding the QRS complex, in which case the tachycardia is supraventricular. His bundle recordings with intracardiac stimulation by programmed, critically timed supraventricular premature beats may establish the supraventricular origin of a tachycardia of unknown cause, but such procedures are indicated only if therapy is ineffective and the prognosis doubtful or if ablation of a bypass tract is contemplated. In troublesome cases, treatment should be directed toward the more serious condition, ventricular tachycardia; lidocaine with or without DC electric shock is helpful in both supraventricular and ventricular tachycardia.

3. TREATMENT OF SUPRAVENTRICULAR TACHYCARDIA

In the treatment of supraventricular tachycardia, drugs should be used unless serious cardiovascular deterioration indicates the need for rapid reversion to sinus rhythm. It is most important for the physician to estimate the degree of urgency. This estimate is made in part by observing how the patient is handling the rapid rate and whether the tachycardia is producing dyspnea, angina, faintness, confusion, hypotension, oliguria or significant hemodynamic abnormalities. In these clinical situations, cardioversion should be performed promptly. The history of previous attacks is most helpful in determining not only their usual duration but also the degree of disability produced. The duration of the attack when the patient is first seen is important, because if arrhythmia has been present for hours or days and the patient is still asymptomatic, the urgency is not great unless the patient's age and the presence of underlying heart disease such as mitral stenosis or coronary heart disease suggest that problems may arise if the attack continues. Therapeutic decisions are also influenced by ineffective treatment that the patient may already have received or by a history of therapeutic agents that have or have not succeeded in stopping previous attacks. If the patient is hypotensive, raising the arterial pressure with pressor agents may stop the attack or allow other therapeutic agents to become effective, and this form of treatment is often the most valuable immediate measure.

A. Underlying Condition: Treatment of underlying metabolic abnormalities such as hypoxia, ischemia, alkalosis, acidosis, or anemia is of first importance. Treatment of ventilatory problems is more important than the use of cardiac drugs in postoperative patients or in patients with chronic lung disease.

B. Sedation: If the ventricular rate is not over 150–180/min in a patient who has no or minimal heart disease with good left ventricular function and who is tolerating the tachycardia without symptoms other than palpitation—and especially if the attack was precipitated by an acute emotional event—sedation may be the initial and only treatment for the first few hours. Secobarbital, 0.1–0.2 g orally; diazepam, 5–10 mg orally; or flurazepam, 30 mg orally, may relax the patient and induce sleep, and the tachycardia may abruptly stop.

C. Stimulation of Vagus Nerve: If sedation fails or if the patient has dyspnea, severe palpitations, cerebral symptoms, polyuria, fall in blood pressure, or angina, stimulation of the vagus nerve should be tried to increase the refractory period of the atrioventricular node, thereby increasing atrioventricular block and delaying atrioventricular nodal transmission of the impulse. If this fails, cardioversion should be considered.

Noninvasive methods of stimulating the vagus may be used first, eg, carotid sinus massage, Valsalva's maneuver (Figure 15–7), breath-holding, squatting, or placing the face in ice water for a few seconds. In one study (Mehta, 1988), the Valsalva maneuver successfully terminated paroxysmal supraventricular tachycardia in 54% of the acute episodes. As with all methods of increasing vagal stimulation, patients may have a few ventricular premature beats or a short run of them at the time of conversion, and, rarely, ventricular fibrillation may develop. For this reason, resuscitative equipment should be immediately available. Gentle unilateral carotid sinus massage should be performed for 5–10 seconds (with the patient's head comfortably supported by a pillow), first on one side and then the other but not on both sides together or continuously. *Caution:* Do not use carotid sinus stimulation if the patient has carotid bruits or a history of transient cerebral ischemic attacks. Pressure on the eyeball should be avoided because of the risk of retinal detachment. Inducing vomiting is an unpleasant measure but may be effective.

D. Drug Treatment:

1. Decrease of atrioventricular conduction– If vagal stimulation fails and the patient is not hemodynamically compromised, thus requiring cardioversion, drugs can be used that directly decrease atrioventricular conduction.

a. Adenosine– Adenosine, because of its ultrashort half-life (10 seconds), is the drug of choice for the acute conversion of supraventricular tachycardia. Its onset of action is within 15–30 seconds after injection (Camm, 1991). It is effective in over 85% of cases, and if hypotension is precipitated, it is of brief duration and is therefore safe even if adenosine is given mistakenly to a patient with ventricular tachycardia or wide QRS tachycardia with Wolff-Parkinson-White conduction, where hypotension precipitated by intravenous verapamil could be fatal (Sharma, 1990). Because adenosine markedly reduces the atrial refractory period, its administration in a patient with supraventricular tachycardia has occasionally resulted in conversion of the rhythm to atrial fibrillation. The dose is 6 mg intravenously initially, followed after 30 seconds by a second dose of 12 mg intravenously. Over 90% of patients will respond to a dose of 10 mg or less. The effects of adenosine are

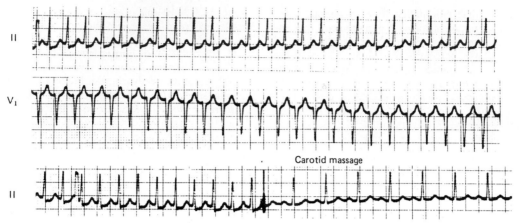

Figure 15–7. Carotid massage abruptly terminates paroxysmal supraventricular tachycardia in a 54-year-old man with carcinoma of the neck. ST ischemic depression is seen just prior to cessation of the attack.

counteracted by aminophylline and potentiated by dipyridamole, which is a potent adenosine receptor inhibitor. Adenosine terminates supraventricular tachycardia faster than intravenous verapamil (DiMarco, 1990).

b. Calcium entry-blocking drugs– Before adenosine, these drugs were the treatment of choice in paroxysmal supraventricular tachycardia. Verapamil has a great inhibiting effect on the atrioventricular node, and diltiazem is intermediate. Nifedipine is likely to be ineffective. Verapamil, 5–10 mg, or diltiazem, 150–300 μg/kg, can be given intravenously over 3–5 minutes (Schugar, 1990). These drugs are successful in terminating the arrhythmia in over 85% of cases. Verapamil decreases atrioventricular nodal conduction and increases the refractory period of the atrioventricular node. It blocks the antegrade pathway of the two most common varieties of supraventricular tachycardia—reentrant atrioventricular nodal and atrioventricular reciprocating tachycardia. It is less likely to be effective in reentrant sinoatrial nodal or atrial tachycardia. Verapamil may be combined with propranolol unless the patient has left ventricular failure. The data are inadequate to determine the value of verapamil combined with digitalis. Bradycardia and hypotension may occur with verapamil, and caution must be used before giving it to patients already receiving digitalis or beta-adrenergic-blocking drugs. The combination may produce various bradycardia syndromes, including sinus arrest.

c. Other drugs– Because of the hypotension, intravenous verapamil is contraindicated and even dangerous in patients with ventricular tachycardia or wide QRS complex supraventricular tachycardias associated with bypass tracts (WPW). The precipitated hypotension increases sympathetic stimulation, which can increase the conduction of impulses to the ventricle over the bypass tract and precipitate ventricular fibrillation. The drop in blood pressure also can increase myocardial ischemia, which could be disastrous in patients with coronary artery disease. Other agents effective in the treatment of paroxysmal supraventricular tachycardia include propranolol, 0.5–1 mg intravenously every 5 minutes, up to a total of 1–5 mg; other beta-adrenergic drugs such as esmolol, 500 μg/kg intravenously over 1 minute, followed by 25 μg/kg/min and increasing by 25–50 μg/kg/min every 5 minutes to desired effect; and digoxin, 0.75–1 mg intravenously. Patients should be monitored closely, and hypotension should be avoided. Caution should be used when giving propranolol if the patient shows evidence of impaired cardiac function, because cardiac failure may result.

Newer drugs such as flecainide, 200–300 mg/d orally, or propafenone, 100–200 mg/d orally, have been successful, especially in the permanent or nearly incessant varieties of supraventricular tachycardia. These are type Ic drugs, which slow the upstroke of phase 0 but do not increase the duration of the action potential. Side effects, however, are common with both, mostly central nervous system symptoms and proarrhythmia (the worsening or precipitation of arrhythmia). These newer drugs may be the treatment of choice in "permanent" supraventricular tachycardia when more conventional drugs have failed.

If these drugs fail, one of the noninvasive methods of stimulating the vagus (such as carotid sinus massage) should be used during the time of drug action to produce additive vagal stimulation. If tachycardia persists, therapeutic agents that reflexly increase vagal stimulation can be used, including such pressor drugs as phenylephrine, 2–4 mg subcutaneously or 0.1–0.2 mg intravenously, which raise blood pressure and stimulate the baroreceptor reflexes. Caution should be used: one should begin with small doses to avoid excess hypertension.

Among the newer drugs, one of the most powerful in treating severe cases of reentrant atrioventricular nodal supraventricular tachycardia unresponsive to conventional therapy is amiodarone, given in a dosage of 5 mg/kg over a 15-minute period, followed by an infusion of 600 mg over a 12- to 24-hour period. Side effects are frequent when the drug is used chronically in dosages of 300–600 mg/d.

2. Decrease of automaticity– (See Tables 15–5 and 15–6.) Drugs that decrease excitability and automaticity may occasionally be helpful in an acute paroxysm of tachycardia. Give quinidine sulfate, 0.2–0.4 g orally every 4 hours; procainamide, 100 mg/5 min intravenously to a total of 1 g; or phenytoin or lidocaine, 50–100 mg of either drug intravenously followed by an infusion of 1–2 mg/min. Quinidine is most effective in atrial arrhythmias but may produce hypotension and ventricular arrhythmias. Propranolol, 20–40 mg two to four times daily orally or in small doses (1–2 mg) intravenously, may be used to increase atrioventricular block. Its mechanism of action is to block beta-adrenergic receptors, increase atrioventricular nodal transmission time, and block the reentry circuit. Begin with 1 mg intravenously every 1–5 minutes until the desired effect is achieved or early toxic manifestations force abandonment of this therapy.

Electrophysiologic testing of the effect of various drugs is advised in resistant or frequently recurring episodes (see Ventricular Tachycardia, below).

E. Cardioversion: In many cases of supraventricular tachycardia, if the conventional drugs are ineffective, cardioversion is the treatment of choice. However, if the patient has digitalis toxicity, cardioversion should be avoided or used in small increments of current beginning with 5–10 J, since it can produce serious ventricular arrhythmias.

F. Rapid Atrial Pacing: If there is digitalis toxicity, if reentrant supraventricular tachycardia occurs following cardiac surgery, or if the patient has automatic atrial tachycardia and fails to revert to sinus rhythm with vigorous pharmacologic therapy, rapid "burst" atrial pacing to produce overdrive suppression of the ectopic focus may be tried (Scheinman, 1988). Since the conditions necessary to sustain a reentrant arrhythmia are conduction delay and unidirectional block, any two conduction pathways that are longitudinally dissociated form the physiologic substrate for reentry. If the pathway can be interrupted by a properly timed impulse or run of impulses, the reentrant rhythm can be interrupted, allowing the sinus node to capture the atrium. Pacing of the atrium at heart rates above that of the tachycardia may terminate the tachycardia during pacing or immediately after pacing is stopped or may induce atrioventricular block, effectively slowing the ventricular rate. Discontinuing the atrial pacing causes transient depression of both the automatic tachycardia and the sinus node; the latter recovers first, restoring sinus rhythm. Atrial pacing not only restores sinus rhythm by this "overdrive suppression"; it may also interrupt the

reentry circuit of the paroxysmal supraventricular tachycardia by depolarizing the atrium so that the reentry pathway is refractory to an oncoming pulse. Occasionally, atrial pacing may induce atrial fibrillation, which may then spontaneously revert to sinus rhythm.

Antitachycardiac pacing must not be used in patients with atrial fibrillation or preexcitation (Wolff-Parkinson-White syndrome) who have short antegrade effective refractory periods (Scheinman, 1988). Patients considered for rapid pacing should have a thorough electrophysiologic study to exclude the likelihood of induction of ventricular fibrillation. Backup defibrillation units are necessary.

Although permanent implantable antitachycardia devices are available that constantly monitor the atrial activity for the onset of atrial tachycardia and then deliver programmed premature beats or bursts of atrial premature beats determined by electrophysiologic study before implantation to be effective in terminating the rhythm, these devices have limited use. These patients have reentrant pathways capable of interruption and are ideal candidates for catheter ablation and permanent cure. Only patients who for some anatomic reason are not amenable to catheter ablation or those who have failed ablation—and who are not responsive to drug suppression—are candidates for implantable antitachycardia devices.

G. Ablation Therapy: Surgical interruption of bypass tracts in the treatment of reentrant supraventricular tachycardias in Wolff-Parkinson-White syndrome has been successful since the initial report by Cobb in 1968. Further experience with surgical ablation resulted in success in ablating the arrhythmia in 95% of cases. The morbidity of thoracotomy and the complications of the large incisions made in the atrioventricular groove led to reservation of surgery for patients in whom medical management has failed and in whom recurrent arrhythmia has resulted in severe disability—or when lifelong antiarrhythmia therapy is unacceptable to the patient.

At the beginning of the last decade, closed-chest electrical ablation of the atrioventricular node and His bundle was accomplished in dogs and shortly thereafter in humans (Gonzalez, 1981; Scheinman, 1982). The first energy used was high-energy direct current (DC) shock with the catheter placed at the anatomic position where the His bundle was recorded. The other electrode was on the body surface. Later, this same technique was used for placing the intracardiac catheter at the point where the earliest appearance of the retrograde atrial depolarization was seen and interrupting the reentrant pathway by creating a lesion. This catheter ablation technique has been successful in treatment of patients with bypass tracts and is now the treatment of choice for the patient with symptomatic Wolff-Parkinson-White reentrant supraventricular tachycardias. Other supraventricular arrhythmias, including atrioventricular reciprocating tachycardia via an accessory pathway, atrioventricular nodal reentrant tachycardia, and atrial flutter, have been successfully treated (Haines, 1992).

The problem with ablation using this energy is the relatively uncontrolled amount of damage created, at times injuring the coronary artery and even causing coronary sinus and myocardial rupture. The discharge is associated with extremely high temperatures at the catheter tip, and with the expanding vapor bubble the tissue expands and collapses in 15 ms, creating a pressure of 70 psi. This barotrauma, together with the heat and direct electrical injury, results in the myocardial lesion and is painful enough to require general anesthesia. Other types of energy that could be delivered through a catheter were investigated, and it was found that alternating current radiofrequency energy (0.3–1 MHz) could create discrete myocardial lesions 8–12 mm in diameter and 5–10 mm in depth, producing myocardial desiccation by means of reactive heating (Lesh, 1992). There is little risk to adjacent structures, including coronary arteries and atrioventricular valves, but the small size of the lesions makes it more difficult to ablate a discrete pathway. This increases the time required to do the procedure, including the catheterization time and radiation exposure to patient and operators. Other forms of energy are being investigated, including microwave energy and laser energy, but at present radiofrequency energy is the most successful. The radiofrequency energy is delivered in unipolar fashion between the electrode tip and a large surface area dispersive electrode on the body surface.

The lesion size created is dependent on the temperature developed at the catheter tip, which is dependent on the power delivered, the electrode size and its contact with the tissue, and the duration of power delivery.

In patients with reentrant supraventricular tachycardia with accessory pathways, radiofrequency catheter ablation has been successful in 89% of 100 cases, and in all but one patient the ablation was accomplished at a single session. Over a mean follow-up period of 10 months, nine patients had some return of accessory pathway conduction, and a repeat ablation procedure was successful in five patients in whom it was attempted. Complications due to catheter placement but not to the ablation itself occurred in four patients (Lesh, 1992). With these results, symptomatic supraventricular tachycardia with an accessory pathway is now treated primarily with catheter ablation rather than chronic drug suppression.

In atrioventricular nodal reentrant tachycardia, the slow and fast atrioventricular nodal pathways are anatomically separate. The retrograde slow pathway is close to the posterior septum near the coronary sinus and can be identified in most patients with electrophysiologic studies showing a small spike just before the retrograde atrial potential. Radiofrequency ablation was performed with the catheter near the coronary sinus in 80 symptomatic patients with atrioventricular

nodal reentrant tachycardia and successfully abolished or modified the slow pathway conduits in 78 patients, eliminating the atrioventricular nodal reentrant tachycardia without affecting atrioventricular nodal conduction. Atrioventricular block occurred in one patient (1.3%). There has been no recurrence of arrhythmia after 15.5 months of follow-up (Jackman, 1992). If the catheter is positioned near the atrioventricular node, the fast pathway can be injured without creating complete atrioventricular block, and the atrioventricular nodal reentrant tachycardia can also be eliminated; however, the frequency of developing complete atrioventricular block is higher, and for that reason this procedure is not as desirable as ablating the slow pathway (Lee, 1991).

H. Paroxysmal Atrial Tachycardia With Block: Paroxysmal atrial tachycardia with block is usually (not always) due to digitalis toxicity. It is wise to stop digitalis and diuretics to minimize potassium loss and, if the situation is not urgent, allow tachycardia with block to gradually disappear over 1–3 days. If the serum potassium is less than 3 meq/L, potassium chloride may be given in a dosage of 40–100 meq orally; or, if the need is or may be urgent, the potassium can be given intravenously in a dosage of 10–20 meq/h. Cardioversion should be avoided in the presence of digitalis toxicity because of the risk of inducing ventricular arrhythmias.

I. Junctional Rhythm With Atrioventricular Dissociation: This rhythm is usually due to increased automaticity (most commonly from digitalis toxicity), acute inferior myocardial infarction, or acute myocarditis or follows cardiac surgery. Treatment is the same as for paroxysmal atrial tachycardia with block. Digitalis and diuretics should be stopped, and if the serum potassium is low, potassium may be given intravenously at a rate of 10–20 meq/L/h. If the abnormal rhythm is due to acute myocardial infarction, treatment should be directed at the acute infarction and should consist of rest, oxygen, and other therapy monitored by frequent determination of hemodynamic indices, noting the response of the patient (see Chapter 8). In the "near-incessant" variety or "permanent" form of paroxysmal junctional reciprocating tachycardia, flecainide, encainide, amiodarone, or aprindine may abolish the arrhythmia, but conventional drugs are usually ineffective. If unresponsive to all drugs, the arrhythmia has been abolished by ablation of the retrograde accessory pathway, which is usually near the coronary sinus in the posterior atrial septum (Scheinman, 1988).

J. Automatic Tachycardias: Automatic atrial tachycardia presents with intermittent or incessant tachyarrhythmias. It frequently results (if of long standing) in tachycardia cardiomyopathy (Hendry, 1990). It cannot be initiated or interrupted by pacing and responds poorly to drugs. Beta-blockers may slow the ventricular response, and type Ic drugs such as flecainide, encainide, and propafenone have been reported to be useful in terminating this arrhythmia (Kuck, 1988; Relmer, 1991). Surgical and catheter ablation can also be successful, but large amounts of myocardial tissue must frequently be ablated, since new foci arise in about 15% of cases (Haines, 1992). Ablation of the atrioventricular node and VVI pacing is a management option when all else fails.

Junctional ectopic tachycardia is a rare arrhythmia occurring in infancy and childhood—often rapid, incessant, and responding poorly to drugs. Since it is an ectopic rhythm probably due to abnormal automaticity, it cannot be precipitated or interrupted by pacing and frequently results in tachycardia cardiomyopathy and sudden death. In adults, ventricular response may be slowed by beta-blockers, but catheter ablation of the atrioventricular node and permanent VVI pacemaker insertion is often necessary (Ruder, 1986).

Multifocal atrial tachycardia is an arrhythmia most often seen with chronic respiratory disease and respiratory failure. The most effective therapy is treatment of the underlying respiratory disease and normalization of blood gases. This tachyarrhythmia is a bad prognostic sign. The mortality rate during the hospital stay ranges from 29% to 59% (Kastor, 1990). The usual antiarrhythmia therapy, including digoxin, is ineffective. Verapamil has been reported as being successful in slowing the atrial rate because of its effect on triggered autoactivity, but calcium channel blockers rarely terminate this arrhythmia. Beta-blockers slow the ventricular response and may suppress the arrhythmia, but they are usually contraindicated in chronic respiratory disease. A short-acting beta-blocker, esmolol, can be used. If esmolol is successful, metoprolol can be gradually started, and success has been reported with this drug (Hazard, 1987). If the rhythm is persistent with hemodynamic deterioration due to rapid ventricular response, atrioventricular nodal ablation and VVI pacemaker insertion is the treatment of choice.

K. Arrhythmias During Cardiac Catheterization: The irritation of the right atrium or the right ventricle may induce atrial or ventricular premature beats. The catheter should be removed from the involved chamber until the premature beats disappear, and the procedure can then be continued.

L. Prevention of Recurrences:

1. Drug treatment– If the paroxysmal supraventricular tachycardia is slow, brief, and asymptomatic, no treatment may be necessary. Recurrences of supraventricular tachycardia can be prevented by long-term administration of digitalis, quinidine, beta-adrenergic-blocking agents, verapamil (Sakurai, 1983), disopyramide, flecainide, encainide, propafenone, or amiodarone. If the paroxysms are of long duration, rapid, or symptomatic, chronic drug therapy can be used. At present, if the supraventricular arrhythmia is chronic and symptomatic, electrophysiologic study should be done to determine the

mechanism and assess whether it can be ablated by catheter.

2. Implantation of pacemakers– Implanted automatic atrial pacemakers, activated by rapid atrial tachycardia, have been used in resistant, recurrent cases associated with considerable hemodynamic deterioration during tachycardia (Boccadamo, 1991). This is now a consideration only if catheter ablation cannot be undertaken or is unsuccessful and medical management has failed.

3. Surgical or catheter cryoablation of the His bundle, atrioventricular node, or perinodal area– When recurrent, disabling episodes of paroxysmal supraventricular tachycardia cannot be controlled by vigorous antiarrhythmic therapy, invasive ablative or destructive procedures have been employed to interrupt the reentry circuit to prevent the arrhythmia as discussed above.

ATRIAL FIBRILLATION & ATRIAL FLUTTER (See Figure 15–8)

Atrial fibrillation consists of rapid (400–650/min) multiple depolarizations of the atria, resulting in an irregular rapid ventricular response to variable block in the atrioventricular node caused by the frequent incoming atrial impulses. It is represented on the ECG as rapid, irregular, usually small undulations of the baseline during the period of atrial contraction and conduction. It is the most common atrial arrhythmia in older people. It can be paroxysmal or established.

Atrial flutter, which can also be paroxysmal or established, occurs less frequently than atrial fibrillation. The atrial depolarizations are slower (approximately 300/min) and usually associated with a 2:1 block with a ventricular rate about 150/min. The ECG shows a characteristic sawtooth appearance with P waves occurring at a rate of 300/min.

1. ATRIAL FIBRILLATION

In atrial fibrillation, paroxysmal attacks usually last hours or days rather than seconds or minutes and almost never longer than 2 or 3 weeks. If the rhythm persists after this period, atrial fibrillation is said to be established, or chronic; this is in contrast to supraventricular tachycardia, which rarely lasts days or weeks and usually lasts minutes or hours. Paroxysmal atrial fibrillation may occur without known heart disease or other obvious reason but most commonly occurs after pulmonary or cardiac surgery or in older individuals with mitral stenosis, atrial septal defect, myocarditis, thyrotoxicosis, or constrictive pericarditis. Atrial fibrillation is common in alcoholism. It can be seen with acute alcohol intoxication, in the course of alcohol withdrawal, or with alcoholic car-

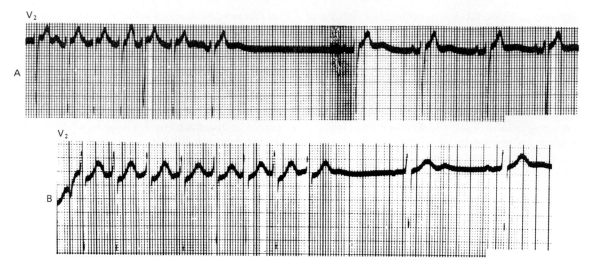

Figure 15–8. Spontaneous changes in atrial arrhythmia. **A:** Spontaneous conversion of atrial fibrillation with rapid irregular ventricular response to sinus rhythm in a 71-year-old woman. **B:** Spontaneous subsidence of supraventricular tachycardia, followed by junctional escape prior to sinus rhythm in a 62-year-old woman.

diomyopathy. Patients with recurrent episodes of atrial fibrillation should be carefully evaluated for alcohol abuse. It is most common in older people with left atrial enlargement due to any cause. It may be precipitated by an acute emotional event even if the patient has underlying cardiac disease such as mitral stenosis. It is not especially common in chronic coronary heart disease and is infrequent in acute myocardial infarction, though continuous monitoring has shown that it may occur. It is common when hypoxia and infection occur in chronic lung disease with cor pulmonale.

Following pulmonary embolism or surgery—perhaps as a result of hypoxia from inadequate ventilation or pericardial injury—as many as one-third of patients may develop paroxysmal atrial fibrillation. Transient atrial fibrillation is also common following cardiac surgery, especially mitral valve surgery. Even if the rhythm reverts to sinus rhythm preoperatively, it often recurs after surgery. It is common during the course of untreated thyrotoxicosis and usually disappears spontaneously when the thyrotoxicosis is treated. It may be precipitated by cardiac catheterization in patients with mitral stenosis or atrial septal defect. Atrial fibrillation may occur after infective endocarditis is established in aortic or mitral valvular heart disease but is uncommon in acute endocarditis occurring in drug users with tricuspid or aortic valve lesions.

Atrial fibrillation is rare in pure aortic valve disease in the absence of heart failure, and its presence should prompt the physician to think of associated mitral valve disease, even if the typical murmurs are not readily heard.

The Framingham study found that in the absence of known heart disease, the incidence of chronic atrial

fibrillation increased with age but still developed infrequently (2% over a period of 20 years). In this study, there was an independent contribution of atrial fibrillation to the risk of stroke as age increased above age 50 even after adjustments were made for hypertension, congestive heart failure, and coronary artery disease. Below age 50, the incidence of atrial fibrillation is low, the incidence of stroke is low in patients with no clinically evident heart disease. The relative risk of stroke in patients with atrial fibrillation above age 50 without known risk factors is four times that of patients without atrial fibrillation (Wolf, 1987). Cardiovascular disease was usually associated with the arrhythmia or developed shortly after the arrhythmia occurred (Kannel, 1982). Isolated or "lone" atrial fibrillation is usually asymptomatic but may result in systemic emboli, though less frequently than in mitral valve disease. Ten percent of the patients in the Framingham study had strokes, some of which may have been due to cerebral emboli.

Another population study involved 3623 patients with atrial fibrillation, including 97 patients who were aged 60 years or younger. In 1440 patient-years of follow-up, there were four cerebrovascular events and four myocardial infarcts in patients without overt coronary artery disease. At 15 years, 1.3% of patients had had a stroke (Kopecky, 1987). This rate of stroke was no different from that in the general population. This low rate of stroke in patients under age 60 with "lone" atrial fibrillation (atrial fibrillation with no clinically apparent heart disease) is supported by two other studies in which the incidence of stroke was less than 0.5% per year. Unfortunately, "lone" or idiopathic atrial fibrillation only occurs in 3–11% of cases of atrial fibrillation. Since the prevalence of atrial fibrillation is low under age 60, these groups of patients with atrial fibrillation with low risk for stroke will be small (Kopecky, 1987; Stein, 1990).

Thyrotoxicosis, either spontaneous or from exogenous thyroid ingestion, should be considered in all patients with atrial fibrillation, especially the "lone" variety. Atrial fibrillation occurs in 9–22% of patients with thyrotoxicosis. It is rare under age 40 and occurs in more than 25% of those over age 60 years (Woeber, 1992). Thirteen percent of 75 patients who had atrial fibrillation with no obvious cardiovascular cause were found to have occult thyrotoxicosis, diagnosed by a failure of thyroid-stimulating hormone (TSH) to respond to thyroid-releasing hormone (TRH), even though serum T_4 was normal. Eighty percent of these patients reverted to sinus rhythm when the thyrotoxicosis was treated (Forfar, 1979). Newer techniques for measuring thyroid-stimulating hormone may show very low or essentially zero values ($< 0.2 \ \mu U/mL$) in thyrotoxicosis. Two subsequent studies matching age controls without atrial fibrillation have shown a similar incidence of failure of thyrotropic response to thyrotropin-releasing hormone. The patients with atrial fibrillation had increased serum T_3 or T_4 or both (Davies, 1985). Another study supports the conclusion that marked thyrotoxicosis with normal serum thyroid hormone concentrations is uncommon in patients with isolated atrial fibrillation (Giladi, 1991). However, atrial fibrillation in the presence of thyrotoxicosis is associated with a high incidence of thromboembolism (Woeber, 1992).

Clinical Course

In the onset of atrial fibrillation, the rapid ventricular rate may impair atrial emptying and left ventricular filling. In the patient with atrial septal defect, this may produce dyspnea and cardiac failure. In the patient with mitral stenosis, it may provoke dyspnea, and the left atrial pressure may rise quickly, producing pulmonary venous congestion, severe dyspnea, and acute pulmonary edema. The atrial transport function of atrial systole may be required to preserve adequate left ventricular filling in patients with low cardiac reserve and especially in patients with left ventricular diastolic dysfunction, eg, patients with hypertrophic cardiomyopathy; the onset of atrial fibrillation and the loss of atrial transport function may produce severely elevated left atrial and pulmonary capillary pressures in these patients. Some individuals merely have palpitations; a few may have no symptoms whatever, and the atrial fibrillation in these cases is discovered accidentally.

Chronic Atrial Fibrillation

In chronic atrial fibrillation—especially if the ventricular rate is controlled with digitalis, beta-blockers, or calcium channel blockers—the patient may be asymptomatic and may be unaware of the atrial fibrillation or its irregularity except when exercising.

Some patients describe what they think are paroxysmal episodes of atrial fibrillation when in fact they have chronic fibrillation but are aware of the rapid, irregular ventricular rate only with exercise or emotion. There is increasing evidence that in patients with atrial fibrillation and rapid ventricular response, congestive heart failure can occur, giving rise to a dilated, poorly contracting left ventricle. If the patient is returned to sinus rhythm or the ventricular rate is controlled, the left ventricle can become normal in size and the systolic function returns to normal (Grogan, 1992). It appears that this is analogous to the tachycardia-induced cardiomyopathy seen in animals.

C. Risk of Systemic Emboli: In addition to the possibility that pulmonary venous congestion and decreased cardiac output may occur when atrial fibrillation supervenes in mitral valve disease, patients with chronic atrial fibrillation have the added risk of systemic emboli, which are uncommon in patients with supraventricular tachycardia. Systemic embolism may be the initial clinical manifestation of mitral stenosis (eg, cerebral embolization with hemiplegia), and a major embolus to an extremity may require surgery. The likelihood that an embolism will develop is greatest in the year following onset of atrial fibrillation, but the course is unpredictable, and patients may develop major emboli after they have had atrial fibrillation for several years. It has been estimated that a third of all patients with atrial fibrillation will eventually suffer a cerebrovascular accident (Halperin, 1988). Systemic emboli are less common in nonrheumatic types of heart disease. The mean frequency of thromboembolism in patients with atrial fibrillation and thyrotoxicosis in five studies in the literature was 19% (Presti, 1989). In four controlled studies of anticoagulants in prevention of stroke in patients with atrial fibrillation, the incidence of stroke in the placebo arm of the study in patients with nonrheumatic atrial fibrillation varied from 3% per year to 7.4% per year. (Petersen, 1989; BAATAF Investigators, 1990; SPAF Investigators, 1991; Connolly, 1991).

Atrial Rate & Ventricular Response

The atrial rate in atrial fibrillation is approximately 400–650/min, and the ventricular response is almost always irregular because of variable "concealed" conduction in the atrioventricular node. Without treatment, the ventricular rate usually varies between 130/min and 160/min, but it may be less than 100/min. So-called F (fibrillation) waves seen on the ECG reflect the circus movements thought to be the cause of the atrial fibrillation, with multiple wave fronts simultaneously exciting the atria. F waves may be obvious on the ECG or may be fine and difficult to see. The differentiation of so-called coarse and fine atrial fibrillation is rarely of clinical importance. When the ventricular rate is rapid and only slightly irregular, the presence of obvious F waves is helpful in diagnosis. When the ventricular rate is rapid or when it is slow as a result of digitalis therapy, the irregularity may not be gross or obvious unless the ventricular rate is timed carefully.

If the ventricular rate is rapid, atrial fibrillation with aberrant conduction may be confused with ventricular tachycardia. As noted above in the differential diagnosis of tachycardia, the presence of a right bundle branch block pattern in lead V_1 is helpful and favors aberrancy of interventricular conduction.

Pulse Deficit

Before digitalis is given, there is a substantial difference between the ventricular rate as determined at the apex of the heart and that felt at the radial pulse—the so-called pulse deficit. This occurs because the more rapid beats may not result in a sufficient stroke output to cause a pulse wave to reach the wrist. Following digitalis therapy, when the ventricular rate is slowed, each beat has a more forceful output and the pulse deficit diminishes.

Treatment

The principal goals of therapy, whether the patient has acute or chronic atrial fibrillation, are to slow the ventricular rate by increasing atrioventricular block with digitalis, beta-blockers, or calcium channel blockers; to restore sinus rhythm; to prevent recurrences; and to prevent thromboemboli.

A. Digitalis: (See Tables 15–5 and 15–6 and Chapter 10 for details of dosage.) When restoration of sinus rhythm is not urgent, because severe symptoms of dyspnea, angina, palpitations, confusion, or hypotension are absent, digitalis—with or without the addition of a beta-adrenergic-blocking drug or a calcium entry-blocking drug such as verapamil—is the treatment of choice and can be used orally or parenterally, depending upon the urgency of the need to slow the ventricular rate by increasing the atrioventricular block. Verapamil may replace both digitalis and beta-blocking drugs as agents to slow the ventricular rate in atrial fibrillation. In the presence of left ventricular dysfunction or frank congestive heart failure, digoxin is the drug of choice. Once the ventricular rate is controlled, the decision to attempt restoration of sinus rhythm can be undertaken in nonurgent circumstances. Since the major action of digitalis is a vagal effect in slowing the ventricular response, with activity and the predominant effect of increased sympathetic tone, the ventricular response, controlled at rest, may accelerate unacceptably. The addition of verapamil or beta-blockers may slow the ventricular rate, especially with exercise, and may be of considerable benefit. Digitalis should never be used to slow ventricular response in rapid atrial fibrillation with a wide QRS complex, since this could be atrial fibrillation in a patient with Wolff-Parkinson-White syndrome and conduction into the ventricle via a bypass tract. Digitalis blocks conduction in the atrioventricular node but facilitates conduction over the cardiac muscle comprising the bypass tract. In some instances, the number of impulses conducted over the bypass tract increases to the rate where the ventricle fibrillates. When atrial fibrillation occurs in the presence of a wide QRS or in a patient with a known bypass tract, the atrioventricular node should be blocked with a beta-blocker or oral verapamil—not digitalis—and the patient should be given a type Ia antiarrhythmic drug that slows myocardial muscle conduction. Intravenous verapamil should be avoided because its vasodilating effect may reflexly increase sympathetic tone, thus facilitating conduction over the bypass tract.

Recently, the use of digitalis as the drug of choice in the patient without congestive heart failure has been challenged (Falk, 1991). A study showed that placebo was as effective as digoxin in preventing recurrences of atrial fibrillation in patients with paroxysmal atrial fibrillation (Rawles, 1990). When atrial fibrillation recurred, the ventricular response of patients taking digoxin was similar to the response in patients receiving placebo, probably because of the sympathetic stimulation present at the onset of the arrhythmia. With digitalis—a poor drug for controlling the ventricular rate during exercise—rate control is probably better achieved with either a combination of digoxin and a beta-blocker or calcium channel blocker or with one of those newer drugs alone. For the elderly patient with a sedentary life-style, digoxin taken once a day is still an excellent drug.

B. Cardioversion: Restoration of sinus rhythm is usually performed by electric shock cardioversion. If an electric defibrillator is not available, quinidine, procainamide or a large number of other antiarrhythmic drugs can be used. Acute conversion of atrial fibrillation and atrial flutter to sinus rhythm has been reported with esmolol, flecainide, propafenone, sotalol, and amiodarone (Haines, 1992). The efficacy of these drugs varies, but on the average conversion is achieved in 70–90% of cases.

Countershock should be used with caution in the presence of digitalis toxicity. If large doses of digitalis have been required to slow the ventricular rate, it is wise to stop digitalis for 1 or more days and to attempt cardioversion with small stimuli such as 5 J, increasing the strength of the shock as necessary. Because atrial fibrillation recurs so often, quinidine or another antiarrhythmic drug is usually begun 2 days before cardioversion to achieve an adequate blood level of the drug in order to prevent recurrence of the arrhythmia. When quinidine (0.3 g four times daily) is given, about 20% of patients revert to sinus rhythm, and countershock is not necessary. This dose of quinidine may produce a blood quinidine concentration of 2–4 μg/mL, which may be sufficient to restore sinus rhythm. It is also a level that is usually adequate to prevent recurrences.

C. Quinidine: Quinidine should rarely be used to reverse atrial fibrillation; cardioversion is the treatment of choice. However, if cardioversion is not available, quinidine may be tried. When quinidine is given to patients receiving digoxin, the mean serum digoxin almost doubles, and some patients develop symptoms of digitalis toxicity (Leahey, 1980). (See below for the use of quinidine to prevent recurrences of atrial fibrillation.)

If quinidine is used to restore sinus rhythm because countershock is not available, it can be started at a dose of 0.2 g every 2 hours for five doses on day 1, with serum levels obtained 2 hours after the last dose. The individual dose can be increased by 0.1 g daily, but it is unwise to increase the dose beyond 3 g/d unless serum concentrations of the drug can be determined and the patient can be seen before each dose. It should be reemphasized that cardioversion is the treatment of choice in attempted conversion of chronic atrial fibrillation and that quinidine is used only if cardioversion is not possible. As the dose of quinidine is increased, there is an average progressive increase in serum quinidine concentration, but there are many departures from the average. A dosage of 2–2.5 g/d may achieve serum levels of 8–10 μg/mL in some patients, but a dosage of 3 g/d achieves levels below 7 μg/mL in others. Myocardial toxicity is more closely related to the serum concentration than to the dose and progressively increases as the serum concentration rises.

If digitalis or verapamil cannot be used (usually because of precxcitation syndromes; see Chapter 14) or are ineffective in the treatment of acute paroxysmal atrial fibrillation, other drugs may sometimes convert the arrhythmia to sinus rhythm. Give procainamide, 50 mg/min intravenously up to a total dose of 1–1.5 g, or, in more critical situations, newer drugs such as flecainide or amiodarone (see above and Ventricular Tachycardia).

D. Anticoagulation Prior to Cardioversion: A controversial area with respect to cardioversion is the necessity for anticoagulation prior to conversion to sinus rhythm. The incidence of systemic emboli following restoration of sinus rhythm without anticoagulation is small—about 0.5%—though some authors have reported rates as high as 2–7% (Stein, 1990). Several recent retrospective studies have indicated a protective effect against embolic events of anticoagulation before cardioversion (Mancini, 1990; Arnold, 1992). In the largest study, in 332 elective cardioversions for atrial fibrillation, there were no embolic events in 153 anticoagulated patients and six such events in 179 patients not anticoagulated before cardioversion (Arnold, 1992). There were no embolic events in 122 patients with atrial flutter, with 90 cardioverted without being anticoagulated. Of the six with emboli, the duration of atrial fibrillation ranged from 3 to 19 days (average: 6 days), and five had atrial fibrillation for less then 1 week. It is our policy

to anticoagulate all patients who have been fibrillating over 48 hours and to cardiovert them after a period of anticoagulation.

Since emboli occur from fresh thrombi, the practice is to anticoagulate the patient with warfarin for 2 weeks before cardioversion to give existing thrombus an opportunity to become organized and adherent. Since atrial mechanical contraction after cardioversion may not return for 3 weeks (Manning, 1989), the recommendation is to continue anticoagulation for 3 weeks postcardioversion. With the low incidence of emboli after cardioversion of patients with atrial flutter—possibly because of the persistent mechanical contraction of the atria in this arrhythmia—we do not anticoagulate these patients prior to conversion.

E. Rapid Atrial Pacing: If atrial flutter with rapid ventricular rates cannot be controlled by conventional pharmacologic therapy—especially following open heart surgery—atrial pacing may induce atrial fibrillation with a slower ventricular rate; digitalis may then increase the atrioventricular block and further slow the ventricular rate. The use of rapid atrial pacing (including safety precautions) for paroxysmal supraventricular tachycardia is discussed elsewhere in this chapter. As with paroxysmal atrial tachycardia, atrial flutter may abruptly stop when rapid atrial pacing is discontinued.)

F. Prevention of Recurrences: Because the recurrence rate following cardioversion is high, especially in patients who have long-standing atrial fibrillation, considerable enlargement of the left atrium or the heart, or arrhythmias that developed following cardiac surgery, it becomes a matter of judgment whether to control the ventricular rate with drugs and leave the patient in chronic atrial fibrillation or to attempt to restore normal sinus rhythm with cardioversion. Successful restoration of sinus rhythm is more likely if atrial fibrillation has been present for less than 12 months and if the left atrium is not enlarged.

1. Quinidine– Quinidine is effective in preventing frequent recurrent attacks of paroxysmal atrial fibrillation of relatively short duration (usually hours to days), the dose and frequency of administration being gradually increased until the attacks no longer occur or are less frequent.

In a patient whose atrial fibrillation has lasted less than 6 months and whose heart and left atrium are normal in size or only slightly enlarged, cardioversion should be tried at least once, combined with an effort to prevent recurrences with oral quinidine therapy, 0.2–0.3 g four times daily, or long-acting quinidine preparations that require only twice-daily dosage. Under these circumstances, about half the patients remain in sinus rhythm for a year or more and are much more comfortable than when they were in atrial fibrillation, primarily because of relief of disproportionate tachycardia with mild exercise. Patients who have been repeatedly converted to sinus rhythm almost always indicate that their cardiac function is much better when they are in sinus rhythm. Quinidine decreases the recurrence rate of atrial fibrillation after restoration of sinus rhythm. In a multicenter study from Stockholm, approximately 50% of patients were still in sinus rhythm a year after treatment of atrial fibrillation or flutter when they received quinidine, whereas only 25% of the control group remained in sinus rhythm (Sodermark, 1975). Similar effectiveness of quinidine in maintaining sinus rhythm over 1 year compared to a control group was found in a meta-analysis of six controlled trials reported in the literature (Coplan, 1990).

Long-acting quinidine is superior to short-acting quinidine in maintaining sinus rhythm after DC cardioversion. After 18 months, 65% of patients remained in sinus rhythm while receiving long-acting quinidine and 30% while receiving short-acting quinidine of comparable dosage (Normand, 1976). In the whole series, sinus rhythm was maintained for 18 months in 50% of patients, which is consistent with the results of the Stockholm study.

Patients with atrial fibrillation who are treated with quinidine go through a transitional phase of atrial flutter prior to the development of sinus rhythm, because quinidine slows the atrial rate. It has a vagolytic action that improves atrioventricular conduction, leading to a more rapid ventricular rate as the atrial rate slows. Digitalis is therefore given before quinidine to prevent a rapid ventricular rate. In these instances, the atrial rate varies from 150/min to 300/min and may be irregular.

Myocardial toxicity may occur with increasing doses of quinidine and is manifested by the presence of ventricular arrhythmias—usually ventricular premature beats but occasionally ventricular tachycardia or even ventricular fibrillation. Ventricular fibrillation occurs infrequently when quinidine is given with the patient in a stable state and receiving no other drug therapy, but the likelihood of fibrillation is enhanced when patients are receiving increasing doses of digitalis with or without diuretic therapy and resultant hypokalemia. When both quinidine and digitalis are given under these circumstances—especially if diuretics are also used—it is an open question whether the ventricular fibrillation is due to digitalis or to quinidine. Prolongation of the QT interval is common and represents the electrophysiologic action of quinidine, delaying repolarization. Intraventricular block or bundle branch block that develops after quinidine is due to a marked conduction defect. When the QRS duration exceeds the value prior to beginning quinidine by 30–50%, it is wise to stop quinidine. Quinidine has a proarrhythmic effect, causing torsade de pointes, a multiform ventricular tachycardia, in up to 5% of patients. The development of this complication, which is potentially fatal, is not dose-related but appears to be an idiosyncratic reaction.

If quinidine is given at regular intervals (eg, four times daily), a blood level plateau is reached in 48–72 hours. A larger dose or administration at shorter intervals is required to achieve higher, more effective blood levels.

A rare complication of quinidine therapy is thrombocytopenia, resulting from the affinity of quinidine and its antibody for a receptor on the surface of platelets, provoking their immunologic destruction. The process usually reverses when quinidine is stopped (Christie, 1982).

The recurrence rate of atrial fibrillation is high after cardioversion in patients with large hearts and a long history of atrial fibrillation, but quinidine is unpleasant for some patients to take because of its side effects: diarrhea, nausea, anorexia, and tinnitus. These symptoms occur in 10–35% of patients. The interaction with digoxin is important, displacing digoxin from tissues and reducing renal clearance, increasing digoxin levels twofold. Digoxin doses should be decreased by half. Amiodarone has a similar effect on digoxin levels.

2. Other drugs– If quinidine is ineffective, the following drugs may be used, alone or in combination: procainamide, 250–500 mg two or three times a day; disopyramide (in the absence of cardiac failure), 0.8–1.2 g/d; propranolol, 10–60 mg two or three times a day (or its equivalent); propafenone, 150–300 mg three times a day; sotalol, 80–480 mg twice a day; flecainide, 200–300 mg/d in divided doses; or encainide, 150–225 mg/d in divided doses. These last two drugs are effective in the treatment of atrial arrhythmias but may cause proarrhythmia, usually mild, in 5–10% of cases, which usually subsides when the drug is decreased in dosage or withdrawn. Because of the higher mortality rate with encainide and flecainide in the Cardiac Arrhythmia Suppression Trial (CAST), there has been concern that proarrhythmic effects may make these drugs too dangerous to use in the treatment of supraventricular arrhythmias. When the mortality rate among patients with supraventricular arrhythmia treated with flecainide was compared with rates among other patients treated with other antiarrhythmic drugs, no excess deaths were reported (Pritchett, 1991). In ventricular tachycardia, these drugs may produce more serious proarrhythmias and should therefore not be used unless the condition is life-threatening.

Amiodarone is probably the most effective of the newer drugs for the prevention of recurrent atrial fibrillation, especially in the presence of Wolff-Parkinson-White syndrome, and can be used in doses of 300–600 mg/d. Side effects are frequent, however (see Table 15–7). Verapamil may not be effective and may be harmful. In chronic atrial fibrillation or in paroxysmal fibrillation when the ventricular rate cannot be controlled with digitalis (especially during exercise), beta-blockers (propranolol, 10–20 mg orally four times daily and increased as needed, or metoprolol, 50–100 mg twice daily) can be added with benefit to slow the ventricular rate during exercise. They should be used with caution if the patient has a history of asthma or left ventricular failure, atrioventricular conduction defects, or bradycardia. Propranolol can be added to quinidine in an effort to prevent recurrences, and there are some data to suggest that the combination is more effective than quinidine alone. If quinidine alone or in combination with propranolol is not tolerated, procainamide, 250–500 mg orally three or four times a day alone or combined with quinidine, is sometimes effective but should be used cautiously.

G. Mitral Stenosis or Coronary Disease: In patients with minimal or moderate mitral stenosis or coronary artery disease, control of atrial fibrillation or flutter is often decisive in determining whether symptoms of dyspnea or angina are due to the arrhythmia or to the anatomic defect. It often happens that control of the ventricular response or conversion to and maintenance of normal sinus rhythm increases exercise capacity and decreases symptoms to the point where surgery is unnecessary.

8. Prevention of thromboembolic events– The danger of thromboembolic events has been recognized for many years in patients with mitral valve disease—especially mitral stenosis—when atrial fibrillation develops. Anticoagulation has been advocated in these patients to prevent this. The evidence that anticoagulation is effective in atrial fibrillation in patients with mitral stenosis is based on nonrandomized, small studies. Yet the belief is so strong that anticoagulation is helpful that mitral stenosis patients have been excluded from all placebo-controlled randomized trials.

Until recently, there was no agreement about whether patients with nonvalvular atrial fibrillation should be anticoagulated. This question has been settled by reports of four randomized, placebo-controlled studies of anticoagulants in patients with nonvalvular atrial fibrillation (BAATAF, 1990; Connolly, 1991; Petersen, 1989; SPAF, 1991). In these studies, the risk reduction for cerebral emboli was decreased from 42% to 86% by warfarin. In the SPAF study, there was an aspirin (325 mg/d) arm that showed a 42% reduction in cerebral embolism compared with placebo. The SPAF study is continuing to randomize patients to warfarin or aspirin, and that study is not yet reported (Table 15–2).

The risk of hemorrhage has always been a problem with anticoagulation. It was finally recognized that the rabbit brain thromboplastin used in determining prothrombin time in the USA was more potent than the human brain thromboplastin used in Europe. With the more potent thromboplastin, it took a higher dose of warfarin to depress the prothrombin time to $2-2\frac{1}{2}$ times control. For this reason, the dosage of warfarin was greater in the United States than in Europe and the incidence of bleeding was also higher. Recognition of these problems led to establishment of the international normalized ratio (INR) as a standard for reporting corrected prothrombin time prolongation following administration of oral anticoagulants. The INR is derived from the prothrombin time ratio related to the relative sensitivity of the local thromboplastin to an international reference thromboplastin. The INR is the prothrombin time ratio that would have been obtained if the reference throm-

Table 15–2. Randomized trials of anticoagulation to prevent cerebral embolism in nonvalvular atrial fibrillation.

	AFASAK	BAATAF	SPAF		CAFA
Number	1007	420	1330		378
Years followed	2	2.2	1.3		15 months[1]
Observed cerebral embolic rate					
Percent per year			**Aspirin Ctrl**		
Placebo	5.5	3.0	7.4	6.3	4.6
Warfarin	2.0	0.4	2.3	...	3.4
Aspirin	5.5	...	...	3.6	...
Risk reduction	60%	86%	67%	42%	42%
(95% CI)	(7 to 81)	(51 to 96)	(21 to 86)		(−68 to 80)
Target INR	2.8–4.2	1.5–2.7	2.0–3.5		2.0–3.0
PT ratio	1.5–2.0	1.2–1.5	1.3–1.8		1.3–1.6
Bleeding		**Major**	**Minor**		**Major**
Placebo	0.4%	1.0%	10.1%	1.6%	0.5%
Warfarin	6.3%	1.9%	17.9%	1.5%	2.5%
Aspirin	0.6%			1.4%	

[1] Trial stopped early because of reports of warfarin's effectiveness.

Key:
AFASAK = Copenhagen Atrial Fibrillation, Aspirin, Anticoagulation Study
SPAF = Stroke Prevention in Atrial Fibrillation
BAATAF = Boston Area Anticoagulation Trial for Atrial Fibrillation
CAFA = Canadian Atrial Fibrillation Anticoagulation Study
CI = Confidence Interval
INR = International Normalized Ratio
PT = Prothrombin time

boplastin had been used for the test. The randomized studies have shown that remarkable protection from thromboembolism is achieved with low-intensity anticoagulation and that the incidence of serious hemorrhage is likewise low, albeit higher than in the control group.

It is now recommended that all patients with atrial fibrillation, including patients with paroxysmal atrial fibrillation—who also, in these studies, had a similar reduction in cerebral emboli—should be chronically anticoagulated. The only exception, which is still not totally agreed upon, is the patient under age 60 years of age with "lone" atrial fibrillation (Cairns, 1991).

2. ATRIAL FLUTTER

Atrial flutter is a rapid, regular series of atrial depolarizations arising from an ectopic focus in the atria. It is thought to be the result of a circus movement with the reentrant circuit around the venae cavae orifices and involving the tricuspid annulus. It is similar to atrial fibrillation in its age distribution and causative factors, but it is less common than atrial fibrillation in mitral valve disease and atrial septal defect. It may be paroxysmal or established, as in atrial fibrillation, but the atrial rate is slower, usually 260–350/min, and the ventricles usually respond to every other atrial excitation wave, so that the pattern is a 2:1 atrioventricular conduction with an atrial rate of about 300/min and a regular ventricular rate of 150/min. In some patients, atrioventricular conduction may be variable and show alternating 2:1, 3:1, or 4:1 conduction with an irregular ventricular rate, simulating atrial fibrillation. At times there may be variable atrioventricular block at what appears to be two functional levels of the atrioventricular node. At one level, the atrioventricular nodal block may be 2:1, and at the lower level each impulse reaching this level is conducted to the ventricles with a 3:1 Wenckebach block. This leads to "group beating" and a regularly irregular ventricular rate. Atrioventricular conduction is less predictable than in atrial fibrillation, and patients may have abrupt changes from 4:1 to 2:1 with postural changes or excitement or while eating. They may have a ventricular rate of 75/min when recumbent and 150/min when sitting. They may then have an abrupt onset of palpitations and symptoms without a change in the basic atrial flutter, reflecting only change in the ventricular response to the flutter.

Under conditions where atrioventricular conduction is facilitated—eg, with sympathetic stimulation or under the influence of quinidine used alone, which has a vagolytic effect—atrioventricular conduction may be facilitated and the atrial flutter may conduct 1:1, resulting in a ventricular rate of 300/min, a marked decrease in cardiac output, and syncope.

For these reasons, atrial flutter is a more unstable and troublesome rhythm than atrial fibrillation. The abrupt jumps in ventricular rate with minor activities may produce pulmonary venous congestion if the patient has underlying cardiac disease such as severe mitral stenosis. This is in contrast to atrial fibrillation, in which there is a more gradual and smaller increase in ventricular response following trivial activity. Atrial flutter, atrial fibrillation, and atrial tachycardia may occur in the same patient on different occasions. Atrial flutter is more commonly seen in diseases that affect the right atrium, whereas atrial fibrillation is seen in diseases affecting the left atrium. For this reason, atrial flutter is commonly seen in people with chronic pulmonary disease and in patients who have had right atrial incisions, such as are made in the course of Fontan or Mustard procedures for tricuspid atresia or for correction of transposition of the great vessels. Atrial fibrillation is seen with mitral valve disease and left ventricular failure for any reason.

Treatment

Paroxysmal atrial flutter responds to cardioversion in about 95% of cases, and this is the treatment of choice in almost all cases. Patients should not be allowed to remain in chronic atrial flutter because of the instability of the rhythm, as noted above. Quinidine by mouth is a relatively ineffective method of acutely converting atrial flutter and should be used only to prevent recurrences. Quinidine should never be used alone to prevent atrial flutter, since it has a vagolytic effect that could allow 1:1 atrioventricular conduction with atrial flutter and cause severe hemodynamic collapse. It should always be used with digoxin, a beta-blocker, or verapamil to provide an atrioventricular nodal blocking action for control of the ventricular response in case atrial flutter recurs.

Systemic emboli are much less frequent than in atrial fibrillation, because atrial systole is made stronger by the slower atrial rate and more uniform atrial contractions, decreasing the likelihood of atrial thrombus formation. As in chronic atrial fibrillation, it is wise to begin quinidine therapy 1–2 days prior to cardioversion if the patient has recurrent episodes of atrial flutter and to realize that an increased ventricular rate may result. The usefulness of digitalis to prevent recurrences should not be overlooked, because it may increase the atrioventricular block. Digitalis is always worth a trial, because if it is successful, the patient can be maintained on a single daily dose, which is tolerated much better than multiple doses of quinidine.

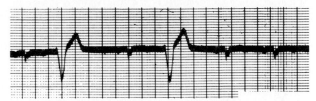

Figure 15–9. Ventricular premature beats with bigeminy in a 48-year-old man not receiving digitalis.

VENTRICULAR ARRHYTHMIAS

VENTRICULAR PREMATURE BEATS (Extrasystoles)

Ventricular premature beats are the most common of all arrhythmias (Figure 15–9). In the absence of heart disease, they are usually not of great clinical significance, but in patients with coronary heart disease, they represent a constant danger of ventricular tachycardia or fibrillation and sudden death. The longer-term prognosis for asymptomatic, healthy subjects with frequent and complex ectopy is similar to that for the healthy United States population (Kennedy, 1980).

Many epidemiologic studies of the incidence and prognostic significance of ventricular premature beats have been performed in recent years in the hope of identifying and perhaps treating a high-risk group liable to sudden death. Whereas in the past a single ECG was used to determine the presence of ventricular premature beats, more recent epidemiologic studies have used 6-, 12-, 24-, or 48-hour ambulatory monitoring of the ECG or continuous ECGs during graded exercise to evaluate the type and frequency of ventricular premature beats in population groups. It has been shown, for example, that multi-hour ambulatory monitoring reveals at least ten times as many premature beats, as well as complex arrhythmias, as does a single routine ECG. Ventricular premature beats may cause concern in as many as one-third of patients convalescing from acute myocardial infarction.

Lown (1971) has devised a grading system for ventricular premature beats (Table 15–3). Since sudden deaths are most apt to occur in people with known coronary disease—especially with ventricular premature beats—efforts have been made to identify those who have frequent or complex premature beats spontaneously or after exercise that might warrant long-term antiarrhythmic therapy, especially if the angiographically identified disease is severe. However, premature beats are capricious and variable in coronary disease, and, just as in normal subjects, they may be present on one occasion and absent on another. In a large study of over 1000 patients who had had a myocardial infarction in the previous year, patients with complex ventricular beats noted in a 1-hour recording showed a threefold incidence of sudden death in 3 years, in contrast to patients who had only single or no arrhythmias during the recording. See Figure 15–10 (Ruberman, 1977). Later follow-up indicates that the effects persist over a 5-year period. Finally, the results of the Cardiac Arrhythmia Suppression Trial (CAST, 1989), which showed an increased mortality rate with the use of flecainide and encainide (believed to be due to a proarrhythmic effect), have created doubt that any asymptomatic non-life-threatening ventricular arrhythmia should be treated with antiarrhythmic drugs—this despite the proved efficacy of these drugs in suppressing the premature contractions.

Premature beats are common in patients with coronary disease (Table 15–4). In the coronary care unit, many arrhythmias are missed as a result of the technical limitations of conventional visual electrocardiographic monitoring. The number of diagnostic errors resulting from such unreliable estimates of the frequency of ventricular arrhythmia and their response to treatment has led to greater reliance on computer

Table 15–3. A grading system for ventricular premature beats.[1,2]

Grade	Characteristics of Beat
0	No ventricular beats
1A	Occasional, isolated ventricular premature beats (less than 30/h): Less than 1/min
1B	Occasional, isolated ventricular premature beats (less than 30/h): More than 1/min
2	Frequent ventricular premature beats (more than 30/h)
3	Multiform ventricular premature beats
4A	Repetitive ventricular premature beats: Couplets
4B	Repetitive ventricular premature beats: Salvos
5	Early ventricular premature beats (ie, abutting or interrupting the T wave)

[1] Reproduced, with permission, from Lown B, Graboys TB: Sudden death: An ancient problem newly perceived. Cardiovasc Med 1977;2:219.
[2] This grading system is applied to a 24-hour monitoring period and indicates the number of hours within that period that a patient has ventricular premature beats of a particular grade.

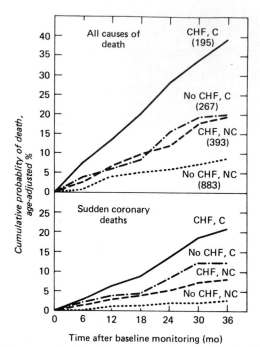

Figure 15–10. Mortality rates over 3 years after baseline monitoring in relation to the presence of complex (C) ventricular premature beats or their absence (NC) and congestive heart failure (CHF). (Reproduced, with permission, from Ruberman W et al: Ventricular premature beats and mortality after myocardial infarction. N Engl J Med 1977;297:750.)

detection and analysis of ventricular arrhythmias in the coronary care unit. The frequency of ventricular arrhythmias, including multiform and complex varieties as well as ventricular tachycardia, has been underestimated.

Table15–4. Incidence of various ventricular arrhythmias in patient population.[1]

Arrhythmias	Number of Cases	Percentage of Total Cases
Premature beats (unifocal)[2]		
<6/min	523	31.3
6–12/min	90	5.4
>12/min	70	4.2
Premature beats (multifocal)[2]		
<6/min	206	12.3
6–12/min	81	4.8
>12/min	69	4.1
Paired premature ventricular contractions	169	10.1
R wave encroaching on the T wave	72	4.3
Tachycardia	69	4.1
Fibrillation	0	0

[1] Reproduced, with permission, from Bleifer SB et al: Diagnosis of occult arrhythmias by Holter electrocardiography. Prog Cardiovasc Dis 1974;16:569.
[2] In *any* 1-minute period.

Many subjects who have complex ventricular premature beats discovered accidentally on Holter monitoring have no significant coronary disease when angiograms are subsequently performed. Most patients with ventricular premature beats in the absence of known coronary disease or symptoms do not, in fact, have coronary disease. On the other hand, 30% of such patients do.

Ventricular premature beats are said to occur during public speaking in 70% of patients with coronary disease but in only 10% of normal subjects (Lown, 1978). The risk of sudden death increases if there are more than ten ventricular premature beats per 1000 complexes (Hinkle, 1969).

Role of Central Nervous System

The role of the central nervous system in ventricular premature beats is particularly important because excitement, anxiety, or fear increases autonomic adrenergic stimuli to the heart and may induce increased automaticity in the Purkinje fibers, leading to premature beats. Increased sympathetic tone and catecholamines can accelerate impulse conduction velocity and shorten the myocardial refractory period as well as increase the amplitude of delayed action potentials by augmenting calcium ion influx into the myocardial cell. All these factors are arrhythmogenic. Ventricular premature beats are common in patients on the day or so preceding elective surgery and disappear spontaneously in the postoperative period after successful surgery. Premature beats may be frequent during the day but less frequent or even absent during sleep. Alcohol, tobacco, and coffee are important causes of increasing the frequency of premature beats. Premature beats may come and go and are apt to occur during periods of emotional stress, even if the source of stress is not clearly defined. In rare cases, ventricular fibrillation may occur.

Significance of Ventricular Premature Beats

The greatest hazards of ventricular premature beats—in contrast to atrial premature beats—are ventricular tachycardia and ventricular fibrillation. Any tachycardia, atrial or ventricular, may have adverse hemodynamic effects if sufficiently rapid. Ventricular tachycardia, because it is most apt to occur in a setting of organic heart disease—particularly coronary heart disease or cardiomyopathy—is feared because of the likelihood of abrupt hemodynamic worsening or of ventricular fibrillation and sudden death.

Ventricular premature beats are common in older people with no heart disease. They increase in frequency with age, and the patients are often asymptomatic; but, as with atrial premature beats, ventricular premature beats may produce symptoms referable to the postpause forceful beat that produces a thump, a sense of skipping or of emptiness in the chest, or a twinge of local pain. The premature beats may be the first sign of coronary heart disease, especially when they occur following exercise, but by themselves they are not a reliable sign of coronary disease. They are apt to occur in patients with slow heart rates because the long diastolic pause slows the subsequent velocity of conduction, increases the likelihood of variable refractory periods among cells, and favors the development of both reentry and automatic ectopic foci.

In coronary disease, there may be scattered areas of ischemia or fibrosis, with different rates of recovery of excitability in neighboring fibers. With ischemia, both early (EAD) and late or delayed (DAD) afterdepolarization can occur, resulting in triggered arrhythmias (January, 1990). This nonuniform recovery of excitability during the relative refractory period as well as the EADs and DADs may induce chaotic propagation of the cardiac impulse and lead to ventricular fibrillation. This may occur with ventricular premature beats or with supraventricular premature beats with aberrant conduction. Aberrantly conducted beats also increase the likelihood of ventricular fibrillation, especially if the premature beats are closely coupled (Yoon, 1975). Prematurity and variable responsiveness are conditions within segments of the cardiac muscle of the ventricle that lead to reentry rhythms. If there is persistent ischemia, hypoxia, ventricular aneurysm, or left ventricular dilation, phase 4 of the action potential may have an increased slope, with resultant increased automaticity. Ventricular premature beats may then be due to increased automatic ectopic firing rather than to reentry. Triggered arrhythmias due to early and delayed afterdepolarization are another possible mechanism for ventricular ectopy and ventricular tachycardia.

Patients whose premature beats occur when the heart rate is slow are often benefited by increasing the rate, as with exercise, but when the rate slows following exercise, the premature beats may reappear. It is generally thought that premature beats are more significant when they occur only during or following exercise, but this requires further validation by prognostic studies. Premature beats occurring at or near peak exercise are believed to be benign. However, in the presence of coronary disease, premature beats occurring at an early stage of exercise may have adverse prognostic significance. Multiform (grade 3) beats occurring during inducement of unifocal ventricular premature beats are associated with left ventricular wall motion abnormality, prior myocardial infarction, and a decreased ejection fraction. The first was the most important factor in distinguishing multiformity from nonmultiformity (Booth, 1982).

Premature beats occurring during acute myocardial infarction are discussed in Chapter 8.

Clinical Findings

A. Symptoms: Patients may be asymptomatic or may complain of a forceful heartbeat that follows the extrasystolic pause. In contrast to atrial premature beats, when there is a normal sequence of conduction via the atrioventricular node through to the ventricles, ventricular premature beats by retrograde activation depolarize the atrioventricular node and interrupt the normal regular rhythm. Patients with coronary disease may have angina pectoris as a result of frequent premature beats.

B. Signs:

1. Cannon waves– (See Chapter 3.) Right atrial systole may find the tricuspid valve closed because of recent intermittent ectopic ventricular systoles and produce, irregularly, a cannon wave in the neck as atrial systole forces blood back into the jugular vein. Cannon waves are presystolic, are of relatively large amplitude, and have a rapid ascent and descent that have suggested the term "venous Corrigan waves." The ventricular premature contractions occur irregularly; the sinus P wave and the ectopic QRS complexes may occur relatively simultaneously, usually with the P wave following the QRS complex, so that atrial contraction finds the tricuspid valve closed. Occasionally, there may be 1:1 synchronous retrograde conduction to the sinus node with ventricular premature beats, and cannon waves do not occur. This pattern of synchronous conduction and absence of cannon waves may also occur if the patient has atrial fibrillation or atrial flutter with a mechanically insignificant or absent atrial systole.

2. Asynchrony of atria and ventricles– The first heart sound may vary in intensity because of the asynchronous contraction of the atria and the ventricles. The pause that follows the premature beat is usually "compensatory" because the basic rhythm is not altered. The premature beat, although it may have retrograde atrioventricular conduction, infrequently depolarizes the sinus node. For this reason, the pause following a ventricular premature beat is prolonged or compensatory, making up for the prematurity of the ectopic beat and keeping the basic sinus rhythm constant. This is in contrast to the usual atrial premature beat, in which the atrial ectopic beat depolarizes the sinus node, resetting its rate so that the pause is not compensatory. The basic rate of sinus rhythm is not altered with ventricular premature beats. If the ventricular premature beats are frequent or occur in irregular runs, the cardiac rhythm may be so irregular that it may be confused with atrial fibrillation. Cannon waves in the neck (see above) may be helpful in the differentiation, as may the recognition of a "quick" premature beat before each pause.

3. Hemodynamic changes– Hemodynamic changes occur infrequently unless the ventricular premature beats are frequent or occur in runs, so that they decrease the cardiac output. When they are frequent and impair cardiac output, coronary perfusion may be reduced, and patients—especially those with coronary disease—may have angina pectoris as a result of the premature beats.

4. Occurrence during anesthesia and surgery– Ventricular premature beats are common during anesthesia and are more apt to be noted in patients whose ECGs are being continuously monitored. They are related to hypoxia, hypotension, ischemia, and alterations in acid-base balance and are usually improved by careful attention to ventilation and arterial pressure. They may occur during intubation, especially if this is traumatic and ventilation is inadequate. Postoperatively, ventricular premature beats may also result from disturbances in ventilation or factors listed previously. Blood gas tensions should be monitored, so that possible causes such as acidosis, alkalosis, hypercapnia, or hypoxia will not be missed, especially in patients who have had pulmonary or cardiac surgery. Hypokalemia resulting from chronic diuretic or corticosteroid therapy combined with excessive digitalis therapy may be the cause of ventricular premature beats during or after surgery. In patients with a central line monitoring central venous pressure, if the catheter advances into the right ventricle, multiple premature ventricular contractions and even ventricular tachycardia can result. Withdrawing the line back into the right atrium or superior vena cava is all that is necessary to stop the ectopy.

5. Beats induced by ambulation or graded exercise– Various studies have shown that ambulatory monitoring and graded treadmill exercise may complement each other in identifying the presence of ventricular premature beats, neither procedure being clearly superior. At least 6 hours are required for ambulatory monitoring. In some patients, exercise is more effective in inducing ectopic beats than ambulation; in others, the opposite is true. Ventricular premature beats should be counted and noted as being univocal, multiform, occurring in pairs or runs, appearing early on the T wave (during the "vulnerable" period), or occurring in short runs of ventricular tachycardia or ventricular fibrillation.

In general, asymptomatic premature ventricular beats either occurring at rest or with exercise are not unusual in the middle-aged and older population. In the absence of clinical cardiac disease, these premature beats, even with nonsustained ventricular tachycardia, appear to be benign and do not require therapy.

Treatment of Ventricular Premature Beats & More Complex Ventricular Ectopy

The indications for treatment of ventricular premature beats are controversial; although patients with ventricular arrhythmias in association with impaired left ventricular function are at increased risk for death, current data are insufficient to establish the effectiveness of treatment in prolonging life. This is especially true after the CAST study. Asymptomatic patients with ventricular premature beats are usually not treated. Patients with sustained ventricular tachy-

cardia are treated—usually guided by electrophysiologic studies—but those with nonsustained ventricular tachycardia are usually not treated unless it occurs spontaneously and is associated with severe heart disease. Nonsustained ventricular tachycardia of five to seven beats can often be induced in electrophysiologic studies in normal individuals. Such a finding indicates that the patient with coronary disease is at increased risk, but further data are required to determine whether treatment will be beneficial. Signal averaging of late potentials may improve our ability to estimate the risk.

Most ambulatory noncoronary patients with only occasional ventricular premature beats require no treatment other than reassurance and elimination of the precipitating cause if it is known to be alcohol, tobacco, anxiety, or digitalis therapy. Treatment is often ineffective.

Holter electrocardiographic 24-hour monitoring was performed in over 3000 survivors of acute myocardial infarction in the BHAT trial. A history of previous myocardial infarction or cardiac failure and advanced age were the major factors associated with the frequency and complexity of the ventricular premature beat. Ventricular ectopic activity was an independent predictor of total mortality (Kostis, 1987).

Premature ventricular beats, especially if they are more frequent than ten per hour or are complex, are independent markers of increased risk for sudden death in survivors of acute myocardial infarction (Lichtstein, 1990). The risk is amplified by decreasing ventricular function. Unfortunately, empiric treatment with antiarrhythmic drugs either has no effect or shows a slight trend toward increase in mortality rate (Furberg, 1983). The CAST study showed that suppression of ventricular premature beats does not improve survival but was associated (in that study) with an increased mortality rate, probably as a consequence of proarrhythmia stimulated by the antiarrhythmic drugs. There is thus no support for the hypothesis that suppressing the ventricular ectopy or "trigger" for sudden death will reduce the number of arrhythmic deaths (Akhtar, 1990). After myocardial infarction, only beta-blockers have been shown to decrease the incidence of sudden death (Singh, 1990). This is true with acebutolol, which even has a mild intrinsic sympathomimetic action (Boissel, 1990).

If the patient has chronic pulmonary disease or is recovering from anesthesia, improvement in ventilation should precede the use of drug therapy. The possible role of cardiac catheters, displacement of a central venous pressure line into the right ventricle, or insertion of pacemakers as causes of arrhythmias should be considered.

Discontinuation of any drugs that may be responsible for the premature beats is part of treatment. Often overlooked as possible causes are aminophylline, beta-agonists, and similar drugs used in chronic obstructive lung disease and the so-called psychotropic drugs, particularly the phenothiazines and tricyclic antidepressants. Thioridazine is particularly important in this respect.

A. Reassurance and Sedation: If premature beats are discovered during routine examination or because of a complaint of a "skipped" beat or palpitations, reassurance and mild sedation are often sufficient. Sedation and relief of anxiety are important therapeutic measures and must never be overlooked. Fatal cardiac arrhythmias have been attributed to central sympathetic influences on cardiac rhythm. Diazepam, 2.5–5 mg two to four times daily, may be very effective but must be used cautiously by ambulatory patients because it may cause undesirable oversedation.

B. Antiarrhythmic Drugs: (Tables 15–5 to 15–7.) There is no present consensus on the best way to treat all forms of ventricular ectopy. There is general agreement that in the asymptomatic patient without evidence of clinical heart disease, treatment of ventricular ectopy, including complex forms and even runs of nonsustained ventricular tachycardia, is not indicated. If the patient is symptomatic because of the ectopy, treatment can be undertaken with digoxin or beta-blockers, both of which can be effective. If these are unsuccessful, one of the class Ia drugs such as quinidine, procainamide, or disopyramide can be tried. Against this view is the meta-analysis of four randomized trials evaluating quinidine, flecainide, and three other antiarrhythmic drugs in the treatment of premature ventricular conduction, where the risk of dying was highest on quinidine (Morganroth, 1991). In the patient with coronary artery disease or cardiomyopathy, although the presence of ectopy increases the risk of death, there is no indication that empiric treatment with antiarrhythmic agents, with the exception of beta-blockers, decreases this risk. With coronary disease or cardiomyopathy and in the absence of contraindications, beta-blockers should be used. If there are complex premature ventricular beats in these patients—especially runs of nonsustained ventricular tachycardia and more especially in the presence of decreased ventricular function, where the risk is highest—low-dose amiodarone may reduce the incidence of death from arrhythmias. One study randomly assigned 312 patients after myocardial infarction with multiform ventricular beats or nonsustained ventricular tachycardia to individualized antiarrhythmic therapy chosen by effectiveness of suppression on the ambulatory ECG, low-dose amiodarone (200 mg/d), or placebo. By 1 year, there were 15 sudden deaths in the placebo group—ten in the individualized antiarrhythmic drug group and five in the amiodarone group ($P < .05$—compared with the placebo group) (Burkart, 1990).

The place of risk stratification by signal-averaged ECG, 24-hour ambulatory ECG, and invasive electrophysiologic studies is still being evaluated, and their role in evaluating these patients is unclear (Nogami, 1992). With sustained or symptomatic ventricular tachycardia, the consensus at present is that antiarrhythmic drugs which suppress induction of ventricular tachycardia should be chosen by electrophysiologic study. The electrophysiologic study versus electrocardiographic monitoring (ESVEM) study, which is now finished but reported only at the American College of Cardiology meeting in 1991, suggests that 24-hour ambulatory ECG is as good as or better than invasive electrophysiologic study in risk stratification and that sotalol, a drug which has class IV activity (prolongs refractory period) as well as beta-blocker activity, will be the best drug for prevention of ventricular tachycardia.

1. Quinidine– Quinidine is effective but may be unpleasant to take over a prolonged period because of side effects of nausea, diarrhea, and tinnitus. Quinidine cardiotoxicity may also result, causing ventricular tachycardia (torsade de pointes) or fibrillation and ventricular conduction defects.

2. Procainamide– Procainamide, 250–500 mg orally every 4–6 hours, is effective for acute tachycardia, but when given over a period of many months for therapy of premature beats, it is likely to cause a lupus-like connective tissue disorder with arthritis and LE cells in the blood. Torsade can be seen with procainamide.

3. Phenytoin– Phenytoin, 300 mg/d orally, is relatively ineffective as an antiarrhythmic agent in ventricular premature beats unless they are induced by digitalis toxicity, but it can be tried if other agents are ineffective.

4. Beta-adrenergic-blocking drugs– Propranolol is the prototype (see Chapters 8 and 9). It is given in a dosage of 80–320 mg/d orally in three doses. It is helpful in controlling ventricular premature beats but may further slow the ventricular rate and in some instances may increase their frequency, especially if they become more frequent with slow heart rates.

5. Digitalis– Digitalis (digoxin) has been helpful in the treatment of ventricular premature beats resulting from heart failure, provided no digitalis has previously been given. It is now recognized that digitalis may also be valuable in the treatment of ventricular premature beats in the absence of heart failure. Treatment of heart failure may improve coronary perfusion and decrease the nonhomogeneous excitability of ventricular fibers that may cause variable refractory periods and be responsible for reentry premature beats. Premature beats may disappear following treatment of heart failure. With digitalis toxicity, there is increased late afterdepolarization, causing triggered activity, premature ventricular contractions, and ventricular tachycardia.

6. Newer antiarrhythmic agents– These include amiodarone, disopyramide, tocainide, verapamil, mexiletine, flecainide, and encainide and are listed in Table 15–7. Other investigational drugs include lor-

Table 15–5. Guide for intravenous administration of antiarrhythmic drugs.[1] See Table 15–7 for newer agents.

Drug	Dose	Therapeutic Plasma Level (µg/mL)	Side Effects	Comments
Lidocaine	100-mg bolus IV over several minutes followed by 2–4 mg/min constant infusion	1.4–6	Focal seizures; grand mal seizures; respiratory arrest; dizziness; heart block (usually associated with preexisting abnormal His-Purkinje conduction); sinoatrial arrest.	Significant reduction in dose in patients with heart failure; moderate reduction in dose in patients with hepatic disease; no oral form available; no significant myocardial depression; toxicity usually seen at high plasma levels; toxicity at low plasma levels may be caused by metabolites.
Digoxin	0.75–1 mg followed by 0.25 mg IV every 2–4 hours	0.8–2 (ng/mL)	Nausea; vomiting; ventricular arrhythmias; conduction defects; atrioventricular dissociation.	Exercise caution if patient is receiving digoxin or any other form of digitalis; then use in smallest doses. Exercise caution in elderly patients and in those with impaired renal function or acute myocardial infarction.
Propranolol	0.1–1 mg/min IV up to 10 mg	40–85 (mg/mL)	Hypotension; bradycardia; prolonged atrioventricular conduction and heart block; myocardial depression; broncho-spasm.	Extreme caution and decreased dose in the presence of heart failure; many of the side effects reversed by large doses of isoproterenol.
Procainamide	100 mg slowly (<50 mg/min) IV every 5 minutes (or more often in life-threatening situations) up to 1000 mg. (May also give 1 g IM.)	4–8	Hypotension; prolonged atrioventricular and His-Purkinje conduction.	Myocardial toxicity usually only at high plasma levels or after rapid administration.
Phenytoin	50–100 mg IV slowly (<50 mg/min) every 5 minutes up to 1000 mg. Additional 500 mg on following day.	10–18	Hypotension; 1:1 conduction in atrial flutter; respiratory arrest; idioventricular rhythm; ventricular fibrillation; asystole; nystagmus.	Administration IM provides erratic blood levels; toxicity usually seen only after rapid administration.
Quinidine	6–10 mg/kg of quinidine gluconate IV slowly over 22–45 minutes or orally 200–400 mg every 2 hours for 5 doses. (May also be given IM.)	2.3–5 (in double extraction assay; higher if protein precipitation assay used.)	Hypotension; prolonged His-Purkinje conduction; ventricular arrhythmias.	Generally given parenterally only in emergencies and is hazardous unless close supervision by an experienced physician is maintained. IM use is preferred. Doubles serum digoxin levels when given along with digoxin and may cause digitalis toxicity.

[1] Modified and reproduced, with permission, from Winkle RA, Glantz SA, Harrison DC: Pharmacologic therapy of ventricular arrhythmias. AM J Cardiol 1975; 36:629.

Table 15–6. Guide for long-term oral administration of antiarrhythmic drugs.[1] See Table 15–7 for newer agents.

Drug	Usual Total Daily Dose	Frequency of Administration	Therapeutic Plasma Level (μg/mL)	Slow Phase Half-Life (hours)	Side Effects	Comments
Propranolol	80–320 mg	Every 8 hours	Uncertain	3–4.6	Myocardial depression; prolonged atrioventricular conduction and heart block; bradycardia; bronchospasm; nausea; vomiting; fatigue; depression; peripheral vascular insufficiency; hyperglycemia; alopecia.	Active metabolites may play a role in clinical effect. Dose chosen empirically. Should be tapered slowly in patients with angina. Caution needed in patients with cardiac function dependent on sympathetic tone.
Procainamide	1–3 g	Every 4–6 hours	4–8	3–4	Nausea; vomiting; agranulocytosis; lupuslike syndrome; myocardial depression; prolonged atrioventricular and His-Purkinje conduction.	Toxic myocardial effect, usually only at toxic plasma levels. Half-life markedly prolonged in renal failure or alkaline urine. Oral absorption erratic after acute myocardial infarction.
Phenytoin	300–400 mg	Once daily	10–18	22	Nystagmus; ataxia; lethargy; nausea; vertigo; rashes; pseudolymphoma; megaloblastic anemia; peripheral neuropathy; hyperglycemia; seizures.	Half-life higher at higher doses. Rate of metabolism affected by many drugs. Clinically significant decrease in plasma binding in azotemia and hypoproteinemia.
Quinidine	1–2.4 g	Every 6 hours	3–5	7	Hypotension; anorexia; nausea and vomiting; diarrhea; tinnitus, vertigo; prolonged His-Purkinje conduction; rash; fever; thrombocytopenia; hepatic dysfunction; hemolytic anemia; ventricular arrhythmias.	Minor gastrointestinal side effects controlled with symptomatic therapy. Clinically significant decrease in plasma binding in hypoproteinemia and hepatic disease. Myocardial toxicity usually only at toxic plasma levels. Protein precipitation drug assay measures inactive metabolites. Accumulation of metabolites in renal disease. Doubles serum digoxin levels when given along with digoxin and may cause digitalis toxicity.
Digoxin	0.125–0.25 mg	Once daily	0.8–2 (ng/mL)	36	Nausea; vomiting; ventricular arrhythmias; conduction defects; atrioventricular dissociation.	Decrease dose when early toxic symptoms or signs appear in order to prevent more serious ones. May require larger daily doses. Use with caution in older patients and in those with impaired renal functions and Wolff-Parkinson-White syndrome.

[1] Modified and reproduced, with permission, from Winkle RA, Glantz SA, Harrison DC; Pharmacologic therapy of ventricular arrhythmias. Am J Cardiol 1975; 36:629.

Table 15–7. Clinical characteristics of newer arrhythmic agents.

Drug	Dose Intravenous	Dose Oral	Effective Serum or Plasma Concentration (μg/mL)	Elimination Half-Life (h)	Absorption	Metabolism Secretion Route	Side Effects	Onset of Action Intravenous (min)	Onset of Action Oral (h)
Amiodarone	5–10 mg/kg.	Maintenance: 200–800 mg.	0.5–1.5	8–14	Fair	Hepatic	Ophthalmologic, endocrine, pulmonary, neurologic, dermatologic, cardiovascular.	5–10	4–6
Disopyramide	2 mg/kg over 15 min; then 2 mg/kg over 1 hour.	Loading: 300 mg. Maintenance: 150 mg every 6 hours.	2–8	5–8	Good	Renal 50%, probably hepatic 50%	Anticholinergic, cardiovascular.	<5	½–3
Encainide	0.6–0.9 mg/kg over 15 min.	25–75 mg every 6–8 hours.	0.48	1.9–3.8	Good	...	Prolongation of PR, HV, and QRS. Proarrhythmia.	15	1½
Flecainide	1–2 mg/kg over 10 m in for paroxysmal supraventricular tachycardia.	200–300 mg/d in 2 divided doses.	0.2–1	12–27 Mean 14	...	Hepatic	Decreased left ventricular function. Proarrhythmia. Conduction defects.	10–15	1–3
Mexiletine	Loading: 1200 mg/12 hours. Maintenance: 250–500 mg/12 hours.	Loading: 400–600 mg. Maintenance: 200–300 mg every 8 hours.	0.5–2	10–26	Good	Probably hepatic	Neurologic, gastrointestinal, cardiovascular.	<5	1–2
Moricizine	...	600–1200 mg/d in 3 divided doses	0.1	1.5–3.5	Good	Hepatic 60%, renal 40%	Neurologic, gastrointestinal.	...	2–3
Propafenone	2 mg/kg over 10 min, then 2 mg/min.	300–900 mg/d in 3 divided doses	0.2–3.0	6–12	Good	Hepatic	Gastrointestinal, neurologic, cardiovascular, dermatologic.	5	2–3
Tocainide	0.5–0.7 mg/kg/min for 15 min.	Loading: 400–600 mg. Maintenance: 400–800 mg every 8 hours.	3.5–10	10–17	Good	Renal 40%, probably hepatic 60%	Neurologic, gastrointestinal, cardiovascular.	5–10	1½
Verapamil	0.075–0.15 mg/kg.	Maintenance: 80–120 mg every 8 hours or every 6 hours.	...	3–7	Good	Hepatic	Neurologic, gastrointestinal, cardiovascular.	<5	1–2

[1]Modified and reproduced, with permission, from Zipes DP, Troup PJ: New antiarrhythmic agents: Amiodarone, aprindine, disopyramide, ethmozin, mexiletine, tocainide, verapamil. Am J Cardiol 1978; 41:1005.

cainide, 100–200 mg orally twice a day or 2 mg/kg intravenously over a 10-minute period (side effects are similar to those of flecainide); and sotalol, intravenous dose between 0.2 mg/kg and 1.5 mg/kg. Oral doses started at 80 mg twice a day and increased to 160–480 mg twice a day. Zipes (1978) and Kupersmith (1985) present a comprehensive review of the newer antiarrhythmic drugs (Table 15–7). Sources for detailed analyses and dosages are listed in the references (Naccarelli, 1991). Most of these drugs are 75–80% effective in suppressing ventricular premature beats or in preventing ventricular tachycardia, but side effects are substantial.

Disopyramide is still used sparingly. It may be an alternative to lidocaine for ventricular arrhythmias in the coronary care unit when given by intravenous infusion in doses of 2–4 mg/g followed by 250–400 mg orally every 6 hours. It has anticholinergic activity, and many patients develop dry mouth and urinary hesitancy. The most important side effect of disopyramide is the development of cardiac failure that occurs in about half of patients with a history of cardiac failure. The drug has significant negative inotropic action; the development of cardiac failure may be delayed, or failure may appear within 48 hours. Cardiac failure is uncommon in patients with no history of cardiac failure.

C. Digitalis Toxicity: The chance that ventricular premature beats due to excessive digitalis will induce ventricular fibrillation increases with more severe heart disease or if there is associated hypokalemia. When digitalis is taken for suicidal purposes by individuals with normal hearts, ventricular arrhythmias are relatively uncommon, whereas bradycardia and atrioventricular block are common. When ventricular premature beats arc absent before treatment and appear after treatment, digitalis toxicity should be considered.

D. Autonomic Discharge Due to Central Nervous System Activity: Treatment of autonomic impulses caused by emotional stress or central nervous system stimulants may prevent ventricular fibrillation in patients with frequent ventricular premature beats. If there is no contraindication and patients appear to be hyperkinetic and excitable (suggesting that autonomic activity may be playing a role), propranolol, 80–320 mg/d orally in divided doses, metoprolol, 50–200 mg/d orally in divided doses, or other beta-blocking drugs may be given a trial. Stimulants such as alcohol, tobacco, and coffee should be used in moderation or should be avoided if their relationship to ventricular arrhythmias can be documented.

E. Coronary Arterial Disease: Goldschlager (1973) found that ventricular premature beats occurred in only 11% of patients with insignificant coronary disease but were three times as common after exercise when there was prior myocardial infarction, an abnormal contractile pattern, and two- or three-vessel dis-

ease. This worker believes that ventricular premature beats in the presence of coronary disease imply an adverse prognosis, presumably because of the likelihood of more severe anatomic disease when premature beats were present. Exercise-induced ventricular premature beats therefore identify a high-risk group of patients with coronary heart disease. Whether antiarrhythmic therapy is indicated in these patients is still being evaluated.

F. Resection of Ventricular Aneurysm: Ventricular premature beats and ventricular tachycardia may be precursors of ventricular fibrillation in patients with ventricular aneurysms following acute myocardial infarction. Identification and resection of the aneurysm in conjunction with intraoperative endocardial mapping to identify the earliest appearance of the ventricular tachycardia (Cox, 1989; Landymore, 1990) in patients with cardiac failure and resistant arrhythmias may sometimes (not always) be followed by disappearance of ventricular arrhythmias and may therefore prevent sudden death. Cardiac failure may be strikingly benefited (Chapter 8). The patients with refractory ventricular tachycardia without ventricular aneurysms and with poor ejection fraction were at the highest risk for operative demise.

G. Prevention of Ventricular Fibrillation: The prevention of ventricular fibrillation is an important goal in the treatment of ventricular premature beats, but there is no unanimity of opinion on how to distinguish the 50% of patients whose premature beats are unimportant prognostically from the other half, in whom ventricular fibrillation or hemodynamic effects are produced. It seems established, however, that in coronary disease, hypertrophic cardiomyopathy, idiopathic dilated cardiomyopathy, aortic valve disease, and connective tissue disorders, sudden death may be precipitated by complex arrhythmias that are frequent, occur in short runs, occur early on the T wave, or are associated with long bursts of ventricular tachycardia. Careful attention should be paid to precipitating factors; ventilation; central nervous system autonomic influences; and iatrogenic factors such as cardiac catheters or pacemakers, sedation, and antiarrhythmic drugs. Graded exercise and long-term monitoring should be used to count the various types of ventricular premature beats as an aid in deciding whether or not to give treatment. Monitoring should be continued during the recovery period after exercise because most premature beats occur during this period. Risk stratification should be done 7–14 days after an acute myocardial infarction. If the patient has frequent premature ventricular beats—especially runs of nonsustained ventricular tachycardia and an ejection fraction of 40% or lower, it is reasonable to start the patient on beta-blockers or even low-dose amiodarone, since these patients are at high risk of sudden death within the ensuing 6–12 months.

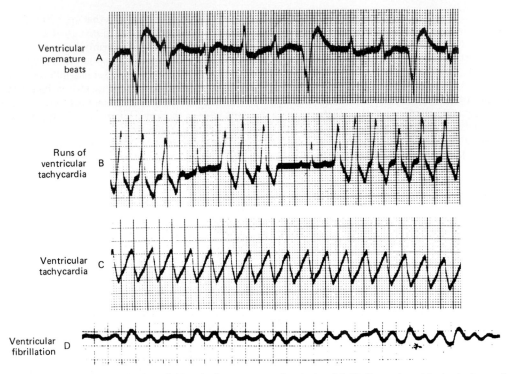

Figure 15–11. Ventricular arrhythmias. **A:** Ventricular premature beats, lead II. **B:** Runs of ventricular tachycardia, lead II. **C:** Ventricular tachycardia, lead V₁. **D:** Ventricular fibrillation, lead II.

VENTRICULAR TACHYCARDIA

Ventricular tachycardia (Figures 15–11 and 15–12) is a rapid, essentially regular (may be slightly irregular) tachycardia of abrupt onset with an average ventricular rate of 150–200/min. Because this rate is similar to that of supraventricular tachycardia, it is not helpful in differential diagnosis. Ventricular tachycardia may occur during complete atrioventricular block and may cause Stokes-Adams attacks. Depending upon the underlying state of the heart and the rapidity and duration of the tachycardia, the patient may develop hemodynamic abnormalities fostered by the decreased ventricular filling and low cardiac output caused by the rapid rate and the lack of an appropriately timed atrial contraction. Patients may de-

velop any of the clinical manifestations noted in this discussion of the hemodynamic significance and impact of arrhythmias in general, with dyspnea, angina, hypotension, oliguria, and syncope. If the ventricular rate is not too rapid (< 160/min), patients may have no symptoms or only mild symptoms of weakness or dizziness. When the more severe symptoms occur in the setting of acute myocardial infarction, ventricular fibrillation is likely.

Some patients with ventricular tachycardia during acute myocardial infarction complain only of weakness and dizziness. The frequency with which ventricular tachycardia degenerates into ventricular fibrillation is not known, but in monitored cases in coronary care units, ventricular tachycardia usually precedes ventricular fibrillation, though the latter

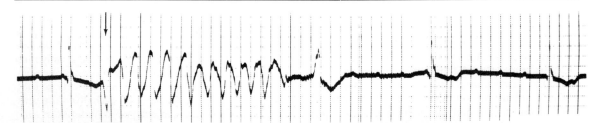

Figure 15–12. Complete atrioventricular block with a run of ventricular tachycardia **(arrow)** initiated by a ventricular premature beat occurring at the end of the T wave (R on T phenomenon).

may occur unexpectedly and de novo early in the course of myocardial infarction.

Mechanisms for the Production of Ventricular Tachycardia (Akhtar, 1990)

(1) Reentry: Usually related to fibrosis in the myocardium, frequently at the border of previous myocardial infarction. Monomorphic ventricular tachycardia implies a reentrant rhythm, where the ventricular depolarization proceeds along the same pathway, repetitively, with the depolarization front always finding repolarized muscle capable of depolarizing ahead of it. Although coronary artery disease is the most common disease associated with monomorphic ventricular tachycardia, dilated cardiomyopathy is also a frequent substrate.

(2) Bundle branch reentry or macro-reentry ventricular tachycardia: (Caceres, 1989.) In up to 30% of patients with dilated cardiomyopathy who have monomorphic ventricular tachycardia, the reentry pathway involves the bundle branches. This medium for the ventricular tachycardia should be suspected if the resting ECG shows evidence of conduction abnormalities—usually PR prolongation and nonspecific QRS widening—and if the ventricular tachycardia has a typical bundle branch block morphology, usually left bundle branch block.

(3) Arrhythmogenic right ventricular dysplasia (Marcus, 1982): (Mehta, 1989; Lemery 1989.) Usually associated with dysplasia of the right ventricle, manifested by fibrosis or replacement with adipose tissue in the right ventricle, usually the outflow tract but occasionally the entire right ventricular free wall. This disease should be suspected if the ventricular tachycardia is of the left bundle branch block type, frequently with a superior axis, and if there is wall motion abnormality, either hypokinesis or akinesis of part or all of the right ventricle. The patients are frequently young (under age 50). The resting ECG frequently shows T wave inversion in the anterior precordial leads (Lemery, 1989).

(4) Ventricular tachycardia without detectable heart disease: (Ohe, 1988; Lemery, 1989.) Seen in young patients, frequently under age 30, frequently precipitated by exercise. The ventricular tachycardia is usually of the right bundle branch morphology, frequently with a superior axis, and apparently originates near the apex of the left ventricle. It appears to be related to calcium-dependent slow conduction defects and is facilitated or accelerated by catecholamines and suppressed by verapamil. The mechanism could be reentry involving the Purkinje system or triggered automaticity.

(5) Exercise-induced ventricular tachycardia: (Sung, 1983; Holt, 1986.) Originating in the right ventricular outflow tract in patients with apparently normal hearts. This type of ventricular tachycardia usually has a left bundle branch block morphology and typically is precipitated by exercise. It is hard to induce in the electrophysiologic laboratory except with isoproterenol infusion. It may be a rhythm precipitated or triggered by automaticity or early delayed depolarization.

(6) Polymorphic ventricular tachycardia: Characterized by beat-to-beat changes in QRS morphology. When the orientation of the QRS seems to change direction during the tachycardia, the term "torsade de pointes" has been applied. One cause is associated with either congenital prolongation of the QT interval (Romano-Ward syndrome) or with long QT interval with congenital deafness (Jervelle and Lange-Nielsen syndrome). Recently, genetic markers have been described in families of patients with the long QT interval syndrome (Vincent, 1992; Moss, 1991; Moss, 1992). Torsade is also seen with acquired long QT interval, seen with certain drugs such as antiarrhythmic agents (especially type Ia and Ic), electrolyte abnormalities, or other medications such as tricyclic antidepressants, neuroleptics, and even antihistamines such as terfenadine. These arrhythmias may be due to early afterdepolarizations associated with prolonged repolarization and bradycardia (Josephson, 1989; Falk, 1992). Polymorphic ventricular tachycardia with normal QT interval occurs most often in the setting of acute ischemia, as with acute occlusion of the coronary artery by thrombus or by spasm.

Diagnosis

By definition, ventricular tachycardia is present when three or more ventricular premature beats occur consecutively. Although this arbitrary definition may seem to include many instances of tachycardia that are not important hemodynamically, it is appropriate in that it does not minimize the potential of this arrhythmia to precipitate ventricular fibrillation. Paroxysms of ventricular tachycardia may occur in the same record with single premature beats.

Ventricular tachycardia is most common in the presence of acute myocardial infarction, usually in the first 1–3 hours, when by continuous monitoring it may be found in as many as 40% of cases. The incidence falls precipitously with the passage of hours, and in only 5% is the onset after the first day. Patients who have ventricular tachycardia early in the course of acute myocardial infarction do not necessarily have recurrences later in the disease or following convalescence, even after exercise. Ventricular tachycardia and ventricular fibrillation occurring early (in the first few minutes or hours) in acute myocardial infarction are thought to be due to myocardial ischemia resulting in reentry or to automatic ectopic ventricular discharge. Patients with large infarcts and cardiac failure are more apt to have ventricular tachycardia and ventricular fibrillation. The former may occur in the setting of sinus bradycardia, associated with hemodynamic deterioration with inferior myocardial infarction, and is less likely to occur when the ventricular rate is increased by administration of small doses of atropine. Large doses of atropine (1 mg or more intravenously) may induce ventricular arrhythmias because of the induced sinus tachycardia and the variable recovery of excitability in different portions of the infarcted heart. Ventricular tachycardia early in the course of acute myocardial infarction must be differentiated from nonparoxysmal junctional tachycardia with aberrant conduction. In the latter, the rate is usually slower (70–120/min), and a careful search for P waves may indicate its supraventricular origin. Accelerated idioventricular rhythm (Figure 15–13) looks the same, but there is atrioventricular dissociation and often capture or fusion beats at the onset and termination of the run of the idioventricular rhythm.

Clinical Findings
(Figure 15–14)

Ventricular tachycardia should be strongly suspected when an abrupt tachycardia with syncope or near-syncope occurs in an older patient with coronary heart disease, especially if the patient had ventricular premature beats before the tachycardia and the QRS complexes are wide and bizarre, with QR or QS complexes in lead V_1, or if the complexes are similar to those seen in the ventricular premature beats present on a prior occasion. The T wave is usually large and in the direction opposite to that of the complex. Prolongation of the QRS complex and atrioventricular dissociation are not absolute criteria to establish the ventricular origin of a tachycardia. (See Tables 15–1 and 15–8.)

A. Asynchrony of Atrial and Ventricular Contractions: The most important clinical feature of ventricular tachycardia is asynchrony of atrial and ventricular contractions, with the atria beating at a slower rate. This is not an absolute criterion because independence of atrial and ventricular activity is occasionally due to junctional atrioventricular rhythms with retrograde atrioventricular block causing atrioventricular dissociation. Furthermore, retrograde activation of the atria may occur in ventricular tachycardia with 1:1 conduction, so that asynchronous atrial and ventricular activity does not occur.

On auscultation, because of the wide QRS complexes and atrioventricular dissociation, there is wide splitting of the first and second heart sounds, beat-to-beat variation in arterial pressure, systolic murmurs,

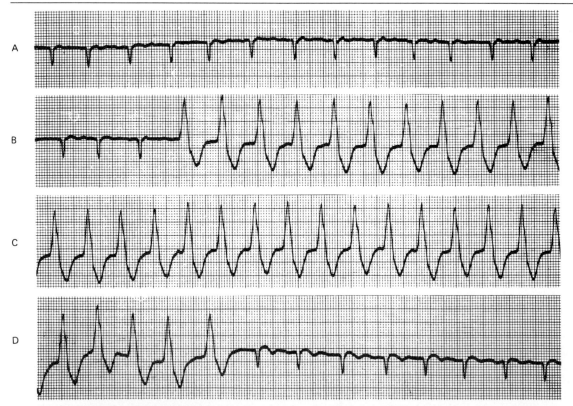

Figure 15–13. Accelerated idioventricular rhythm. Continuous recording of lead V_1 in a patient with acute myocardial infarction. **A:** Atrial fibrillation with irregular ventricular response, rate = 100. **B** and **C:** Appearance of idioventricular rhythm, which initially has a rate of 100 and then increases to 120. **D:** Spontaneous reversion. (Reproduced, with permission, from Goldman MJ: *Principles of Clinical Electrocardiography,* 12th ed. Lange, 1986.)

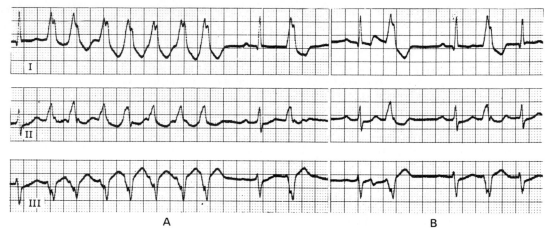

Figure 15–14. Ventricular tachycardia and ventricular premature beats. **A:** Following one sinus beat, there are 7 consecutive ventricular premature beats, indicating ventricular tachycardia. The ventricular rate is 150, and the rhythm is irregular. **B:** The above is followed by sinus rhythm with ventricular bigeminy. The configuration of the ventricular ectopic beats is identical to that of the tachycardia. This indicates that both are arising from the same ventricular focus. (Reproduced, with permission, from Goldschlager N, Goldman MJ: *Principles of Clinical Electrocardiography*, 13th ed. Appleton & Lange, 1989.)

changing intensity of the first heart sound depending upon the relation of the P wave to the QRS complex, and intermittent, large cannon *a* waves in the jugular venous pulse. When the atria contract with the tricuspid valve closed, large cannon waves appear in the jugular venous pulse unless the patient has atrial fibrillation or flutter or 1:1 retrograde conduction to the atria. When the relationship between atrial and ventricular contraction is such that the mitral and tricuspid valves are wide open at the onset of ventricular systole, they close with a snap and the first heart sound is louder. When the atria and the ventricle contract close together, the mitral valve leaflets are relatively closed and the first sound is soft. The systolic blood pressure varies from beat to beat depending upon the sequence of the atrial and ventricular contraction and the contribution of atrial systole to ventricular filling. If ventricular excitation is transmitted backward to the atrium or sinoatrial node, the result is 1:1 ventriculoatrial conduction with no variation in the intensity of the first heart sound and no cannon waves in the jugular venous pulse.

Table 15–8. Some mechanisms causing widening of the QRS complex in supraventricular rhythms. (After Puech, 1970.)

- Preexisting bundle branch block.
- Aberrant ventricular conduction (functional bundle branch block).
  1. Short coupling interval with long preceding cycle.
  2. Different rates of recovery of excitability in the ventricular conduction system.
- Drug-induced intraventricular conduction delay.
- Ectopic activity of supranodal origin, with conduction through an accessory pathway in Wolff-Parkinson-White syndrome.
- Other more complex mechanisms.

B. Electrocardiography:

1. Capture and fusion beats and supraventricular tachycardia with aberrant conduction– A "capture" beat is a supraventricular impulse that is conducted across the atrioventricular node in the presence of a wide QRS tachycardia, activating ("capturing") the ventricle and creating a normal QRS duration. The appearance of capture beats suggests ventricular tachycardia and indicates the presence of atrioventricular dissociation rather than atrioventricular block.

Supraventricular tachycardia can only be diagnosed with confidence when P waves are found with the same frequency as the QRS complexes unless ventricular tachycardia with retrograde atrioventricular conduction is present, with one-to-one atrial and ventricular activity.

Fusion beats (Dressler beats) are those in which, intermittently during tachycardia, an impulse from the sinoatrial node fortuitously activates an independent ventricular beat to produce a QRS complex that is from two different foci—a fusion of both atrial and ventricular depolarizations. This fusion indicates that tachycardia is ventricular in origin.

Carotid sinus pressure or edrophonium may impair atrioventricular conduction and allow P waves to be seen in supraventricular tachycardia with aberration.

Rapid (> 250/min) tachycardia with wide, slightly irregular QRS complexes should suggest atrial fibrillation with Wolff-Parkinson-White conduction and lead to a search for slurred initial delta waves.

2. Careful search for P waves– Review of long strips of the ECG in different leads with double sensitivity and a careful search for P waves may show independent atrial beats at a rate slower than the ventricular tachycardia. These are often not seen or may be buried in the QRS complex. The absence of P waves on a routine ECG does not exclude ventricular tachycardia. Furthermore, in junctional or ventricular tachycardia there may be retrograde activation of the atria that prevents independent sinus beats. Onset of tachycardia with an ectopic P wave is strong evidence of supraventricular tachycardia with aberrant conduction.

C. Electrophysiologic Studies: His bundle recordings may establish the diagnosis by noting the relationship of the His spike and the P wave to the QRS complexes. In supraventricular arrhythmia, the P wave and the His spike preceded the QRS complex, whereas in ventricular tachycardia the QRS complex with retrograde conduction precedes the His potential.

D. Comparison of Previous Premature Beats and Tachycardia: The diagnosis can be clarified in retrospect if, after cessation of tachycardia, ventricular premature beats can be seen that have a configuration similar to that seen during tachycardia. As mentioned in the discussion of supraventricular arrhythmias, if the initial or first few QRS complexes of tachycardia are normal in configuration and later ones become bizarre, this favors a supraventricular over a

ventricular origin. Monitoring of the ECG during graded exercise may produce short bursts of ventricular tachycardia as well as ventricular premature beats and clarify the nature of the preceding tachycardia.

E. Accelerated Idioventricular Rhythms: Accelerated idioventricular rhythms (Figure 15–15) may "escape" when there is suppression of higher pacemakers due to sinoatrial and atrioventricular block but may also represent "slow" ventricular tachycardia due to reentry or increased automaticity due to ischemia. Norris (1974), in his experience with 61 patients with accelerated idioventricular tachycardia in acute myocardial infarction, noted that the attacks of tachycardia consisted of paroxysms of relatively short duration which were relatively slow (< 100/min), often beginning with sinus bradycardia or sinoatrial block, and therefore were probably escape rhythms because the sinoatrial node was depressed. The first beat almost always occurs after a long diastolic pause; the initial and final beats of a paroxysm may have a normal, nonpremature P wave and a QRS configuration combining sinus and ventricular origin (fusion beats). The incidence of ventricular fibrillation is only about one-fourth that of ectopic (nonescape) ventricular tachycardia with a more rapid rate. Atrioventricular dissociation occurs in most patients with acceler-

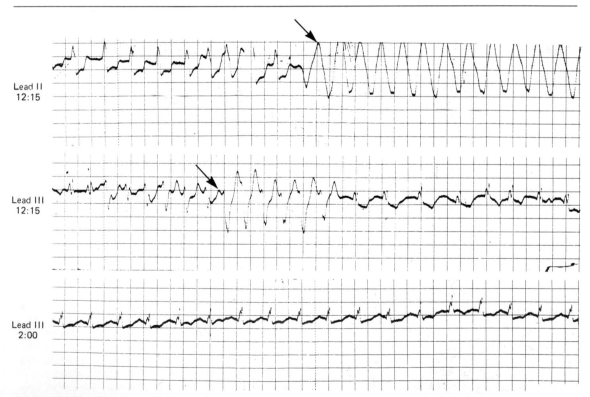

Figure 15–15. Woman age 30 years with myocarditis and runs of ventricular tachycardia **(arrows)** at 12:15 PM. Quinidine gluconate (0.8 g) was given intramuscularly at 12:30 PM. Sinus rhythm without premature beats noted at 2:00 PM. Blood quinidine level at this time was 4.8 μg/mL.

ated idioventricular rhythms because although the ventricular rhythm is usually "escape" in nature, the sinus node still discharges at a slower rate.

Accelerated idioventricular rhythms must be differentiated from idioventricular rhythm that occurs in complete atrioventricular block. In the latter, the ventricular rate is slower (< 40/min), and evidence of complete atrioventricular block is found on the ECG and in the clinical features noted in the discussion above.

The differentiation may be more difficult in congenital atrioventricular block because the ventricular rate is faster than in noncongenital cases (approximately 60–70/min), but the presence of complete block still identifies the rhythm as nonaccelerated idioventricular rhythm.

Atrioventricular dissociation is always present in complete atrioventricular block. In accelerated idioventricular rhythm, in which there is no atrioventricular block, atrioventricular dissociation still occurs, with independent atrial and ventricular pacemakers.

F. Polymorphous Ventricular Tachycardia, Including Torsade de Pointes: Polymorphous ventricular tachycardia is ventricular tachycardia with a varying morphology of the QRS complex in a rapid ventricular tachycardia and includes torsade de pointes. Torsade is considered separately because of the bizarre orientation of the QRS complexes, its association with a prolonged QT interval, and poor prognosis. Torsade often begins with a long-short sequence (Kay, 1983). The QRS complex of the tachycardia varies in polarity and twists around the isoelectric line in irregular bursts. It is found particularly in patients who have a long QT interval, in those receiving drugs such as quinidine, in those with acute myocardial ischemia or hypokalemia, or spontaneously in those with congenital QT syndrome. The changing configuration of the QRS complex is thought to be an ominous sign of imminent ventricular fibrillation when the QRS widens in response to antiarrhythmic drugs, and the drugs should be stopped. However, some effective drugs prolong the QT interval without producing torsade de pointes.

Bradycardia in association with atypical ventricular tachycardia is a warning sign. Prolongation of the QT_c interval is usually substantial, with a mean of 0.59 s (Kay, 1983).

The treatment of torsade de pointes depends on the cause. In the congenital long QT syndromes, since torsade is precipitated in the setting of increased sympathetic stimulation, beta-blocking drugs are successful in preventing the ventricular tachycardia. When this is ineffective, left stellate ganglionectomy has been effective. If torsade is caused by sudden ischemia, beta-blockers or, preferably, revascularization is indicated. If the torsade is related to a precipitating drug, the offending drug must be stopped. Any electrolyte abnormalities should be corrected. Since bradycardia increases the QT interval and the tempo-

ral dispersion of ventricular refractoriness, temporary atrial or ventricular pacing or isoproterenol, 1–4 μg/min, can stop these episodes. Other drugs have been used with varying success, including lidocaine, phenytoin, bretylium, and atropine. Recently, magnesium sulfate, 1–2 g given intravenously over 10 minutes, even in patients with normal serum magnesium, has been reported to be very successful in stopping torsade and, together with temporary pacing, is now the treatment of choice (Tzivoni, 1988; Keren, 1990).

Treatment of Ventricular Tachycardia*

A. Emergency Treatment: In the patient who has minimal symptoms and no hemodynamic abnormality, treatment can be started with procainamide, 750–1000 mg(or 10 mg/kg total dose) intravenously at a rate of 50 mg/min, or lidocaine, 50–100 mg as an intravenous bolus. If the patient is hemodynamically unstable or having marked symptoms due to angina, congestive heart failure, or hypotension, immediate electrical cardioversion under diazepam or midazolam anesthesia is indicated. Figure 15–15 shows the effects of intramuscular quinidine gluconate. If 50–100 mg of intravenous lidocaine does not terminate the arrhythmia and the patient is hemodynamically stable, a second injection can be given in 2–5 minutes with the hope of achieving blood levels of 1.5–4 μg/mL. If the patient does not respond to the increased lidocaine dosage, other drugs (see Table 15–5) can be given. If drug therapy is still ineffective or if the patient has important clinical symptoms, cardioversion preceded by intravenous anesthesia, usually diazepam, 5–15 mg, should be accomplished promptly; almost all patients revert to sinus rhythm, often with low-energy currents. A thump over the chest should be tried prior to electrical external countershock and may be successful in restoring sinus rhythm. Most instruments for defibrillation deliver 10 J as the lowest dose. If this amount of energy is insufficient, repetitive and larger amounts of energy— up to 400 J—should be given as soon as possible to convert the arrhythmia to sinus rhythm. In patients with recurrent attacks, hypoxia and metabolic or electrolyte factors should all be corrected, since they may be predisposing factors. Bedside hemodynamic monitoring with appropriate treatment may also help improve the function of the left ventricle and eliminate factors that predispose to ventricular tachycardia. Management of these hemodynamic abnormalities revealed by hemodynamic monitoring is discussed in detail in Chapter 8.

Since ventricular tachycardia can be mistaken for supraventricular tachycardia with aberrancy or bundle branch block, there is a possibility that inappropriate

---

*The details of dosage and other information about antiarrhythmic drugs are presented in Tables 15-5, 15–6, and 15-7.

and even dangerous therapy can be given. Although intravenous verapamil is an excellent drug with which to convert supraventricular tachycardia to sinus rhythm, it can be disastrous in ventricular tachycardia because of the vasodilation that causes blood pressure to drop, resulting in a sympathetic reflex response and hemodynamic decompensation (Morady, 1985). For this reason, intravenous verapamil should never be used in wide QRS tachycardia unless it is certain that the rhythm is supraventricular, conducted antegrade to the ventricle through the atrioventricular node.

B. Prevention of Recurrences: Pharmacologic therapy should be employed to prevent recurrence. Following cardioversion, the patient should be given prophylactic intravenous infusions of lidocaine, 1–4 mg/min, which, if ineffective, should be supplemented with quinidine, 0.2–0.6 g orally three to five times daily, or procainamide, 250–500 mg orally every 4 hours. One should avoid large doses of lidocaine over long periods because the patient may develop central nervous symptoms, with dizziness, blurred vision, and excitement. Lidocaine blood levels are linearly dose-related and can be very helpful in avoiding toxicity. Lidocaine is metabolized in part by the liver, and smaller doses should be used in the presence of impaired liver function. If doses greater than 3–4 mg/min in an infusion must be exceeded or continued, one should consider combining lower doses of lidocaine with drugs such as quinidine and procainamide or consider the drugs listed in Table 15–7.

B. Overdrive Suppression by Rapid Pacing: If drugs and attention to precipitating factors are unsuccessful in preventing ventricular tachycardia, overdrive suppression of the ectopic focus by pacing may help prevent attacks (Figure 15–16). One should attempt to stop the initial attack and then use pacing at a rate somewhat faster than the ordinary sinus rate to prevent subsequent attacks. Overdrive suppression is ordinarily useful only temporarily, though long-term pacing has been used with success. Electrophysiologic study should be performed before permanent insertion of a long-term pacing unit. One must be certain that the tachycardia can be terminated by rapid pacing, and one must exclude Wolff-Parkinson-White syndrome to avoid ventricular fibrillation.

Treatment of Recurrent Ventricular Tachycardia

Most cases of recurrent ventricular tachycardia—especially frequent recurrences—are due to coronary heart disease and follow acute myocardial infarction, often with life-threatening clinical and hemodynamic features. Activity triggered by late ventricular potentials arising at the border of previous myocardial infarction is a rare cause of ventricular tachycardia and is thought to be caused by late ventricular potentials after myocardial infarction (Breithardt, 1987). Ventricular tachycardia may deteriorate to ventricular fibrillation and sudden death (see Chapter 8).

When ventricular tachycardia occurs spontaneously and is not associated with acute myocardial infarction, an electrophysiologic study is necessary to determine the most effective treatment. Treatment is often difficult and may require the newer antiarrhythmic drugs (eg, amiodarone), which have important side effects. Because of the serious clinical manifestations of recurrent ventricular tachycardia, patients may visit the emergency room repeatedly. The frequency of recurrent ventricular tachycardia and the urgent need for treatment results to a certain extent from the survival of patients in the coronary care unit who in earlier days would have died. These patients often have poor left ventricular function, cardiac failure, and recurrent myocardial ischemia; treatment is taxing for both the clinician and the patient. An aggressive approach, including electrophysiologic study and surgical or catheter ablation or implanted pacemakers or automatic defibrillators, may be required.

A. Drug Treatment: All patients with ventricular tachycardia or cardiac arrest not associated with a known precipitating cause such as acute myocardial infarction or torsade de pointes due to a drug should have an electrophysiologic study to determine the most effective and rational drug to prevent recurrence. Programmed electrical stimulation in the electrophysiology laboratory in patients with spontaneous episodes of tachycardia allows the physician to initiate and terminate ventricular tachycardia by critically timed atrial or ventricular stimuli. Individual antiarrhythmic drugs can then be given to determine whether or not they prevent induction of tachycardia. Drugs found to be effective in preventing ventricular

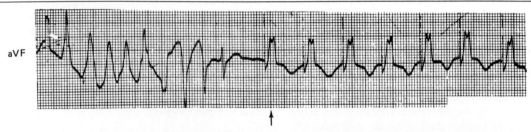

aVF

Figure 15–16. Short runs of ventricular tachycardia abolished **(arrow)** by transvenous pacemaker in a 43-year-old man following the replacement of a mitral valve.

tachycardia in the laboratory have been found to be effective in preventing spontaneous occurrences of the arrhythmia. The induced and spontaneous arrhythmias are said to be identical in about 80–90% of patients. The method allows a more rational and rapid selection of the most potent antiarrhythmic agent (Zipes, 1989). If an antiarrhythmic drug results in the ventricular tachycardia being noninducible during the electrophysiologic study, there is an 80% chance that the patient will do well. However, if the ventricular tachycardia is still inducible, there is an 80% chance of recurrence within 1 year (Rickenberger, 1991). Wellens (1986) emphasized that these stimulation studies were primarily of value when clinically documented sustained ventricular tachycardia could be induced. Chronic oral therapy with the same drug proves to be effective in most patients. In some instances, especially with amiodarone, the drug may be effective clinically even though ventricular tachycardia can still be induced in the laboratory while the patient is receiving the drug. There is presently a study designed to determine whether serial antiarrhythmia drug testing is better evaluated by electrophysiologic studies or by electrocardiographic end points (ESVEM, 1989). Preliminary reports show that ambulatory ECG evaluation is as effective as electrophysiologic studies in evaluating the effects of antiarrhythmic therapy.

Complex ventricular arrhythmias following myocardial infarction are an independent high-risk finding for cardiac or sudden death, especially when associated with left ventricular dysfunction, decreased ejection fraction ($\leq 40\%$), and the presence of late potentials in the signal-averaged ECG, a special technique that records low-amplitude signals in the terminal QRS complex (Gomes, 1987; Odemuyiwa, 1992). Late potentials may result from delayed left ventricular conduction and may induce ventricular tachycardia—and therefore indicate a patient at high risk of cardiac death (Breithardt, 1987).

Unfortunately, currently available antiarrhythmic agents are of limited effectiveness in ventricular arrhythmias, and newer ones such as encainide and flecainide are associated with a substantial incidence of side effects, usually related to the central nervous system but including proarrhythmia (the worsening or new appearance of ventricular tachycardia or fibrillation that may increase fatality) in 10–20% of cases. The incidence of proarrhythmia increases as the ventricular function worsens. The value of beta-blockers following a myocardial infarction has been established, but it is not known how their beneficial effect is mediated.

Asymptomatic patients do not require treatment for ventricular arrhythmias when they occur with an ejection fraction exceeding 40% and in the absence of signal-averaged late potentials (Epstein, 1990).

Symptomatic patients with postinfarction complex ventricular arrhythmias or ventricular tachycardia associated with left ventricular dysfunction require antiarrhythmic treatment, but there is no convincing evidence that such treatment prolongs life (Hallstrom, 1991). Treatment with drugs such as amiodarone can be tried, guided by electrophysiologic studies. A recent study (Pfisterer, 1992) showed a significantly lower mortality rate without arrhythmic events in survivors of myocardial infarction with asymptomatic complex ventricular arrhythmias with left ventricular ejection fractions of 40% or more when given low-dose amiodarone (200 mg/d) compared with a control group (1.5% versus 8.9%; $P < .03$). There was no difference in the group with the left ventricular ejection fraction less than 40%. If drugs prove ineffective in recurrent resistant ventricular tachycardia, surgical treatment can be considered after localizing the electrical focus of origin of the arrhythmia by electrophysiologic mapping, confirmed in the operating room. Resection of a ventricular aneurysm or of the endocardial tissue where the first endocardial breakthrough of the ventricular tachycardia QRS occurs, usually adjacent to a myocardial scar, may prevent recurrent arrhythmia but has a high mortality rate, especially with decreased left ventricular function (Bourke, 1990; Landymore, 1990). The good late results make surgical therapy an important option, but obviously surgery should not be performed until antiarrhythmic therapy has been vigorously applied. Hemodynamic and clinical improvement of congestive failure may result from surgical resection and therefore may increase survival when ventricular arrhythmias and congestive failure coexist (Josephson, 1986).

B. Implantation of Antitachycardia Devices and Automatic Cardioverter-Defibrillators:

Electrical pacemaker devices with external monitoring that can sense and then deliver stimuli to terminate ventricular tachyarrhythmias have been implanted with some success in patients with frequently recurring ventricular tachycardia or fibrillation (Mirowski, 1985; Scheinman, 1988). The devices represent a major advance in the treatment of these difficult arrhythmias, reducing the arrhythmic 1-year mortality rate to 2% or less (Klein, 1991). Variations of technique, including miniaturization and transvenous implantation, have been attempted to eliminate the need for thoracotomy. These devices have had encouraging results, especially in inducible monomorphic ventricular tachycardia (Miles, 1986). Problems and complications remain, such as false-positive electrical discharges in which the pacemaker senses electrical activity that is not a ventricular tachycardia, the short life of the battery, the lack of programmability, the relatively large size of the devices, the continuing need for thoracotomy, and the localized myocardial injury under patch electrodes (found at autopsy) (Gabry, 1987; Singer, 1987). Further experience is required, though initial results are better than with other forms of therapy (Newman, 1992).

The newer devices monitor rate as well as other parameters—such as QRS width—that define ventricular tachycardia as opposed to other types of tachycardia. When the criteria for ventricular tachycardia occur, after a programmed lag to ensure that the arrhythmia is sustained, a low-energy depolarization or series of depolarizations is induced that is designed to terminate a reentrant ventricular tachycardia by the extra stimuli entering the "excitable gap." Since it is possible to accelerate a ventricular tachycardia by this technique in up to one-third of patients (Waldecker, 1986), a back-up defibrillating mode is mandatory.

Devices with combined antitachycardia pacing, pacemakers for bradyarrhythmia, and defibrillation capability are currently available. Most sustained monomorphic ventricular tachycardia is due to reentry. Such an arrhythmia can be terminated by low-energy shock (< 0.05–2.0 J) synchronized with the QRS to avoid precipitating ventricular fibrillation. If ventricular fibrillation occurs, higher-energy shock (30 J) must be delivered, usually across electrode patches placed via thoracotomy—one on the right ventricle and the other on the left ventricle. Detection of ventricular fibrillation depends on the "probability density function," which analyzes the proportion of the cardiac cycle that the ventricular electrogram spends on the isoelectric line, thus distinguishing ventricular fibrillation from ventricular tachycardia and from wide QRS supraventricular tachycardia. Future detection will probably involve detecting atrioventricular dissociaton and even biosensors to detect hemodynamic deterioration.

The currently available device is the AICD (Cardiac Pacemakers Co.). More than 7000 nonprogrammable AICDs have been implanted worldwide. This device is activated when the rate counter has recorded eight beats, fulfilling the rate detection criteria. A charging cycle is initiated after a less than 2.5 s delay to ensure that the ventricular tachycardia is sustained. Charging time is 6–7 seconds, so that the total duration that the arrhythmia lasts prior to delivery the defibrillating shock is under 25 seconds. Once the device charges the capacitors, it is committed and will fire even if sinus rhythm is restored. If the arrhythmia fails to be terminated with the first shock, a second detection interval begins and the capacitors recharge. Up to five shocks can be delivered for a single arrhythmic event. At least 35 seconds of a rate not satisfying the detection criteria (ie, normal sinus rhythm) must elapse before the device can deliver another defibrillating shock.

The North American Society of Pacing and Electrophysiology (NASPE) has developed criteria for implantation of cardioverter-defibrillators. In essence, there is a consensus that implantation is indicated when the patient has ventricular tachycardia or ventricular fibrillation for which no other therapy is successful because of drug inefficacy, natural intolerance, or noncompliance; when surgical or ablation therapy is contraindicated or fails; or when no satisfactory end point exists by which to judge therapeutic efficacy (when the ventricular tachycardia remains inducible despite therapy at electrophysiologic study) (Klein, 1991).

The efficacy of these implantable pacemaker-cardioverter-defibrillators is being evaluated in a number of studies. One study (Saksena, 1992) reported a series of 200 patients with sustained ventricular tachycardia, ventricular fibrillation, or prior cardiac arrest where a programmable device was implanted. They were followed for a mean of 12 months, and during this time there was a 1% arrhythmia mortality rate, a 6.5% cardiac mortality rate, and a 10.5% total mortality rate. A European Multicenter Study of 102 implanted devices reported an actuarial 12-month survival of 91% and one sudden arrhythmic death. Over a thousand spontaneous ventricular tachycardia episodes were detected and treated in 43 patients, and the overall defibrillation efficacy was 97.6% (Fromer, 1992). Only one study (Newman, 1992), however, reported the survival of 60 consecutive patients with the implanted cardioverter-defibrillator compared with a matched case-control group of 120 patients treated medically over the same time period. At 3 years, the actuarial survival was significantly higher for the device-implanted patients (65%) compared with the control patients (49%). Others have found significant survival improved only in those with left ventricular ejection fractions of 30% or more. With lower ejection fractions, although the incidence of sudden death may be decreased, the cardiac and total mortality rate, including the surgical mortality rate, is high (Kim, 1992). The proof of overall effectiveness in terms of total mortality rate may require a randomized trial (Connolly, 1992).

C. Surgical or Catheter Ablation of the Focus (Resection of Ventricular Aneurysm, Ischemic Zone of Increased Excitability or Both): If episodes of ventricular tachycardia occur frequently (some patients have 75–100 attacks over a period of days or weeks), the possibility of ventricular aneurysm should be considered. Two-dimensional echocardiography, radionuclide angiography, and cardiac catheterization with left ventricular angiography should be considered in order to establish the presence of a localized expansile pulsation of the left ventricle that might be treated surgically. Recurrent ventricular tachycardia unrelieved by other measures may be prevented in some cases by resection of the ventricular aneurysm, and cardiac failure may be reversed (see Chapter 8).

Before resection of an aneurysm for complex ventricular tachycardia that recurs despite vigorous medical therapy, electrophysiologic studies should be employed to define the focus of origin of the arrhythmia (Page, 1989). The initial electrical activity of the focus usually occurs in the border between the edge of the aneurysm and the neighboring viable myocardium but occasionally can be in multiple areas, at times at some distance from the aneurysm. At surgery, intraoperative mapping should also be performed, and encircling endocardial resection (which includes the area of earliest electrical activity in the border zone) should be combined with resection of the ventricular aneurysm. When this localized endocardial area was resected in patients with recurrent ventricular tachycardia, the arrhythmia could no longer be induced by electrical stimulation, and the disabling ventricular tachycardia and complex ventricular premature beats were usually abolished (Josephson, 1982). Electrophysiologic studies, including electrical stimulation and mapping at the time of surgery, require experienced specialists in the field and cooperation between cardiologists and surgeons.

Patients accepted for resection should have recurrent severe ventricular tachycardia with failure of antiarrhythmic drugs now available, including amiodarone. Cardiac mapping can be done preoperatively with an electrode catheter and ventricular tachycardia initiated. Endocardial foci of activity are located, and their timing is compared with that of the surface ECG. The endocardial site of origin of the arrhythmia is the location whose activity is earliest in relation to activity on the ECG. Intraoperative electrophysiologic mapping is also performed to more accurately localize the site of the endocardium to be resected. The surgical mortality rate of resection is approximately 15%. In most centers, electrode patches for an automatic internal cardioverter-defibrillator will be placed in case the ventricular tachycardia returns. Some patients have continued to have recurrent tachycardia because satisfactory intraoperative endocardial maps were not possible and apparently not resected. The most important independent predictor of postoperative survival was the systolic function of the nonaneurysmal ventricular segments of the left ventricle (Garan, 1986).

As an alternative to surgical resection, a newer technique of catheter electrical ablation of the focus of ventricular tachycardia has been developed. Administration of 1–4 shocks of 100–300 J, each delivered to the endocardial exit site of ventricular tachycardia, as determined by endocardial mapping, was successful in about half the patients in a substantial series. None died during the procedure (Morady, 1987). Others have reported less success with catheter ablation attempts at eliminating ventricular tachycardia. A report of 164 patients who underwent catheter ablation for a ventricular tachycardia focus reported 18% completely successful and another 41% to be improved with drug therapy. There was a high incidence of procedure-related complications, with a total of 11 deaths, intractable arrhythmias, myocardial infarction, and intractable heart failure (Evans, 1988).

The use of radiofrequency catheter ablation does not improve success with ventricular tachycardia ablation in patients with structural heart disease unless the mechanism of the ventricular tachycardia was bundle branch reentry, where it is highly successful. The reason for this is probably the smaller volume of myocardium and the shallow depth of the lesion created by radiofrequency energy (Klein, 1992). However, in the more unusual patient with ventricular tachycardia without structural heart disease, radiofrequency catheter ablation guided by electrophysiologic mapping appears to be very successful, with 94% success in one small series of patients (Klein, 1992).

At the present time, catheter ablation for patients with ventricular tachycardia and structural heart disease should be reserved for situations where the ventricular tachycardia is mappable and the patient is not a candidate for cardiac surgery or insertion of an automatic defibrillator (Scheinman, 1991).

VENTRICULAR FIBRILLATION

Ventricular fibrillation (shown in Figure 15–17) is the most feared arrhythmia because of its relationship to sudden cardiac death.

Uncoordinated cardiac impulses spread rapidly across the ventricle from multiple areas of reentry and through pathways that vary in size and direction. As a result, there is failure of the normal sequential contraction of the heart. A heart in ventricular fibrillation is seen as a mass of multiple small twitches. The pressure within the ventricle does not rise, and the peripheral tissues are not perfused because there is no effective cardiac output. In effect, the heart is in a state equivalent to cardiac arrest. The random reentry pathways of the excitatory wave result in perpetuation of the dysrhythmia. Spontaneous episodes of ventricular fibrillation may terminate without therapy. If the ventricular fibrillation persists for more than a few minutes, perfusion of the heart and brain essentially stops, and even if the patient is subsequently resuscitated, irreversible brain damage may have occurred. As a result, efforts have been made to recognize the high-risk patient susceptible to ventricular fibrillation and to alert everyone concerned to the need for immediate treatment should the arrhythmia occur. As indicated in the sections on ventricular tachycardia and ventricular premature beats, most instances of ventricular fibrillation are preceded by less severe varieties of ventricular arrhythmia, but some patients—particularly in the early minutes or hours of acute myocardial infarction—may have ventricular fibrillation without warning arrhythmias. Furthermore, in patients who were fortuitously being monitored when an acute myocardial infarction developed, the immediate phase of the infarction was not associated with ventricular arrhythmias, which developed later—within minutes to an hour. The frequency of ventricular arrhythmias—especially ventricular fibrillation—is well established in coronary heart disease (see Chapter 8) but is a matter of dispute in prolapsed mitral valve syndrome.

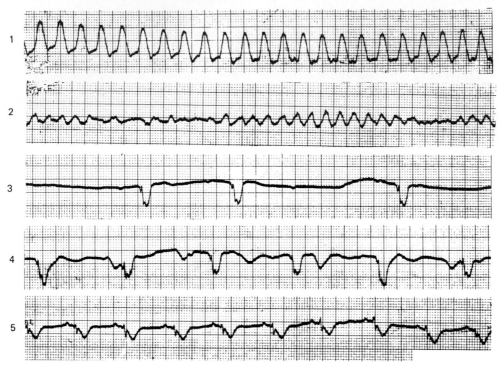

Figure 15–17. Sequential changes after cardiac arrest in a 55-year-old woman with unstable angina: Strip 1 shows ventricular tachycardia. Strip 2 shows ventricular fibrillation. Strip 3 shows sinus bradycardia with atrioventricular Wenckebach and bundle branch block. Strip 4 shows ventricular premature beats; idioventricular rhythm cannot be excluded. Strip 5 shows sinus rhythm. (Courtesy of K Gershengorn.)

On physical examination, the patient with ventricular fibrillation is usually unconscious, pulseless, with obvious poor perfusion and cold skin, and apparently dead.

Background of Patients Who Develop Ventricular Fibrillation

Most patients who develop ventricular fibrillation have known coronary heart disease or a history of hypertension, hypercholesterolemia, ventricular premature beats, or some other evidence of heart disease. Since approximately 60% of all coronary deaths are sudden and since most sudden deaths occur in patients with known coronary disease, identification of coronary patients at greatest risk of cardiac arrest and preventive treatment must take precedence over treatment of cardiac arrest itself if one hopes to decrease the mortality rate from sudden cardiac death.

Although many patients have seen their physician within the month preceding the ventricular fibrillation—and about one-fifth on the day of the arrest because of chest pain, dyspnea, or palpitations—most patients collapse instantaneously and therefore cannot be saved by a mobile team but only by a trained person who witnesses the episode and can immediately institute resuscitative measures. Many patients who develop ventricular fibrillation have un-witnessed episodes that may be instantaneous or last only minutes, and death occurs before medical help can be obtained.

In many communities, efforts are under way to train lay persons to perform resuscitative measures, with the hope that external cardiac massage and artificial respiration will be instituted pending the arrival of a trained ambulance or fire department rescue team. The American Heart Association makes available a film for the purpose of encouraging people—especially relatives or coworkers of patients who have once been defibrillated or are known to have coronary heart disease—to take special courses in resuscitation. Cobb (1975) has analyzed the types of activities immediately preceding ventricular fibrillation and notes that only about one-sixth have had unusual physical or mental stress. About one-third of cases occur during sleep, and the great majority of cases of ventricular fibrillation occur during ordinary activities at work or at home.

In some communities, paramedical teams can reach a stricken individual within 5 minutes. Experience with out-of-hospital onset of ventricular fibrillation has shown that only about one-fourth of patients will have unequivocal evidence of acute myocardial infarction by electrocardiographic criteria—perhaps half if one includes enzyme changes. Forty to 60

Table 15–9. Hospital follow-up data on surviving patients who had defibrillation.[1]

	Hospital Deaths (Percent)	Discharged Survivors (Percent)	Totals Prehospital Ventricular Fibrillation (Percent)
Acute myocardial infarction	37	31	35
Ischemia without infarction	34	29	32
No acute electrocardiographic change	10	26	17
Complete left bundle branch block[2]	19	14	17
Complete right bundle branch block	24	7	17
Repeat ventricular fibrillation	50	24	40
Congestive heart failure	69	53	63
Cardiogenic shock	39	5	25
Severe pulmonary complications[3]	41	44	42
Severe neurologic deficit	95	12	61
Partial neurologic deficit	5	28	15
No neurologic deficit	. . .	60	25

[1] Reproduced, with permission, from Liberthson RR et al: Prehospital ventricular defibrillation: Prognosis and follow-up course. N Engl J Med 1974; 291:317.
[2] Possibly masking an acute myocardial change.
[3] Aspiration pneumonia or flail chest.

percent of patients are resuscitated, and about 30% of resuscitated victims leave the hospital alive (see also Table 15–9). The resuscitation efforts are therefore clearly worthwhile. Some prehospital cardiac arrests are found by mobile teams to be due to asystole rather than ventricular fibrillation, but it is not known whether or not the asystole followed a period of ventricular fibrillation. These patients rarely survive hospitalization.

Treatment

A. Emergency Treatment: Treatment consists of immediate emergency resuscitative measures (see Chapter 7) to restore the circulation by external cardiac massage combined with mouth-to-mouth breathing. Chest compression is applied by means of a sharp downward thrust over the lower sternum at a rate of approximately 80–100/min, combined with two or three quick breaths with the nose closed and the neck extended, and quick breaths are continued at a rate of 18/min until help arrives. If two people are available, the inflations and the chest compression

should be continued without interruption until help arrives. The patient must be intubated and defibrillated at the earliest possible moment.

In the coronary care unit, with electrocardiographic monitoring, resuscitation should be accomplished within 30 seconds after the onset of fibrillation. Specially trained nurses in the coronary care unit should defibrillate the patient if a doctor is unavailable. Defibrillation is accomplished with 400 J, repeated if necessary. In current practice, it is held that routine administration of sodium bicarbonate is contraindicated and that one should control arterial pH by adequate ventilation. The accumulation of pyruvic and lactic acids and hypercapnia from absent ventilation lead to a low pH, which in turn may induce further arrhythmias and interfere with defibrillation by electric countershock. If severe acidosis persists, sodium bicarbonate, 44 meq intravenously, can be administered.

In the coronary care unit, defibrillation is almost always successful, at least initially, but fibrillation may be recurrent, usually within the first day or so, and antiarrhythmic therapy such as lidocaine, 1–4 mg/min by infusion, should be started promptly after the patient is resuscitated.

B. Bypass Coronary Surgery: Because of the extensive coronary disease found on coronary arteriography in most patients recovered from ventricular fibrillation, bypass surgery has been recommended to prevent recurrence. The data are limited, but it is not established that bypass surgery can prevent recurrent attacks of ventricular fibrillation.

C. Prophylactic Drugs to Prevent Recurrences: The same can be said for antiarrhythmic drugs such as quinidine, procainamide, and phenytoin (especially in digitalis toxicity). A number of studies have shown that these drugs may decrease the number of simple or complex ventricular premature beats seen on 24-hour monitoring, but the side effects are significant and there is as yet only minimal evidence that they will in fact prevent sudden cardiac death even though the number of ventricular premature beats seems to be decreased.

The incidence of primary ventricular fibrillation in acute myocardial infarction appears to be declining. Meta-analysis of a series of reports in the literature found the incidence of primary ventricular fibrillation to have fallen from 4.51% in 1970 to 0.35% in 1990. The reason for this decrease is not evident, though the increased use of beta-blockers during acute myocardial infarction has been suggested. This decline in incidence of primary ventricular fibrillation is one of the reasons for the decreased evidence that prophylactic lidocaine is useful in decreasing the mortality rate in acute myocardial infarction.

Table 15–7 summarizes the clinical characteristics of some newer agents. The most promising appear to be amiodarone, flecainide, and encainide. Further clinical data are awaited. The unpredictability of ventricular fibrillation is an especially devastating aspect of this fatal arrhythmia, and efforts are being made to preselect a high-risk group from the coronary heart disease population in which various forms of therapy can be prospectively tested.

Beta-adrenergic-blocking agents are the only drugs that have decreased the incidence of sudden death when used prophylactically. Almost all such drugs tried have reduced the incidence of sudden death and cardiac death when used on a long-term basis following myocardial infarction. The value of beta-blocking drugs emphasizes the role of adrenergic central nervous system stimuli in causing ventricular arrhythmias. Decreasing these adrenergic stimuli with drugs such as tranquilizers, diazepam, or beta-blockers may prove to be more valuable than using purely antiarrhythmic drugs such as quinidine and procainamide.

D. Implanted Automatic Defibrillators: Implanted automatic pacemakers may sense ventricular fibrillation and spontaneously fire a defibrillatory impulse. Further study with modifications of the implanted defibrillator is under way in a number of centers.

E. Control of Risk Factors: Control of risk factors that increase the likelihood of clinical coronary events—especially control of hypertension and hyperlipidemia and cessation of smoking—has been shown to decrease the incidence of sudden death in patients with known coronary heart disease with or without ventricular fibrillation. Patients who have had ventricular fibrillation and have been resuscitated should be strongly advised to stop smoking. It is of considerable interest that overt diabetes is uncommon in this group of patients; however, diabetes should be treated if present.

Holter monitoring at intervals following recovery from acute myocardial infarction or from an episode of ventricular fibrillation may identify some individuals in whom spontaneous cardiac pain occurs coincidentally with the development of complex ventricular arrhythmias. This group may benefit from antiarrhythmic therapy with amiodarone or beta-adrenergic-blocking agents.

Prognosis

Although about one-half to two-thirds of patients with ventricular fibrillation outside the hospital are satisfactorily defibrillated, most of these patients die in the hospital. However, 30% are discharged alive, often with only mild evidence of cardiac failure or pulmonary complications. Subsequent coronary arteriography almost always shows extensive coronary disease, and approximately half have left ventricular wall motion abnormalities. Severe neurologic deficits are uncommon in patients who are promptly defibrillated. Impaired memory is described by Cobb (1975) as the most common late neurologic sequela. The high incidence of recurrence of fibrillation within the months following release from the hospital indicates that chronic myocardial ischemia is still present. The incidence of recurrence of ventricular fibrillation is greater among persons who show no evidence of myocardial infarction than among those who do.

Without treatment, the patient with acute myocardial infarction who develops ventricular fibrillation almost always dies. Prospective follow-up of patients who have been resuscitated is unfavorable, with a 30% 1-year mortality rate and a 50% 3-year mortality rate. Most of the recurrences of "sudden cardiac death" occur within the first few months. These patients should have coronary arteriography and evaluation by myocardial perfusion study to identify vessels supplying viable myocardium that can be revascularized. If they have recurrent episodes of ventricular tachycardias uncontrolled by antiarrhythmics selected by electrophysiologic study, they should be considered for implantation of an automatic defibrillator.

REFERENCES

Pathophysiology & Mechanisms

Califf RM et al: Relationships among ventricular arrhythmias, coronary artery disease, and angiographic and electrocardiographic indicators of myocardial fibrosis. Circulation 1978;57:727.

Commerford PJ, Lloyd EA: Arrhythmias in patients with drug toxicity, electrolyte, and endocrine disturbances. Med Clin North Am 1984;68:1051.

Dimarco JP, Garan H, Rusin JN: Complications in patients undergoing cardiac electrophysiologic procedures. Ann Intern Med 1982;97:490.

Han J: Mechanisms of ventricular arrhythmias associated with myocardial infarction. Am J Cardiol 1969;24:800.

Hoffman BF, Rosen MR, Wit AL: Electrophysiology and pharmacology of cardiac arrhythmias. 3. The causes and treatment of cardiac arrhythmias. (Part A.) Am Heart J 1975;89;115.

Horowitz LN et al: Risks and complications of clinical cardiac electrophysiologic studies: A prospective analysis of 1000 consecutive patients. J Am Coll Cardiol 1987;9:1261.

Josephson ME et al: Comparison of endocardial catheter mapping with intraoperative mapping of ventricular tachycardia. Circulation 1980;61:395.

Lown B, Verrier RL, Rabinowitz SH: Neural and psychologic mechanisms and the problem of sudden cardiac death. Am J Cardiol 1977;39:890.

Malliani A, Schwartz PJ, Zanchetti A: Neural mechanisms in life-threatening arrhythmias. Am Heart J 1980;100:705.

Myerburg RJ: Electrocardiographic analysis of cardiac arrhythmias. Hosp Pract (June) 1980;15:51.

Ochs HR et al: Single and multiple dose pharmacokinetics of oral quinidine sulfate and gluconate. Am J Cardiol 1978;41:770.

Podrid PJ, Schocneberger A, Lown B: Congestive heart failure caused by oral disopyramide. N Engl J Med 1980;302:614.

Schwartz PJ et al (editors): *Neural Mechanisms in Cardiac Arrhythmias*. Vol 2 in: *Perspectives in Cardiovascular Research*. Raven Press, 1979.

Vaughn Williams EM: Classification of antiarrhythmic drugs. In: *Symposium on Cardiac Arrhythmias*. Sandoe E, Flensted-Jensen E, Olesen KH (editors). Astra, 1970.

Vera Z, Mason DT: Reentry versus automaticity: Role in tachyarrhythmia genesis and antiarrhythmic therapy. Am Heart J 1981;101:329.

Wellens HJJ, Bär FWHM, Lie KI: The value of the electrocardiogram in the differential diagnosis of a tachycardia with a widened QRS complex. Am J Med 1978;64:27.

WHO/ISC Task Force: Definition of terms related to cardiac rhythm. Am Heart J 1978;95:796.

Wit AL, Hoffman BF, Rosen MR: Electrophysiology and pharmacology of cardiac arrhythmias. 9. Cardiac electrophysiologic effects of beta adrenergic receptor stimulation and blockade. (Three parts.) Am Heart J 1975;90:521, 665, 795.

Wit AL, Rosen MR, Hoffman BF: Electrophysiology and pharmacology of cardiac arrhythmias. 8. Cardiac effects of diphenylhydantoin. Am Heart J 1975;90:265.

Supraventricular Arrhythmias

Akhtar M et al: Wide QRS complex tachycardia: Reappraisal of a common clinical problem. Ann Intern Med 1988;109:905.

Barold SS, Coumel P: Mechanisms of atrioventricular junctional tachycardia: Role of reentry and concealed accessory bypass tracts. Am J Cardiol 1977;39:97.

Betriu A et al: Beneficial effect of intravenous diltiazem in the acute management of paroxysmal supraventricular tachyarrhythmias. Circulation 1983;67:88.

Josephson ME, Horowitz LN, Kastor JA: Paroxysmal supraventricular tachycardia in patients with mitral valve prolapse. Circulation 1978;57:111.

Josephson ME, Kastor JA: Supraventricular tachycardia in Lown-Ganong-Levine syndrome: Atrionodal versus intranodal reentry. Am J Cardiol 1977;40:521.

Keefe DL, Mirua D, Somberg JC: Supraventricular tachyarrhythmias: Their evaluation and therapy. Am Heart J 1986;111:1150.

Morady F, Scheinman MM: Paroxysmal supraventricular tachycardia. 1. Diagnosis. Mod Concepts Cardiovasc Dis 1982;51:107.

Narula OS, Narula JT: Junctional pacemakers in man: Response to overdrive suppression with and without parasympathetic blockade. Circulation 1978;57:880.

Pick A, Dominguez P: Nonparoxysmal A-V nodal tachycardia. Circulation 1957;16:1022.

Pritchett ELC et al: Supraventricular tachycardia dependent upon accessory pathways in the absence of ventricular preexcitation. Am J Med 1978;64:214.

Puech P et al: The diagnosis of supraventricular arrhythmias and the differentiation between supraventricular tachycardia with aberrant conduction and ventricular tachycardias. In: *Symposium on Cardiac Arrhythmias*. Sandoe E, Flensted-Jensen E, Olesen KH (editors). Astra, 1970.

Tchou P et al: Useful clinical criteria for the diagnosis of ventricular tachycardia. Am J Med 1988;84:53.

Waxman MB et al: Effects of respiration and posture on paroxysmal supraventricular tachycardia. Circulation 1980;62:1011.

Wellens HJJ: Brugada P, Stevenson WG: Programmed electrical stimulation of the heart in patients with life-threatening ventricular arrhythmias: What is the significance of induced arrhythmias and what is the correct stimulation protocol? Circulation 1985;72:1.

Treatment of Supraventricular Arrhythmias

Anderson JL, Pritchett ELC (guest editors): International symposium on supraventricular arrhythmias: Focus on flecainide. Am J Cardiol 1988;62:1D.

Abrams J et al: Efficacy and safety of esmolol vs propranolol in the treatment of supraventricular tachyarrhythmias: A multicenter double-blind clinical trial. Am Heart J 1985;110:913.

Boccadamo R et al: Prevention and interruption of supraventricular tachycardia by antitachycardia pacing. In: *Interventional Electrophysiology*. Underitz B, Saksena S (editors). Futura, 1991.

Brugada P et al: Suppression of incessant supraventricular tachycardia by intravenous and oral encainide. J Am Coll Cardiol 1984;4:1255.

Camm AJ, Garratt CJ: Adenosine and supraventricular tachycardia. N Engl J Med 1991;325:1621.

Cobb FR et al: Successful surgical interruption of the bundle of Kent in a patient with Wolff-Parkinson-White syndrome. Circulation 1968;38:1018.

Crozier IG et al: Flecainide acetate for conversion of acute supraventricular tachycardia to sinus rhythm. Am J Cardiol 1987;59:607.

DiMarco JP et al: Adenosine for paroxysmal supraventricular tachycardia: Dose ranging and comparison with verapamil in placebo-controlled, multicenter trials. Ann Intern Med 1990;113:104.

Gillette PC et al: Treatment of atrial automatic tachycardia by ablation procedures. J Am Coll Cardiol 1985;6:405.

Gonzalez R et al: Closed-chest electrode-catheter techniques for His bundle ablation in dogs. Am J Physiol 1981;241:H283.

Haines DE, DiMarco JP: Current therapy for supraventricular arrhythmias. Curr Probl Cardiol 1992;17:415.

Hazard PB et al: Treatment of multifocal atrial tachycardia with metoprolol. Crit Care Med 1987;15:20.

Hendry FJ et al: Surgical treatment of automatic atrial tachycardias. Ann Thorac Surg 1990;49:253.

Jackman WM et al: Treatment of supraventricular tachycardia due to atrioventricular nodal reentry by radiofrequency catheter ablation of slow-pathway conduction. N Engl J Med 1992;327:313.

Kastor JA: Multifocal atrial tachycardias. N Engl J Med 1990;322:1713.

Klein GJ et al: Cryosurgical ablation of the atrioventricular node-His bundle: Long-term follow-up and properties of the junctional pacemaker. Circulation 1980;61:8.

Kuck KH et al: Encainide versus flecainide for chronic atrial and junctional ectopic tachycardia. Am J Cardiol 1988;322:1713.

Lee MA et al: Catheter modification of the atrioventricular junction with radiofrequency energy for control of atrioventricular nodal reentry tachycardia. Circulation 1991;83:827.

Lerman BB, Belardinelli L: Cardiac electrophysiology of adenosine: Basic and clinical concepts. Circulation 1991;83:1499.

Lesh MD et al: Curative percutaneous catheter ablation using radiofrequency energy for coronary pathways in all locations: Results in 100 consecutive patients. J Am Coll Cardiol 1992;19:1303.

Lie KI et al: Long-term efficacy of verapamil in the treatment of paroxysmal supraventricular tachycardias. Am Heart J 1983;105:688.

Mehta, D et al: Relative efficacy of various physical manoeuvres in the termination of junctional tachycardia. Lancet 1988;1:1181.

Nacarelli GV, Wellens HJJ (guest editors): A symposium: The use of encainide in supraventricular tachycardias. Am J Cardiol 1988;62:1L.

Pritchett ELC et al: Mortality in patients treated with flecainide and encainide for supraventricular arrhythmias. Am J Cardiol 1991;67:976.

Relmer A et al: Efficiency and safety of intravenous and oral preparations in pediatric cardiac dysrhythmias. Am J Cardiol 1991;68:741.

Rosen KM: Junctional tachycardia: Mechanisms, diagnosis, differential diagnosis, and management. Circulation 1973;47:654.

Ruder MA et al: Clinical and electrophysiological characterization of automatic junctional ectopic tachycardia in adults. Circulation 1986;73:930.

Sakurai M et al: Acute and chronic effects of verapamil in patients with paroxysmal supraventricular tachycardia. Am Heart J 1983;105:619.

Scheinman MM: Nonpharmacologic treatment of life-threatening cardiac arrhythmias. Cardiovasc Rev Re 1988;9:27.

Scheinman MM et al: Catheter-induced ablation of the atrioventricular function to control refractory supraventricular arrhythmias. JAMA 1982;248:851.

Scheinman MM et al: Current role of catheter ablation procedures in patients with cardiac arrhythmias. Circulation 1991;83:2146.

Schugar CD et al: Clinical management of patients with atrioventricular nodal reentrant tachycardia. Cardiol Clin 1990;8:491.

Sharma AD et al: Intravenous adenosine triphosphate during wide QRS complex tachycardia: Safety, therapeutic efficacy, and diagnostic utility. Am J Med 1990;88:337.

Spurrell RJ et al: Implantable automatic scanning pacemaker for termination of supraventricular tachycardia. Am J Cardiol 1982;49:753.

Woosley RL, Wood AJJ, Roden DM: Encainide. N Engl J Med 1988;318:1107.

Zipes DP: A consideration of antiarrhythmic therapy. (Editorial.) Circulation 1985;72:949.

Atrial Fibrillation & Atrial Flutter

Arnold AZ et al: Role of prophylactic anticoagulation for direct current cardioversion in patients with atrial fibrillation or atrial flutter. J Am Coll Cardiol 1992;19:851.

Atwood JE et al: Effect of beta-adrenergic blockade on exercise performance in patients with chronic atrial fibrillation. J Am Coll Cardiol 1987;10:314.

BAATAF Investigators: The effect of low-dose warfarin on the risk of stroke in patients with nonrheumatic atrial fibrillation. N Engl J Med 1990;323:1505.

Barold SS et al: Implanted atrial pacemakers for paroxysmal atrial flutter: Long-term efficacy. Ann Intern Med 1987;107:144.

Brand FN et al: Characteristics and prognosis of lone atrial fibrillation: 30-year follow-up in the Framingham Study. JAMA 1985;254:3449.

Brodsy MA et al: Amiodarone for maintenance of sinus rhythm after conversion of atrial fibrillation in the setting of a dilated left atrium. Am J Cardiol 1987;60:572.

Cairns JA, Connolly SJ: Nonrheumatic atrial fibrillation: Risks of stroke and role of antithrombotic therapy. Circulation 1991;84:469.

Campbell RWF et al: Atrial fibrillation in the preexcitation syndrome. Am J Cardiol 1977;40:514.

Christie DJ, Aster RH: Drug-antibody-platelet interaction in quinine- and quinidine-induced thrombocytopenia. J Clin Invest 1982;70:989.

Connolly SJ: Canadian atrial fibrillation anticoagulation (CAFA) study. J Am Coll Cardiol 1991;18:349.

Coplen SE et al: Efficacy and safety of quinidine therapy for maintenance of sinus rhythm after cardioversion. Circulation 1990;82:1106.

Davies AB et al: Diagnostic value of thyrotropin releasing hormone in elderly patients with atrial fibrillation. Br Med J 1985;291:773.

Falk RH, Leavitt JI: Digoxin for atrial fibrillation: A drug whose time has gone? Ann Intern Med 1991;114:573.

Flegel KM, Shipley MJ, Rose G: Risk of stroke in nonrheumatic atrial fibrillation. Lancet 1987;1:526.

Forfar JC, Miller HC, Toft AD: Occult thyrotoxicosis: A correctable cause of "idiopathic" atrial fibrillation. Am J Cardiol 1979;44:9.

Giladi M et al: Is idiopathic atrial fibrillation caused by occult thyrotoxicosis? A study of one hundred consecutive patients with atrial fibrillation. Int J Cardiol 1991;30:309.

Grogan M et al: Left ventricular dysfunction due to atrial fibrillation in patients initially believed to have idiopathic dilated cardiomyopathy. Am J Cardiol 1992;69:1570.

Halperin JL, Hart RG: Atrial fibrillation and stroke: New ideas, persisting dilemmas. Stroke 1988;19:937.

Hinton RC et al: Influence of etiology of atrial fibrillation on incidence of systemic embolism. Am J Cardiol 1977;40:509.

Kannel WB et al: Epidemiologic features of chronic atrial fibrillation. N Engl J Med 1982;306:1018.

Klein HO, Kaplinsky E: Verapamil and digoxin: Their respective effects on atrial fibrillation and their interaction. Am J Cardiol 1982;50:894.

Kopecky SL et al: The natural history of lone atrial fibrillation: A population-based study over three decades. N Engl J Med 1987;317:669.

Leahey EB Jr et al: The effect of quinidine and other oral antiarrhythmic drugs on serum digoxin: A prospective study. Ann Intern Med 1980;92:605.

Mancini GBJ, Weinberg DM: Cardioversion of atrial

fibrillation: A retrospective analysis of the safety and value of anticoagulation. Cardiovasc Rev Rep 1990;11:18.

Manning WF et al: Pulsed Doppler evaluation of atrial mechanical function after electrical conversion of atrial fibrillation. J Am Coll Cardiol 1989;13:617.

Miles WM et al: Evaluation of the patient with wide QRS tachycardia. Med Clin North Am 1984;68:1015.

Morady F et al: Electrophysiologic testing in the management of patients with the Wolff-Parkinson-White syndrome and atrial fibrillation. Am J Cardiol 1983;51: 1623.

Normand JP et al: Comparative efficacy of short-acting and long-acting quinidine for maintenance of sinus rhythm after electrical conversion of atrial fibrillation. Br Heart J 1976;38:381.

Petersen P et al: Placebo-controlled, randomized trial of warfarin and aspirin for prevention of thromboembolic complications in chronic atrial fibrillation. (The Copenhagen AFASAK Study.) Lancet 1989;1:175.

Presti CF et al: Thyrotoxicosis, atrial fibrillation, and embolism revisited. Am Heart J 1989;117:976.

Rawles JM et al: Time of occurrence, duration, and ventricular rate of paroxysmal atrial fibrillation: The effect of digoxin. Br Heart J 1990;63:225.

Södermark T et al: Effect of quinidine on maintaining sinus rhythm after conversion of atrial fibrillation or flutter: A multicentre study from Stockholm. Br Heart J 1975;37:486.

SPAF Investigators: Stroke Prevention in Atrial Fibrillation Study. Circulation 1991;84:527.

Stein B et al: Should patients with atrial fibrillation be anticoagulated prior to and chronically following cardioversion? In: *Dilemmas in Clinical Cardiology.* Cheitlin MD (editor). Davis, 1990.

Steinberg JS et al: Efficacy of oral diltiazem to control ventricular response in chronic atrial fibrillation at rest and during exercise. J Am Coll Cardiol 1987;9:405.

Woeber K: Thyrotoxicosis and the heart. N Engl J Med 1992;327:94.

Wolf PA et al: Atrial fibrillation: A major contributor to stroke in the elderly. The Framingham study. Arch Intern Med 1987;147:1561.

Zipes DP, Prystowsky EN, Heger JJ: Amiodarone: Electrophysiologic actions, pharmacokinetics and clinical effects. J Am Coll Cardiol 1984;3:1059.

Ventricular Arrhythmias

Akhtar M: Clinical spectrum of ventricular tachycardia. Circulation 1990;82:1561.

Akhtar M et al: CAST and beyond: Implications of the Cardiac Arrhythmia Suppression Trial. Eur Heart J 1990;11:194.

Bär FW et al: Differential diagnosis of tachycardia with narrow QRS complex (shorter than 0.12 second). Am J Cardiol 1984;54:555.

Benditt DG, Pritchett EL, Gallagher JJ: Spectrum of regular tachycardias with wide QRS complexes in patients with accessory atrioventricular pathways. Am J Cardiol 1978;42:828.

Booth D, Popio KA, Gettes LS: Multiformity of induced unifocal ventricular premature beats in human subjects: Electrocardiographic and angiographic correlations. Am J Cardiol 1982;49:1643.

Caceres J et al: Sustained bundle branch reentry as a mechanism of clinical tachycardia. Circulation 1989;79:256.

The Cardiac Arrhythmia Suppression Trial (CAST) Investigators: Preliminary report: Effect of encainide and flecainide on mortality in a randomized trial of arrhythmia suppression after myocardial infarction. N Engl J Med 1989;321:406.

Falk RH: Proarrhythmia in patients treated for atrial fibrillation or flutter. Ann Intern Med 1992;117:141.

Fisher JD: Role of electrophysiologic testing in the diagnosis and treatment of patients with known and suspected bradycardias and tachycardias. Prog Cardiovasc Dis 1981;24:25.

Furberg CD: Effects of anti-arrhythmic drugs on myocardial infarction. Am J Cardiol 1983;53:32C.

Hinkle LE Jr, Carver ST, Stevens M: The frequency of asymptomatic disturbances of cardiac rhythm and conduction in middle-aged men. Am J Cardiol 1969;24: 629.

Holt PM et al: Right ventricular outflow tract tachycardia in patients without apparent structural heart disease. Int J Cardiol 1986;10:99.

January CT, Makielski JC: Triggered arrhythmias: New insights into basic mechanisms. Curr Opin Cardiol 1990;5:65.

Josephson ME: Antiarrhythmic agents and the danger of proarrhythmic events. Ann Intern Med 1989;111:191.

Kay GN et al: Torsade de pointes: The long-short initiating sequence and other clinical features: Observations in 32 patients. J Am Coll Cardiol 1983;2:806.

Kennedy HL et al: Coronary artery status of apparently healthy subjects with frequent and complex ventricular ectopy. Ann Intern Med 1980;92:179.

Kostis JB et al: Prognostic significance of ventricular ectopic activity in survivors of acute myocardial infarction: BHAT Study Group. J Am Coll Cardiol 1987;10: 231.

Lemery R et al: Nonischemic ventricular tachycardia: Clinical course and long-term follow-up in patients without clinically overt heart disease. Circulation 1989;79:990.

Levy D et al: Risk of ventricular arrhythmias in left ventricular hypertrophy: The Framingham Heart Study. Am J Cardiol 1987;60:560.

Lichtstein E et al: Relation between beta-adrenergic blocker use, various correlates of left ventricular function and the chance of developing congestive heart failure. J Am Coll Cardiol 1990;16:1327.

Lown B, DeSilva RA, Lenson R: Roles of psychologic stress and autonomic nervous system changes in provocation of ventricular premature complexes. Am J Cardiol 1978;41:979.

Lown B, Temte JV, Arter WJ: Ventricular tachyarrhythmias: Clinical aspects. Circulation 1973;47: 1364.

Lown B, Wolf MA: Approaches to sudden death from coronary heart disease. Circulation 1971;44:130.

Marcus FI et al: Right ventricular dysplasia: A report of 24 adult cases. Circulation 1982;65:384.

Marriott HJL: Differential diagnosis of supraventricular and ventricular tachycardia. Geriatrics 1970;25:91.

Mehta, D et al: Echocardiographic and histologic evaluation of the right ventricle in ventricular tachycardia of left bundle branch block morphology without overt cardiac abnormality. Am J Cardiol 1989;63:939.

Moss AJ et al: The long QT syndrome: Prospective longitudinal study of 328 families. Circulation 1991;84:1136.

Moss AJ, Robinson J: Clinical patterns of the long QT syndrome. Circulation 1992;85:I–140.

Nogami A et al: Combined used of time and frequency domain variables in signal-averaged ECG as a predictor of inducible sustained monomorphic ventricular tachycardia in myocardial infarction. Circulation 1992;86:780.

Norris RM, Mercer CJ: Significance of idioventricular rhythms in acute myocardial infarction. Prog Cardiovasc Dis 1974;16:455.

Ohe T et al: Idiopathic sustained left ventricular tachycardia: Clinical and electrophysiologic characteristics. Circulation 1988;77:560.

Podrid PJ et al: Prognostic implications of asymptomatic ventricular arrhythmia. Cardiovasc Rev Rep 1988;9:49.

Reynolds EW, Vander Ark CR: Quinidine syncope and the delayed repolarization syndromes. Mod Concepts Cardiovasc Dis 1976;45:117.

Rodstein M, Wolloch L, Gubner RS: Mortality study of the significance of extra-systoles in an insured population. Circulation 1971;44:617.

Ruberman W et al: Ventricular premature beats and mortality after myocardial infarction. N Engl J Med 1977;297:750.

Ryan M, Lown B, Horn H: Comparison of ventricular ectopic activity during 24-hour monitoring and exercise testing in patients with coronary heart disease. N Engl J Med 1975;292:224.

Stratmann HG, Kennedy HL: Torsades de pointes associated with drugs and toxins: Recognition and management. Am Heart J 1987;113:1470.

Van Durme JP: Tachyarrhythmias and transient cerebral ischemic attacks. Am Heart J 1975;89:538.

Vincent GM et al: The spectrum of symptoms and QT intervals in carriers of the gene for the long-QT syndrome. N Engl J Med 1992;327:846.

Wellens HJJ, Fritz WHM, Lie KI: The value of the electrocardiogram in the differential diagnosis of a tachycardia with a widened QRS complex. Am J Med 1978;64:27.

Yoon MS, Han J, Fabregas RA: Effect of ventricular aberrancy on fibrillation threshold. Am Heart J 1975;89:599.

Treatment of Ventricular Arrhythmias

Antman EM, Berlin JA: Declining incidence of ventricular fibrillation in pericardial infection: Implications for the prophylactic use of lidocaine. Circulation 1992;86:764.

Bauman JL et al: Long-term therapy with disopyramide phosphate: Side effects and effectiveness. Am Heart J 1986;111:654.

Boissel J-P et al: Efficacy of acebutolol after acute myocardial infarction (the APSI Trial). Am J Cardiol 1990;66:24C.

Bourke JP et al: Surgery for control of recurrent life-threatening ventricular tachyarrhythmias within 2 months of myocardial infarction. J Am Coll Cardiol 1990;16:42.

Breithardt G, Borggrefe M: Recent advances in the identification of patients at risk of ventricular tachyarrhythmias: Role of ventricular late potentials. Circulation 1987;75:1091.

Burkart F et al: Effect of antiarrhythmic therapy on mortality in survivors of myocardial infarction with asymptomatic complex ventricular arrhythmias: Basel Antiarrhythmia Study of Infarct Survival (BASIS). J Am Coll Cardiol 1990;16:1711.

Connolly SJ, Yusuf S: Evaluation of the inflatable cardioverter defibrillator in survivors of cardiac arrest: The need for randomized trials. Am J Cardiol 1992;69:959.

Cox JL: Patient selection criteria and results of surgery for refractory ischemic ventricular tachycardia. Circulation 1989;79(Suppl I):I–163.

DiBianco R: Chronic ventricular arrhythmias: Which drug for which patient? Am J Cardiol 1988;61:83A.

Echt DS et al: Mortality and morbidity in patients receiving encainide, flecainide, or placebo. N Engl J Med 1991;324:781.

The Electrophysiologic Study Versus Electrocardiographic Monitoring (ESVEM) Investigators: Electrophysiologic monitoring for selection of antiarrhythmic therapy of ventricular tachyarrhythmias. Circulation 1989;79:1354.

Epstein LM, Scheinman MM: Should asymptomatic patients with coronary artery disease and nonsustained ventricular tachycardia be treated with antiarrhythmic drugs? In: *Dilemmas in Clinical Cardiology.* Cheitlin MD (editor). Davis, 1990.

Evans JT et al: The Percutaneous Cardiac Mapping and Ablation Registry: Final summary of results. PACE 1988;11:1621.

Evans SJL et al: High dose oral amiodarone loading: Electrophysiologic effect and clinical tolerance. J Am Coll Cardiol 1992;19:169.

Fromer M et al: Efficacy of automatic multinodal device therapy for ventricular tachyarrhythmias as delivered by a new inflatable pacing cardioverter-defibrillator. Circulation 1992;86:363.

Gabry MD et al: Automatic implantable cardioverter-defibrillator: Patient survival, battery longevity and shock delivery analysis. J Am Coll Cardiol 1987;9:1349.

Gallagher JJ et al: Surgical treatment of arrhythmias. Am J Cardiol 1988;61:27A.

Gallagher JJ et al: Techniques of intraoperative electrophysiologic mapping. Am J Cardiol 1982;49:221.

Garan H et al: Perioperative and long-term results after electrophysiologically directed ventricular surgery for recurrent ventricular tachycardia. J Am Coll Cardiol 1986;8:201.

Garson A et al: Amiodarone treatment of critical arrhythmias in children and young adults. J Am Coll Cardiol 1984;4:749.

Goldschlager N, Cake D, Cohn K: Exercise-induced ventricular arrhythmias in patients with coronary artery disease: Their relation to angiographic findings. Am J Cardiol 1973;31:434.

Gomes JA et al: A new noninvasive index to predict sustained ventricular tachycardia and sudden death in the first year after myocardial infarction: Based on signal-averaged electrocardiogram, radionuclide ejection fraction and Holter monitoring. J Am Coll Cardiol 1987;10:349.

Graboys TB et al: Long-term survival of patients with malignant ventricular arrhythmia treated with antiarrhythmic drugs. Am J Cardiol 1982;50:437.

Guiraudon G et al: Encircling endocardial ventriculotomy: A new surgical treatment for life-threatening ventricular tachycardias resistant to medical treatment following myocardial infarction. Ann Thorac Surg 1978;26:438.

Haines DE et al: Surgical ablation of ventricular tachycardia with sequential map-guided subendocardial resection: Electrophysiologic assessment and long-term follow-up. Circulation 1988;77:131.

Hallstrom AP et al: An antiarrhythmic drug experience in 941 patients resuscitated from a mitral cardiac arrest between 1970 and 1985. Am J Cardiol 1991;68:1025.

Hartzler GO: Treatment of recurrent ventricular tachycardia by patient-activated radiofrequency ventricular stimulation. Mayo Clin Proc 1979;54:75.

Hess DS, Morady F, Scheinman MM: Electrophysiologic testing in the evaluation of patients with syncope of undetermined origin. Am J Cardiol 1982;50:1309.

Hohnloser SH et al: Short-and long-term therapy with tocainide for malignant ventricular tachyarrhythmias. Circulation 1986;73:143.

Horowitz LN, Josephson ME, Kastor JA: Intracardiac electrophysiologic studies as a method for thc optimization of drug therapy in chronic ventricular arrhythmia. Prog Cardiovasc Dis (Sept–Oct) 1980;23:81.

Horowitz LN, Zipes DP (editors): Perspectives on proarrhythmia. (Symposium.) Am J Cardiol 1987;59:1E. .

Josephson ME: Treatment of ventricular arrhythmias after myocardial infarction. Circulation 1986;74:653.

Josephson ME et al: Role of catheter mapping in the preoperative evaluation of ventricular tachycardia. Am J Cardiol 1982;49:207.

Keren A, Tzivoni D: Magnesium therapy in ventricular arrhythmias. PACE 1990;13:937.

Kim SG et al: Influence of left ventricular function on outcome of patients treated with inflatable defibrillators. Circulation 1992;85:1304.

Kim SG et al: Rapid suppression of spontaneous ventricular arrhythmias during oral amiodarone loading. Ann Intern Med 1992;117:197.

Klein LS et al: Antitachycardia devices: Realities and promises. J Am Coll Cardiol 1991;18:1349.

Klein LS et al: Radiofrequency catheter ablation of ventricular tachycardia in patients without structural heart disease. Circulation 1992;85:1666.

Kreeger RW, Hammill SC: New antiarrhythmic drugs: Tocainide, mexiletine, flecainide, encainide, and amiodarone. Mayo Clin Proc 1987;62:1033.

Kupersmith J, Reder RF, Slater W: New antiarrhythmic drugs. Cardiovasc Rev Rep 1985;6:35.

Landymore RW et al: Surgical intervention in drug-resistant ventricular tachycardia. J Am Coll Cardiol 1990;16:37.

Marchlinski FE et al: The automatic implantable cardioverter-defibrillator: Efficacy, complications, and device failures. Ant Intern Med 1986;104:481.

Mason JW: Amiodarone. N Engl J Med 1987;316:455.

Mason JW, Winkle RA: Accuracy of the ventricular tachycardia-induction study for predicting long-term efficacy and inefficacy of antiarrhythmic drugs. N Engl J Med 1980;303:1073.

McGiffin DC et al: Relief of life-threatening ventricular tachycardia and survival after direct operations. Circulation 1987;76(Suppl V):V–93.

Miles WM et al: The implantable transvenous cardioverter: long-term efficacy and reproducible induction of ventricular tachycardia. Circulation 1986;74:518.

Mirowski M: The automatic implantable cardioverter-defibrillator: An overview. J Am Coll Cardiol 1985;6:461.

Mitchell LB et al: A randomized clinical trial of the noninvasive and invasive approaches to drug therapy of ventricular tachycardia. N Engl J Med 1987;317:1681.

Morady F et al: Catheter ablation of ventricular tachycardia with intracardiac shocks: Results in 33 patients. Circulation 1987;75:1037.

Morady F et al: Intravenous amiodarone in the acute treatment of recurrent symptomatic ventricular tachycardia. Am J Cardiol 1983;51:156.

Morady F et al: A prevalent misconception regarding wide complex tachycardias. JAMA 1985;254:2790.

Morganroth J: Treatment of life-threatening ventricular tachycardia with encainide hydrochloride in patient with left ventricular dysfunction. Am J Cardiol 1988;62:571.

Morganroth J, Goin JE: Quinidine-related mortality in the short- to medium-term treatment of ventricular arrhythmias. Circulation 1991;84:1977.

Naccarelli GV et al: Pharmacological therapy of arrhythmias. In: *Cardiac Arrhythmias: A Practical Approach*. Nacarelli GV (editor). Futura, 1991.

Newman D et al: Survival after implantation of the cardioverter defibrillator. Am J Cardiol 1992;69:899.

Nguyen PT, Scheinman MM, Seger J: Polymorphous ventricular tachycardia: Clinical characterization, therapy, and the QT interval. Circulation 1986;74:340.

Odemuyiwa O et al: Differences between predictive characteristics of signal-averaged electrocardiographic variables for postinfarction sudden death and ventricular tachycardia. Am J Cardiol 1992;69:1186.

Opie LH: Drugs and the heart. 4. Antiarrhythmic agents. Lancet 1980;1:861.

Page PL et al: Surgical treatment of ventricular tachycardia: Regional cryoablation guided by computerized epicardial and endocardial mapping. Circulation 1989;80(Suppl I):I–124.

Pfisterer M et al: Beneficial effect of amiodarone on cardiac mortality in patients with asymptomatic complex ventricular arrhythmias after acute myocardial infarction and preserved but not impaired left ventricular function. Am J Cardiol 1992;69:1399.

Platia EV et al: Treatment of malignant ventricular arrhythmias with endocardial resection and implantation of the automatic cardioverter-defibrillator. N Engl J Med 1986;314:213.

Podrid PJ et al: Ethmozin: A new antiarrhythmic drug for suppressing ventricular premature complexes. Circulation 1980;61:450.

Pratt CM et al: Asymptomatic telephone ECG transmissions as an outpatient surveillance system of ventricular arrhythmias: Relationship to quantitative ambulatory ECG recordings. Am Heart J 1987;113:1.

Prystowsky EN (editor): Arrhythmia therapy: Controversies, directions and challenges. (Symposium.) Am J Cardiol 1988;61:1A.

Prystowsky EN et al: Clinical efficacy and electrophysiologic effects of encainide in patients with Wolff-Parkinson-White syndrome. Circulation 1984;69:278.

Puech P: Ectopic ventricular rhythms: Ventricular tachycardia and His bundle recordings. In: *His Bundle Electrocardiography and Clinical Electrophysiology.* Narula O (editor). Davis, 1975.

Reid PR et al: Clinical evaluation of the internal automatic cardioverter-defibrillator in survivors of sudden cardiac death. Am J Cardiol 1983;51:1608.

Rickenberger RL et al: Indications for electrophysiologic testing in patient with cardiac arrhythmias. In: *Cardiac Arrhythmias: A Practical Approach.* Naccarelli GV (editor). Futura, 1991.

Rosenbaum MS et al: Immediate reproducibility of electrically induced sustained monomorphic ventricular tachycardia before and during antiarrhythmic drug therapy. J Am Coll Cardiol 1991;17:133.

Saksena S, Camm AJ: Clinical investigation of implantable antitachycardia devices: Report of the Policy Conference of the North American Society of Pacing and Electrophysiology. J Am Coll Cardiol 1987;10:225.

Saksena S et al: Long-term multicenter experience with a second generation inflatable pacemaker-defibrillator in patients with malignant ventricular tachyarrhythmias. J Am Coll Cardiol 1992;19:490.

Scheinman MM et al: Current role of catheter ablative procedures in patient with cardiac arrhythmias. Circulation 1991;83:2146.

Scheinman MM: Nonpharmacologic treatment of life-threatening cardiac arrhythmias. Cardiovasc Rev Rep 1988;9:27.

Singer I et al: Pathologic findings related to the lead system and repeated defibrillations in patients with the automatic implantable cardioverter-defibrillator. J Am Coll Cardiol 1987;10:382.

Singh BN: Advantages of beta blockers versus antiarrhythmic agents and calcium antagonists in secondary prevention after myocardial infarction. Am J Cardiol 1990;16:9C.

Singh BN (moderator): Recent trends in the management of life-threatening ventricular arrhythmias. (Conference.) West J Med 1984;141:649.

Singh BN, Zipes DP (guest editors): The role of oral mexiletine in the management of ventricular arrhythmias.(Symposium.) Am Heart J 1984;107:1053.

Smith WM, Gallagher JJ: "Les torsades de pointes": An unusual ventricular arrhythmia. Ann Intern Med 1980;93:578.

Sung RJ et al: Electrophysiologic mechanism of exercise-induced sustained ventricular tachycardia. Am J Cardiol 1983;51:525.

Surawicz B: Prognosis of ventricular arrhythmias in relation to sudden cardiac death: Therapeutic implications. J Am Coll Cardiol 1987;10:435.

Tzivoni D et al: Treatment of torsade de pointes with magnesium sulfate. Circulation 1988;77:392.

Velebit V et al: Aggravation and provocation of ventricular arrhythmias by antiarrhythmic drugs. Circulation 1982;96:337.

Waldecker B et al: Importance of nodes of electrical termination of ventricular tachycardia for the selection of implantable antitachycardia devices. Am J Cardiol 1986;57:150.

Waldo AL, Arciniegas JG, Klein H: Surgical treatment of life-threatening ventricular arrhythmias: The role of intraoperative mapping and consideration of the presently available surgical techniques. Prog Cardiovasc Dis 1981;23:247.

Wellens HJ, Brugada P, Stevenson WG: Programmed electrical stimulation: Its role in the management of ventricular arrhythmias in coronary heart disease. Prog Cardiovasc Dis 1986;29:165.

Winkle RA: Ambulatory electrocardiography and the diagnosis, evaluation, and treatment of chronic ventricular arrhythmias. Prog Cardiovasc Dis 1980;23:99.

Winkle RA et al: Practical aspects of automatic cardioverter/defibrillator implantation. Am Heart J 1984;108:1335.

Woosley RL, Wood AJ, Roden DM: Encainide. N Engl J Med 1988;318:1107.

Zipes DP et al: Guidelines for clinical intracardiac electrophysiologic studies. Circulation 1989;80:1925.

Zipes DP (guest editor): Symposium on cardiac arrhythmias. (Two parts.) Med Clin North Am 1984;68:783, 1013.

Zipes DP, Rahimtoola SH (editors): State-of-the-art consensus conference on electrophysiologic testing in the diagnosis and treatment of patients with cardiac arrhythmias. Circulation 1987;75(Suppl 3):III–1.

Zipes DP, Troup PJ: New antiarrhythmic agents: Amiodarone, aprindine, disopyramide, ethmozin, mexiletine, tocainide, verapamil. Am J Cardiol 1978;41:1005.

Zoll PM, Linenthal AJ: Termination of refractory tachycardia by external countershock. Circulation 1962;25:596.

Ventricular Fibrillation & Sudden Death

Cobb LA, Werner JA, Trobaugh GB: Sudden cardiac death. 1. A decade's experience with out-of-hospital resuscitation. Mod Concepts Cardiovasc Dis 1980;49:31.

Cobb LA et al: Resuscitation from out-of-hospital ventricular fibrillation: Four year follow-up. Circulation 1975;52(Suppl 3):223.

Eldar M, Sauve MJ, Scheinman MM: Electrophysiologic testing and follow-up of patients with aborted sudden death. J Am Coll Cardiol 1987;10:291.

Freedman RA et al: Prognostic significance of arrhythmia inducibility or noninducibility at initial electrophysiologic study in survivors of cardiac arrest. Am J Cardiol 1988;61:578.

Guarnieri T et al: Success of chronic defibrillation and the role of antiarrhythmic drugs with the automatic implantable cardioverter/defibrillator. Am J Cardiol 1987;60:1061.

Lewis BH, Antman EM, Graboys TB: Detailed analysis of 24-hour ambulatory electrocardiographic recordings during ventricular fibrillation or torsade de pointes. J Am Coll Cardiol 1983;2:426.

Lie KI et al: Observations on patients with primary ventricular fibrillation complicating acute myocardial infarction. Circulation 1975;52:755.

Lown B, Verrier RL, Rabinowitz SH: Neural and psychologic mechanisms and the problem of sudden cardiac death. Am J Cardiol 1977;39:890.

Myerburg RJ et al: Clinical, electrophysiologic and hemodynamic profile of patients resuscitated from prehospital cardiac arrest. Am J Med 1980;68:568.

Standards and guidelines for cardiopulmonary resuscitation (CPR) and emergency cardiac care (ECC). JAMA 1986;255:2905.

Reid PR et al: Clinical evaluation of the internal automatic cardioverter-defibrillator in survivors of sudden cardiac death. Am J Cardiol 1983;51:1608.

Schaffer WA, Cobb LA: Recurrent ventricular fibrillation and modes of death in survivor of out-of-hospital ventricular fibrillation. N Engl J Med 1975;293:259.

Selzer A, Wray HW: Quinidine syncope: Paroxysmal ventricular fibrillation occurring during treatment of chronic atrial arrhythmias. Circulation 1964;30:17.

Swerdlow CD, Winkle RA, Mason JW: Determinants of survival in patients with ventricular tachyarrhythmias. N Engl J Med 1983;308:1486.

Weaver WD et al: Factors influencing survival after out-of-hospital cardiac arrest. J Am Coll Cardiol 1986;7:752.

Wilber DJ et al: Out-of-hospital cardiac arrest: Use of electrophysiologic testing in the prediction of long-term outcome. N Engl J Med 1988;318:19.

16 Infective Endocarditis

Infective endocarditis is infection of the endocardium, occurring on valve leaflets, congenital or acquired lesions, a prolapsed mitral valve, walls of the heart cavities, or tissue surrounding prosthetic valves. Infections of arteriovenous fistulas or the shunts used for renal dialysis are more properly called infective endarteritis (see Chapter 20). The term "infective endocarditis" is now generally preferred to "bacterial endocarditis," because many different microorganisms other than bacteria (fungi, rickettsiae, viruses, animal parasites) can also cause the disease.

The infection may be acute or subacute (chronic), depending largely on the susceptibility of the host, occurrence in intravenous drug abusers, and the virulence of the organism. Because an acute fulminant course may occur from disruption or rupture of any valve from any organism, some authorities do not organize their discussion of endocarditis around the distinction between acute or subacute endocarditis but around the differing characteristics of the organisms. However, we follow the distinction between acute and subacute endocarditis because of the differences in clinical course, as well as for historical reasons.

Subacute disease usually occurs in patients with an underlying cardiac abnormality and has a less traumatic clinical course than acute disease. Acute infection usually occurs in persons with normal hearts following intravenous drug abuse or cardiovascular surgery due to acute development of valve disease. Rapid destruction of valves and a fulminant clinical course follow unless antibiotic therapy is quickly administered.

Infective endocarditis is often an insidious disease not diagnosed during life that tends to occur in patients already acutely or chronically ill from other causes. Early diagnosis and effective antibiotic therapy are vital not only for eradication of infection but also to prevent or minimize damage to heart valves, which becomes more severe the longer infection is uncontrolled. Changing patterns of disease have necessitated changes in treatment regimens.

Complexity of Management

Infective endocarditis is one of the most difficult of all cardiac diseases to manage. Not only is the diagnosis often difficult, but the choice of antibiotic, its route of administration, and the assessment of its effects cause problems. Effective drug treatment requires penetration of the vegetation in order to reach the bacteria in sufficient concentration to kill them.

Surgical drainage in addition to antibiotics may be required for metastatic abscesses.

Close observation of the patient during therapy is essential because of the likelihood of development of acute heart failure due to acute valvular damage. Acute cardiac catastrophes, such as dislodgment of valve leaflets or prosthetic valves, perforation of valve cusps, rupture of aneurysms, or abscesses of the myocardium into other cardiac chambers with fistula formation—as well as the ever-present threat of serious systemic embolism—make the management of infective endocarditis a difficult and worrisome task. Since emergency cardiac surgery may become necessary at a few hours' notice, it is an advantage to treat the patient at a center where facilities and personnel for open heart surgery are available. The period during which the patient is at risk is long, because in some cases with infection the valve may be weakened but tearing and rupture may not occur until later, after the infection has been cured.

A. Benefits and Complications of Antibiotic Therapy: Before penicillin became available, subacute infective endocarditis was uniformly fatal within months to about 2 years. Acute infective endocarditis was rare, because patients with overwhelming septicemic infections did not live long enough to develop clinical manifestations of cardiac involvement, although vegetations were often seen on the heart valves at autopsy. Penicillin usually eradicated the infection but did not prevent damage to heart valves. Patients with preexisting valvular disease—even minimal disease—were likely to have increased incompetence following antibiotic treatment for subacute infection. Patients with acute infection were likely to suffer severe valvular incompetence following successful antibiotic therapy, leading to acute heart failure that was often fatal. Thus, prevention of valvular damage and surgical techniques for valvular repair have become almost as important as control of infection.

B. Differentiation of Acute From Subacute Infective Endocarditis: Although acute infective endocarditis is more fulminant, usually occurs in intravenous drug abusers, and requires more urgent treatment, it may be caused by organisms that in the past have produced subacute clinical pictures, and treatment of the two conditions is similar. The course of acute infective endocarditis is measured in days or weeks, rather than months as in subacute infective endocarditis. *Staphylococcus aureus* rather than *Streptococcus viridans* is most apt to be the responsible organism, and valve destruction and perforation are more likely to occur quickly, leading to rapidly developing cardiac failure. Prompt treatment with specific anti-infective drugs is essential. Surgical treatment is more often required, because rapid destruction of valves may occur. The prognosis is better in subacute than in acute infective endocarditis, because valve destruction occurs more slowly. Acute infective endocarditis may be overlooked because it frequently occurs on a normal valve, whereas subacute infective endocarditis often occurs on previously damaged valves.

PATHOGENESIS & PATHOLOGY

Hosts Likely to Develop Infective Endocarditis

Infective endocarditis most frequently occurs in patients who have undergone cardiac surgery, in those with prosthetic heart valves, in those receiving prolonged intravenous therapy, and in persons who are intravenous drug abusers. In this last group, the condition is apt to be acute and fulminant. It also occurs in patients with staphylococcal septicemia, atherosclerotic changes, immunosuppression due to drugs or disease (though endocarditis rarely develops as a result of immunosuppression alone, as in patients with AIDS), and in patients undergoing complex diagnostic or therapeutic procedures (eg, peritoneal dialysis, hemodialysis). In the latter, the disease is properly called endarteritis. The incidence of the disease is increasing owing to increased numbers of people in each of these groups.

A cooperative study of infective endocarditis by the American Heart Association in 1978 indicated that almost one-fourth of patients developed the infection following cardiovascular surgery, usually with insertion of a prosthetic valve or creation of a systemic to pulmonary artery shunt in congenital heart disease. One-fourth of these patients were about 20 years of age, and most of this group were intravenous drug abusers. There was no recognizable prior heart disease in a third of the patients. There were recurrent episodes in 10%. Three-fourths of the infected patients were alive 2 years following institution of antibiotic therapy (Kaplan, 1979).

The age distribution is bimodal, with younger individuals most apt to have acute infective endocarditis, because they are more likely to be intravenous drug abusers, and older ones subacute endocarditis, probably because older patients with valvular disease due to different causes have more opportunity to develop bacteremia—and therefore endocarditis—from a variety of causes. Current data indicate that the median age at onset of the subacute cases is 45 years, that 25% of patients are over 60 years, and that onset before age 20 is less frequent.

Microorganisms Causing Infective Endocarditis

Microorganisms in the bloodstream may be deposited on damaged, roughened valves, such as congenital or rheumatic lesions; the organisms become enmeshed in deposits of fibrin and platelets on the endothelium of the valve to form irregular vegetations. The pathogens most often responsible for infective endocarditis are those with surface capsules which make their surfaces "sticky." This is a characteristic of streptococci and staphylococci. *E coli* and other gram-negative organisms do not have this property and therefore are much less likely to cause infective endocarditis. Pathogens may invade the endothelium but are usually relatively superficial. A typical infected rheumatic aortic valve is seen in Figure 16–1. The microorganisms multiply within the fibrin-platelet matrix to incredible concentrations. Products of their metabolism act to disrupt the connective tissue of the valve, thus weakening the collagen structure, which under the hemodynamic stresses acting on the valve results in tearing of the valve, leading to valvular incompetence. In patients who have died of infective endocarditis, autopsy can reveal local attempts at repair and local macrophage infiltration that were not adequate to clear the infection.

Widespread, sometimes almost casual use of antibiotics has led to an increase in cases involving drug-resistant microorganisms rarely seen in the past. Fewer cases are now caused by pathogens highly susceptible to antibiotics. In the past, *Streptococcus viridans* and group D streptococci were responsible for 90–95% of cases of subacute infective endocarditis, but these organisms are now responsible for only about one-third of all cases of infective endocarditis. The relative frequency of infection with *Staphylococcus aureus*, *Staphylococcus epidermidis*, *Enterococcus faecalis*, gram-negative organisms both aerobic and anaerobic, and fungi is increasing. Each of these organisms may cause either acute or subacute endocarditis. Infections with certain organisms (eg, *Bacteroides*) are still infrequent, but all rare organisms must now be considered possible causative agents (Wilson, 1977). Subacute infection of chronically diseased rheumatic valves due to *S viridans* is less common now. More frequently seen is infection of calcified valves in elderly patients or in patients with prosthetic valves.

Vegetations vary in size and may become quite large and friable in fungal infections. They may occur on the downstream side of the jet, in an area of low pressure. Small fragments may break off, causing embolization to the systemic circulation in left-sided mitral or aortic valve lesions and to the lungs in right-sided lesions, usually on the tricuspid valve. Embolism is responsible for many of the clinical features.

A precipitating cause of infection should always be sought. Dental procedures (extraction or deep scaling), recent instrumentation of the genitourinary tract,

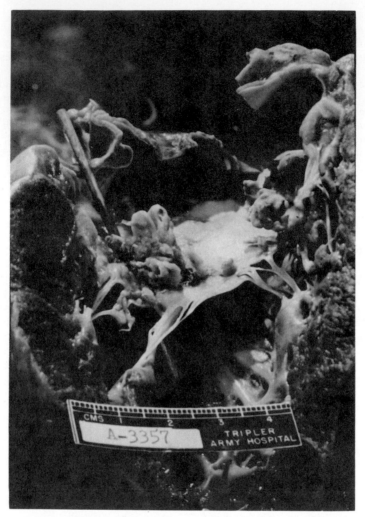

Figure 16–1. Vegetation on the aortic leaflet of the mitral valve in a patient who died with staphylococcal infective endocarditis. The probe is through a perforation in the leaflet.

gynecologic procedures, or inflammatory gastrointestinal disease sometimes precedes the illness. In about half of subacute cases, no cause can be established; fewer cases of acute endocarditis are of unknown cause.

Involvement of Heart Valves

A. Normal Valves: Bacteria and fungi from intravenous injection of infective material (as in intravenous drug abuse), from indwelling venous catheters, from infection of arteriovenous shunts, or from bacteria that gain entry during renal dialysis may settle on normal valves. As the infective organisms become embedded in the fibrin-platelet matrix, further growth of organisms enlarges the vegetation and makes the organisms inaccessible to normal cellular host defenses. Massive bacteremia and infection may

weaken or tear the valves, causing perforation of the leaflets, progressive gross incompetence or destruction of the involved valves, and rapid development or worsening of cardiac failure.

The tricuspid valve is involved almost exclusively in intravenous drug users. The frequency of left- or right-sided lesions in such patients varies in different cities and institutions.

B. Diseased Valves: Endocarditis is more apt to occur in patients with mild to moderate valvular disease. Pulmonary stenosis, patent ductus arteriosus, ventricular septal defect, and bicuspid aortic valve are the most common congenital cardiac lesions in which endocarditis develops. Infective endocarditis is rare in atrial septal defect (especially in ostium secundum defects) and severe mitral stenosis and infrequent in patients with established atrial fibrillation. Mitral valve prolapse is being seen more frequently as the site of endocarditis, although endocarditis is rare in the overall population with mitral valve prolapse.

Pathogenesis

The clinical picture of infective endocarditis arises from the consequences of infection of a cardiac valve:

(1) Infection causes inflammation, fever, malaise, and leukocytosis and an increase in acute phase reactants such as C-reactive proteins. Eventually, the anemia of chronic disease results.

(2) The presence of a foreign antigen stimulates antibody formation, and binding complement results in immune complex injury to basement membranes in the kidneys and capillaries, resulting in glomerulonephritis.

(3) Disruption of the valve results in valvular incompetence and eventually congestive heart failure.

(4) Vegetations embolize, causing systemic and pulmonary emboli and metastatic infection.

CLINICAL FEATURES

1. SUBACUTE INFECTIVE ENDOCARDITIS

Diagnosis

The onset of endocarditis may be slow and insidious, and unless one searches for infections due to bacteria or fungi in every patient with fever and valvular lesions, the diagnosis can be missed for months. The presenting symptoms are nonspecific and are often attributed to a febrile illness (eg, "flu"), with fever, malaise, arthralgia, fatigue, and anemia. If short-term antibiotic treatment is given, the clinical picture is that of recurrent "flu." In subacute cases, left-sided valvular involvement is more frequent than right-sided involvement; by contrast, in acute endocarditis, right-sided valvular involvement may occur as an isolated lesion or in combination with left-sided lesions.

The diagnostic features of endocarditis are given below. If the diagnosis is suspected, blood cultures must be obtained. The diagnosis may be difficult if antibiotics have been given earlier.

A. Fever: Subacute endocarditis is an important cause of fever of unknown origin in patients in whom cardiac disease is overlooked. Fever is the most frequent presenting sign and may appear without apparent predisposing cause or may follow a surgical procedure. Prostatic and other urogenital operations in men and dilation and curettage of the uterus, abortion, and other gynecologic procedures in women are sometimes precursors of endocarditis. Weakness, malaise, and loss of weight without fever may occur in debilitated or elderly patients, especially if antibiotics have been given or sometimes because of renal failure secondary to endocarditis. Fever may be sub-

tle with some microorganisms, perhaps being present only in the afternoon or even disappearing for several days in sequence, only to recur. The symptoms may be overlooked and the diagnosis made only at autopsy. In the elderly patient, endocarditis is often missed despite the fever because systolic murmurs are common and the fever may be less obvious or even absent. In these patients, unexplained systemic embolism, anemia, renal failure, confusion, or dementia should suggest the presence of endocarditis. Blood cultures should be obtained to exclude the diagnosis.

B. Emboli: The presenting symptom may be acute systemic embolism (especially to the brain, spleen, or kidney), which may occur at any time during the course of the disease. Emboli are usually small except in fungal or *Serratia* infections and may produce only microscopic hematuria or petechiae. Osler's nodes are painful erythematous nodules on the skin, chiefly of the hands and feet. These cutaneous manifestations are probably caused by minute emboli, or they might be due to an immune mechanism with vasculitis. Nontender plaques on the soles of the feet and the palms of the hands (Janeway's lesion) are probably a deposit of immune complexes with inflammation or are due to arteriolitis. Emboli to the systemic circulation are rare in right-sided endocarditis; the right-sided manifestations are recurrent pulmonary infiltrates, pneumonia, or pulmonary embolism.

1. Small emboli— In left-sided lesions, emboli to the skin may produce splinter hemorrhages in the nails of the fingers or toes (but these may occur in persons doing manual labor). Petechiae (usually on the conjunctiva or hard palate or around the neck and upper trunk) are more definite evidence of embolism. At first they are red and small, but over a period of days they become brown and gradually fade. Hemorrhagic areas with white centers may be seen in the fundi owing to emboli in the nerve fiber retinal layer (Roth spots). Emboli to the kidney may cause flank pain or hematuria.

2. Large emboli— Large emboli may involve (1) the cerebral arteries, causing hemiplegia, other central nervous system deficit, neurologic syndromes including headache, psychiatric symptoms, confusion, or sterile meningitis; (2) the coronary arteries, resulting in acute myocardial infarction; or (3) the vasa vasorum, leading to mycotic aneurysms. Mycotic aneurysms may appear anywhere, often in branches of the renal artery and cerebral vessels. Rupture is infrequent, and these lesions are often missed.

C. Septic Abscesses: If staphylococci are the infecting organisms in either acute or subacute cases, septic abscesses may develop, especially in the liver, heart, kidney, brain, and spleen. Septic abscesses may contribute to continued fever and require surgical incision even though the organisms on the endocardium of the valves have been eradicated. Abscesses around valve rings may cause so-called ring abscesses, which may involve the atrioventricular node, causing atrioventricular block and even Stokes-Adams attacks. Surgery is usually necessary in these cases.

D. Splenomegaly and Clubbed Fingers: These are usually late signs in untreated patients and, although they were common in the preantibiotic era, are much less common today (approximately 10% of cases). As in any systemic infection, splenomegaly may occur, although it is less frequent when antibiotic therapy is given early in the course of the disease.

E. Immune Complex Nephritis and Renal Emboli: Glomerulonephritis and renal failure frequently occur in infective endocarditis and were formerly thought to be embolic in origin. However, renal lesions are now usually considered to be due to the deposit of antigen-antibody complexes and complement on the glomerular basement membrane. The antigen in glomerular deposits corresponds to the organism found in blood cultures. Petechiae can be due also to immune complex disease.

F. Anemia: Normocytic anemia is common, especially in long-standing infection, and probably accounts in part for the weakness and lassitude seen in patients with chronic infective endocarditis.

G. Cardiac Findings: Symptoms of heart disease such as dyspnea or palpitations develop late in subacute (in contrast to acute) infective endocarditis, and the cardiac origin of the illness may only be suspected if a valvular lesion or murmurs are present or if embolic manifestations appear. Left heart failure is the rule in subacute cases, because right-sided valvular lesions are infrequent, in contrast to acute endocarditis (see below).

In subacute infective endocarditis, a murmur is almost always present, either because of previous valvular disease or as a result of valvular insufficiency due to the infective endocarditis. The valve involvement is usually mild, and patients may not know they have a cardiac lesion. Careful search for such a lesion is mandatory in suspicious cases.

Changing murmurs occur but are rarely helpful in the diagnosis of subacute infective endocarditis, because the murmurs are often due in large part to anemia, tachycardia, or other hemodynamic variables. The abrupt appearance of a diastolic murmur, such as that of aortic insufficiency, is more helpful in diagnosis of infective endocarditis.

Valvular diseases that have become more important as predisposing factors in infective endocarditis are mitral valve prolapse and mitral and aortic calcification in elderly people. The patients with mitral valve prolapse who are most predisposed to infective endocarditis are those with the murmur of mitral regurgitation and the thickened myxomatous valve. This disease can be recognized by echocardiography, as can other predisposing valve diseases such as rheumatic valvular insufficiency and bicuspid aortic valve. Echocardiography may also be helpful in recognizing

valvular vegetations (> 2–3 mm), and especially if they are large, as in fungal infections, and are mobile and protruding into the cardiac chamber.

Cardiac failure formerly was a late occurrence, as was the development of atrial fibrillation. Untreated patients often died of infection before cardiac failure could develop. In subacute cases, cardiac failure may not occur until months after bacteriologic cure, as infection heals and valve lesions worsen (especially aortic valve lesions). Pericarditis is infrequent but can result either as an irritative phenomenon or, disastrously, as a purulent pericarditis.

Laboratory Findings:
Blood Cultures

In 90–95% of cases, definitive diagnosis is based on positive blood culture. Organisms are discharged into the circulation independently of the time of the fever. Only 3–5% of cases of infective endocarditis are culture-negative.

Important principles regarding blood cultures for investigation of infective endocarditis are as follows:

(1) For subacute cases, three separate cultures from different veins should be obtained over a period of several hours.

(2) Both aerobic and anaerobic bacteria and fungi should be sought with appropriate techniques. When cultures remain negative, consultation should be obtained from the microbiologist concerning the use of special cultures (special media, environments). Involving the bacteriologist as a colleague results in a higher yield of positive cultures.

(3) The cultures must be incubated long enough (2–3 weeks) to allow slow-growing organisms to emerge, and appropriate subcultures must be performed. Venous blood is adequate.

(4) At least two cultures should yield the same organism to rule out contamination.

(5) Blood cultures must be obtained before antibiotics are started. Alternatively, antimicrobials should be stopped for 3–7 days before blood is drawn for cultures.

(6) If cultures are positive, the sensitivity of the organism to various antibiotics, singly and in combination, should be determined as a guide to treatment (see below). Bactericidal effects are essential.

Echocardiography

Echocardiography is extremely valuable in determining what valve is involved and the severity of the regurgitation. Doppler valvular regurgitation can be detected before a regurgitant murmur can be detected. In patients presenting early, after only a few days of infection, there may be no pathologic murmur present. Valvular disruption can take up to 10 days to 2 weeks to occur, and if a vegetation can be detected, the diagnosis of infective endocarditis can be made early. Vegetations larger than 2 mm can be detected in over 80% of patients with infective endocarditis.

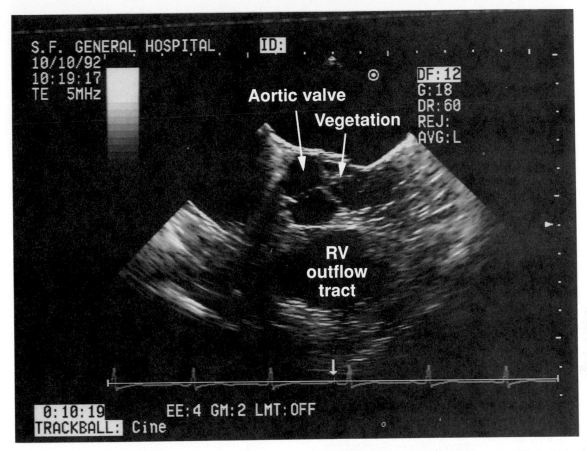

Figure 16–2. Transesophageal echocardiogram at the level of the aortic valve in a 66-year-old woman with staphylococcal septicemia showing a vegetation in the left posterior aortic cusp. The transthoracic echocardiogram was normal.

The presence of vegetations increases the risk of death, congestive heart failure, and embolism and the frequency with which patients are sent to surgery (Buda, 1986). In one study, the incidence of complications listed above was significantly increased depending on the mobility of the vegetation and the presence of extravalvular extension of the infection. Contrary to other studies, vegetative size was not significantly related to complications in this study (Sanfillipo, 1989).

Transesophageal echocardiography can provide a detailed magnified view of the left atrium, mitral valve, and aortic valve and the left ventricular outflow tract. Since the transducer is posterior to the heart and the echoes are not absorbed by other structures, valvular regurgitation and vegetations can be seen that cannot be detected by transthoracic echocardiography (Figure 16–2).

Transesophageal echocardiography is particularly indicated when infective endocarditis is suspected but the transthoracic echocardiogram is normal. It is also indicated where a ring abscess must be ruled out—ie, in the majority of patients with aortic valve endocar-

ditis or where endocarditis is present in a patient with a prosthetic valve (Bansal, 1992; Zabalgoitia, 1992).

2. ACUTE INFECTIVE ENDOCARDITIS

This section emphasizes the differences between acute and subacute endocarditis, including the causative organisms, the involved valves, and the hemodynamic effects.

Diagnosis

The infection is apt to be more abrupt, with higher fever, chills, and the presence of septic abscesses, because the predominant organism is often *S aureus* (about 90% of cases in intravenous drug abusers). The symptoms of infection usually predominate, and organisms are more easily cultured and identified than in subacute cases. However, when the lesion is on the tricuspid valve (which is common in acute and uncommon in subacute cases), pulmonary complications of "pneumonia," pulmonary embolism, and pulmonary abscess are dominant. X-rays of the chest

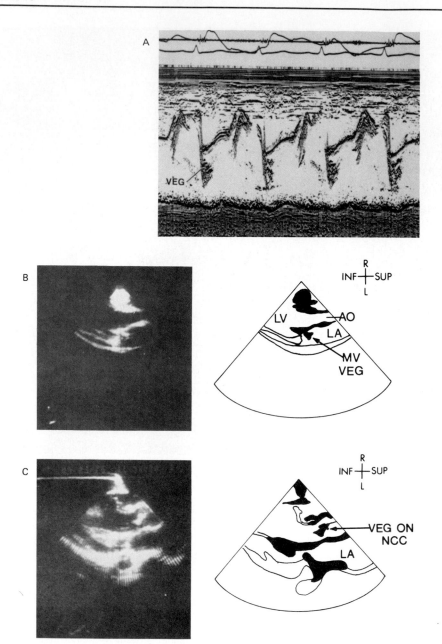

Figure 16–3 (above and at right). **A:** Dense echoes below the tricuspid valve in a patient with acute endocarditis of the tricuspid valve. M mode echocardiogram. (VEG, vegetation.) (Courtesy of NB Schiller.) **B:** Vegetation (VEG) on the mitral valve (MV). Real-time two-dimensional echocardiogram. (LV, left ventricle; AO, aorta; LA, left atrium.) (Courtesy of NB Schiller and NH Silverman.) **C:** Vegetation (VEG) on the aortic valve. (NCC, noncoronary cusp; LA, left atrium.) Real time two-dimensional echocardiogram. (Courtesy of NB Schiller and NH Silverman.) **D:** Vegetation on the aortic valve shown with anatomic lesion at autopsy. M mode echocardiogram. (CW, chest wall; RVAW, right ventricular anterior wall; RVO, right ventricular outflow tract.) (Reproduced, with permission of the American Heart Association, Inc., from Hirschfeld DS, Schiller N: Localization of aortic valve vegetations by echocardiography. Circulation 1976;53:280.)

reveal pleural effusions and changing pulmonary infiltrates of variable size and shape that may recur. There are geographic differences with respect to both the infecting organisms and the valves involved.

A. Emboli: In fungal endocarditis, emboli are more frequent and can be large and disabling. Cerebral embolism may produce hemiplegia, and the possibility of endocarditis must always be considered in patients who develop acute stroke. The lower frequency of systemic embolism in acute infective endo-

D

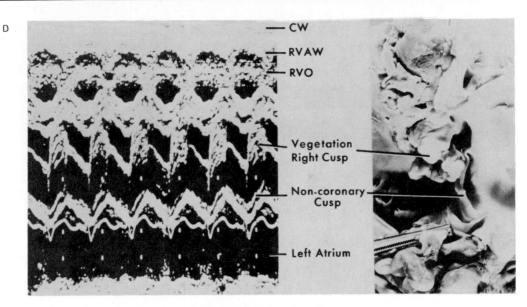

CW
RVAW
RVO

Vegetation
Right Cusp

Non-coronary
Cusp

Left Atrium

Figure 16–3 (Continued)

carditis is due to the frequency of right-sided lesions as well as to the rapid downhill course.

B. Cardiac Findings:

1. Changing murmurs and valve findings– The frequency with which acute infective endocarditis occurs on normal cardiac valves makes serial examination more rewarding than in subacute endocarditis. Murmurs may be absent at the onset of acute infective endocarditis, but valve lesions may result in gross insufficiency of the involved valve even though the infection is controlled by antibiotic therapy. With left-sided lesions, the murmurs of valvular regurgitation may be absent at the onset but eventually occur, almost always within 2 weeks of the onset of the disease. With tricuspid valve involvement, a typical regurgitant murmur may never develop.

The development of murmurs and evidence of valvular involvement may be noted if the patient is under close observation as the vegetations become larger. This is especially true of tricuspid insufficiency in heroin addicts. The progressive appearance and lengthening of a tricuspid systolic murmur can be noted and are made louder by inspiration as right atrial inflow increases. A right-sided gallop rhythm may appear, as may the progressive development of a prominent *v* wave in the jugular venous pulse and enlargement of a tender, pulsating liver, with right-sided failure. Valvular vegetations can be demonstrated by echocardiography (Figure 16–3). When acute infective endocarditis involves the aortic valve, the diastolic murmur may be long and soft and the first sound may be soft because of early closure of the mitral valve (see below). The diastolic pressure may be maintained by reflex peripheral arteriolar vasoconstriction, and early mitral valve closure may be a sign of increasing aortic insufficiency (Figure 16–4). As the magnitude of the aortic regurgitant flow increases, there is a rapid early diastolic rise in left ventricular pressure and left atrial pressure before the onset of systole, are a prominent Austin Flint diastolic murmur (see Chapter 13). If hemodynamic measurements are made, the crossover of left ventricular end-diastolic pressure and left atrial pressure precedes the Q wave of the ECG instead of slightly following it at the peak or downstroke of the R wave. Early closure of the mitral valve can be clearly demonstrated on echocardiography, when the anterior and posterior leaflets approximate each other well before the onset of the Q wave of the ECG with a normal PR interval (Figure 16–5). The presence and severity of aortic incompetence can be evaluated by two-dimensional echocardiography with Doppler. Color Doppler helps in visualizing the area of the left ventricular outflow tract disturbed by increased regurgitant velocity and turbulence. By continuous Doppler, the shape of the regurgitant high-velocity jet gives some clue to the severity of the leak. As the regurgitation becomes more severe, the pressure in the aorta in diastole approaches the pressure in the left ventricle. The gradient between aorta and left ventricle therefore decreases rapidly. This is mirrored by the shape of the jet, which drops off rapidly from high to low velocity during diastole. This ominous sign is a harbinger of severe left ventricular failure. The magnitude of the acute aortic insufficiency can also be shown by supra-aortic cineangiography, which shows the left ventricle fully opacified in a single beat of the regurgitant flow.

2. Cardiac failure– Cardiac failure is the most feared complication of acute infective endocarditis and may occur with startling rapidity in left-sided

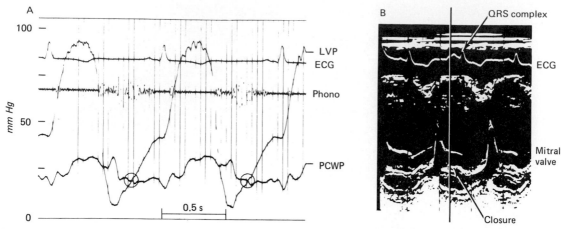

Figure 16–4. A: Early closure of the mitral valve. Simultaneous ECG, left ventricular pressure (LVP) and pulmonary capillary wedge pressure (PCWP), and phonocardiogram. Mitral valve closure (circled) occurs when LVP exceeds PCWP, clearly preceding electrocardiographic QRS complex. Phonocardiogram obtained at the cardiac apex demonstrates a middiastolic Austin Flint murmur. (Adapted and reproduced, with permission of the American Heart Association, Inc., from Botvinick EH et al: Echocardiographic demonstration of early mitral valve closure in severe aortic insufficiency: Its clinical implications. Circulation 1975;51:836.) **B:** Echocardiogram showing mitral valve closure **(line)** preceding the QRS complex. (Courtesy of NB Schiller.)

lesions, whether mitral or aortic. One cannot use the width of the pulse pressure, the loudness of the murmur, or the size of the left ventricle as a guide to the severity or imminence of left ventricular failure. With sudden rupture of the valve, the aortic diastolic pressure falls to 50–60 mm Hg and equilibrates with the markedly elevated diastolic pressure in the left ventricle. The diastolic murmur is therefore short, and with tachycardia it may be inaudible. The left ventricle is often only slightly enlarged, and the ECG may not reveal left ventricular hypertrophy in acute as compared to chronic aortic insufficiency because of the

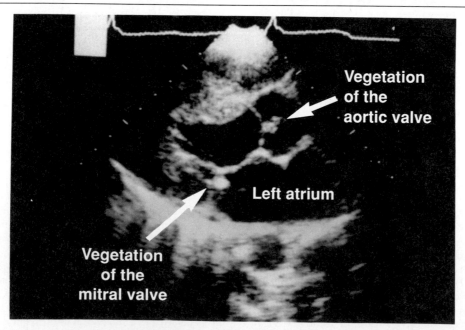

Figure 16–5. Two-dimensional echocardiogram. Parasternal long axis view showing vegetation of the aortic valve and the mitral valve in a patient with staphylococcal infective endocarditis involving both valves. Picture taken in diastole.

rapid development of aortic or mitral insufficiency (see Chapter 13).

Symptoms of pulmonary edema and echocardiographic evidence of marked early closure of a mitral valve lead the physician to suspect perforation or destruction of the aortic valve and indicate the need for valve replacement. Vigorous medical treatment may be needed while the infection subsides so that the sutures will hold. The hazard of death is so imminent that a prosthetic valve must be inserted without substantial delay. Because of the low perfusion pressure gradient across the myocardium as well as the increased myocardial oxygen demand, myocardial ischemia is present and may result in sudden death. In these cases, it may still be necessary to maintain vigorous medical treatment for 12–24 hours before replacing the valve. Careful judgment is required to determine the timing of operation if cardiac failure worsens despite control of the infection.

3. Ventricular septum and muscle involvement– The infection on the aortic valve may spread to the ventricular septum, and abscesses may develop and rupture into the right heart or may interfere with conduction of the cardiac impulse and cause atrioventricular block with or without syncope.

4. Septic abscesses– Septic abscesses can be suspected if there is sudden development of atrioventricular block, hemiblock, or bundle branch block (Figures 16–6 and 16–7). Mitral valve infections may cause septic abscesses of the papillary muscles or destruction of the mitral ring, resulting in flail mitral valves that require prompt surgical correction.

DIFFERENTIAL DIAGNOSIS

Infective endocarditis must be differentiated from all other causes of prolonged and obscure fever. The diagnosis is based on a positive blood culture in conjunction with the presence of a valve lesion and the absence of diagnostic signs or tests supporting an alternative diagnosis. The diagnosis should be made presumptively in any patient with an organic murmur and unexplained fever persisting for over 1 week. This combination is an indication for drawing blood for culture. Infection, neoplasm, and connective tissue disorders are the most common causes of fever of unknown origin (40%, 20%, and 20%, respectively), and these must be excluded.

The major difficulty in diagnosis occurs when blood cultures are negative, which means that reliance must be placed on associated diagnostic features. This emphasizes the importance of optimally obtained and examined blood cultures. In difficult cases, two-dimensional or transesophageal echocardiograms may reveal vegetations, establishing the diagnosis.

Transesophageal echo-Doppler has proved to be

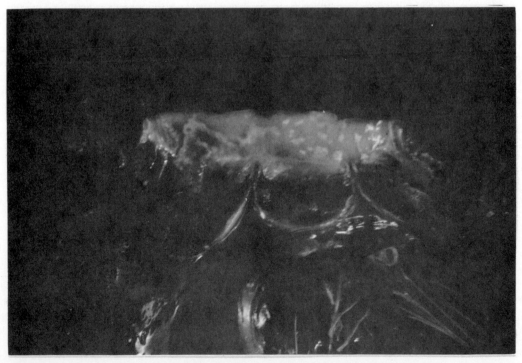

Figure 16–6. Root abscess involving the right coronary cusp of the aortic valve in a patient with pneumococcal infective endocarditis.

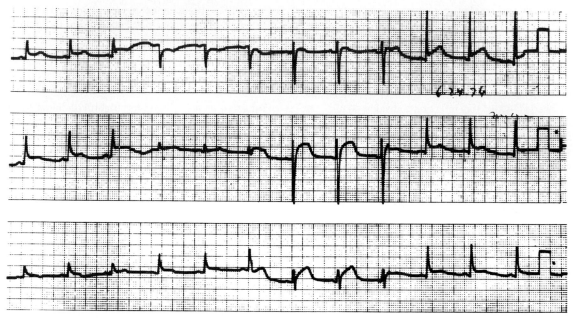

Figure 16–7. ECG in a patient with staphylococcal endocarditis involving the aortic and mitral valves. The patient developed chest pain and a pericardial friction rub. Note ST segment elevations in I, II, aVF, and V_{1-6} consistent with pericarditis. At postmortem, the patient had purulent pericarditis.

more sensitive in finding vegetative and regurgitant mitral and aortic jets than transthoracic echo-Doppler. This is especially important when endocarditis is suspected in the presence of a mechanical valve, where transesophageal echocardiography is definitely superior. Transesophageal echo-Doppler is also more sensitive in detecting ring abscesses and fistulous connections of the aorta to other chambers. When extravalvular infection is suspected, transesophageal echocardiography is indicated.

A. Bacteremia: Bacteremia may be due to pneumonia, septic thrombophlebitis, meningitis, cellulitis, or infected fistulas. There must be evidence of valve lesions as well as emboli before septicemia can be considered to have originated in the heart. When bacteremia occurs in a patient with an indwelling catheter, the catheter should be removed and the tip cultured. If there is no pathologic murmur, the patient should be treated for bacteremia presumably transmitted from an infected catheter. This diagnostic supposition is supported by a positive culture from the catheter tip and permanent subsidence of fever. If the fever recurs or if the blood culture becomes positive again, a diagnosis of probable infective endocarditis should be made and the patient treated on that basis. Miliary tuberculosis must be kept in mind and serial chest x-rays obtained.

B. Acute Rheumatic Fever: Rheumatic fever occasionally is confusing, but only if blood cultures are negative. In acute rheumatic fever, the arthralgia or arthritis responds rapidly to salicylates, and there may be erythema marginatum, chorea, or previous beta-streptococcal infection which can be documented by increasing antistreptolysin O titers in the serum.

C. Neoplasm: Neoplasm can be diagnosed by appropriate measures or by biopsy of lymph nodes or bone marrow. Atrial myxoma can mimic infective endocarditis. The myxoma can act as a foreign antigen, and the patient develops fever, murmurs, immune complex disease, and emboli. If atrial myxoma is suspected, echocardiography and angiography can be diagnostic. (See Chapter 21 for discussion of atrial myxoma.)

D. Connective Tissue Disorders: Connective tissue disorders must be suspected and diagnosed on the basis of skin or renal lesions, a positive LE cell preparation or antinuclear antibody test, renal biopsy, and negative blood cultures.

PREVENTION OF BACTERIAL ENDOCARDITIS

Prevention of infective endocarditis involves prevention or early treatment of all causes of bacteremia; social and educational programs for control of "mainline" drug abuse; and early recognition of systemic infection in the compromised host. The American Heart Association has recommended chemoprophylaxis when bacteremia is likely, as with dental extraction or deep scaling, genitourinary instrumentation, and similar procedures. Some dentists believe that prophylaxis is futile, because vigorous chewing may also produce transient bacteremia, and continuous prophylaxis to prevent infective endocarditis is ineffective or unreasonable.

The following recommendations are from "A Statement for Health Professionals by the Committee on Rheumatic Fever, Endocarditis, and Kawasaki Disease of the Council on Cardiovascular Disease in the Young" (1990) and are published with the permission of the American Heart Association, Inc.

Dental, Oral, & Upper Respiratory Tract Procedures

A. Standard Penicillin Regimen: For patients at risk, including those with prosthetic heart valves and other high-risk patients.

1. Amoxicillin, 3 g orally 1 hour before the procedure, and then 1.5 g 6 hours after the initial dose.

2. Alternatives–

a. Patients unable to take oral medications– Ampicillin, 2 g intravenously or intramuscularly, 30 minutes before the procedure, and then ampicillin, 1 g intravenously or intramuscularly 6 hours after the initial dose.

b. For patients considered at high risk who are not candidates for the standard regimen– Ampicillin, 2 g intravenously or intramuscularly, plus gentamicin, 1.5 mg/kg intravenously or intramuscularly (not to exceed 80 mg), 30 minutes before the procedure, followed by amoxicillin, 1.5 g orally 6 hours after the initial dose. Alternatively, the parenteral regimen may be repeated 8 hours after the initial dose.

B. Standard Regimen for Patients Allergic to Penicillin: For patients at risk, including those with prosthetic heart valves and other high-risk patients.

1. Erythromycin ethyl succinate, 800 mg, or erythromycin stearate, 1 g, orally 2 hours before the procedure, then half the dose 6 hours after the initial dose; or clindamycin, 300 mg orally 1 hour before the procedure, and 150 mg 6 hours after the initial dose.

2. Patients unable to take oral medications– Clindamycin, 300 mg intravenously 30 minutes before the procedure, and 150 mg intravenously 6 hours after initial dose.

C. For Patients at High Risk But Allergic to Amoxicillin, Ampicillin, and Penicillin: Vancomycin, 1 g intravenously over 1 hour, starting 1 hour before the procedure. No repeat dose is necessary.

Genitourinary & Gastrointestinal Tract Surgery & Instrumentation

A. Standard Penicillin Regimen: Ampicillin, 2 g intravenously or intramuscularly, plus gentamicin, 1.5 mg/kg intravenously or intramuscularly (not to exceed 80 mg), 30 minutes before the procedure, followed by amoxicillin, 1.5 g orally 6 hours after the initial dose. Alternatively, the parenteral regimen may be repeated once 8 hours after the initial dose.

B. Patients Allergic to Penicillin: Vancomycin, 1 g intravenously administered over 1 hour, plus gen-

tamicin, 1.5 mg/kg intravenously or intramuscularly (not to exceed 80 mg), 1 hour before the procedure. May be repeated once 8 hours after the initial dose.

C. Oral Regimen for Low-Risk Patients: Amoxicillin, 3 g orally 1 hour before the procedure, then 1.5 g 6 hours after the initial dose.

Pediatric Doses of Antibiotic

Initial doses are listed below. Follow-up doses are half the initial doses.

Amoxicillin, 50 mg/kg, *or–*
  < 15 kg, 750 mg
  15–30 kg, 1500 mg
  > 30 kg, 3000 mg
Clindamycin, 10 mg/kg
Erythromycin ethyl succinate or stearate, 20 mg/kg
Ampicillin 50 mg/kg
Vancomycin, 20 mg/kg
Gentamicin, 2 mg/kg

TREATMENT OF INFECTIVE ENDOCARDITIS

General Principles

The cardinal principles of treatment of infective endocarditis are as follows:

(1) Isolate the infecting organism by obtaining at least two positive blood cultures.

(2) Determine susceptibility of the organism to various antibiotics, alone and in combination.

(3) Choose antimicrobial therapy that is bactericidal and not merely bacteriostatic.

(4) Continue therapy long enough to totally eradicate the infection.

If septic abscesses are present and do not respond to appropriate antibiotic therapy given long enough, surgical drainage is required if technically feasible. If severe valvular insufficiency develops, along with symptoms of progressive cardiac failure, surgical excision of the involved valve and insertion of a prosthesis must be undertaken with proper timing. The results are less good with tricuspid than with mitral or aortic prostheses.

A. Choice of Antibiotic: The choice of antibiotic is based on experience, the results of laboratory sensitivity tests, the status of renal function, and the presence or absence of allergic hypersensitivity to any particular antibiotic, eg, penicillin. Prior to the identification of the infecting organism, antibiotic therapy should be given intravenously in acutely ill patients, using a combination of antibiotics that appear most appropriate on the basis of experience and knowledge of the organisms usually responsible for acute endocarditis.

When the physician does not know which organism

is causing the endocarditis, the "best guess" method is employed. A combination of penicillin, 20–40 million units, and tobramycin, 5–7 mg/kg/d intramuscularly, is given, because the most common organisms are *S viridans* and *S faecalis*. This combination may also be effective in *S epidermidis* endocarditis. If the patient fails to improve in 1–2 weeks, a trial of other bactericidal drugs is indicated, eg, vancomycin, 0.5 g every 4 hours intravenously. Because of its great frequency in autopsied cases, endocarditis must be assumed to be present in staphylococcal septicemia even if its clinical diagnosis is not certain.

The least toxic but most effective antibiotics, such as the penicillins, are preferable; tetracyclines, erythromycins, lincomycins, and chloramphenicol generally cannot eradicate the infection even if the organism appears to be susceptible in vitro. Aminoglycosides are rarely single drugs of choice but participate in synergistic drug combinations that provide optimal bacterial action. The objective should be total eradication of the infection. One should choose a regimen shown by experience to result in the highest percentage of cures and lowest percentage of relapses, rather than one which may be more convenient to use or require a shorter course of therapy but has a lower percentage of cures.

Eradication of infection is almost always possible with one drug or a combination of drugs. Deaths are usually due to delayed or inadequate treatment, exotic organisms, septic abscesses, perforation of mycotic aneurysms, or destruction of valves, requiring surgery. Table 16–1 shows drug selections for various organisms and Table 16–2 their dosage when renal failure is present.

B. Steps in Management:

1. Obtaining positive blood culture– For subacute endocarditis, presumptive therapy with antibiotics that cover the usual organisms (alpha-hemolytic streptococci, enterococci, and staphylococci) can be initiated and continued until a positive blood culture is obtained. Any complications that occur within a few days before the report of the blood culture are apt to be embolic and probably will not be influenced by immediate therapy.

2. Parenteral therapy– The antimicrobial agent is best injected as a bolus over a 20-minute period (by Volutrol) into the tubing of a continuous intravenous infusion of 5% dextrose and water. Injections should be given every 4–6 hours to avoid deterioration of the antibiotic as well as irritation of the venous endothelium. Some drugs (eg, vancomycin) cause severe pain if given intramuscularly or if extravasation outside the vein occurs. Patients receiving therapy over a period of 4–6 weeks usually tolerate a slow intravenous drip of glucose and water and intermittent injection of a bolus of antibiotic. The patient can be ambulatory (in the hospital).

3. Duration of therapy– The duration of therapy for infective endocarditis has always been in some dispute. In general, infection with organisms such as sensitive *S viridans* can be cured in 3–4 weeks, whereas infections with *S aureus* require 5–6 weeks of therapy. In intravenous drug abusers with tricuspid endocarditis, there have been studies showing that the infection can be eradicated with 2 weeks of intravenous antibiotics followed by 2 weeks of oral antibiotics. This has been done only with right-sided endocarditis and is complicated by the difficulty of keeping patients in the hospital for the entire course of therapy.

In patients with very sensitive organisms (alpha-hemolytic streptococci sensitive to $\leq 0.1\mu g/mL$), 2 weeks of combined penicillin and an aminoglycoside is successful in eradicating the infection. In order to reduce the costs of hospitalization, patients have been started on antibiotics in the hospital and then sent home after 1 or 2 weeks to complete the intravenous course with the aid of a specially trained visiting nurse. The aim of treatment is to cure as many infections as possible, and it is advisable to err on the side of overtreating rather than risk the dangers of stopping too soon and allowing the infection to regain a foothold. Organisms that are more difficult to eradicate, such as *Candida*. *Serratia*, or *Pseudomonas*, require early surgical excision of the involved valve because drug therapy alone is ineffective.

4. Testing for bactericidal activity– When antimicrobial agents are used singly or in combination, it is wise to determine if bactericidal concentrations have been achieved by determining the level of serum dilution that is bactericidal for the infecting organism 2 hours after the last dose of the antibiotic. It is believed that a dilution of at least 1:8 is desirable in order to assure a satisfactory result. Patients may continue to have occasional fever or embolic phenomena, yet the antibiotic program may be completely effective. Knowing that the serum dilution of 1:8 or higher is bactericidal for the organism gives the physician the confidence to continue the antibiotic regimen without changing drugs. Bacteriostatic drugs have not been successful in eradicating endocarditis. Once a course of treatment has been chosen on the basis of all the evidence, it should not be changed without a good reason.

5. Observations during the course of treatment– If a satisfactory antimicrobial regimen has been selected, patients usually begin to feel well within a few days even though occasional fever may continue for 7–10 days or embolic phenomena may occur. A negative blood culture and serum bactericidal activity in adequate dilution ($\geq 1:8$) are important prognostic features. If the patient continues to have fever, especially with chills, after the start of a regimen that should be effective, the possibility of septic abscesses should be considered; radioactive isotope scans of the liver, kidney, and spleen may be helpful. Drug fever is another possibility.

a. Daily examination– The patient should be ex-

Table 16–1. Anti-infective chemotherapeutic agents against suspected or proved causes of infective endocarditis.[1,2]

Suspected or Proved Etiologic Agent	Drug(s) of First Choice	Alternative Drug(s)
Gram-negative cocci		
Gonococcus	Amoxicillin + probenecid, ceftriaxone	Spectinomycin, cefoxitin
Gram-positive cocci		
Pneumococcus (*Streptococcus pneumoniae*)	Penicillin[3]	Erythromycin[5], cephalosporin[6]
Streptococcus, hemolytic, groups A, C, G	Penicillin[5]	Erythromycin[5], cephalosporin[6]
Streptococcus viridans	Penicillin[3] ± aminoglycosides[7]	Cephalosporin[6], vancomycin
Staphylococcus, non-penicillinase-producing	Penicillin[3]	Cephalosporin[6], vancomycin
Staphylococcus, penicillinase-producing	Penicillinase-resistant penicillin[8]	Vancomycin, cephalosporin[6]
Streptococcus faecalis; streptococcus, hemolytic, group B	Ampicillin + aminoglycoside[7]	Vancomycin
Gram-negative rods		
Bacteroides, oropharyngeal strains	Penicillin[3], clindamycin	Metronidazole, cephalosporin[6,10]
Bacteroides, gastrointestinal strains	Metronidazole, clindamycin	Cefoxitin, chloramphenicol
Enterobacter	Newer cephalosporins[10]	Aminoglycoside[7], TMP-SMZ[9]
Escherichia coli (sepsis)	Aminoglycoside[7] ± ampicillin	Newer cephalosporins[10], TMP-SMZ[9]
Haemophilus (meningitis, respiratory infections)	Ampicillin + chloramphenicol	Newer cephalosporins[10]
Klebsiella	Newer cephalosporins,[10] aminoglycoside[7]	Chloramphenicol, TMP-SMZ[9]
Proteus mirabilis	Ampicillin	Newer cephalosporins,[10] aminoglycoside[7]
Proteus vulgaris and other species	Newer cephalosporins[10]	Aminoglycosides[7]
Pseudomonas aeruginosa	Aminoglycoside[7] + ticarcillin	Newer cephalosporins[10] ± aminoglycoside
Serratia, Providencia	Newer cephalosporins,[10] aminoglycoside	
Gram-positive rods		
Listeria	Ampicillin ± aminoglycoside[7]	TMP-SMZ,[9] erythromycin[5]
Acid-fast rods		
Nocardia	Sulfonamide[4]	Minocycline
Rickettsiae	Tetracycline[11]	Chloramphenicol

[1] Modified and reproduced with permission from Schroeder SA et al (editors): *Current Medical Diagnosis and Treatment 1989.* Appleton & Lange, 1989.

[2] ± = alone or combined with.

[3] Penicillin G is preferred for parenteral injection; penicillin V for oral administration—to be used only in treating infections due to highly sensitive organisms.

[4] Oral sulfisoxazole and trisulfapyrimidines are highly soluble in urine; parenteral sodium sulfadiazine can be injected intravenously in treating severely ill patients.

[5] Erythromycin estolate is best absorbed orally but carries the highest risk of hepatitis; erythromycin stearate and erythromycin ethylsuccinate are also available.

[6] Older cephalosporins are cephalothin, cefazolin, cephapirin, and cefoxitin for parenteral injection; cephalexin and cephradine can be given orally.

[7] Aminoglycosides—gentamicin, tobramycin, amikacin, netilmicin—should be chosen on the basis of local patterns of susceptibility.

[8] Parenteral nafcillin or oxacillin; oral dicloxacillin, cloxacillin, or oxacillin.

[9] TMP-SMZ is a mixture of 1 part trimethoprim and 5 parts sulfamethoxazole.

[10] Newer cephalosporins (1988) include cefotaxime, cefuroxime, ceftriaxone, ceftazidime, cefitizoxime, and others.

[11] All tetracyclines have similar activity against microorganisms. Dosage is determined by rates of absorption and excretion of various preparations.

amined daily for the appearance of new murmurs, evidence of cardiac enlargement or cardiac failure, and evidence of embolic manifestations. The development of pain and friction rub in the left upper quadrant suggests an embolus to the spleen. Pain in the flank associated with hematuria suggests an embolus to the kidney. If aminoglycosides are used, hearing should be checked intermittently by audiometer. If the patient develops central nervous system symp-

toms with headache and somnolence, the possibility of brain abscess or mycotic aneurysm of a cerebral artery should be considered; if the symptoms are severe and progressive, cerebral angiography or CT scan should be performed with a view toward localizing an aneurysm whose rupture is imminent.

b. Checking laboratory work– Renal function should be monitored frequently, because it may deteriorate either as a result of renal emboli or because of

Table 16–2. Use of antibiotics in patients with renal failure.[1]

	Principal Mode of Excretion or Detoxification	Approximate Half-Life in Serum		Proposed Dosage Regimen in Renal Failure		Significant Removal of Drug by Dialysis (H = Hemodialysis; P = Peritoneal Dialysis)
		Normal	Renal Failure[2]	Initial Dose[3]	Give Half of Initial Dose at Interval of	
Penicillin G	Tubular secretion	0.5 h	6 h	4 g IV	8–12 h	H, P no
Ampicillin	Tubular secretion	1 h	8 h	6 g IV	8–12 h	H yes, P no
Carbenicillin, ticarcillin	Tubular secretion	1.5 h	16 h	3–4 g IV	12–18 h	H, P yes
Nafcillin	Liver 80%, kidney 20%	0.5h	2 h	2 g IV	4–6 h	H, P no
Amikacin	Glomerular filtration	2.5 h	2–3 d	15 mg/kg IM	3 d	H, P yes
Tobramycin, gentamicin	Glomerular filtration	2.5 h	2–4 d	3 mg/kg IM	2–3 d	H, P yes[4]
Vancomycin	Glomerular filtration	6 h	6–9 d	1 g IV	5–8 d	H, P no
Tetracycline	Glomerular filtration	8 h	3 d	1 g orally or 0.5 g IV	3 d	H yes, P no
Chloramphenicol	Mainly liver	3 h	4 h	1 g orally or IV	8 h	H, P no
Erythromycin	Mainly liver	1.5 h	5 h	1 g orally or IV	8 h	H, P no
Clindamycin	Glomerular filtration and liver	2.5 h	4 h	600 mg IV or IM	8 h	H, P no

[1] Modified and reproduced with permission from Schroeder SA et al (editors): *Current Medical Diagnosis and Treatment 1989.* Appleton & Lange, 1989.
[2] Considered here to be marked by creatinine clearance of 10 mL/min or less.
[3] For a 60-kg adult with a serious systemic infection. The "initial dose" listed is administered as an intravenous infusion over a period of 1–8 hours, or as 2 intramuscular injections during an 8-hour period, or as 2–3 oral doses during the same period.
[4] Aminoglycosides are removed irregularly in peritoneal dialysis. Gentamicin is removed 60% in hemodialysis.

drug toxicity. The drug regimen should be adjusted to take account of renal failure (Table 16–2). Frequent blood counts should be performed to note the development of progressive anemia or a marked elevation of the white count that might suggest septic abscess. Frequent ECGs are desirable to detect intraventricular conduction defects or atrioventricular block suggesting abscess of the ventricular septum.

Course of the Disease

A. Valvular Changes:

1. Aortic insufficiency– If endocarditis involves the aortic valve, attention must be paid to signs suggesting worsening of aortic insufficiency. Frequent examination is required to measure diastolic blood pressure, to note the duration of the diastolic murmur, and to assess the possibility of early mitral valve closure and progressive enlargement of the heart or signs of left ventricular failure (eg, frank pulmonary edema or episodic dyspnea). Many of these patients are young adults with no previous valvular disease. In intravenous drug users with aortic valve involvement, the regurgitant murmur may become shorter and

rougher, as the aortic insufficiency worsens. The murmur may completely disappear as severe failure causes tachycardia and an increase in diastolic pressure.

2. Mitral insufficiency– Progressive enlargement of the left atrium as shown by echocardiographic or radiologic examination, as well as progressive enlargement of the left ventricle, may signify serious dysfunction of the mitral valve (see Chapter 12).

3. Tricuspid insufficiency– In acute endocarditis involving the tricuspid valve, the patient should be examined daily for the appearance of signs of tricuspid insufficiency (see Diagnosis, above). (See also Figure 16–3A.)

B. Heart Failure: Progressive destruction of any of the valves associated with either left or right ventricular failure should force serious consideration of cardiac surgery, because many of these patients have perforation of the valve leaflets, septal abscess, or rupture of a mycotic aneurysm from the aortic sinus (sinus of Valsalva) into the right heart, and they can be helped by surgical repair. When heart failure occurs in a patient in whom the infection has not been controlled, a serious dilemma arises; surgery should be considered any time that an optimal anti-infectious program is under way and cardiac failure cannot be controlled medically.

Specific Antimicrobial Regimens*
(See Tables 16–1 and 16–2.)

A. Subacute Endocarditis Due to *Streptococcus viridans:* Viridans streptococci (usually originating in the oropharynx) are the infecting organism in more than 60% of spontaneously arising cases of typical slow-onset endocarditis. A majority of such organisms are susceptible to 0.1–1 unit/mL penicillin G in vitro. Penicillin G, 5–10 million units daily (in divided doses given as a bolus every 4 hours in an intravenous infusion of 5% dextrose in water), continued for 3–4 weeks, is generally curative. Enhanced bactericidal action is obtained if an aminoglycoside (eg, gentamicin, 3–5 mg/kg/d intramuscularly) is added during the first 10–14 days of treatment. More resistant organisms may require daily doses of penicillin G of 20–50 million units. Probenecid, 0.5 g three times daily orally, further enhances blood levels of penicillin by interfering with its tubular excretion. A cephalosporin and vancomycin are alternative drugs.

A short (2-week) course of therapy with penicillin alone or combined with an aminoglycoside (streptomycin or gentamicin) is being advised increasingly in selected cases. These include cases in which the infecting organism is very sensitive to penicillin (< 0.1 µg/mL), those without complications, and those not associated with a cardiac prosthesis. Treatment should be parenteral—oral therapy is *not* advised. Some reports indicate that relapses are slightly more common than in the 4-week treatment course. The advantage is the decreased stay in the hospital; the disadvantages (if aminoglycosides are added) include the possibility of auditory or vestibular damage or renal impairment (Wilson, 1985; Bisno, 1989).

Because of the risk of new infection with local organisms, the catheter site must be cleaned carefully and changed every 2 days during prolonged intravenous infusions. To avoid phlebitis, the daily dose should be divided and given at the appropriate intervals over a half-hour period in a continuous infusion of 5% glucose in water. The potassium content of potassium penicillin G (1.7 meq/million units) must be kept in mind if renal impairment is present.

B. Endocarditis Due to *Streptococcus faecalis:* This organism causes about 5–10% of cases of spontaneously occurring endocarditis and occasionally also follows abuse of intravenous drugs. Treatment is with ampicillin or penicillin, plus an aminoglycoside. Penicillin G, 20–40 million units daily, or ampicillin, 6–12 g daily, is given in divided doses

as bolus injections every 2–3 hours in an intravenous infusion of 5% dextrose in water. An aminoglycoside (kanamycin, 15 mg/kg/d; gentamicin, 5 mg/kg/d) selected by appropriate laboratory test for ribosomal susceptibility is injected intramuscularly two or three times daily in divided doses. The cell wall inhibitory drug (penicillin) enhances entry of the aminoglycoside and permits killing of enterococci. This treatment must be continued for 4–5 weeks. Cephalosporins cannot be substituted for penicillins in this regimen.

C. Endocarditis Due to Staphylococci *(Staphylococcus aureus, Staphylococcus epidermidis):* If the infecting staphylococci are not penicillinase producers, penicillin G, 10–20 million units in divided doses as an intravenous bolus, is the treatment of choice. If the staphylococci produce penicillinase, nafcillin, 8–12 g daily, given as a bolus every 2 hours in an intravenous infusion, as the first-choice alternative drug. In probable or established hypersensitivity to penicillin, the alternative drug is vancomycin or a cephalosporin, 2–3 g daily in divided doses every 4 hours intravenously. Alternatively, an intravenous cephalosporin such as cefazolin (0.5–1 g every 12 hours) or cefuroxime (0.75–1.5 g every 8 hours) can be used. (See Table 16–1). The dosage should be reduced in impaired renal function. This treatment must usually be continued for 5–6 weeks, and a frequent careful check for metastatic lesions or abscesses must be conducted to avoid reseeding of cardiac lesions from such reservoirs of infectious organisms.

D. Endocarditis Due to Gram-Negative Bacteria: The susceptibility of these organisms to antimicrobial drugs varies so greatly that effective treatment must be based on laboratory tests. Aminoglycosides (gentamicin, 5–7 mg/kg/d; kanamycin, 15 mg/kg/d; amikacin, 15 mg/kg/d; or tobramycin, 5–7 mg/kg/d) are often combined with a cell wall-inhibitory drug (cephalothin, 6–12 g/d; cefazolin, 4 g/d; ampicillin, 6–12 g/d; ticarcillin 10–18 g/d; or cefotaxime or cefoperazone, 12 g/d) to enhance penetration by the aminoglycoside. (See Table 16–1.) Laboratory guidance is essential not only for drug susceptibility tests but also for establishment of the presence of sufficient bactericidal activity in serum obtained during treatment. All aminoglycosides may not be equally effective in any given patient; if the clinical response and the laboratory tests warrant, one can, for example, switch from gentamicin to amikacin. The dosage of aminoglycosides must be adjusted if renal function is impaired as determined by serum creatinine levels and creatinine clearance. Suggested modifications in time-dose regimens for aminoglycosides and other nephrotoxic drugs are given in Table 16–2. Each of these drugs also is capable of causing eighth nerve damage, and the patient should be monitored daily for hearing loss and vestibular function. Auditory toxicity with either gentamicin or tobramycin occurred in

---

*With the assistance of Ernest Jawetz, MD.

about 10% of patients, whereas nephrotoxicity may be less after tobramycin (Smith, 1980).

E. Endocarditis Due to Fungi: These organisms rarely arise spontaneously but are seen with increasing frequency in abusers of intravenous drugs, after cardiac surgery, or in immunosuppressed individuals. *Candida albicans, Candida parapsilosis,* and *Torulopsis glabrata* are among those encountered most commonly, but virtually any fungus, including *Aspergillus* and even *Histoplasma,* can be seen. Candidal endocarditis is often associated with bulky, friable vegetations that tend to produce massive emboli in large arteries. Candidal endocarditis has occurred early after the insertion of prosthetic valves, and the diagnosis may be based on the finding of pseudohyphae in emboli surgically removed from large vessels. It may take 1–3 weeks to grow these organisms in blood cultures.

The drugs most active against fungi are amphotericin B (0.4–0.8 mg/kg/d intravenously, and flucytosine, 150 mg/kg/d orally, alone or in combination). However, these drugs rarely eradicate fungal endocarditis. Early surgical excision of the involved valve tissue during antifungal therapy and the continuation of the latter for several weeks offer the best opportunity for cure.

Medical & Surgical Treatment for Infective Endocarditis

After diagnosis, treatment with appropriate antibiotics in the appropriate amounts designed to achieve a blood level capable of killing the organism is the primary indispensible element in therapy. In about 90% of cases, bacteriologic cure can be achieved, with failure occurring in only the most resistant organisms such as fungi, *Pseudomonas,* and *Serratia marcescens* infections. The long-term outcome is most frequently determined by the valvular damage that eventually occurs or by the complications of the endocarditis such as aortic ring abscess, cerebral or coronary emboli, or ruptured mycotic aneurysms.

In general, medical management is indicated as long as the hemodynamic effects of the valvular insufficiency are not severe. The most common reason for operation is the development of congestive heart failure, whereas multiple emboli and the persistence of a resistant infection are less common indications. The incidence of complications, especially systemic emboli, is increased with the presence of large, mobile vegetations, but it is questionable whether the presence of vegetations alone should be an indication for valve replacement. When the vegetation is very large (> 1–2 cm) and mobile, surgery is usually recommended, especially if there is already moderate to severe valvular insufficiency even in the absence of heart failure. At times the vegetation can be removed and the valve repaired without valvular replacement. This is especially true with tricuspid valve endocarditis. The usual indications for surgery are listed in Table 16–3.

Table 16–3. Considerations for possible surgical treatment of endocarditis.

- Severe cardiac failure unresponsive to vigorous medical treatment, especially perforated aortic valve with hemodynamic deterioration and early mitral valve closure.
- Faulty prosthetic valve with paravalvular leak or obstruction.
- Extension of infection, forming a ring or septal abscess.
- Recurrent major emboli to the vital organs, especially if echocardiography reveals large vegetations (Figure 16–3).
- Failure of antibiotic therapy with persistent positive blood cultures and organisms known to be resistant to various antibiotics used alone or in combination, especially if the clinical situation is deteriorating.
- Endocarditis from fungal or other organisms for which there is no effective bactericidal antibiotic.

When there is acute rupture of the aortic valve, with a sudden drop in aortic diastolic pressure, an S_3 gallop, pulmonary congestion, shortening or even disappearance of the aortic insufficiency murmur, decrease in the first heart sound, and early mitral valve closure by echocardiography, surgery should be done as soon as possible, since sudden death as a result of subendocardial ischemia is not uncommon. This can occur even if the patient appears to be compensating for the severe aortic insufficiency and is not in pulmonary edema. Another reason for considering surgery in the absence of heart failure is the presence of a ring abscess.

Many studies have shown that after 12–24 hours of appropriate antibiotics in sufficient dosage to achieve bactericidal serum levels, the mortality rate is decreased by immediate surgery rather than medical management and that patients will survive surgery without reinfecting their prosthetic valve.

Rupture of the mitral valve can result in acute pulmonary edema. However, medical management with digitalis, diuretics, and vasodilators can stabilize the patient. Since the afterload burden is not as great in mitral valve regurgitation as it is in aortic regurgitation and the danger of sudden death from ischemia is not present, the patient with acute mitral regurgitation can be treated with the expectation that with eccentric hypertrophy the left valvular wall stress will be reduced and the patient will develop the hemodynamics of chronic mitral regurgitation. In this case, surgery can be postponed. If symptoms continue in spite of medical management or if left ventricular function deteriorates, valve replacement should be performed.

Another reason for valvular surgery after appropriate antibiotic therapy is begun is the presence of a resistant organism, especially if there is recurrence of the septicemia after a course of therapy. In fungal endocarditis, with removal of the valve under appropriate antifungal therapy, the survival rate can be increased from virtually nil to about 50%.

While the patient is still hospitalized and receiving

appropriate antibiotic therapy, a complete dental evaluation should be offered, with correction of any potential sources of dental or gum infection, in order to reduce the chance of a repeat episode of infective endocarditis.

Prosthetic Valve Endocarditis

Endocarditis on tissue surrounding a prosthetic valve occurs at a rate of about 0.5–1% per year and is one of the most serious postoperative complications of prosthetic valve surgery. Most cases have involved the aortic valve, but the mitral valve may be infected as well. Infection may occur early, within 2–8 weeks after operation, or late, as with any diseased valve. Early-onset infections are caused by organisms introduced at the time of surgery from such sources as an infected pump oxygenator, contaminated intravenous lines used during the procedure, or infected personnel. A postoperative wound infection, especially of the sternum, may be a source of infection of the prosthetic valve. Although only one-third of all infections of prosthetic valves occur early (within the first 2 months), the mortality rate is high (70–80%) in early-onset cases as compared to the more frequent late-onset endocarditis (often many months to a year or so after the valve was introduced); the overall mortality rate of all cases of prosthetic valve endocarditis approximates 50–60%. The causes of early death in Wilson's 1975 series were prosthetic valve dysfunction, infection, cardiac failure, and emboli.

Early-onset endocarditis of a prosthetic valve is usually due to S epidermidis or S aureus; gram-negative bacilli are the next most common cause. Late-onset endocarditis is usually due to streptococci (S viridans or S faecalis), although staphylococci are also frequent (Table 16–4).

Late-onset endocarditis usually follows one of the common predisposing causes of endocarditis on a damaged valve and pathologically involves the neo-endothelium that grows over cloth-covered valves.

On pathologic examination, all patients with prosthetic valve endocarditis have infection located behind the site of attachment of the prosthesis to the valve ring, with spread to the neighboring structures. Severe regurgitation through the involved valve follows the prosthetic detachment and may require urgent surgery.

A. Medical and Surgical Treatment: Medical treatment of prosthetic valve endocarditis is most disappointing, and it may be necessary to resect the valve, introduce a new one, and combine the procedure with effective antimicrobial therapy. It is generally agreed that in the patient with prosthetic valve endocarditis, anticoagulation should be continued rather than stopped. There is evidence that continuing anticoagulation decreases the incidence of clinically important systemic emboli—especially cerebral emboli. The mortality rate is 50–60% even in properly treated patients.

Table 16–4. Microbiology of prosthetic valve infective endocarditis.[1]

	Early Endocarditis[2]	Late Endocarditis[2]
Number of cases[3]	146	140
Infecting organisms		
Staphylococcus epidermidis	40 (27.4%)	32 (22.9%)
Staphylococcus aureus	28 (19.2%)	16 (11.4%)[4]
Streptococci	11 (7.5%)	52 (37.1%)
Gram-negative bacilli	30 (20.5%)	19 (13.6%)
Fungi	14 (9.6%)	6 (4.3%)
Miscellaneous bacteria	15 (10.3%)	7 (5.0%)
Mixed organisms	8 (5.5%)	8 (5.7%)

[1] Reproduced, with permission, from Watanakunakorn C: Prosthetic valve infective endocarditis. Prog Cardiovasc Disease 1979;22:181.
[2] Early endocarditis: occurring within 2 months after operation; late endocarditis: occurring 2 months or more after operation.
[3] From multiple references.
[4] $P < .001$ (χ^2 test with Yates correction).

The high mortality rate may be a function of delayed surgery, since delay allows destruction of the valve, progressive development of renal and cardiac failure, and development of emboli (especially cerebral) before the patient is operated on again. Early surgical replacement of the infected valve is required if the infection is not rapidly controlled by aggressive antibiotic therapy or if there is evidence of destruction of the involved valve, with progressive cardiac failure or valvular regurgitation.

B. Prevention: Preventing infection is obviously better than treating prosthetic valve endocarditis; it is most important to ensure adequate antibacterial prophylaxis when prosthetic valves are inserted, because the fatality rate is high when the prosthetic valve becomes infected. Since the most common bacteria that cause early-onset prosthetic valve endocarditis are S aureus and gram-negative organisms, vigorous therapy with combined drugs is recommended, eg, nafcillin, 8–12 g/d intravenously, and gentamicin, 3–5 mg/kg/d intramuscularly, in three equal doses for 3 or 4 postoperative days. The results with cephalothin have been poor, and the toxicity of amphotericin B makes its use to prevent the uncommon Candida infections unwise. Good studies to establish the most effective prophylactic regimen are not available, but vigorous prophylaxis against the most likely organisms is indicated.

For prophylaxis of late-onset endocarditis, antimicrobials are used as in patients with known rheumatic or congenital heart lesions. The predisposing factors are similar, and *S viridans* is the most common organism.

Penicillin Hypersensitivity

For many forms of endocarditis, penicillins have the best record of cure. A history of allergic reaction to penicillin is notoriously unreliable. Only 5–10% of patients with such a history cannot be given penicillin in a situation where it is clearly the drug of choice. All penicillins are cross-reactive, and cephalosporins have a much less successful record than penicillins in the treatment of endocarditis. Therefore, in spite of a history of penicillin reaction—except one of anaphylaxis—it may be desirable to attempt penicillin treatment in cases of endocarditis where a penicillin-susceptible organism has been recovered.

The following steps are advisable:

(1) Skin tests with penicilloyl-polylysine, native penicillin (1–10 units), and penicillin degraded after prolonged storage in a refrigerator. Unless strongly positive reactions are observed within 1 hour, proceed with treatment.

(2) An available airway and a person skilled in its insertion and the use of resuscitation must be at the bedside (preferably in the intensive care unit) for 40–45 minutes. An intravenous infusion of 5% dextrose in water must be in place and running. A syringe with 5 mL of epinephrine 1:1000 must be available at the bedside. A test dose of 100 units of penicillin G is injected into the intravenous tubing with close observation for a possible immediate reaction. If none has occurred in 45 minutes, inject 50,000 units of penicillin G into the tubing and again observe for 40 minutes. Absence of a reaction permits beginning of regular penicillin dosage with the assurance that an immediate life-threatening anaphylactic reaction will not occur.

Delayed, serum sickness type reactions, with skin rashes, angioneurotic edema, fever, or arthritis, may develop in such individuals. Administration of corticosteroids or antihistamines can often suppress these reactions and permit completion of the planned treatment. In extremely penicillin-hypersensitive patients, vancomycin is the best drug.

Persistent & Resistant Infection or Development of Cardiac Failure

If effective antibiotic therapy fails to eradicate the infection and positive blood cultures persist or recur, or if adequate combinations of drugs are not bactericidal, one should change the antibiotics, as mentioned previously, and hope to find the combination that will eradicate the organism. This may be difficult in the case of gram-negative or unusual organisms, especially fungi, or if the patient has a prosthetic valve. Cardiac failure may develop late as a result of progressive damage of the valve, especially the aortic valve. The development of severe aortic insufficiency may be rapid, and surgical replacement with a prosthetic valve is essential. At times, the urgency of surgical replacement is such that patients must be operated on within hours of arrival at the hospital. Such patients have been cured by antibiotic therapy combined with surgical removal of the infected valve, though the mortality rate approaches 20%. Cardiac failure may progressively worsen even though the infection is eradicated; the physician is then faced with a different situation—cardiac failure produced by a valve that has been destroyed and must therefore be replaced.

Patient Follow-Up

The physician's responsibility does not end with completion of the course of therapy. The only proof of cure is persistence of good health, absence of relapse, and repeatedly negative blood cultures. The patient should be observed at weekly intervals and should keep a daily temperature record. Blood for culture should be taken once a week for one month. The patient should be examined carefully for evidence of embolic phenomena, splenomegaly, clubbed fingers, and microscopic hematuria. If after 2 months there are no clinical symptoms or signs and the blood cultures have been consistently negative, it is safe to consider that cure has been achieved. The patient is then seen every month for another 3 or 4 months. It is always advisable to keep the cultures of the organism, because in case of relapse or recurrence, a question will arise about whether the same organism is responsible.

PROGNOSIS

Antibiotic therapy has reduced the mortality rate of infective endocarditis from almost 100% in all untreated cases to about 10–20% in subacute cases and 20–30% in acute cases. This remarkable achievement is best appreciated by physicians who had to deal with endocarditis prior to the antibiotic era. The residual high mortality rate in acute staphylococcal infections is due to the destruction of valves and to occurrence of septic abscess that may be inaccessible to drainage. The prognosis in sub acute infective endocarditis depends upon the time elapsed before diagnosis, the organism involved and its sensitivity to antibiotic agents, the presence of an artificial valve, and the delay in beginning effective treatment. In sensitive *S viridans* infections, for example, the mortality rate is about 10%. However, with more resistant *S viridans, S aureus,* or gram-negative organisms, the mortality rate increases to 30–40%.

The prognosis depends also upon the class of patient being reported. Deaths are more frequent in elderly debilitated patients, in whom fever may be absent or minimal in the subacute variety and in whom the diagnosis may be delayed or missed because of atypical features of the disease. In *S aureus* endocarditis, for example, there may be a two- to threefold higher mortality rate in older patients as compared to younger ones; most of the unsuspected fatal cases have been in the age group over 70.

The significant residual mortality rate in acute and subacute endocarditis means that the physician should actively seek the diagnosis, obtain blood cultures whenever fever occurs in a patient with valvular disease, and look for septic abscesses that can be surgically drained. Cooperation between the infectious disease specialist and the cardiologist is necessary both to eradicate the infection and to recognize when the complications of valve destruction require surgical therapy.

The incidence of endocarditis following placement of an aortic homograft valve (frequently used in En-

gland, Australia, and some centers in the USA) was 2.6% in 539 patients in the experience of Barratt-Boyes of New Zealand (1972). Early endocarditis occurred in less than 1% and was almost universally fatal. The mortality rate was almost 50% in patients with late endocarditis associated with development of an aortic leak. This incidence of endocarditis is about the same as that following the insertion of Starr-Edwards prostheses.

Continuous prophylactic antibiotics are not required in patients with homograft valves, but "antibiotic cover" is recommended when dental or surgical procedures are required in patients with plastic valves.

If endocarditis presents with renal failure, the prognosis is good for return of renal function.

REFERENCES

Pathology

Bayer AS, Theofilopoulos AN: Immunopathogenetic aspects of infective endocarditis. Chest 1990;97:204.

Caputo GM et al: Native valve endocarditis due to coagulase-negative staphylococci: Clinical and microbiologic features. Am J Med 1987;83:619.

Ivert TSA et al: Prosthetic valve endocarditis. Circulation 1984;69:223.

Wilkowske CJ: Enterococcal endocarditis. Mayo Clin Proc 1982;57:101.

Wilson WR, Washington JA II: Infective endocarditis: A changing spectrum? Mayo Clin Proc 1977;52:254.

Diagnosis

Alpert JS et al: Pathogenesis of Osler's nodes. Ann Intern Med 1976;85:471.

Arber N et al: Native valve *Staphylococcus epidermidis* endocarditis: Report of seven cases and review of the literature. Am J Med 1991;90:758.

Berger M et al: Two-dimensional echocardiographic findings in right-sided infective endocarditis. Circulation 1980;61:855.

Botvinick EH et al: Echocardiographic demonstration of early mitral valve closure in severe aortic insufficiency: Its clinical implications. Circulation 1975; 51:836.

Cliff MM, Soulen RL, Finestone AJ: Mycotic aneurysms: A challenge and a clue. Arch Intern Med 1970;126:977.

Cohen PS, Maguire JH, Weinstein L: Infective endocarditis caused by gram-negative bacteria: A review of the literature, 1945–1977. Proc Cardiovasc Dis 1980; 22:205.

Durack DT, Kaplan EL, Bisno AL: Apparent failures of endocarditis prophylaxis: Analysis of 52 cases submitted to a national registry. JAMA 1983;250:2318.

Hermans PE: The clinical manifestations of infective endocarditis. Mayo Clin Proc 1982;57:15.

Johnson DH, Rosenthal A, Nadas AS: A forty-year review of bacterial endocarditis in infancy and childhood. Circulation 1975;51:581.

Kaplan EL et al: A collaborative study of infective endocarditis in the 1970's: Emphasis on infections in patients who have undergone cardiovascular surgery. Circulation 1979;59:327.

Lowy FD, Hammer SM: *Staphylococcus epidermidis* infections. Ann Intern Med 1983;99:834.

MacMahon SW et al: Risk of infective endocarditis in mitral valve prolapse with and without precordial systolic murmurs. Am J Cardiol 1986;59:105.

Pesanti EL, Smith IM: Infective endocarditis with negative blood cultures: An analysis of 52 cases. Am J Med 1979;66:43.

Pringle TH et al: Clinical, echocardiographic, and operative findings in active infective endocarditis. Br Heart J 1982;48:529.

Pruitt AA et al: Neurologic complications of bacterial endocarditis. Medicine 1978;57:329.

Rubenson DS et al: The use of echocardiography in diagnosing culture-negative endocarditis. Circulation 1981; 64:641.

Sanfillipo AJ: Prediction of risk for complications in patients with left sided infectious endocarditis. J Am Coll Cardiol 1989;13:72A.

Shapiro SM, Bayer AS: Transesophageal and Doppler echocardiography in the diagnosis and management of infective endocarditis. Chest 1991;100:1125.

Terpenning MS, Buggy BP, Kauffman CA: Infective endocarditis: Clinical features in young and elderly patients. Am J Med 1987;83:626.

Tobin MF et al: Q fever endocarditis. Am J Med 1982; 72:396.

Washington JA II: The role of the microbiology laboratory in the diagnosis and antimicrobial treatment of infective endocarditis. Mayo Clin Proc 1982;57:22.

Welton DE et al: Recurrent infective endocarditis: Analysis of predisposing factors and clinical features. Am J Med 1979;66:932.

Welton DE et al: Value and safety of cardiac catheterization during active infective endocarditis. Am J Cardiol 1979;44:1306.

Zabalgoitia M: Echocardiographic assessment of prosthetic heart valves. Curr Probl Cardiol 1992;17:265.

Prevention

Antibiotic prophylaxis of infective endocarditis: Recommendations from the Endocarditis Working Party of the British Society for Antimicrobial Chemotherapy. Lancet 1990;335:88.

Kaye D: Infective endocarditis: An overview. Am J Med 1985;78(Suppl 6B):107.

Prevention of bacterial endocarditis: A statement for health professionals by the Committee on Rheumatic Fever, Endocarditis, and Kawasaki Disease of the Council on Cardiovascular Disease in the Young. JAMA 1990;264:2919.

Sipes JN, Thompson RL, Hook EW: Prophylaxis of infective endocarditis: A reevaluation. Annu Rev Med 1977;28:371.

Sugrue D et al: Antibiotic prophylaxis against infective endocarditis after normal delivery: Is it necessary? Br Heart J 1980;44:499.

Treatment

Alsip SG et al: Indications for cardiac surgery in patients with active infective endocarditis. Am J Med 1985; 78(Suppl B):138.

Appel GB, Neu HC: The nephrotoxicity of antimicrobial agents. (Three parts.) N Engl J Med 1977;296:633, 722, 784.

Bennett WM et al: Guidelines for drug therapy in renal failure. Ann Intern Med 1977;86:754.

Bisno AL et al: Antimicrobial treatment of infective endocarditis due to viridans streptococci, enterococci, and staphylococci. JAMA 1989;261:1471.

Brandenburg RO et al: Infective endocarditis: A 25-year overview of diagnosis and therapy. J Am Coll Cardiol 1983;1:280.

Brooks GF, Barriere SL: Clinical use of the new beta-lactam antimicrobial drugs: Practical consideration for physicians, microbiology laboratories, pharmacists, and formulary committees. Ann Intern Med 1983; 98:530.

Calderwood SB et al: Risk factors for the development of prosthetic valve endocarditis. Circulation 1985;72:31.

Donowitz GR, Mandell GL: Beta-lactam antibiotics. (Two parts.) N Engl J Med 1988;318:419, 490.

Edwards J (moderator): Severe candidal infections: Clinical perspective, immune defense mechanisms, and current concepts of therapy. (UCLA Conference.). Ann Intern Med 1978;89:91.

Galgiani JN et al: *Bacteroides fragilis* endocarditis, bacteremia and other infections treated with oral or intravenous metronidazole. Am J Med 1978;65:284.

Geraci JE et al: *Haemophilus* endocarditis: Report of 14 patients. Mayo Clin Proc 1977;52:209.

Green GR, Peters GA, Geraci JE: Treatment of bacterial endocarditis in patients with penicillin hypersensitivity. Ann Intern Med 1967;67:235.

Hermans PE: Antifungal agents used for deep-seated mycotic infections. Mayo Clin Proc 1977;52:687.

Hermans PE (editor): Symposium on antimicrobial agents. (Two parts.) Mayo Clin Proc 1987;62:788, 901.

Hubbell G, Cheitlin MD, Rapaport E: Presentation, management, and follow-up evaluation of infective endocarditis in drug addicts. Am Heart J 1981;102: 85.

Jacobs RA: Anti-infective chemotherapeutic and antibiotic agents. In: *Current Medical Diagnosis & Treatment 1993.* Tierney LM Jr et al (editors). Appleton & Lange, 1992.

Karchmer AW: Staphylococcal endocarditis: Laboratory and clinical basis for antibiotic therapy. Am J Med 1985;78(Suppl 6B):116.

Korzeniowski O, Sande MA: Combination antimicrobial therapy for *Staphylococcus aureus* endocarditis in patients addicted to parenteral drugs and in nonaddicts. Ann Intern Med 1982;97:496.

Kumin GD: Clinical nephrotoxicity of tobramycin and gentamicin: A prospective study. JAMA 1980;244: 1808.

Mayer KH, Schoenbaum SC: Evaluation and management of prosthetic valve endocarditis. Prog Cardiovasc Dis 1982;25:43.

McAnulty JH, Rahimtoola SH: Surgery for infective endocarditis. JAMA 1979;242:77.

Moellering RC Jr, Siegenthaler WE (editors): Aminoglycoside therapy: The New Decade: A worldwide perspective. (Symposium.) Am J Med 1986;80(Suppl 6B):1.

Moore RD et al: Risk factors for nephrotoxicity in patients treated with aminoglycosides. Ann Intern Med 1984;100:352.

Sande MA, Scheld WM: Combination antibiotic therapy of bacterial endocarditis. Ann Intern Med 1980; 92:390.

Sorrell TC et al: Vancomycin therapy for methicillin-resistant *Staphylococcus aureus.* Ann Intern Med 1982;97:344.

Stinson EB: Surgical treatment of infective endocarditis. Prog Cardiovasc Dis 1979;22:145.

Symposium on antimicrobial agents. (Two parts.) Mayo Clin Proc 1987;62:788 and 901.

Tumulty PA: Management of bacterial endocarditis. Geriatrics 1967;22:122.

Varma MPS, Adgey AAJ, Connolly JF: Chronic Q fever endocarditis. Br Heart J 1980;43:695.

Watanakunakorn C: Prosthetic valve infective endocarditis. Prog Cardiovasc Dis 1979;22:181.

Weinstein MP et al: Multicenter collaborative evaluation of a standardized serum bactericidal test as a prognostic indicator in infective endocarditis. Am J Med 1985;78:262.

Wilson WR, Geraci JE: Treatment of streptococcal infective endocarditis. Am J Med 1985;78(Suppl 6B):128.

Wilson WR et al: Cardiac valve replacement in congestive heart failure due to infective endocarditis. Mayo Clin Proc 1979;54:223.

Wilson WR et al: Prosthetic valve endocarditis. Ann Intern Med 1975;82:751.

Working Party of the British Society for Antimicrobial Chemotherapy: The antibiotic prophylaxis of infective endocarditis. Lancet 1982;2:1323.

Myocardial Disease (Myocarditis & Cardiomyopathy)

17

This chapter discusses myocarditis, cardiomyopathy, and various disease and clinical states of which disease of the myocardium may be a manifestation. The common known causes of chronic myocardial disease (ischemic, hypertensive, valvular, congenital, as well as infective endocarditis and syphilis) are discussed in other chapters.

OVERVIEW OF MYOCARDIAL DISEASE

The myocardium is susceptible to diseases of various causes, not all of them known. Any virus, bacteria, or other organism can cause myocarditis, which may lead to dilated cardiomyopathy. The clinical manifestations vary from mild illness to cardiac failure and death. Myocarditis may be acute or chronic, and acute myocarditis may be benign or fulminant. The terms "chronic myocarditis" and "chronic cardiomyopathy" are often used interchangeably. Myocarditis may be a primary disorder, or it may be secondary to systemic diseases such as connective tissue disorders.

The clinical diagnosis of myocardial disease is often one of exclusion. The physician must consider common diseases with unusual clinical features in the differential diagnosis. As hypertensive heart disease and rheumatic heart disease in adults become less common, cardiomyopathy and the acute myocarditides have come to form a larger percentage of cases of cardiac disease. Some forms of myocardial disease are inexplicably more common in tropical and subtropical areas than in temperate climates.

Myocarditis is often associated with pericarditis, especially in viral infections. The endocardium and the valves are less often involved except in acute rheumatic fever or endocardial fibrosis. Myocardial disease due to drug toxicity is becoming increasingly common with the use of many cardiotoxic drugs (eg, the phenothiazines, doxorubicin). Some drugs have been shown to cause cardiomyopathy that is reversible upon withdrawal (eg, interleukin-2 and alpha interferon).

ETIOLOGY & CLASSIFICATION

A working classification of the myocardial disorders is given in Table 17–1. All classifications are arbitrary and none are completely satisfactory, because of the many unknown causes and overlapping among the cardiomyopathies (Abelmann, 1984). Many of the diseases are of unknown cause. In such cases the diagnosis must be inferred from the associated systemic features, as in secondary cardiomyopathy and primary viral myocarditis. Infiltrative diseases such as primary amyloidosis may be difficult to diagnose, but newer immunoelectrophoretic techniques and procedures such as endomyocardial, rectal, abdominal fat, or gum biopsy may be helpful. In sarcoidosis, chest x-ray may reveal characteristic hilar adenopathy or pulmonary infiltration or, in advanced disease, right ventricular hypertrophy and cor pulmonale.

PATHOLOGY

The pathologic features of cardiomyopathy associated with systemic disease are rarely specific. They may be relatively minor and discovered only at autopsy. One should distinguish myocarditis recognized only postmortem from clinically significant disease that produces cardiac symptoms and dysfunction.

Inflammatory changes often occur during viral infections and are often unassociated with cardiac symptoms. Varying degrees of myofibrillary hypertrophy, fibrosis, or inflammation involving the myocardial cells or conduction system may be found in any type of cardiomyopathy. Cardiac failure may be evident, including chronic passive congestion. Evidence of the primary systemic disease may be apparent in other organs.

The pathologic processes in cardiomyopathy and myocarditis may be focal or diffuse; may be a pathologic curiosity at autopsy; or may cause fatal cardiac failure, arrhythmias, or conduction defects.

Percutaneous transvenous endomyocardial biopsy is a simple, safe technique when performed by expe-

Table 17–1. Classification of diseases of the myocardium.

I. Acute or subacute myocarditis:
  A. Infectious: Usually acute but may be subacute.
    Viral (especially coxsackie, echo, or poliomyelitis)
    Mycotic (eg, histoplasmosis, *Candida*)
    Parasitic (eg, schistosomiasis, toxoplasmosis, trichinosis, trypanosomiasis [acute Chagas' disease])
    Rickettsial (eg, epidemic typhus, scrub typhus, Q fever)
    Bacterial (eg, pneumonia, diphtheria)
  B. Acute rheumatic fever

II. Acute or subacute myocardial damage due to drugs:
  Alpha interferon
  Antiarrhythmic agents (eg, disopyramide)
  Catecholamines
  Antimony
  Corticosteroids
  Doxorubicin
  Emetine
  Hydralazine
  Interleukin-2
  Methysergide
  Phenothiazines
  Phenytoin
  Tricyclic antidepressants (eg, amitriptyline, imipramine)
  Drug-induced connective tissue disorders

III. Chronic cardiomyopathy (pathophysiologic classification):
  Dilated (congestive) cardiomyopathy
  Hypertrophic obstructive cardiomyopathy
  Restrictive cardiomyopathy

IV. Cardiomyopathy associated with specific metabolic diseases:
  Thyrotoxicosis
  Myxedema
  Alcoholic cardiomyopathy
  Beriberi heart
  Nutritional cardiomyopathy
  Keshan disease (selenium deficiency)
  Acromegaly
  Inherited metabolic disorders

V. Cardiomyopathy associated with recognized chronic diseases, often of unknown cause:
  Sarcoidosis
  Connective tissue disorders (systemic lupus erythematosus, progressive systemic sclerosis [scleroderma], rheumatoid arthritis, polyarteritis nodosa)
  Hemochromatosis
  Amyloid disease
  Endomyocardial fibrosis
  Sickle cell disease
  Chagas' disease
  Peripartum disease
  Neurologic disorders (eg, Friedreich's ataxia)

rienced personnel. Biopsy permits anatomic diagnosis of conditions such as acute myocarditis, drug toxicity, cardiac graft rejection, amyloidosis, sarcoidosis, hemochromatosis, and endomyocardial fibrosis (Fowles, 1984; Marboe, 1988). Myocardial biopsy has proved to be most useful in detecting cardiac transplant rejection. About 20% of patients with cardiomyopathy of recent onset on biopsy show inflammatory changes, mainly round cell infiltration, presumably as a result of myocarditis. Biopsy has not been helpful either in diagnosis or in planning therapy in most patients with cardiomyopathy. Most patients with secondary cardiomyopathy can be diagnosed because of the other manifestations of the underlying disease. Until recently, it was believed that the finding of focal myocarditis on biopsy was useful in deciding to use steroids or antimetabolites. Since there is good evidence that these drugs with serious side effects are not useful in patients with "myocarditis," the indications for myocardial biopsy have markedly decreased.

Common Specific Pathologic Pictures

The following are common pathologic changes seen at autopsy with some examples of the underlying causes that may be responsible. Most cases of cardiomyopathy ($\approx$ 80%) are of unknown cause. When the cause is known, the condition is usually identified as cardiomyopathy due to whatever the underlying cause may be (eg, "cardiomyopathy due to amyloidosis").

(1) Infiltration of the myocardium with inflammatory cells of a variety of types, disorganizing their structure; the intracellular changes are best seen by electron microscopy. Light microscopy may show myocardial cell necrosis with loss of striations. (Acute myocarditis, connective tissue disorders.)

(2) Infiltration with infecting organisms. (Acute viral myocarditis, *Candida* infections, Chagas' disease.)

(3) Focal or diffuse fibrosis of any part of the myocardium or conduction system. (Scleroderma, sarcoidosis, endocardial fibrosis.) In connective tissue disease, when the fibrosis affects the vascular bed of the lungs, pulmonary hypertension, cor pulmonale, and right heart failure may occur.

(4) Vasculitis in the walls of small arteries as well as perivascular and intestinal infiltration of cells with or without granuloma formation. (Systemic lupus erythematosus.)

(5) Injury to myocardial cells as a result of excessive deposition of various substances. (Immune complexes in lupus erythematosus, fibrils of light chain immunoglobulins in amyloid disease, glycogen in von Gierke's disease, calcium in renal failure, iron in hemochromatosis, products of abnormal metabolism, invasive tumors.)

(6) Metabolic changes caused by biochemical substances produced by tumor.

(7) Direct injury of myocardial cells from drugs. (Doxorubicin, disopyramide phosphate, sympathetic amines, alcohol, methysergide, and others.)

Pathology of Conduction System

In all cases of myocardial disease, the damage to cardiac muscle may include the conduction system, causing destruction of the sinoatrial or atrioventricular node or large portions of the Purkinje system. Stokes-Adams attacks, arrhythmias, and sudden death occur in such disorders as scleroderma, sarcoidosis, and Chagas' disease. Inflammatory or fibrotic lesions may be localized and interrupt the ventricular conduction system, so that patients may have symptoms of the conduction defect in the absence of cardiac enlargement or cardiac failure.

GENERAL PATHOPHYSIOLOGY

Diseases of the myocardium have been classified pathophysiologically as follows:

(1) Dilated (congestive) cardiomyopathy.
(2) Hypertrophic obstructive cardiomyopathy.
(3) Restrictive cardiomyopathy.

Specific diseases (see Table 17–1) most commonly present in one of these pathophysiologic forms; eg, viral myocarditis frequently presents as dilated cardiomyopathy. Alcoholic cardiomyopathy also usually presents as dilated cardiomyopathy, but early forms can present with only arrhythmias or conduction defects, before dilation or poor left ventricular function. At a later stage, systolic dysfunction can occur without dilation. Other diseases, such as glycogen storage disease or myocardial amyloidosis, usually present as restrictive cardiomyopathy, ie, with a normal-sized left ventricular cavity, frequently with well-preserved left ventricular contractility but with a stiff left ventricle requiring a high diastolic filling pressure to achieve a normal left ventricular diastolic volume. Finally, hypertrophic cardiomyopathy usually presents as restrictive cardiomyopathy but presents signs, such as systolic ejection murmurs, of left ventricular outflow tract obstruction. The diastolic left ventricular cavity is usually normal or small, and systolic function is well preserved.

Occasionally, there may be increased cardiac output insufficient to meet physiologic demands, as in thyrotoxicosis, severe anemia, or Paget's disease of bone. (See High-Output Failure, Chapter 10.) When impairment of left ventricular function is sufficiently great, the ejection fraction falls below 30%, and progressive cardiac failure usually ensues.

In restrictive cardiomyopathy, there is restricted filling of both ventricles due to a fibrotic or infiltra-

tive lesion; this leads to pulmonary and systemic congestive phenomena.

ACUTE MYOCARDITIS

In acute myocarditis, there is frequently an acute febrile illness, with fever, malaise, arthralgias, chest pain, dyspnea, syncope, and palpitations. The patient may have associated pericarditis.

Signs

A. Cardiac Signs: Tachycardia out of proportion to the degree of fever suggests myocarditis. The cardiac impulse may be displaced to the left. Palpation may disclose left ventricular heave. The blood pressure is usually normal. Auscultation may reveal equalization of the first and second sounds (**tic-tac rhythm**), and a systolic murmur of tricuspid or mitral regurgitation due to cardiac dilation may be present. Paradoxically, a split second sound may be present, especially when left bundle branch block is present. There may be a gallop rhythm with an S_3 and S_4. If definite cardiac failure is present, a raised pulmonary venous or jugular venous pressure and pulsus alternans may be seen. Various ventricular arrhythmias or atrioventricular conduction defects may be found.

Acute circulatory collapse, with hypotension, oliguria, and obtundation, may occur when myocardial damage is severe (eg, in severe infections). Emboli may form, and sudden death may occur.

B. Signs of Associated Disease: Signs of an underlying disease may be present in the lungs, skin, liver, kidneys, or elsewhere.

Electrocardiographic Findings

Nonspecific ST–T changes, often in the inferior leads, are the most common abnormalities. If the conduction system is involved, there may be conduction defects, including partial atrioventricular block. In a young person with acute viral infection, the development of ST–T abnormalities, partial atrioventricular block, and conduction defects (especially left bundle branch block) suggests myocarditis; in an older person, ischemic cardiomyopathy must be excluded.

Imaging Studies

The radiologic findings are also nonspecific. The heart may be enlarged and globular with signs of pericardial effusion. With gross cardiac failure there may be pulmonary venous congestion, and with cor pulmonale there may be radiologic signs of pulmonary hypertension and right ventricular enlargement. If the patient has sarcoidosis, there may be hilar adenopathy and pulmonary infiltration. In lymphomatous and malignant disease, tumor in various parts of the body may be evident.

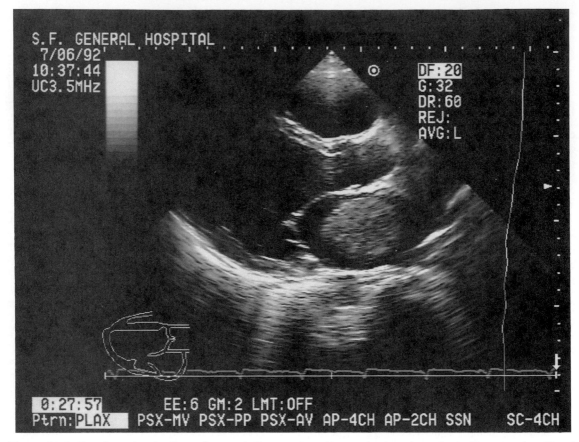

Figure 17–1. Two-dimensional echocardiogram in the parasternal long axis view of a patient with congestive dilated cardiomyopathy with a large ball thrombus in the left atrium. Picture taken in early systole.

Echocardiographic Findings

Echocardiography with Doppler studies may demonstrate pericardial thickening or effusion, enlargement of specific chambers of the heart, wall motion abnormalities, left ventricular ejection fraction, valvular and septal abnormalities, and findings characteristic of other diseases. In pericardial effusion, the echocardiogram shows an echo-free zone between the epicardium of the left ventricle and the chest wall (see Chapter 18). On two-dimensional echocardiography, ventricular mural thrombosis, especially in the apex, may be detected (Figure 17–1).

Cardiac Catheterization

Cardiac catheterization is usually done to rule out surgically treatable lesions in dilated cardiomyopathy (see below) or to differentiate the latter from hypertrophic cardiomyopathy or constrictive pericarditis (see Chapter 18). Two-dimensional echocardiography and Doppler examination make catheterization rarely necessary to make a diagnosis of dilated cardio-

myopathy. Catheterization and angiography in dilated cardiomyopathy will show a left ventricle of increased volume in diastole with poor pulsations; a decreased ejection fraction (< 40%); normal coronary arteries; and symmetric, decreased wall motion without aneurysm or marked segmental contraction abnormalities.

Prognosis

The cardiac failure of myocardial disease may differ from that due to ischemic cardiomyopathy or severe valvular disease depending upon the cause. In alcoholic cardiomyopathy, with abstention from alcohol, about one-third of patients improve. The longer they remain with a dilated, poorly contracting left ventricle, the less likely it is that improvement will occur. In acute viral myocarditis or peripartum cardiomyopathy, cardiac failure may be completely reversible over a period of 1–2 months. Viral myocarditis may be recurrent. The prognosis for survival is much less favorable when the ejection fraction is low—especially when it is less than 20%.

ACUTE & SUBACUTE MYOCARDITIS ASSOCIATED WITH SPECIFIC DISEASES

Acute myocarditis most commonly follows group A streptococcal infection leading to acute rheumatic fever or infection caused by type B coxsackievirus but may also be caused by infection due to type A coxsackievirus, echovirus, adenovirus; by other viral diseases such as poliomyelitis, varicella, mumps, and hepatitis; or by infection due to other organisms such as *Chlamydia trachomatis*. In one series, one-third of the patients with acute myocarditis developed IgM responses specific to type B coxsackievirus (El-Hagrassy, 1980). Most patients with myocarditis seen in infectious disease services in general hospitals are free of cardiac symptoms, and signs are discovered only by careful clinical examination (including ECG). The acute exanthems rarely cause cardiac failure or cardiac dysfunction. In adults, clinical myocarditis and especially death from myocarditis are infrequent.

Controversy continues about how the cardiotropic virus causes myocarditis and especially prolonged chronic myocardial dysfunction after the stage of viremia has passed. There is evidence that the virus can be recovered from the myocardium for only a few days—probably not more than a week after onset. After the viremia clears, either viral RNA remains in the myocardial cell, incapable of replicating but capable of stimulating an antibody response, or a false autoantigen forms that has cross-reactivity to some component of the myocardial cell. Through the immune system, perhaps via the mediation of macrophages releasing cytokines, chronic changes take place in the myocardium, resulting in chronic cardiomyopathy.

Clinical Findings

A. Myocarditis Due to Type B Coxsackieviruses: These viruses are the most common agents causing viral myocarditis (Herskowitz, 1987). Susceptibility to these viruses is genetically determined in mice; to our knowledge, data are not available regarding genetic determination in humans. Cardiac involvement occurs in 5–10% of coxsackievirus infections (Grist, 1974), and the histologic effects are shown in Figures 17–2 and 17–3. The disease may be mild or severe.

1. Symptoms and signs– Types B3 and B5 are most commonly associated with myocarditis in adults. Coxsackievirus myocarditis is usually suspected in adults on the basis of an acute febrile illness with lethargy, chest pain, dyspnea, enlargement of the heart, ventricular premature beats, ventricular tachycardia, atrioventricular block, and nonspecific ST–T changes. There may be obvious signs of cardiac failure in severe cases. Patients often have associated pericarditis; the presence of a pericardial rub in asso-

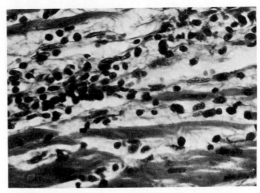

Figure 17–2. Focus of inflammatory cell infiltration in the myocardium in viral myocarditis. (H&E stain.) (Courtesy of O Rambo.)

ciation with electrocardiographic abnormalities demonstrates pericardial involvement and distinguishes coxsackievirus infection with myocarditis from other influenza-like syndromes (Sainani, 1975).

The illness usually lasts 1–4 weeks but may persist for months and may recur over a period of 1–2 years, but rarely is the condition severe, fulminant, or fatal. Patients are usually completely well months later, but chronic cardiac failure has continued over a period of 2–3 years in 5–10% of patients. There is increasing evidence that coxsackievirus myocarditis may be a cause of dilated cardiomyopathy later in life. In 42 patients with coxsackievirus myocarditis supported by a fourfold rise in complement-fixing antibodies, 15-year follow-up revealed death in ten patients (24%), all with evidence of cardiomyopathy (Levi, 1988). A relationship between coxsackievirus myocarditis and chronic constrictive pericarditis has also been proposed, but only a few well-documented examples of such patients have been reported.

2. Laboratory findings– The diagnosis of viral infection is confirmed by virus isolation from throat washings or feces or by a fourfold increase in neutralizing antibody in paired sera during the course of the disease. In the presence of documented viral infection in the patient with the clinical picture of myocardial disease, one infers the infection to be the cause of the myocarditis.

3. X-ray findings– The chest film may demonstrate significant cardiac enlargement, often with pleural or pericardial effusion. If the latter is suspected, echocardiography can then establish its presence and magnitude (see Chapter 18).

4. Special investigations– Echocardiography is a more accurate way of establishing individual chamber size and wall motion activity and identifying intraventricular clots and other specific diseases. E-point separation, ie, poor opening of the mitral and aortic valve leaflets and poor motion of the aortic

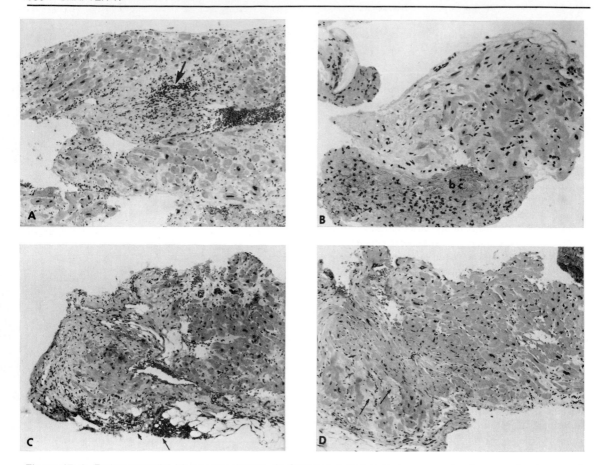

Figure 17–3. Endomyocardial biopsy specimens. **A:** Obtained before immunosuppressive therapy, showing an obvious lymphocytic infiltrate **(arrow)** that was present in each biopsy specimen. (H&E × 120.) **B:** Obtained after 4 months of immunosuppressive therapy; there is now complete absence of cell infiltrate. Blood clot (bc) is attached to the biopsy specimen. (H&E × 192.) **C:** After discontinuation of immunosuppressive therapy. There is a return of the lymphocytic infiltrate and, in addition, considerable pericardial infiltrate is present **(arrows).** (H&E × 120.) **D:** The final biopsy, taken 1 full year after initiation of immunosuppressive therapy, shows considerable fibrosis **(arrows),** but absence of cell infiltrate. (H&E × 120.) (Reproduced, with permission, from Mason JW, Billingham ME, Ricci DR: Treatment of acute inflammatory myocarditis assisted by endomyocardial biopsy. Am J Cardiol 1980;45:1037.)

root, is a sign of decreased stroke volume. Echocardiographic abnormalities are common in acute myocarditis. In one study, left ventricular dysfunction was seen in 69% and in patients with congestive heart failure in 88%, often without cavity dilation or with only minor dilation. Additional findings include "left ventricular hypertrophy," reversible and perhaps due to edema, left ventricular thrombi, and restrictive ventricular filling by Doppler (Pinamonti, 1988). Indium 111-monoclonal antimyosin antibody imaging can be used to detect myocardial necrosis, following which endomyocardial biopsy may be performed (Yasuda, 1987).

5. Endomyocardial biopsy– Biopsy of the right ventricular endocardium occasionally establishes the specific diagnosis of the myocarditis. More commonly, the biopsy shows a nonspecific inflammatory infiltrate that establishes the diagnosis of myocarditis

but not its cause. In patients with sudden onset of congestive heart failure, biopsy will show myocarditis in about 10–20% of cases. Serial biopsies have been advocated to determine the value of treatment with corticosteroids or immunosuppressive drugs. However, in recently reported studies, the value of these drugs in acute myocarditis has been seriously questioned (Latham, 1989; Kishimoto, 1990). Furthermore, histologic resolution of the myocarditis during immunosuppressive treatment is not a prerequisite to improvement in left ventricular function, which is the most important determinant of prognosis (Dec, 1988).

B. Myocarditis Due to Other Viruses: Myocarditis has been noted frequently, usually by electrocardiographic changes or some alteration of heart sounds, as an incidental feature of other viral diseases such as echovirus infection, mumps, varicella, poliomyelitis, infectious mononucleosis, measles, and hepatitis. Human immunodeficiency virus (HIV) has been associated with myocarditis. Although focal myocarditis identified by myocardial biopsy or at postmortem is seen in about 20% of hearts of people who die with AIDS, it is not clear whether this represents infection with HIV, infection with an opportunistic virus or other organisms, or myocardial damage due to some other mechanism, such as drug toxicity (Acierno, 1989; Kaul, 1991). Gallop rhythm, enlargement of the heart, or other signs of cardiac failure (see Chapter 10) may be present. Focal myocardial infiltration may be found on pathologic examination of the heart from patients with many types of viral infections who had no clinical evidence of heart disease during life.

C. Acute Myocarditis in Rickettsial Diseases: In rickettsial diseases, infection may result in cardiac or circulatory failure in the second week of disease, but this is rarely a prominent feature. In typhus epidemics of 1915, cardiac failure was thought to be the cause of death in one-third of cases autopsied. In Q fever, there may be tachycardia out of proportion to the degree of fever, as well as dyspnea, fatigue, or chest pain suggesting myocardial involvement.

Rocky Mountain spotted fever may rarely cause myocarditis. Serologic confirmation can only be made late in the disease, and the diagnosis can be made earlier only on epidemiologic and clinical evidence.

Scrub typhus myocarditis in US military personnel during World War II was characterized by persistent fatigue, tachycardia, and electrocardiographic and radiologic evidence of cardiac involvement requiring prolonged convalescence even in otherwise healthy young men. Eventually, all patients recovered completely.

D. Acute Myocarditis in Trypanosomiasis: In Chagas' disease, the initial skin and eye lesions may be associated with acute myocarditis, but the dominant feature is late chronic cardiac failure, conduction defects, or apical aneurysm. African trypanosomiasis can cause chronic pancarditis as well as valvulitis and lesions of the conduction system. The usual presenting symptoms are neurologic rather than cardiac, because meningoencephalitis is a frequent complication. The histologic pattern is similar to that of Chagas' disease, but myocarditis is less frequent in infections due to *Trypanosoma gambiense* than in those due to *Trypanosoma cruzi*. Cases of idiopathic hypertrophy occurring in African countries might be due to undiagnosed trypanosomiasis.

E. Diphtheritic Myocarditis: Diphtheria is rare in the USA as a result of widespread immunization with diphtheria toxoid, but it is a substantial health problem in some other countries. The disease occurs chiefly in children and is usually transmitted by nasopharyngeal secretions, but any underlying skin lesion may become infected. The diagnosis is made by bacteriologic examination of a grayish-green adherent membrane that may involve the nares, pharynx, larynx, bronchi, or skin. An exotoxin secreted by the bacilli causes the acute clinical disease.

Myocarditis occurs in 10–25% of cases, usually in the first few weeks, and is manifested by clinical features and by ST–T changes in the ECG. In more severe cases, acute circulatory or cardiac failure may occur, associated with various arrhythmias or conduction defects, especially ventricular tachycardia and atrioventricular block (Halvadar, 1989).

Prevention by immunization in infancy with booster injections every 10 years is the most effective form of control.

Treatment consists of early intramuscular or intravenous injection of diphtheria antitoxin, combined with antibiotic treatment with penicillin, erythromycin, or ampicillin to eradicate the organism. Intensive care nursing may be necessary, especially if there is airway obstruction requiring tracheostomy or bronchoscopy. Bed rest and supportive care may be necessary for several weeks. Digitalis is rarely of value. Antitoxin is usually ineffective once myocarditis has occurred. Large doses of corticosteroids have been given in severe cases, but their therapeutic value has not been established.

The course of the disease varies from a mild illness to a fulminant, fatal process. In severe cases, with circulatory failure or atrioventricular block, the mortality rate approaches 60–70%, emphasizing the importance of preventive immunization and early treatment with antitoxin. Carrier states are relatively common and should be sought and treated with antibiotics after the patient has recovered. Permanent partial atrioventricular block may occur, but cardiac failure or complete heart block is rare in the years following the acute attack.

F. Acute Myocarditis in Trichinosis: *Trichinella spiralis* in inadequately cooked pork may cause disease leading to myocarditis. The parasite frequently invades the heart, but it rarely encysts there. The myocardial injury may be due to the toxic effects of the host's reaction to the parasite. Disease is suspected in a patient with fever, periorbital edema, muscle pains, and eosinophilia who has eaten inadequately cooked meat. The larvae spread through the body, but focal inflammatory myocarditis and endocarditis with thrombosis are responsible for some deaths.

Myocarditis occurs 3–8 weeks after infection and is suspected on the basis of dyspnea, tachycardia, and electrocardiographic demonstration of ST–T changes, sinus tachycardia, and ventricular premature beats. Congestive failure occurs rarely. The diagnosis is strongly suspected on the basis of severe eosinophilia (often ≥ 50%) and splinter hemorrhages of the nails, and it is confirmed by serologic tests and skeletal muscle biopsy.

Treatment is supportive, with corticosteroid ther-

ing. There is no evidence that they have any effect on the natural course of the disease. Note: The salicylates should be continued as long as necessary to relieve pain, swelling, or fever. If withdrawal results in recurrence of symptoms, treatment should be reinstituted immediately.

a. Sodium salicylate is the most widely used of this group of drugs. The maximum adult dose is 1 g orally every 4 hours to allay symptoms and fever; 4 g/d suffice in most adults. In an occasional patient, maximum doses may not be completely effective. There is no evidence that intravenous administration has any advantage over the oral route. Early untoward reactions to the salicylates include tinnitus, nausea and vomiting, and gastrointestinal bleeding. Salicylates may be used with antacids, after meals, or with milk to reduce gastric irritation. Caution: Do not use sodium salicylate or sodium bicarbonate in patients with acute rheumatic fever who have associated cardiac failure.

b. Aspirin may be substituted for sodium salicylate. A satisfactory daily dose for children is usually 15–25 mg/kg given in divided doses every 4 hours during the day for a week, with the dose then decreased by half. Adults initially may require 0.6–0.9 g every 4 hours during the day. Hyperpnea may occur with large doses. Other anti–inflammatory agents (eg, indomethacin) have not been used in large–scale studies.

2. Penicillin– Penicillin is given at the outset of disease to eradicate streptococcal infections.

3. Corticosteroids– A short course of corticosteroids usually causes rapid improvement in the acute manifestations of rheumatic fever and is indicated in severe cases. Give prednisone, 5–10 mg orally every 6 hours for 3 weeks, and then gradually withdraw over a period of 3 weeks. In severe cases, the dosage should be increased, if necessary, to levels adequate to control symptoms. There is, however, no evidence that either corticosteroids or salicylates prevent or reduce permanent myocardial damage.

B. General Measures: Bed rest should be enforced until all signs of active rheumatic fever have disappeared (ie, normal temperature with the patient at bed rest and without medications, normal resting pulse rate [< 100/min in adults], and normal heart function or fixed abnormalities on ECG). Several months should elapse before return to full activity, unless the disease was very mild. Maintain good nutrition.

C. Treatment of Complications:

1. Congestive heart failure– Treat as for congestive heart failure due to other causes, with the following variations:

a. Digitalis is usually not as effective in congestive heart failure due to acute rheumatic fever as in other forms of congestive failure. It may accentuate myocardial irritability, producing arrhythmias, and should therefore be given with care.

b. Corticosteroids– Congestive failure and pericarditis may respond dramatically to corticosteroids, but the anti-inflammatory action may fail to modify subsequent valvular damage. When sodium–retaining drugs are employed, sodium intake is restricted and thiazide diuresis is used.

2. Pericarditis– Treat as for any acute nonpurulent pericarditis. The rheumatic effusion is sterile, and antibiotics are of no value. The general principles include relief of pain, by opiates if necessary, and removal of fluid by pericardiocentesis if tamponade develops. This, however, is rarely necessary. Corticosteroids and salicylates should be continued or started, as they aid resorption of fluid.

Prognosis

Initial episodes of rheumatic fever last months in children and weeks in adults. Twenty percent of children have recurrences within 5 years. Recurrences are uncommon after 5 years of well-being and rare after age 21. The immediate mortality rate is 1–2%. Persistent rheumatic activity with a greatly enlarged heart, heart failure, and pericarditis indicate a poor prognosis as shown in Table 17–3; 30% of children thus affected die within 10 years of the initial attack. Table 17–4 shows causes of death. Otherwise, the prognosis for life is good. (More recent data on a comparable series are not available.) Approximately one-third of young patients have detectable valvular damage after the initial episode, most commonly involving the mitral valve. After 10 years, two-thirds of surviving patients will have detectable valvular disease. In adults, residual heart damage occurs in less than 20% and is generally less severe (Engleman, 1954). Aortic incompetence is more common in adults than in children. Twenty percent of patients who have chorea develop valvular deformity even after a long latent period of apparent well-being.

Table 17–3. Fatalities in rheumatic fever in patients with special features.[1]

Onset (Number of Cases)	10 Years (Fatalities)	20 Years (Fatalities)
Greatly enlarged heart 70	56 (80%)	57 (81%)
Congestive failure 207	148 (71%)	152 (80%)
Pericarditis 130	73 (56%)	77 (63%)
Nodules 88	34 (38%)	37 (43%)
Arthritis 410	91 (22%)	109 (27%)
Chorea 518	49 (9.4%)	63 (12%)

[1] Reproduced, with permission, from the American Heart Association, Inc., Bland EF, Jones TD: Rheumatic fever and rheumatic heart disease: A 20-year report on 1000 patients followed since childhood. Circulation 1951; 4:836.

Table 17–4. Causes of death in 301 cases of rheumatic fever and heart disease among 1000 patients after 20 years.[1]

Rheumatic Heart Disease		
Rheumatic fever		231	(77%)
Congestive failure			
Subacute infective endocarditis	26	30	(10%)
Acute infective endocarditis	4		
Other causes:			
Cerebral embolism	3		
Sudden and unexpected	10	30	
Uncertain	8		(10%)
Unrelated disease or accident	9		
Possible Rheumatic Heart Disease		
Unrelated disease or accident		10	(3%)

[1] Modified and reproduced, with permission, from the American Heart Association, Inc., Bland EF, Jones TD: Rheumatic fever and rheumatic heart disease: A 20-year report on 1000 patients followed since childhood. Circulation 1951;4:836.

ACUTE MYOCARDIAL DAMAGE DUE TO DRUG TOXICITY

Acute myocardial damage is seen after the use of a variety of drugs, notably cytotoxic agents, emetine, sympathomimetic drugs, arsenic, antimony, amphetamines, tricyclic antidepressants, and cocaine. About one-fourth of patients (4 out of 15) receiving high-dose multiple chemotherapy may die of acute myocardial failure during treatment as a result of endothelial injury, pericardial effusion, cardiac failure, and cardiac arrhythmias (Appelbaum, 1976).

Cocaine blocks the reuptake for norepinephrine at sympathetic nerve endings, thus producing a hyperadrenergic state. This has resulted in coronary artery spasm and myocardial infarction, intracoronary thrombosis, and cardiomyopathy (Rezkalla, 1990; Kloner, 1990).

Cytotoxic agents, eg, cyclophosphamide and doxorubicin, may produce clinical as well as pathologic myocardial disease; the toxic effects are dose-related and more apt to occur when cytotoxic drugs are used in combination (Fu, 1990). As with any variety of acute myocardial disease or toxicity, the clinical presentation may be with arrhythmias or conduction defects rather than predominant cardiac failure (with systolic or diastolic dysfunction) (Lee, 1987). Postural hypotension or electrocardiographic T wave abnormalities may also occur. MRI has shown proton relaxing abnormalities as myocardial disease worsens (Thompson, 1987).

Cautious restriction of total dosage, using a weekly schedule (Torti, 1983), or continuous intravenous infusion of doxorubicin (Legha, 1982) may decrease toxicity (see above). Close clinical observation for early evidences of cardiac involvement is advised. Serial ECGs, chest films, echocardiograms, and in selected cases, endomyocardial biopsy, may reveal early signs of myocardial toxicity. Decrease in the height of the R wave is an early sign of cardiac toxicity, and the risk:benefit ratio of continued therapy must be assessed. Cardiac enlargement and cardiac failure may develop slowly or rapidly. With rapid withdrawal, doxorubicin cardiomyopathy has been reported to be reversible (Saini, 1987).

Patients receiving emetine (for amebiasis) may demonstrate electrocardiographic abnormalities without clinical symptoms or signs; it is then desirable to use alternative drugs or proceed with smaller dosages.

Interleukin-2 and alpha interferon have been reported to cause reversible severe cardiomyopathy (Samlowski, 1989).

Many drugs may cause myocarditis through a hypersensitivity reaction. The onset of myocarditis may occur within hours after taking the drug or may be delayed up to months later. Symptoms clear and residua may be minimal if the drug is rapidly withdrawn (Taliercio, 1985).

Treatment

Withdraw cardiotoxic drugs and treat cardiac failure and arrhythmias as outlined in Chapters 10 and 15.

Prognosis

The prognosis is good if appropriate measures are taken before severe cardiac failure occurs, poor if the offending drug is continued after early cardiac toxicity is manifest. Mild to moderate cardiac failure subsides gradually after the cardiotoxic drug is stopped.

DRUG-INDUCED CONNECTIVE TISSUE DISORDERS

A variety of drugs such as procainamide, hydralazine, phenytoin, and some of the phenothiazines may cause a syndrome indistinguishable from lupus erythematosus (see below), with pericarditis, arteritis, and characteristic serologic changes (Table 17–5). In practically all instances, the syndrome subsides after withdrawal of the drug.

The worst offender is procainamide; at least half of all patients receiving this drug for about 6 months develop positive serologic changes and ultimately clinical signs of the lupus-like syndrome, which disappear slowly when the drug is stopped. The skin and kidneys are usually spared, and the first manifestations may be serologic and hematologic ones. The high frequency with which procainamide produces the syndrome prevents its use in chronic therapy of arrhythmias; however, since it may take months for the syndrome to appear, the drug may be used during the acute phase for short periods.

The lupus-like syndrome occurs less commonly

Table 17–5. Drugs implicated (in descending order of importance) in the induction of a lupus-like syndrome.[1]

Procainamide	Penicillamine
Hydralazine	Oral contraceptive agents
Isoniazid	Phenothiazines
Sulfonamides	Quinidine
Penicillin	Ethosuximide
Tetracycline	Phenylbutazone
Streptomycin	Phenytoin
Aminosalicylic acid	Mephenytoin
Griseofulvin	Trimethadione

[1] Reproduced, with permission, from Bardana EJ, Pirofsky B: Recent advances in the immuno-pathogenesis of systemic lupus erythematosus. West J Med 1975; 122:130.

with hydralazine, particularly in the doses ordinarily prescribed. In patients receiving 200 mg/d or less, the syndrome is uncommon; it is much more common with doses of 600–800 mg/d.

CHRONIC CARDIOMYOPATHIES

This is a miscellaneous group of diseases of unknown cause (not related to known causes such as coronary, hypertensive, valvular, or congenital heart diseases), classified on the basis of clinical and hemodynamic features into three types: (1) dilated (congestive) cardiomyopathy, with clinical features of cardiac enlargement, increased cardiac volume, and symptoms and signs of congestive failure with poor systolic pump function; (2) hypertrophic obstructive cardiomyopathy; and (3) restrictive cardiomyopathy, with infiltrative myocardial disease associated with endomyocardial fibrosis, amyloid disease, scleroderma, hemochromatosis, and other disorders that interfere with left ventricular filling and emptying (impaired diastolic function).

The clinical division into these three types is imperfect because of overlap (eg, amyloid heart disease may be both restrictive and congestive). Conduction defects may be predominant in some cardiomyopathies (eg, Chagas' disease; sarcoid).

1. DILATED (CONGESTIVE) CARDIOMYOPATHY

Idiopathic dilated cardiomyopathy has become an increasingly common disease with an estimated annual incidence of 7.5 cases per 100,000 population (Torp, 1980).

Dilated cardiomyopathy is a nonspecific diagnosis. The predominant feature, dilation of either ventricle, can be caused by many conditions, of which it may be the end stage leading to cardiac failure. Possible causes are (1) excessive alcohol intake over a period of many years; (2) ischemic cardiomyopathy (see

Chapter 8); (3) acute viral myocarditis; (4) diabetes mellitus affecting the small vessels of the heart, causing vasculitis, heart failure, and anginal pains similar to those of large–vessel coronary disease, but with the main coronary arteries often remaining normal; and (5) deficiencies of thiamine and other nutrients (Manolio, 1992). The frequency of viral myocarditis as a cause is controversial, but it has been shown increasingly that unexplained dilated cardiomyopathy may follow acute myocarditis (Dec, 1985). Endomyocardial biopsy has demonstrated myocarditis and other conditions in dilated cardiomyopathy (Parrillo, 1984).

There is evidence that the development of dilated cardiomyopathy is related to a previous episode of viral myocarditis. The prevalence of idiopathic dilated cardiopathy in the general population is 0.005%, whereas in patients with a history of viral myocarditis it is between 4% and 9% (Hosenpud, 1988). Studies using in situ hybridization techniques show enterovirus-specific RNA in the myocardial cells of 18–50% of patients (Tracy, 1990). It is unlikely that the dilated cardiomyopathy is the result of chronic myocarditis but more likely that changes incited by the viral myocarditis have resulted in an immunologically mediated myocardial injury. As evidence for the immunologic mechanism, abnormalities of both the cellular and the humoral arms of the immune system have been reported in patients with cardiomyopathy. Abnormalities in the CD4 (helper lymphocyte) and CD8 (suppressor lymphocyte) ratio have been reported, along with T cell abnormalities (Koike, 1989). Circulating autoantibodies against a variety of myocardial cell proteins such as actin, myosin, tropomyosin, and ADP/ATP carrier protein of the mitochondrial membrane have been described (Schultheiss, 1989; Beisel, 1988). Although these findings do not establish a causal relationship with chronic dilated cardiomyopathy, they support the hypothesis that dilated cardiomyopathy is an "autoimmune" disease.

Although it is believed that most cases of idiopathic cardiomyopathy are sporadic, families have been described with several members affected. In the past, 5–10% of patients with cardiomyopathy have had a family history of the disease. A recent report of systematic examination of relatives of patients with idiopathic cardiomyopathy disclosed an incidence of 20% with familial disease (Michels, 1992).

Clinical Findings

A. Symptoms: The disease is suspected early in patients who have dyspnea, chest pain, or palpitations. Dyspnea may progress from dyspnea on exertion to orthopnea, paroxysmal nocturnal dyspnea, and pulmonary edema. When right heart failure supervenes, peripheral edema may be a prominent symptom.

The chest pain is nondescript and may be related to pulmonary congestion or, if pleuritic, to pulmonary embolism. Occasionally, the patient will present with typical pericarditis, including fever and chest discomfort aggravated by inspiration, coughing, and lying down. In addition, the patient will have signs of cardiomyopathy with dilated, poorly contracting ventricles and congestive heart failure.

Patients who complain of palpitations may have chronic atrial fibrillation or paroxysmal atrial or ventricular arrhythmia. Ventricular premature beats occur in about half of cases; ventricular tachycardia or fibrillation usually occurs late. Recognition of arrhythmias is increased if ambulatory monitoring or exercise electrocardiographic tests are used. Complex arrhythmias or conduction defects can be identified in at least one-third of symptomatic patients and may explain some cases of sudden death.

Dizziness or syncope may occur from bradyarrhythmia or ventricular conduction defects secondary to fibrosis.

Symptoms of pulmonary or systemic emboli may occur, sometimes dominating the clinical features.

B. Signs: The signs are those of cardiac hypertrophy or cardiac failure (see Chapter 10). The cardiac failure is usually left ventricular with pulmonary rales, left ventricular gallop rhythm, and left ventricular heave that is displaced downward and to the left. If the disease is more advanced, right ventricular enlargement and congestive heart failure are found with a raised venous pressure and pulsating neck veins and liver, an enlarged tender liver, and dependent edema of the legs or sacrum. Thirty to 40 percent of patients with cardiomyopathy have a history of hypertension, and patients who have severe congestive heart failure can have markedly elevated blood pressure when first seen as a result of marked elevation of circulating catecholamines and sympathetic stimulation.

Signs of pulmonary emboli (see Chapter 19) or systemic emboli (see Chapter 20) may be found.

C. Laboratory Findings: There are no specific laboratory findings unless the dilated cardiomyopathy is due to specific diseases such as hemochromatosis or thyroid disorders.

D. Electrocardiographic Findings: Changes on the ECG include left ventricular hypertrophy (see Chapter 9), ventricular and atrial arrhythmias (see Chapter 15), conduction defects (see Chapter 14)—both atrioventricular block and bundle branch block—and nonspecific ST–T abnormalities.

E. Imaging Studies: X-ray findings include cardiac enlargement, chiefly left ventricular, with a large cardiac volume and with pulmonary congestion but without disproportionate left atrial enlargement, calcified valves, or abnormalities of the aorta (see Chapter 10). Echocardiography is particularly helpful in excluding pericardial effusion (see Chapter 18), aortic stenosis (when murmur is not heard because of severely decreased cardiac output) (see Chapter 13), and mitral valve disease (see Chapter 12) and in estimating left ventricular volume and ejection fraction

(see Chapter 10). Massive increases in diastolic volume or decreases in ejection fraction ($< 20\%$) are of bad prognostic import. Recently, patients with mild left ventricular dilation and low ejection fraction have been reported to have a poor prognosis. Endomyocardial biopsy in these patients showed only mild myofibrillary loss, probably accounting for the nearly normal heart size (Keren, 1990).

F. Hemodynamic Findings and Angiography: With the development of echo-Doppler techniques, catheterization is rarely necessary to make the diagnosis of congestive cardiomyopathy. It is most often done to rule out coronary artery disease in patients abnormal calcium kinetics related to an increased number of calcium channel receptors, abnormal adrenergic hypersensitivity, and myocardial ischemia due to abnormality of the microcirculation, resulting in sequestration of small amounts of calcium on the contractile mechanism (Wagner, 1989; Brush, 1989).

Differential Diagnosis

A. Ischemic Cardiomyopathy: Increased left ventricular volume with decreased ejection fraction and generalized hypokinesia are seen on angiography in both dilated and ischemic cardiomyopathy. The latter may also exhibit greatly increased cardiac volume, segmental defects in contraction rather than symmetric hypokinesis, and myocardial ischemia during exercise. Coronary artery disease can be suspected in patients with angina or in those with abnormal thallium or sestamibi perfusion tests, although patients with congestive cardiomyopathy can also have these findings.

B. Other Disorders: Other forms of cardiac disease (eg, valvular heart disease), hypertension, and secondary cardiomyopathies are discussed elsewhere in this book.

Treatment

There are no specific measures for congestive cardiomyopathy. Treat cardiac failure as outlined in Chapter 10.

Beta-adrenergic blocking agents starting with very small doses have been recommended in the treatment of cardiac failure secondary to dilated cardiomyopathy. Decrease in symptoms, increase in exercise tolerance, increase in ejection fraction, and decrease in heart size have been reported (Waagstein, 1989). There is evidence that the beta-blockers can increase the depressed beta receptors at the cell membrane, making the cell more responsive to catecholamines.

In severe cardiac failure, vasodilators are valuable, and there is excellent evidence that ACE inhibitors prolong life. Perhaps as a result of chronic enhanced catecholamine stimulation, there may be myocellular calcium accumulation that may cause hemodynamic deterioration. Calcium entry blockade may be useful for reversing this effect, and in one small prospective study it was shown that long-term diltiazem treatment was helpful in improving ejection fraction and survival (Figulla, 1989). Inotropic agents should be considered. There is no evidence that the new phosphoesterase inhibitors such as milrinone or xamoterol will be better than digoxin and much evidence that they will increase the mortality rate (German and Austrian Xamoterol Study Group, 1988). Anticoagulant and antiarrhythmic treatment may be valuable in some cases. Amiodarone in doses of 200–400 mg/d is effective in suppressing arrhythmias in patients in chronic congestive heart failure. There was little adverse effect on hemodynamics and a low incidence of side effects (Cleland, 1987).

Cardiac transplantation is the treatment of choice in the patient with class III or class IV heart failure and an ejection fraction below 20%. The optimal time for transplantation is still being investigated. Patients who are minimally symptomatic tend to live longer when the ejection fraction is under 20%. Transplantation is warranted within 6 months to 1 year. If the ejection fraction is 10%, transplantation is indicated even if the patient is not in class III or IV (Keogh, 1988) (see Chapter 14).

The newest approach to the patient with cardiomyopathy and severe congestive heart failure is "dynamic cardiomyoplasty," or wrapping a skeletal muscle flap—usually the latissimus dorsi—electively synchronized with the cardiac contraction, around the heart. In early studies in patients with class III or IV heart failure in a follow-up of almost 11 months, there was improvement in seven of eight patients to class I or II status and small improvements in ejection fraction and left ventricular stroke volume (Moreira, 1990).

Prognosis

Without treatment, the prognosis for dilated cardiomyopathy is generally poor, but exceptions do occur. Two-thirds of deaths occur within 2 years. The 5-year mortality rate is about 50%; roughly one-third to one-fourth of patients survive for 10 years (Fuster, 1981). Frequent episodes of ventricular arrhythmias occur in patients with dilated cardiomyopathy and significantly impaired left ventricular function and may result in sudden death (Meinertz, 1984). In fact, death is sudden in about half of patients with idiopathic cardiomyopathy who die (Anderson, 1987). Endomyocardial biopsies are of prognostic value; survival is twice as long if the biopsy is normal as when it shows abnormalities (Shirey, 1980). Myofilament loss at endomyocardial biopsy predicted a poor outcome independent of clinical class or ejection fraction (Hammond, 1987). Afterload reduction and intensive treatment of cardiac failure and arrhythmias may improve the prognosis. In patients referred for cardiac transplantation, functional class III or IV, low ejection fraction, high pulmonary artery wedge pressure, elevated plasma catecholamines, and the presence of

ventricular tachycardia all had negative prognostic implications (Keogh, 1990).

2. HYPERTROPHIC CARDIOMYOPATHY

The best clinical definition of hypertrophic cardiomyopathy is that of unexplained left ventricular hypertrophy (Brandenburg, 1980). The cardinal features are illustrated in Figure 17–5. The considerable hypertrophy, which involves chiefly the septum but can involve the mid ventricle or apex or may even be generalized and include the right ventricle, leads to decreased compliance of the left ventricle, decreased left ventricular diastolic filling, and increased left ventricular filling pressure to maintain adequate flow; the latter consequence causes dyspnea and decreased exercise tolerance. In some patients with systole, the anterior leaflet of the mitral valve comes into apposition with the septal muscle, and narrowing of the outflow tract gives rise to the characteristic systolic murmur. Systolic outflow obstruction is not essential to the diagnosis, and there is doubt that it has prognostic significance. When present, the severity of the obstruction varies with the level of the peripheral resistance, the adequacy of the central blood volume, and the degree of ventricular emptying. In some cases, septal hypertrophy involves the right side of the heart in addition to or instead of the left, and a picture resembling that of infundibular pulmonary stenosis is then seen.

Symptoms of heart failure are related to decreased compliance of the left ventricle because of abnormalities of left ventricular relaxation and filling. These diastolic abnormalities are not related to the degree of left ventricular hypertrophy. Diagnostic filling abnormalities by Doppler are common in patients with diffuse hypertrophy and in patients with mild localized hypertrophy (Spirito and Maron, 1990) can further impair diastolic function (Cannon, 1985; Vatner, 1990).

Etiology

There is a high familial incidence if enough family members are studied. Search for the genetic abnormality in hypertrophic cardiomyopathy has intensified with localization of the gene to a specific site on chromosome 14 in one large French Canadian family (Jarcho, 1989). Subsequent in situ hybridization studies have confined the locus to a region of the long arm of chromosome 14, now designated FHC-1 (Solomon, 1990). This gene is responsible for encoding for myosin heavy chains. There is genetic heterogeneity, since studies of other families have localized the gene to other chromosomes, so that it may be difficult to find genetic markers that will reliably predict a familial predisposition to hypertrophic cardiomyopathy (Epstein, 1992). There are also patients with

DIASTOLE   Aorta   SYSTOLE   Aorta

Right atrium   Left atrium   Left atrium

Left ventricle

Cardinal features: *Left ventricular (especially septal) hypertrophy; diastolic dysfunction; systolic outflow obstruction; systolic anterior motion of mitral valve; excessive left ventricular emptying.*

Variable factors: *Severity; level of peripheral resistance; low resistance and low blood volume lead to obstruction.*

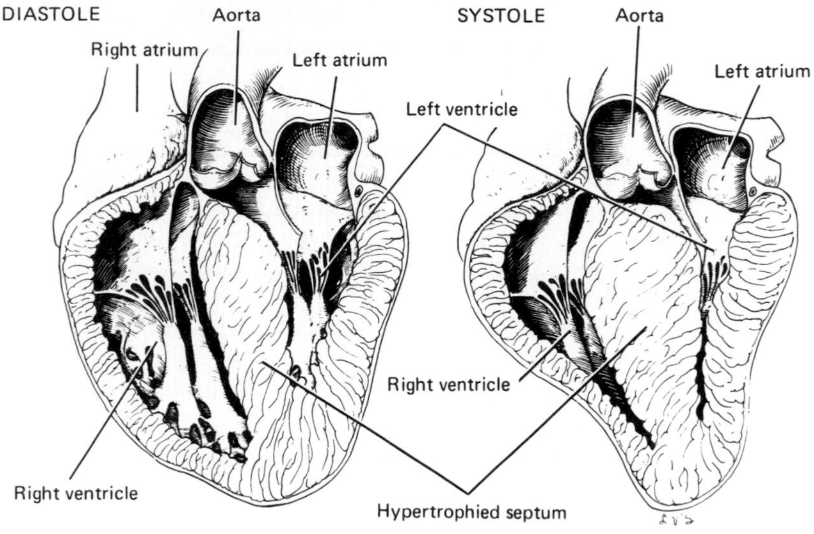

Right ventricle

Right ventricle

Hypertrophied septum

Figure 17–5. Hypertrophic cardiomyopathy (left lateral view). The cardinal features are displayed.

hypertrophic cardiomyopathy who appear to be sporadic cases with no familial association. In other patients, especially elderly ones, the disease appears to develop late in life in association with hypertension.

Although the cause is unknown, congenitally determined myocardial fiber disarray is probably related to the genetic abnormality and results in the hypertrophy and diastolic functional abnormalities that characterize this disease. The genetic abnormality may also result in other possible abnormalities leading to hypertrophic cardiomyopathy. There are data suggesting abnormal calcium kinetics related to an increased number of calcium channel receptors, abnormal adrenergic hypersensitivity, and myocardial ischemia due to abnormality of the microcirculation, resulting in sequestration of small amounts of calcium on the contractile mechanism (Wagner, 1989; Brush, 1989).

Age & Sex Incidence

The disease occurs with equal frequency in both sexes and is seen in all age groups. The age- and sex-adjusted prevalence rate for hypertrophic cardiomyopathy is 18.8 per 100,000 population in the USA (Codd, 1989). The possibility of associated skeletal muscle disease has been raised.

Criteria for Diagnosis

The criteria required for diagnosis are controversial but include left ventricular hypertrophy, frequently asymmetrically in the septum but at times in the mid ventricle or the apex of the left ventricle. In other cases, the hypertrophy can be generalized and may even involve the right ventricle. There may be variable obstruction in the body of the left ventricle, decreased distensibility and impaired diastolic function

and relaxation of the left ventricle, and a propensity to sudden death, especially after severe exertion. The outflow tract obstruction, which is of variable severity, can be demonstrated by observing a significant pressure difference as an end-hole catheter is withdrawn from the body of the left ventricle into the outflow tract. There is no gradient on crossing the aortic valve (Figures 17–6 and 17–7).

This gradient can be demonstrated by Doppler echocardiography. Systolic anterior motion (SAM) of the anterior leaflet of the mitral valve is also a sign of potential or actual obstruction.

Evidence of hypertrophy can also be obtained in other ways (ECG, echocardiogram, or angiogram), but the results are often inconsistent. Emptying of the ventricle that is more complete than normal on echo-

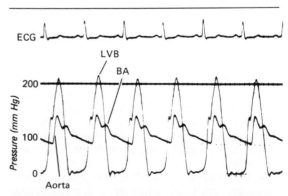

Figure 17–6. Simultaneous brachial arterial (BA) and left ventricular body (LVB) pressure tracings and ECG in a patient with hypertrophic obstructive cardiomyopathy.

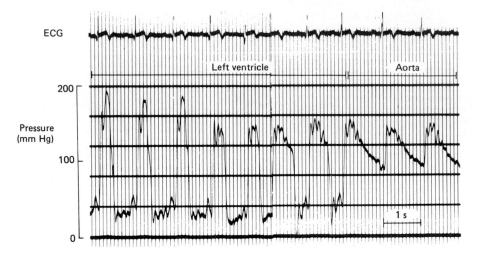

Figure 17–7. Withdrawal pressure tracing from left ventricle to aorta in a patient with hypertrophic obstructive cardiomyopathy. The pressure difference of 50 mm Hg is in the ventricle and not between the ventricle and the aorta.

cardiography or angiocardiography is an important feature of the disease. Abnormalities in left ventricular diastolic function (impaired relaxation) have been described in most patients (Wigle, 1987).

There are wide differences of opinion about the minimum abnormality required to establish the diagnosis. The finding of left ventricular hypertrophy on echocardiography or on an ECG that shows left ventricular hypertrophy or abnormal Q waves in a patient with a family history of hypertrophic cardiomyopathy justifies the diagnosis. The dangers of creating cardiac neurosis by warning patients with minor or subclinical findings of the possibility of sudden death are obvious.

Clinical Findings

A. Symptoms:

1. History of heart murmur– The presence of a heart murmur is not an uncommon reason for referral to a cardiologist. A spurious history of rheumatic fever is sometimes given because the murmur was heard in childhood, perhaps in association with an episode of sore throat.

2. Dyspnea and chest pain– Dyspnea on exertion and chest pain are the commonest presenting symptoms. The pain is a dull, aching, substernal discomfort and radiates to the arm like angina pectoris. At times, it is closely associated with dyspnea. In many patients, the discomfort described is classic angina pectoris, and one may even see the clinical picture of unstable angina.

3. Other symptoms– Fatigue, dizziness, palpitations, and syncope are often reported. Syncope may be related to ventricular arrhythmias but may also be associated with bradycardia incompatible with an activated baroreflex (Gilligan, 1992). Sudden death oc-

curs, especially in familial cases with marked septal hypertrophy, but the frequency of this outcome is not well documented, and it is not directly related to severity. Ventricular arrhythmias are common and may be responsible for symptoms or sudden death. Sudden death is more apt to occur in individuals under the age of 30 with a positive family history, and it even occurs in infants. Its occurrence cannot be predicted by symptoms, hemodynamic variables, or left ventricular septal thickness. However, the degree of left ventricular hypertrophy may be a potential marker for identifying patients at risk of sudden death. Marked diffuse hypertrophy in asymptomatic or mildly symptomatic patients was eight times more common in patients who died suddenly (Spirito and Maron, 1990). Forty percent of cases of sudden death occur during or immediately after vigorous exercise (Maron, 1982; Maron, 1987).

4. Factors influencing symptoms– The severity of obstruction to left ventricular outflow varies with the state of the circulation. Anything that reduces peripheral resistance, such as a hot environment, pregnancy, standing up suddenly, exercise, or amyl nitrite inhalation, may induce or exaggerate outflow obstruction and bring on symptoms. Left ventricular failure occurs late and may follow the onset of atrial fibrillation. Severe dyspnea and even pulmonary edema can occur solely as a consequence of diastolic dysfunction with normal systolic function. With atrial fibrillation and loss of atrial contraction and the shortened diastolic filling period, left ventricular filling pressure rises markedly, and the patient can develop pulmonary edema.

In patients with severe left ventricular relaxation abnormality, especially if given diuretics or preload reducing agents such as nitrites, the filling pressure

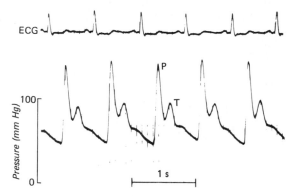

Figure 17–8. Bifid brachial arterial pulse in a patient with hypertrophic obstructive cardiomyopathy. The early percussion wave (P) is followed by a smaller tidal wave (T).

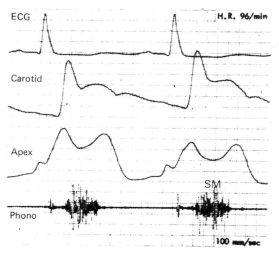

Figure 17–9. ECG, carotid pulse, apexcardiogram (Apex), and phonocardiogram (Phono) of a 36-year-old man with clinical and hemodynamic features of hypertrophic obstructive cardiomyopathy. Blood pressure was 120/50 mm Hg. Note the a wave and double humped apical impulse in the apexcardiogram, as well as the position of the systolic murmur (SM) late in systole. (Reproduced, with permission, from Burchell HB: Hypertrophic obstructive type of cardiomyopathy: Clinical syndrome. In: *Ciba Foundation Symposium: Cardiomyopathies.* Wolstenholme GEW, O'Connor M [editors]. Little, Brown, 1964.)

may be insufficient to develop a normal left ventricular volume, the stroke volume can decrease, and the patient may develop postural hypotension.

B. Signs:

1. Carotid pulse– The pulse has a bifid quality. The rapid initial upstroke is followed by a small tidal wave (Figure 17–8). However, this is frequently difficult to detect by palpation. The outflow obstruction develops after the start of systole, and the initial ejection of blood through an unobstructed outflow tract is responsible for the sharp rise in the pulse wave. As the obstruction develops during systole, it cuts down the rate of ejection and the pulse wave falls off, only to rise again later in systole. The characteristic carotid pulse can be helpful in elderly individuals whose systolic murmur may resemble aortic stenosis or mitral regurgitation.

2. Cardiac impulse– The same mechanism accounts for the findings on palpation at the apex of the heart in some cases, where a bifid impulse is felt during systole. The apical impulse may be bifid for another reason. The hypertrophied ventricle is less compliant than normal, and there is an abnormally forceful left atrial contraction. This produces a palpable presystolic impulse that gives a double apical impulse. When both of these factors are present, there is a triple cardiac impulse ("triple ripple") that is virtually pathognomonic of the condition (Figure 17–9).

3. Systolic murmur– Since obstruction is variable, the systolic murmur is variable also—from none at all to a loud, long systolic murmur similar to that of ventricular septal defect. The mechanism by which systolic obstruction occurs is still debated. Because of the hypertrophied septum, there is narrowing of the left ventricular outflow tract. The velocity of blood flow in systole and the outflow tract may create a Venturi effect on the anterior leaflet of the mitral valve, causing it to be pushed toward the septum and thus increasing the obstruction. The murmur is usu-

ally harsh and long, at times sounding like a systolic ejection murmur similar to that of aortic stenosis and at times like a regurgitant murmur in that it sounds almost holosystolic. The murmur can be soft, becoming loud only on standing, thus pooling venous return and making the ventricle smaller in diastole and collapsing the left ventricular outflow tract. Because the anterior leaflet of the mitral valve moves toward the septum, variable degrees of mitral regurgitation are frequent.

4. Other signs– Third and fourth heart sounds are commonly heard, but ejection clicks and aortic diastolic murmurs are rare. Mitral incompetence is often also present. The murmur may be best termed a **holosystolic ejection murmur.** Mitral diastolic murmurs may also occur. Left ventricular contraction may be prolonged, and paradoxic splitting of the second sound is sometimes present. The obstruction and therefore the gradient and loudness of the murmur are variable, which is characteristic of hypertrophic cardiomyopathy. The variable obstruction is related to any maneuver that decreases ventricular volume and therefore brings the anterior leaflet of the mitral valve closer to the septum. This occurs with any maneuver than increases contractility, decreases preload, or decreases afterload. Posture has a marked effect on the murmur, and sudden squatting, increas-

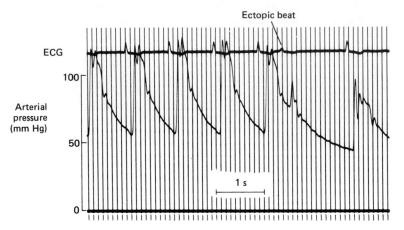

Figure 17–10. Bifid arterial pulse in a patient with hypertrophic obstructive cardiomyopathy showing Brockenbrough's sign, ie, decrease in pulse pressure in a beat following an ectopic beat.

ing ventricular volume, often abolishes it or lessens its intensity, as it does the obstruction. Valsalva's maneuver increases the murmurs of mitral regurgitation and of obstruction to the outflow of the left ventricle during the strain by decreasing the size of the left ventricle as a result of the reduced venous return.

The increase in loudness of murmur with Valsalva's maneuver is specific for hypertrophic cardiomyopathy but not very sensitive. The decrease in loudness of the murmur on squatting and the increase on standing are both sensitive and specific signs of the disorder (Lembo, 1988).

5. Effect of an ectopic beat– The peripheral arterial pulse pressure is often lower after a long diastolic pause following an ectopic beat (Brockenbrough's sign; Figure 17–10). The more forceful ventricular contraction (postectopic potentiation) increases the degree of outflow obstruction and therefore decreases the stroke volume.

6. Effect of amyl nitrite– Amyl nitrite inhalation and isoproterenol induce or exaggerate the outflow obstruction murmur, whereas phenylephrine relieves obstruction (Figure 17–11). Such studies may help in determining the degree of associated mitral incompetence. Amyl nitrite also brings out the murmur of aortic stenosis, but this murmur is shorter and associated with a slowly rising pulse and should not lead to confusion.

C. Electrocardiographic Findings: An abnormal ECG is always present. Electrocardiographic evidence of left ventricular hypertrophy or left or (less often) right bundle branch block is common, and the diagnosis is suspect if the ECG is normal. Arrhythmias are common, and Wolff-Parkinson-White forms of abnormality are sometimes seen. The frequency of ventricular tachycardia with ambulatory electrocardiographic monitoring suggests vigorous treatment of arrhythmias with amiodarone as one possible approach to prevention of sudden death (Mc-

Kenna, 1988). The apical form of hypertrophic cardiomyopathy can be suspected if the ECG shows marked T wave inversion in the precoridal leads, usually with QT prolongation.

D. Imaging Studies: Left ventricular enlargement can be seen on chest x-ray, but the cardiac silhouette is often not much enlarged, because the hypertrophy takes place at the expense of left ventricular cavity. Left atrial enlargement is frequent, and pulmonary congestion may be present if left ventricular failure has occurred. Calcification in the mitral ring is found in about one-fourth of cases.

1. Noninvasive investigations– Doppler echocardiography is the principal tool for clinical diagnosis, which is strongly suggested by a normal aortic valve, asymmetric hypertrophy of the interventricular septum, and the characteristic systolic anterior motion of the anterior cusp of the mitral valve (Figure 17–12). Systolic anterior motion of the mitral valve can be seen in other situations where the left ventricle is hyperdynamic. In normal people, systolic anterior motion can be seen after amyl nitrite inhalation. Asymmetric hypertrophy with disproportionate thickness of the septum compared with the posterior wall, with a ratio of thickness of the septum and posterior wall of 1.3 or greater, is characteristic. However, hypertrophy can involve the midventricular and apical regions of the left ventricle, the entire left ventricle, and even the right ventricle. Another characteristic finding of hypertrophic cardiomyopathy is midsystolic closure and reopening of the aortic valve. This usually occurs when the obstruction is severe, and it can also occur in other forms of subvalvular aortic stenosis such as discrete membranous subaortic stenosis (Figure 17–13).

The left ventricular cavity is small or "crowded," and with systole the ventricle is hypercontractile, tending to obliterate the left ventricular cavity, especially at the apex and the papillary muscle level. It is char-

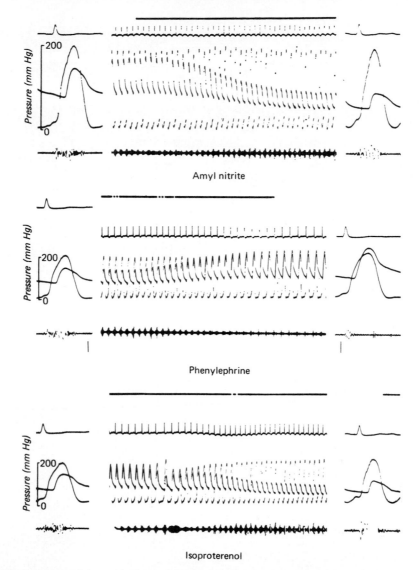

Figure 17–11. Simultaneous left ventricular and femoral artery pressure and phonocardiogram. **_Top:_** Increase of pressure gradient and systolic murmur with inhalation of amyl nitrite. **_Middle:_** Abolition of murmur and gradient with phenylephrine. **_Bottom:_** Increase of gradient and murmur with isoprenaline (isoproterenol). (Reproduced, with permission, from Nellen M in: *Hypertrophic Obstructive Cardiomyopathy.* Wolstenholme G, O'Connor M [editors]. Churchill Livingstone, 1971.)

acteristic in the face of an apparent hypercontractile ventricle that the septum does not thicken normally with systole, perhaps because of the disorganized fiber arrangement. Doppler color flow imaging demonstrates a turbulent flow in mid systole and the greatest degree of mitral regurgitation in late systole, creating a "dagger-like" jet envelope (Figure 17–14). The late–peaking flow supports the concept of outflow obstruction. Mitral regurgitation is related to the degree of systolic anterior motion of the mitral valve (Nishimura, 1986). The diastolic abnormality resulting from delayed relaxation of the left ventricle re-

sults in the characteristic change: Doppler mitral valve flow with a decrease in the early "E" wave and an increase in the late "A" wave (Figure 17–14).

2. Invasive investigations– Doppler echocardiographic study alone is sufficient to diagnose hypertrophic cardiomyopathy, without cardiac catheterization. The only indication for catheterization would be to rule out concomitant coronary artery disease in an older patient.

a. Pressure tracings– In patients with clear evidence of obstruction, there is a pressure difference between the body of the left ventricle and the sub-

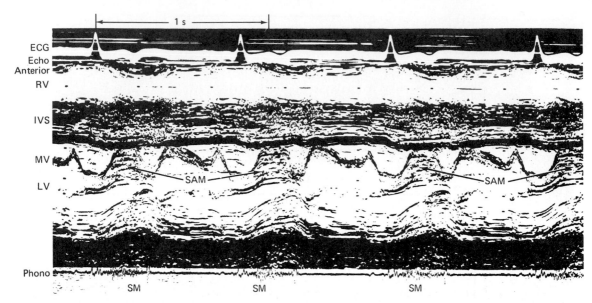

Figure 17–12. Echocardiogram showing systolic anterior motion (SAM) of mitral valve in a patient with hypertrophic obstructive cardiomyopathy. Septal (IVS) thickening and a long systolic murmur (SM) can also be seen. (MV, mitral valve; RV, right ventricle; LV, left ventricle.) (Courtesy of NB Schiller.)

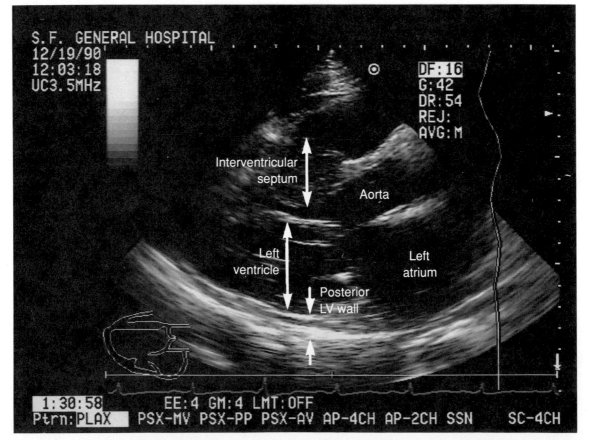

Figure 17–13. Two-dimensional echocardiogram. Parasternal long axis view of patient with hypertrophic cardiomyopathy. Note thick interventricular septa and their posterior left ventricular wall with narrow left ventricular outflow tract. Peak systolic gradient across left ventricular outflow tract was 50 mm Hg.

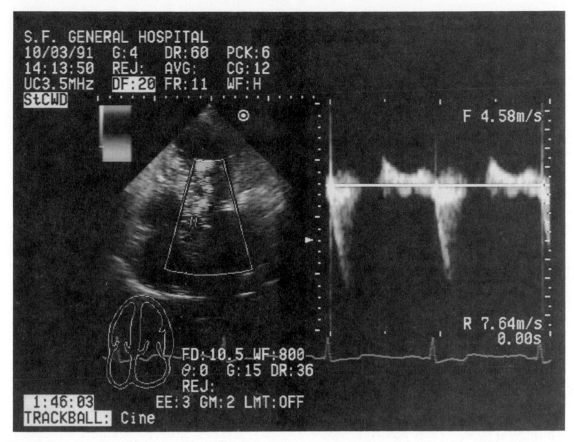

Figure 17-14. Two-dimensional color Doppler echocardiogram in the four-chamber view. Patient has hypertrophic obstructive cardiomyopathy. In the Doppler window, note the high-velocity jet which originates in the left ventricular outflow tract. The high-velocity jet has a "dagger-like" shape owing to the gradual development of the gradient, which reaches a peak of 5.5 m/s, or about 120 mm Hg.

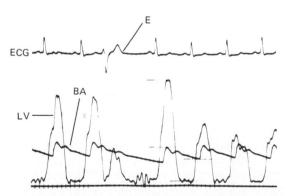

Figure 17-15. Pressure tracings in the left ventricle (LV) and brachial artery (BA) in a patient with hypertrophic obstructive cardiomyopathy. The pressure difference is greater after an ectopic beat (E).

valvular chamber. A closed-tip sidehole (Lehman) catheter should be used for studies in which the diagnosis is suspected. The outflow chamber distal to the obstruction can often be recognized by violent systolic oscillations of pressure. Withdrawal of the catheter from the body of the left ventricle to the outflow area ordinarily shows a pressure difference of 30–100 mm Hg, and no further pressure difference is seen on withdrawal across the aortic valve (Figure 17–7).

b. Provocative tests– The hemodynamic findings can vary from moment to moment, even when provocative measures are not employed. The effects of ectopic beats on the pressure difference across the obstruction are shown in Figure 17–15. In cases in which there is little or no pressure difference within the ventricle, amyl nitrite inhalation can be used to reduce the peripheral resistance, encourage ventricular emptying, and induce obstruction. Similarly, an infusion of isoproterenol can be used to increase the force of cardiac contraction and decrease the peripheral vascular resistance and bring about the physical signs. Valsalva's maneuver decreases venous return and increases or induces obstruction.

c. Angiography– On left ventricular angiocardiography, the hypertrophied left ventricular muscle mass can be seen to narrow the waist of the ventricle in early systole. At times at end-systole, the tips of the mitral valve may be seen narrowing the left ventricular outflow tract. The body of the left ventricle is almost completely empty because of the exaggerated "muscle-bound" contraction that has expelled almost all of its contents. The base of the cone is the aortic valve; the posterior surface is the anterior cusp of the mitral valve; and the anterior surface is the hypertrophied interventricular septum. The tip of the cone is the site of the obstruction. Left ventricular angiography also shows mitral incompetence, but care must be taken to exclude spurious incompetence associated with ectopic beats. Angiography can also delineate rings and shelves of tissue that may be present in some cases and which are located below the aortic valve. Coronary angiography should be done in patients with angina, since these patients can have coexistent coronary artery disease.

d. Electrophysiologic studies– Because of the frequency of arrhythmias and conduction defects, intracardiac electrophysiologic studies have been advocated. Signal-averaged electrocardiography in hypertrophic cardiomyopathy has shown abnormalities that correlated with the occurrence of nonsustained ventricular tachycardia on 48-hour ambulatory electrocardiography (Cripps, 1990). Whether electrophysiologic studies are warranted in the asymptomatic patient is doubtful. In one study, polymorphic ventricular tachycardia could be induced in a third of patients, but there was no difference between patients with previous syncope or cardiac arrest and those without such histories (Kuck, 1988). A more recent study showed that 80% of the patients had an abnormal electrophysiologic study, most having sinoatrial dysfunction. Sustained ventricular tachycardia could be induced in two-thirds of patients with a history of syncope or spontaneous ventricular tachycardia compared with 10% of hypertrophic cardiomyopathy patients without such activity. Certainly, in patients with a history of syncope or sustained ventricular tachycardia, electrophysiologic studies are indicated to select a proper antiarrhythmic therapy (Fananapazir, 1989).

Differential Diagnosis

The physical signs of hypertrophic obstructive cardiomyopathy may resemble those of mitral incompetence or ventricular septal defect. However, marked left ventricular hypertrophy is not seen in either of the latter, and in a patient with a long, harsh systolic murmur, especially if there is a history of angina pectoris or syncope, obstructive cardiomyopathy should be suspected.

Aortic stenosis also enters into the differential diagnosis. There is left ventricular outflow obstruction in both valvular and subvalvular lesions, though the jerky, bifid pulse of hypertrophic cardiomyopathy is readily distinguished from the anacrotic, slow-rising pulse of aortic stenosis. Poststenotic dilation and ejection clicks are seen in valvular aortic stenosis but not in hypertrophic cardiomyopathy; and cinefluoroscopy in the latter does not show calcification of the aortic valve. In valvular and discrete membranous subvalvular aortic stenosis, a murmur of aortic regurgitation is common, whereas it is rare in hypertrophic cardiomyopathy.

Complications

Atrial fibrillation and ventricular arrhythmias are important complications, and sudden death may occur. Young patients with familial disease seem most prone to these complications. Sudden death may be the first manifestation of hypertrophic cardiomyopathy, and it often occurs during or immediately after moderate or severe physical exertion (Maron, 1982). It may be related to ventricular arrhythmias or conduction defects. Another mechanism for sudden death may be related to the vicious cycle initiated by intramural myocardial ischemia. This results in increased diastolic stiffness, thus decreasing left ventricular filling and resulting in decreased left ventricular stroke volume. With ischemia, systolic function is also impaired, further decreasing stroke volume. With decreased stroke volume, aortic and coronary artery perfusion pressures drop, thus increasing ischemia and finally resulting in electromechanical dissociation.

Left ventricular failure with pulmonary edema may occur while in sinus rhythm or may follow the onset of atrial fibrillation. Mitral incompetence may be the result of movement of the anterior leaflet of the mitral valve in the left ventricular outflow tract during ejection. Endocardial fibrosis and thickening are seen in this area and are thought to be due to mechanical trauma.

Occasionally at the end stage, poor systolic and diastolic left ventricular function is seen with no or minimal dilation of the left ventricular cavity. This may be the result of increasing intramural fibrosis and loss of myocytes (Oakley, 1990).

Treatment

A. Medical Treatment: Medical treatment may relieve symptoms, decrease the left ventricular outflow gradient, and prevent or decrease ventricular arrhythmias, but it has not unequivocally prevented progression of disease or affected survival rates (Anderson, 1984; Goodwin, 1982). Propranolol and other beta-adrenergic blocking drugs have been the mainstay of treatment for years. Sudden death or progression of left ventricular hypertrophy is not prevented by treatment with propranolol (McKenna, 1982). In some cases, the drug did not relieve the symptoms or left ventricular obstruction, and myectomy was performed (see below).

Calcium entry-blocking agents have been employed before myotomy or myectomy is attempted. Verapamil or nifedipine may benefit patients with hypertrophic cardiomyopathy by improving diastolic filling, increasing exercise capacity, and relieving symptoms, even when beta-blocking drugs have failed (Chatterjee, 1982). Not all studies, however, have shown this benefit (Yamakado, 1990).

Ventricular arrhythmias including ventricular tachycardia are relatively common and may play a role in the sudden death that occurs in these patients. Disopyramide has been used both for its antiarrhythmic and its negative inotropic effect (Pollick, 1988). Amiodarone (see Chapter 15) has controlled many of these arrhythmias and may decrease the incidence of sudden death. It is an important therapeutic advance in high-risk patients with ventricular arrhythmias (McKenna, 1988; McKenna, 1989; Gill, 1992).

Beta-blockers such as propranolol are usually started first. The bradycardia increases the time for diastolic filling and decreases the systolic contractile force. Propranolol is especially helpful in patients with angina pectoris. The initial dose is 20–40 mg three times a day, and the dose is then increased until a satisfactory effect is obtained or side effects develop. Verapamil is usually begun at a dosage of 40 mg orally every 8 hours, and this may be increased to tolerance. Nifedipine has been used in a dosage of 10 mg sublingually twice daily. Both verapamil and nifedipine increase the peak rate of left ventricular diastolic filling without affecting systolic function (Chatterjee, 1982; Lorell, 1982). Amiodarone, 400–600 mg/d, abolishes ventricular tachycardia in most patients who have it and is significantly superior to verapamil; its important side effects are described in Chapter 15. It remains to be seen whether amiodarone decreases the incidence of sudden death thought to be due to the arrhythmia. McKenna (1988) believes it does. A recent study of 50 patients with hypertrophic cardiomyopathy refractory to calcium antagonists and beta-blockers who were treated with amiodarone still had an incidence of sudden death despite the ablation of ventricular tachycardia on 24-hour ambulatory electrocardiographic monitoring (Fananapazir, 1991).

Verapamil, especially intravenously, may produce significant adverse effects, particularly hypotension, sinoatrial block with junctional rhythms, and atrioventricular block resulting from inhibition of atrioventricular nodal conduction (Epstein, 1981). Pulmonary edema has occurred but usually only in patients with left ventricular failure and pulmonary edema prior to therapy. Nifedipine lacks the sinoatrial and atrioventricular inhibitory effects of verapamil, but because it is a more potent vasodilator, it is more likely to produce hypotension.

B. Surgical Treatment: Surgical incision and resection of hypertrophied muscle bundles in the ventricular outflow tract is advocated in some centers, mitral valve replacement has been recommended in others, and even the production of bundle branch block has been suggested as a mode of therapy. Surgery is advocated in symptomatic patients with a systolic resting gradient of 50 mm Hg or more (McIntosh, 1988). There are some institutions that recommend surgery when there is lesser resting gradient but a provocable gradient of 50 mm Hg or more. However, it is controversial whether the systolic gradient has any prognostic significance (Romeo, 1990). It seems likely that the wide spectrum of cases accounts for the differences of opinion about treatment. Surgery is not advocated until medical treatment has been given a thorough trial. Muscular incision and resection are then recommended (McIntosh, 1988; Williams, 1987). The operative mortality rate in an accumulated series of 1700 operations was about 5%. In a report of 123 patients operated on at the National Institutes of Health, with a mean follow-up of 11–15 years, of 102 survivors of the surgery, 48% were still living and about two-thirds continued to be symptomatically improved in comparison with their preoperation states. Of the 53 deaths, 55% were due to causes related to the cardiopathy, with most deaths occurring suddenly (McIntosh, 1988). The patient most likely to achieve benefit from surgery in the form of increased exercise tolerance is one who preoperatively had decreased exercise tolerance and postoperatively had a decrease in resting left ventricular outflow tract gradient and a decrease in left ventricular filling pressure (Diodati, 1992). About the same results have been reported with mitral valve replacement (Krajcer, 1988).

Recently, the effect of dual-chamber pacing (DDD pacemaker) has been reported—ie, reducing the left ventricular outflow tract obstruction by making the septum move away from the left ventricular wall and opening the outflow tract. Left ventricular outflow tract gradients are decreased and exercise tolerance increased in such patients, and the benefits appear to persist after pacing is acutely discontinued (Fananapazir, 1992). This approach to therapy will have to be confirmed by further studies.

The two major complications of surgery are complete heart block and the creation of a ventricular septal defect. Transesophageal electrocardiography before or at the time of surgery is very helpful in visualizing the exact site of septal hypertrophy. If the hypertrophy is minimal, mitral valve replacement is preferred in order to avoid creating a ventricular septal defect. With all these considerations, surgery is indicated only in symptomatic patients failing medical management.

The question whether to give digitalis often arises in patients with evidence of left ventricular failure. Digitalis has been thought to aggravate obstruction because it increases the force of cardiac contraction. However, in most cases, congestive heart failure is related to diastolic dysfunction, not to systolic dysfunction. Digitalis should not be used except for the unusual circumstance when the left ventricle is beginning to develop systolic impairment, the ejection fraction is falling, and the ventricle is beginning to dilate.

Prognosis

The long-term prognosis of hypertrophic obstructive cardiomyopathy is not fully established. The annual mortality rate is approximately 3% per year; most deaths are sudden, especially in young patients. In children and adolescents, the mortality rate can be as high as 6% per year (McKenna, 1988). Most patients live for years; heart failure, systemic emboli, infective endocarditis, and arrhythmias occur gradually in older patients over a period of years (Hecht, 1992). The course is more benign when abnormal muscular hypertrophy develops later in life. In some patients, the characteristic murmur disappears with the onset of left ventricular failure, and the evidence of obstruction disappears as the failing ventricle dilates. High-risk patients appear to be those who are young, have a family history of sudden death, or have had syncope. A study investigating the prognostic significance of indices of diastolic function by radionuclide angiography in 161 patients showed no correlation with those patients who either die suddenly or demonstrate electrical contractility. The study did demonstrate both systolic and diastolic abnormalities in those who died from cardiac failure (Chikamori, 1990).

Pregnancy is well tolerated in young women with the disease unless cardiac failure is present.

3. RESTRICTIVE CARDIOMYOPATHY

This is the third and least common general category of Goodwin's classification of cardiomyopathy. It frequently overlaps the category of hypertrophic cardiomyopathy where hypertrophic changes decrease compliance of the ventricles and simulate some of the findings of restrictive cardiomyopathy. (See also Endomyocardial Fibrosis.) The term "restrictive" is used because a characteristic feature of the condition is a restriction in ventricular filling resulting from a noncompliant, less distensible ventricle with essentially normal systolic function. An infiltrative pathologic process is responsible for the decreased compliance and other clinical features.

Restrictive cardiomyopathy can be classified as follows:

Primary: Of unknown cause.

(1) With eosinophilia, eg, hypereosinophilic syndrome, eosinophilic myocarditis, endomyocardial fibrosis.

(2) Without eosinophilia, with myocardial fibrosis.

Secondary: Entities with restrictive hemodynamics due to specific diseases, eg, amyloidosis, hemochromatosis, pseudoxanthoma elasticum, systemic sclerosis, sarcoidosis, post-transfusion rejection.

Pathology

The pathology is that of the underlying infiltrative process, occasionally of unknown cause but often due to amyloid disease, hemochromatosis, glycogen storage disease, sarcoidosis, or endomyocardial fibrosis with or without the idiopathic hypereosinophilic (Löffler's) syndrome. Eosinophilia from any cause can result in endocardial damage, probably related to a direct toxic effect of the eosinophilic granule protein on endocardial tissues. This can frequently cause mural thrombus formation, entrapping chordae and resulting in mitral or tricuspid valvular insufficiency (or both). The two ventricles may not be enlarged, but there is systemic venous congestion of the liver and peripheral tissues.

Criteria for Diagnosis

The diagnosis is usually made in a patient who has symptoms and signs of congestive heart failure and a raised venous pressure but in whom the heart is not significantly enlarged and who has echocardiographic findings of normal left and right ventricular dimensions, a relatively normal ejection fraction, and echoes representing fibrosis that do not correspond to vascular regions (Acquatella, 1983). The absence of considerable hypertrophy of the left ventricle is in contrast to the clinical features of systemic congestive (right heart) failure.

Restriction of ventricular filling with preservation of systolic function is characteristic of this group of diseases.

Abnormalities in diastolic function can be evaluated by two-dimensional echo-Doppler techniques as well as by radionuclide angiography.

Diastolic filling abnormalities are of two types: (1) abnormality of relaxation and (2) restrictive filling. With abnormal relaxation, early diastolic filling is prolonged, deceleration time of early diastolic filling is also prolonged, and this decreased early filling is compensated for by increased filling at the time of atrial contraction. Doppler study shows that the transmitral velocity at the time of atrial contraction (the *a* wave) is greater than the transmitral velocity at the time of early filling (the "E" wave). This type of diastolic abnormality is characteristic of ventricular fibrosis, ventricular hypertrophy, and hypertrophic cardiomyopathy.

The second type of diastolic abnormality is that of restrictive physiology, where most diastolic filling is early, resulting in an increased "E" wave. Because the ventricle is already at its restricted maximum volume at the time of atrial contraction, the transmitted velocity is low, resulting in a low *a* wave. This is similar to the abnormality of filling seen in constrictive pericarditis and results in the ventricular pressure "dip and plateau."

The manifestations of the disease vary in the early and late stages; in full–blown cases, the disease may be indistinguishable from chronic constrictive pericarditis (see Chapter 18). Endomyocardial biopsy may identify the specific cause of the restrictive cardiomyopathy (Schoenfeld, 1987).

Clinical Findings

A. Symptoms: The earliest symptoms may be fatigue, peripheral edema, enlargement of the abdomen owing to ascites, and occasionally dyspnea resulting from pulmonary congestion but not acute pulmonary edema. The symptoms may be severe in the later stages.

B. Signs: The dominant features are raised venous pressure with prominent x and y descents and signs of systemic venous congestion, with enlarged, pulsating liver, slight or moderate ascites, and dependent edema. There may be a third heart sound later in the disease. Cardiac murmurs are usually minimal or absent. The carotid pulse is usually normal. Right or left ventricular heaves are usually absent, indicating no significant cardiac hypertrophy. Premature beats (usually ventricular) may occur, but cardiac arrhythmias (including ventricular tachycardia or fibrillation) or conduction defects may be late manifestations.

C. Laboratory Findings: The laboratory findings are those of the underlying disease. A striking eosinophilia characteristic of Löffler's syndrome should always be sought.

D. Electrocardiographic Findings: The electrocardiographic changes are usually nonspecific, with slight ST–T changes not characteristic of any particular condition. Considerable left ventricular hypertrophy is uncommon, but many different kinds of conduction defects or arrhythmias may occur.

E. Imaging Studies: Concentric left ventricular hypertrophy and dilation may be seen on the chest x-ray, but it is rarely marked. Pulmonary venous congestion may occur, but it is usually not severe. Calcification of the pericardium is absent, but intracardiac calcification may occasionally be present.

1. Noninvasive investigations– Echocardiography provides one of the chief means of diagnosing the disease (see Criteria for Diagnosis, above). In addition to the Doppler diastolic abnormalities outlined above with early rapid filling and decreased late ventricular filling, the two-dimensional echocardiogram can reveal echogenic densities in the left and right ventricular apex that may represent endocardial fibrosis or thrombus obliterating the apices, which can involve the papillary muscle and chordae, causing valvular regurgitation. The left ventricular wall thickness is normal, and systolic function is relatively preserved. Biatrial enlargement is usually present.

2. Invasive investigations– Cardiac catheterization and left ventricular angiography are helpful. The absence of segmental akinesia or of significant enlargement of one ventricular cavity is helpful in excluding congestive cardiomyopathy or old scars from myocardial infarction. Coronary arteriograms are usually normal. The characteristic hemodynamic feature of restrictive cardiomyopathy consists of elevation of the filling pressure of both ventricles, associated with a prominent x and rapid y descent, producing an M-shaped pattern. Left and right atrial pressures are also increased. The ventricles display the early diastolic dip and late plateau characteristic of restriction of ventricular filling, often indistinguishable from chronic constrictive pericarditis.

Differential Diagnosis

The main diseases that must be ruled out are chronic constrictive pericarditis and occasionally dilated cardiomyopathy, which may produce identical clinical, radiologic, and hemodynamic findings. Diastolic filling differences on radionuclide angiography and transvalvular flow velocities by Doppler echocardiography may help differentiate restrictive cardiomyopathy from constrictive pericarditis (Aroney, 1989; Hatle, 1989). In patients with constrictive pericarditis, there are marked changes with the onset of inspiration and expiration in left ventricular isovolumic relaxation time and in early mitral and tricuspid flow velocities. Although the deceleration time of early mitral and tricuspid flow velocity is shorter than normal in both diseases, only in restrictive cardiomyopathy is there a further shortening of tricuspid deceleration time with inspiration. The basis of these differences is the fact that in constrictive pericarditis, left ventricular compliance is normal early in diastole but there is a limitation by the constricted pericardium to cardiac filling that includes both atria and ventricles. With inspiration, the increase in filling of the right heart interferes with left ventricular filling by displacement of the interventricular septum, thus explaining the reciprocal effect of inspiration on the velocity of flow through tricuspid and mitral valve during inspiration and expiration. In constrictive pericarditis, with atrial contraction, blood can be moved from the atria to the ventricles because total intrapericardial volume does not increase. In restrictive cardiomyopathy, however, there is a marked decrease in left ventricular chamber compliance that limits cardiac filling. The impedance to filling increases throughout diastole, leading to a reduction in the proportion of ventricular filling seen with atrial contraction. With inspiration and an increase in venous return into the right ventricle, there is an abrupt rise in early diastolic pressure and an inspiratory shortening of the tricuspid flow deceleration time. Since there is no pericardial constriction, there is less interventricular interdependence and less inspiratory effect on left ventricular filling.

In severe dilated cardiomyopathy, the ejection fraction is usually decreased below 30% and ventricular

take, either as medication or during radiologic studies using iodine-containing contrast media.

Treatment

The treatment of thyrotoxic heart disease is similar to the treatment of thyrotoxicosis in the absence of cardiac disease, consisting usually of antithyroid drugs such as propylthiouracil or methimazole followed in several weeks by radioiodine. If the thyroid gland is very large, substernal, or multinodular, subtotal thyroidectomy may be the treatment of choice.

If the cardiovascular manifestations, especially tachycardia, are dominant and severe, beta-adrenergic blocking agents such as propranolol may be used to control the rapid heart rate and decrease the cardiac output with exercise (Geffner, 1992). They do not affect the underlying excess thyroid secretion. Oral propranolol is usually adequate in doses of less than 160 mg/d; it can be given intravenously at a rate no faster than 1 mg/min if the clinical situation dictates rapid reversal of the cardiac symptoms—especially if thyroid storm is thought to be imminent. Younger individuals, however, require larger doses—up to 320 mg/d—and usually require more definitive treatment. Overall thyroid function is not affected by administration of propranolol, which should be considered an adjunct to other definitive therapeutic methods (Ingbar, 1981).

Prognosis

The early diagnosis of thyrotoxicosis may influence the subsequent therapeutic results. Twenty percent of the patients studied by Sandler (1959) died of congestive heart failure within 1–7 years after starting therapy; complete relief of symptoms occurred in only 40% and was directly related to the disappearance of atrial fibrillation after treatment. In patients in whom sinus rhythm followed treatment with radioiodine, no deaths occurred and all patients with cardiac failure were improved. In patients in whom atrial fibrillation persisted, 20% died. Electric cardioversion for the treatment of atrial fibrillation should improve these results if atrial fibrillation persists after treatment of thyrotoxicosis with radioiodine.

MYXEDEMA & MYXEDEMA HEART

Myxedema heart is a well-known entity described by Zondek in 1918. In most myxedema patients, pericardial effusion and not cardiac failure is responsible for the enlarged cardiac shadow seen radiologically. Investigations using echocardiography have shown that some patients have dilation of the left ventricle without significant pericardial effusion, whereas others have dominant pericardial effusion with an essentially normal cardiac shadow, and a third group have a combination of both. The cause of the effusion

is not clearly understood. There is evidence that in myxedema increased capillary permeability to protein causes pericardial effusion (Zimmerman, 1983). There is clear evidence for depressed myocardial contractility in some patients with hypothyroidism (Lee, 1990).

In one large series of cases of myxedema, the disease occurred spontaneously in 40% of patients, but in the remaining 60% it followed either ^{131}I therapy or thyroidectomy. At present, many more cases of myxedema are seen following successful ^{131}I therapy, and it is feared that with the passage of time the numbers will increase. Amiodarone has a high iodine content and thus antagonizes thyroid hormone action on pituitary cells and inhibits peripheral conversion of T_4 to T_3. For these reasons, hypothyroidism and at times hyperthyroidism can occur as a side effect of amiodarone administration (Gammage, 1987; Wilson, 1991).

Clinical Findings

A. Symptoms: The symptoms of myxedema include weakness; fatigue; paresthesias; dry, puffy skin; hoarseness; thick tongue; and slow pulse. Patients with myxedema heart characteristically complain of exertional fatigue more than of dyspnea, angina, and periorbital and peripheral edema. The pulse volume has a small amplitude, with a weak carotid upstroke—in contrast to what would be expected in bradycardia. Paresthesias, deafness, and a husky hoarse voice may be prominent.

B. Signs: The cardiac manifestations of myxedema are usually due to pericardial effusion rather than cardiac failure. Orthopnea, raised venous pressure, enlargement of the liver, gallop rhythm, and pulmonary venous congestion are often absent. Following the removal of pericardial fluid, cardiac size is often found to be normal.

The slow pulse may be only relative in patients with myxedema. For example, the heart rate may be only 60–70 beats/min, which would be an unusual finding in a patient with cardiomegaly and presumed congestive heart failure.

Patients may have effusions in the pericardial, pleural, and peritoneal cavities; because of the slow development of effusion, large amounts of pericardial fluid may be found (2000–4000 mL).

C. Electrocardiographic Findings: Low voltage of the QRS complex as well as of the T and P waves suggests cardiac failure in patients with myxedema. A typical ECG showing the development and regression of T wave abnormalities in myxedema is presented in Figure 17–16.

D. Imaging Studies: (Figure 17–17.) The cardiac shadow may be enlarged and may be due to cardiac failure, pericardial effusion, or a combination of the two. Echocardiograms can differentiate between enlarged cardiac shadows due to pericardial effusion and those due to left ventricular dilation. Following

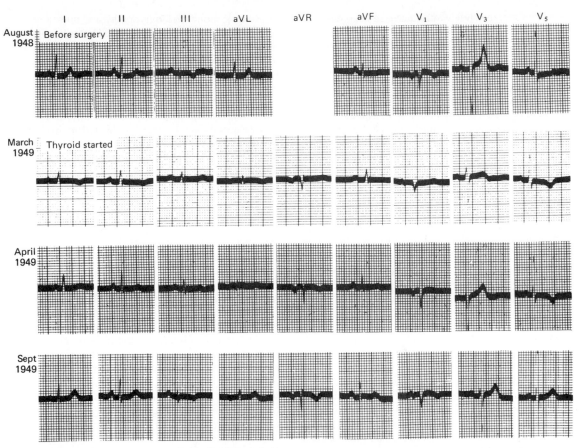

Figure 17–16. Hypothyroidism in a 47-year-old woman following thyroidectomy for hyperthyroidism in September 1948. The BMR was −51 in March 1949. Note progressive improvement in T waves after thyroid replacement was started in March 1949.

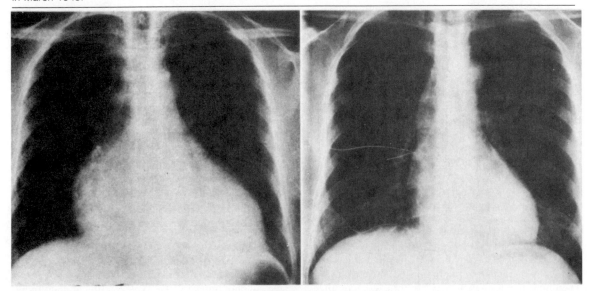

Figure 17–17. Chest x-ray studies of patient with hypothyroid cardiomyopathy. **Left:** Before therapy, showing pronounced cardiomegaly. **Right:** Six months after institution of thyroxine therapy, the heart size has returned to normal. (Reproduced, with permission, from Reza MJ, Abbasi AS: Congestive cardiomyopathy in hypothyroidism. West J Med 1975;123;228.

thyroxine therapy, left ventricular size becomes normal on chest films as well as echocardiograms.

E. Hemodynamic Data: Patients with myxedema heart do not require cardiac catheterization. The arteriovenous oxygen difference and response of cardiac output, peripheral resistance, and right atrial pressure to exercise are all normal. The cardiac index is low but increases normally with exercise. The cardiac index in myxedema is one-third that seen in patients with thyrotoxicosis.

Differential Diagnosis

The diagnosis of myxedema is frequently missed because the clinical manifestations occur slowly and subtly and may be attributed to aging, as the patient tires more easily and becomes slower in thought and movement. Periorbital nonpitting edema, collections of serous fluid, and proteinuria may suggest nephritis. The diagnosis of cardiomyopathy is often made in myxedematous patients because of the presence of presumed cardiomegaly on radiologic examination.

Treatment

The response to treatment with thyroid hormone is dramatic, but severe angina, acute myocardial infarction, cardiac failure, psychotic reactions, and ventricular tachycardia may develop within 24–72 hours if the initial dose is too large. Treatment should be started with 12.5–25 μg of synthetic thyroxine and should be increased slowly by increments of 12.5 μg over a period of weeks. Improvement may occur within days. If the patient has severe myxedema and develops angina pectoris following small-dose thyroid replacement therapy, coronary revascularization can be considered if a coronary arteriogram shows localized stenosis, in order to make thyroxine therapy feasible.

Prognosis

The enlarged heart shadow usually returns to normal after thyroid therapy with complete clinical resolution, often within a month, but relapses may occur rapidly if thyroid therapy is stopped.

ALCOHOLIC CARDIOMYOPATHY*

Excessive intake of alcohol may produce cardiomyopathy by a primary toxic effect on the heart, by associated nutritional deficiency (especially of thiamine, as in beriberi heart disease), or as a result of additives (cobalt in cobalt-beer cardiomyopathy). Chronic alcoholics may have intermittent thiamine deficiency or excessive requirements for thiamine, as when they develop fever owing to infections, or after a high-carbohydrate diet; therefore, a mixed picture

---

*See also Beriberi Heart Disease and Nutritional Heart Disease, below.

of toxic alcoholic cardiomyopathy and nutritional beriberi heart disease may be found. Dietary deficiency of protein or calories infrequently causes dilated cardiomyopathy. In populations afflicted by famine and in prisoners of war examined after a weight loss of about 20 kg, cardiac enlargement, hypoproteinemia, and cardiac failure are rarely seen; cardiac atrophy is much more common (Ramalingaswami, 1968). Endomyocardial fibrosis may be related to inadequate nutrition. The myocardial pathology in alcoholic cardiomyopathy is nonspecific and similar to that seen with dilated cardiomyopathy.

Alcoholic cardiomyopathy is common in persons who drink excessive alcohol daily, even though they may be receiving adequate nutrition and vitamins (Urbano-Marquez, 1989). Most cases of alcoholic cardiomyopathy in the USA are probably due to a direct toxic action of alcohol or its metabolites on the myocardium (Diamond, 1989). Depression of myocardial contractility can be demonstrated even in normal individuals given alcohol acutely.

Involvement of the Liver

Alcohol not only affects the cells of the myocardium by direct toxic action; it also affects the cells of the liver, even in patients receiving good diets with adequate vitamins. As a result, patients may present with hepatic involvement as well as cardiac disease, although some patients tolerate large amounts of alcohol for many years without evident harm.

Relationship of Beriberi Heart Disease to Alcoholic Cardiomyopathy

In beriberi heart disease related to thiamine deficiency, high output failure is the predominant clinical feature. In contrast, the patient with alcoholic cardiomyopathy has signs of low cardiac output, weak pulses of small volume, and cold extremities. The heart is large and bulky, with a markedly decreased ejection fraction. In the early stages of alcoholic cardiomyopathy, the left ventricle can be normal in size and hypocontractile. In contrast to beriberi heart disease, large doses of thiamine are ineffective in treatment of alcoholic cardiomyopathy.

Beriberi heart disease was formerly common in developing countries and found occasionally in the USA before it was realized that thiamine supplements were necessary in patients receiving deficient diets.

Clinical Findings

The criteria for the diagnosis of alcoholic cardiomyopathy are similar to those of dilated cardiomyopathy, with the exception of the history of excessive alcohol intake. The typical clinical picture is cardiac failure in a middle-aged person without coronary heart disease, hypertension, valvular heart disease, or congenital heart disease. There is a history of excessive alcohol intake over a period of many years;

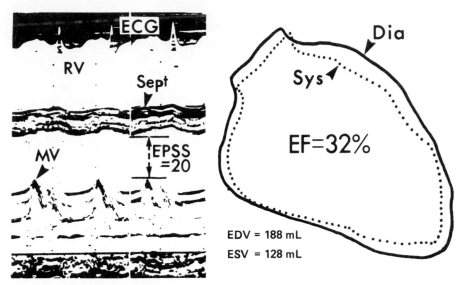

Figure 17–18. Echocardiogram of patient with alcoholic cardiomyopathy, demonstrating a decreased ejection fraction of 32%, a large end-diastolic volume, and a wide separation between the anterior portion of the mitral valve leaflet and the ventricular septum. (EF, ejection fraction; EDV, end-diastolic volume; ESV, end-systolic volume; MV, mitral valve; RV, right ventricle; Sept, septum; EPSS, end [E] point of mitral valve separated from septum; Sys, systole; Dia, diastole.) (Reproduced, with permission, from Massie BM et al: Mitral-septal separation: A new echocardiographic index of left ventricular function. Am J Cardiol 1977;39:1008.)

most patients have drunk more than 250 mL of whiskey or its equivalent every day for at least 10 years. Some believe that alcohol plays a role in at least half of all cases of chronic congestive cardiomyopathy.

A. Symptoms: The onset is usually insidious, with nonspecific fatigue, dyspnea, palpitations, and possibly edema.

B. Signs: There may be cardiac enlargement and left ventricular failure. When cardiac failure develops, it is low-output failure, with all its clinical features. The cardiac failure is chiefly left ventricular, but there may be right ventricular failure as well, with raised venous pressure, tricuspid insufficiency, a left or right ventricular heave, gallop rhythm, murmurs of functional mitral or tricuspid insufficiency and pulmonary rales, enlarged tender liver, and dependent edema. The arterial blood pressure may be elevated during severe failure; the pressure falls to normal when failure is improved with cardiac therapy.

C. Electrocardiographic Findings: Abnormalities, especially low voltage of QRS complexes, ST–T abnormalities, and left ventricular hypertrophy, may be present before the development of cardiac failure. Arrhythmias and conduction defects are common.

D. X-Ray Findings: Cardiac enlargement, cardiac failure, and pulmonary congestion may be present.

E. Special Investigations: In addition to left ventricular hypertrophy and a low cardiac output, patients have enlarged hearts with pulmonary venous engorgement; on coronary angiography and left ventricular cineangiography, the coronary arteries are normal and the ejection fraction is decreased, so that

the heart is a large, boggy organ. Echocardiography can demonstrate the large left ventricle with decreased ejection fraction and the mitral valve floating within the left ventricular cavity (Figure 17–18). Doppler echocardiography demonstrates diastolic dysfunction, possibly as one of the earliest manifestations of functional impairment due to alcoholic cardiomyopathy. Thus, diastolic abnormalities can occur before left ventricular dilation or abnormalities in systolic function (Kupari, 1990).

Differential Diagnosis

Alcoholic cardiomyopathy must be distinguished from other dilated cardiomyopathies in patients with long-term excessive alcohol intake. Hypertension is excluded by normal blood pressure after restoration to the compensated state; coronary artery disease by the absence of angina pectoris or myocardial infarction; valvular heart disease by the decrease of murmurs when compensation is restored. Congenital heart disease is excluded by a negative history and no abnormalities on cineangiograms.

Treatment

If cardiomyopathy is discovered early, complete abstinence from alcohol may be beneficial, but later, abstinence may have only marginal benefit (Milgaard, 1990). Bed rest, intravenous thiamine (50 mg), and conventional treatment for heart failure are the mainstays of management (see Chapter 10). If the disease is not too far advanced, improvement but not complete reversal may be achieved.

Prognosis

The heart may become much smaller and all cardiac symptoms may disappear following complete abstinence from alcohol in up to one-third of patients. The longer the patient has had a dilated, poorly contractile heart, the less likely it is that recovery of normal function will occur. Prolonged bed rest increases the hazard of multiple episodes of thromboembolism and has psychologic and economic consequences. With severe heart failure, the prognosis is poor—approximately a 50% mortality rate in 2 years (see Chapter 10).

BERIBERI HEART DISEASE

In the USA, beriberi heart disease is uncommon because thiamine deficiency severe enough to result in beriberi is rare. It is usually seen in malnourished alcoholics, as described above. Beriberi is most common in populations and individuals (as in the Orient) who eat thiamine–deficient diets (Kawai, 1980).

Clinical Findings

Beriberi is one cause of high-output heart failure. The high cardiac output is in response to the low peripheral vascular resistance. Heart failure can occur very suddenly, with death in 48 hours. This Shoshin beriberi is characterized by hypotension, lactic acidosis, and fulminant pulmonary edema (Naidoo, 1987).

Patients with beriberi have dyspnea, edema, and biventricular heart failure in combination with warm extremities and bounding pulses characteristic of the high cardiac output state. Later, when severe congestive heart failure occurs, the peripheral vessels may constrict. A third heart sound is almost always present.

Treatment & Prognosis

Beriberi heart disease improves rapidly when large doses (50 mg) of thiamine are given orally or parenterally. The skin temperature falls in hours after parenteral thiamine therapy. Enlargement of the heart and right heart failure subside within a matter of days to 1–2 weeks, and the syndrome does not occur when adequate thiamine supplements are given.

Beriberi heart disease is reversed by thiamine only when the process is relatively acute. Chronic alcoholic cardiomyopathy does not respond to thiamine.

NUTRITIONAL HEART DISEASE

As discussed above, malnutrition with selective deficiency of thiamine may cause beriberi heart disease and is in part responsible for the clinical features of alcoholic cardiomyopathy.

Deficiency of Calories, Proteins, Fats, & Vitamins (Total Malnutrition)

Under conditions of famine or semistarvation in which there are combined dietary deficiencies and not selective ones (as with thiamine), the heart responds with atrophy, interstitial edema, and disappearance of all pericardial fat, but the patient does not develop cardiac failure of either the beriberi type or the chronic alcoholic type (although the ECG may show nonspecific ST–T changes). Protein deficiency may cause kwashiorkor, a disease of children due to deficiency of protein relative to calories and characterized by hypoproteinemia and generalized edema. This is seen in underdeveloped countries and is a major cause of death in those areas. Cardiac failure due to protein starvation is uncommon both in children and (especially) in adults, although cardiac output may be decreased. When the diet is abruptly improved, as in liberated prisoners of war, generalized edema simulating cardiac failure may develop because of the abrupt increase in sodium intake associated with the normal diet; diuresis occurs spontaneously in weeks, aided by small amounts of diuretics. There are no short-term cardiac sequelae.

Patients with anorexia nervosa can produce symptoms similar to those seen in kwashiorkor. Electrolyte abnormalities, including hypokalemia, hypocalcemia, and hypomagnesemia, can result in heart failure and even sudden death (Isner, 1985).

The coincidence of chronic nutritional deficiency and endomyocardial fibrosis in developing tropical countries in Africa suggests that the latter may be due in part to malnutrition. However, in a famine in India in 1967, no mural thrombi or other abnormalities of the endocardial wall were found at autopsy (Ramalingaswami, 1968).

Obesity

Obesity is the commonest form of malnutrition seen in the United States and Western Europe. Obesity affects the heart by increasing metabolic demands and the requirement for increased cardiac output. There is also an increased incidence of hypertension and diabetes mellitus. The metabolic consequences of obesity are a decreased sensitivity to insulin and hyperinsulinemia, glucose intolerance, hypercholesterolemia, and hypertriglyceridemia, leading to accelerated coronary atherosclerosis.

Massive obesity, also called **morbid obesity,** can lead to increased blood volume and cardiac output, ventricular and atrial dilation, eccentric ventricular hypertrophy, and cardiac failure. With exercise, there may be a marked increase in left ventricular filling pressure and eventually chronic congestive heart failure. This is referred to as the **cardiomyopathy of obesity.**

Morbid obesity can lead to hypoventilation, causing hypoxemia, hypercapnia, and respiratory acidosis, each a powerful constrictor of the pulmonary vascular bed. Hypoventilation can be aggravated by sleep apnea in these patients. Severe pulmonary hypertension leads to right ventricular hypertrophy and eventually to right heart failure, the so-called **Pickwickian syndrome.**

Weight reduction is exceedingly difficult in these morbidly obese patients but can achieve remarkable reversal of the cardiovascular abnormalities. At times, such extreme measures as jejunoileal bypass operations are necessary to achieve adequate weight loss.

Problems seen with very rapid weight loss consist of the development of cardiac arrhythmias and even sudden death. First recognized with liquid protein diets, these arrhythmias are probably the result of electrolyte abnormalities resulting in prolongation of the QT interval, ventricular tachycardia, and sudden death (Pringle, 1983).

CARDIAC INVOLVEMENT IN INHERITED DISORDERS OF METABOLISM

These constitute a group of genetically determined enzymatic abnormalities and are only mentioned here for completeness. A comprehensive paper by Blieden (1974) classifies the inherited metabolic disorders and discusses them from the point of view of genetics, biochemistry, and clinical features. Attention is called to the fact that the cardiac manifestations may be the presenting features.

CHRONIC CARDIOMYOPATHY DUE TO SPECIFIC DISEASE ENTITIES

SARCOIDOSIS

Sarcoidosis is a chronic granulomatous disease of unknown cause affecting chiefly young persons (average age about 25). Many organ systems are affected, but especially the liver, lungs, and heart. The disease may cause cardiac failure (with or without diastolic dysfunction), cor pulmonale, ventricular arrhythmias, heart block, and sudden death; autopsy studies show involvement of the heart in about 25% of fatal cases (Figure 17–19). Granulomas in patients with cardiac involvement are most commonly seen in the left ventricle, ventricular septum, and papillary muscles. Occasionally, massive cardiac involvement has resulted in ventricular aneurysm formation.

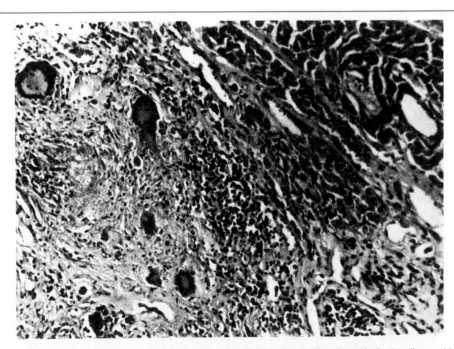

Figure 17–19. Sarcoid granuloma in myocardium with epithelioid cells, multinucleated giant cells, and lymphocytes. (× 350.) (Reproduced, with permission, from Fawcett FJ, Goldberg MJ: Heart block resulting from myocardial sarcoidosis. Br Heart J 1974;36:220.)

Clinical Findings

The clinical findings can be the result of direct myocardial involvement by the sarcoid granulomas. If massive involvement occurs, signs of systolic and diastolic dysfunction can appear, causing the clinical picture of congestive heart failure. If the conduction system is involved, the only evidence of sarcoid cardiac involvement may be complete atrioventricular block and sudden death. Ventricular arrhythmias can also cause sudden death.

The most common cardiac feature is cor pulmonale secondary to fibrosis of the interstitial tissues of the lung and small pulmonary arteries resulting in pulmonary hypertension, right ventricular hypertrophy, and ultimately right ventricular failure (see Chapter 19).

A. Symptoms and Signs: The onset is with general symptoms of fatigue and malaise, acute uveitis, hilar adenopathy and nodular and fibrous pulmonary infiltrates on the chest film, and skin lesions, most characteristically erythema nodosum. Other systemic manifestations include hypercalcemia, hyperglobulinemia, and generalized adenopathy. Cardiac failure is uncommon in sarcoidosis in general but occurs in a third of patients with cardiac sarcoidosis. There may be pericardial effusion, ventricular arrhythmias, syncope, or sudden death—especially upon exertion. Biopsy of the skin or lymph nodes shows extensive fibrosis and noncaseating granulomatous infiltration without organisms; the same process may affect the heart. In the majority of patients with active sarcoidosis, the serum angiotensin-converting enzyme concentration is elevated. This probably reflects the increased secretory activity of epithelioid cells in the sarcoid granulomas and is a nonspecific finding. Kveim-Siltzbach skin tests are positive in 80% of cases but are of limited value in diagnosis. The endocardium and valves are rarely involved.

B. Observations Leading to Treatment:

1 Pulmonary function studies and serial chest films demonstrate pulmonary fibrosis. If pulmonary function studies show progressive abnormalities, corticosteroid therapy may be tried, particularly if the patient has pulmonary hypertension, atrial gallop, a palpable pulmonary artery, or evidence on the ECG of right ventricular hypertrophy; but the evidence of benefit is controversial.

2. Serial ECGs can detect progressive right ventricular hypertrophy, as well as involvement of the conduction system, in which case insertion of a pacemaker may prevent Stokes-Adams attacks and sudden death. Corticosteroids are usually ineffective when conduction defects and ventricular arrhythmias predominate in the clinical picture.

3. Thallium 201 scans may demonstrate perfusion defects due to granulomas; echocardiography may demonstrate impaired cardiac function even in asymptomatic patients (Kinney, 1980), but these findings do not influence treatment. Since sarcoid in-

volvement of the heart is localized, regional wall motion abnormalities occur, resembling those seen with coronary artery disease (Burstow, 1989). MRI has shown myocardial masses with increased signal intensity compared with the normal myocardium (Riedy, 1988).

4. Endomyocardial biopsy may establish the diagnosis of myocardial sarcoma by demonstrating the typical granulomas.

C. Asymptomatic Features: Most patients, even with obvious sarcoid disease elsewhere, do not exhibit cardiac dysfunction, although electrocardiographic abnormalities (usually atrioventricular conduction delay, right ventricular hypertrophy, or ST–T changes) may be found. In proved sarcoidosis of the heart, complete atrioventricular block and atrioventricular and intraventricular conduction defects occur in approximately 25% of cases (Figure 17–20).

Treatment & Prognosis

Once cardiac symptoms and signs appear, the prognosis is generally poor, but there are exceptions. Sudden death is responsible for most fatal cases. Early recognition of conduction defects and treatment with pacemakers may improve the prognosis. In patients with aborted sudden death, implantation of an automatic internal defibrillator may be indicated.

SYSTEMIC LUPUS ERYTHEMATOSUS

Lupus erythematosus is a systemic disease probably due to vasculitis secondary to autoimmunity and is characterized by deposition of immune complexes in the small arteries (0.1–1 mm in diameter) of visceral organs. The disease is characterized by the production of a number of antinuclear antibodies (ANA) as well as antibodies against phospholipids. The disorder affects the heart in the majority of cases studied at autopsy, causing an inflammatory reaction that may be widespread or focal and that may involve the pericardium, the myocardium, and the valves. Often this reaction is silent, and clinical manifestations of cardiac involvement are present in only about one-third of cases. As more sophisticated diagnostic techniques are developed, most patients will be found to have cardiac involvement. In a recent study (Nihoyannopoulos, 1990), there was echocardiographic evidence of cardiac involvement in 54% of 93 patients. In patients with anticardiolipin antibodies, cardiac involvement was present in 78%. Chronic renal failure is common, but patients may have pericardial effusion or cardiac failure. Systemic lupus erythematosus is a common cause of pericardial effusion in tertiary care centers in the USA.

Clinical Findings

A. Symptoms and Signs: In serologic surveys designed to identify early manifestations of lupus

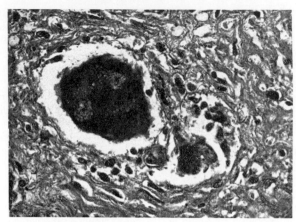

Figure 17–20. Atrioventricular bundle destroyed and replaced by dense fibrous tissue containing numerous giant cells in sarcoidosis. (H&E × 365.) (Reproduced, with permission, from Porter GH: Sarcoid heart disease. N Engl J Med 1960;263:1350.)

erythematosus, the disease is often found to be chronic, mild, and characterized by a rash, slightly raised arterial pressure, arthritis, Raynaud's phenomenon, myopericarditis, and prompt response to corticosteroid therapy.

Cardiac involvement in active cases is suspected by enlargement of the heart, pericardial effusion, and changes on the ECG. Pericarditis is the most frequent type of clinical involvement. Tamponade is rare. A typical example of T wave inversions characteristic of

myopericarditis in systemic lupus erythematosus is shown in Figure 17–21. Hypertension is common and may lead to left ventricular hypertrophy and left ventricular failure.

Other manifestations include a characteristic butterfly malar rash, photosensitivity reaction, Raynaud's phenomenon, arthritis resembling rheumatoid arthritis, and lupus nephritis (focal or diffuse proliferative glomerulitis, membranous glomerular nephropathy). The patient may have pleural effusion as well as

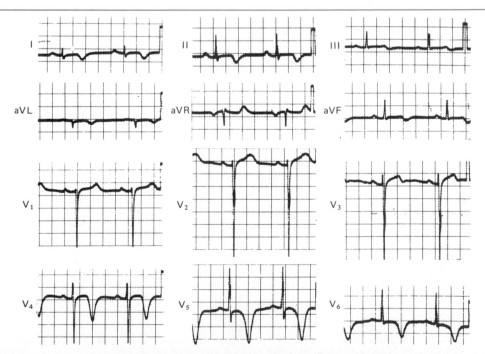

Figure 17–21. T wave inversions characteristic of myopericarditis in a 27-year-old woman with classic clinical lupus erythematosus.

central nervous system involvement, with seizures, chronic organic brain syndrome (dementia, confusion), aseptic meningitis, reversible psychosis, and peripheral neuritis. Libman-Sacks endocarditis may be found pathologically but is rarely a clinical problem. Libman-Sacks valvular lesions are usually small (up to 3–4 mm in diameter) and wart-like ("verrucous"). On occasion, severe mitral regurgitation and rarely aortic regurgitation can occur with healing and retraction of leaflets.

B. Laboratory Findings: The diagnosis is confirmed by finding lupus erythematosus cells in the blood and pericardial fluid, a chronic false-positive serologic test for syphilis, antinuclear and other autoantibodies in the serum, hypergammaglobulinemia, an increased erythrocyte sedimentation rate, and reduced serum complement. Urinalysis reveals proteinuria and the characteristic "telescopic" findings (Krupp, 1943) in which all varieties of cells and casts are found simultaneously in the urinary sediment. Anemia, leukopenia, lymphopenia, and thrombocytopenia are common.

C. Imaging Studies: Two-dimensional echocardiography may reveal left ventricular dysfunction or pericardial effusion. In one two-dimensional echocardiographic study of 93 patients with lupus erythematosus, 28% had valvular lesions, 20% had pericardial thickening, and 5% had regional or global hypokinesis (Nihoyannopoulos, 1990). Compared with age-matched normal controls, patients with lupus have a lower ejection fraction, more diastolic dysfunction, and more mitral, tricuspid, and pulmonary valvular regurgitation (Crozier, 1990).

Treatment

Although mild forms of systemic lupus erythematosus may be treated symptomatically, myocarditis and other serious complications of the disease require judicious use of corticosteroids. Prolonged careful clinical and laboratory follow-up is necessary. Cytotoxic drugs such as cyclophosphamide, azathioprine, or chlorambucil are used in resistant cases but are apt to cause renal failure.

Early steroid therapy makes it less likely that the kidneys will become involved, so that much longer survival is now possible. The disease may be intermittently active but at times is fulminant. Large doses of corticosteroids are beneficial but also often cause adverse side effects.

Prognosis

Sepsis is the most common cause of death in systemic lupus erythematosus and often occurs as a side effect of corticosteroid therapy. Other causes of death are heart disorders (myocardial infarction, arrhythmias, cardiac failure; mitral or, rarely, aortic valve regurgitation), progressive renal disease, and central nervous system involvement (see above).

PROGRESSIVE SYSTEMIC SCLEROSIS (Scleroderma)

The diffuse fibrosis and vasculitis so obvious in the skin, gastrointestinal tract, and lungs in generalized scleroderma may also involve the heart. The predominant pathophysiologic feature is spasm of the small visceral arteries, including those of the myocardium, resulting in fibrosis. The clinical cardiac abnormalities in patients with scleroderma are tabulated in Table 17–7. Figure 17–22 shows the typical pathologic features of scleroderma involving the kidney. Similar changes are seen in the heart. Perivascular fibrosis is

Table 17–7. Clinical cardiac abnormalities in 47 patients with scleroderma.[1,2]

Myocardial Lesion	Severe (13 patients)		Mild (10 patients)		Absent (24 patients)	
Congestive heart failure	11 (85%)		3 (30%)		8 (33%)	
Congestive heart failure without renal or lung involvement	4 (31%)		0		0	
Angina pectoris	3 (23%)		0		0	
Ventricular irritability	8 (62%)		1 (10%)		1 (4%)	
Conduction abnormality	8 (62%)		3 (30%)		6 (25%)	
Right bundle block		5		1		3
Left anterior hemiblock		2		2		5
First-degree heart block		1		1		1
Complete heart block		3		0		0
Cardiac death	8 (62%)		2 (20%)		1 (4%)	
Sudden death	5 (38%)		1 (10%)		0	
Congestive heart failure	3 (23%)		1 (10%)		1 (4%)	
Constrictive pericarditis	0		0		1 (4%)	
Total with clinical cardiac abnormalities →	11 (79%)		4 (40%)		10 (42%)	

[1] Five patients excluded because of coexisting severe epicardial coronary artery disease.
[2] Reproduced, with permission, from the American Heart Association, Inc., Bulkley BH et al; Myocardial lesions of progressive systemic sclerosis: A cause of cardiac dysfunction. Circulation 1976; 53:483.

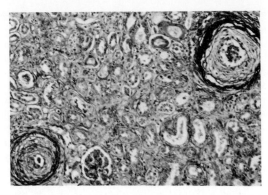

Figure 17–22. Pathologic features of scleroderma of the kidney (similar to myocardium). (Courtesy of O Rambo.)

Table 17–8. Frequency of cardiac symptoms and signs in 254 patients with rheumatoid arthritis and 254 controls.[1]

Cardiac Abnormality	Patients With Arthritis	Controls
Congestive heart failure	25	3
Angina pectoris	16	4
Enlargement of left ventricle	48	28
Enlargement of right ventricle	5	0
Atrial enlargement	6	1
Aortic systolic murmur	7	1
Aortic diastolic murmur	4	0
Mitral diastolic murmur	7	1
Totals	118	38

[1] Reproduced, with permission, from Cathcart ES, Spodick DH: Rheumatoid heart disease: A study of the incidence and nature of cardiac lesions in rheumatoid arthritis. N Engl J Med 1962; 266:959.

clearly shown. Congestive heart failure is rare in mild cases. In severe systemic scleroderma, cardiac failure, arrhythmia, and conduction defects are common. Involvement of the pulmonary vasculature leads to severe pulmonary hypertension and cor pulmonale. In cases without diffuse skin changes but with other features such as calcinosis, Raynaud's phenomenon, esophageal dysfunction, sclerodactyly, and telangiectasia, the term "CREST syndrome" has been applied.

The major cardiac lesion is fibrotic destruction of the conduction system and the small coronary arteries. The fibrotic lesions may also involve the myocardial cells, sometimes causing necrosis and angina pectoris. Despite the myocardial necrosis and fibrosis, the coronary arteries may be patent. Six of eight patients studied postmortem by James (1974) died suddenly as a result of fibrous destruction of the sinoatrial and atrioventricular nodes. Cardiac arrhythmias were frequent in these patients. Electrocardiographic and clinical features of atrioventricular block, Stokes-Adams attacks, and sudden death are similar to those seen in cardiac sarcoidosis. Serial ECGs may determine when conduction defects have progressed, making it advisable to insert an artificial pacemaker to prevent sudden death. The presence of clinical cardiac involvement is an extremely bad prognostic sign, and most of these patients are dead within 5 years.

There is no specific treatment. Supportive treatment includes pacing for conduction defects and use of antiarrhythmic agents for complex ventricular arrhythmias and ventricular tachycardia, which may be documented by ambulatory electrocardiographic monitoring. Recently, an encouraging observation has been made suggesting improved perfusion of the heart and lungs and a decrease in incidence of Raynaud's phenomenon following use of calcium channel blockers and angiotensin-converting enzyme inhibitors (Kahan, 1986; Kahan, 1990). Vasodilators have also been demonstrated occasionally to decrease pulmonary vascular resistance in this disease. Whether this will lead to long-term improvement in symptoms or increased longevity is not yet known.

RHEUMATOID ARTHRITIS

Rheumatoid arthritis is a form of connective tissue disorder. Rheumatoid factor and other autoantibodies are present in the serum. The frequency of cardiac symptoms and signs in a large group of patients with rheumatoid arthritis is shown in Table 17–8. Rheumatoid arthritis may cause inflammatory changes in the pericardium, myocardium, and mitral and aortic valve, producing pericardial effusion and aortic and mitral insufficiency as the most common cardiac manifestations. The frequency with which pericarditis is detected is increased if echocardiograms are done on all patients with rheumatoid arthritis. A typical histologic example of rheumatoid vasculitis of the myocardium is shown in Figure 17–23. The process may involve the coronary arteries and the myocar-

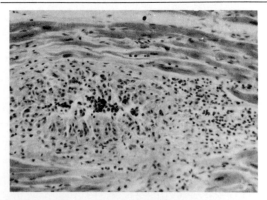

Figure 17–23. Inflammatory infiltrate of the myocardium in rheumatoid arthritis. (Courtesy of O Rambo.)

dium. At autopsy, about a third of all patients with rheumatoid arthritis have evidences of pericarditis, conduction system abnormalities, or aortic and mitral valve disease. Clinically, however, only a small percentage of patients—probably less than 5%—have active cardiac disease. Rheumatoid arthritis may be a precursor of amyloid disease of the heart (see below).

Treatment

There is no specific treatment for cardiac disease in rheumatoid arthritis. Treat cardiac manifestations as indicated elsewhere in this book.

HEMOCHROMATOSIS

Hemochromatosis, an excess iron storage disease, can be classified as primary (idiopathic) or secondary (transfusion) hemosiderosis. Idiopathic hemochromatosis is genetic, transmitted as an autosomal dominant trait. Iron storage is increased because of enhanced intestinal absorption of iron from the normal 1 mg to 3 mg/d. The increased absorption ultimately leads to overloading of the body cells with iron (Finch, 1982).

Idiopathic genetic hemochromatosis is much commoner in men. Excessive amounts (10–40 g instead of the normal 1–2 g) of iron are retained and stored in the cells in the tissues, especially the liver cells, and provoke a variable fibrotic reaction that may involve the myocardium, interfering with left ventricular function. A typical example of iron deposition in the heart is shown in Figure 17–24. Ordinary myocardial cells are affected more than the cells of the conductive system.

Secondary hemochromatosis is more common and usually due to multiple blood transfusions (100 or more) in chronic aplastic or hemolytic anemias of thalassemia. The 250 mg of iron in each unit of blood (500 mL) is stored in the body because excretion of iron cannot be increased. Iron is deposited as hemosiderin, leading to the alternative name **transfusion siderosis.** Rarely, iron loading results from excessive oral intake for many years or from congenital abnormalities of iron metabolism (eg, thalassemia major, transferrinemia, pyridoxine-responsive anemia) (Crosby, 1974; Crosby, 1977).

Iron is deposited in the liver, pancreas, heart, spleen, thyroid, lymph nodes, adrenals, anterior pituitary, joints, gonads, lungs (to a lesser extent), and central nervous system (rarely). It presents clinically as "bronze" diabetes in association with cirrhosis, pituitary insufficiency, testicular atrophy, involvement of the heart, and arthropathy with chondrocalcinosis. Occasionally, chronic arthritis due to chondrocalcinosis suggests the possibility of the disease, especially in the relatives of patients with hemochromatosis.

The presenting symptoms and signs of cardiac deposition of iron may be similar to those of any infiltrative cardiac disease, with fatigue, dyspnea, gallop rhythm, atrial or ventricular arrhythmias, conduction defects, and signs of heart failure. The deposition of iron in the myocardium results in fibrosis, which can present either as a dilated or restrictive cardiomyopathy. In general, the extent of ventricular dysfunction is related to the amount of iron deposition in the sarcoplasm (Olson, 1989).

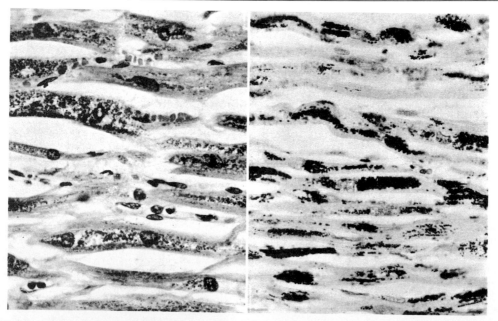

Figure 17–24. Histologic sections of left ventricular myocardium showing extensive iron depositions (dark areas). **Left:** H&E × 560. **Right:** Iron stain × 560. (Reproduced, with permission, from Arnett EN et al: Massive myocardial hemosiderosis: A structure-function conference at the National Heart and Lung Institute. Am Heart J 1975;90:777.)

The diagnosis can be established by biopsy of the liver, kidney, heart, or skin and the use of stains for stainable iron (hemosiderin) appropriate to the tissues obtained.

Screening Tests

Various screening tests have been used to detect preclinical disease. These have included determinations of serum ferritin, serum iron, transferrin saturation, or deferoxamine-chelatable iron. All are helpful, but direct demonstration of increased tissue iron is the definitive finding. Serum ferritin, the storage form of iron, was found to be increased in almost all relatives of patients with hemochromatosis who had increased iron stores, whereas it was rarely increased in relatives of those with normal iron stores (Halliday, 1977).

Cardiac involvement consists of atrial and ventricular arrhythmias, conduction defects, cardiac enlargement, and cardiac failure.

The course of the disease is usually unfavorable unless excess iron stores are removed early by frequent phlebotomies (see below). Early diagnosis can be made if the disease is suspected in every case of unexplained cardiomyopathy, cirrhosis, or diabetes, especially if the skin is an unusual bronze or a grayish tan color. Plasma iron is usually elevated, saturation of transferrin is 60–70% (often more) instead of the normal 20–40%, and serum ferritin is elevated. The diagnosis is established by finding abnormal iron deposits in tissues such as the skin, liver, or myocardium.

Echocardiography has shown decreased systolic function and abnormal diastolic function in these patients. Increased ventricular wall thickness has been described in hemochromatosis, but this appears to be true only in patients with transfusion-related secondary hemochromatosis. In the primary idiopathic type of hemochromatosis, patients are more likely to have a nonrestrictive, dilated systolic dysfunctional ventricle (Olson, 1987).

Noninvasive radionuclide angiography has been used to determine the response of the ejection fraction to exercise in these patients. Changes in the ejection fraction may be the earliest manifestation of left ventricular dysfunction prior to the development of cardiac failure (Leon, 1979).

Treatment & Prognosis

Treatment consists of repeated phlebotomy and, over a period of 6–24 months, continuous subcutaneous administration of a chelating agent, deferoxamine, to decrease organ damage and prevent fibrosis (Weatherall, 1983). Removal of the deposition of iron in the heart by serial phlebotomies can reverse the abnormal cardiac findings and reverse cardiac failure. It has been estimated that 100 phlebotomies of 500 mL of blood once a week will eliminate the excess iron within 2 years. More rapid removal of blood may produce hypotension or cardiac arrhythmias. The condition can subsequently be controlled by intermittent phlebotomies that maintain the hemoglobin at about 11 g/dL.

In secondary hemochromatosis, phlebotomies are unsatisfactory. Deferoxamine, whether given subcutaneously or intravenously, has been shown to increase urinary iron excretion. A method for 12- to 24-hour subcutaneous infusion has been devised using a portable infusion pump and administration of the drug through a No. 27 needle placed in the subcutaneous tissues of the anterior abdominal wall (Propper, 1982). Long-term subcutaneous deferoxamine infusions are effective in enhancing iron excretion but have caused optic neuropathy with visual loss and a high-frequency hearing deficit in some patients. Vision and hearing improved again when the drug was stopped. Serial monitoring of vision and hearing is advised to regulate the dosage. An orally active chelating agent for removing iron may be as effective as intravenous or subcutaneous deferoxamine and has the advantage of ease of administration (Kontoghiorges, 1987).

Serial determination of deferoxamine-chelatable iron is a safe and practical way of assessing the effect of phlebotomy as well as infusions of deferoxamine (Baldus, 1978). The results of regular blood transfusions in patients with beta-thalassemia are satisfactory for 2 or 3 decades, but most patients ultimately die of the effects of iron overload from the transfused blood (Pippard, 1977).

AMYLOID DISEASE

Amyloid disease of the heart is estimated to be responsible for about 5–10% of cases of cardiomyopathy due to causes other than coronary artery disease. It is more common in men than women and rarely is seen before age 30. It is usually primary in the heart but may be secondary to other conditions, eg, multiple myeloma, chronic infections, regional ileitis, chronic disorders of connective tissues such as rheumatoid arthritis, or periodic fever (familial Mediterranean fever). The cause is obscure, but a faulty immunologic response may be responsible for increased production by plasma cells and deposition of amyloid protein in the heart, kidney, and other organs of the body. In primary amyloidosis, this abnormal amyloid protein is composed of portions of immunoglobulin light chains (designated AL) produced by a monoclonal plasma cell population that is often associated with multiple myeloma. Secondary amyloidosis is due to the production of a nonimmunoglobulin protein called AA. In familial amyloidosis, a DNA mutation has been described, the histidine-58 transthyretin (TTR) mutation, which may be responsible for the cardiomyopathy (Benson, 1992; Gertz, 1992). In familial amyloidosis and senile amyloidosis, the amyloid protein is a prealbumin protein. The

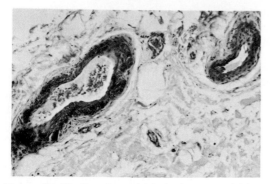

Figure 17–25. Rectal amyloidosis from rectal biopsy. (Congo red × 40.) The dark areas are deposits of amyloid in the walls of blood vessels. (Courtesy of O Rambo.)

heart has a "glassy" appearance, and there may be generalized vasculitis involving the liver, spleen, and kidneys as well as the heart. The small vessels of the heart may have amyloid deposits in their walls that produce occlusive disease from the vasculitis as well as restrictive disease from the deposition of amyloid. Above the age of 80 years, the majority of hearts show some senile amyloid deposition. Figure 17–25 is a typical Congo red stain preparation of amyloidosis from a rectal biopsy.

Clinical Findings

A. Symptoms and Signs: Amyloid disease of the heart is a restrictive cardiomyopathy and may be confused with constrictive pericarditis. Cardiac amyloidosis can present as systolic dysfunction causing congestive heart failure. Clinically apparent heart involvement occurs in 25–50% of patients with amyloidosis. Amyloid disease should be considered in all patients with plasma cell leukemia, multiple myeloma, chronic infections, and long-standing periodic fever.

Other clinical presentations are orthostatic hypotension, possibly due to involvement of the autonomic nervous system or the vessels themselves. Arrhythmias and involvement of the conduction system are the least common presentation, though sudden death is not uncommon in cardiac amyloidosis.

Definitive diagnosis is based on finding amyloid deposits in endomyocardial biopsies or in biopsies of the abdominal fat, rectum, liver, or gums; of these sites, rectal and abdominal fat biopsy are the most reliable of the simple and well-tolerated procedures and most likely to be positive (Duston, 1987). The oral lesions, in addition to papules, may include macroglossia with a large, firm tongue resulting from amyloid deposition. The details of the present status of Bence Jones protein and the light chains of the immunoglobulins are discussed by Kyle (1983), and Sleisinger (1987). Cardiac involvement is a common cause of death in amyloidosis.

Amyloid deposits consisting of fibrils of light chain immunoglobulins may be found anywhere in the myocardium; if large and extensive, they may produce restrictive cardiomyopathy; if small and scattered, especially in older individuals, they may not give rise to any cardiovascular symptoms or signs. If the amyloid deposits involve the conduction system (eg, the sinoatrial node or the atrioventricular node), the patients may have ventricular arrhythmias or conduction defects, heart block, and syncope. The severity of amyloid involvement varies greatly.

Chronic skin infections secondary to repeated subcutaneous injection of heroin can cause so-called "skin popper's amyloidosis." These patients may also present with nephrosis. Renal biopsies in drug abusers for the evaluation of proteinuria revealed systemic amyloidosis in a fourth to three-fourths of patients (Neugarten, 1986).

Progressive renal failure may occur as excess protein is deposited in the basement membrane of the glomeruli.

B. Laboratory Findings: Bence Jones proteinuria is usually associated with multiple myeloma or secondary amyloidosis, although it occurs to a lesser degree in primary amyloid disease, neoplastic diseases, and immunologic disorders such as Waldenström's macroglobulinemia. Bence Jones protein was discovered because it precipitates when heated to moderate temperatures (50–60 °C) but redissolves on further heating to 100 °C and then reprecipitates upon cooling. Other proteins (eg, albumin) precipitate upon heating but do not redissolve.

Bence Jones proteins are homogeneous light chain polypeptides of immunoglobulins that can be found in both urine and blood; the light chains can be found by electron microscopy or quantitative immunochemistry of the urinary sediment. The autoimmune nature of amyloid disease is supported by the finding that the characteristic protein represents the light chains of immunoglobulins (Gertz, 1989).

The distinction between primary and secondary amyloidosis has become blurred because of the lower incidence of chronic infections and the availability of more precise immunochemical methods (immunoelectrophoresis, immunoassay) of quantifying the light chain polypeptides in the urine and serum that characterize amyloid disease. Levels of light chain polypeptide immunoglobulins vary in different patients and at different times in the course of the disease.

C. Electrocardiographic Findings: The ECG sometimes arouses suspicion of an infiltrative process in the heart because of low voltage of the QRS complexes.

D. Imaging Studies: Echocardiographic examination can assess left ventricular function and also demonstrate decreased diastolic filling with prolonged left ventricular relaxation. The decreased left ventricular function may be associated with normal left ventricular cavity size. Doppler echocardiography has clarified the types of diastolic dysfunction seen in amyloidosis. Early, there is abnormal relaxation with a prominent c wave and a high A/E ratio of the mitral valve flow velocity signal. In later stages, there is stiffening of the ventricle by amyloid replacement, and fibrosis and myocardial restriction occur where there is normalization of the A/E ratio (Kline, 1989). The appearance of the thickened left ventricular wall in amyloidosis is characteristic. There is a bright, sparkling granular texture that highlights the wall, probably due to the amyloid pattern.

Treatment

The only treatment is that of the underlying condition causing the amyloidosis, eg, chronic infection. Attempts to treat primary amyloidosis with cytotoxic agents and corticosteroids have not been convincing. Two-year survival rates are 30–50% after the onset of cardiac symptoms.

ENDOMYOCARDIAL FIBROSIS & LÖFFLER'S ENDOCARDITIS (Idiopathic Hypereosinophilic Syndrome) (See also Restrictive Cardiomyopathy.)

These uncommon conditions of unknown cause may be a single entity or different entities. Whether or not endomyocardial fibrosis and Löffler's endocarditis are identical or distinct pathologic processes, the cardiac lesion consists of endomyocardial fibrosis, myocarditis, endocardial thrombosis, and eosinophilic infiltration (Fauci, 1982). With Löffler's endocarditis, persistent eosinophilia with 1500 or more eosinophils per microliter is the rule. Endomyocardial fibrosis and eosinophilic endocarditis are infrequent in the Western world but are common in developing countries. The cases with eosinophilia are often associated with leukemia and lymphoma, and these disorders should be sought. It is postulated that Löffler's endocarditis and endomyocardial fibrosis are different phases of the same disease. The early phase is characterized by eosinophilic myocarditis. The eosinophilic granules are cardiotoxic, releasing substances that damage the myocardium. Thrombus is deposited on the endocardium, and finally fibrous tissue and scarring result. Endomyocardial fibrosis produces a plaque-like thickening of the endocardium that appears grossly as a white lining of the entire endocardium, frequently associated with mural thrombi and systemic or pulmonary emboli. The disease usually affects the endocardium and myocardium of the left more than the right ventricle. There is interference with cardiac filling, and the patient may present with clinical features of restrictive cardiomyopathy and may be diagnosed as having chronic constrictive pericarditis (Parrillo, 1979; Cherian, 1983).

The onset of the disease is usually vague and insidious. It occurs in teenagers and young adults in developing countries and in older adults in developed ones. Some patients present with fever, suggesting a viral infection as the basic cause of the process.

Clinical Findings

When restriction of filling and emptying of the ventricles occurs because of the thick lining of endomyocardial fibrosis, the patient presents with cardiac failure of unknown cause. When the process affects predominantly the right ventricular endocardium, the patient may have systemic venous hypertension and right ventricular failure. With endocardial thrombus and fibrosis, the papillary muscle and chordae can be involved, resulting in mitral and tricuspid regurgitation. This must be differentiated from mitral valve disease and chronic pulmonary disease—as well as from congenital heart disease in children and teenagers. Pericardial effusion followed by heart failure requires exclusion of tuberculous pericarditis. When the process involves the left ventricle, left ventricular failure may occur (see Chapter 10). In advanced cases, both right and left ventricular endocardiums are involved with both right and left ventricular failure and pulmonary hypertension. The diagnosis is suspected on the basis of the clinical features, including intracardiac calcification, but often cannot be distinguished from congestive cardiomyopathy.

Treatment & Prognosis

Treatment is generally only supportive, with conventional therapy for cardiac failure. Prednisone may be tried and occasionally produces a remission. Anticoagulation may be helpful in preventing thromboembolism. In some instances, the thrombus can be surgically removed, which enlarges the ventricular chamber and increases distensibility. In general, the prognosis is poor, and the patient usually lives only a few years.

SICKLE CELL DISEASE & CHRONIC ANEMIA

Sickle cell disease is an infrequent cause of cardiovascular manifestations. The anemia may increase the cardiac output (high-output failure), and the tendency of sickle cells to occlude small vessels may narrow the pulmonary or coronary arteries and produce cor pulmonale or angina. Thrombus in the coronary arteries and acute myocardial infarction are rare in sickle cell disease. When the hemoglobin is less than 6 or 7 g/dL in any type of anemia, cardiac output is increased at rest (see Chapter 10), but the maximal cardiac output with exercise is still less than normal. The left ventricular ejection fraction is usually normal, and the systemic vascular resistance is decreased (Denenberg, 1983). Because of thrombotic obliteration of the pulmonary arteries that occurs in sickle

It is not clear whether pregnancy is a precipitating cause of possible preexisting cardiomyopathy or whether this is a distinct clinical entity. A possible viral or immunologic disorder is supported by the consistency with which clinical reports describe the time of onset and the absence of any known preexisting cardiac disease prior to peripartum cardiac failure.

The clinical manifestations may be alarming, with the rapid development of cardiac failure and pericardial effusion shortly after delivery. Severe dyspnea, orthopnea, tachycardia, chest pain, cardiac enlargement, gallop rhythm, pulmonary rales, and pulmonary congestion on the chest film attest to the presence of severe left ventricular failure. Raised venous pressure indicates right ventricular failure as well. Systemic embolism may occur. Preeclampsia-eclampsia and acute glomerulonephritis must be excluded. The ECG shows primary T wave inversions (not secondary to conduction defects) in the left ventricular leads, suggesting acute myopericarditis, with which this disorder is frequently confused.

The clinical course usually lasts 3–6 months, and most patients recover following conventional treatment for cardiac failure, but some progress to dilated cardiomyopathy. Gilchrist (1963) found no evidence of residual cardiac symptoms or signs in seven patients studied 1–10 years after congestive heart failure. Figure 17–27 illustrates the course in a 32-year-old woman who developed cardiac failure 4 months following delivery of a normal child. X-rays of the chest show decrease in size of the heart shadow, and ECGs showed regression of electrocardiographic abnormalities.

NEUROPATHIC DISORDERS & HEART DISEASE

Neuropathic disorders are a rare cause of heart disease. Patients with Friedreich's ataxia, pseudohypertrophic muscular (Duchenne) dystrophy, dystrophia myotonica, and other neuropathic disorders may develop cardiac failure, arrhythmias, and conduction defects with Stokes-Adams attacks.

REFERENCES

General

Abelmann WH: Classification and natural history of primary myocardial disease. Prog Cardiovasc Dis 1984; 28:73.

Fowles RE, Mason JW: Role of cardiac biopsy in the diagnosis and management of cardiac disease. Prog Cardiovasc Dis 1984;27:153.

Marboe CC, Fenoglio JJ: Biopsy diagnosis of myocarditis. Cardiovasc Clin 1988;18:137.

McNulty CM: Active viral myocarditis: Application of current knowledge to clinical practice. Heart Dis Stroke 1992;1:135.

Roberts WC, Ferrans VJ: Pathologic anatomy of the cardiomyopathies: Idiopathic dilated and hypertrophic types, infiltrative types and endomyocardial disease with and without eosinophilia. Hum Pathol 1975;6:287.

Wahr DW, Schiller NB: Evaluating myopericardial disease with echocardiography. J Cardiovasc Med 1982;7:799.

Acute Myocarditis Associated With Specific Diseases

Acierno LJ: Cardiac complications in acquired immunodeficiency syndrome (AIDS): A review. J Am Coll Cardiol 1989;13: 1144.

Andy JJ et al: Trichinosis causing extensive ventricular mural endocarditis with superimposed thrombosis. Am J Med 1977;63:824.

Binak K et al: Coronary changes in acute glomerulonephritis at rest and during exercise. Br Heart J 1975;37:833.

Bowles NE et al: Detection of coxsackie-B-virus-specific RNA sequences in myocardial biopsy samples from patients with myocarditis and dilated cardiomyopathy. Lancet 1986;1:1120.

Dec GW Jr et al: Relation between histological findings on early repeat right ventricular biopsy and ventricular function in patients with myocarditis. Br Heart J 1988;60:332.

El-Hagrassy MMO, Banatvala JE: Coxsackie-B-virus-specific IgM responses in patients with cardiac and other diseases. Lancet 1980;2:1160.

Grist NR, Bell EJ: A 6-year study of coxsackievirus B infections in heart disease. J Hyg (Camb) 1974;73: 165.

Halvadar PV et al: Fulminant diphtheritic myocarditis. Indian Heart J 1989;41:265.

Herskowitz A et al: Coxsackievirus B3 murine myocarditis: A pathologic spectrum of myocarditis in genetically defined inbred strains. J Am Coll Cardiol 1987;9:1311.

Kaul S et al: Cardiac manifestations of acquired immune deficiency syndrome: A 1991 update. Am Heart J 1991;122:535.

Kishimoto C, Thorp KA, Abelmann WH: Immunosuppression with high doses of cyclophosphamide reduces the severity of myocarditis but increases the mortality in murine coxsackievirus B3 myocarditis. Circulation 1990;82:982.

Latham RD et al: Recently diagnosed idiopathic dilated cardiomyopathy: Incidence of myocarditis and efficacy of prednisone therapy. Am Heart J 1989;117: 876.

Lee MG et al: Cardiac involvement in severe leptospirosis. West Indian Med J 1986;35:295.

Levi G et al: Coxsackie virus heart disease: 15 years after. Eur Heart J 1988;9:1303.

Lieberman EB et al: Clinicopathologic description of myocarditis. J Am Coll Cardiol 1991;18:1617.

Mason JW, Billingham ME, Ricci DR: Treatment of

acute inflammatory myocarditis assisted by endo-myocardial biopsy. Am J Cardiol 1980;45:1037.

Matsumori A et al: Treatment of viral myocarditis with ribavirin in an animal preparation. Circulation 1985; 71:834.

McAlister HF et al: Lyme carditis: An important cause of reversible heart block. Ann Intern Med 1989;110:339.

O'Connell JB, Mason JW: Immunosuppressive therapy in experimental and clinical myocarditis. Pathol Immunopathol Res 1988;7:292.

Pinamonti B et al: Echocardiographic findings in myocarditis. Am J Cardiol 1988;62:285.

Remes J et al: Clinical outcome and left ventricular function 23 years after acute Coxsackie virus myopericarditis. Eur Heart J 1990;11:182.

Reyes MP, Lerner AM: Coxsackievirus myocarditis—with special reference to acute and chronic effects. Prog Cardiovasc Dis 1985;27:373.

Ruskin J, Remington JS: Toxoplasmosis in the compromised host. Ann Intern Med 1976;84:193.

Sainani GS, Dekate MP, Rao CP: Heart disease caused by coxsackie virus B infection. Br Heart J 1975;37:819.

Salvi A et al: Immunosuppressive treatment in myocarditis. Int J Cardiol 1989;22:329.

Yasuda T et al: Indium 111-monoclonal antimyosin antibody imaging in the diagnosis of acute myocarditis. Circulation 1987;76:306.

Rheumatic Fever

Agarwal BL: Rheumatic heart disease unabated in developing countries. Lancet 1981;2:910.

American Heart Association Committee on Rheumatic Fever and Bacterial Endocarditis. Circulation 1988; 78:1082.

Bland EF: Rheumatic fever: The way it was. Circulation 1987;76:1190.

Combined Rheumatic Fever Study Group: A comparison of short-term, intensive prednisone and acetylsalicylic acid therapy in the treatment of acute rheumatic fever. N Engl J Med 1965;272:63.

Dajani AS et al: Prevention of rheumatic fever. Heart Dis Stroke 1992;1:108.

Disciascio G, Taranta A: Rheumatic fever in children. Am Heart J 1980;99:635.

Engleman EP, Hollister LE, Kolb FO: Sequelae of rheumatic fever in men: Four to eight year follow-up study. JAMA 1954;155:1134.

Gordis L: The virtual disappearance of rheumatic fever in the United States: Lessons in the rise and fall of disease. (T. Duckett Jones Memorial Lecture.) Circulation 1985;72:1155.

Gotsman MS: Rheumatic fever in the 80s. (2 parts.) Cardiovasc Rev Rep 1985;6:861, 935.

Jones Criteria (Revised) for guidance in the diagnosis of rheumatic fever. Circulation 1965:32:664.

Kaplan EL: The carditis/cardiomyopathy of rheumatic fever: Relationship to pathogenesis. Postgrad Med 1992;68(Suppl I):S21.

Krause RM: The influence of infection on the geography of heart disease. Circulation 1979;60:972.

Massell BF et al: Penicillin and the marked decrease in morbidity and mortality from rheumatic fever in the United States. N Engl J Med 1988;318:280.

Schieken RM, Kerber RE: Echocardiographic abnormalities in acute rheumatic fever. Am J Cardiol 1976;38:458.

Stollerman GH: *Rheumatic Fever and Streptococcal Infections.* Grune & Stratton, 1975.

Stollerman GH: Rheumatogenic group A streptococci and the return of rheumatic fever. Adv Intern Med 1990;35:1.

Veasy LG et al: Resurgence of acute rheumatic fever in the intermountain area of the United States. N Engl J Med 1987;316:421.

Yoshinoya S, Pope RM: Detection of immune complexes in acute rheumatic fever and their relationship to HLA-B5. J Clin Invest 1980;65:136.

Zabriskie JB: Rheumatic fever: The interplay between host, genetics, and microbe. Circulation 1985;71:1077.

Acute Myocardial Damage
Due to Drug Toxicity

Albert SG, Alves LE, Rose EP: Thyroid dysfunction during chronic amiodarone therapy. J Am Coll Cardiol 1987;9:175.

Appelbaum FR et al: Acute lethal carditis caused by high-dose combination chemotherapy: A unique clinical and pathological entity. Lancet 1976;1:58.

Brennan FJ: Electrophysiologic effects of imipramine and doxepin on normal and depressed cardiac Purkinje fibers. Am J Cardiol 1980;46:599.

Elkayam U, Frishman W: Cardiovascular effects of phenothiazines. Am Heart J 1980;100:397.

Fu LX et al: A new insight into Adriamycin-induced cardiotoxicity. Int J Cardiol 1990;29:15.

Kantrowitz NE, Bristow MR: Cardiotoxicity of antitumor agents. Prog Cardiovasc Dis 1984;27:194.

Kloner RA et al: The effects of acute and chronic cocaine use on the heart. Circulation 1992;85:407.

Lee BH et al: Alterations in left ventricular diastolic function with doxorubicin therapy. J Am Coll Cardiol 1987;9:184.

Legha SS et al: Reduction of doxorubicin cardiotoxicity by prolonged continuous intravenous infusion. Ann Intern Med 1982;96:133.

Marshall JB, Forker AD: Cardiovascular effects of tricyclic antidepressant drugs: Therapeutic usage, overdose, and management of complications. Am Heart J 1982;103:401.

Rezkalla SH et al: Cocaine-induced heart disease. Am Heart J 1990;120:1403.

Saini J et al: Reversibility of severe left ventricular dysfunction due to doxorubicin cardiotoxicity. Ann Intern Med. 1987;106:814.

Samlowski EW et al: Severe myocarditis following high-dose interleukin-2 administration. Arch Pathol Lab Med 1989;113:838.

Schwartz RG et al: Congestive heart failure and left ventricular dysfunction complicating doxorubicin therapy: Seven-year experience using serial radionuclide angiocardiography. Am J Med 1987;82:1109.

Taliercio CP et al: Myocarditis related to drug hypersensitivity. Mayo Clin Proc 1985;60:463.

Thompson RC et al: Adriamycin cardiotoxicity and proton nuclear magnetic resonance relaxation properties. Am Heart J 1987;113:1444.

Torti FM et al: Reduced cardiotoxicity of doxorubicin delivered on a weekly schedule: Assessment by endomyocardial biopsy. Ann Intern Med 1983;99:745.

Dilated (Congestive) Cardiomyopathy

Anderson KP et al: Sudden death in idiopathic dilated cardiomyopathy. Ann Intern Med 1987;107:104.

Beahrs MM et al: Hypertrophic obstructive cardiomyopathy: Ten- to 21-year follow-up after partial septal myectomy. Am J Cardiol 1983;51:1160.

Beisel KW: Immunogenetic basis of myocarditis: Role of fibrillary antigens. Springer Semin Immunopathol 1989;11:31.

Brigden W: Uncommon myocardial diseases: The noncoronary cardiomyopathies. (2 parts.) Lancet 1957; 2:1179, 1243.

Cleland JGF et al: Clinical hemodynamic and antiarrhythmic effects of long-term treatment with amiodarone of patients with heart failure. Br Heart J 1987;57:436.

Dec GW et al: Active myocarditis in the spectrum of acute dilated cardiomyopathies: Clinical features, histologic correlates, and clinical outcome. N Engl J Med 1985;312:885.

Eisenberg JD, Sobel BE, Geltman EM: Differentiation of ischemic from nonischemic cardiomyopathy with positron emission tomography. Am J Cardiol 1987;59: 1410.

Figulla HR et al: Beneficial effects of long-term diltiazem treatment in dilated cardiomyopathy. J Am Coll Cardiol 1989;13:653.

Fuster V et al: The natural history of idiopathic dilated cardiomyopathy. Am J Cardiol 1981;47:525.

German and Austrian Xamoterol Study Group: Double-blind placebo controlled comparison of digoxin and xamoterol in chronic heart failure. Lancet 1988;1: 489.

Greenwood RD, Nadas AS, Fyler DC: The clinical course of primary myocardial disease in infants and children. Am Heart J 1976;92:549.

Griffin ML et al: Dilated cardiomyopathy in infants and children. J Am Coll Cardiol 1988;11:139.

Hamby RI: Primary myocardial disease. Medicine 1970;49:55.

Hammond EH et al: Predictive value of immunofluorescence and electron microscopic evaluation of endomyocardial biopsies in the diagnosis and prognosis of myocarditis and idiopathic dilated cardiopathy. Am Heart J 1987;1141:1055.

Harvey WP, Segal JP, Gurel T: The clinical spectrum of primary myocardial disease. Prog Cardiovasc Dis 1964;7:17.

Hosenpud JD: Classic idiopathic myocarditis: Controversies in causes and therapy. Cardiovasc Res Rep 1988;95:32.

Johnson RA, Palacios I: Dilated cardiomyopathies of the adult. (2 parts.) N Engl J Med 1982;307:1051, 1119.

Kawai C, Takatsu T: Clinical and experimental studies on cardiomyopathy. N Engl J Med 1975;293:592.

Keough AM et al: Timing of cardiac transplantation in idiopathic dilated cardiomyopathy. Am J Cardiol 1988;61:418.

Keough AM et al: Prognostic guides in patients with idiopathic or ischemic dilated cardiomyopathy as-sessed for cardiac transplantation. Am J Cardiol 1990;65:903.

Keren A et al: Mildly dilated congestive cardiomyopathy. Circulation 1990;81:506.

Koike S: Immunologic disorders in patients with dilated cardiomyopathy. Jpn Heart J 1989;30:799.

Manolio TA et al: Prevalence and etiology of idiopathic dilated cardiomyopathy (summary of a National Heart, Lung, Blood Institutes Workshop). Am J Cardiol 1992;69:1458.

Massie BM et al: Mitral-septal separation: A new echocardiographic index of left ventricular function. Am J Cardiol 1977;39:1008.

Meinertz T et al: Significance of ventricular arrhythmias in idiopathic dilated cardiomyopathy. Am J Cardiol 1984;53:902.

Michels VV et al: The frequency of familial dilated cardiomyopathy in a series of patients with idiopathic dilated cardiomyopathy. N Engl J Med 1992;326:77.

Moreira LFP et al: Latissimus dorsi cardiomyoplasty in the treatment of patients with dilated cardiomyopathy. Circulation 1990;82:257.

Olsen EGJ: Fundamentals of clinical cardiology: The pathology of cardiomyopathies: A critical analysis. Am Heart J 1979;98:385.

Parrillo JE et al: The results of transvenous endomyocardial biopsy can frequently be used to diagnose myocardial diseases in patients with idiopathic heart failure. Circulation 1984;69:93.

Report of the WHO/ISFC task force on the definition and classification of cardiomyopathies. Br Heart J 1980;44:672.

Shirey EK, Proudfit WL, Hawk WA: Primary myocardial disease: Correlation with clinical findings, angiographic and biopsy diagnosis. Am Heart J 1980;99: 198.

Shultheiss HP: The significance of autoantibodies against the ADP/ATP carrier for the pathogenesis of myocarditis and dilated cardiomyopathy: Clinical and experimental data. Springer Semin Immunopathol 1989;11:15.

Stevenson LW et al: Poor survival of patients with idiopathic cardiomyopathy considered too well for transplantation. Am J Med 1987;83:871.

Torp A: Incidence of congestive cardiomyopathy. In: *Congestive Cardiomyopathy.* Goodwin JF, Hjalmarson A, Olsen EGF (editors). AB Håassel, 1980.

Tracy S et al: Molecular approaches to enteroviral diagnosis in idiopathic cardiomyopathy myocarditis. J Am Coll Cardiol 1990;15:1088.

Waagstein F et al: Long-term beta-blockade in dilated cardiomyopathy: Effects of short- and long-term metoprolol treatment followed by withdrawal and readministration of metoprolol. Circulation. 1989;80:551.

Zee-Cheng C-S et al: High incidence of myocarditis by endomyocardial biopsy in patients with idiopathic congestive cardiomyopathy. J Am Coll Cardiol 1984; 3:63.

Hypertrophic Cardiomyopathy

Anderson DM et al: Hypertrophic obstructive cardiomyopathy: Effects of acute and chronic verapamil treatment on left ventricular systolic and diastolic function. Br Heart J 1984;51:523.

Brush JE Jr et al: Cardiac norepinephrine kinetics in hypertrophic cardiomyopathy. Circulation 1989;79: 836.

Brandenburg RO et al: Report of the WHO/IFSC Task Force on the Definition and Classification of Cardiomyopathies. Br Heart J 1980;44:672.

Cannon RO et al: Myocardial ischemia in hypertrophic cardiomyopathy: Contribution of inadequate vasodilator reserve and elevated ventricular filling pressure. Circulation 1985;71:234.

Chatterjee K et al: Hypertrophic cardiomyopathy: Therapy with slow channel inhibiting agents. Prog Cardiovasc Dis 1982;25:193.

Chikamori T et al: Prognostic significance of radionuclide assessed diastolic function in hypertrophic cardiomyopathy. Am J Coll Cardiol 1990;65:478.

Codd MB et al: Epidemiological features of the idiopathic cardiomyopathies: A population-based study. Br Heart J 1989;61:80.

Cripps R et al: Signal-averaged electrocardiography in hypertrophic cardiomyopathy. J Am Coll Cardiol 1990;15:956.

Diodati JG et al: Predictors of exercise benefit after operative relief of left ventricular outflow obstruction in the myotomy-myectomy procedure in hypertrophic cardiomyopathy. Am J Cardiol 1992;69:1617.

Epstein ND et al: Evidence of genetic heterogeneity in five kindreds with familial hypertensive cardiomyopathy. Circulation 1992;85:635.

Epstein SE, Rosing DR: Verapamil: Its potential for causing serious complications in patients with hypertrophic cardiomyopathy. Circulation 1981;64:437.

Fananapazir L et al: Electrophysiologic abnormalities in patients with hypertrophic cardiomyopathy: A conservative analysis of 155 patients. Circulation 1989;80: 1259.

Fananapazir L et al: Impact of dual-chamber permanent pacing in patients with obstructive hypertrophic cardiomyopathy with symptoms refractory to verapamil and β-adrenergic blocker therapy. Circulation 1992; 85:2149.

Fananapazir L, Epstein SE: Value of electrophysiologic studies in hypertrophic cardiomyopathy treated with amiodarone. Am J Cardiol 1991;67:175.

Frank S, Braunwald E: Idiopathic hypertrophic subaortic stenosis: clinical analysis of 126 patients with emphasis on the natural history. Circulation 1968;37: 759.

Gill J et al: Amiodarone: An overview of its pharmacologic preparations, and review of its therapeutic use with cardiac arrhythmias. Drugs 1992;43:69.

Gilligan DM et al: Investigation of a hemodynamic basis for syncope in hypertrophic cardiomyopathy. Circulation 1992;85:2140.

Goodwin JF: The frontiers of cardiomyopathy. Br Heart J 1982;48:1.

Hecht EM et al: Clinical course of middle-aged asymptomatic patients with hypertrophic cardiomyopathy. Am J Cardiol 1992;69:935.

Henry WL et al: Mechanism of left ventricular outflow obstruction in patients with obstructive asymmetric septal hypertrophy (idiopathic hypertrophic subaortic stenosis). Am J Cardiol 1975;35:337.

Jarcho JA et al: Mapping a gene for familial hypertrophic cardiomyopathy to chromosome 14q1. N Engl J Med 1989;321:1372.

Krajcer Z et al: Mitral valve replacement and septal myomectomy with hypertrophic cardiomyopathy: Ten year follow-up in 80 patients. Circulation 1988;78:I-35.

Kuck K-H et al: Programmed electrical stimulation in hypertrophic cardiomyopathy: Results in patients with and without cardiac arrest or syncope. Eur Heart J 1988;9:177.

Lembo NJ et al: Bedside diagnosis of systolic murmur. N Engl J Med 1988;318:1572.

Lorell BH et al: Modification of abnormal left ventricular diastolic properties by nifedipine in patients with hypertrophic cardiomyopathy. Circulation 1982;65:499.

Maron BJ, Roberts WC, Epstein SE: Sudden death in hypertrophic cardiomyopathy: A profile of 78 patients. Circulation 1982;65:1388.

Maron BJ et al: Hypertrophic cardiomyopathy: Interrelations of clinical manifestations, pathophysiology, and therapy. (2 parts.) N Engl J Med 1987;316:780, 844.

McIntosh CL, Maron BJ: Current operative treatment of obstructive hypertrophic cardiomyopathy. Circulation 1988;78:487.

McKenna WJ et al: Long-term survival with amiodarone in patients with hypertrophic cardiomyopathy and ventricular tachycardia. Br Heart J 1989;61:472.

McKenna WJ et al: Arrhythmia and prognosis in infants, children and adolescents with hypertrophic cardiomyopathy. J Am Coll Cardiol 1988;11:147.

McKenna WJ et al: The natural history of left ventricular hypertrophy in hypertrophic cardiomyopathy: An electrocardiographic study. Circulation 1982;66:1233.

Morrow AG et al: Left ventricular myotomy and myectomy in patients with obstructive hypertrophic cardiomyopathy and previous cardiac arrest. Am J Cardiol 1980;46:313.

Nishimura RA et al: Evaluation of hypertrophic cardiomyopathy by Doppler color flow imaging: Initial observations. Mayo Clin Proc 1986;61:631.

Oakley CM: Cardiomyopathies. Curr Opin Cardiol 1990; 5:300.

Pollick C et al: Disopyramide in hypertrophic cardiomyopathy: I. Hemodynamic assessment after intravenous administration. II. Noninvasive assessment after oral administration. Am J Cardiol 1988;62:1248.

Popp RL, Harrison DC: Ultrasound in the diagnosis and evaluation of therapy of idiopathic hypertrophic subaortic stenosis. Circulation 1969;40:905.

Romeo F et al: Hypertrophic cardiomyopathy: Is a left ventricular outflow tract gradient a major prognostic determinant? Eur Heart J 1990;11:233.

Sasson Z et al: Doppler echocardiographic determination of the pressure gradient in hypertrophic cardiomyopathy. J Am Coll Cardiol 1988;11:752.

Solomon SD et al: A locus for familial hypertrophic cardiomyopathy is closely linked to the cardiac myosin heavy chain genes, CRI-L436 and CRI-L329 on chromosome 14 at q11–q12. Am J Hum Genet 1990;47: 389.

Spirito P: Left ventricular hypertrophy and occurrence of sudden cardiac death in hypertrophic cardiomyopathy. J Am Coll Cardiol 1990;15:1521.

Spirito P, Maron BJ: Relation between extent of left ventricular hypertrophy and diastolic filling abnormalities in hypertrophic cardiomyopathy. J Am Coll Cardiol 1990;15:808.

Stewart WJ et al: Intraoperative Doppler echocardiography in hypertrophic cardiomyopathy: Correlations with the obstructive gradient. J Am Coll Cardiol 1987;10:327.

Vatner SR et al: Reduced subendocardial coronary reserve: A potential mechanism for impaired diastolic function in the hypertrophied and failing heart. Circulation 1990;81:IV–8.

Wagner JA et al: Calcium-antagonist receptors in atrial tissue of patients with hypertrophic cardiomyopathy. N Engl J Med 1989;320:755.

Watson RM et al: Inducible polymorphic ventricular tachycardia and ventricular fibrillation in a subgroup of patients with hypertrophic cardiomyopathy at high risk for sudden death. J Am Coll Cardiol 1987;10:761.

Wigle ED: Hypertrophic cardiomyopathy 1988. Mod Concepts Cardiovasc Dis 1988;57:1.

Wigle ED: Hypertrophic cardiomyopathy: A 1987 viewpoint. Circulation 1987;75:311.

Wigle ED et al: Hypertrophic cardiomyopathy: The importance of the site and the extent of hypertrophy. A review. Prog Cardiovasc Dis 1985;28:1.

Williams WG et al: Results of surgery for hypertrophic obstructive cardiomyopathy. Circulation 1987;76 (Suppl 5):V–104.

Yamakado T et al: Effects of nifedipine on left ventricular diastolic function in patients with asymptomatic or minimally symptomatic hypertrophic cardiomyopathy. Circulation 1990;81:593.

Restrictive Cardiomyopathy

Acquatella H et al: Value of two-dimensional echocardiography in endomyocardial disease with and without eosinophilia: A clinical and pathologic study. Circulation 1983;67:1219.

Aroney CN et al: Differentiation of restrictive cardiomyopathy from pericardial constriction: Assessment of diastolic function by radionuclide angiography. J Am Coll Cardiol 1989;13:1007.

Gottdiener JS et al: Two-dimensional echocardiographic assessment of the idiopathic hypereosinophilic syndrome. Circulation 1983;67:572.

Graham JM et al: Management of endomyocardial fibrosis: Successful surgical treatment of biventricular involvement and consideration of the superiority of operative intervention. Am Heart J 1981;102:771.

Gupta PN et al: Clinical course of endomyocardial fibrosis. Br Heart J 1989;62:450.

Hatle LK, Appleton CP, Popp RL: Differentiation of constrictive pericarditis and restrictive cardiomyopathy by Doppler echocardiography. Circulation 1989; 79:357.

Hirota Y et al: Spectrum of restrictive cardiomyopathy: Report of the National Survey in Japan. Am Heart J 1990;120:188.

Lorell BH, Grossman W: Profiles in constrictive pericarditis, restrictive cardiomyopathy, and cardiac tamponade. In: Cardiac Catheterization and Angiography, 3rd ed. Grossman W (editor). Lea & Febiger, 1986.

Olson LJ et al: Echocardiographic features of idiopathic hemochromatosis. Am J Cardiol 1987;60:885.

Schoenfeld MH et al: Restrictive cardiomyopathy versus constrictive pericarditis: Role of endomyocardial biopsy in avoiding unnecessary thoracotomy. Circulation 1987;75:1012.

Spry CJF: Restrictive cardiomyopathy. Curr Opin Cardiol 1991;6:397.

Thyrotoxic Heart Disease & Myxedema

Ciaccheri M: Occult thyrotoxicosis in patients with chronic and paroxysmal isolated atrial fibrillation. Clin Cardiol 1984;7:413.

Davis PJ, Davis FB: Hyperthyroidism in patients over the age of 60 years. Medicine 1974;53:161.

Feldman T et al: Myocardial mechanics in hyperthyroidism: Importance of left ventricular loading conditions, heart rate, and contractile state. J Am Coll Cardiol 1986;7:967.

Forfar JC, Miller HC, Toft AD: Occult thyrotoxicosis: A correctable cause of "idiopathic" atrial fibrillation. Am J Cardiol 1979;44:9.

Forfar JC et al: Abnormal left ventricular function in hyperthyroidism. N Engl J Med 1982;307:1165.

Gammage MD, Franklyn JA: Amiodarone and the thyroid. Q J Med 1987;62 83.

Geffner DL, Hershman JM: β-Adrenergic blockade for the treatment of hyperthyroidism. Am J Med 1992; 93:61.

Ingbar SH: The role of antiadrenergic agents in the management of thyrotoxicosis. Cardiovasc Rev Rep 1981;2:683.

Keating FR et al: Treatment of heart disease associated with myxedema. Prog Cardiovasc Dis 1960;3:364.

Kerber RE, Sherman B: Echocardiographic evaluation of pericardial effusion in myxedema: Incidence and biochemical and clinical correlations. Circulation 1975; 52:823.

Lee RT et al: Depressed left ventricular systolic ejection force in hypothyroidism. Am J Cardiol 1990;65:526.

Nixon JV, Anderson RJ, Cohen ML: Alterations in left ventricular mass and performance in patients treated effectively for thyrotoxicosis: A comparative echocardiographic study. Am J Med 1979;67:268.

Olshausen K et al: Cardiac arrhythmias and heart rate in hyperthyroidism. Am J Cardiol 1988;63:930.

Sandler IG, Wilson GM: The nature and prognosis of heart disease in thyrotoxicosis: A review of 150 patients treated with 131I. Q J Med 1959;28:347.

Santos AD et al: Echocardiographic characterization of the reversible cardiomyopathy of hypothyroidism. Am J Med 1980;68:675.

Wilson JS, Podrid PJ: Side effects from amiodarone. Am Heart J 1991;14:158.

Woeber K: Thyrotoxicosis and the heart. N Engl J Med 1992;327:94.

Zimmerman J et al: Clinical spectrum of pericardial effusion as the presenting feature of hypothyroidism. Am Heart J 1983;106:770.

Alcoholic Cardiomyopathy

Alexander CS: Cobalt-beer cardiomyopathy: A clinical and pathologic study of twenty-eight cases. Am J Med 1972;53:395.

Diamond I: Alcoholic myopathy and cardiomyopathy. (Editorial.) N Engl J Med 1989;320:458.

Kupari M et al: Left ventricular filling impairment in asymptomatic chronic alcoholics. Am J Cardiol 1990; 66:1473.

Massie BM et al: Mitral-septal separation: A new echocardiographic index of left ventricular function. Am J Cardiol 177;39:1008.

McCall D: Alcohol and the cardiovascular system. Curr Probl Cardiol 1987;12:351.

Milgaard H et al: Importance of abstention from alcohol in alcoholic heart disease. Int J Cardiol 1990;26:373.

Ramalingaswami V: Nutrition and the heart. Cardiologia 1968;52:57.

Urbano-Marquez A et al: The effects of alcoholism on skeletal and cardiac muscle. N Engl J Med 1989;320: 409.

Beriberi & Nutritional Heart Disease

Alexander JL: The cardiomyopathy of obesity. Prog Cardiovasc Dis 1985;27:325.

Isner JM et al: Anorexia nervosa and sudden death. Ann Intern Med 1985;102:49.

Foster WR, Burton T: Health complications of obesity: NIH Consensus Development Conference. Ann Intern Med 1985;103:979.

Naidoo DP: Beriberi heart disease in Durban. S Afr Med J 1987;72:241.

Kawai C et al: Reappearance of beriberi heart disease in Japan: A study of 23 cases. Am J Med 1980;69:383.

Pringle TH et al: Prolongation of the QT interval during therapeutic starvation: A substrate for malignant arrhythmias. Int J Obes 1983;7:253.

Shocken MD et al: Weight loss and the heart: Effects of anorexia nervosa and starvation. Arch Intern Med 1989;149:878.

Sarcoidosis

Burstow DJ: Two-dimensional echocardiographic findings in systemic sarcoidosis. Am J Cardiol 1989;63: 478.

Kinney EL et al: Thallium-scan myocardial defects and echocardiographic abnormalities in patients with sarcoidosis without clinical cardiac dysfunction. Am J Med 1980;68:497.

Lemery R et al: Cardiac sarcoidosis: A potentially treatable form of myocarditis. Mayo Clin Proc 1985;60: 549.

Riedy K et al: MR imaging of myocardial sarcoidosis. AJR Am J Roentgenol 1988;151:915.

Roberts WC, McAllister HA Jr, Ferrans VJ: Sarcoidosis of the heart: A clinicopathologic study of 35 necropsy patients (group I) and review of 78 previously described necropsy patients (group II). Am J Med 1977;63:86.

Swanton RH: Sarcoidosis of the heart. Eur Heart J 1988;9(Suppl G):169.

Valantine H et al: Sarcoidosis: A pattern of clinical and morphological presentations. Br Heart J 1987;57:256.

Young JB, Kumpuris AG: Sarcoidosis: Cardiac complications. Primary Cardiol 1981;7:111.

Systemic Lupus Erythematosus

Ansari A, Larson PH, Bates HD: Cardiovascular manifestations of systemic lupus erythematosus: Current perspective. Prog Cardiovasc Dis 1985;27:421.

Bidani AK et al: Immunopathology of cardiac lesions in fatal systemic lupus erythematosus. Am J Med 1980; 69:849.

Crozier IF et al: Cardiac involvement in systemic lupus erythematosus detected by echocardiography. Am J Cardiol 1990;65:1145.

Decker JL (moderator): Systemic lupus erythematosus: Evolving concepts. (NIH conference.) Ann Intern Med 1979;91:587.

Enomoto K et al: Frequency of valvular regurgitation by color Doppler echocardiography in systemic lupus erythematosus. Am J Cardiol 1991;67:209.

Galve E et al: Prevalence, morphologic types and evolution of cardiac valvular disease in systemic lupus erythematosus. N Engl J Med 1988;319:817.

Krupp MA: Urinary sediment in visceral angiitis (periarteritis nodosa, lupus erythematosus,Libman-Sachs disease): Quantitative study. Arch Intern Med 1943; 71:54.

Leung WH et al: Doppler echocardiographic evaluation of left ventricular diastolic function in patients with systemic lupus erythematosus. Am Heart J 1990;120: 82.

Nihoyannopoulos P et al: Cardiac abnormalities in systemic lupus erythematosus: Association with raised anticardiolipin antibodies. Circulation 1990;82:369.

Progressive Systemic Sclerosis (Scleroderma)

Clements PJ et al: The relationship of arrhythmias and conduction disturbances to other manifestations of cardiopulmonary disease in progressive systemic sclerosis (PSS). Am J Med 1981;71:38.

James TN: De subitaneis mortibus. 8. Coronary arteries and conduction system in scleroderma heart disease. Circulation 1974;50:844.

Morgan JM et al: Hypoxic pulmonary vasoconstriction in systemic sclerosis and primary pulmonary hypertension. Chest 1991;99:581.

Kahan A et al: The effect of captopril on thallium 201 myocardial perfusion in systemic sclerosis. Clin Pharmacol Ther 1990;47:483.

Kahan A et al: Nifedipine and thallium-201 myocardial perfusion in progressive systemic sclerosis. N Engl J Med 1986;314:1397.

Kostis JB et al: Prognostic importance of cardiac arrhythmias in systemic sclerosis. Am J Med 1988;84: 1007.

Smith JW et al: Echocardiographic features of progressive systemic sclerosis (PSS): Correlation with hemodynamic and postmortem studies. Am J Med 1979; 66:28.

Rheumatoid Arthritis

Kelly CA et al: Chronic pericardial disease in patients with rheumatoid arthritis: A longitudinal study. Q J Med 1990;75;461.

Lie JT: Rheumatoid arthritis and heart disease. Primary Cardiol 1982;8:137.

Morris PB et al: Rheumatoid arthritis and coronary arteritis. Am J Cardiol 1986;57:689.

Rapoport RJ et al: Cutaneous vascular immunofluorescence in rheumatoid arthritis: Correlation with circulating immune complexes and vasculitis. Am J Med 1980;68:325.

Hemochromatosis

Arnett EN et al: Massive myocardial hemosiderosis: Structure-function conference at National Heart and Lung Institute. Am Heart J 1975;90:777.

Baldus WP et al: Deferoxamine-chelatable iron in hemochromatosis and other disorders of iron overload. Mayo Clin Proc 1978;53:157.

Candell-Riera J, Permanyer-Miralda G, Soler-Soler J: Cardiac hemochromatosis. Prim Cardiol 1986;12: 123.

Crosby WH: Current concepts in nutrition: Who needs iron? N Engl J Med 1977;297:543.

Dabestani A et al: Primary hemochromatosis: Anatomic and physiologic characteristics of the cardiac ventricles and their response to phlebotomy. Am J Cardiol 1984;54:153.

Easley RM et al: Reversible cardiomyopathy associated with hemochromatosis. N Engl J Med 1972;287:866.

Finch CA, Huebers H: Perspectives in iron metabolism. N Engl J Med 1982;306:1520.

Freeman AP et al: Sustained normalization of cardiac function by chelation therapy in thalassemia major. Clin Lab Haematol 1989;11:299.

Halliday JW et al: Serum ferritin in diagnosis of haemochromatosis. Lancet 1977;2:621.

Kontoghiorges GT et al: 1,2-Dimethyl-3-hydroxypyrid-4-one, an orally active chelator for treatment of iron overdose. Lancet 1987;1:1294.

Leon MB et al: Detection of early cardiac dysfunction in patients with severe beta-thalassemia and chronic iron overload. N Engl J Med 1979;301:1143.

Niederau C et al: Survival and causes of death in cirrhotic and noncirrhotic patients with primary hemochromatosis. N Engl J Med 1985;313:1256.

Olivieri NF et al: Visual and auditory neurotoxicity in patients receiving subcutaneous deferoxamine infusions. N Engl J Med 1986;314:869.

Olson LJ, Baldus WP, Tajik AJ: Echocardiographic features of idiopathic hemochromatosis. Am J Cardiol 1987;60:885.

Olson LJ et al: Endomyocardial biopsy in hemochromatosis: Clinicopathologic correlates in six cases. J Am Coll Cardiol 1989;13:116.

Pippard MJ et al: Iron absorption in iron-loading anaemias: Effect of subcutaneous desferrioxamine infusions. Lancet 1977;2:737.

Propper R, Nathan D: Clinical removal of iron. Annu Rev Med 1982;33:509.

Rosenqvist M et al: Prevalence of hemochromatosis among men with clinically significant bradyarrhythmias. Eur Heart J 1989;10:473.

Short EM, Winkle RA, Billingham ME: Myocardial involvement in idiopathic hemochromatosis. Am J Med 1981;70:1275.

Weatherall DJ, Pippard MJ, Callender ST: Iron loading in thalassemia: Five years with the pump. (Editorial retrospective.) N Engl J Med 1983;308:456.

Amyloid Disease

Benson MD: Hereditary amyloidosis and cardiomyopathy. Am J Med 1992;93:1.

Duston MA et al: Diagnosis of amyloidosis by abdominal fat aspiration: Analysis of four years' experience. Am J Med 1987;82:412.

Falk Rh et al: Sensitivity and specificity of the echocardiographic features of cardiac amyloidosis. Am J Cardiol 1987;59:418.

Gertz MA et al: Familial amyloidosis: A study of 52 North American-born patients examined during a 30-year period. Mayo Clin Proc 1992;67:428.

Gertz MA, Kyle RA; Primary systemic amyloidosis: A diagnostic primer. Mayo Clin Proc 1989;64:1505.

Hongo M et al: Early identification of amyloid heart disease by technetium-99m-pyrophosphate scintigraphy: A study with familial amyloid polyneuropathy. Am Heart J 1987;113:654.

Hongo M et al: Radionuclide angiographic assessment of left ventricular diastolic filling in amyloid heart disease: A study of patients with familial amyloid polyneuropathy. J Am Coll Cardiol 1989;13:48.

Isobe T, Osserman EF: Patterns of amyloidosis and their association with plasma-cell dyscrasia, monoclonal immunoglobulins and Bence-Jones proteins. N Engl J Med 1974;290:473.

Kline AL et al: Doppler characterization of left ventricular diastolic function in cardiac amyloidosis. J Am Coll Cardiol 1989;13:1017.

Kline AL et al: Prognostic significance of Doppler measures of diastolic function in cardiac amyloidosis: A Doppler echocardiography study. Circulation 1991; 83:808.

Kyle RA, Greipp PR: Amyloidosis (AL): Clinical and laboratory features in 229 cases. Mayo Clin Proc 1983;58:665.

Lie JT: Amyloidosis and amyloid heart disease. Primary Cardiol 1982;8:75.

Neugarten J et al: Amyloidosis in subcutaneous heroin abusers ("skin poppers' amyloidosis"). Am J Med 1986;81:635.

Pinamonti B et al: Qualitative texture analysis in two-dimensional echography: Application to the diagnosis of myocardial amyloidosis. J Am Coll Cardiol 1989; 14:666.

Plehn JF, Friedman BJ: Diastolic dysfunction in amyloid heart disease: Restrictive cardiomyopathy or not? J Am Coll Cardiol 1989;13:54.

Sleisinger MH, Havlir D, Tierney LM Jr: Biochemical and clinical aspects of amyloidosis. West J Med 1987;147:65.

Endomyocardial Fibrosis & Löffler's Endocarditis

Acquatella H, Schuler NB: Echocardiographic recognition of Chagas' disease and endocardial fibrosis. J Am Soc Endocardiogr 1988;1:60.

Cherian G et al: Endomyocardial fibrosis: Report on the hemodynamic data in 29 patients and review of the results of surgery. Am Heart J 1983;105:659.

Fauci et al: The idiopathic hypereosinophilic syndrome. Ann Intern Med 1982;97:78.

Metras DJ et al: Recent trends in surgical treatment of endomyocardial fibrosis. J Cardiovasc Surg 1987;28: 607.

Olsen EGJ, Spry CJF: Relation between eosinophilia and endomyocardial disease. Prog Cardiovasc Dis 1985; 27:241.

Parrillo JE et al: The cardiovascular manifestations of the hypereosinophilic syndrome: Prospective study of 26 patients, with review of the literature. Am J Med 1979;67:572.

Shah AM et al: Eosinophils from hypereosinophilic patients damage endocardium of isolated feline heart muscle preparations. Circulation 1990;81:1081.

Webb-Peploe MM: Obliterative and restrictive cardiomyopathies. Eur Heart J 1985;9(Suppl G):159.

Sickle Cell Disease
& Chronic Anemia

Denenberg BS et al: Cardiac function in sickle cell anemia. Am J Cardiol 1983;51:1674.

Falk RH, Hood WB Jr: The heart in sickle cell anemia. Arch Intern Med 1982;142:1680.

Simmons BE et al: Sickle cell heart disease: Two-dimensional echo and Doppler ultrasonographic findings in the hearts of adult patients with sickle cell anemia. Arch Intern Med 1988;148:1526.

Chagas' Disease

Acquatella H et al: Long-term control of Chagas' disease in Venezuela: Effects on serologic findings, electrocardiographic abnormalities, and clinical outcome. Circulation 1987;76:556.

Acquatella H et al: M-mode and two-dimensional echocardiography in chronic Chagas' heart disease: A clinical and pathologic study. Circulation 1980;62:787.

Andrade ZA et al: Histopathology of the conducting tissue of the heart in Chagas' myocarditis. Am Heart J 1978;95:316.

Carrasco Guerra HA et al: Clinical, histochemical, and ultrastructural correlation in septal endomyocardial biopsies from chronic chagasic patients: Detection of early myocardial damage. Am Heart J 1987;113:716.

Carrasco Guerra HA et al: Ventricular arrhythmias and left ventricular myocardial function in chronic chagasic patients. Int J Cardiol 1990;28:35.

dePaola AAV et al: Angiographic and electrophysiologic substrates of ventricular tachycardia in chronic chagasic myocarditis. Am J Cardiol 1990;65:360.

Morris SA et al: Pathophysiologic insights into the cardiomyopathy of Chagas' disease. Circulation 1990;82:1900.

Oliveira JSM et al: Cardiac thrombosis and thromboembolism in chronic Chagas' heart disease. Am J Cardiol 1983;52:147.

Prata A: Chagas' heart disease. Cardiologia 1968;52:79.

Peripartum Cardiomyopathy

Carvalho A et al: Prognosis in peripartum cardiomyopathy. Am J Cardiol 1989;64:540.

Cole P et al: Longitudinal changes in left ventricular architecture and function in peripartum cardiomyopathy. Am J Cardiol 1987;60:871.

Gilchrist AR: Cardiological problems in younger women, including those of pregnancy and the puerperium. Br Heart J 1963;1:209.

Homans DC: Peripartum cardiomyopathy. N Engl J Med 1985;312:1432.

Julian DG, Szekely P: Peripartum cardiomyopathy. Prog Cardiovasc Dis 1985;27:223.

Lee W, Cotton DB: Peripartum cardiomyopathy: Current concepts and clinical management. Clin Obstet Gynecol 1989;32:57.

Medei MG et al: Peripartum myocarditis and cardiomyopathy. Circulation 1990;81:922.

Melvin KR et al: Peripartum cardiomyopathy due to myocarditis. N Engl J Med 1982;307:731.

O'Connell JB et al: Peripartum cardiomyopathy: Clinical, hemodynamic, histologic and prognostic characteristics. J Am Coll Cardiol 1986;8:52.

Sullivan JM et al: Management of medical problems with pregnancy: Severe cardiac disease. N Engl J Med 1985;313:304.

Walsh JJ et al: Idiopathic myocardiopathy of the puerperium (postpartal heart disease). Circulation 1965;32:19.

Neuropathic Disorders
& Inherited Disorders of Metabolism

Blieden LC, Moller JH: Cardiac involvement in inherited disorders of metabolism. Prog Cardiovasc Dis 1974;16:615.

Forseberg H et al: Cardiac involvement in congenital myotonic dystrophy. Br Heart J 1990;63:119.

Gottdiener JS et al: Characteristics of the cardiac hypertrophy in Friedreich's ataxia. Am Heart J 1982;103:525.

Roberts WC, Honig HS: The spectrum of cardiovascular disease in the Marfan syndrome: A clinicomorphologic study of 18 necropsy patients and comparison to 151 previously reported necropsy patients. Am Heart J 1982;104:115.

Pericarditis

Pericardial disease usually involves the epicardium, often spreading to or from the myocardium. It almost always produces inflammatory changes, which include irritative and mechanical effects in addition to those caused by bacterial, viral, and fungal infections. Pericardial disease exhibits a wide spectrum of clinical manifestations and varies in importance from an inconsequential associated finding to a major cardiovascular problem, as in acute myopericarditis.

Causes of Pericardial Disease

The pericardium may be involved in acute bacterial or viral infections such as pneumonia, when infection spreads from the lungs or mediastinum, and in chronic infections such as tuberculosis. Other generalized conditions such as uremia, systemic lupus erythematosus, scleroderma, serum sickness, radiation therapy, rheumatoid arthritis, or different varieties of lymphoma or other malignant disorders, usually lung or breast cancer, may involve the pericardium. Although the involvement of the pericardium in these disorders is usually incidental, all of these conditions may occasionally cause significant hemodynamic changes (about 10% of cases). Pericarditis as manifested by a pericardial friction rub occurs in 15–20% of patients after acute myocardial infarction (Tofler, 1989). Uremia has become an important factor in pericardial disease now that renal dialysis is widely used in the palliative treatment of chronic renal disease. The commonest primary pericardial infections are those due to viruses (eg, coxsackie B virus), but these infections usually also affect the myocardium. The relative frequency of other causes depends upon the type of clinical practice of the physician. Oncologists see malignant pericarditis; nephrologists see uremic pericarditis; rheumatologists see lupus or rheumatoid pericarditis. The relative incidence of pericardial disease from each cause is unknown. When myocarditis predominates, the clinical picture is as described in Chapter 17.

Aseptic inflammatory changes are seen following acute myocardial infarction. They are especially noticeable in anteroseptal infarcts in which the necrosis of cardiac tissue involves the surface of the heart and causes changes that are indistinguishable from those due to inflammation. Another form of aseptic inflammation, postpericardiotomy syndrome, occurs both after myocardial infarction (3–6 weeks) and following cardiac surgery, with low-grade, probably autoimmune, self-limiting inflammation involving the pericardium and pleura. It was first seen after mitral commissurotomy and was originally thought to represent a recurrence of rheumatic fever. However, it is also seen after operations for congenital lesions and is believed to be an autoimmune response to pericardial and epicardial injury.

Blunt or penetrating trauma such as that associated with stab wounds or rib fracture may damage the pericardium and lead to hemopericardium. Hemopericardium also occurs when vascular structures such as the heart or the aorta rupture into the pericardium.

Malignant disease also affects the pericardium, usually causing effusion. Neoplastic involvement of the pericardium may occur either by direct spread from the breast or lung or, more rarely, by blood-borne means, and the effusion is often large and recurrent. Tumor usually spreads directly by way of the mediastinum, but secondary deposits and even primary tumors of the pericardium (mesoendothelioma and sarcoma) can occur. The accumulation of fluid in the pericardial cavity seen in heart failure is due to transudation. In myxedema, enlargement of the cardiac silhouette is usually due to pericardial fluid but may be due to myocardial enlargement. In tuberculous cases, the infection is more chronic and effusion is relatively common. In some cases, other serous cavities (pleura or peritoneum) are also affected. The disease runs a chronic course, and pain, fever, and myocardial involvement are less prominent than in viral cases.

Pericarditis presents a spectrum of cases ranging from fibrinous (dry) pericarditis through pericardial effusion, with or without evidence of cardiac tamponade, to seroconstrictive and classic chronic pericardial constriction. These different manifestations are interrelated, as shown in Figure 18–1. Spread of the disease to involve the myocardium is not infrequent.

FIBRINOUS (DRY) PERICARDITIS

Clinical Findings

A. Symptoms: Fibrinous pericarditis most commonly occurs in the course of some other disease; thus, the symptoms depend on the cause, and pain is not necessarily a feature. In primary pericarditis

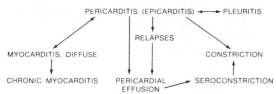

Figure 18–1. Spectrum of pericardial disease. (Reproduced, with permission, from Goldman MJ: Pericarditis. West J Med 1975;123:467.)

caused by viral infection, the usual presenting symptoms are pain, malaise, fever, and myalgia. The pain is often worse with breathing, swallowing, or belching, and it may radiate to the shoulder. It is often substernal and associated with cough. The patient may obtain relief by sitting up and leaning forward or by kneeling on all fours. Pain characteristically decreases or disappears when effusion develops.

The pericarditis that occurs in about 15% of cases of acute myocardial infarction is not generally painful. It is noted about the third day after infarction, is usually transient, and is of little hemodynamic significance except when anticoagulants cause hemorrhage into the pericardial cavity. Postpericardiotomy syndrome, which occurs about 3–6 weeks after cardiac surgery or myocardial infarction, also believed to be an autoimmune phenomenon, causes pericardial or pleural pain and may be associated with fever. It may be confused with hemorrhagic pericardial effusion due to anticoagulant therapy or postoperative infection.

B. Signs: The most important and often the only sign of fibrinous pericarditis is the development of a pericardial friction rub. A friction rub is also the only sign of pericardial involvement in most cases of pericarditis secondary to a generalized disease; this rub is often transient and variable. Pericardial friction produces a rough, scratchy one-, two-, or three-component superficial sound that is unrelated to other heart sounds. The components are associated with atrial systole, ventricular systole, and ventricular diastole. Friction rubs can be confused with extraneous stethoscope sounds, with noise caused by hair on the chest, and with murmurs, especially to-and-fro murmurs. Both the bell and the diaphragm of the stethoscope are used to listen for friction rubs, and the patient should not breathe during auscultation.

C. Electrocardiographic Findings: Like the friction rub, electrocardiographic signs of pericarditis may be the only evidence indicative of pericardial involvement. Initially, electrocardiographic changes consist of ST–T segment elevation in leads I, II, aVL, aVF, and V_2–V_6 (Figure 18–2), with preservation of the upward concavity, in contrast to the acute injury of acute myocardial infarction, in which the ST segment has upward convexity. Return of the ST segment (Figure 18–3) to the baseline in a few days is

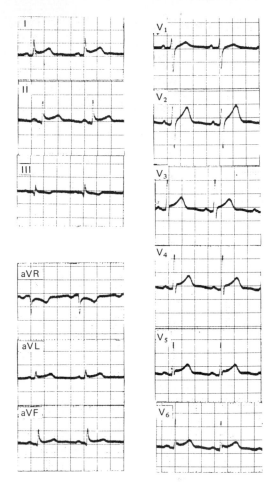

Figure 18–2. Acute pericarditis. ST segment elevation with concave upward curvature is seen in leads I, II, aVL, aVF, and V_{2-6}. Reciprocal ST segment depression is seen in cavity lead aVR. (Reproduced, with permission, from Goldschlager N, Goldman MJ: *Principles of Clinical Electrocardiography,* 13th ed. Appleton & Lange, 1989.)

followed by symmetric T wave inversion. Reciprocal changes are absent except in aVR, and Q waves do not occur. P wave abnormalities are common. It may be difficult to differentiate pericarditis from non-Q wave infarction at the stage of T wave inversion because epicarditis is present; the presence of other diagnostic features, especially elevated serum enzymes (myocardial band creatine phosphokinase), is required to make a diagnosis of myocardial infarction.

D. Imaging Studies: The heart is not necessarily enlarged on x-ray. Any radiologic changes should be attributed to the underlying disease.

Fibrinous (dry) pericarditis has no hemodynamic effects per se. If and when effusion of more than about 15 mL develops, or when the inflammatory process heals, causing thickening of the pericardium, echocardiographic changes develop.

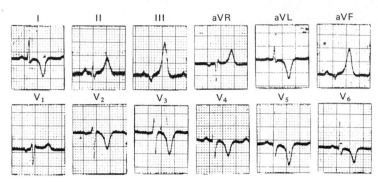

Figure 18–3. Pericarditis (late pattern). Deep, symmetrically inverted T waves in I, aVL, and V_{2-6}. The marked T wave abnormalities, unusual in pericarditis, may indicate concomitant myocarditis. (Reproduced, with permission, from Goldschlager N, Goldman MJ: *Principles of Clinical Electrocardiography*, 13th ed. Appleton & Lange, 1989.)

E. Laboratory Findings: Leukocytosis of 10,000–20,000U/UµL is usually seen in viral pericarditis. A raised sedimentation rate is also found regardless of cause. Serologic abnormality due to generalized disease may be present (eg, positive LE cell preparation, presence of antinuclear antibody, or elevated serum creatinine).

Differential Diagnosis

Acute viral pericarditis must be distinguished from acute myocardial infarction. In pericarditis, pain, fever, and electrocardiographic changes are present from the onset of illness. In myocardial infarction, pain comes first and is followed more than 24 hours later by fever and friction rub. Q waves are not seen in pericarditis. It is almost always possible to make the diagnosis by following the serial changes on the ECG, unless the patient is first seen after the third or fourth day and has non Q wave infarction. Serial examination of ECGs as well as specific myocardial enzyme studies (myocardial band creatine kinase) should be used to decide whether the electrocardiographic changes seen in a patient who is suffering from some generalized disease are due to infarction. The diagnosis of associated myocarditis may prove difficult, and the distinction between pleural and pericardial inflammation is likewise difficult: The friction rub is related to inspiration in pleural inflammation but is heard during held respiration in pericardial inflammation, but in many cases the friction rub is pleuropericardial and shares the features of both entities.

Viral pericarditis is sometimes difficult to distinguish from tuberculous pericarditis. Viral cases tend to be more acute and are less likely to lead to effusion. Because tubercle bacilli are difficult to find, the fluid should be cultured. Diagnostic pericardiocentesis is indicated, although the yield is low; and pericardial biopsy may be needed. A positive tuberculin skin test, especially in a person under age 50, is excellent evidence favoring tuberculosis as a cause of pericarditis (Sagrista-Sauleda, 1988).

Complications

Myocardial involvement is almost inevitably present on microscopic examination. Clinical evidence of myocarditis is most frequently seen in viral pericarditis. Relapses and recurrences are also common, perhaps owing to autoimmune mechanisms. Progression of the disease, leading to effusion, seroconstriction, and classic chronic pericardial constriction, can occur in pericarditis due to any cause.

Treatment

The underlying disease should be treated and symptomatic therapy given for the pericarditis. In acute viral pericarditis, salicylates, nonsteroidal anti-inflammatory agents, and expectant treatment with bed rest during the acute febrile phase are usually all that is needed, but corticosteroids may be helpful in severe cases. Corticosteroids should usually be given for not more than a week and then gradually tapered, because of the risk of side effects. Corticosteroids are not indicated in tuberculous cases unless given with antituberculosis drugs. In postpericardiotomy syndrome, symptomatic treatment is also all that is necessary in most cases. If the pericarditis fails to clear in a week to 10 days, or if the infection is severe, corticosteroids are often utilized. Although there is no conclusive evidence that they are effective, a trial of treatment may be worthwhile. The development of pericarditis in a patient with uremia is an indication to start or increase the frequency of dialysis. If fever persists and purulent pericarditis is suspected, pericardiocentesis should be performed, and antibiotic therapy should be instituted, tailored to the organism. Thorough bacteriologic study is required to exclude acid-fast bacteria, fungi, and anaerobic organisms (see Pericardial Effusion, below). Detailed treatment for specific organisms is beyond the scope of this book; consult a text on infectious diseases.

Prognosis

The prognosis in most cases of acute viral pericarditis is excellent, provided that myocardial involvement is minimal. Tuberculous cases respond to specific treatment, which must sometimes be administered without proof of the cause. The relative incidence of viral and tuberculous lesions varies in different areas, and viral lesions are now more common than tuberculous ones in the USA. In rare cases, the disease persists or recurs, and signs of pericardial constriction can develop in a period of weeks to months. In most cases of fibrinous pericarditis, the prognosis depends more on the underlying disease, and pericardial involvement is only a minor part of the clinical picture. Relapses are common and may constitute a major problem. Rarely with multiple recurrences of pericarditis, immunosuppressive therapy has been necessary, using azathioprine. Recently, colchicine (1 mg/d) has been effective in recurrences in patients who had suffered at least three relapses while receiving other therapy (Guindo, 1990). Occasionally, surgical pericardiectomy is necessary to prevent recurrences.

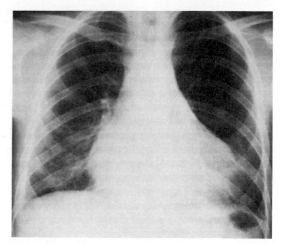

Figure 18–4. Chest x-ray of a patient with pericardial effusion.

PERICARDIAL EFFUSION WITHOUT TAMPONADE

If pericardial fluid accumulates slowly, the pericardium stretches, and there is little rise in pressure and little or no interference with cardiac filling.

Clinical Findings

A. Symptoms: Pericardial effusion per se causes no specific symptoms. The pain of pericarditis may disappear when effusion develops. On the other hand, pain may develop with hemopericardium as blood irritates the pericardium.

B. Signs: The physical signs of pericardial effusion depend on the amount of effusion. In the absence of evidence of tamponade, the pulse, pulse pressure, and blood pressure are normal, but the patient may appear anxious, and there is usually some tachycardia.

The cardiac impulse is usually difficult to detect but may be palpable. Heart sounds are often distant, and a friction rub may still be audible even though the pain has disappeared and significant effusion has occurred. Murmurs are usually absent.

C. Electrocardiographic Findings: The T waves are usually low, biphasic, inverted, or flat, and the overall voltage is low in the limb leads in pericardial effusion associated with myxedema. There are no specific electrocardiographic changes, but electrical alternans is sometimes seen in pericardial effusion when the position of the heart changes excessively during the cardiac cycle.

D. Imaging Studies: The cardiac x-ray silhouette is enlarged in pericardial effusion and may reach enormous proportions in chronic lesions without affecting cardiac function. The principal problem is to decide whether the heart itself is enlarged. The shape of the cardiac silhouette in pericardial effusion is triangular on posteroanterior view (Figure 18–4). An acute right cardiophrenic angle, clear lung fields, and associated pleural effusion are common. Left-sided pleural effusion is common in pericardial disease, whereas in heart failure effusion is usually bilateral. Serial examinations may be useful to determine changes in heart size. The lack of signs of specific chamber enlargement may be helpful. It is important not to confuse the massive cardiac enlargement seen in giant left atrium with pericardial effusion. Since the left atrium forms the right border of the heart in giant left atrium, right heart catheterization and right atrial angiography can produce misleading results and lead to an unnecessary and dangerous attempt at pericardiocentesis, with inadvertent puncture of the heart.

1. Noninvasive techniques– Two-dimensional echocardiography demonstrates the echo-free space surrounding the heart in pericardial effusion. Very small effusions can be demonstrated by this technique. Abnormal swinging of the heart within this echo-free space can be seen. Fibrin strands can be seen in the echo-free space and, in the case of tumor, epicardial masses. With fibrin deposition and fibrosis, thickening of the epicardium-pericardium can be seen (Figure 18–5).

CT and MRI can also show pericardial effusion and a thickened pericardial wall.

2. Invasive techniques–

a. Catheterization and angiography– Right heart catheterization and right atrial angiography with contrast or intravenous injection of CO_2 gas to demonstrate the density of the fluid beyond the right atrial wall were used in the past to help in the diagnosis of pericardial effusion, but they are seldom necessary now that echocardiography has become available. The finding of a significant gap ($\geq$ 1 cm) between the catheter tip or the border of the contrast material in

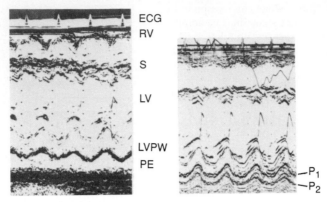

Figure 18–5. Serial echocardiograms 3 weeks apart in a patient with pericardial effusion, showing development of pericardial thickening and fibrosis when the effusion is absorbed. (RV, right ventricle; S, septum; LV, left ventricle; LVPW, left ventricular posterior wall; PE, pericardial effusion; P_1 and P_2, visceral and parietal pericardial layer.) (Courtesy of NB Schiller.)

the atrium and the edge of the cardiac silhouette suggests the presence of fluid.

b. Pericardiocentesis– Although echocardiography is extremely valuable in indicating the presence and site of pericardial effusion, the ultimate diagnostic procedure is pericardiocentesis. The procedure is described in Chapter 7. The data provided by echocardiography help the physician decide whether to tap the pericardium, and pericardiocentesis is not indicated if echocardiography is negative or shows only a small effusion.

E. Laboratory Findings: Specific diagnostic tests such as LE cell preparations or antinuclear antibody tests, thyroid function tests, and renal function tests are indicated in some cases. Tuberculin testing and bacteriologic examination are required if an infective cause is suspected.

Differential Diagnosis

Enlargement of the heart due to dilation or hypertrophy is virtually the only condition that must be distinguished from pericardial effusion, although primary tumor (angiosarcoma, thymoma, or thymosarcoma) may rarely enter into the differential diagnosis. In some cases there may be effusion in addition to cardiac enlargement. In these cases, the introduction of air or CO_2 into the pericardium at the time of pericardiocentesis serves to indicate heart size and the thickness of the pericardium. Echocardiographic examination provides definitive differentiation between pericardial effusion and cardiac enlargement.

Complications

Cardiac tamponade is the most important complication of pericardial effusion. It can occur with surprising speed, because the compliance of the pericardial cavity can be markedly nonlinear, and the accumulation of a small additional amount of fluid can cause a marked rise in intrapericardial pressure.

This is especially important in trauma, where 200–300 mL of blood can cause tamponade without obvious enlargement of the cardiac silhouette.

Treatment

The treatment of pericardial effusion depends on the cause and on the severity of the hemodynamic effects. If effusion is not great and there are no symptoms, supportive treatment is all that is needed, but if effusion is considerable or recurrent or if signs and symptoms of tamponade are developing, a pericardial tap should be performed. Purulent pericardial effusion should be drained and smear and culture of the fluid obtained for examination; thoracotomy is often necessary to achieve adequate drainage. Open drainage of the pericardium also allows biopsy, which can be most helpful in establishing the cause of the pericarditis. This can be done through a subxiphoid approach as a local procedure (Wall, 1992). Serous effusion that occurs in such diseases as tuberculosis, uremia, or cancer may need to be tapped repeatedly. In this circumstance, a short pigtail catheter can be introduced percutaneously into the pericardium and constant drainage obtained over a period of several days. With heparinized saline flushes, the catheter can be kept patent during this time. This is especially true if malignant disease is the cause of the effusion. Chemotherapeutic agents may be instilled into the pericardial cavity after tapping to prevent recurrence of effusion. Tetracycline and nonabsorbable steroid compounds have also been used for this purpose.* Dialysis may help to control effusions in patients with renal disease, but many kinds of effusion require no

---

*Tetracycline for this purpose is no longer available from its only manufacturer (Lederle Laboratories), though stocks on hand are still being used. Possible substitutes such as doxycycline are being investigated.

treatment other than measures treating the underlying cause.

In tuberculous pericarditis, even with appropriate antituberculous therapy, constrictive pericarditis can still develop. In a study of 240 patients, surgical pericardial drainage and pericardiocentesis were compared, and patients were randomly assigned to prednisolone or a placebo. Compared with pericardiocentesis, open drainage neither decreased the mortality rate nor affected progression to constriction. Prednisolone reduced the mortality rate in the first 2 years as well as the need for repeated pericardiocenteses but did not significantly reduce the incidence of constriction—although there was a trend in favor of prednisolone (Strang, 1988).

Prognosis

The prognosis in pericardial effusion per se depends on the cause of the disease. Pericardial effusion is seldom a dangerous condition in the absence of tamponade, and repeated pericardiocentesis is seldom necessary for more than a few weeks except in malignant or other major systemic disease.

CARDIAC TAMPONADE

The time necessary for fluid to accumulate in the pericardial cavity can vary from seconds (in rupture of a major structure) to weeks or months in chronic infections. It is the rate of rise of intrapericardial pressure that is the most important factor in determining the development of the hemodynamic and clinical features of cardiac tamponade. When the fluid accumulates rapidly, or if effusion occurs into a pericardium thickened and noncompliant because of fibrosis, serious interference with cardiac filling can occur with remarkable speed. The compliance of the pericardial cavity is markedly nonlinear, so that although significant amounts of fluid can sometimes accumulate without much rise in pressure, a further slight increase in fluid may produce a considerable rise in pressure as well as symptoms and signs of cardiac tamponade.

Cardiac tamponade develops when the pressure in the pericardial cavity rises to a level equal to that in the heart during diastole. Because the right atrium and ventricle have the lowest diastolic pressures, they are the first structures to be compressed by the increasing pericardial pressure, and the compression is mainly diastolic. The venous pressure and the intracardiac and intrapericardial pressures rise together as pericardial tamponade progresses, and soon the diastolic pressures in both the left and right sides of the heart are raised. At this stage, respiration has a marked hemodynamic effect, and pulsus paradoxus develops. The increased negative intrathoracic pressure produced by inspiration stretches the right heart and opens up the compressed right ventricle, increasing its output and filling the lungs with blood. At the same time, the pulmonary veins are dilated, dropping pressure in the pulmonary venous bed and reducing the return of blood to the left heart. In severe cases, the interventricular septum may bulge to the left on inspiration. All these events interfere with left ventricular filling and cause an inspiratory fall in arterial pressure and left ventricular output. Conversely, on expiration, the right ventricular volume decreases and the blood stored in the lungs returns to the left heart, increasing its output. The reciprocal effects of inspiration and expiration on the right and left heart are not seen when there is an atrial septal defect, nor do they occur unless the diastolic pressures in both sides of the heart are equal. Thus, pulsus paradoxus is not seen when the left ventricle is hypertrophied and stiff, as occurs in some cases of chronic renal disease and hypertension; in these instances, left atrial pressure is higher than right atrial pressure, and the right ventricle is compressed before the left heart is.

Clinical Findings

A. Symptoms: Acute cardiac tamponade may cause symptoms ranging from anxiety, sweating, dyspnea, dizziness, and syncope to frank shock. The clinical picture ranges from slight circulatory and hemodynamic abnormalities to circulatory collapse.

B. Signs: Venous pressure is raised in cardiac tamponade except when severe dehydration or blood loss has caused a reduction in circulating blood volume. The venous pressure does not usually show an increase with inspiration (Kussmaul's sign). The rise in pericardial pressure interferes with cardiac filling throughout the whole of the cardiac cycle, and the rapid y descent seen in the jugular venous pulse in pericardial constriction is absent. With systole, there is descent of the base of the atria and a brief drop in venous pressure is seen, forming the x descent. The cardiac impulse is classically not palpable, the heart sounds are distant, and murmurs are absent. Since filling is impaired throughout diastole, the rapid filling phase of early diastole seen in pericardial constriction is not prominent, and a pericardial third sound ("knock") is seldom heard.

The pulse rate is rapid, and the blood pressure and pulse pressure are low. Pulsus paradoxus, defined as a fall of more than 10 mm Hg or 10% in systolic arterial blood pressure on normal inspiration, can be detected when the blood pressure is measured either indirectly or directly (Figure 18–6). The term pulsus paradoxus is a misnomer, because the condition is basically an exaggeration of the normal finding of a decrease in arterial pressure with inspiration and therefore is not actually "paradoxic" (see Chapter 3).

C. Electrocardiographic Findings: There are no specific electrocardiographic changes of cardiac tamponade, but the ECG is seldom normal. Low voltage and flat or inverted T waves are commonly seen. Electrical alternans can be seen, caused by the swing-

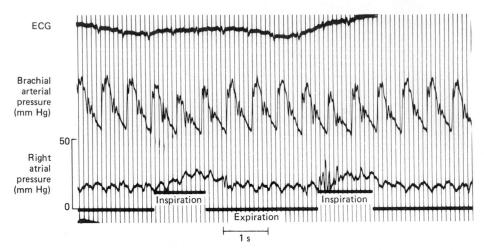

Figure 18-6. Brachial arterial and right atrial pressures showing pulsus paradoxus in a patient with constrictive pericarditis and an increase in right atrial pressure on inspiration (Kussmaul's sign). Both the systolic and diastolic atrial pressures rise with inspiration.

ing of the heart with each beat, and when it involves QRS and T waves it is nearly pathognomonic.

D. Imaging Studies: The heart may be small in patients with acute tamponade, but since all combinations of effusion and constriction can occur, heart size is not of diagnostic value. The lung fields are usually clear, and the pulmonary vessels are not prominent.

1. Noninvasive techniques– The development of cardiac tamponade can be detected on the basis of diastolic collapse of the right atrium and right ventri-

cle and narrowing of the outflow tract of the right ventricle seen on echocardiography. As the intrapericardial pressure becomes equal to the right atrial pressure, diastolic collapse of the right atrium and right ventricle can be seen. Later, left atrial collapse at end-diastole occurs. There is also marked dilation of the inferior vena cava, which fails to collapse with inspiration. On Doppler flow studies, marked reciprocal changes in tricuspid and mitral inflow velocities occur during the respiratory cycle, as well as

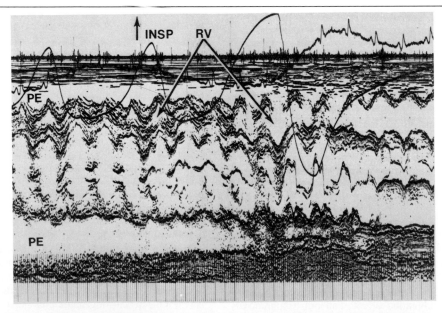

Figure 18-7. Echocardiogram showing cardiac tamponade in a patient with substantial pericardial effusion (PE). The right ventricular cavity (RV) is compressed and almost obliterated; it is seen to enlarge during inspiration. Inspiration (INSP) is upward. (Courtesy of NB Schiller.)

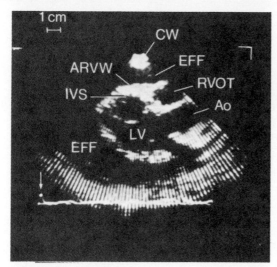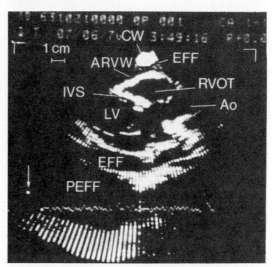

Figure 18–8. Two-dimensional echocardiograms before *(left)* and after *(right)* pericardiocentesis. These images, obtained in the long-axis view, encompass all portions of the heart seen in the standard M mode echocardiographic sweep. Before drainage, the right ventricular cavity is barely discernible below the aortoseptal junction, narrowing abruptly at this level. Following pericardiocentesis, the right ventricle expands and is well visualized to the midseptal level. Note diminished effusion size after drainage. Both studies were performed at end-expiration and at end-diastole (R + 0.00). The bright spot (arrow) represents the timing of camera gating at end-diastole. The calibration factor is the same for the two studies. However, the posterior gain setting is reduced in the initial study, obscuring the pleural effusion (PEFF) seen later. (LV, left ventricular cavity; CW, chest wall; ARVW, anterior right ventricular wall; EFF, effusion; IVS, interventricular septum; RVOT, right ventricular outflow tract; Ao, aorta.) (Reproduced, with permission of the American Heart Association, Inc., from Schiller NB, Botvinick EH: Right ventricular compression as a sign of cardiac tamponade: Analysis of echocardiographic ventricular dimensions and their clinical implications. Circulation 1977;56: 774.)

marked reciprocal variations in ventricular chamber size (Reeder, 1989).

In the example shown in Figure 18–7, the right ventricular cavity is almost obliterated during expiration and only opens up on inspiration. Two-dimensional echocardiograms demonstrate this important sign of cardiac tamponade. Figure 18–8 shows a sector scan in the long-axis view before and after pericardiocentesis. The change in size of the right ventricular outflow tract (RVOT) is clearly visible.

2. Invasive techniques– Management of cardiac tamponade is facilitated by monitoring systemic arterial, central venous, and pericardial pressures during pericardiocentesis. The procedure can be conveniently carried out in the cardiac catheterization laboratory. When intracardiac pressures are measured in tamponade, the diastolic pressures in the two ventricles and the pericardial cavity are equal. As fluid is withdrawn from the pericardium and tamponade is relieved (see Figure 18–9), these pressures at first fall together as cardiac output and arterial pressure increase and heart rate and pulsus paradoxus decrease. Ultimately, pericardial pressure falls below ventricular diastolic pressure, and at that point tamponade is relieved. Further withdrawal of fluid then leads to little or no hemodynamic improvement.

Differential Diagnosis

Cardiac tamponade must be distinguished from other acute cardiac emergencies such as hemorrhage, myocardial infarction, and pulmonary embolism. Signs of a falling arterial pressure and cardiac output and a rising venous pressure and heart rate should alert the physician to the possibility of cardiac tamponade, and pulsus paradoxus strongly suggests the diagnosis. Echocardiography is the most helpful diagnostic investigation.

Complications

The complications of cardiac tamponade include those of circulatory collapse, with inadequate perfusion of any organ system, but most commonly the brain and the kidneys. Early recognition and prompt treatment are essential, especially in acute cases.

Treatment

Acute cardiac tamponade is always an emergency, and the physician must always remain on the alert to prevent its recurrence. Whenever jugular venous pressure is elevated in the course of pericarditis, tamponade is beginning and the patient must be closely monitored. Pericardiocentesis is indicated as soon as the diagnosis is made. The procedure is described in Chapter 7 (p 137). The response to the removal of the

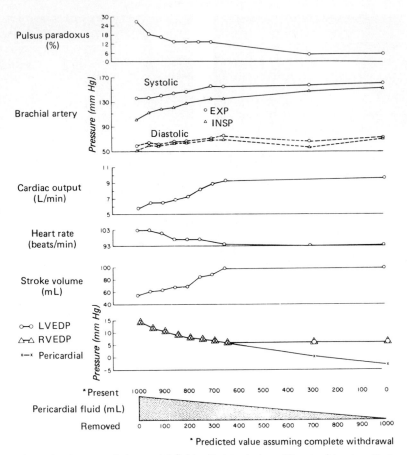

Figure 18–9. Hemodynamic changes during serial fluid withdrawals in a 22-year-old man with tamponade resulting from uremic pericarditis. Diagnostic levels of pulsus paradoxus persist as long as left ventricular end-diastolic pressure (LVEDP) remains equilibrated with pericardial pressure. (RVEDP, right ventricular end-diastolic pressure; EXP, expiration; INSP, inspiration.) (Reproduced, with permission of the American Heart Association, Inc., from Reddy PS et al: Cardiac tamponade: Hemodynamic observations in man. Circulation 1978;58:265.)

first 25–50 milliliters of fluid is usually dramatic, but residual abnormalities in venous and pericardial pressures may be seen if both effusion and fibrosis were initially responsible for the tamponade.

Resection of a portion or all of the pericardium to allow free communication with the pleura may be needed if repeated pericardiocentesis fails to prevent recurrence. It is possible that the mechanism by which a surgical "pericardial window" eliminates recurrent pericardial effusion is obliteration of the pericardial space (Sugimoto, 1990). Instillation of chemotherapeutic agents into the pericardial cavity can also be used to prevent recurrence.

Prognosis

Acute cardiac tamponade is a life-threatening complication of pericardial disease, but the immediate prognosis is good with efficient treatment, provided that rupture of a major structure into the pericardium has not occurred. The long-term prognosis depends on the underlying cause of the pericardial disease.

PERICARDIAL CONSTRICTION

The term pericardial constriction is used to describe both the classic chronic disease (constrictive pericarditis) that mimics right heart failure, and the subacute condition, in which a rigid pericardium and pericardial fluid combine to compress the heart and interfere with its late diastolic filling (subacute effusive constrictive pericarditis). With the improved diagnostic techniques now available, more subacute cases are being recognized. Although tuberculosis is the classic cause of constrictive pericarditis, at present the cause of most cases is unknown. Fungal, traumatic, and probably even viral pericarditis can all result in constrictive pericarditis. A relatively new form of constrictive pericarditis is seen after open heart surgery, especially coronary bypass surgery, probably related to either intrapericardial bleeding or to pericardium-mediated bleeding, and occurs within weeks or months after surgery (Killian, 1989). Inflammatory (viral, associated with idiopathic mediastinal fibrosis, or sarcoidosis), uremic, neoplastic, and traumatic (including postcardiotomy and irradiation) pericardial diseases are more likely to cause the subacute form than classic chronic constrictive pericarditis, in which no evidence of effusion is ordinarily detectable.

The chronic inflammatory changes in the pericardial cavity surround the heart with a sheath of tough, unyielding fibrous tissue that interferes with cardiac filling. The actual, or effective, intrapericardial pressure rises, and the pressure in all heart chambers at the end of diastole rises. The heart is immobilized because it is encased in an unyielding fibrous cage that interferes with its excursion during contraction and relaxation. The more compliant chambers, the atria and the right ventricle, bear the brunt of the burden, but end-diastolic pressures in all cardiac chambers tend to be the same: about 15–25 mm Hg in severe cases. The encasement does not necessarily involve all chambers, but the effective intrapericardial pressure rises on both sides of the heart. Although the effects of the disease are more severe in the more distensible right heart, the left side is almost invariably involved also. Since decrease in stroke volume and cardiac output occurs before the pulmonary venous and capillary pressure reaches 25 mm Hg, pulmonary edema rarely occurs with isolated constrictive pericarditis.

Clinical Findings

A. Symptoms: Swelling of the abdomen and legs is the symptom suggesting a diagnosis of constrictive pericarditis. Dyspnea is not generally prominent but is usually present in all cases to some degree. Anorexia, weakness, wasting, and dyspepsia are seen in advanced cases that have not been properly diagnosed. These symptoms are due to a combination of low cardiac output and marked hepatic congestion. A history of a previous attack of acute or subacute pericarditis is an important feature. The absence of a history of other forms of heart disease is also valuable. Pain is not a prominent feature of the disease. The patient is usually able to lie flat without any problem and does not suffer from paroxysmal nocturnal dyspnea.

B. Signs: The patient appears chronically ill in advanced cases.

1. Pulse and heartbeat– The pulse is usually rapid and the blood pressure low. Pulsus paradoxus is present in classic cases of the disease, but in only about one-third of cases. The heartbeat is irregular in about 30% of cases because of atrial fibrillation. The onset of arrhythmia is related to the age of the patient and the severity of the disease.

2. Venous pulse and pressure– Venous pressure and the nature of the venous pulse are important in pericardial constriction. The neck veins are distended, the venous pressure is markedly raised, and there is a rapid x and y descent. The neck veins usu-

ally show a major negative wave at the time of the y descent. This constitutes diastolic collapse of the veins and is caused by rapid filling of the right heart in early diastole at a time when intracardiac pressure is at its lowest after the end of systole. The sign is not specific for pericardial disease and can be seen in any form of severe right heart failure. There is no consistent difference in venous pulse between tamponade and constriction, though classically the presence of a rapid x and prominent y descent characterizes constriction and the absence of a rapid y descent signifies tamponade (Figures 18–10 and 18–11). Another nonspecific physical sign associated with pericardial disease is Kussmaul's sign, an inspiratory increase in venous pressure (Figure 18–6). When right heart filling is excessive, the increase in venous pressure occurring on inspiration cannot be accommodated in the restricted right atrium, and atrial pressure consequently rises.

4. Palpation and heart sounds– In pericardial constriction, cardiac filling stops abruptly when the heart meets the limits of the unyielding pericardial cavity. This shock is felt as a palpable diastolic impulse in some cases. It is associated with the pericardial "knock," or filling sound, that generally occurs after the time of the opening snap and before the time of the usual third sound (Figure 18–12). It can be the loudest sound in the cardiac cycle. There is usually no cardiac murmur, and the heart sounds are soft.

5. Signs in other organs– Rales may be present at the base of the lung, and the liver is usually markedly enlarged and tender but not pulsating. Liver function abnormalities may be present because of congestive hepatopathy, and the patient may even be jaundiced. Ascites tends to be more prominent than ankle edema, and the combination of wasting and edema resembles that seen in advanced right heart failure or cirrhosis of the liver.

C. Electrocardiographic Findings: There are no specific electrocardiographic changes. The voltage in the limb and precordial leads tends to be low, and T wave inversion is common. The presence of significant right or left ventricular hypertrophy on the ECG contradicts a diagnosis of constrictive pericarditis.

D. Imaging and Hemodynamic Studies: The heart is classically not significantly enlarged on x-ray and shows no specific chamber enlargement. The pulmonary artery is not enlarged, and pulmonary congestion is seldom marked. Redistribution of pulmonary blood flow to the apexes speaks against the diagnosis. X-rays provide the most useful sign distinguishing myocardial disease from pericardial constriction, namely intrapericardial calcification, shown in Figure 18–13. This sign is most commonly seen in tuberculous cases, but it can occur in cases with viral origins. Signs of calcification on x-ray do not necessarily mean that constriction is always present, but if calcification is found, a primary myocardial cause for

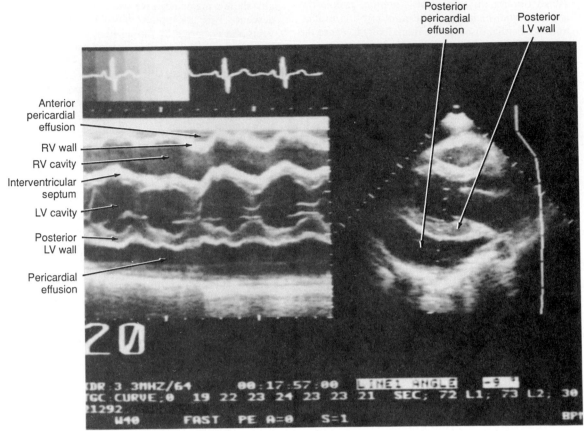

Figure 18–10. Two-dimensional echocardiogram in a patient with a large pericardial effusion. The left panel is an M-mode echogram showing an echo-free space anterior to the right ventricle and posterior to the left ventricle. Note the gentle undulation of the heart in the pericardial fluid. The right panel represents a long axis view of the same patient showing the large posterior echo-free space. See Figure 18–11 also.

the patient's disease is unlikely except in tropical (African) endomyocardial fibrosis.

1. Noninvasive techniques– Venous pulse tracings and echocardiography are helpful in making the distinction between constrictive pericarditis and primary myocardial disease, but they are not absolutely diagnostic. The abrupt cessation of ventricular filling can be seen on echocardiography and contrasts with the ventricular dilation and slowed ejection rate seen in cardiomyopathy. The thickness of the pericardium can be measured using CT or MRI (Figure 18–14). By this means, the thickened pericardium in patients with constriction can be distinguished from the normal pericardium in patients with restrictive cardiomyopathy.

Hemodynamic differences between constrictive pericarditis and restrictive cardiomyopathy may also differentiate these conditions. In restrictive cardiomyopathy with respiration, the right and left ventricular systolic and diastolic pressures tend to fall with inspiration and rise with expiration, while in constrictive pericarditis there is a reciprocal relationship be-

tween the right and left ventricle during the respiratory cycle. In constrictive pericarditis with inspiration, the left ventricular systolic and diastolic pressures fall while the right ventricular pressure rises. With expiration, the left ventricular pressure rises and the right ventricular pressure falls (Hatle, 1989).

Doppler echocardiographic features parallel the hemodynamics. With pericardial constriction, there is a significant ($> 25\%$) reciprocal respiratory variation in early diastolic filling velocity across the mitral and tricuspid valves during the respiratory cycle. With inspiration, tricuspid flow velocity increases and mitral flow velocity decreases. With expiration, the opposite occurs. In patients with restrictive cardiomyopathy, there are only minor variations in Doppler atrioventricular valve flow velocities with respiration. Isovolumic relaxation times also show significant variations during the respiratory cycle in constrictive pericarditis but not in restrictive cardiomyopathy.

2. Invasive techniques– Cardiac catheterization is often performed in an attempt to confirm the diagnosis. Unfortunately, there are no absolute diagnostic

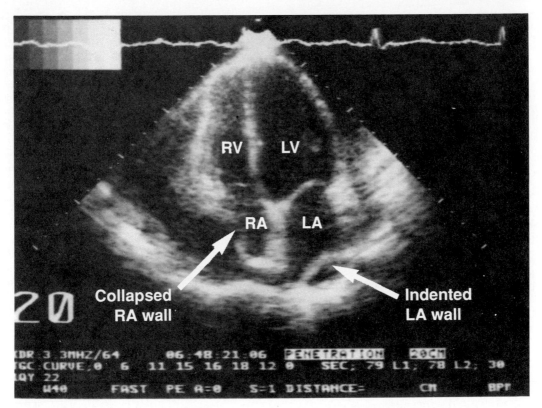

Figure 18–11. Two-dimensional echocardiogram of a patient with pericarditis, pericardial effusion, and cardiac tamponade. Four-chamber view taken in diastole. Note collapse of right lateral atrial wall with mild indentation in left atrial wall.

hemodynamic features that can help distinguish between constrictive pericarditis and restrictive cardiomyopathy, the principal condition with which constrictive pericarditis is confused. The problem of diagnosis is greatest when the level of diastolic pressure in all cardiac chambers is equal. There is little hemodynamic difference between interference with filling resulting from causes outside the heart, those in the heart wall, and those within the cardiac chambers. The hemodynamic features of impaired cardiac filling are shown in Figure 18–15 and include a marked diastolic dip and plateau in the right ventricular pressure tracing (square root sign), a marked diastolic drop in venous pressure, and equalization of

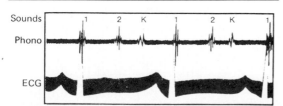

Figure 18–12. Phonocardiogram of typical sharp, early diastolic pericardial knock (K). (Courtesy of Roche Laboratories Division of Hoffman-La Roche, Inc.)

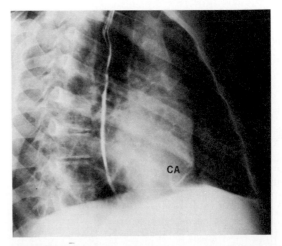

Figure 18–13. Chest x-ray of a patient with constrictive pericarditis showing calcification (CA) in the pericardium. Right anterior oblique view.

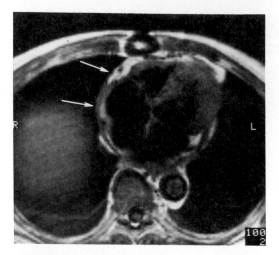

Figure 18–14. Magnetic resonance image of cross-section of thorax showing pericardial thickening (arrows) in a patient with constrictive pericarditis. (Courtesy of C Higgins.)

end-diastolic pressure in all cardiac chambers. The square root sign is caused by limitation of cardiac filling, and the start of the plateau coincides with the audible filling sound. Pulsus paradoxus is not a specific sign of pericardial disease, and all the hemodynamic manifestations can be seen in patients with restrictive cardiomyopathy as well. These signs also occur in patients with endomyocardial fibrosis of the type seen in tropical Africa. In this condition, there is endocardial rather than pericardial calcification.

Although it is true that the distinction between pericardial and myocardial disease cannot be made with certainty on hemodynamic grounds, there are some features that strongly suggest primary myocardial disease. They are disproportionate increase in wedge pressure, low cardiac output, raised pulmonary vascular resistance, marked cardiac enlargement, raised pulmonary arterial pressure (systolic > 50 mm Hg), atrial gallop, marked pulmonary congestion, and a diastolic right ventricular pressure plateau less than 30% of systolic pressure.

The heart in constrictive pericarditis fills most rap-

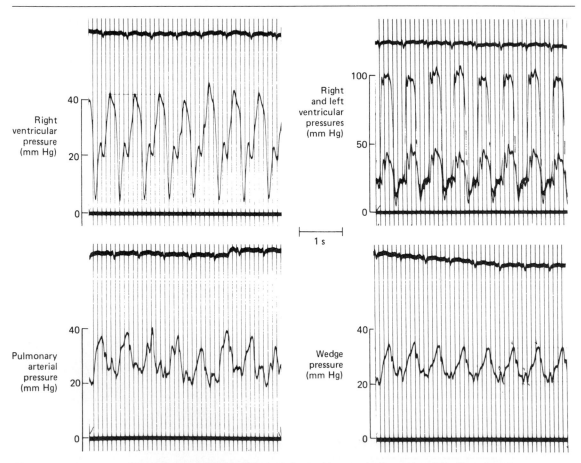

Figure 18–15. Intracardiac pressure tracings from a patient with constrictive pericarditis. The diastolic pressure is elevated to about 20 mm Hg in every chamber. The right ventricular pressure tracing shows a marked diastolic dip followed by a plateau (square root sign).

idly in early diastole, and in some cases the distinction between pericardial and myocardial disease can be made from cineangiographic measurements of the rate of cardiac filling. In patients with myocardial disease, the heart fills more slowly than normally. Unfortunately, some patients with pericardial constriction also have myocardial disease, and the distinction based on the rate of ventricular filling is not clear-cut.

Differential Diagnosis

In difficult cases involving differential diagnosis of amyloidosis or myocarditis, endomyocardial biopsy may help.

Superior vena caval obstruction with hepatic enlargement and ascites, in which venous pulsation and evidence of inferior vena caval obstruction, are absent, should not be confused with constrictive pericarditis. Similarly, cirrhosis of the liver, in which the jugular venous pressure is not raised, should be readily distinguished. The principal entities with which constrictive pericarditis can be confused are restrictive cardiomyopathy (eg, due to amyloidosis) and endomyocardial fibrosis. The distinction is extremely difficult to make; furthermore, pericardial, myocardial, and endocardial fibrosis tend to influence one another because the fibrotic process tends to spread from one structure to the other. Pericardial fibrosis tends to involve the muscle of the thin-walled right ventricle; similarly, endocardial fibrosis tends to spread to the underlying cardiac muscle. A thickened pericardium noted on CT or MRI is strong evidence favoring constrictive pericarditis over restrictive cardiomyopathy. Although exploratory thoracotomy may be indicated in difficult cases, it is harmful in patients with cardiomyopathy and should be avoided if possible.

The response to treatment with digitalis and its derivatives can be helpful in the diagnosis. The venous pressure may fall to normal in patients with right heart failure. In contrast, the venous pressure remains high in spite of medical therapy in constrictive pericarditis. Diuretics can be dangerous in constrictive pericarditis because a decrease in ventricular filling pressure may markedly diminish cardiac output.

Complications

Involvement of the myocardium is such an inevitable consequence of pericardial constriction that it can hardly be called a complication. The effects are most clearly seen after surgery, when the heart (especially the right ventricle) may dilate when the constricting pericardium is removed, with subsequent cardiac dilation and failure.

Treatment

Surgical resection of the shell of fibrous tissue around the heart is always indicated in symptomatic cases, preferably before marked hepatic enlargement has occurred. The operation is almost always palliative rather than curative, since some evidence of restricted motion of the heart is evident after operation, even though symptoms and signs may no longer be present. The operation can be either one of the easiest or one of the most difficult facing the cardiac surgeon. If there is a well-defined plane of cleavage between the fibrotic pericardium and the heart, or even a thin layer of fluid between the thickened pericardium and the heart, pericardial resection can be relatively simple. In most cases, however, especially when the disease is of long standing, the pericardium and the wall of the right ventricle form a single mass of dense fibrous tissue, and dissection is hazardous because of the danger of perforating the right ventricle. The left side of the heart may also be involved; if so, this side should be freed first to avoid pulmonary edema. Considerable judgment is necessary to decide when sufficient tissue has been resected to relieve the obstruction to filling. Intraoperative measurement of right atrial pressure is a help in determining the effects of surgery. If resection of the parietal pericardium does not result in a fall in venous pressure, epicardial resection is needed. The aim of the operation is to resect enough pericardial tissue to free the heart and lower the venous pressure significantly. If too much is removed, the right ventricle tends to dilate, and right heart failure results. Resection of fibrous tissue around the back of the heart is also often needed, and this may be technically difficult. The surgical mortality rate is about 5-10% and varies with the stage of the disease. It is higher in advanced cases. Any resected tissue should be examined histologically, and tubercle bacilli should be sought. If tuberculosis is not diagnosed by pathologic examination, specific diagnosis by other means is indicated, eg, tuberculin testing, sputum examination, or culture of gastric washings.

Restoration of sinus rhythm after operation is indicated in patients with atrial fibrillation or flutter.

Prognosis

The prognosis in constrictive pericarditis is reasonably good. The disease runs a chronic course. In patients in whom the disease is not diagnosed, the chronically raised venous pressure may be tolerated surprisingly well. Cardiac cirrhosis of the liver eventually develops. The principal determinant in prognosis is the success of the surgical treatment.

REFERENCES

General

Chandraratna PAN, Aronow WS: Detection of pericardial metastases by cross-sectional echocardiography. Circulation 1981;63:197.

Fowler NO: Pericardial disease. Heart Dis Stroke 1992;1: 85.

Hancock EW: Pericarditis and other pericardial diseases. Curr Opin Cardiol 1991;6:428.

Moncada R et al: Diagnostic role of computed tomography in pericardial heart disease: Congenital defects, thickening, neoplasms, and effusions. Am Heart J 1982;103:263.

Shabetai R: Pericardial and cardiac pressure. Circulation 1988;77:1.

Pericarditis

Arsenian MA: Cardiovascular sequelae of therapeutic thoracic radiation. Prog Cardiovasc Dis 1991;33:299.

Guindo J et al: Recurrent pericarditis: Relief with colchicine. Circulation 1990;82:1117.

Hall IP: Purulent pericarditis. Postgrad Med J 1989;65: 444.

Hara KS et al: Rheumatoid pericarditis: Clinical features and survival. Medicine 1990;69:81.

Kumar S, Lesch M: Pericarditis in renal disease. Prog Cardiovasc Dis 1980;22:357.

Permanyer-Miralda G, Sagrista-Sauleda J, Soler-Soler J: Primary acute pericardial disease: A prospective series of 231 consecutive patients. Am J Cardiol 1985; 56:623.

Sagrista-Sauleda J, Permanyer-Miralda G, Soler-Soler J: Tuberculous pericarditis: Ten-year experience with a prospective protocol for diagnosis and treatment. J Am Coll Cardiol 1988; 11:724.

Tofler GH et al: Pericarditis in acute myocardial infarction: Characterization and clinical significance. Am Heart J 1989;117:86.

Pericardial Effusion & Tamponade

Eisenberg MJ, Schiller NB: Bayes' theorem and the echocardiographic diagnosis of cardiac tamponade. Am J Cardiol 1991;68:1242.

Grose R et al: Left ventricular volume and function during relief of cardiac tamponade in man. Circulation 1982;66:149.

Himelman RB et al: Inferior vena cava plethora with blunted respiratory responses: A sensitive echocardiographic sign of cardiac tamponade. J Am Coll Cardiol 1988;12:1470.

Kopecky SL et al: Percutaneous pericardial catheter drainage: Report of 42 consecutive cases. Am J Cardiol 1985;58:633.

Kronzon I, Cohen ML, Winer HE: Diastolic atrial compression: A sensitive echocardiographic sign of cardiac tamponade. J Am Coll Cardiol 1983;2:770.

Levine MJ et al: Implications of echocardiography assisted diagnosis of pericardial tamponade in contemporary medical patients: Detection before hemodynamic embarrassment. J Am Coll Cardiol 1991;17: 59.

Reddy PS et al: Spectrum of hemodynamic changes in cardiac tamponade. Am J Cardiol 1990;66:1487.

Reeder GS: Pericardial disease: Echocardiographic and hemodynamic aspects. Curr Opin Cardiol 1989;4: 417.

Sugimoto JT et al: Pericardial window: Mechanisms of efficacy. Ann Thorac Surg 1990;50:442.

Wall TC et al: Diagnosis and management by subxiphoid pericardiotomy of large pericardial effusions causing cardiac tamponade. Am J Cardiol 1992;69:1075.

Constrictive Pericarditis

Byrd BF III, Linden PW: Superior vena cava Doppler flow velocity patterns in pericardial disease. Am J Cardiol 1990;65:2404.

Cimino JJ, Kogan AD: Constrictive pericarditis after cardiac surgery: Report of three cases and review of the literature. Am Heart J 1989;118:1292.

Garrett J, O'Neill H, Blake S: Constrictive pericarditis associated with sarcoidosis. Am Heart J 1984;107: 394.

Hanley PC, Shub C, Lie JT: Constrictive pericarditis associated with combined retroperitoneal and mediastinal fibrosis. Mayo Clin Proc 1984;59:300.

Hatle LK et al: Differentiation of constrictive pericarditis and restrictive cardiomyopathy by Doppler echocardiography. Circulation 1989;79:357.

Isner JM et al: Differentiation of constrictive pericarditis from restrictive cardiomyopathy by computed tomographic imaging. Am Heart J 1983;105:1019.

Killian DM et al: Constrictive pericarditis after cardiac surgery. Am Heart J 1989;118:563.

Lipton MJ et al: Clinical applications of dynamic computed tomography. Prog Cardiovasc Dis 1986;28:349.

Ribiero P et al: Constrictive pericarditis as a complication of coronary artery bypass surgery. Br Heart J 1984;51:205.

Strang JIG et al: Controlled clinical trial of complete open surgical drainage and of prednisolone in treatment of tuberculous pericardial effusion in Transkei. Lancet 1988;2:759.

Tyberg TI et al: Left ventricular filling in differentiating restrictive amyloid cardiomyopathy and constrictive pericarditis. Am J Cardiol 1981;47:791.

Disease of the Pulmonary Circulation

19

The principal site of involvement in diseases of the pulmonary circulation is the pulmonary vascular bed. The pulmonary blood vessels, arterioles, capillaries, and veins may be affected by heart disease, leading to pulmonary parenchymal involvement, or by pulmonary disease, leading to cardiac involvement, mainly affecting the right heart.

PULMONARY HYPERTENSION

The most important response of pulmonary blood vessels to disease is the development of increased pulmonary arterial pressure—pulmonary hypertension. It may result from primary parenchymal disease of the lungs, changes in the walls of the blood vessels, or obstruction to the lumen caused by thrombosis or embolization. **Cor pulmonale**—right heart involvement—is said to be present when any right-sided abnormality can be demonstrated; frank right heart failure does not have to be present.

Pulmonary circulation in the adult seems to be almost completely passive when compared to the systemic circulation. It behaves as an unreactive, low-pressure, low-resistance, short, high-flow pathway from the heart via the pulmonary arteries to the pulmonary capillary bed, which constitutes the large (100 m²) site of gas exchange.

Mechanism of Production of Pulmonary Hypertension

The principal stimuli evoking a response in the pulmonary arterioles are (1) alveolar hypoxia, as occurs with exposure to high altitude; (2) pulmonary venous hypertension; and (3) acidosis. The site of reaction in these three instances is the smooth muscle of the pulmonary arterioles. Both stimuli cause arteriolar vasoconstriction that is at first functional, spasmodic, and reversible; with time, however, the vasoconstriction develops into organic muscular hypertrophy, which is ultimately irreversible. The age at which the patient is first exposed to these stimuli and their magnitude and duration play an important role in determining the response of the pulmonary circulation. Since responsiveness decreases with age, stimuli that have been present since birth or infancy cause more severe and less readily reversible changes. With high-flow, high-pressure pulmonary hemodynamics,

as seen in large ventricular septal defects and patent ductus arteriosus, there is shear force injury to the endothelium, resulting in fibrous intimal hyperplasia. Furthermore, as the lung grows, the vasculature does not divide as normally as does the bronchial system, so there are fewer arterioles than normal in the mature lung. These changes are irreversible.

Hypoxia and raised pulmonary venous pressure interact; consequently, pulmonary hypertension is more severe in patients living at higher altitudes who have disorders causing raised pulmonary venous pressure. Similarly, patients with diseased pulmonary vessels are prone to pulmonary embolism, thrombosis, and infarction, all of which aggravate the development of pulmonary hypertension. With pulmonary embolism, platelet-related vasoactive substances which are both vasoconstrictive and bronchoconstrictive are released (eg, serotonin, histamine, and thromboxane A_2). These humoral factors increase pulmonary vascular resistance directly and through increased hypoxia.

Effects of Loss of Lung Tissue

The normal pulmonary circulation is capable of handling increased blood flow without much concomitant rise in pressure. The pressure/flow characteristics of pulmonary circulation are thus highly nonlinear, and the use of a single value (in mm Hg/L/min) to describe its resistance is overly simplistic. Increasing flow without increasing pressure implies the opening up of parallel circulatory pathways. It follows that loss of lung tissue, eg, following pneumonectomy or with pulmonary fibrosis, decreases the reserve capacity of the pulmonary vascular bed and increases the tendency for pulmonary hypertension to develop. As progressively larger amounts of lung tissue are removed, the capacity of the pulmonary vascular bed is ultimately reduced to a level at which the normal cardiac output cannot be accommodated without an increase in pulmonary arterial pressure. In chronic lung disease, alveolar hypoxia, the effects of which are potentiated by hypercapnia and acidosis, causes an additional (potentially reversible) element of pulmonary hypertension.

Effects of Increased Left Atrial Pressure

The most important cause of pulmonary hypertension and right heart failure in patients with heart disease is pulmonary arterial vasoconstriction in response to a rise in left atrial pressure. The mechanism of this response is unknown, although it is known that increased pulmonary interstitial fluid can compress small vessels and small airways, causing local alveolar hypoxia and vasoconstriction. The magnitude of the response varies considerably in different patients, but younger persons usually show greater changes. Although mitral stenosis is the classic example of a lesion causing raised pulmonary vascular resistance in adults, any long-standing moderate or severe increase in left atrial pressure—eg, left atrial myxoma, aortic valve disease, systemic hypertension, cardiomyopathy, or any combination of causes—can result in raised pulmonary vascular resistance. Severe pulmonary hypertension does not inevitably follow raised left atrial pressure. In some cases, chronic left atrial hypertension causes marked dyspnea and recurrent pulmonary edema without provoking any vasoconstrictive reaction in the pulmonary arterioles.

Pulmonary Hypertension in Patients With Lung Disease

Patients with parenchymal lung disease tend to develop pulmonary hypertension during acute exacerbations of their disease. Thus, during acute episodes of asthma, bronchitis, or pneumonia, the combination of lung disease and alveolar hypoxia leads to an acute rise in pulmonary arterial pressure. The pulmonary arterial pressure may fall to normal when the acute illness subsides, but with time some permanent changes occur, and ultimately the pulmonary hypertension becomes permanent.

Pulmonary Hypertension in Schistosomiasis (Bilharziasis)

Bilharzial heart disease is due to the deposition of ova of *Schistosoma* (*Schistosoma japonicum*, *Schistosoma mansoni*, or *Schistosoma haematobium*) in the lung. The condition arises from urinary or intestinal tract infection, and the disease is common in Egypt in agricultural workers in the Nile delta. The ova lodge in the pulmonary arterioles during their migration through the body and produce an inflammatory change that on healing leaves a nodule. The change leads to pulmonary hypertension, right ventricular hypertrophy, and right heart failure. The classic radiologic signs include a large pulmonary artery and diffuse mottling of the lung parenchyma.

The clinical picture is one of right heart failure without lung disease and is similar to that in primary pulmonary hypertension. It is not uncommon to see aneurysmal dilatation of the pulmonary artery and marked enlargement of the right ventricle.

There is no satisfactory treatment when cor pulmonale develops. Prevention of bilharziasis consists of avoiding wading or swimming in stagnant fresh water in which the snail vector *(Planorbis)* lives.

Primary Pulmonary Hypertension

Pulmonary arterial vasoconstriction can occur without a rise in left atrial pressure, giving rise to a disease known as primary, or idiopathic, pulmonary hypertension. The condition is commonest in premenopausal women but can occur at any age and in men. The onset is insidious and the course usually relentlessly progressive, leading to death in 2–8 years after diagnosis from intractable right heart failure or cardiac arrhythmia. A familial incidence has been reported, and the condition is more prevalent in persons living at high altitude.

Pulmonary Hypertension Due to Vascular Disease

Thromboembolic pulmonary hypertension can occur as a separate identifiable disease in patients who have such frequent episodes of pulmonary embolism that complete resolution between attacks is impossible. It is difficult to differentiate between vasospasm and thromboembolism in the genesis of primary pulmonary hypertension because multiple small pulmonary emboli can trigger reflex changes and may also produce pulmonary vasoconstriction.

Any disease affecting the pulmonary vasculature can result in pulmonary hypertension. This is especially common in systemic sclerosis but can occur also in other collagen vascular diseases such as systemic lupus arteriosus.

An epidemic of toxic arteriolitis caused by contaminated rapeseed oil recently reported in Spain resulted in fatal pulmonary hypertension; in the United States, toxicity due to ingestion of contaminated L-tryptophan has caused pulmonary hypertension.

Pulmonary Hypertension Due to Congenital Heart Left-to-Right Shunts (see Chapter 11)

PULMONARY ARTERIOVENOUS FISTULA

Pulmonary arteriovenous fistula is a rare but specific form of pulmonary vascular disease. This condition, which is often associated with hereditary hemorrhagic telangiectasia (Osler-Rendu-Weber disease), consists of congenital arteriovenous malformations in the lungs that give rise to cyanosis, clubbing of the fingers, and a high output state. Venous blood passing through the abnormal channels often causes a bruit; in addition, the blood is not exposed to oxygen in the lungs, so that arterial desaturation occurs that is exaggerated on exercise. Cardiac output may be increased, and polycythemia and increased blood volume follow. Since the arteriovenous fistulas are low-resistance shunts, there is no increase in pulmonary vascular resistance and the pulmonary arterial pressure remains normal. The condition is most frequently seen in young adults and tends to mimic

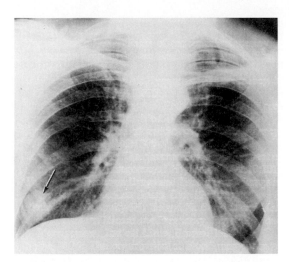

Figure 19–1. Chest x-ray showing a pulmonary arterio-venous fistula in the lower lobe of the right lung.

congenital heart disease. Hemoptysis is a common complication. Resection of the lobe of the lung that is the malformation site is the principal treatment. Unfortunately, the lesions are often multiple, and if this is not detected preoperatively, a second lesion may sometimes enlarge and cause a recurrence of the condition after operation. The lesions usually show up on plain chest x-rays, as shown in Figure 19–1, and their vascular nature can be readily determined by pulmonary angiography (Figure 19–2).

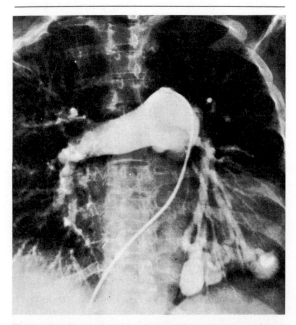

Figure 19–2. Angiogram showing three large arteriovenous fistulas in left lower lobe of the lung. (Reproduced, with permission, from Dines DE et al: Pulmonary arteriovenous fistulas. Mayo Clin Proc 1974;49:460.)

PULMONARY EMBOLISM

Pulmonary embolism is an important complication of heart disease, but its incidence and significance are extremely difficult to determine. Data based on autopsy findings indicate that pulmonary embolism is extremely common, some studies having found thrombus in pulmonary vessels in over half of patients, but the distinction between antemortem and postmortem thrombus may be difficult to make. Agonal embolism and thrombosis in situ in the slow-moving blood in the lungs of moribund patients almost certainly account for many of the thrombi seen at autopsy.

The significance of the thrombotic material found at autopsy is difficult to determine. In massive pulmonary embolism in which a large mass of red cells, fibrin, and platelets impacts in a main pulmonary artery and causes a sudden fatal obstruction to the circulation, the importance of the event is plainly evident. However, in chronically ill patients with wasting diseases who are comatose for several days, the episode is likely to be masked.

These considerations should not lead one to underestimate the importance of pulmonary embolism as a complication. They are presented to show that autopsy studies may not provide a realistic view of the incidence and clinical picture. Pulmonary embolism is insidious, often missed on physical examination, and often misdiagnosed as pneumonia, atelectasis, pleurisy, pulmonary congestion, or edema.

Obstruction of the pulmonary vascular bed involving the lumen of blood vessels—pulmonary embolism or thrombosis—is more common in patients with heart disease than those with lung disease. The nature and amount of embolic material, the site of obstruction, and the rate of removal of embolic material all play a part in determining the clinical picture, and the previous state of the pulmonary circulation determines whether the lung undergoes infarction or not. Normal lungs obtain their blood supply from both pulmonary and bronchial arteries. When the lungs are congested, as occurs in heart failure or in prolonged immobilization of comatose patients, bronchial blood flow is not ordinarily sufficient to maintain the viability of lung tissue that has been deprived of its pulmonary arterial blood supply. In such cases of congestion, the affected area of lung is infarcted and consolidated, which deprives it of air and causes a temporary loss of function.

The manifestations of pulmonary embolism vary greatly. Acute massive impaction of several hundred grams of thrombus in the main pulmonary artery can cause acute circulatory collapse or shock, with almost instantaneous death. There can also be repeated showers of multiple microscopic emboli, eg, schistosome ova in bilharziasis. Small emboli lodge in the pulmonary arterioles far out in the lungs and cause much more insidious pulmonary changes; in rare cases, right heart failure is the first clinical manifestation. The site of origin of the embolic material is commonly the veins of the legs and pelvis, but the right atrium is an important source of emboli in patients with atrial fibrillation. Fat emboli from the bone marrow also occur following fracture of the long bones. Here the mechanism of injury to the lung is not only obstruction by fat but also a chemical inflammatory reaction generated by the chemical breakdown of the fat into fatty acids.

Soft, recently formed thrombus is much more readily lysed than well-organized old thrombus. Thus, the ability of the thrombolytic processes of the body to dispose of embolic material by breaking it up into smaller pieces that lodge in more peripheral parts of the lung constitutes an important and highly variable factor in the clinical course of pulmonary embolism. The cross-sectional area of the pulmonary arterial bed increases with each division of the pulmonary artery. Consequently, as embolic material moves farther out in the lungs, pulmonary blood flow progressively increases, pulmonary arterial pressure progressively falls, and right ventricular overload is relieved.

Acute overload of the right heart, like acute overload of the left heart, tends to produce a different clinical picture from that observed in chronic obstruction of pulmonary blood flow. The magnitude of the overload can also vary because the pulmonary embolism may be massive or only moderate. The release of vasoactive substances also complicates the problem. There is thus a wide variation in severity of the clinical effects of pulmonary embolism, further complicated by variations in the state of the preexisting pulmonary circulation and the efficiency of the thrombolytic mechanisms. It may be several weeks before hypertrophy occurs in the right heart in response to sudden severe pulmonary vascular obstruction. A sudden acute rise in systemic venous pressure, without marked increase in pulmonary arterial or right ventricular pressure, is thus the principal effect of an acute lesion on the right side of the heart. Inadequate left-sided venous return,with an acute fall in left ventricular output, tachycardia, hypotension, shock, and circulatory collapse, dominates the clinical picture,and it may be difficult to determine whether the basic lesion is right-sided or left-sided. In more chronic, less rapidly developing, less severe lesions, right ventricular output can be maintained and the compensatory changes—right ventricular hypertrophy and dilatation—are more obvious.

Massive Pulmonary Embolism; Acute Right Heart Failure (Acute Cor Pulmonale)

Acute cor pulmonale is seen almost exclusively in association with massive pulmonary embolism. Massive pulmonary embolism usually occurs in apparently healthy persons who may be of any age. The disease affects females more often than males. Patients have usually been recently subject to some minor trauma. Recent normal delivery, hernia operation, minor gynecologic or urologic surgery, varicose vein operation, or some other procedure involving the legs or pelvis is ordinarily the precipitating factor. Prolonged bed rest and the presence of malignant disease predispose to pulmonary embolism. Loosely adherent, soft, friable thrombus forms undetected in the veins of the legs or pelvis (phlebothrombosis). The thrombus suddenly breaks loose and lodges at or near the bifurcation of the main pulmonary artery. The patient complains of sudden, severe central chest pain and collapses, often with loss of consciousness. Death can occur within a few minutes if the thrombus is large and does not dislodge. If the thrombus is smaller or moves more peripherally, either spontaneously or in response to pounding on the chest or chest compression, acute cor pulmonale rather than sudden death is seen, and the condition may run a subacute course.

Dyspnea, cyanosis, anxiety, impaired consciousness, and all the manifestations of an acute circulatory catastrophe are present. The diagnosis is difficult to confirm in the face of simultaneous emergency and supportive treatment and the general hectic activity involved in managing an acute life-threatening situation. Physical examination may not reveal any specific diagnostic signs. The ECG and chest x-ray may not be diagnostic in the earliest stages. The ECG will not necessarily show the changes of acute myocardial infarction, the disorder that must be considered most frequently in the differential diagnosis. The electrocardiographic changes of acute right ventricular overload can mimic myocardial infarction. Evidence of oligemic lungs, perhaps with an asymmetric increase in translucency, may be seen on chest radiographs in patients who survive the initial episode by 30 minutes or more. Evidence of arterial hypoxia ($PO_2 < 70$ mm Hg) is nonspecific.

The place of surgical removal of embolic material in the treatment of massive pulmonary embolism has been the subject of controversy in recent years. A confirmed diagnosis of massive pulmonary embolism with accessible thrombus in the main pulmonary artery or its branches is required before surgery is performed. This necessitates emergency pulmonary angiocardiography, preferably done in an operating room in a center equipped to perform cardiopulmonary bypass. Since such facilities are not widely available, less drastic measures must also be instituted. Anticoagulation with heparin (5000–10,000 units intravenously, repeated every 3 hours) prevents further accumulation of thrombus while the body's own defenses lyse the thrombus. Any factor that moves the obstructing thrombus farther down the pulmonary artery may promote the patient's recovery. Even a small increase in the flow of blood to the lungs will sometimes help to provide a venous return to the left heart and will also avoid the development of secondary thrombosis around the embolus. Suction embolectomy via a special catheter may be successful, or manipulation of a cardiac catheter in the pulmonary artery may serve to move the thrombus farther down the vessel; turning the patient into various positions and striking forceful blows to the precordium may also help (Essop, 1992).

PULMONARY HEART DISEASE

Streptokinase, urokinase, recombinant alteplase (tissue plasminogen activator; rt-PA), and anistreplase are enzymes that have been extensively tested as therapeutic agents for the lysis rather than the prevention of thrombi. Extreme care is needed in their use, because they may induce hemorrhage in patients who have wounds that are healing. They are contraindicated in patients who have undergone surgery, childbirth, liver or kidney biopsy, or arterial puncture in the preceding 10 days. Recent cerebrovascular accidents, any bleeding tendency, and severe hypertension also contraindicate their use.

Prevention of massive pulmonary embolism is clearly preferable to treatment. Patients with a history of pulmonary embolism, deep venous thrombosis, cerebral thrombosis, or thrombophlebitis should not use oral contraceptives. The morbidity and mortality rate from pulmonary embolism is 4-8 times higher in women who take oral contraceptive drugs. Encouraging patients to move about in bed and allowing them to walk about in their rooms as soon as possible after minor surgery or childbirth have helped to reduce the incidence of massive pulmonary embolism. Subcutaneous heparin injections in low doses (2500–3000 units every 6–8 hours) in the postoperative period or intravenous dextran 70 administered with intravenous fluids after surgery has reportedly been effective in reducing the incidence of fatal massive pulmonary embolism in double-blind studies. The results have been best in patients undergoing abdominal surgery.

Low-dose heparin has not proved to be valuable in hip replacement or prostatic surgery, because of the prevalence of postoperative hemorrhage and because it does not decrease the incidence of deep vein thrombosis. Fat embolism, following fractures of the long bones, is an indication for steroid therapy. In thrombophlebitis (which is a much more common condition), smaller, more adherent thrombi occur that provoke local pain, swelling, and signs of inflammation. These seldom if ever break loose, and prophylactic measures other than avoiding oral contraceptives are of doubtful value.

Moderate Pulmonary Embolism

The description of massive pulmonary embolism given above concerns cases in which no prior heart or lung disease is present, cardiopulmonary reserve is large, and bronchial arterial blood supply is good. In most cardiac patients, however, these conditions do not exist. The clinical picture in such patients is different. Relatively small emboli that would pass unnoticed in a healthy person cause serious problems, with exacerbation of congestive heart failure or pulmonary infarction, with pain, pleural irritation, hemoptysis, and effusion. The venous stasis and congestion seen in heart failure predispose to thrombus formation not only in the legs but also in the right heart and even in the lungs themselves, so that pulmonary thromboembolic complications are especially common in cardiologic practice. Pulmonary embolism in which a moderate-sized embolus lodges in the lungs and is sufficiently large to occlude the artery leading to a lobe or a lobule is an insidious condition that is often overlooked. Data obtained at autopsy indicate a surprisingly high incidence of thrombi in the lungs ($> 50\%$ of cases), and this suggests that agonal lesions may be common.

Clinical Findings
A. Symptoms: The classic symptoms of a chest pain that is often worse on inspiration, dyspnea, cough, and hemoptysis in susceptible patients such as those with congestive heart failure, mitral valve disease, or myocardial infarction should strongly suggest a diagnosis of pulmonary embolism. Unfortunately, the classic clinical picture of pulmonary embolism is uncommon. Not infrequently, unexplained dyspnea, fever, tachycardia, increase in venous pressure, or worsening of venous congestion provides a clue to the diagnosis, but in many cases the acute episode passes unnoticed.

B. Signs: Tachypnea and tachycardia are the most frequent signs of pulmonary embolism. Physical signs in the lungs depend on the development of consolidation or pleural involvement. Pleural friction rub, impaired movement, dullness to percussion, diminished air entry, and bronchial breathing can be heard, and signs of pleural effusion may develop. Signs of increased pulmonary arterial pressure such as increased right ventricular impulse, increased intensity of the pulmonary valve closure sound, or palpable pulmonary artery pulsation should be sought.

C. Electrocardiographic Findings: The signs of pulmonary embolism on the ECG are variable. A peaked right atrial P wave may be seen, and atrial arrhythmias, especially fibrillation or flutter, can occur. A change in electrical axis toward the right; right bundle branch block, either complete or incomplete (Figure 19–3); and T wave inversions in the anterior chest leads (V_{1-3}) are seen in about 10–15% of patients. In some cases, Q waves in leads II, III, and aVF mimic posterior myocardial infarction. In many cases, nonspecific ST changes and slight right axis deviation are seen. Patients with associated coronary disease may show changes indicative of myocardial ischemia.

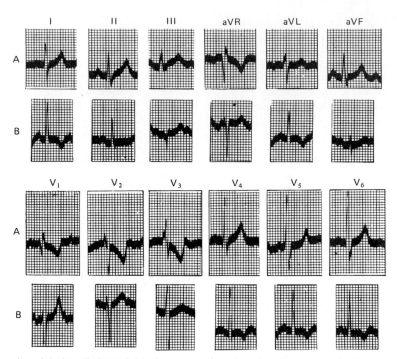

Figure 19–3. Incomplete right bundle branch block as a manifestation of acute right ventricular strain. **A:** The pattern is that of an incomplete bundle branch block (rsR complexes with depressed ST segments and inverted T waves in V_{1-3}). **B:** Five days after **(A)**, there has been a marked change. The incomplete right bundle branch block is no longer present. In the interval the T waves have become inverted in leads I, aVL, and V_{4-6}. **Clinical status:** At **(A)** the patient had an episode of acute pulmonary infarction. Five days later he had markedly improved. The ECG in **(A)** was a reflection of acute right ventricular strain. The pulmonary hypertension had clinically subsided by **(B)**, and the second ECG demonstrated the abnormalities associated with the basic heart disease, beriberi. (Reproduced, with permission, from Goldman MJ: *Principles of Clinical Electrocardiography,* 12th ed. Lange, 1986.)

D. Imaging Studies:

1. X-ray– The patient may be too ill for anything except a bedside x-ray, which is often unsatisfactory. Significant pulmonary embolism can occur even with completely clear lung fields, and radiologic evidence of consolidation following pulmonary infarction takes up to 12 hours to develop. The diaphragm tends to be high on the side of the lesion, which is commonly at the base of the lung. A wedge-shaped shadow extending out to the pleural surface (Figure 19–4) is a classic but uncommon manifestation. The lesion may cavitate later, and pleural effusion at the costophrenic angles or in the interlobular fissures is not uncommon.

2. Ventilation/perfusion scans– External radioactive scanning following injection of radionuclides such as radioiodinated or ^{99m}Tc-labeled human serum albumin has proved valuable in patients who have no history of prior lung disease. The results of lung scans must be interpreted together with simultaneous or near-simultaneous chest x-rays and ventilation scans must be interpreted together with simultaneous or near-simultaneous chest x-rays and ventilation scans using ^{133}Xe. Pulmonary lesions other than emboli can give rise to clear, unperfused

areas on the lung scan, and only the finding of an unperfused area in a segment of lung that is clear on the chest x-ray is significant. Pulmonary emboli can clear so rapidly and can move to the periphery of the lungs so readily that confusion may occur when the radioactive scan and chest x-ray are obtained even a few hours apart.

Ventilation/perfusion scans are characterized as implying low, intermediate, or high probability for pulmonary embolism. Low-probability scans are those demonstrating multiple subsegmental perfusion defects without ventilation defects or larger subsegmental defects with corresponding ventilation defects. Intermediate-probability scans are those showing multiple subsegmental defects with normal ventilation scans or segmental or larger perfusion defects without ventilation studies. High-probability scans are those showing segmental or large perfusion defects with normal ventilation scans or those with multiple perfusion defects substantially larger than either ventilation defects or chest x-ray abnormalities. Intermediate-probability scans are those where chest x-ray shows chronic obstructive pulmonary disease or abnormalities in the region of the perfusion defect.

The sensitivity of the ventilation/perfusion lung

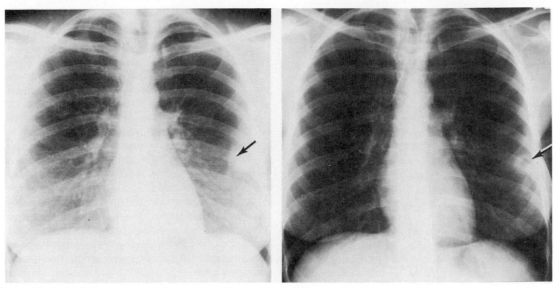

Figure 19–4. Serial chest x-rays of a woman with pulmonary infarction. The infarct has formed a cavity in the second (right-hand) x-ray. (Courtesy of G Gamsu.)

scan has recently been well delineated in a multi-hospital study entitled Prospective Investigation of Pulmonary Embolism Diagnosis (PIOPED) (PIOPED Investigators, 1990). In this study, the results of ventilation/perfusion scans were compared, with pulmonary angiography used as the standard against which results were evaluated. This study showed that 98% of patients with pulmonary embolism had an "abnormal" lung scan of either high, intermediate, or low probability. However, the specificity was low (10%), meaning that most patients without pulmonary embolism also had abnormal lung scans. Of patients with high-probability scans, 88% had pulmonary embolisms, whereas in patients with intermediate-probability scans, only 33% had embolisms. In patients with low-probability scans, 12% had embolisms. If the lung scan was normal, only 4% had embolisms. The sensitivity and specificity were increased if the clinical probability was also used together with the lung scan probability.

In reviewing studies of lung scans in the literature, a normal lung scan rules out the presence of pulmonary emboli with 95% certainty. High- and low-probability lung scans have about a 15% error rate in diagnosing or ruling out pulmonary embolism. The accuracy of the ventilation/perfusion scan improves when the clinical suspicion of pulmonary embolism is consistent with the lung scan result (Kelley, 1991).

With the addition of evidence of lower extremity deep vein thrombosis by serial impedance plethysmography or duplex ultrasonic study, the sensitivity of a high or intermediate probability scan can be markedly increased.

Even with high-probability ventilation/perfusion scans, where there is discrepancy between the clinical picture and the scan, pulmonary angiography should be performed before the patient is committed to a protracted course of oral anticoagulants.

3. Pulmonary angiography– Pulmonary angiography can be used to demonstrate blockage of the pulmonary vasculature, which may be present although it does not appear on a chest radiogram, as shown in Figure 19–5. It provides the clearest, most definitive evidence for the diagnosis of pulmonary embolism. Abrupt pulmonary artery cutoff and visualization of intrapulmonary arterial thrombosis are definite evidence of pulmonary emboli. Angiography carries a small but definite risk of death or morbidity and is expensive in terms of manpower and equipment. Protagonists of angiography point out that unnecessary anticoagulant therapy probably carries an equal or greater risk because of hemorrhagic complications. It is logical, therefore, to reserve angiography for patients with significant symptoms in whom lung scans give equivocal results; for patients with some contraindication to anticoagulation; or for situations in which interruption of the inferior vena cava is contemplated. A normal lung scan effectively excludes serious pulmonary embolism, and a clearly positive perfusion scan with a normal chest x-ray and a normal ventilation scan provides adequate evidence on which to base anticoagulant therapy (PIOPED Investigators, 1990; Cheely, 1981). With this approach, pulmonary angiography can probably be restricted to fewer than 20% of patients in whom the diagnosis is seriously in question.

E. Laboratory Findings: Leukocytosis, increased sedimentation rate, increased serum enzymes (lactate dehydrogenase and aspartate aminotransferase), and slight increase in indirect bilirubin concentration are

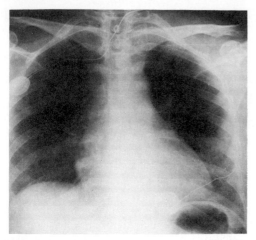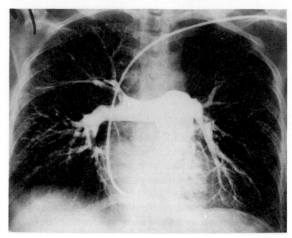

Figure 19–5. Normal chest x-ray *(left)* obtained on the same day as a pulmonary angiogram *(right).* The angiogram shows significant obstruction to the right and left upper lobes, even though the chest x-ray was normal. (Courtesy of G Gamsu.)

seen in many cases. Arterial PO_2 is often reduced (< 70 mm Hg), but the finding is nonspecific. An increased alveolar-arterial oxygen gradient has been said to be more sensitive than a low PO_2 in the diagnosis of pulmonary embolism. However, studies have shown that a normal alveolar-arterial oxygen gradient does not rule out pulmonary embolism (Overton, 1988).

Complications

Secondary thrombus with further blockage of pulmonary vessels, inadequate recanalization, and secondary infection of infarcted lung tissue are the principal complications of pulmonary embolism. Recurrence of pulmonary embolism is always possible. However, complete recovery with full recanalization is the usual outcome, and the complication of chronic thromboembolic pulmonary hypertension is rare—certainly less than 5% of patients with pulmonary embolism. Such chronic hypertension develops only after a long period of several months or perhaps years of repeated embolization, possibly with some associated impairment of the thrombolytic mechanisms. Occasionally, patients can be found with cor pulmonale who have chronic pulmonary thromboembolism without ever having had a clinical pulmonary embolism.

Differential Diagnosis

The diagnosis of pulmonary embolism can be extremely difficult, especially in patients who are ill from other causes and in postoperative patients. The condition is so insidious that it should be suspected in any sick patient in whom unexplained deterioration or failure to thrive is detected. The physician must maintain a high index of suspicion in order to make the correct diagnosis. In many cases the diagnosis can be made in retrospect from careful examination of the chart of the vital signs. A sudden increase in heart rate or respiratory rate, followed by an unexplained rise in temperature on the following day, may have occurred in a patient with an obvious pulmonary infarct that was not previously apparent. Intercurrent lower respiratory tract infections can be readily mistaken for pulmonary emboli and vice versa. Likewise, minor, short-lived episodes of acute pulmonary congestion may cause a similar clinical picture. Repeated episodes of embolism tend to differ slightly in their manifestations, whereas recurrent pulmonary congestion tends to produce a series of similar episodes.

Pulmonary embolism enters into the differential diagnosis of almost all forms of lung disease and many varieties of heart disease. It occurs during the course of these diseases and may also be confused with the diseases themselves. Thus, pneumonia and atelectasis (especially if they occur postoperatively) and pleurisy with or without effusion may all be confused with pulmonary infarction. Hemorrhage into the lung is an important feature of pulmonary infarction that is also seen in other conditions such as bronchial carcinoma, tuberculosis, or any disease causing hemoptysis. Acute chest pain in pulmonary embolism can be confused with that occurring in myocardial infarction, spontaneous pneumothorax, pericarditis, aortic dissection, and even upper abdominal disease such as cholecystitis or perforated peptic ulcer.

Treatment

Acute pulmonary embolectomy has been advocated in patients with massive pulmonary embolism and hemodynamic collapse. The perioperative mortality rate is 30% (Gray, 1988). Most patients with massive pulmonary emboli and shock die before any surgical procedure can be done. If they survive long enough so that surgery can be considered, most will survive with medical management. At present, patients with massive pulmonary emboli are candidates for thrombolytic therapy. Under investigation are catheter techniques for extracting or breaking up emboli (Feitelberg, 1987; Stein, 1990). If patients have a contraindication to thrombolytic therapy—or in situations where thrombolytic therapy has failed—emergency pulmonary embolectomy should be considered. Another circumstance where open heart surgery should be considered is when the patient has thrombosis in the right atrium or right ventricle with recurrent emboli in spite of thrombolysis and anticoagulant therapy.

The principal decision in treatment is whether to use anticoagulant therapy. Anticoagulant therapy is more generally accepted in pulmonary embolism than in any other disorder. Anticoagulation for established pulmonary embolism is preventive therapy. It does not dissolve thrombus but prevents extension. Heparin is given intravenously as a bolus of 5000–10,000 units, followed by a continuous infusion of 1000–1500 units/h. The activated partial thromboplastin time is determined 4–6 hours after the start of treatment and is maintained at $1\frac{1}{2}$–2 times the control time. The platelet count is determined every 2–3 days, as heparin may cause thrombocytopenia.

Oral anticoagulant therapy with warfarin is started either immediately or after 1–3 days of heparin. It takes 5–7 days for warfarin to have its full effect. The daily dose of 5–15 mg by mouth is given until the prothrombin time is $1\frac{1}{2}$–2 times normal or reaches an International Normalized Ratio (INR) of 2–3. The INR is a method of reporting prothrombin times that adjusts for the different thromboplastins used in different laboratories to measure prothrombin time. If the risk factors predisposing to pulmonary embolism are slow to resolve, anticoagulation should be maintained for 3 months. Patients who have had recurrent episodes of venous thrombosis or pulmonary embolism and those whose risk factors are not reversible—ie, patients with protein C or S deficiency, those with antithrombin III deficiency, and those with recurrent venous or arterial thrombosis who have a circulating antiphospholipid antibody—should be anticoagulated indefinitely (NIH Consensus Development Statement, 1986).

The place of fibrinolysis is still uncertain, since studies have not been large enough to prove a decrease in mortality rate with this treatment (Goldhaber, 1991; Meyer, 1992; Dalla-Volta, 1992). The major advantages of fibrinolysis over anticoagulation alone in the studies that have been reported are earlier resolution of the clinical picture with a more rapid drop in the pulmonary arterial pressure, a probable increase in the mass of the surviving pulmonary vas-

cular bed, and—perhaps most importantly—a decrease in the residuals of severe chronic venous obstruction in the legs ("milk leg"). For this reason, fibrinolysis is indicated if the embolism is large, with a drop in blood pressure or right heart failure, or in the presence of significant leg edema indicative of iliac venous thrombosis.

Which fibrinolytic agent is best and what the dosage should be are matters still being investigated (Goldhaber, 1992; Meyer, 1992). The present FDA-approved regimens for pulmonary embolism thrombolysis are as follows: (1) Streptokinase, 250,000 IU as loading dose over 30 minutes, then 100,000 IU/h for 24 hours. Since this is the least expensive drug, it probably should be used until some evidence of advantage for one of the other fibrinolytics justifies the increased cost. (2) Urokinase, 2000 IU/lb as loading dose over 10 minutes, then 2000 IU/lb/h for 12–24 hours. (3) Alteplase, recombinant (rt-PA), 100 mg given as 60 mg in the first hour (of which 6–10 mg are given as a bolus over the first 1–2 minutes), 20 mg over the second hour, and 20 mg over the third hour.

The partial thromboplastin time (PTT) should be determined every 4 hours after thrombolysis; when it reaches twice normal or less, intravenous heparin is begun to maintain the PTT at $1\frac{1}{2}$–$2\frac{1}{2}$ times normal. Warfarin is started with a dose of 10 mg to achieve a prothrombin time between $1\frac{1}{2}$ and 2 times normal.

There are no measures that absolutely prevent the development of pulmonary embolism in cardiac patients, but initiating active leg exercises and breathing exercises, avoiding long periods of bed rest (especially with pressure on the popliteal fossa), and discontinuing the use of oral contraceptives are useful. The physician must exercise care in treating cardiac patients who are in a sitting position. Excessive flexing of the knee and sitting in cramped positions in automobiles and on airplanes predispose to venous stasis. In patients with embolism that recurs in spite of anticoagulant treatment, insertion of a filter into the inferior vena cava or partial or complete ligation of the inferior vena cava has been advocated (Grassi, 1989). These are not totally satisfactory because they do not necessarily prevent embolism and may even provide another site for thrombus formation or lead to edema of the legs. The thrombolytic process is generally so effective that the long-term (6- to 12-week) prognosis depends on the underlying cardiac condition rather than on the embolism. No specific treatment is needed for pulmonary infarction. Control of pain and antibiotics for the treatment of secondary lung infection may be required. If infarction results in severe hemoptysis, anticoagulant therapy may have to be withdrawn.

There is a place for surgical treatment late in the course of pulmonary thromboembolic disease. In some cases, the patient is left with severe and disabling dyspnea due to pulmonary hypertension resulting from blockage of large pulmonary arteries. Exploring the pulmonary arteries, with cardiopulmonary bypass and hypothermia, in an attempt to extract old endothelialized embolic material has proved valuable in some cases (Moser, 1990). Percutaneous catheter-contained endoscopy is a new technique whereby the thrombi can be visualized and the extent and chronicity of the embolism assessed. The value of this procedure is still under investigation. The mortality rate of the operation is about 15%, and the principal complication is reperfusion pulmonary edema (Daily, 1990). This problem can persist for up to 3 months postoperatively. While surgery is palliative rather than curative, the pulmonary vascular resistance can fall dramatically, and symptomatic improvement can be gratifying.

Prognosis

Pulmonary embolism seldom leads to chronic lung disease. If the patient survives the acute episode, whether it is a massive embolism or a moderate-sized one involving pulmonary infarction, the lesion almost invariably heals completely without leaving a scar. The prognosis in acute massive embolism improves with the passage of time; however, most patients die within the first hour. This important cause of death in previously healthy people accounts for over 40,000 fatalities per year in the USA. In those who survive the first hour, the prognosis improves, partly because of the opportunity for treatment and partly because the embolic material may have broken up and moved to a more peripheral area of the lungs. Chronic pulmonary hypertension occurs when there are frequent recurrent episodes of embolism with inadequate time between episodes for resolution of the disease process or when there are inadequate thrombolytic mechanisms.

RIGHT HEART FAILURE DUE TO LUNG DISEASE

1. ADULT RESPIRATORY DISTRESS SYNDROME (ARDS)

An acute, life-threatening form of pulmonary edema can develop after acute lung injury and put a severe acute load on the right ventricle. The clinical picture of adult respiratory distress syndrome (ARDS) can be precipitated by smoke injury, drowning, gastric aspiration, viral infections, fat embolism, surgical shock, sepsis, or direct trauma to the chest and lungs. The syndrome varies little with the underlying cause.

The two essential features of ARDS are hypoxia that is not relieved by oxygen inhalation and retention of carbon dioxide. Dyspnea, cyanosis, and circulatory collapse are prominent. At the onset, the patient is often also severely ill from the underlying cause of

the syndrome. Acute cardiopulmonary failure usually develops insidiously over 24–48 hours. Most patients require artificial ventilation with high pressures and high oxygen concentration to maintain levels of P_{O_2} and P_{CO_2} compatible with life in the presence of poorly compliant (stiff) lungs. The pulmonary circulation is inevitably compromised; the pulmonary vascular resistance is raised and the cardiac output low. Measurements by Swan-Ganz catheter show a normal or slightly raised ($<$ 12 mm Hg) wedge pressure. Surface tension-lowering agents containing phospholipids are being used in treatment of newborns with respiratory distress syndrome and, by analogy, show promise for treatment of ARDS.

2. CHRONIC COR PULMONALE

Chronic cor pulmonale is defined as heart *disease* (rather than heart *failure*) that is secondary to disease of the respiratory system, but right heart failure is often involved. Right ventricular enlargement secondary to chronic disease of the respiratory system is most commonly due to parenchymal lung diseases such as fibrosis, emphysema, or pneumonia. The clinical picture is little influenced by the underlying cause, which may be pulmonary granuloma, sarcoidosis, scleroderma, pneumoconiosis, or any form of fibrosis, including idiopathic lesions (Hamman-Rich disease) or repeated episodes of *Pneumocystis carinii* pneumonia in patients with AIDS. Usually, one of the recurrent episodes of pulmonary infection or bronchial obstruction leads to temporary increases in the load on the right heart and right heart failure. Any lesion producing alveolar hypoxia causes a vicious circle because of increased pulmonary arterial pressure due to pulmonary vasoconstriction. This mechanism is involved in alveolar hypoventilation due to weakness or paralysis of the respiratory muscles and also in central nervous system disease leading to inadequate pulmonary ventilation. Both can cause chronic cor pulmonale even when the lungs themselves are normal. Massive obesity, as in the Pickwickian syndrome, can also cause right heart failure; it is another cause of alveolar hypoventilation in which the lungs are normal. Chest wall disorders such as kyphosis and scoliosis may occasionally lead to heart failure but usually only when pulmonary infection is present. Arterial hypoxia increases cardiac output by causing systemic vasodilation and especially by increasing the heart rate. These factors tend to aggravate right heart failure. Since patients with chronic lung disease are often middle-aged and have smoked cigarettes for many years, associated atherosclerotic heart disease is common, and an element of left heart failure is frequently present in addition to right heart failure. Some feel that right heart failure can lead to left heart failure as the enlarging right ventricle inside a normal pericordial sac interferes with the filling of the left ventricle.

Clinical Findings

A. Symptoms: Dyspnea is the primary symptom in patients with chronic cor pulmonale. Coexisting pulmonary and cardiac disease may make it difficult to determine the cause of dyspnea. In the usual case of chronic cor pulmonale, dyspnea is most commonly due to the increased work of breathing resulting from the mechanical effects of the lung disease causing the right heart overload.

However, dyspnea is also seen in the rarest form of chronic cor pulmonale—primary pulmonary hypertension. In this condition, the mechanical properties of the lungs are normal, and some other explanation must be sought to explain the dyspnea. An inadequate systemic cardiac output is thought to cause alveolar hyperventilation, and excessive ventilation, especially during exercise, is thought to be responsible for the dyspnea. Edema of the ankles, abdominal swelling, and right upper quadrant pain due to hepatic congestion are often seen. Palpitations, weakness, syncope, and coldness of the hands and feet with Raynaud's phenomenon also occur in primary pulmonary hypertension.

B. Signs:

1. Noncardiac signs– Patients with arterial hypoxia due to bronchitis tend to exhibit hypervolemia

and vasodilatation rather than the vasoconstriction and low output state seen in patients with emphysema or primary pulmonary hypertension. Patients with chronic lung disease have been divided into "blue bloaters," in whom hypoxia, hypervolemia, recurrent bronchitis, and cor pulmonale are prominent, and "pink puffers," in whom hypoxia is absent, hypovolemia and emphysema are common, and cor pulmonale is rare. Cor pulmonale has also been classified as either hypoxic or pulmonary hypertensive, depending on whether a high output or a low output state predominates. Such generalizations are useful in delineating the different mechanisms involved but must not be taken as definitive, mutually exclusive categories.

Cyanosis and clubbing of the fingers are often seen. The cyanosis may be peripheral, due to the low cardiac output in patients with pulmonary hypertension, or central and associated with significant arterial hypoxemia ($Po_2 < 60$ mm Hg) and hypercapnia ($Pco_2 > 50$ mm Hg) in patients with chronic lung disease or alveolar hypoventilation. At times, elevation of right atrial pressure may blow open a patent foramen ovale and cause a right-to-left shunt at the atrial level. Clubbing of the fingers is most frequently seen in patients with chronic pulmonary infections or bronchial carcinoma. Tachycardia and a raised jugular venous pressure with *a* and *v* waves occur. Hepatomegaly, ascites, and edema of the ankles are seen if the patient is in right heart failure.

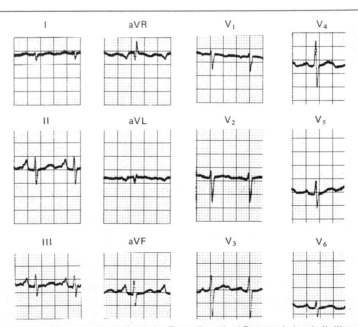

Figure 19–6. Pulmonary emphysema and cor pulmonale. The tall peaked P waves in leads II, III, and aVF are consistent with right atrial hypertrophy. There are small initial QRS forces to the left (r in lead I) with greater terminal forces to the right (S in I). These terminal forces are directed superiorly (S in II, III, and aVF). This is an example of the S_1, S_2, S_3 syndrome. The tracing is consistent with pulmonary emphysema. The prominent P waves are the only positive evidence of right heart overload. (Reproduced, with permission, from Goldschlager N, Goldman MJ: *Principles of Clinical Electrocardiography,* 13th ed. Appleton & Lange, 1989.)

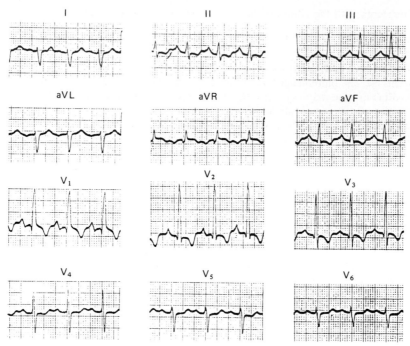

Figure 19–7. ECG from a patient with primary pulmonary hypertension, showing severe right ventricular hypertrophy. Note the monophasic tall R preceded by a small Q in V_1 and the small R and deep S in V_6. The P wave in V_1 is upright and directed anteriorly, indicating right atrial hypertrophy, and there is also right axis deviation with a deep S in lead I and a tall R in lead III.

2. Cardiac signs– Cardiac manifestations depend on the nature of the lung disease. In patients with emphysema, bronchitis, or bronchial obstruction, the cardiac impulse may be difficult to palpate because of overlying lung tissue. The sounds may be distant and murmurs absent. Conversely, in primary pulmonary hypertension, signs include a prominent right ventricular heave below the sternum, a loud pulmonary valve closure component of a closely split second heart sound and ejection click, and a short pulmonary systolic murmur, often with a pulmonary diastolic (Graham Steell) murmur due to pulmonary incompetence. Prominent right-sided S_4 and S_3 sounds, often increased with inspiration, can be heard. In later stages, a pansystolic high-pitched murmur of tricuspid incompetence is often easily detected.

C. Electrocardiographic Findings: Sinus rhythm is the rule, and the ECG shows evidence of right atrial or ventricular predominance. In patients with severe obstructive lung disease, right atrial hypertrophy may be all that is apparent. Electrocardiographic changes of right ventricular hypertrophy (Figure 19–6), like the physical signs, are sometimes masked. In patients with marked pulmonary hypertension, the reverse is true, and clear evidence of right ventricular hypertrophy, with P pulmonale, tall R waves, and ST depression with T wave inversion in the right-sided chest leads, is prominent, as shown in Figure 19–7 (Shah, 1992).

D. Imaging Studies: Enlargement of the main pulmonary artery is the most reliable radiologic indication of chronic cor pulmonale. The degree of cardiac enlargement, although obvious in serial radiograms, may be unimpressive, especially in emphysema. Right ventricular and right atrial enlargement are seen in primary pulmonary hypertension, as shown in Figure 19–8. Pulmonary congestion is not seen unless associated left-sided disease is present. In practice, many patients with chronic lung disease have associated left ventricular disease, and it may be difficult to ascertain how much damage has been done by cardiac disease and how much by pulmonary disease. Superimposed pulmonary congestion and intercurrent pulmonary infection further complicate the differentiation of the effects of heart disease from those of lung disease.

Echocardiography can be extremely helpful in assessing right and left ventricular function. Doppler echocardiography can detect pulmonary and tricuspid valvular regurgitant jets even in the absence of murmurs. By calculating the pressure gradient using the modified Bernoulli equation (gradient $= 4 \times$ jet velocity^2) and adding to it the estimated jugular venous pressure, an estimate of right ventricular and pulmonary arterial systolic pressure can be obtained. By

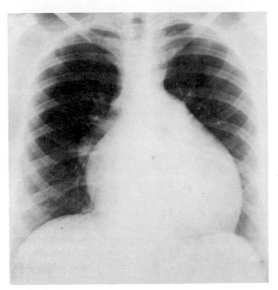

Figure 19–8. Chest x-ray cardiac enlargement, with prominence of the pulmonary artery, right atrium, and right ventricle, in a patient with primary pulmonary hypertension. The lung fields are abnormally translucent in association with reduced pulmonary blood flow.

injecting agitated saline as a contrast agent, the systolic jet of tricuspid insufficiency can be enhanced. Calculating the right-sided systolic pressure during exercise by echo-Doppler can reveal marked elevation in pulmonary arterial pressure when resting pressure is normal or only mildly elevated, indicating advanced disease and loss of pulmonary vascular reserve. In chronic cor pulmonale, the left ventricular volume and systolic function are usually normal. Mitral stenosis can also be ruled out. If echocardiography is unsatisfactory, a radioisotope study can demonstrate the absence of left ventricular dysfunction as well as dilation of the right ventricle with or without normal function.

E. Laboratory Findings: Polycythemia with hematocrit levels above 50% is usually present in hypoxic patients. Measurement of arterial blood gas tensions and pH is necessary in acutely ill patients in order to assess the severity of pulmonary failure. Right heart catheterization is indicated in patients with pulmonary hypertension in order to confirm the diagnosis by determining wedge pressure. Such investigations are extremely important, because lesions repairable by surgery, such as mitral stenosis and left atrial myxoma, can easily be overlooked during examination. With the development of echo-Doppler techniques, this is far less likely now than in the past. However, catheterization is frequently preferred to test the effect of oxygen and vasodilators on the pulmonary artery pressure and vascular resistance (see below).

Differential Diagnosis

Disorders to be differentiated from right heart failure due to lung disease include mitral stenosis, thromboembolic pulmonary hypertension, and pulmonary hypertension in association with congenital heart lesions (Eisenmenger's syndrome). The presence of right-to-left shunting causing arterial desaturation does not necessarily indicate congenital heart disease, since a foramen ovale can open up in chronic cor pulmonale when right atrial pressure rises above left atrial pressure. When coincidental pulmonary disease is present, the differential diagnosis can be extremely difficult. Cardiac catheterization is indicated when clear evidence of pulmonary hypertension is found. This diagnosis is suspected more commonly than it is proved, and clinical signs of right heart failure (palpable pulmonary arterial pulsation and loud pulmonary valve closure) tend to be unreliable signs of pulmonary hypertension.

Complications

Right heart failure is such an integral part of chronic cor pulmonale that it is hardly a complication. Similarly, pulmonary infection, pulmonary thrombosis, embolism, and alveolar hypoxia occur so frequently in the course of the disease that they are not really considered complications. Atrial arrhythmias—especially atrial flutter and multifocal atrial tachycardia—are relatively common in acute exacerbations of pulmonary infection, but chronic atrial fibrillation is rare. Pulmonary valvular incompetence causing an immediate diastolic (Graham Steell) murmur over the pulmonary artery is more a part of the disease than a complication. In severe pulmonary hypertension, chest pain similar to angina pectoris, arrhythmias, and syncope are described. Sudden death occurs, presumably due to ventricular arrhythmia. It is possible that right ventricular myocardial ischemia or fibrosis of the right ventricle is the cause.

Treatment

The prevention of heart failure is of the utmost importance in patients with lung disease. Prevention involves early and vigorous treatment of chest infections, vaccination against influenza, and avoidance of contact with persons who have upper respiratory tract infections. Cigarette smoking is extremely likely to have a serious effect on cardiopulmonary function in patients with cor pulmonale. Every effort should be made to persuade the patient to stop smoking.

The most important principles of therapy are to improve respiratory function, relieve arterial hypoxemia, reduce pulmonary hypertension, and improve right ventricular function.

The patient must first be treated vigorously and effectively for any intercurrent chest infection that is clearly present, or such infection must be carefully ruled out if there are no apparent symptoms. Relief of arterial hypoxia by oxygen therapy with a mask or nasal catheter as described in Chapter 7 is of great help. The dangers of oxygen therapy—abolition of the patient's hypoxic ventilatory drive and hypoventilation with serious CO_2 retention—have been exaggerated. Any tendency toward hypoventilation with oxygen should be remedied by the use of assisted or artificial ventilation via an endotracheal tube, with clearing of the air passages. Opinions differ about the indications for intensive artificial ventilation via an endotracheal tube, with clearing of the air passages. Opinions differ about the indications for intensive artificial ventilation in patients in pulmonary failure (which is defined as a Pco_2 level $>$ the Po_2 level). Tracheostomy and artificial ventilation with frequent endotracheal suction and fiberoptic bronchoscopy are readily performed in some centers.

The present trend is toward long-term intubation rather than tracheostomy. Improvements in the design of endotracheal tubes and low pressure cuff inflation have made it possible to continue intubation for as long as 2 or 3 months, with hoarseness as the only long-term complication. Intubation is less likely than tracheostomy to result in infection, hemorrhage, mediastinal emphysema, and tracheal stenosis.

The treatment of right heart failure with digitalis and diuretics is of secondary importance and is seldom effective as a sole treatment regimen. Digitalis has a reputation for ineffectiveness in patients with cor pulmonale, but there is no evidence that it is harmful except when excessive doses are administered in the hope of slowing the heart rate. In older patients in whom there is associated left ventricular disease, digitalis is often of value and should always be tried. Chronic anticoagulant therapy may be of value for patients with obvious thromboembolic complications. Such therapy is also used in patients with primary pulmonary hypertension but without evidence of benefit. The treatment of primary pulmonary hypertension is particularly unsatisfactory, and the patient develops increasingly severe right heart failure in spite of all measures, including corticosteroid therapy, which is often given as a last resort in the hope that some form of collagen disease is responsible for the pulmonary hypertension. Diazoxide in doses starting at 200 mg three times a day has been advocated. It can sharply reduce pulmonary vascular resistance and must be used with caution because it also lowers systemic vascular resistance. Calcium channel-blocking drugs in large doses, especially nifedipine (240 mg/d) and diltiazem (720 mg/d), have been successful in some cases in reducing pulmonary resistance, increasing cardiac output, and lowering pulmonary artery pressure. Resolution of right ventricular hypertrophy has been documented (Rich, 1987). In 64 patients with primary pulmonary hypertension treated with high-dose calcium channel-blocking agents, 17 (27%) responded with a decrease in pulmonary arterial pressure and pulmonary vascular resistance. After 5 years, 16 (94%) of the respond-

ing patients were still alive, compared with the 55% of those who did not respond (Rich, 1992). Care must be exercised in giving vasodilator drugs to patients with primary pulmonary hypertension, as fatalities have occurred during pharmacologic studies undertaken in the course of cardiac catheterization. Vasodilator drugs other than diazoxide have been tried (eg, hydralazine, phentolamine, isoproterenol) with varying results. Other agents such as indomethacin, epoprostenol (prostacyclin, PGI_2), and verapamil or nifedipine may also prove beneficial in some cases. Vasodilator drugs must be tested during right heart catheterization to find the drug that may result in decreased pulmonary artery pressure with no decrease or increase in cardiac output. This requires hospitalization with an indwelling balloon flotation catheter in the pulmonary artery—usually for several days, while each vasodilator is carefully tested. Corticosteroids may be of value in the treatment of chronic cor pulmonale associated with connective tissue disorders (eg, scleroderma), but they do not generally help patients who are in right heart failure.

End-stage pulmonary hypertension is becoming a prime indication for heart-lung transplantation. The patients are generally young, and the prognosis with conventional treatment is gloomy and reasonably predictable. The initial results are encouraging. By the end of 1991, over 1000 heart-lung transplants and over 500 single- or double-lung transplants had been reported. The 1- and 3-year survival figures are 65% and 55%, respectively (Kreitt, 1991). In a report of 96 single-lung transplants, there was a 75% 1-year survival rate (Yacoub, 1991). A major problem in lung transplantation is the integrity of the tracheal anastomosis, but this may be improved by bronchial artery revascularization. Immunosuppression is necessary, and chronic rejection is manifested by obliterative bronchiolitis, which occurs in 40–50% of recipients. The most important problems in lung transplantation are the short time ($<$ 6 hours) the lung can be kept after separation from the donor before transplantation and, of course, the shortage of donors.

Prognosis

Cor pulmonale is such a late manifestation of pulmonary disease that the prognosis is poor. Pulmonary reserve has been severely compromised by the time a patient develops either hypercapnia secondary to inadequate ventilation or right ventricular enlargement. The prognosis is best in patients who have a severe pulmonary infection but little or no chronic underlying lung disease. Because such patients cannot be positively identified until after the acute infection has been treated, intensive measures are indicated in emergency situations for patients who have not previously been under the care of a physician. The prognosis in primary pulmonary hypertension is poor. Death in 2-8 years is the rule. In 194 patients with primary pulmonary hypertension, the survival rate at

1 year was 68%; at 3 years, 48%; and at 5 years, 34%. The median survival time was 2.8 years (D'Alonzo, 1991). Patients with thromboembolic disease live longer because favorable factors such as lysis and organization of thrombi may influence the clinical picture.

The prognosis in patients with pulmonary hypertension who develop the disease while taking birth control pills is better than in those in whom this possible etiologic factor is absent, since stopping oral contraceptives may prevent further progress of the disease and improve the prognosis.

DIFFERENTIATION OF HEART DISEASE & LUNG DISEASE

Lung disease and heart disease often coexist. The harmful effects of cigarette smoking predispose to chronic bronchitis and emphysema and also to carcinoma of the bronchus. They also increase the risk of premature coronary artery disease. In consequence, many patients suffer from both cardiac and pulmonary disease, and the 2 compound each other. Whereas the distinction between pure lung disease and pure heart disease is relatively easy, separating the pulmonary and cardiac elements in mixed lesions is extremely difficult.

Clinical Findings Common to Both Lung & Heart Disease

A. Symptoms: Dyspnea is an important symptom in both heart and lung disease. The dyspnea of lung disease tends to be episodic, being worse at some times than others. It is not infrequently present at rest, when attacks of asthma, bronchospasm, or acute bronchitis occur. It may also be worse on exercise, especially when asthma or bronchospasm is induced by effort. The dyspnea of emphysema produces a basic, permanent, irreversible level of dyspnea. Although the patient's dyspnea may be worse at times, it never remits completely. It is thus important in obtaining a history of dyspnea to find out how much the patient's breathlessness varies from day to day and to concentrate on the level of dyspnea on the patient's 'best day." If significant emphysema is present, dyspnea will be present even on the 'best day." Conversely, if the patient has a normal exercise tolerance on the best day, then emphysema is less likely.

Chest pain occurs in both heart and lung disease. The patient with lung disease complains of a tight constricting feeling across the chest on exertion or at rest when bronchitis or bronchospasm is present. This can usually be distinguished from anginal pain, because it usually neither radiates like angina nor is so quantitatively related to exertion. As previously stated, typical angina pectoris can be seen in patients with severe pulmonary hypertension. Pleural pain suggests lung disease but can occur in heart disease

when pulmonary embolism leads to pulmonary infarction.

Cough occurs both in heart disease and lung disease. Its presence is much more common in lung disease, but pulmonary congestion secondary to raised left atrial pressure can also cause cough. The cough in heart disease is dry and unproductive unless pulmonary edema develops, when profuse watery, frothy sputum occurs. The cough of pulmonary congestion often comes on with exercise. Cough with purulent, mucopurulent, rusty, or tenacious sputum is indicative of lung disease. Hemoptysis occurs in both heart and lung disease, and its presence is not often of value in distinguishing heart and lung disease.

B. Signs: In comparison with symptoms, there is much less overlap in physical signs between heart and lung disease. Pleural friction rubs and rales and rhonchi can occur in both. The pulmonary signs associated with pulmonary congestion and edema can be mistaken for those of asthma or bronchospasm, but 'cardiac asthma" is not often confused with asthma or bronchitis, because of the history of previous attacks in asthma and the presence of obvious signs of mitral or left ventricular disease in patients with pulmonary congestion.

C. Electrocardiographic Findings: The ECG is particularly helpful in distinguishing between heart and lung disease in cigarette smokers. The presence of evidence of left ventricular predominance with ST–T wave changes in the left-sided leads indicates that there is some heart disease. Atrial arrhythmias occur in both varieties of disease, but chronic atrial fibrillation is more common in heart disease.

D. Imaging Studies: Cardiac enlargement is difficult to interpret. The heart is often smaller than normal in patients with emphysema, and hearts of apparently normal size may in fact be enlarged for those particular patients.

E. Special Investigations: One of the principal uses of pulmonary function tests is to distinguish between heart and lung disease. Whereas the vital capacity is reduced in patients with pulmonary congestion, the maximum expiratory flow rates are relatively normal, and the flow-volume curves do not indicate significant obstruction. The percentage of the vital capacity expelled in the first second is greater than 70 in heart disease but is less than 70 in patients with significant obstruction due to lung disease. In difficult cases, the measurements of lung compliance, lung and airway resistance , and lung volume may be required to detect the large lung volumes, high resistance, and normal or increased compliance in emphysema. The variation in the values of compliance and resistance with the respiratory rate, characteristic of chronic lung disease, is also helpful in diagnosis. Air trapping on expiration and large closing volumes are also characteristic of obstructive lung disease.

Arterial blood gas measurements should be made if there is any doubt. The hypoxia and hypercapnia (PO_2

< 70 mm Hg, Pco_2 > 45 mm Hg) often seen in lung disease are rare in heart disease except when pulmonary edema is present. Echocardiography and radioisotope multiple-gated scanning can frequently reveal abnormalities in left ventricular volume or systolic function indicating left ventricular disease. In difficult cases, cardiac catheterization with measurement of pulmonary vascular resistance and full pulmonary function studies are likely to be needed to separate the effects of lung disease from those of heart disease.

REFERENCES

Bell WR, Simon TL: Current status of pulmonary thromboembolic disease: Pathophysiology, diagnosis, prevention, and treatment. Am Heart J 1982:103:239.

Carson JL et al: The clinical course of pulmonary embolism. N Engl J Med 1992;326:1240.

Cheely R et al: The role of noninvasive tests versus pulmonary angiography in the diagnosis of pulmonary embolism. Am J Med 1981;70:17.

Daily PO et al: Risk factors for pulmonary thromboendarterectomy. J Thorac Cardiovasc Surg 1990;49:670.

Dalla-Volta S et al: PAIMS 2: Alteplase combined with heparin versus heparin in the treatment of acute pulmonary embolism. Plasminogen activator Italian multicenter study 2. J Am Coll Cardiol 1992;20:520.

D'Alonzo GE et al: Survival in patients with primary pulmonary hypertension. Ann Intern Med 1991;115:343.

Dawkins KD et al: Long-term results, hemodynamics, and complications after combined heart and lung transplantation. Circulation 1985;71:919.

Essop MR et al: Simultaneous mechanical clot fragmentation and pharmacologic thrombolysis in acute massive pulmonary embolism. Am J Cardiol 1992;69:427.

Feitelberg SP et al: Transfemoral embolectomy for massive pulmonary embolism and associated myocardial infarction. Am Heart J 1987;113:819.

Flick MR, Murray JF: High-dose corticosteroid therapy in the adult respiratory distress syndrome. JAMA 1984;251;1054.

Fowler AA et al: Attack-rates and mortality of the adult respiratory distress syndrome in patients with known predispositions. (Abstract.) Am Rev Respir Dis 1983; 125 (4):77.

Goldhaber SZ: Thrombolysis for pulmonary embolism. Prog Cardiovasc Dis 1991;34:113.

Goldhaber SZ et al: Recombinant tissue-type plasminogen activator versus a novel dosing regimen of urokinase in acute pulmonary embolism: A randomized controlled multicenter trial. J Am Coll Cardiol 1992;20:24.

Grassi CJ, Goldhaber SZ: Interruption of the inferior vena cava for prevention of pulmonary embolism: Transvenous filter devices. Herz 1989;14:182.

Gray HH et al: Pulmonary embolectomy for acute massive pulmonary embolism: An analysis of 71 cases. Br Heart J 1988;60:196.

Hall RJC et al: Subacute massive pulmonary embolism. Br Heart J 1981;45;681.

Harris P, Heath D: *The Human Pulmonary Circulation*, 3rd ed. Churchill Livingstone, 1986.

Heijbeer H et al: Deficiencies of coagulation: Embolism and fibrinolytic problems in outpatients with venous thrombosis. N Engl J Med 1990;323:1572.

Kelley MA et al: Diagnosing pulmonary embolism: New tests and strategies. Ann Intern Med 1991;114:300.

Kreitt JM, Kaye MP: The registry of the International Society for Heart and Lung Transplantation: Eighth Official Report. J Heart Lung Transpl 1991;10:491.

Mahmoud AA: Schistosomiasis. N Engl J Med 1977;297:1329.

McGoon MD, Edwards WD: Primary pulmonary hypertension: Current status. Mod Concept Cardiovasc Dis 1985;545:29.

Meyer G et al: Effects of intravenous urokinase versus alteplase on total pulmonary resistance in acute massive pulmonary embolism: A European multicenter double-blind trial. J Am Coll Cardiol 1992;19:239.

Moser KM et al: Chronic major-vessel thromboembolic pulmonary hypertension. Circulation 1990;81:1735.

Moser KM et al: Thromboendarterectomy for chronic, major-vessel thromboembolic pulmonary hypertension: Immediate and long-term results in 42 patients. Ann Intern Med 1987;107:560.

NIH Consensus Development Statement: Prevention of venous thrombosis and pulmonary embolism. JAMA 1986;256:744.

Overton DT, Bocka JJ: The alveolar-arterial oxygen gradient in patients with documented pulmonary embolism. Ann Intern Med 1988;148:1617.

Packer M: Vasodilator therapy for primary pulmonary hypertension: Limitations and hazards. Ann Intern Med 1985;103:258.

Petty TL, Fowler AA III: Another look at ARDS. Chest 1982;82:98.

PIOPED Investigators: Value of the ventilation/perfusion scan in acute pulmonary embolism. JAMA 1990;263:2753.

Rozkovec A, Montanes P, Oakley CM: Factors that influence the outcome of primary pulmonary hypertension. Br Heart J 1986;55:449.

Rich S: Primary pulmonary hypertension. Prog Cardiovasc Dis 1988;31:205.

Rich S, Brundage BH: High-dose calcium channel-blocking therapy for primary pulmonary hypertension: Evidence of long-term reduction in pulmonary arterial pressure and regression of right ventricular hypertrophy. Circulation 1987;76:135.

Rich S et al: The effect of high doses of calcium-channel blockers on survival in primary pulmonary hypertension. N Engl J Med 1992;327:76.

Rosenow EC III, Osmundson PJ, Brown ML: Pulmonary embolism. Mayo Clin Proc 1981;56:161.

Rosove MH, Brewer PM: Antiphospholipid thrombosis: Clinical course after the first thrombotic event in 70 patients. Ann Intern Med 1992;117:303.

Schrader BJ et al: Comparison of the effects of adenosine

and nifedipine in pulmonary hypertension. J Am Coll Cardiol 1992;19:1060.

Shah NS et al: Electrocardiographic patterns of restrictive pulmonary disease and comparison with those of obstructive pulmonary disease. Am J Cardiol 1992;70:394.

Stein PD, Willis PW III, DeMets DL: History and physical examination in acute pulmonary embolism in patients without preexisting cardiac or pulmonary disease. Am J Cardiol 1981;47:218.

Stein PD et al: Complications and validity of pulmonary angiography in acute pulmonary embolism. Circulation 1992;85:462.

Stein PD et al: Mechanical disruption of pulmonary thromboemboli in dogs with a flexible rotating-tip catheter (Kensey catheter). Chest 1990;98:994.

Uren NG et al: Response of the pulmonary circulation to acetylcholine, calcitonin, gene-related peptide, substance P, and oral nicardipine in patients with primary pulmonary hypertension. J Am Coll Cardiol 1992;19: 835.

Weisman IM, Rinaldo JE, Rogers RM: Positive end-expiratory pressure in adult respiratory failure. N Engl J Med 1982;307:1381.

Yacoub M et al: Single lung transplantation for obstructive airways disease. Transpl Proc 1991;23:1213.

Diseases of the Aorta & Systemic Arteries

20

The diseases discussed in this chapter include aneurysm of the abdominal aorta, syphilitic aortitis and aneurysm, arteritis involving arteries of different sizes, systemic embolism, and systemic arteriovenous fistula. Arteritis and systemic embolism occur in a wide variety of diseases, and the accounts in this chapter deal mainly with the cardiologic aspects. Aortic dissection is considered a complication of systemic hypertension (see Chapter 9).

ANEURYSM OF THE ABDOMINAL AORTA

Ninety percent of aneurysms of the abdominal aorta are atherosclerotic in origin and arise below the takeoff of the renal arteries. The aneurysms are usually fusiform and may involve the aortic bifurcation.

Abdominal aortic aneurysm occurs most frequently in elderly men with hypertension, coronary artery disease, or peripheral vascular disease. In these high-risk groups, the diagnosis of abdominal aortic aneurysm can usually be suspected by finding a pulsatile and expansile mass on physical examination if the patient is of normal weight or is thin. If the patient is obese, the presence of an abdominal aortic aneurysm can be missed at least half the time. In this group, screening with abdominal ultrasound for the presence of an aneurysm is important.

Clinical Findings

A. Symptoms: Most patients are symptom-free when the aneurysm is discovered. The patient may be aware of a painless, throbbing mass in the mid abdomen. Pain is the most important presenting symptom. It may be felt in the back or in the anterior abdomen. Intermittent claudication can occur due to peripheral vascular involvement or embolism from thrombotic lesions in the aneurysm. Pain may be episodic and associated with expansion or dissection within the wall of the lesion. Rupture occurs late in the course of the condition. Severe abdominal pain of sudden onset is the usual manifestation, and rupture usually causes hemorrhage into the retroperitoneal tissues. Circulatory collapse and shock almost inevitably follow rupture, but there may be a short period of relatively good circulatory function early after rupture.

B. Signs: A diffuse, pulsating, mid-abdominal mass

is the most important physical finding. The exact size of the aneurysm is difficult to determine on physical examination. After rupture, the abdomen is extremely tender, and extravasation of blood may lead to ecchymosis in the flank or groin.

C. Electrocardiographic Findings: The ECG shows no specific findings. It may show changes due to associated coronary disease or hypertension.

D. Imaging Studies: Calcification in the wall of the aneurysm shown on x-ray is common and helps to delineate the size of the lesion. A lateral abdominal x-ray is most helpful in demonstrating the presence of calcification of the abdominal aorta. Ultrasonography (Figure 20–1), CT scan, and MRI can all help to determine the size of the aneurysm, eliminating the need for aortography.

Complications

Renal perfusion is likely to be compromised. Ischemia of the lower bowel or lower extremities may occur, as blood supply to these areas may be reduced. Distal emboli to the extremities arise from the mural thrombi which are commonly found in patients with abdominal aortic aneurysms. The incidence of myocardial infarction is high in older men.

Treatment

The size and rate of expansion of the aneurysm determine the form of treatment. Small aneurysms (< 6 cm in diameter) in asymptomatic patients should be followed, especially if there is associated cardiac, cerebral, renal, or peripheral vascular disease that makes the patient a poor risk for surgery. Follow-up should be done using ultrasonography. In the asymptomatic patient with a small aneurysm, this can be done every year. As the aneurysm approaches 5 cm in diameter, the examination should be repeated every 4–6 months. Surgical excision and grafting of the resulting defect is recommended for aneurysms 6 cm or more in diameter, in symptomatic patients and in those in whom the aneurysm is known to have increased in size recently. Surgery is mandatory if rupture has occurred. If carried out early, it is often successful; if delayed, the mortality rate increases. Without operation, rupture is fatal.

Prognosis

The mortality following surgery before rupture occurs is about 5%. Once rupture has occurred, the

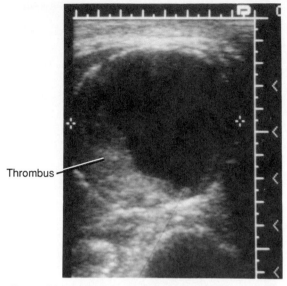

Figure 20–1. Ultrasound of abdomen showing a 6-cm abdominal aneurysm with thrombus.

Thrombus

mortality rate at surgery exceeds 50%. The 5-year survival rate after diagnosis is over 50%, and myocardial infarction is the commonest cause of death.

SYPHILITIC CARDIOVASCULAR DISEASE

Pathology

The basic lesion in the tertiary form of syphilis that affects the cardiovascular system is endarteritis obliterans. The primary site of disease is the thoracic aorta, and endarteritis of the vasa vasorum weakens the media and causes swelling and scarring of the intima, giving rise to the characteristic "crow's foot" or "tree bark" markings seen at autopsy. The changes in the intima can narrow the ostia of the coronary vessels and also affect the aortic valve commissures. The weakening of the media leads to dilation of the aorta that, in addition to causing fusiform or saccular aneurysms in the thoracic aorta, leads to aortic valve ring dilation, commissural separation, and progressive aortic incompetence.

Clinical Findings

Syphilitic heart disease has become much rarer in the past 50 years since effective treatment of primary syphilis has been widely available. When it does occur, the disease is less florid, and instead of causing symptoms in persons 40–60 years of age, cardiovascular syphilis now affects older persons. Consequently, atherosclerotic lesions almost always coexist with syphilitic lesions. Atherosclerotic aneurysms are described in Chapter 9. In contrast to syphilitic aneurysms, they are usually fusiform rather than saccular

and are much more likely to involve the descending aorta. Syphilitic aneurysms of the thoracic aorta act as space-occupying, expanding, cardiovascular "tumors" that compress and erode surrounding structures. They occur more commonly in men by a factor of 3:1. Their clinical manifestations vary with the site of the aneurysm. Aneurysms of the ascending aorta classically produce physical signs; aneurysms of the arch of the aorta cause symptoms; and aneurysms of the descending aorta cause pain or are asymptomatic.

A. Symptoms: Symptoms appear late in cardiovascular syphilis, and significant abnormalities may be found in asymptomatic patients. The latent period after the initial infection is usually 10–25 years but may be as long as 40 years. Pain in the chest is the most important symptom of aortic aneurysm. In descending thoracic aortic lesions, pain is caused by erosion of the vertebral column, and it is constant, boring, severe, and worse at night. Ascending aortic lesions involving coronary ostia may cause angina pectoris, with pain at rest or during exercise. The angina occurs as the result of interference with coronary blood flow. Ascending aortic lesions may occur with or without aortic incompetence. Pain may also arise from aortic lesions that do not involve the coronary vessels; this pain is attributed to stretching of aortic tissue. The symptoms associated with aneurysms of the arch of the aorta stem from pressure on surrounding structures and include cough due to pressure on the trachea or left bronchus, hoarseness due to pressure on the left recurrent laryngeal nerve, dysphagia due to pressure on the esophagus, swelling of the neck and face due to superior vena caval compression, left-sided cervical venous dilation due to obstruction of the left innominate vein, and hemoptysis. This last manifestation may be the final symptom when the aneurysm ruptures into the bronchial tree.

B. Signs: The signs of aortic aneurysm may be attributable to the lesion, as in visible or palpable pulsation localized to the right of the sternum, which is more specific than the pulsation in the suprasternal notch seen with minor aortic dilation. Signs caused indirectly by involvement of neighboring structures include the wide pulse pressure and water-hammer pulse of aortic incompetence, jugular venous distention and facial edema due to superior vena caval obstruction, Horner's syndrome (enophthalmos, miosis, and ptosis) due to sympathetic nerve compression, and tracheal tug. This latter sign is elicited by standing behind the patient and pulling the larynx upward; the "tug" of the aneurysm pulls the cervical structures down with each heartbeat. Cardiac enlargement, which is often massive, results from aortic incompetence. The high pitched diastolic murmur of aortic incompetence is heard to the right of the sternum and typically is louder in the third interspace to the right of the sternum, compared with the left of the sternum. This right parasternal radiation of the murmur is typical for that associated with a dilated aortic root,

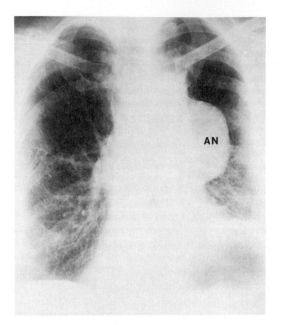

Figure 20–2. Chest x-ray showing a syphilitic aneurysm of the arch of the aorta (AN).

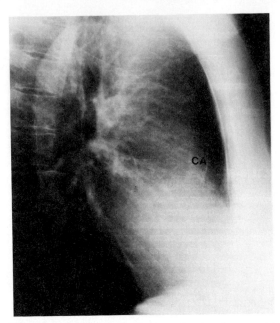

Figure 20–3. Lateral chest x-ray showing linear calcification (CA) of the ascending aorta in a patient with syphilitic aortitis

compared with the murmur of aortic regurgitation due to aortic valvular disease. The aortic valve closure sound is often high-pitched and has a tambour musical quality even in the absence of an aneurysm or aortic incompetence, possibly due to stretching and tensing of the aortic cusps. Aortic systolic murmurs are commonly heard, both with and without aortic incompetence, and they should not be taken as evidence of aortic stenosis. Signs of left ventricular failure may be present in patients with severe aortic incompetence. Associated neurologic signs of central nervous system syphilis are common and help point out the syphilitic cause of the aortic aneurysm.

C. Electrocardiographic Findings: There are no specific syphilitic changes on the ECG. Left ventricular hypertrophy occurs in response to aortic incompetence. Left bundle branch block and ischemic ST and T wave changes can occur in older persons.

D. Imaging Studies: Aortic dilation is often visible in patients with aortitis without aneurysm formation. Aortic aneurysms give rise to abnormal shadows on the chest x-ray that vary enormously from case to case. An example of an aneurysm of the arch of the aorta is shown in Figure 20–2. To distinguish between aneurysms and other tumors is difficult. Transmitted pulsations are not readily distinguished from the direct expansile pulsation of an aneurysm. Lack of pulsation does not exclude the possibility of an aneurysm, because thrombus formation may obliterate the cavity and leave a solid tumor. Calcification should be sought in the wall at the origin of the ascending aorta, where it is virtually pathognomonic of a syphilitic lesion, though thin calcification of the

ascending aorta has been described in other aortic diseases such as Takayasu's disease. Calcification in the aortic arch and knuckle is much more common and is indicative of atherosclerosis. Syphilitic calcification is thin, beaded, and eggshell-like. It is usually seen best on the left anterior oblique or lateral view, as shown in Figure 20–3. When the descending aorta is involved, erosion of the thoracic vertebral column should be sought on the lateral view. Syphilis virtually never involves the abdominal aorta.

Echocardiography—especially transesophageal echocardiography—may help in the diagnosis. CT scan with contrast and MRI are excellent for demonstrating the presence and extent of aortic aneurysms. Angiography may be needed to precisely define which vessels of the aorta are involved or to evaluate the presence and extent of coronary arterial involvement; the procedure is generally well tolerated.

E. Laboratory Findings: Positive routine serologic tests for syphilis (Wasserman, Kahn, VDRL), either past or present, are most helpful in the diagnosis, but negative tests, which can be negative in 15–30% of patients, do not exclude the possibility of syphilitic disease any more than a positive test indicates that a given lesion is syphilitic. Serologic tests identifying a specific treponemal antigen such as the *Treponema pallidum* immobilization test (TPI) or the fluorescent treponemal antibody absorption test (FTA-ABS) are almost always positive. An elevated blood sedimentation rate is almost always seen when syphilitic cardiovascular disease is active and untreated. The possibility of associated neurosyphilis should not be overlooked. Lumbar puncture should be performed in order to detect cerebrospinal fluid abnormalities associated with tertiary syphilis, tabes, or general paresis.

Differential Diagnosis

The differential diagnosis of syphilitic lesions is often difficult. Syphilitic aneurysms can be confused with intrathoracic tumors and cysts, and their syphilitic origin cannot always be proved. Atherosclerotic aneurysms can also occur; these are more likely to dissect than syphilitic aneurysms. Although positive serologic tests are of great value, they do not always indicate the true cause of the lesion. Furthermore, mixed lesions also occur.

Treatment

If syphilitic disease is active or progressive and especially if serologic tests are positive, antisyphilitic treatment with penicillin is indicated before any surgical measures are undertaken. Penicillin treatment for syphilitic cardiovascular disease should be undertaken in the hospital, if possible, because of the possibility of a Jarisch-Herxheimer reaction. This involves a sudden acute allergic response attributed to massive death of spirochetes. It causes swelling of the aortic endothelium and may occlude the coronary ostia. Initial treatment should use a small (10,000 units) test dose of penicillin combined with corticosteroids (eg, prednisone, 10–20 mg every 6 hours) for the first few doses. The treatment of choice for cardiovascular syphilis is benzathine penicillin G, 7.2 million units total, divided into weekly doses of 2.4 million units by intramuscular injection for 3 successive weeks. Alternative treatment consists of aqueous procaine penicillin G, 9 million units total, administered as 600,000 units a day by intramuscular injection for 15 days. In patients who are allergic to penicillin, doxycycline, 200 mg orally twice daily for 21 days, or tetracycline, 500 mg orally four times a day for 30 days, is recommended, or erythromycin, 500 mg orally four times a day for 30 days. Although antibiotic treatment of syphilis is mandatory, there is no evidence that treatment alters the progression of aortic aneurysm formation or aortic regurgitation.

Surgical resection of syphilitic aneurysms and aortic valve replacement for aortic incompetence should always be considered. Direct surgery for ostial coronary lesions may be necessary. If the patient is asymptomatic and the disease shows no evidence of progression, the patient's progress should be monitored. The results of valve replacement in syphilitic lesions are similar to those obtained in operation on lesions due to other causes. The aorta in patients with syphilis holds sutures securely, and the tissues tend to be less friable than in Marfan's syndrome.

Complications

Almost all of the manifestations of syphilitic cardiovascular disease can be regarded as complications,

since endarteritis obliterans of the vasa vasorum, which is the basic lesion, has no direct effects, and expansion of the aorta is a secondary effect. Rupture of the aorta into any hollow thoracic structure is a late complication that is inevitably fatal. Thrombosis in association with stasis is common, but secondary embolism is rarer than in atherosclerotic lesions. Cardiac arrhythmias, complete atrioventricular block, infective endocarditis, and acute aortic dissection seldom occur. It should be remembered that the primary lesion is aortic and that cardiac involvement is almost always secondary, although gummatous myocarditis may be seen at autopsy.

Prognosis

The prognosis in syphilitic cardiovascular disease has greatly improved with better treatment of primary and secondary syphilis. Inadequately treated patients rather than untreated ones form the majority of cases. In partially arrested syphilitic disease, the patient develops a lesion in later life that progresses more slowly and carries a better prognosis. When the aortic valve is diseased, with significant aortic incompetence, the prognosis is worse. It is also worse when the aortic arch is involved in aneurysm formation because of the large number of vital structures that can be readily affected. The cause of death in patients with cardiovascular syphilis is now usually atherosclerotic in origin, and death in middle age (age 40–60) is rare.

ARTERITIS

Arteries of various sizes may be involved in an inflammatory process that can be either idiopathic or part of some generalized systemic disease.

Classification

A clinical classification of the various vasculitis syndromes is presented in Table 20–1. The three types of lesions that produce arteritis as their main manifestation are temporal arteritis, aortic arch arteritis (Takayasu's disease), and polyarteritis nodosa. In the other diseases, either the other manifestations predominate or the arteritis is a pathologic feature found on histologic examination.

A. Temporal Arteritis: The term "temporal arteritis"—other terms are granulomatous arteritis and giant cell arteritis—is not specific but refers to a form of arteritis that is usually associated with giant cell formation and involves the cranial arteries of older persons, usually Caucasian women in the age group from 65 to 75. Although the temporal arteries are a readily accessible site of lesions, their involvement is not inevitable, and the clinical picture overlaps that of Takayasu's disease.

B. Takayasu's Disease: Takayasu's disease ("pulseless disease") is a form of arteritis that classi-

Table 20–1. Clinical classification of vasculitis syndromes, indicating the wide variety of conditions in which the syndromes may occur.[1]

Usually characterized by necrotizing vasculitis
Temporal arteritis
Wagener's granulomatosis
Aortic arch aortitis
Henoch-Schönlein purpura
"Classic" polyarteritis nodosa

Occasionally complicated by necrotizing vasculitis
Rheumatic diseases
Rheumatoid arthritis
Systemic lupus erythematosus
Dermatomyositis
Ankylosing spondylitis
Rheumatic fever
Infections
Hepatitis B
Acute respiratory infections
Streptococcal infections
Poststreptococcal glomerulonephritis
Infective endocarditis
Respiratory diseases
Löffler's syndrome
Asthma
Serous otitis media
Hypersensitivity
Serum sickness
Drug allergy
Amphetamine abuse
Paraproteinemias
Essential cryoglobulinemia
Multiple myeloma
Macroglobulinemia
Others
Dermal vasculitis
Ulcerative colitis
Cogan's syndrome
Colon carcinoma

[1] Modified and reproduced, with permission, from Christian CL, Sergent JS: Vasculitis syndromes: Clinical and experimental models. Am J Med 1976;61:385.

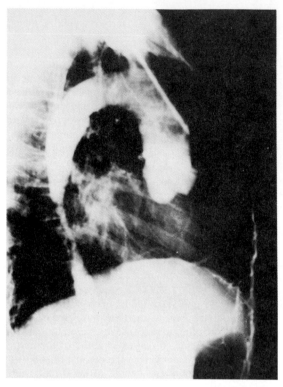

Figure 20–4. Aortogram showing narrowing of the descending aorta due to Takayasu's disease in a child. (Courtesy of Dai Ru-ping.)

cally affects the aorta and its major branches, especially those leading to the head and upper limbs in young Oriental women. In some cases other vessels such as the descending aorta, renal arteries, and even pulmonary arteries may be involved (Figure 20–4). Four types of Takayasu's disease have been described. Type I involves the aortic arch and its branches; type II involves chiefly the thoracic abdominal aorta and its branches; type III combines features of both type I and type II; and type IV involves the pulmonary arteries. In our experience, types I and III are most common. The cause is unknown, and although specific pathogens such as tuberculosis and syphilis have been suggested, the probable cause is an autoimmune response, perhaps to a number of different antigens. Giant cell formation may be seen histologically, and smaller arteries can also be involved. Occlusion of major vessels, at times with thrombosis, accounts for the major manifestations. After several major aortic branches have been occluded, the proximal pressure in the remaining vessels rises, because the heart

pumps into a restricted vascular bed. If the descending aorta or renal arteries are involved, renal hypertension can develop through the renin-angiotensin system. This leads to cardiac hypertrophy and ultimately to left ventricular failure.

C. Polyarteritis Nodosa: Polyarteritis nodosa is a multisystem disease of unknown cause that is usually considered one of the connective tissue disorders but is primarily a diffuse necrotizing vasculitis with aneurysm formation involving the muscular arteries, adjacent veins, and occasionally smaller vessels throughout the body. Diffuse vasculitis may occur as a variant of polyarteritis nodosa. James (1977) has noted that small coronary arteries varying from 0.1 to 1 mm in diameter may be involved, producing angina pectoris, myocardial infarction, and left ventricular failure with ventricular arrhythmias. The lesions in polyarteritis nodosa can occur anywhere in the body. The kidney, heart, gastrointestinal tract, lungs, and central nervous system are commonly affected. Most patients are hypertensive. Because of the variability of the site and severity of the individual lesions, the clinical features can mimic almost any disease.

D. Kawasaki Disease: Kawasaki disease, or mucocutaneous lymph node syndrome, is an inflammatory disease of unknown cause affecting children, usually at an early age, and manifested by fever and ocular and oral inflammation, followed by a polymorphous exanthem and edema and erythema of the palms and feet, and finally by cutaneous desquamation. There is multiple organ involvement, with arthritis, pulmonary infiltration, hepatitis, and cervical adenopathy. Cardiovascular system manifestations include myocarditis, coronary arteritis with aneurysm formation and occlusion, and pericarditis, causing the 1–3% mortality rate associated with this disease. The coronary aneurysms that are present in 20–40% of patients can be visualized by two-dimensional echocardiography or arteriography; it has been documented by angiography 1 or 2 years later that the aneurysms resolve in about half the patients.

Treatment is unsatisfactory. High-dose aspirin (50–100 mg/kg/d) is recommended during the acute illness. Later, low-dose aspirin (3–5 mg/kg/d) is recommended indefinitely to prevent platelet aggregation in patients with coronary aneurysm. Corticosteroids may actually be harmful and should not be used during the acute illness. Intravenous gamma globulin in high doses (400 mg/kg/d for 4 days) administered during the acute illness has been most impressive in reducing coronary arterial involvement.

Whether we will see the coronary residuals of this disease in adults is as yet unclear.

E. Other Arteritis Syndromes: Other arteritis syndromes manifested by joint involvement of the aortic root and ascending aorta include Reiter's syndrome, ankylosing spondylitis, psoriatic arthritis, relapsing polychondritis, and ulcerative colitis. The pathologic picture consists of inflammatory infiltration of the aortic wall, subendothelial fibrosis, and dilation of the aortic root. The usual clinical presentation is that of aortic regurgitation in the clinical setting of the underlying disease.

F. Other Forms of Diffuse Vasculitis With Cardiovascular Complications:

1. Churg-Strauss vasculitis (allergic granulomatosis) is similar to polyarteritis nodosa except that there are granulomas with giant cells and eosinophilia. Asthma is a prominent feature, as is a striking peripheral eosinophilia. Pericarditis, myocardial infarction, and myocarditis with failure are seen.

2. Behçet's syndrome is characterized by a diffuse vasculitis and clinically by oral and genital ulcerations and uveitis. Pericarditis, aortic and mitral valvular regurgitation, right ventricular endomyocardial fibrosis, and arterial aneurysms can be seen.

3. Wegener's granulomatosis is distinguished by necrotizing granulomas that cause destructive ulcerations in the upper respiratory tract, including the paranasal sinuses, the nasopharynx, the middle ear, and the bronchi. Inflammatory changes occur in smaller vessels such as the pulmonary artery branches and the renal arteries. The cardiovascular manifestations may consist of high-degree atrioventricular block and pericarditis. Especially important are the dramatic remissions seen with cyclophosphamide therapy.

4. Hypersensitivity (leukocytoblastic) vasculitis is the commonest form of immune complex disease. Antigen-antibody complexes are present in all lesions and are similar to those seen in infective endocarditis or lupus erythematosus. Pericarditis is the commonest cardiovascular manifestation.

Clinical Findings

A. Symptoms: The symptoms of arteritis vary widely with the site of the lesion. In temporal arteritis, the principal presenting symptom is headache with a throbbing swelling over the affected artery. Pain on mastication (jaw claudication), fever, malaise, visual disturbance—blurring of vision or even sudden blindness—or neurologic disturbances are commonly seen. In other cases, the disease is more general, and arthralgia, abdominal pain, or chest pain may be the presenting symptom. In Takayasu's disease, the effects of sudden occlusion of a major vessel may be the first manifestation, eg, limb pain, hemiplegia, or sudden blindness. The presenting symptoms of polyarteritis nodosa are extremely variable.

B. Signs: The signs of arteritis, like the symptoms, vary widely. Loss of the pulse of a major vessel and a bruit over a vessel are the commonest signs, and systemic hypertension, which may be secondary to renal ischemia, is also a prominent feature. Systemic hypertension is very common in polyarteritis nodosa; in consequence, cardiac enlargement, fundal changes, and proteinuria are often seen. The age of the patient varies in the different forms of arteritis. Temporal arteritis commonly occurs in women over age 65, whereas Takayasu's disease is most frequently seen in women 20-30 years of age. Polyarteritis nodosa is more common in men than in women and occurs at any age.

C. Electrocardiographic Findings: Electrocardiographic changes resulting from hypertension with left ventricular hypertrophy and ST-T wave changes, may be seen. In some cases, actual myocardial infarction occurs, with consequent changes on the ECG.

D. Imaging Studies: The heart is not infrequently enlarged on x-ray, and signs of pulmonary congestion or infarction may develop. In difficult cases, help can sometimes be obtained from selective angiography. For example, mesenteric angiography may demonstrate multiple small aneurysms on the arteries to the gut. In Takayasu's disease, aortography is extremely helpful in demonstrating the extent of involvement of the aorta and its branches and the pulmonary arteries. Because the involvement is segmental, there are areas of stenosis, other areas that are aneurysmal, and still others that are normal.

E. Laboratory Findings: Leukocytosis, perhaps with eosinophilia, is not uncommon. The sedimentation rate is raised, and tests of renal function often show impairment. Biopsy of an early accessible lesion constitutes the most important means of establishing the diagnosis, and if giant cell arteritis is suspected it is worthwhile to biopsy the temporal artery even if it is not clinically involved. The classic picture of arteritis may be found in any organ, and biopsy of a small sensory nerve (eg, the sural nerve at the ankle) may provide diagnostic information, especially in polyarteritis nodosa. Skin, muscle, and renal biopsy are often used.

Differential Diagnosis

The differential diagnosis of arteritis covers almost the entire range of medicine. The possibility of arteritis must be borne in mind with any patient in whom more than one organ system is involved.

Complications

Blindness, hemiplegia, myocardial infarction, left heart failure, renal failure, and systemic embolization are some of the more severe complications of arteritis. Almost any complication can occur, and the diseases generally run a steadily progressive course.

Treatment

The treatment of arteritis is unsatisfactory. Corticosteroids are commonly used, and there is evidence that they can prevent and even reverse blindness in temporal arteritis. If hypertension is a feature, the blood pressure should be reduced with antihypertensive drugs (see Chapter 9), and surgery to relieve renal arterial obstruction should be considered. Vascular bypass grafts can effectively revascularize proximally obstructed vessels causing ischemia. Angioplasty has been successful in some highly obstructed arteries in Takayasu's disease. Immunosuppressive drugs (eg, cyclophosphamide or azathioprine) have been used, particularly in polyarteritis nodosa, but their effectiveness is not established.

Prognosis

The prognosis is poor, especially when renal or left heart failure occurs. Most patients die within 5 years.

SYSTEMIC EMBOLISM

Systemic embolism is an important complication of a number of heart diseases, including valvular and congenital heart disease, infective endocarditis, and myocardial infarction, which have been discussed elsewhere in this book. This section deals with embolism that is apparently unrelated to heart disease as well as embolism that has an established cardiac cause. It also deals more extensively with the manifestations and treatment of systemic embolism affecting particular parts of the systemic arterial bed.

Factors Promoting Thrombosis

The three factors promoting thrombosis in the left side of the heart and great vessels are stasis, changes in composition of the blood, and endothelial damage. Stasis is associated both with dilation of such chambers as the left atrium, left ventricle, and aorta and with ineffective contraction, as occurs in atrial fibrillation and myocardial infarction. Changes in composition of the blood may be due to hemoconcentration, polycythemia, or an increase in the number or stickiness of platelets, as occurs in certain blood diseases. Endothelial damage is usually the result of inflammation (using the term in its widest sense to include trauma, ischemic necrosis, mechanical damage, and infections). The role of drugs, especially oral contraceptive agents, is also important in the development of thrombosis. Such drugs increase blood lipids and platelet stickiness and have been demonstrated to increase the chances of thromboembolism.

The Nature of Embolic Material

Not all embolism is due to the accumulation of thrombotic material. Emboli composed of microorganisms, especially fungi from exuberant vegetations, can cause important damage. Valve tissue, artificial valve material, pieces of tumor (as in left atrial myxoma), foreign bodies (eg, in drug addicts), calcium, and aggregates of platelets and fibrin from heart valves or atheromatous lesions may cause embolism.

The clinical consequences of embolism vary widely. This fact is explained by the great variety of materials that form the emboli by the differences and the size and location of the artery embolis in the age and size of the thrombus that breaks off. Fresh red thrombus is the commonest form of embolic material. Because it is often readily lysed by the defense mechanisms of the body, in many cases the clinical effects of embolism, although severe and dramatic at onset, are relatively short-lived and are followed by complete or almost complete recovery.

In contrast, if organized thrombus, calcium, tumor material, or a large mass of Candida organisms constitutes the embolus, the obstruction to the blood vessel will be permanent.

The State of the Arterial Bed

The state of the arterial bed where the embolus lodges is an important variable in the clinical picture. Healthy young persons with normal blood vessels and a well-marked capacity to develop good collateral circulation withstand embolism better than do older, more atherosclerotic persons in whom degenerative changes have already occurred. Paradoxically, older patients with chronic arterial disease causing obstruction may have developed collateralization before the embolus. In the young patient without preformed collaterals, the acute embolus causes severe ischemia and even gangrene. In the patient with preformed collaterals, there may be little change in symptoms with only a worsening of ischemia. Thus, age and age-related disease influence the clinical effects of embolism. Local spasm of the embolized vessel can also suddenly occur in response to the impact of the embolus, and such spasms aggravate the acute manifestations of an embolism. The role played by secondary thrombosis in exacerbating the damage also varies, and in some cases thrombosis of the vein accompanying the embolized artery leads to secondary pulmonary embolism. If the embolus contains viable virulent organisms, abscesses may occur. If the organisms are less virulent, they may simply weaken the wall of the artery, and a mycotic aneurysm may form, as in infective endocarditis.

Clinical Manifestations & Treatment According to Specific Sites of Embolism

Many emboli lodge in sites where they provoke no clinical manifestations. Skeletal muscles harbor emboli without any signs of disease. The kidneys are also capable of accommodating emboli, and scars from infarcts that have occurred at various times are occasionally seen at autopsy in patients who have died of congestive heart failure. The liver with its double arterial blood supply is seldom if ever the site of infarction except in polyarteritis nodosa. The visceral manifestations of embolism generally occur as infarction, with death and necrosis of tissue, which is clinically recognizable only when the infarction is large or strategically placed or when it interferes with organ function. The central nervous system is the prime site for embolism that is likely to cause symptoms and signs. Even here, however, areas of infarction are found at autopsy in patients who had no clinical manifestations of any lesion.

A. Cerebral Embolism:

1. In patients with heart disease– Embolic material lodged in the brain produces the most serious and dramatic clinical manifestations of embolism. The onset is instantaneous, often with loss of consciousness or convulsions. Neurologic damage is most severe at onset. Hemiplegia, aphasia, and loss of vision are the commonest acute severe manifestations. Almost any clinical neurologic picture can occur, but an instantaneous, dramatic onset is the most characteristic feature. Spasm of the cerebral vessels and cerebral edema tend to make initial damage seem greater than it is, and recovery of function, although variable, is frequently remarkably rapid and surprisingly complete.

The physician's course of action in treating a patient who has just suffered a cerebral embolism depends on the certainty of the diagnosis of cerebral embolism. If the physician has not seen the patient before, the heart should be examined carefully for evidence of valvular disease, and a history of possible heart disease should be elicited from relatives. Head injury, subarachnoid hemorrhage, cerebral thrombosis, and intracerebral hemorrhage must be ruled out, and the patient must be closely watched for evidence of clinical deterioration or recovery. The foot of the bed should be raised and oxygen administered by face mask. The addition of CO_2 to act as a cerebral

vasodilator has been advocated, but there is little or no evidence that this procedure is beneficial. Systemic vasodilators should be avoided because they tend to reduce cerebral perfusion pressure. Lumbar puncture is indicated if there is any doubt about the diagnosis. The cerebrospinal fluid is seldom if ever hemorrhagic in cases of embolism. CT scan with contrast enhancement is valuable in establishing the presence and location of cerebral infarction and distinguishing infarction with edema from intracerebral hemorrhage. Cerebral angiography is not indicated, since embolectomy is never performed in cases of spontaneous cerebral embolism involving intracranial vessels.

The place of anticoagulant therapy in the treatment of acute cerebral embolism is not clear. Hemorrhage into the area of infarction and secondary thrombosis around the site of embolism can occur and exacerbate neurologic damage. The most logical course is to continue anticoagulant therapy if the patient has already been given anticoagulants and to withhold it in all other cases. In comparison with the prognosis in cerebral hemorrhage or cerebral thrombosis, the prognosis in cerebral embolism without anticoagulant therapy is sufficiently good that striking evidence of therapeutic benefit would be necessary to justify the use of anticoagulants in all patients. It is our practice to anticoagulate all patients with cerebral embolism where the infarction is not hemorrhagic as soon as the neurologist permits. This is usually 48 hours after acute episode.

Rehabilitation of the patient should be started as soon as possible. Improvement in nervous system function tends to occur at an exponentially decreasing rate over a 2-year period after the episode of embolism. Complete or almost complete recovery occurs in over 80% of patients with mitral valve disease who suffer cerebral embolism from left atrial thrombus. However, recovery seldom occurs if endocarditis is the cause of the embolus. The management of patients with mitral disease in whom cerebral embolism has occurred is not altered by the embolus. Mitral valve surgery is performed if indicated but not solely because of the embolus. The indications for restoration of sinus rhythm by cardioversion are similar to those in patients without embolism.

Embolism is, if anything, more common after valve replacement than before the operation, and restoration of sinus rhythm is likely to be only temporary unless the atrial fibrillation is of recent onset. Another embolism may well occur when atrial fibrillation recurs. Anticoagulant therapy is recommended but does not always prevent embolism.

2. In patients without heart disease– A different form of cerebral embolism frequently occurs in patients with atherosclerotic lesions involving the vessels of the head. In this case, the clinical picture is different from that seen in patients with heart lesions. The emboli are smaller and much more likely to be multiple, and the entire clinical picture is much more insidious, causing symptoms that have been labeled as transient ischemic attacks. Small aggregations of platelets and thrombi form on ulcerative atherosclerotic lesions in moderate-sized arteries such as the internal carotid or vertebral artery and even the ascending aorta. Pieces of these thrombi dislodge and move to other areas, giving rise to repeated episodes that resemble one another and always involve vessels distal to the lesion. Dizziness, sudden vertigo, weakness or paralysis, faintness, loss of speech, and sudden blindness are the common presenting features. A systolic bruit should be listened for in the neck and a full neurologic examination performed. Every attempt should be made to see the patient during an attack, when central nervous system abnormalities are more likely to be detected. The clinical picture is likely to be confused with that of arrhythmia, aortic stenosis, senile dementia, or central nervous system disease rather than that associated with embolism from thrombotic material accumulated in the heart.

Doppler blood velocity measurements and ultrasonic imaging of the vessels in the neck are helpful in diagnosis, and cerebral angiography is required for diagnostic purposes if surgical treatment of extracranial lesions is contemplated. Autopsy studies have shown that ulcerated atherosclerotic plaques are very common, increasing in frequency with age and five times more common in patients with cerebral infarction of unknown cause compared with patients who have cerebral infarctions of known cause (Amerenco, 1992). Furthermore, transesophageal echocardiography can show atherosclerotic plaques in the ascending aorta and can identify intraluminal thrombi in some cases (Karalis, 1991). Whether this will be useful clinically requires further study.

B. Coronary Embolism: (See also Chapter 8.) Coronary embolism presents a clinical picture that is indistinguishable from that of myocardial infarction due to atherosclerosis. Embolism presumably can occur without infarction and pass unnoticed in persons with excellent collateral blood supply. The onset of coronary embolism is instantaneous, and syndromes in which there is a gradual onset of chest pain are not seen. Electrocardiographic changes develop in the usual manner, and the clinical course may be benign if the source of the embolus is a recent left atrial thrombus. The reason is that in such cases, the embolic material (fresh red thrombus) is readily lysed. Embolism with calcific material in patients with aortic valve disease carries a much poorer prognosis. The treatment is similar to that in patients with lesions due to an atherosclerotic cause; in most instances, a period of rest under observation is the only thing that is required. Where the left atrial or ventricular thrombus is the source of the embolism, anticoagulation is required.

C. Peripheral Embolism Involving the Extremities: It is rare for embolism involving the arms to cause symptoms sufficient to warrant treatment. Ex-

ceptions occur when the embolic material is not thrombus. In such cases embolectomy may be indicated. The commonest sites of embolization requiring urgent treatment are the external iliac and femoral arteries. The development of symptoms and the clinical picture depend on the presence of collateral circulation and the suddenness with which the occlusion occurs. In patients with previous high-grade arterial obstruction, extensive collateral circulation may already be present, and an embolism suddenly obstructing the main artery cause no acute symptoms. If the embolus lodges farther down the leg, collateral circulation through the profunda femoris artery is usually sufficient to maintain adequate circulation unless significant atherosclerosis is also present. Femoral arterial occlusion usually causes an acute, severe pain in the leg, with loss of sensation, pallor, and a cold, pulseless limb.

The severe ischemic pain provides the most important indication for surgical treatment. The femoral artery is readily accessible in the groin, and the dangers of damaging distal tissues are negligible. Although angiography is usually done, it is not necessary to localize the site of the embolus accurately by means of angiography because balloon-tipped (Fogarty) catheters can be passed up and down the vessel and used to extract thrombus from areas not directly accessible through the incision. Any embolic material should always be saved for bacteriologic and histologic examination. The diagnosis of atrial myxoma has occasionally been accomplished by this means, and the nature of the infecting organism in endocarditis has been established by analysis of embolic material.

Surgical exploration should be undertaken as soon as possible after diagnosis. It can be conveniently carried out under local anesthesia. In the period before operation the limb should be kept dependent to maximize blood flow past the obstruction and kept cool in order to slow the metabolic processes. Meperidine (50–150 mg intramuscularly) should be given for relief of pain. Problems may arise if the patient is not seen until some time after an acute episode. Embolectomy can be beneficial even as long as a week after an acute episode, and the length of time that has elapsed since the embolism should not necessarily be taken as a contraindication to surgical exploration. In cases seen shortly after the acute episode, anticoagulation can be delayed until after operation. If surgery is not to be undertaken, anticoagulation with heparin should be given (5000–10,000 units intravenously every 4–6 hours), followed by warfarin, 10–15 mg for 2 days and a maintenance dose of 5–15 mg, depending on the prothrombin time, on later days. The heparin should be stopped on the third day when the prothrombin time is prolonged.

The prognosis following embolism in the leg depends mainly on the degree of atherosclerosis and consequently on the age of the patient. The prognosis is worse in patients with mural thrombi following myocardial infarction and in those with endocarditis. Intermittent claudication following the acute episode occurs occasionally, but in younger patients in whom the source of embolus is left atrial thrombus, recovery is usually complete.

D. Other Sites of Embolism: Mesenteric embolism causes severe epigastric pain of acute onset, with or without acute circulatory collapse. Mesenteric embolism must be differentiated from other acute abdominal emergencies. Melena occurs within a few hours, followed by paralytic ileus with vomiting and abdominal distention. Surgical exploration with bowel resection is often performed, but the results are not uniformly good. If ischemia progresses to intestinal infarction even with surgery, the reported mortality rate is in the range of 60–80%. As with all other forms of systemic embolism, expectant treatment can sometimes give good results, especially if the embolus moves to a more distal site and blood flow is thereby restored. Anticoagulant therapy is contraindicated because hemorrhage into the gut is almost always present.

Renal embolism seldom causes significant difficulties. The commonest manifestations are hematuria and renal colic associated with the passage of blood clots or dull flank pain due to the embolus itself. Acute renal failure is rarely seen. Renal embolism may be followed by hypertension (see Chapter 9). Studies of renal function and renal angiography in patients with mitral stenosis and systemic hypertension have shown evidence of segmental renal ischemia, and embolism should be considered when systemic hypertension is seen in association with mitral valve disease—especially when atrial fibrillation is present.

Splenic embolism may cause left upper quadrant pain and tenderness and may be associated with perisplenitis, a friction rub, and pain that is worse on inspiration. Mild analgesics are usually all that is required.

Investigation of Causes of Embolism

It is not uncommon for the patient to present with one or more acute episodes and symptoms highly suggestive of embolism. There may be no obvious signs of heart disease to account for the episodes. Careful examination of the heart reveals no evidence of valvular disease. The heart is not enlarged, and the ECG is within normal limits. In such cases, two-dimensional echocardiography is performed, especially in order to rule out a lesion that is amenable to surgery, such as left atrial myxoma. Transthoracic echocardiography can show left ventricular aneurysms with or without mural thrombi. Rarely is thrombus seen in the left atrium. However, with transesophageal echocardiography, the atrial appendage is well visualized, and thrombus can be seen. Stasis of blood in the atrium causes echocardiographic signals resembling microbubbles, probably resulting from echoes off rouleau formations of red cells, called "spontaneous echo contrast." This finding has been correlated with the presence of thrombus and the occurrence of thromboembolism (Daniel, 1988). Its clinical usefulness is not yet determined. In the presence of a normal echocardiogram, cardiac catheterization is rarely necessary.

Ulcerative atheromatous lesions in the aorta or in the carotid artery should also be considered as possible causes. If the lesions are confined to some specific part of the circulation, a lesion in the artery supplying that area (eg, a vessel in the head) may be suspected as the cause. In most cases in which the cause is not immediately obvious and emboli involve more than one area, an explanation is not found. Paradoxic embolism via a patent foramen ovale is sometimes suggested as a cause, but this is difficult to prove or disprove until autopsy. Two-dimensional echocardiography with injection of agitated saline microbubble "contrast" can demonstrate right-to-left shunting through a patent foramen ovale and thus establish the possibility of paradoxic embolism. Embolism has always been a common postmortem finding in both the systemic and the pulmonary circulations. In dying patients circulation is often extremely sluggish in the period just before death. Small nodular thrombotic (marantic) lesions are not uncommonly found on the heart valves at autopsy, particularly in patients dying of malignant disease. Occasionally, marantic endocarditis presents as an embolism and is found by two-dimensional echocardiography.

SYSTEMIC ARTERIOVENOUS FISTULA

A systemic arteriovenous fistula provides a low-resistance pathway through which blood can flow from the high-pressure arterial bed into the low-pressure venous system. The volume flow rate through the fistula depends on the size of the communication and on the height of the arterial pressure above the venous pressure. If a normal blood flow is to be maintained to perfuse the body in the presence of a fistula, the cardiac output must be increased by an amount equal to the fistula flow. The fistula flow thus constitutes a constant unremitting load on the heart, and if the fistula is large or if cardiac function is impaired, heart failure is likely to develop.

Systemic arteriovenous fistulas may be congenital, as in hemangiomatous lesions, or traumatic. The trauma may be due to stab or gunshot wounds that establish a communication between an artery and its adjacent vein, often in a limb. In some cases the trauma is surgical, and a fistula forms after an operation. Iatrogenic trauma causing arteriovenous fistulas occurs during percutaneous catheterization of arteries and is being increasingly reported (Marsan, 1990). Nephrectomy, cholecystectomy, and laminectomy are among the more common operations in which this complication occurs. In other cases, the systemic arteriovenous fistula is purposely created to provide ready access to a blood vessel with high flow for the treatment of renal failure by hemodialysis.

Pathophysiology

A systemic arteriovenous fistula is a prime cause of a high-output state (see Chapter 10). The extra load on the heart resulting from a high-output state gives rise to a number of secondary effects that become more important as the patient becomes older or cardiac function deteriorates.

When there is a systemic arteriovenous fistula, the baroreceptor mechanisms act to maintain a normal arterial blood pressure. The tendency for the arterial pressure to fall as blood leaks out of the arterial bed leads to tachycardia, increased cardiac output, and vasoconstriction in other beds that, unlike the fistula, are capable of responding to sympathetically mediated peripheral vasoconstriction. The increased cardiac output constitutes a constant extra load on the heart that varies with the size of the fistula. Although the load is well tolerated if the fistula is small and the patient is young, problems arise when the fistula is large (30% increase in resting output) or when age-related changes such as atherosclerosis or hypertension are present. When the load on the heart is so great that adequate perfusion of the body—especially the kidneys—cannot be maintained, a form of heart failure called high-output failure develops.

High-output failure. Some increase in blood volume occurs in any arteriovenous fistula that is large enough to increase the resting cardiac output significantly. When renal perfusion is inadequate, further increase in blood volume with salt retention and edema occurs. This increases the load on the heart. The left ventricular and later the right ventricular end-diastolic pressures rise, and the patient develops heart failure. The resulting signs—a bounding pulse, a hyperdynamic cardiac impulse, warm moist palms, warm limbs, and pink skin—contrast markedly with those of low-output failure—peripheral vasoconstriction, weak pulse, hypodynamic cardiac impulse, cool extremities, and peripheral cyanosis. The acuteness of the onset of the load, its magnitude, and its duration are important variables determining the clinical picture.

Clinical Findings

A. Symptoms: The patient is sometimes aware of the flow through the fistula, which gives rise to a buzzing sensation localized to the affected area. Palpitations, fatigue, and dyspnea are seen, but, in general, exercise tolerance is well maintained, because the fall in systemic resistance with exercise tends to decrease the fistula flow. The patient may notice that the skin near the fistula is warmer than normal and notice overgrowth of blood vessels around the site of the lesion.

B. Signs: The pulse is bounding and the heart rate increased. The pulse pressure is increased and the skin warm and moist. If the fistula is in a limb, that limb often grows to be longer than the opposite one, and tortuous varicose veins develop near the site of the fistula. Increased venous pressure occurs late in the disease. The heart is often enlarged, with a hyperdynamic cardiac impulse and a loud first sound. Third and fourth heart sounds may be heard, and a systolic murmur not infrequently develops in association with the increased stroke volume. A palpable and audible continuous bruit is also detectable over the site of the fistula. This sign is of most help when the fistula is in the abdomen or back. If the fistula is accessible and can be occluded by manual compression, its clinical significance can be assessed. If the fistula is significant, its occlusion raises the systemic vascular resistance and provokes a baroreceptor response. This consists of bradycardia and peripheral vasodilation. The fall in heart rate on occlusion and the increase on release (Branham's sign) constitute the best means of assessing a fistula at the bedside. In older patients and those with renal failure, this simple test is less reliable, and a significant fistula can be present in a patient in whom Branham's sign is negative.

C. Electrocardiographic Findings: Tachycardia and minor changes indicative of left ventricular overload (high-voltage QRS complexes and ST–T wave changes in the left ventricular leads) are seen. Significant hypertensive changes may be present in patients undergoing dialysis.

D. Imaging Studies: The heart is usually enlarged on x-ray, with a left ventricular configuration, and serial chest x-rays are valuable in demonstrating progressive enlargement. Pulmonary congestion is only seen in the late stages, when heart failure is present. Echocardiography shows the left ventricle to be dilated and overactive, with evidence of excessive wall motion. Angiography demonstrates the site and extent of fistula and the presence of multiple fistulas.

Doppler blood velocity measurements can be used to determine the hemodynamic significance of the fistula. Cardiac catheterization is not indicated for diagnosis, but if it is performed, the intracardiac pressures are found to be relatively normal and the cardiac output raised.

E. Laboratory Findings: Blood volume is increased in most cases of fistula of significant degree, and mild anemia is seen because it is the plasma volume that is raised.

Differential Diagnosis

Systemic arteriovenous fistula must be distinguished from other forms of high-output state, eg, pregnancy, thyrotoxicosis, beriberi, anemia, and Paget's disease. Heart failure due to hypertensive or atherosclerotic disease or cardiomyopathy may be confused with or associated with the effects of a fistula, especially in patients undergoing hemodialysis. The possibility that the fistula is playing a part in cardiac problems must always be kept in mind in such patients, especially when the stress of anemia is added. In addition, the development of heart failure after a surgical operation should raise the possibility that an arteriovenous fistula has been accidentally created.

Complications

A fistula may become infected, leading to endarteritis with subsequent sepsis, hemorrhage, or embolism. The fistula may progressively increase in size as the abnormal blood vessels grow in response to increased flow through them, or spontaneous thrombosis of the fistula may occur. Heart failure is the most important complication, and the purpose of treatment is to prevent its development.

Treatment

Any arteriovenous fistula that is of clinical significance—one causing bradycardia on occlusion or one large enough to increase heart size—should be closed if possible. Traumatic fistulas and those accidentally created at surgery are usually readily dealt with surgically, but hemorrhage may be difficult to control at operation. Congenital malformations with arteriovenous fistulas often recur after surgical attempts to eradicate them. In congenital cases, there are often multiple potential fistulas that enlarge and become evident only after a surgical attempt to eradicate the obvious ones. Catheter embolization of arterial venous fistulas with metal coils, detached reabsorbable balloons or other material can eradicate the fistulas or markedly reduce the size of the shunt. Fistulas that are created to facilitate hemodialysis may have to be reduced in size if they cause too large a cardiac load; if they become thrombosed, another fistula may have to be created.

Digitalis and diuretics are generally less effective in the treatment of high-output failure than in the treatment of low-output failure, and elimination of the fistula or at least reduction of its size is the treatment of choice.

Prognosis

The prognosis of systemic arteriovenous fistula depends on the ease with which its cardiovascular effects can be eliminated. The results are worst in patients with large congenital malformations. The prognosis of patients with renal failure undergoing hemodialysis should not be influenced by the fistula. A fistula large enough to provide an adequate route for dialysis can be achieved without compromising cardiac function in almost every case.

REFERENCES

Amarenco P et al: The prevalence of ulcerated plaques in the aortic arch in patients with stroke. N Engl J Med 1992;326:221.

Aronow WS, Schoenfeld MR, Gutstein H: Frequency of thromboembolic stroke in persons greater than or equal to 60 years of age with extracranial carotid arterial disease and/or mitral annular calcium. Am J Cardiol 1992;70:123.

Cohen RD, Corn DL, Ilstrup DM: Clinical features, prognosis, and response to treatment in polyarteritis. Mayo Clin Proc 1980;55:146.

Crawford ES et al: Aortic dissection and dissecting aortic aneurysm. Ann Surg 1988;208:254.

Crawford ES et al: Infrarenal abdominal aortic aneurysm: Factors influencing survival after operation performed over a 25-year period. Ann Surg 1981;193:699.

Cupps TR, Fauci AS: The vasculitis syndromes. Adv Intern Med 1982;27:315.

Daniel WG et al: Left atrial spontaneous echo contrast in mitral valve disease: An indicator for an increased thromboembolic risk. J Am Coll Cardiol 1988;11:1204.

Erbel R et al: Echocardiography in diagnosis of aortic dissection. Lancet 1989;1:457.

Fauci AS et al: Cyclophosphamide therapy of severe systemic necrotizing vasculitis. N Engl J Med 1979;301:235.

Fogarty TJ, Cranley JJ: Catheter technic for arterial embolectomy. Ann Surg 1965;161:325.

Fortner G, Johansen K: Abdominal aortic aneurysms. West J Med 1984;140:50.

Hamza M et al: [Arterial involvement in Behçet's disease.] J Mal Vasc 1988;13:245. (In French.)

Hashimoto S et al: Assessment of transesophageal Doppler echocardiography in dissecting aortic aneurysm. J Am Coll Cardiol 1989;14:1253.

Hasley PS et al: Cardiac manifestations of Churg-Strauss syndrome: Report of a case and review of the literature. Am Heart J 1990;120:996.

Hull RG, Asherson RA, Rennie JAN: Ankylosing spondylitis and an aortic arch syndrome. Br Heart J 1984;51:663.

Huston KA, Hunder GG: Giant cell (cranial) arteritis: A clinical review. Am Heart J 1980;100:99.

Ishikawa K: Diagnostic approach and proposed criteria for the clinical diagnosis of Takayasu's arteriopathy. J Am Coll Cardiol 1988;12:964.

Ishikawa K: Patterns of symptoms and prognosis in occlusive thromboaortopathy (Takayasu's disease). J Am Coll Cardiol 1986;8:1041.

James TN: Small arteries of the heart. Circulation 1977;56:2.

Karalis DG et al: Recognition and embolic potential of intraaortic atherosclerotic debris. J Am Coll Cardiol 1991;17:73.

Kersting-Sommerhoff BA et al: Aortic dissection: Sensitivity and specificity of MR imaging. Radiology 1988;166:651.

Lagneau P et al: Surgical treatment of Takayasu's disease. Ann Surg 1987;207:157.

Marsan RE et al: Iatrogenic femoral arteriovenous fistula. Cardiovasc Intervent Radiol 1990;13:314.

Moore P, Fauci AS: Neurologic manifestations of systemic vasculitis: A retrospective and prospective study of the clinicopathologic features and responses to therapy in 25 patients. Am J Med 1981;71:517.

Nishihara S et al: Intravenous gamma globulin and reduction of coronary artery abnormalities in children with Kawasaki disease. Lancet 1988;2:972.

O'Hara PJ: Acute mesenteric ischemia. Curr Opin Cardiol 1991;6:762.

Parrillo JE, Fauci AS: Necrotizing vasculitis, coronary angiitis, and the cardiologist. Am Heart J 1980;99:547.

Pyeritz RE, McKusick VA: The Marfan syndrome: Diagnosis and management. N Engl J Med 1979;300:771.

Reed D et al: Are aortic aneurysms caused by atherosclerosis? Circulation 1992;85:205.

Rubin DC et al: Intraaortic debris as a potential source of embolic stroke. Am J Cardiol 1992;69:819.

Schrader ML et al: The heart in polyarteritis nodosa: A clinicopathologic study. Am Heart J 1985;109:1353.

Shelhamer JH et al: Takayasu's arteritis and its therapy. Ann Intern Med 1985;103:121.

Strachan RW, How J, Bewsher PD: Masked giant-cell arteritis. Lancet 1980;1:194.

Suzuki A et al: Myocardial ischemia in cardiac catheterization and coronary angiography. Pediatr Cardiol 1988;9:1.

Vecht RJ et al: Acute dissection of the aorta: Long-term review and management. Lancet 1980;1:109.

Walker DH, Mattern WD: Rickettsial vasculitis. Am Heart J 1980;1:896.

Wees SJ, Sunwoo IN, Oh SJ: Sural nerve biopsy in systemic necrotizing vasculitis. Am J Med 1981;71:525.

Miscellaneous Forms of Heart Disease: Cardiac Tumors, Hypotension, Neurocirculatory Asthenia, & Traumatic Heart Disease

21

CARDIAC TUMORS

Cardiac tumors are rare and more frequently metastatic than primary. Although pathologic evidence of cardiac or pericardial involvement can be found in about 10% of autopsies in patients with malignant disease, the incidence of clinical manifestations is less. The site of the primary tumor is most often in the lung or the breast, indicating that the tumor is likely to spread locally to involve the heart or pericardium. Various types of lymphoma also tend to involve the heart, again mainly by spread from the mediastinum. Metastases seldom affect left ventricular function, although when pericardial effusion occurs, the patient may show manifestations of pericardial tamponade. The most common primary malignant tumors involving the heart are sarcomas. The most common benign tumor is a myxoma—usually left atrial myxoma—although the right atrium may be involved and, more rarely, the ventricles. It occurs in more than one chamber in about 10% of cases.

Clinical Findings

A. Symptoms: The presenting symptoms in patients with cardiac tumors are often bizarre and confusing. Posturally variable dyspnea, cough, and syncope can occur. Chest pain is not infrequent, and evidence of systemic or pulmonary congestion, with dyspnea or edema, is sometimes seen. The clinical picture can resemble that of infective endocarditis, with fever, immune complex vascular injury with petechiae, and embolism. In patients with metastases, there is often no clinical clue to involvement of the heart in the patient's history.

B. Signs: Evidence of pericardial involvement may be found with a pericardial friction rub or increased jugular venous pressure. In myxoma there are often changing murmurs, perhaps influenced by posture. The tumor is often pedunculated and mobile, and the degree of obstruction to blood flow varies with posture and varying hemodynamic events. The patient may thus have a diastolic murmur in one body position but not in another. There may be a filling sound resembling a third heart sound that occurs when a mobile tumor hits the mitral valve in early diastole ("tumor plop") and suddenly checks diastolic flow through the mitral valve. Careful search for evidence of embolism is always important, and the recovery of embolic material for histologic examination is sometimes of diagnostic value. In some cases of myxoma, systemic signs such as fever, tachycardia, and clubbing of the fingers are seen.

C. Electrocardiographic Findings: There are no specific electrocardiographic changes in cardiac tumors. High-voltage P waves have been reported in rare cases of myxoma, and P mitrale is sometimes seen. If pulmonary hypertension develops, there may be right ventricular hypertrophy on the ECG. Myocardial invasion can lead to atrial or ventricular tachyarrhythmias.

D. Imaging Studies: Bizarre x-ray outlines of the cardiac shadow and enlargement of the heart shadow due to pericardial effusion should be sought. Left atrial enlargement is seen in left atrial myxoma in many cases (see Chapter 12).

Echocardiography can be helpful in showing dense multiple echoes posterior to the anterior mitral valve leaflet in diastole. Pre- and postoperative echocardiograms in a patient with left atrial myxoma are shown in Figure 21–1. The results of echocardiography are not always so dramatic, and the tumor can be missed. Two-dimensional echocardiography (Figure 21–2) is more likely to provide a correct diagnosis. It can reveal the pedunculated mass in the left atrium, prolapsing down through the mitral valve in diastole. With catheterization, raised atrial or venous pressures on the right or left side are usually found, and in left atrial myxoma pulmonary congestion with perhaps a raised pulmonary vascular resistance is common. The tumors are usually slow-growing, and the disease is therefore insidious. CT scan and MRI are helpful in establishing the diagnosis. Angiography is most useful in diagnosis. Left atrial myxoma can often be seen on left ventricular angiography. The small amount of

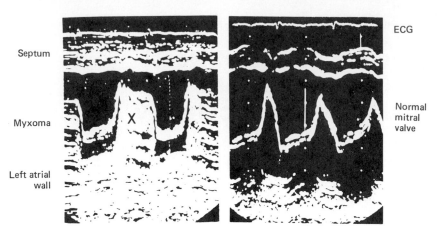

Figure 21–1. **Left:** Preoperative echocardiogram showing mass of echoes (X) posterior to the anterior mitral valve cusp and continuous with the left atrial wall in diastole. In systole, no such echoes are present. Posterior descent of anterior mitral cusp is restricted. **Right:** In postoperative echocardiogram, mass of echoes posterior to the anterior mitral valve cusp is no longer present, and descent of the cusp in diastole is normal. Atrial fibrillation is present. (Reproduced, with permission, from Srivastava TN, Fletcher E: The echocardiogram in left atrial myxoma. Am J Med 1973;54:136.)

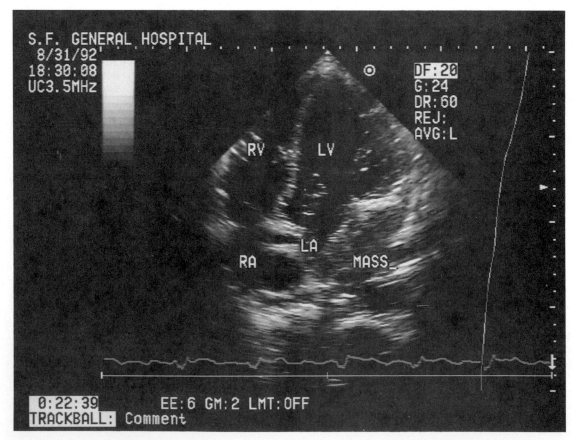

Figure 21–2. Two-dimensional echocardiogram in the four-chamber view of a patient with AIDS who presented with dyspnea on exertion. The mass compressing the lateral wall of the left atrium was found to be a lymphoma. (RV, right ventricle; LV, left ventricle; LA, left atrium; RA, right atrium.)

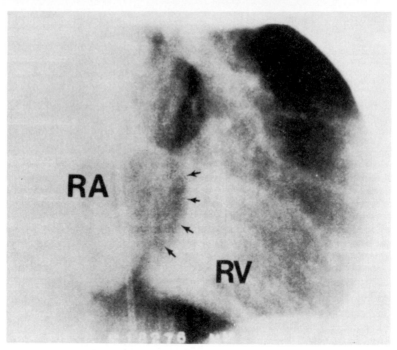

Figure 21–3. Right atrial angiocardiogram in 30-degree right anterior oblique view. Arrows indicate edge of filling defect. (RA, right atrium; RV, right ventricle.) (Reproduced, with permission, from Berman ND et al: Angiographic demonstration of blood supply of right atrial myxoma. Br Heart J 1976;38:764.)

mitral incompetence that often accompanies left ventricular injections of contrast material may outline the tumor, and the motion of the myxoma as it moves up and down with the heartbeat can sometimes be seen. An angiogram in a patient with right atrial (Figure 21–3) myxoma shows how a filling defect can be demonstrated.

E. Laboratory Findings: A raised sedimentation rate, anemia, and raised serum globulin are sometimes seen in myxomas. Large pericardial effusions, frequently with tamponade, are seen with tumors involving the pericardium; pericardial fluid is often hemorrhagic. In patients with other forms of primary or secondary tumors, pericardiocentesis is often responsible for the establishment of the diagnosis when malignant cells are demonstrated in the fluid.

Differential Diagnosis

Left atrial myxoma is most likely to be confused with rheumatic disease of the mitral valve. The episodic nature of the symptoms and signs and the presence of systemic manifestations are the most useful features in diagnosis. Other primary or secondary tumors involving the heart can be confused with pericardial disease, with myocarditis or cardiomyopathy, or with valvular heart disease in some instances. The systemic manifestations of myxoma bring to mind many differential diagnoses, eg, infective endocarditis, connective tissue disorders, occult malignant disease, and chronic infections.

Treatment

Surgical removal of a right or left atrial myxoma is usually curative, although the tumor may rarely recur. Malignant cardiac tumors are usually fatal whether they are metastatic or primary angiosarcomas. In 21 patients with cardiac sarcomas treated by chemotherapy, surgical resection, or both, the survival was 14% at 24 months after resection (Putnam, 1991). Malignant pericardial effusion from metastatic disease usually requires systemic chemotherapy combined with local instillation of chemicals or radiotherapy (or both) to the pericardium. Malignant pericardial effusions tend to be large and to recur. Multiple pericardiocenteses, prolonged drainage, or pericardiectomy is often necessary to keep pericardial tamponade from recurring. Instillation of an irritative substance such as tetracycline* into the pericardium can obliterate the pericardial space and stop recurrence of effusion.

Prognosis

Without treatment, patients with atrial myxoma may gradually develop worsening symptoms of pulmonary or systemic venous congestion as the tumor grows. Sudden death may occur if the mitral valve

---

*This agent is no longer available for this purpose from its only manufacturer (Lederle Laboratories), though stocks on hand are still being used. Possible substitutes such as doxycycline are being investigated.

becomes totally obstructed. Pulmonary emboli in right atrial myxoma may lead to severe pulmonary symptoms and, if repeated, to pulmonary hypertension and right heart failure. Systemic emboli from left atrial myxoma may lead to hemiplegia, loss of a limb, or other severe vascular occlusions. Systemic symptoms of fever, arthralgia, and fatigue may cause chronic invalidism until one of the major cardiac or embolic catastrophes occurs.

HYPOTENSION

Hypotension should be regarded as a symptom rather than a disease.

Hypotension cannot be defined in terms of a specific level of arterial blood pressure—systolic or diastolic. The adequacy of the level of blood pressure is indicated by the patient's symptoms and in particular by the response to changes in posture. Remarkably low pressures can be tolerated in the supine position; and, conversely, when patients who have been hypertensive suffer a fall in pressure, symptoms may occur at surprisingly high pressure levels. The prevalence of orthostatic hypotension increases with age. In a study of over 5000 men and women aged 65 years or older, 16.2% experienced a fall in systolic pressure greater than 20 mm Hg—or in diastolic blood pressure greater than 10 mm Hg—on standing for 3 minutes. The prevalence increased with age and was greater in those with isolated systolic hypertension and carotid artery stenosis by ultrasonography (Rutan, 1992).

Causes of Hypotension

Hypotension results from inadequate cardiac output, as in myocardial infarction; from inadequate circulating blood volume; or from failure of the normal reflex mechanisms that maintain a constant arterial pressure. All these factors operate in a number of disorders, and several may combine in a given patient to cause the primary symptom of hypotension— dizziness or faintness that is made worse when the patient suddenly stands up.

Disturbances of blood volume are clinically more common than disturbances of reflex control of the circulation, and they stem from two factors. One is a decrease in plasma or red cell volume due to hemorrhage, fluid loss, diarrhea, vomiting, unrecognized internal hemorrhage, dehydration, excessive diuresis, or excessive sweating; the other is a change in capacity of a blood-filled compartment (heart, arteries, capillaries, or veins).

Decreased blood volume as a cause of hypotension is particularly striking in adrenal insufficiency disorders, eg, Addison's disease and hypopituitarism. Wasting disorders of the bowel associated with diarrhea and anemia are also commonly associated with hypotension, and a sudden episode of faintness with

hypotension is often the first manifestation of gastrointestinal hemorrhage.

Abnormalities of reflex control of arterial pressure usually result from disease of the central nervous system and its autonomic pathways. Peripheral parts of the autonomic nervous system that innervate blood vessels may also be affected and are particularly susceptible to the effects of drugs, especially the alpha-blocking and beta-blocking drugs.

Clinical Features

The clinical picture of hypotension associated with an inadequate blood volume is dominated by the effects of the compensatory mechanisms that are mediated by the autonomic nervous system. These effects cause anxiety, weakness, palpitations, tachycardia, restlessness, vasoconstriction, sweating, pallor, and cold extremities. In contrast, in hypotension associated with autonomic nervous system disease, the patient faints, with few or no accompanying symptoms. Recovery is rapid when cerebral blood flow is restored with the patient in the recumbent position.

Hypotension Associated With Inadequate Blood Volume

A. Vasovagal Attacks and Fainting: The commonest form of hypotension is that seen in simple fainting. Sudden vasodilation of the muscular arterioles and veins mediated by cholinergic sympathetic nerves results in an acute fall in effective blood volume owing to sudden pooling of blood in peripheral areas of the body (normally the legs). Vasovagal fainting may be preceded by an increase in sympathetic activity shortly before loss of consciousness. The blood pressure and heart rate may remain unchanged or may increase suddenly, followed by hypotension and bradycardia. The reason for the hypotension is vasodilation mediated by a withdrawal of sympathetic vasoconstrictor activity. This is thought to be brought about by stimulation of mechanoreceptors in the myocardium by the increased reflex sympathetic stimulation in the setting of a reduced ventricular filling. This understanding has led to the development of the tilt-table test, in which the patient is suddenly passively tilted upright on a tilt table. In some patients, the bradycardia and drop in blood pressure are preceded by sympathetic-mediated tachycardia. In others, hypotension can be precipitated only after an infusion of isoproterenol. In patients with unexplained syncope and negative electrophysiologic studies, hypotension was provoked in 27–67% of those not given isoproterenol and 87% of patients of those who received isoproterenol. In controls, the incidence of provoked hypotension was 10% (Almquist, 1989; Raviele, 1990).

Simple fainting occurs in normal subjects and may also be provoked by disease, especially myocardial infarction with or without pain. Fainting may also occur during cardiologic investigations. The vagus nerve plays an important part in the mechanism of fainting, and simple faints are sometimes called vasovagal attacks. The primary stimulus to simple fainting may be physical or psychic. Trauma, pain, or stimulation of vagal afferents—especially in the ascending aorta near the right coronary ostium—may cause hypotension, even in recumbent subjects. Fear, the sight of blood, observing trauma to others, or seeing other people faint may all cause hypotension. Premonitory symptoms include feeling alternately hot and cold, yawning, sweating, and an uneasy or sinking feeling in the epigastrium. The patient looks pale and develops bradycardia before the ultimate sudden acute arteriolar vasodilation occurs.

Hypotension and syncope can be stimulated in a number of different physiologic situations, such as postmicturition, postdefecation, and after paroxysms of coughing. The pathophysiology leading to hypotension results from contraction of vagal reflex vasodilation, retarding venous return and incipient hypovolemia. Occasionally, syncope after swallowing occurs in patients with structural abnormalities of either the esophagus or the heart and occurs as result of reflex stimulation with afferent input from the esophagus to the central nervous system, causing efferent vasodilation and bradycardia.

B. Prevention and Treatment of Fainting Attacks: Fainting attacks can be aborted by lying down or raising the legs or by administration of intravenous atropine (0.4–0.8 mg). A tendency to faint is aggravated by all the factors causing low blood volume and also by a hot environment, prolonged standing, an empty stomach, pregnancy, suddenly standing up, nervousness, and novel surroundings. Fainting seldom occurs spontaneously in supine subjects, but it can readily be provoked during arterial puncture or coronary artery catheterization. If the patient has lost consciousness, recovery may take 15–45 minutes. The earlier restorative measures are instituted, the sooner recovery occurs. Raising the legs and administering atropine are specific remedies. Vasoconstrictive drugs such as norepinephrine and angiotensin have no place in treatment.

In patients who on a tilt-table test have sinus tachycardia preceding the hypotension, beta-blocking drugs to prevent stimulation of the left ventricular mechanoreceptors have been successful in preventing recurrent syncope.

Bradycardia is the most important indication that reflex factors are involved in syncope in patients with hypotension. Dramatic improvement occurs after the administration of atropine in patients with myocardial infarction in whom reflex hypotension has occurred. A short period of cerebral and cardiac hypoperfusion is relatively harmless in healthy young subjects, but disastrous consequences may result in older atherosclerotic patients with cerebral or coronary arterial disease and in those with aortic or pulmonary stenosis. Cerebral and myocardial infarction may result,

and ventricular arrhythmia may occur during periods of marked vagal bradycardia. The role of simple vasovagal attacks in causing sudden death in patients with heart disease is not known.

Hypotension Associated With Abnormal Reflex Control Mechanisms

A. Autonomic Insufficiency: Postural (orthostatic) hypotension due to disturbances of autonomic nervous system control is seldom seen in patients under age 50. It occurs in patients with diabetes mellitus or uremia associated with peripheral neuropathy, in tabes dorsalis, and in various types of degenerative central nervous system disease involving the basal ganglia. The Shy-Drager syndrome, which resembles parkinsonism, is associated with autonomic failure and involvement of the corticospinal, cerebellar, and extrapyramidal tracts. At least two of the classic triad of symptoms—postural hypotension, impaired sweating, and loss of sexual function, with impotence in men—are usually present. In these patients, supine norepinephrine serum levels are normal, but unlike the normal subject they do not rise on standing, suggesting an inability to stimulate normally functioning peripheral neurons. No associated disease is found in about one-third of cases. The diagnostic physical finding is a progressive fall in arterial pressure when the patient is standing or when the lower body is subjected to suction, as shown in Figure 21–4. There is little or no accompanying increase in heart rate. In the lower body suction procedure, the subject lies flat, with the legs and pelvis enclosed in an airtight box. Pressure in the box is reduced by sucking air out of the system at a rate sufficient to maintain a desired level of pressure around the legs.

A lack of overshoot in arterial pressure also occurs after Valsalva's maneuver, as shown in Figure 21–5. This finding should be sought in direct arterial pressure tracings because it cannot always be accurately assessed in noninvasive bedside studies using indirect methods. After release of the Valsalva maneuver, systolic pressure overshoot can be inferred at the bedside by observing a reflex slowing of the pulse mediated by the vagal reflex as a result of the sudden increase in blood pressure. Sympatholytic (antihypertensive) drugs, diuretics, tranquilizers, calcium channel-blocking drugs, potassium depletion, and primary aldosteronism also impair circulatory reflex reactivity. In some cases, myocardial infarction causes unexplained loss of autonomic nervous system function; in rare cases, autonomic insufficiency is seen in acute viral infections.

B. Treatment of Autonomic Insufficiency: The treatment of postural hypotension due to autonomic insufficiency consists of eliminating any factors that tend to reduce blood volume or impair circulatory reactivity. In addition, active measures to expand blood volume should be instituted. Such simple

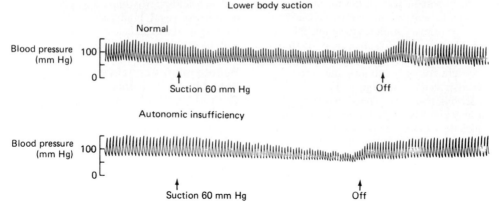

Figure 21–4. Arterial pressure tracings from a normal subject and a patient with autonomic insufficiency showing the effects of negative pressure applied to the lower body. There is a progressive fall in blood pressure and no overshoot when the pressure is released in the patient with autonomic insufficiency.

remedies as increasing salt intake and raising the head of the bed to provide a constant stimulus to the autonomic nervous system control mechanisms during sleep often help. Avoiding sudden changes in posture and stopping or decreasing medication such as antihypertensive drugs, sedatives, tricyclic antidepressants, and alcohol, which impair circulatory reactivity, may also improve symptoms. Wearing two pairs of support panty hose may be as effective as and cheaper than wearing elastic surgical stockings. Blood volume expansion by means of fludrocortisone acetate should be reserved for patients in whom simple measures have failed. It should be remembered that the primary function of autonomic nervous system reflex control is to limit rises in arterial pressure and that patients with autonomic insufficiency are frequently hypertensive in the supine or head down position. The measures taken to prevent hypo-

tension in the standing position often result in hypertension in the supine position.

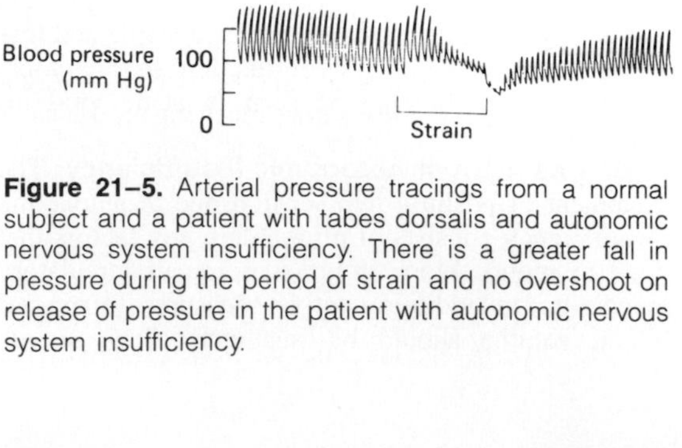

When autonomic insufficiency is due to central nervous system disease, paralysis of the nervous control system is almost inevitably irreversible. Treatment is basically palliative, but indomethacin (75–150 mg/d) is worth trying. Alpha-adrenergic agonists, eg, dihydroergotamine and midodrine, can help but are likely to cause supine hypertension. The prognosis depends on the underlying pathologic process. Patients whose heart rates change in response to posture, exercise, and other stimuli live longer than those with fixed heart rates.

NEUROCIRCULATORY ASTHENIA (Cardiac Neurosis)

The functional cardiac disorder known as neurocirculatory asthenia is also called "effort syndrome," "disordered action of the heart," "soldier's heart," and DaCosta's syndrome. This condition causes the most difficulty during wartime, when conscription mobilizes apparently healthy men who develop symptoms either during military training or during actual combat that make them entirely unfit for military service. DaCosta first described the condition in the American Civil War; Thomas Lewis in World War I and Paul Wood in World War II were both involved in defining and diagnosing the condition. A similar clinical picture is seen in civilian life, but in that context the symptoms vary from patient to patient, and the four classic symptoms of dyspnea, palpitations, chest pain, and fatigue seen in wartime are supplemented by other complaints.

Clinical Findings

The spectrum of cases is wide, with incapacity varying from mild to severe. The condition has usu-

Figure 21–5. Arterial pressure tracings from a normal subject and a patient with tabes dorsalis and autonomic nervous system insufficiency. There is a greater fall in pressure during the period of strain and no overshoot on release of pressure in the patient with autonomic nervous system insufficiency.

ally been present before military service and is found in men, women, and children. Wood stressed the psychologic aspects of the disorder and considered the condition to be a form of anxiety neurosis. Physicians sometimes unwittingly contribute to the patient's neurotic tendency by stressing the need for rest in patients with heart disease. The patient becomes fearful of exercise, and the combination of anxiety and inactivity is particularly likely to produce the clinical picture of cardiac neurosis. Occasionally, prolonged enforced bed rest in suspected cases of rheumatic fever may lead to cardiac neurosis. The physician must guard against the possibility of causing or aggravating neurotic tendencies, especially in young persons.

A frequent precipitator of cardiac neurosis is the finding of an "abnormality" by a physician. The patient being told of a murmur or an abnormal finding, such as mitral valve prolapse on Doppler echocardiography, can become a cardiac cripple with all the patient's attention and concern focused on the "cardiac disease." The physician must assess the emotional stability of the patient and the impact that such information might have before announcing a diagnosis of a possible cardiac problem. The patient is often better served by having the possible abnormality noted in the record along with a statement explaining the reason for not reaching a definite diagnosis and not informing the patient of the possible echocardiographic abnormality.

A. Symptoms: Dyspnea on exertion or on exposure to threatening situations is the predominant symptom, and all symptoms are aggravated by mental or physical stress. The breathlessness often involves an inability to get a deep enough or satisfying breath. The patient takes deep sighing breaths that reduce alveolar and arterial CO_2, resulting in respiratory alkalosis. This provokes cerebral arterial vasoconstriction. Increased anxiety, headaches, dizziness, faintness, and even loss of consciousness can result. In addition, the ionized calcium level decreases with respiratory alkalosis; this can provoke numbness and tingling in fingers and lips, tetany, carpopedal spasm, and convulsions (hyperventilation syndrome). The vicious cycle of anxiety, hyperventilation, and cerebral symptoms that in turn increase anxiety is extremely common and can be broken by the old-fashioned remedy of having the patient breathe expired air from a bag. Another effective means of aborting the process is to have the patient begin to exercise at the first sensation of inability to take a deep enough breath. Other symptoms, in the order of frequency, are weakness, palpitations, noncardiac pain in the left chest, fatigue, cold sweating (especially of the palms), nervousness, dizziness, headache, tremulousness, sighing, flushing, cramps, paresthesias, dryness of the mouth, vasovagal fainting, insomnia, increased frequency of micturition, diarrhea, and anorexia. Although some of these symptoms may be indicative of organic cardiac disease in certain circumstances, they are also readily recognized as symptoms of an anxiety state.

B. Signs: The patient is often thin and of asthenic build. A distaste for physical activity and a rapid resting heart rate are usually present. Blood pressure may be increased if the patient is excited when examined, but persistent hypertension is not found. The heart rate increases readily with exercise or when the patient stands up after lying down or squatting. Return of the heart rate to normal after exercise is delayed. Hyperventilation and tachypnea are common, particularly with stress, but no abnormal physical signs other than occasional systolic ejection or late systolic murmurs or clicks are found on examination. The presence of hemodynamically insignificant organic heart disease, a trivial "functional" murmur, or insignificant electrocardiographic changes may complicate the picture, and it may be extremely difficult to decide which problems are functional.

C. Electrocardiographic Findings: The ECG is usually normal apart from sinus tachycardia, although ST segment changes simulating ischemia may be seen. An exercise test may be useful in demonstrating disproportionate tachycardia, hyperventilation, and tachypnea.

D. Imaging Studies: Chest x-ray shows a normal or reduced heart size. Cardiac catheterization reveals normal pressures and a cardiac output that is often raised.

Differential Diagnosis

Active rheumatic fever, rheumatic carditis, anemia, thyrotoxicosis, systemic arteriovenous fistula, tuberculosis, pleurisy, influenza, or any high-output state must be differentiated from neurocirculatory asthenia. The diagnosis of effort syndrome probably includes more than one condition; with time, various different syndromes will probably be identified. There is almost certainly a relationship between effort syndrome and poor physical conditioning. Modern life in the Western world has meant a low average level of physical activity for the general population. Physical inactivity tends to produce a physiologic state resembling that seen in effort syndrome. Prolonged bed rest, debilitating illness, or simple inactivity all reduce exercise tolerance, cause disproportionate tachycardia, and result in marked tiredness after effort. Physical training programs are capable of altering the response to exercise.

The physiologic "defect" in untrained persons is a failure in the mechanisms distributing cardiac output to different parts of the systemic circulation. Muscular exercise involves a marked increase in muscle blood flow. As a compensatory mechanism, perfusion of nonessential parts of the systemic circulation (skin, kidneys, other viscera, and nonexercising muscles) is ordinarily reduced. If nonessential perfusion is maintained, the total cardiac output for a given work load is greater than normal; a higher pulse rate and limited exercise tolerance result. Training programs can reduce both cardiac output and heart rate at submaximal loads and increase the subject's maximal exercise performance. The arteriovenous oxygen difference at a given work load consequently increases. The statement that training increases the amount of oxygen extracted by the muscles is not correct. The arteriovenous oxygen difference is increased because a larger proportion of cardiac output perfuses the exercising muscles, and blood draining exercising muscles is low in oxygen content.

Treatment

Like patients with any form of neurosis, those with cardiac neurosis respond poorly to treatment such as exercise training programs, and they are not generally treated sympathetically by physicians. It is possible that some patients will be shown to have enzymatic defects in their muscles and that the present consensus that the condition is entirely psychologic will be proved false. The clinical manifestations so closely resemble those of sympathetic nervous system overactivity that propranolol should be given a trial in gradually increasing doses up to 200 mg/d.

Prognosis

Patients with cardiac neurosis can usually lead relatively normal lives if they are not subject to stress. There is no evidence that cardiac neurosis shortens life. Patients who develop symptoms while in the armed forces usually recover when they return to civilian life. However, some patients persist in self-imposed chronic invalidism.

TRAUMATIC HEART DISEASE

Many of the ways in which trauma can affect the heart have been mentioned in the chapters dealing with coronary disease, hypertension, congenital heart disease, valvular disease, arrhythmias, and pericarditis. Cardiac trauma can be due to either penetrating or nonpenetrating injury. Any cardiac structure can be injured, and, although the frequencies may be different, the types of injuries to the heart are similar in penetrating and nonpenetrating trauma.

In penetrating injuries, the degree of trauma depends on the energy released to the heart by the penetrating missile. This energy depends on the velocity, the mass, and the tumbling characteristics of the object. Thus, a low-velocity missile, such as shrapnel or a penetrating knife, causes damage in the path of the missile's penetration. A high-velocity bullet, on the other hand, releases energy that causes damage to tissues at a distance from its direct path and thus is far more damaging. Nonpenetrating injury, such as sudden deceleration, chest compression, or a blast, injures the heart by suddenly compressing it, moving it violently from its anatomic location in the mediastinum or forcefully smashing it against the rib cage or vertebral column.

The most important cause of cardiac trauma in peacetime is automobile accidents. Injury to the heart is not usually foremost in the minds of physicians dealing with acutely injured persons, and the manifestations of cardiac trauma can be easily overlooked when other more obvious injuries are present. The anterior aspect of the right ventricle is subject to damage in sudden deceleration injuries. Thus, when a person is thrown forward onto the steering wheel of an automobile, the myocardium may be bruised, the anterior descending coronary artery may be damaged, and myocardial infarction or hemopericardium may result. Myocardial infarction after trauma results most commonly from myocardial contusion or underlying coronary artery disease and least commonly from injury to the coronary arteries.

Damage to the mitral, aortic, and tricuspid valves may give rise to acute valvular incompetence. In the case of the mitral valve, rupture of the chordae tendineae or acute disruption of an already abnormal (prolapsing) valve may cause or aggravate mitral incompetence. Papillary muscle rupture can also cause acute mitral or tricuspid regurgitation.

A particularly important insidious injury is localized rupture of the aorta in motorcyclists who are thrown from their machines. In deceleration trauma, the aorta tends to rupture at the point of greatest torque—the aortic isthmus, just distal to the origin of the left subclavian artery. A tear in the intima can result in hemorrhage that is confined to the adventitia and does not spread to the pleural space or mediastinum. Rising pressure around the vessel can occlude the aorta and produce a false aneurysm, shutting off the blood flow to the lower body. Renal ischemia, acute hypertension, and renal failure can occur insidiously, and the lesion is easily missed. The false aneurysm thus formed becomes chronic in about 15% of cases. Because this false aneurysm can unfortunately rupture, even after many years of quiescence, it should always be repaired.

Stabbings and gunshot wounds of the heart may result in hemopericardium and tamponade, ventricular perforation, or late cardiac rupture at the site of a myocardial contusion. Ventricular septal defects and intracardiac damage may result. Injury to the left ventricle can weaken the ventricular wall, resulting in a false ventricular aneurysm. Not all direct cardiac trauma is immediately fatal, and the fall in arterial pressure associated with shock may limit hemorrhage.

Systemic arteriovenous fistula is an important cause of problems in the weeks following trauma. The close relationship between arteries and veins in different areas of the body makes fistula formation an important complication of stab and gunshot wounds. Surgical trauma may also cause similar lesions. Fistulas have developed after cholecystectomy, nephrectomy, and laminectomy; and fistulas at the elbow and groin have been seen following cardiac catheterization. If the fistula is due to a wound and is close to the surface, the diagnosis is relatively easy, but more deeply situated fistulas may not be detected until high-output cardiac failure develops (see Chapter 10).

Minor forms of trauma associated with straining or lifting heavy objects may be the precipitating cause of acute cardiac events such as mitral valve disruption (see Chapter 12) or aortic dissection.

Unfortunately, the form of cardiovascular trauma which is increasing in incidence most rapidly is iatrogenic trauma. The invasive techniques of needle puncture of arteries and organs and the placing of catheters intravenously has resulted in arterial and cardiac laceration, arteriovenous fistulas, false aneurysms, cardiac tamponade, lost catheters, and fatal arrhythmias.

Clinical Findings

A. Symptoms: Symptoms of cardiac damage are often absent, either because the patient is unconscious or because trauma to other areas dominates the picture. Chest pain can be due to myocardial ischemia or pericardial involvement, and dyspnea and pulmonary edema can occur with acute valvular incompetence. In arteriovenous fistula formation, the patient often notices local warmth and a buzzing sensation in the neighborhood of the fistula.

B. Signs: Examination of the cardiovascular system in injured persons is always important. The jugular venous pressure will be raised if there is tamponade. The pulses in the legs will be diminished or absent and urinary output decreased or absent if there is a ruptured aorta. Murmurs will be present if valvular damage has occurred. Listening for bruits in the abdomen or back may disclose deep-seated fistulas. About 20% of the time, there is no external evidence of thoracic trauma in patients who have aortic rupture following an automobile accident. The absence of such external trauma thus does not rule out serious cardiovascular trauma.

C. Electrocardiographic Findings: Electrocardiographic changes are often the first indication that cardiac damage has occurred. ST–T wave changes due to pericardial involvement or even indications of myocardial infarction can be seen, and all patients with chest injuries should have an ECG recorded as soon as possible after injury.

D. Imaging Studies: Chest x-ray can demonstrate pericardial effusion and rib fractures that may have caused cardiac damage. Chest x-ray does not detect localized aortic rupture but can detect hemothorax, widening of the mediastinum, and mediastinal emphysema.

Cardiac catheterization and angiocardiography are essential in diagnosing and qualifying the various abnormalities seen after trauma. They are especially important if the patient has hemodynamically significant lesions causing cardiac failure or symptoms due to inability to increase cardiac output. Angiography is the most effective means of diagnosing localized aor-

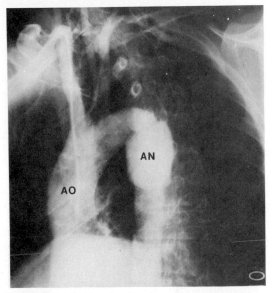

Figure 21–6. Angiogram showing a left anterior oblique view of the aorta. A traumatic false aneurysm (AN) is shown at the isthmus of the aorta (AO). The lesion resulted from an automobile accident and caused acquired coarctation.

tic rupture. An angiogram of a traumatic false aneurysm of the aorta is shown in Figure 21–6.

E. Laboratory Findings: Myocardial contusion or infarction may cause release of myocardial enzymes.

Differential Diagnosis

A high index of suspicion and an awareness of the possibility of cardiac trauma in injured persons are the most important factors in diagnosis. The longer the interval between injury and the development of cardiac symptoms, the more difficult the recognition of a traumatic cause.

Treatment

Emergency surgical treatment, with exploration of the injured area, must always be considered after emergency measures have stabilized the patient's condition sufficiently to permit operation. Pericardiocentesis may be needed to treat cardiac tamponade, and operative treatment of direct cardiac trauma can be remarkably successful. If the patient is severely hypotensive after penetrating chest injury, immediate thoracotomy in the emergency room with suture of the cardiac laceration can be life-saving.

Most patients admitted for observation for myocardial contusion do very well. Only those with obvious and definite myocardial contusion manifested by an ECG showing changes of acute myocardial infarction; congestive heart failure; or pericardial effusion, rub, or tamponade have the potential for serious complications. It is still prudent for medicolegal reasons to observe the patient suspected of myocardial contusion in the hospital for 12–24 hours.

Prognosis

The prognosis following cardiac trauma is surprisingly good if the patient survives the first few hours. Trauma usually involves healthy young persons who can withstand injury well and have great powers of recuperation. The long-term prognosis for specific lesions is similar to that when more usual causes are responsible.

REFERENCES

Cardiac Tumors

Barakos JA et al: MR imaging of secondary cardiac and pericardial lesions: AJR Am J Roentgenol 1989;153: 47.

Fyke FE et al: Primary cardiac tumors: Experience with 30 consecutive cases since the introduction of two-dimensional echocardiography. J Am Coll Cardiol 1985;5:1465.

Godwin JD et al: Computed tomography: A new method for diagnosing tumor of the heart. Circulation 1981;63:448.

Larsson S et al: Atrial myxomas: Results of 25 years' experience and review of the literature. Surgery 1989;105: 695.

Mugge A et al: Diagnosis of noninfective cardiac mass lesions by two-dimensional echocardiography: Comparison of the transthoracic and transesophageal approaches. Circulation 1991;83:70.

Murphy MC et al: Surgical treatment of cardiac tumors: A 25-year experience, discussion. Ann Thorac Surg 1990;49:612.

Putnam JB Jr et al: Primary cardiac sarcomas. Ann Thorac Surg 1991;51:906.

Salcedo EE et al: Cardiac tumors: Diagnosis and management. Curr Probl Cardiol 1992;17:79.

Hypotension

Almquist A et al: Provocation of bradycardia and hypotension by isoproterenol and upright position in patients with unexplained syncope. N Engl J Med 1989;320: 346.

Bannister R (editor): *Autonomic Failure*. Oxford Univ Press, 1983.

Biglieri EG, McIlroy MB: Abnormalities of renal function and circulatory reflexes in primary aldosteronism. Circulation 1966;33:78.

Bradbury S, Eggleston C: Postural hypotension: A report of three cases. Am Heart J 1925;1:73.

Brigden W, Sharpey-Schafer EP: Postural changes in peripheral blood flow in cases with left heart failure. Clin Sci 1950;9:93.

Brignole M et al: A controlled trial of acute and long-term medical therapy in tilt-induced neurally mediated syncope. Am J Cardiol 1992;70:339.

Grubb BP et al: Head-upright tilt-table testing in evaluation and management of the midgut vasovagal syndrome. Am J Cardiol 1992;69:904.

Jacobsen TN et al: Contrasting effects of propranolol on sympathetic nerve activity and vascular resistance during orthostatic stress. Circulation 1992;85:1072.

Kroenke K: Orthostatic hypotension. West J Med 1985;143: 253.

Raviele A et al: Usefulness of head-up tilt test in evaluating patients with syncope of unknown origin and negative electrophysiologic study. Am J Cardiol 1990;65: 1322.

Schatz IJ: Orthostatic hypotension. Arch Intern Med 1984;144:773.

Sharpey-Schafer EP: Circulatory reflexes in chronic disease of the afferent nervous system. J Physiol (Lond) 1956;134:1.

Sheldon R, Killam S: Methodology of isoproterenol-tilt table testing in patients with syncope. J Am Coll Cardiol 1992;19:773.

Shy GM, Drager GA: A neurological syndrome associated with orthostatic hypotension. Arch Neurol 1960;2:511.

Sra JS et al: Use of intravenous esmolol to predict efficacy of oral beta-adrenergic blocker therapy in patients with neurocardiologic syncope. J Am Coll Cardiol 1992;19:402.

Valsalva AM: *De Aure Humana: Traj ad Rhenum.* Utrecht. G. Vand Water 84, 1707.

Wagner HN Jr: Orthostatic hypotension. Bull Johns Hopkins Hosp 1959;105:322.

Neurocirculatory Asthenia

Cohen ME, White PD: Neurocirculatory asthenia: 1972 concept. Milit Med 1972;137:142.

DaCosta JM: On irritable heart: A clinical study of a form of functional cardiac disorder and its consequences. Am J Med Sci 1871;61:17.

Grant RT: Observations on the after-histories of men suffering from the effort syndrome. Heart 1925;12:121.

Lewis T: *The Soldier's Heart and the Effort Syndrome.* Hoeber, 1919.

Wood PH: DaCosta's syndrome. (Three parts.) Br Med J 1941;1:767, 805, 845.

Traumatic Heart Disease

Bellotti P et al: Myocardial contusion after a professional boxing match. Am J Cardiol 1992;69:709.

Cheitlin MD: The internist's role in the management of the patient with traumatic heart disease. Cardiol Clin 1991;9:675.

Symbas PN: Cardiac trauma. Am Heart J 1976;92:387.

Heart Disease in Pregnancy

22

Heart disease in pregnancy has become less important in developed countries because valvular and congenital heart diseases are now recognized and treated prior to childbearing age. Rheumatic heart disease, especially mitral stenosis, accounts for about 90% of cases of heart disease in pregnant women but is usually mild because those with more severe disease have had surgical treatment. Acute rheumatic fever, the precursor of rheumatic valvular heart disease, is much less common today than was the case 20–30 years ago, in part because of prompt treatment of streptococcal infections. In developing countries, cardiac surgery is less frequently performed and the clinical problems of pregnancy in women with severe mitral stenosis still arise. Recent immigration into the USA has increased the number of young women with severe valvular rheumatic disease or congenital heart disease; physicians should look for these conditions in pregnancy.

Congenital heart disease is now recognized at a much earlier age as a result of greater availability of neonatal and pediatric cardiac care units. With the exception of the infrequent Eisenmenger syndrome, in which shunt defects are associated with severe pulmonary hypertension, severe congenital heart disease is treated surgically before childbearing age. Immunization against rubella before pregnancy occurs has resulted in a marked decrease in the incidence of rubella in early pregnancy, one of the important causes of congenital heart disease. The prevalence of congenital heart disease has not decreased in recent years, but even before the advent of open heart surgery, untreated congenital heart disease was responsible for only 3–5% of all cases of heart disease in pregnancy.

CLASSIFICATION

Pregnant women with heart disease can be divided into two general categories. The first category consists of women with preexisting heart disease in whom the physiologic load imposed by pregnancy increases the work of the heart. In such cases, if the reserve capacity of the heart is compromised, the heart may fail. Preexisting heart disease is usually valvular or congenital, but hypertensive heart disease, mitral valve prolapse, and hypertrophic cardiomyopathy may also occur in women of childbearing age. Coronary heart disease is very rare at this age except in women with severe type I (insulin-dependent) diabetes mellitus or homozygous genetic hypercholesterolemia.

The second category is made up of women with disease induced by pregnancy, eg, preeclampsia-eclampsia, peripartum cardiomyopathy, thromboembolic disease causing multiple pulmonary emboli and pulmonary hypertension, and dissection of the aorta or of a coronary artery.

PHYSIOLOGIC CHANGES DURING PREGNANCY, LABOR, & THE PUERPERIUM

Pregnancy

The most striking cardiovascular change in pregnancy is an increase in the cardiac output of about 30% by the third or fourth month, usually owing to increased stroke volume. The heart rate increases only slightly (Table 22–1), as does oxygen consumption. Systemic vascular resistance decreases despite the raised cardiac output because of the arteriovenous fistula-like pregnant placenta and possibly as a result of increased prostaglandin production. There is a marked increase in total body water, of which 75% is extracellular, reaching a maximum in the second trimester. Plasma volume and red cell volume also increase in normal pregnancy (Table 22–1). The increased extracellular fluid is in part the result of estrogen-mediated stimulation of renin, which increases aldosterone secretion, as well as increased deoxycorticosterone (DOC) (Ehrlich, 1980). Plasma renin and angiotensin are substantially increased, yet blood pressure in most normal pregnancies actually falls, especially in the first two trimesters. Body weight increases an average of 10 kg. The increased renin secretion in the first trimester may be due to prostaglandins or changes in sodium and water balance, or both.

The glomerular filtration rate increases in normal pregnancy, which results in a greatly increased load of sodium, all of which is reabsorbed or excreted except for a small amount that is progressively retained, so that by the end of pregnancy approximately 500 meq of sodium is retained in the extracellular fluid volume and in the developing fetus.

Table 22–1. Effect of pregnancy on maternal circulatory and respiratory functions.[1]

Function	Change
Heart rate	Slow increase of 10 beats/min from 14 to 30 weeks. Rate maintained at this level to 40 weeks.
Arterial blood pressure	Systolic unchanged until the 30th week. Diastolic slightly reduced (period of maximal pulse pressure).
Venous blood pressure	Arms: No change. Legs: Gradual marked increase between 8 and 40 weeks.
Cardiac output	Increase of 30–50% by the 32nd week; decline to 20% increase at 40 weeks.
Total body water	Increased between 10 and 40 weeks.
Plasma and blood volume	Rise of 15% between 12 and 32 weeks; slight decline to 40 weeks.
Red cell mass	Increased 15% between 16 and 40 weeks.
Vital capacity	Rises 15% by the 20th week; decline of 5% by 40 weeks.
Oxygen consumption	Increased 10–15% between 8 and 40 weeks.
Circulation time	Decreases from 13 to 11 s by 32nd week, then returns to 13 s by 40th week.
Glomerular filtration	Increases 30–50% by second trimester.

[1] Modified and reproduced, with permission, from Benson RC: Handbook of Obstetrics & Gynecology, 8th ed., Lange, 1983.

The relative increase in plasma and blood volume in comparison to red cell mass accounts for the hemodilution and fall in hemoglobin during pregnancy; this is often confused with true anemia.

Patients with cardiac disease may develop symptoms of cardiac failure early in pregnancy if their cardiac reserve is severely limited. If the problem causing cardiac failure is due to a primary myocardial disease and not to a remediable condition such as mitral stenosis, therapeutic abortion can still be performed vaginally. Some patients may tolerate pregnancy well until the last 1–2 months, despite the fact that the load has been present all through pregnancy.

The maximum cardiac output in normal pregnancy occurs at about 28 weeks. The peak cardiac output exceeds the normal nonpregnant cardiac output by 30–50%. In the latter part of pregnancy, posture has an important influence on the cardiac output, which is reduced in the supine position (by mechanical obstruction of the inferior vena cava and decreasing venous return) and increased in the lateral position. This obstruction to venous return with decrease in cardiac output in the supine position late in pregnancy can lead to episodes of nausea, light-headedness, and faintness which is relieved by rolling over into the lateral position.

Oxygen consumption at rest increases progressively during pregnancy, whereas cardiac output increases in the first and second trimesters and for unknown reasons—perhaps because of the postural effect of the gravid uterus on venous return—falls in the last several weeks of pregnancy. The high cardiac output may be due to hormonal vasodilation and the arteriovenous fistula-like function of the placenta. The high output state resembles that seen in arteriovenous fistulas, and the patient has a hyperdynamic cardiac impulse, dilated and pulsating digital arteries, warm skin, and decreased systemic vascular resistance.

Labor & the Puerperium

In addition to marked changes in arterial and pulse pressure and in pulse rate with uterine contractions during labor, cardiac output increases with each contraction up to 50%, especially in the supine position. There is a marked increase (up to threefold) in oxygen consumption during labor. Strong uterine and cardiac contractions and decreased preload due to blood loss may enhance left ventricular obstruction in hypertrophic cardiomyopathy. These factors may produce chest pain or dyspnea.

Most of the hemodynamic changes return to normal by 10 days after delivery. With the exception of peripartum cardiomyopathy, cardiac complications of pregnancy are rare after that time.

CARDIAC DISEASE IN PREGNANCY

The cardiovascular load of normal pregnancy is large, but most normal women and women with mild valvular or congenital heart disease or hypertension tolerate pregnancy without difficulty. If cardiac function is impaired in the prepregnant state or worsens in the first trimester of pregnancy, cardiac complications progressively increase. Patients who have had cardiac failure in a previous pregnancy are more apt to develop cardiac failure in the current pregnancy. The most serious varieties of heart disease complicating pregnancy are severe mitral or aortic stenosis, Eisenmenger's syndrome, cyanotic congenital heart disease (especially if not corrected by previous surgery) (see Chapter 11), primary pulmonary hypertension, and severe coarctation of the aorta. In the presence of these varieties of cardiac disease, cardiac failure or arrhythmias may be anticipated as pregnancy continues and may cause serious problems at the time of delivery. Patients with Marfan's syndrome have an increased incidence of aortic dissection, especially if they have a dilated arch.

Diagnosis

The recognition of cardiac disease or of early cardiac failure may be difficult in pregnant women, especially if they have not been seen prior to pregnancy.

Even in normal patients, the increased blood volume, cardiac output, and hyperdynamic cardiac state may cause systolic ejection murmurs, hyperdynamic cardiac impulse, physiologic S_3, symptoms of dyspnea, and, especially later in pregnancy, edema resulting from sodium retention or venous obstruction by the large uterus. In late pregnancy, with the large uterus elevating the diaphragm and interfering with inspiration in the supine position, orthopnea and even paroxysmal nocturnal dyspnea can be seen. These normal physiologic changes of pregnancy must be recognized as such and not attributed to cardiac failure. Vital capacity does not normally change during pregnancy, and a decrease indicates developing pulmonary venous congestion. Basal vital capacity should be determined early in pregnancy so that changes can be assessed; a single test is not useful. An abnormally raised jugular venous pressure suggests early ventricular failure.

Treatment

If possible, the presence and severity of cardiac disease should be determined before a woman becomes pregnant, in order to evaluate the risks of pregnancy and to initiate therapeutic measures. Cardiac failure is uncommon in patients who, before pregnancy, had minimal symptoms and good cardiac reserve, with class I or II impairment (New York Heart Association criteria; see Chapter 2). If the limitation was more severe prior to pregnancy and patients were in class III or IV, if they had a history of cardiac failure in a previous pregnancy, or if they had one of the severe varieties of cardiac disease mentioned above—and especially if symptoms increase in the first trimester of pregnancy and are not controlled by medical therapy—surgical correction of the lesion (if possible) or therapeutic abortion is advised.

A. General Measures: Pregnant women with heart disease should have adequate rest and a nutritious diet. It is important to correct anemia and thyrotoxicosis. Patients should give up alcohol and stop smoking and avoid excessive sodium intake or weight gain. If cardiac symptoms are not severe or if they appear late in pregnancy, treatment consists of bed rest, restriction of sodium intake, digitalis, and antihypertensive agents if indicated. Bed rest throughout the remainder of pregnancy may allow a woman to maintain the pregnancy and avoid the development of cardiac failure. The fetal mortality rate is increased in patients who develop cardiac symptoms during pregnancy, possibly because of impaired uterine and placental perfusion, and management of the pregnant cardiac patient should also include careful examination of the fetal heart sounds and fetal movements.

The Medical Letter on Drugs and Therapeutics (1987) provides a useful table of antimicrobial drugs known to be safe or unsafe during pregnancy. It covers almost all antimicrobial agents available in 1987 and indicates when they are contraindicated, when they should be used with caution, and when they are probably safe. A more recent paper updates this information (Lynch, 1991).

Mitral valve prolapse, which occurs in 5–10% of women, requires no special treatment during pregnancy. In one prospective study, there were no cardiac complications in the mother or abnormalities in the infants. Labor and delivery are safe in mitral valve prolapse, but prophylactic antibiotics are advised during delivery (Shapiro, 1985). Prophylactic antibiotics to prevent infective endocarditis in patients undergoing procedures likely to provoke bacteremia should be given to those who would receive such prophylaxis in the nonpregnant state. Since bacteremia during normal labor and vaginal delivery is unusual (0–5%), the need for antibiotic prophylaxis is questionable. Certainly patients with a suspected genitourinary infection or at high risk—eg, those with prosthetic valves—should receive prophylaxis even with normal labor and delivery. The antibiotics recommended by the American Heart Association Committee (1990) are ampicillin, 2 g intravenously or intramuscularly, plus gentamicin, 1.5 mg/kg intravenously or intramuscularly (not to exceed 80 mg), on going into labor, followed by amoxicillin, 1.5 g orally, 6 hours after the initial dose. Alternatively, the parenteral regimen can be repeated one time 8 hours after the initial dose. For patients allergic to penicillin, vancomycin, 1 g intravenously given over 1 hour, plus gentamicin in the above dose, on going into labor and repeated 8 hours after the initial dose, may be substituted. The second doses of vancomycin and gentamicin can be omitted if renal function is depressed.

The factors that increase obstruction in hypertrophic cardiomyopathy, such as vasodilation, hypotension, or greatly increased cardiac contractions, should be avoided. The use of diuretic agents is controversial in patients who gain excessive weight or develop edema, because thiazides decrease plasma volume, which may decrease plasma and uterine blood flow. In general, it is best for patients to avoid drugs and rely on diet and a low sodium intake to prevent excessive weight gain and edema (see below).

Iron therapy should not be given for the hemodilution of pregnancy unless the hemoglobin is less than 10–11 g/dL. In patients who have valvular or congenital heart disease, antibiotic prophylaxis to prevent infective endocarditis should be given before delivery. In older pregnant patients with mitral stenosis, adequate treatment of atrial fibrillation with digitalis may prevent pulmonary venous congestion.

B. Surgical Treatment: In patients with surgically curable cardiac lesions such as severe mitral stenosis or severe aortic stenosis, it is preferable to delay definitive surgery until after delivery or, even better, to perform it before pregnancy. When the patient is first seen during pregnancy with severe cardiac failure, surgery may be undertaken then. Because medical treatment of cardiac failure has improved, the need for cardiac surgery in pregnancy has become considerably less. However, when a patient with mitral stenosis is seen and is already NYHA class III in the final trimester, surgical mitral valvuloplasty is indicated. One study (Becker, 1983) reported 101 pregnant patients undergoing closed mitral commissurotomy with no maternal deaths and the loss of three fetuses. Open mitral commissurotomy and mitral valve replacement with the patient on extracorporeal bypass is attended by a higher fetal loss but is still indicated when the mother is class III or class IV early in pregnancy.

Whether balloon valvuloplasty is as safe as surgical commissurotomy has yet to be proved. The marked hemodynamic changes that occur during balloon valvuloplasty and the high radiation exposure make it questionable that this procedure will replace surgery. Patients with severe aortic stenosis, especially if they are symptomatic, should have surgical repair even during pregnancy.

Patients with congenital heart disease who are NYHA class I or class II can tolerate pregnancy without surgical repair. This is especially true in the most common congenital cardiac lesion seen in this age group, ie, interatrial septal defect (Wooley, 1992).

C. Hypertension: (See below.) The management of hypertension due to hypertensive disease of pregnancy (preeclampsia), preexisting hypertension, or the hypertension of coarctation is important because of the hazard of eclampsia, aortic dissection and cardiac failure. It is estimated that half of all cases of dissection of the aorta in women occur during pregnancy, not all of them in women with hypertension. Less than 5% of all pregnancies in Western Europe are complicated by elevated blood pressure; but in cases that are, the risk of perinatal morbidity and mortality is increased (Svensson, 1985; Cunningham, 1992).

D. Management of Delivery: In the past there has been controversy over whether cardiac patients should be delivered by cesarean section or vaginal delivery. Physiologic studies are difficult during labor because of the rapid fluctuations of cardiac output, blood pressure, pulse rate, and adrenergic impulses associated with anxiety. In most patients with cardiac disease, the vaginal delivery, with deliberate rupture of the membranes if the cervix is dilated, combined with the use of low forceps, causes less physiologic disturbance and is tolerated better than cesarean section. Although the physiologic and circulatory changes of cesarean section are often relatively slight with skilled anesthesia and surgery, it is better to avoid an abdominal operation if possible.

Sterilization is advisable for the patient with an inoperable underlying disease and cardiac failure during pregnancy. If the patient has a cardiac condition that is amenable to cardiac surgery and operation can be performed after delivery, or if the cardiac symptoms have been precipitated by reversible and perhaps nonrecurrent situations, sterilization should not be performed, because many women deliver normal infants after the underlying cardiac condition has been corrected surgically.

E. Management of Patients With Cardiac Prostheses: Patients with valvular prostheses may tolerate pregnancy well. The decision whether to stop anticoagulant therapy may be difficult. If anticoagulants are stopped, systemic emboli may develop, even with cloth-covered prostheses. If warfarin is continued, there is a greater risk of spontaneous abortion, stillborn fetuses, central nervous system abnormalities in liveborn infants, and maternal hemorrhage following spinal or epidural block or during delivery. Despite the risks, some women have continued to receive oral anticoagulants throughout pregnancy. The proper treatment is not agreed on (Iturbe-Alessio, 1986), but in general the use of warfarin during pregnancy is contraindicated.

An alternative method of anticoagulation that is being used in some centers is deep subcutaneous administration of heparin, twice daily, in full dosage during the first trimester and before delivery. Although the danger of warfarin is less during mid pregnancy, if deep subcutaneous heparin is used, it should be continued throughout pregnancy. Deep subcutaneous heparin does not cross the placenta as does warfarin. At the time of labor, the heparin should be discontinued until after delivery. After delivery, heparin can be restarted once hemostasis is achieved, and warfarin can be restarted simultaneously. The two drugs should be continued together for 4 days before the heparin is stopped. This may be a successful compromise method that avoids the teratogenic effects of warfarin. Women who wish to become pregnant and who require valve replacement should be offered a bioprosthesis, which is less thrombogenic than a mechanical valve and can be managed without anticoagulation. The drawback to this approach is the high incidence of prosthetic valve calcification and disruption after 5–15 years, requiring a second valve replacement.

F. Management of Cardiac Arrhythmias: The incidence of cardiac arrhythmias during pregnancy has been increasing, because women who had corrective surgery for heart disease as children are now surviving to reproductive age and more women are delaying pregnancy until age 30 or older. If the underlying cardiac disease does not cause hemodynamic abnormalities and cardiac function is good, most arrhythmias are well tolerated and can be treated as outlined in Chapter 15. Most conventional drugs can be given without damage to the fetus. Digitalis, quinidine, beta-adrenergic blockers, lidocaine, and verapamil can be considered relatively safe, but phenytoin has caused birth defects. Table 22–2 summarizes antiarrhythmic drug therapy during pregnancy.

Table 22–2. Guide to the use of antiarrhythmic drugs in pregnancy.[1]

Drug	Route of Administration	Clinical Application	Therapeutic Concentration	Comments
Digoxin	Oral, IV	Paroxysmal supraventricular tachyarrhythmias; rate control in chronic atrial fibrillation and flutter	1–2 μg/mL	Adjust dosage when quinidine or verapamil are given concomitantly.
Quinidine	Oral	Prophylaxis in atrial and ventricular tachyarrhythmias	2–5 μg/mL	Excessive doses may lead to premature labor.
Procaina-mide	Oral, IV	Termination and prophylaxis in atrial and ventricular tachyarrhythmias	4–8 μg/mL	High incidence of maternal antinuclear antibodies and lupuslike syndrome with chronic use.
Disopyra-mide	Oral, IV	Atrial and ventricular tachyarrhythmias	3–7 μg/mL	One report documents uterine contractions.
Mexiletene	Oral	Symptomatic ventricular arrhythmias	1–2 μg/mL	Fetal bradycardia, hypoglycemia; low Apgar score.
Amiodarone	Oral	Life-threatening ventricular arrhythmias when other drugs fail. Also used in supraventricular arrhythmias.	1–2.5 μg/mL	Fetal hypothyroidism, hypotonia, bradycardia.
Beta-adrenergic blocking agents	Oral, IV	Termination and prophylaxis in atrial and ventricular tachyarrythmias; rate control in chronic atrial fibrillation	Variable	Chronic administration may be associated with intrauterine growth retardation.
Phenytoin	Oral, IV	Digitalis toxicity; refractory ventricular tachyarrhythmias	10–18 μg/mL	High risk of malformations ("fetal hydantoin syndrome").
Verapamil	Oral, IV	Paroxysmal supraventricular tachycardia; rate control in chronic atrial fibrillation	15–30 ng/mL	Rapid intravenous injection may occasionally cause maternal hypotension and fetal distress.
Lidocaine	IV	Drug of choice in ventricular tachyarrhythmias; digitalis toxicity	2–4 μg/mL	Toxic doses and fetal acidosis may cause central nervous system and cardiovascular depression in newborns.

[1] Modified and reproduced, with permission, from Rotmensch HH, Elkayam U, Frishman W: Antiarrhythmic drug therapy during pregnancy. Ann Intern Med 1983; 98:487.

Almost all antiarrhythmic drugs are excreted in the breast milk, but rarely in sufficient amounts to affect the infant.

G. Peripartum Cardiomyopathy: See Chapter 17.

Prognosis

Most patients with cardiac disease tolerate pregnancy surprisingly well if modern methods of treating cardiac failure and arrhythmias are available. The exceptions are severe mitral or aortic stenosis, severe coarctation of the aorta, primary pulmonary hypertension, Eisenmenger's syndrome, and cyanotic congenital heart disease. In Eisenmenger's syndrome, a maternal mortality rate in the range of 30–50% is reported (Gleicher, 1979). There is also a poor fetal outcome. In the same study, only one-fourth of all pregnancies reached term. More than half the infants were premature, and perinatal death occurred in 28%. Women with residual cyanotic congenital heart disease not corrected by previous surgery whose prepregnancy cardiac function was only fair or poor have a substantial incidence of cardiac failure or arrhythmias and deliver fewer live infants (Whittemore,

1982). Good prenatal care, awareness of the cardiac functional capacity of the patient prior to pregnancy, and appropriate surgical treatment may prevent cardiac problems during pregnancy. Unpredictable factors such as respiratory infections, atrial fibrillation, and other arrhythmias may complicate a straightforward clinical situation. These complications should be treated promptly and appropriately. Severe cardiac complications are uncommon today and probably will become even less so.

The prognosis for pregnancy in patients with hypertrophic cardiomyopathy is good. No deaths occurred in mothers or infants in a large series reported by Oakley (1979).

HYPERTENSIVE DISORDERS OF PREGNANCY

Hypertension during pregnancy may occur independently of pregnancy, as in essential hypertension, renal disease, pheochromocytoma, or coarctation of the aorta, or it may be a complication of pregnancy, as in preeclampsia or eclampsia. In essential hypertension, raised arterial pressure either precedes pregnancy or occurs early in pregnancy, whereas preeclampsia is characterized by normal blood pressure prior to pregnancy or early in pregnancy but a rise in pressure in the last trimester. Preeclampsia may complicate essential hypertension, in which case the blood pressure is raised early in pregnancy, and later the pressure increases substantially and is associated with proteinuria and edema. Pheochromocytoma and coarctation of the aorta are independent processes diagnosed and treated as discussed in Chapters 9 and 11.

ESSENTIAL HYPERTENSION

Essential hypertension is relatively uncommon (about 5%) in the USA and elsewhere in the Western world in young women, as contrasted with a prevalence of about 20% for individuals in their 40s and 50s. Pregnancies complicated by elevated blood pressure have an increased risk of perinatal morbidity and mortality (Svensson, 1985). Repeated blood pressures exceeding 140/90 mm Hg before the 20th week or a history of chronic hypertension prior to pregnancy distinguishes essential hypertension from preeclampsia. Multiple readings are required for diagnosis of hypertension, because pressures frequently vary over a period of time (Chapter 9). Diagnosis may be complicated in pregnant women because vasodilation produces a fall in pressure in the second trimester. Individuals seen for the first time in the second trimester may be considered to be normotensive even though observations before and after pregnancy indicate that the individual is indeed hypertensive. The diagnosis of essential hypertension must be based only on the arterial pressure, because in the age range of the usual pregnant patient, vascular complications are uncommon, and the ECG and examination of the ocular fundi and heart usually show no abnormalities. If the hypertension is severe, and if vascular complications are present during the first few months of pregnancy, the resulting increased likelihood of preeclampsia and an increased probability of fetal death may be an indication for therapeutic abortion.

Essential hypertension in pregnancy does not differ greatly from essential hypertension in nonpregnant women, and the decision regarding treatment depends on the severity of the hypertensive disorder. Slight elevations of pressure in the absence of vascular abnormalities require observation, but the decision regarding drug treatment can be delayed until after delivery. Fetal death is more frequent in patients with more severe hypertension, but it is possible to control the elevated blood pressure and improve maternal and fetal prognosis. Antihypertensive treatment should be given if the diastolic blood pressure is consistently greater than 100 mm Hg.

Treatment

The medical treatment of hypertension in pregnant women is similar to that in nonpregnant women (see Chapter 9). Treatment must begin at an early stage. Rest and sodium restriction may be sufficient to lower the pressures to normal in mild to moderate hypertension (Lowe, 1992). If the hypertension is more severe, methyldopa, beta-adrenergic-blocking drugs, and hydralazine can be used. Methyldopa has been used extensively during pregnancy, with excellent control of blood pressure and with only a 10% fetal mortality rate in severely hypertensive women. Hydralazine can be used orally or parenterally; in the latter instance, the blood pressure falls in 15–30 minutes. Hydralazine can be combined with methyldopa and beta-adrenergic blocking drugs. Atenolol has also been used with good results (Rubin, 1983). There is concern that beta-blocking drugs may cause fetal growth retardation. Data are insufficient regarding the side effects of newer antihypertensive agents in pregnancy. Labetalol may be hepatotoxic, and converting enzyme inhibitors have been associated with oligohydramnios and neonatal renal failure. These drugs are therefore contraindicated in pregnancy (Rosa, 1989). Preeclampsia occurs in 10–20% of cases. Unless the hypertension is severe, it is advisable to discontinue or decrease antihypertensive drugs 2–3 days before delivery. Data on the effects of treatment of hypertension on the newborn infant are limited, but adverse effects are uncommon.

Induction of labor and management of delivery should be similar to techniques used in cardiac disease in pregnancy. Vaginal delivery is usually satisfactory, with early rupture of the membranes and the use of low forceps to shorten the duration of labor. A few patients first develop raised arterial pressure in the postpartum period. The course of the condition is usually benign, and treatment should be withheld for 3–6 months unless complications occur or the diastolic pressure rises alarmingly (to about 110–120 mm Hg).

Prognosis

The prognosis of essential hypertension in pregnancy is usually good unless preeclampsia is severe or eclampsia with convulsions develops. Control of blood pressure with modern antihypertensive drugs has made therapeutic abortion unnecessary in most cases, although immediate delivery vaginally or by cesarean section late in pregnancy is preferable to drug therapy if severe preeclampsia or convulsions occur. Malignant hypertension or cardiac or renal failure discovered early in pregnancy may warrant therapeutic abortion, especially if the patient has preexisting renal disease. The differentiation of renal disease due to chronic glomerulonephritis or chronic pyelonephritis from essential hypertension is difficult if renal impairment is present when the patient is first seen. In addition to benefit to the mother, antihypertensive therapy with methyldopa results in a significantly improved fetal outcome. In terms of both birth weight and general health, the surviving infants of mothers treated with antihypertensive agents were similar to those of untreated mothers. Diuretics are usually avoided because of the possible decrease in plasma volume and uterine and placental blood flow.

PREECLAMPSIA-ECLAMPSIA

Preeclampsia, the clinical syndrome of hypertension, edema, and proteinuria developing in the last trimester of pregnancy, progresses as a continuum at various rates and extends from mild preeclampsia to eclampsia, in which the syndrome includes convulsions. Preeclampsia occurs in about 5% of pregnancies. The disorder has gradually declined in incidence in the past several decades (see Prognosis), possibly as a consequence of better prenatal care. Eclampsia is much less frequent and, for reasons that are not clear, is less frequent than it formerly was, is occurring in about 0.1% of pregnant women.

Pathophysiology

The cause of preeclampsia is unknown, and many theories have been offered. The condition is more frequent in the first pregnancy, in patients with preexisting hypertension, in twin pregnancies, in patients with a history of preeclampsia, in patients with hydatidiform mole, and in some populations of black women. Preeclampsia may result from impaired uteroplacental perfusion; this is supported by the observation that during preeclampsia, plasma volume, glomerular filtration rate, and uterine and placental blood flow decrease about 25% in recumbency. The gravid uterus has a poorer arterial blood supply in preeclampsia as compared to the nongravid or normal pregnant uterus. Preeclampsia has been produced in animals by constricting the uterine arteries to reduce the uterine blood flow.

Elevated blood pressure is not the only manifestation of preeclampsia; at autopsy and renal biopsy, thromboses and immunoglobulin deposits have been found in the kidney, liver, and elsewhere (see below).

A. Hemodynamic and Volume Changes: In preeclampsia, as compared to normal pregnancy, systemic vascular resistance is increased; plasma and red cell volume, glomerular filtration rate, and renal blood flow are decreased; sodium retention is enhanced; and uric acid clearance falls (Lindheimer, 1981; Cunningham, 1992).

B. Role of Prostaglandins and the Renin-Angiotensin-Aldosterone System: Prostaglandin E (PGE) can be synthesized by the uterus. The reduced uteroplacental blood flow may decrease PGE synthesis and increase the secretion of renin, setting in motion the sequence of events leading to increased production of angiotensin and hypertension (Remuzzi, 1991) (Figure 22–1).

Renin is produced by the uterus and chorion as well as by the kidney; plasma renin and aldosterone are lower in pregnancy associated with hypertension than in normal pregnancy (Pedersen, 1983).

Serum concentration of atrial natriuretic factor (ANF) was found in one study to be greater in healthy pregnant than in normal nonpregnant women, but higher still in preeclampsia despite the plasma volume expansion and low pulmonary capillary wedge pressures seen in preeclampsia. Why ANF is increased is not known; factors other than atrial pressure may determine the release of the ANF in preeclampsia (Thomsen, 1987).

Prostacyclin biosynthesis increases during normal pregnancy and in pregnancy-induced hypertension of preeclampsia but increases less in the latter. The difference persists throughout gestation, suggesting that the decreased synthesis of prostacyclin plays a pathophysiologic role related to the hypertension (Fitzgerald, 1987). Aspirin, 20–60 mg daily, resulted in a significantly lower incidence of the pregnancy-induced hypertension of preeclampsia among otherwise normal pregnant women. No adverse effects of treatment were observed in the mother or the infant. Low-dose aspirin may restore prostacyclin thromboxane imbalance, which seems to add to the evidence that the imbalance is important in preeclampsia (Wallenburg, 1986). In a meta-analysis of 13 trials of low-dose aspirin, a significant decrease in the incidence of proteinuric preeclampsia was found (Collins, 1989).

C. Renal and Hepatic Changes in Preclampsia; Possible Immunologic Mechanisms: The proteinuria that occurs as part of the characteristic triad of hypertension, edema, and proteinuria in preeclampsia is considered to be of glomerular origin. Renal biopsies have shown endothelial swelling, narrowing of the lumen of the capillaries, deposits of fibrin in the glomeruli, evidences of intravascular coagulation, and "glomerular endotheliosis" (Lindheimer, 1981). About one-fourth of patients with preeclampsia show evidence of chronic renal disease (nephrosclerosis, chronic glomerulonephritis, or chronic pyelonephritis). There may be a correlation between the clinical severity of preeclampsia and the density and pattern of IgM and IgG deposits in the glomeruli of the kidney. The typical electron microscopic appearance of renal biopsy specimens in preeclampsia is fibrin and immunoglobulin deposition in the capillary loops, especially deposition of IgM and complement. Complement deposits occur within the walls of afferent and efferent arterioles (Petrucco, 1974). Similar deposits of fibrin, immunoglobulins, and complement were found in the livers of preeclamptic but not normal pregnant women by means of immunofluorescence (Figure 22–2).

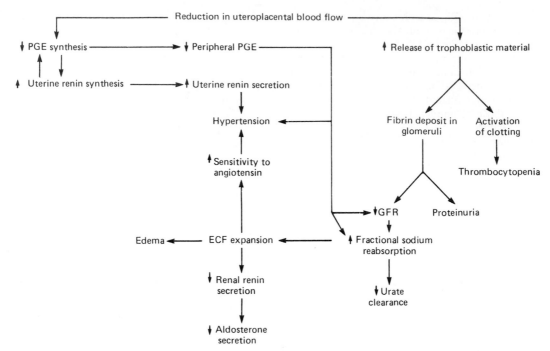

Reduction in uteroplacental blood flow

↓ PGE synthesis ────────→ ↓ Peripheral PGE ──────→ ↑ Release of trophoblastic material

↑ Uterine renin synthesis ────────→ ↑ Uterine renin secretion

Hypertension ←────────

↑ Sensitivity to angiotensin

Edema ←──── ECF expansion ←────

↓ Renal renin secretion

↓ Aldosterone secretion

Fibrin deposit in glomeruli   Activation of clotting

Thrombocytopenia

↓ GFR   Proteinuria

↑ Fractional sodium reabsorption

↓ Urate clearance

Figure 22–1. Hypothesis for the pathophysiology of preeclampsia-eclampsia. Diminished uteroplacental blood flow leads to a possible decrease in uterine synthesis of PGE but an increase in renin synthesis. In addition, fibrin deposits in the glomeruli cause a reduction in GFR and an increase in sodium retention. (PGE, prostaglandin E; GFR, glomerular filtration rate; ECF, extracellular fluid.) (Reproduced, with permission, from Ferris TF: Toxemia of pregnancy: A model of human hypertension. Cardiovasc Med 1977;2:877.)

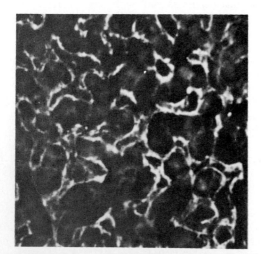

Figure 22–2. Diffuse staining of hepatic sinusoids with fluorescent antiserum to fibrinogen. (Reproduced, with permission, from Arias F, Mancilla-Jimenez R: Hepatic fibrinogen deposits in preeclampsia: Immunofluorescent evidence. N Engl J Med 1976;295:578.)

Thus, an immunologic mechanism may be responsible for the renal and hepatic lesions of preeclampsia, with a primary vascular disorder similar to the transplant rejection mechanism involving the antibody system. Antiplacental antibodies may be produced that result in deposition of immunoglobulins and complement in the kidney. Because of the familial occurrence of preeclampsia, genetic factors are being actively investigated.

The severity of preeclampsia and eclampsia may be related to the magnitude of the deposition of the immunoglobulins, but the mechanism by which this is accomplished is at present obscure.

Clinical Findings

Preeclampsia is defined as a syndrome encountered in the last trimester of pregnancy that is characterized by at least two of three cardinal manifestations (Page, 1953):

(1) A rather abrupt increase of blood pressure amounting to 30 mm Hg or more systolic and 15 mm Hg or more diastolic after the 26th week of pregnancy.

(2) The appearance (or sudden increase) of proteinuria of at least 0.5 g/d.

(3) Edema in the upper half of the body.

Any two of these signs must be manifest on two occasions at least 6 hours apart. If convulsions occur in addition to the above criteria, the case is classified as eclampsia.

Generalized edema is common in pregnancy and when present in the lower half of the body is not considered diagnostic of heart failure. The increased tubular reabsorption of sodium and water causes edema in the upper half of the body that may precede the appearance of proteinuria and hypertension. About 6% of all pregnant women in the USA develop preeclampsia, and one in 20 of this total group develops the convulsions of eclampsia. Approximately 5% of patients with eclampsia die of the disease. There are about 1500 maternal deaths each year and about 15,000 fetal deaths. Deaths from preeclampsia are rare.

Apart from weight gain, edema in the upper half of the body, proteinuria, and hypertension, patients with preeclampsia may develop headache, drowsiness, visual disturbances, dyspnea, and, if the hypertension is severe, pulmonary edema and cardiac failure. Cerebral hemorrhage causes 10% of deaths in eclampsia. Acute tubular necrosis rarely causes death but may occur in severe eclampsia. Hypotension may develop in severe eclampsia with hemorrhage and necrosis in the adrenal glands.

Clinical Course

The onset of preeclampsia may be gradual or sudden, and the diagnosis may be difficult to establish in the early stages because the pathophysiologic changes may be present before clinical symptoms or signs appear. Women who later develop preeclampsia may show differences in their response to angiotensin before proteinuria and a rise in blood pressure occur. Patients may develop edema similar to the edema of normal pregnancy. The proteinuria may be slight, and the elevation of blood pressure may be slight and variable. In mild cases, restriction of activity and sodium intake may be sufficient to reverse the process by increasing uterine, renal, and placental blood flow. If proteinuria increases, if blood pressure rises, or if symptoms such as blurred vision, decreased urine output, a rise in serum creatinine, enzyme changes reflecting hepatic dysfunction, or rapid gain in weight develop, the patient should be hospitalized. Papilledema, hemorrhages, and exudates are rare. The development of a generalized boring headache signals an impending convulsion and should be the immediate indication for more intensive hospital therapy, including termination of pregnancy (Working Group: National High Blood Pressure Education Program, 1990).

Prevention

Prevention depends on good prenatal care, good nutrition, education so that patients recognize the earliest development of preeclampsia, bed rest and sodium restriction when manifestations first appear, recommendations against subsequent pregnancies in patients who have had severe preeclampsia, and antihypertensive drugs to control preexisting hypertension in patients who become pregnant.

When signs of impending convulsions (see above) appear, delivery is the best preventive treatment for eclampsia. Eclampsia does not occur after the uterus is emptied.

Treatment

A. Preeclampsia: Bed rest and sodium restriction usually reverse the process in mild preeclampsia. In severe preeclampsia, antihypertensive drugs are used. Hydralazine intravenously, starting with 5 mg and repeating 5–10 mg every 20–30 minutes, is excellent for severe hypertension. If convulsions appear imminent, intravenous magnesium sulfate may be given in addition to keep the serum level at 4–6 meq/L. Thiazides should not be used because they may exaggerate the diminished plasma volume in patients with preeclampsia. Nitroprusside should not be used, since it crosses the placenta and can result in accumulation of fetal cyanide and fetal death (Dicke, 1985). Pharmacologic agents lower blood pressure but do not affect the pathophysiology of the condition and do not decrease the fetal mortality rate. If preeclampsia does not subside after a few days of hospital care, the pregnancy should be interrupted by cesarean section or, if the patient is near term, labor should be induced. The infant mortality rate is greater the longer preeclampsia persists. In severe preeclampsia, the infant mortality rate is five times the normal rate. The transition from severe preeclampsia to eclampsia with convulsions is one of degree rather than of kind. It is preferable to interrupt the pregnancy by cesarean section if convulsions, muscular twitching, severe headache, epigastric pain (vascular crisis), or visual disturbances are imminent. Interruption of pregnancy is the most reliable means of preventing the transition from preeclampsia to eclampsia.

B. Eclampsia: Prevention of convulsions is a cardinal goal of therapy. If convulsions occur, the clinical situation is much worse; the maternal mortality rate is 5% and the fetal mortality rate about 20–25%. Convulsions should be managed by use of intravenous magnesium sulfate, absolute rest in bed, constant nursing care, and avoidance of anything that disturbs the patient and may precipitate a convulsion. Delivery should be postponed until the convulsions can be stopped. Magnesium toxicity (blood levels > 6 meq/L) may occur when use is prolonged. Magnesium toxicity is suggested clinically by absent patellar reflexes and low urine output (< 30–40 mL/h). Both urine output and patellar reflexes should be monitored before each dose of magnesium sulfate is given. In a consecutive series of 154 cases managed by this method, there were no maternal deaths and all infants weighing more than 4 lb survived (Pritchard,

1975). Antihypertensive drugs should be used if the diastolic blood pressure is elevated to 110 mm Hg or more. Some patients with eclampsia have cerebral edema rather than hypertension as the mechanism of their convulsions, and magnesium sulfate therapy is therefore preferred. If the patient is oliguric, intravenous fluids should be used with caution.

Pregnancy should not be terminated unless the patient has had no convulsions for 24–48 hours.

Prognosis

Maternal deaths are now rare in preeclampsia. Preeclampsia is more frequent in patients with preexisting essential hypertension or renal disease than in patients who were normotensive before pregnancy. About 25% of patients who develop hypertension in late pregnancy have unsuspected chronic renal disease on renal biopsy and not preeclampsia.

Infants of mothers with preeclampsia have a mortality rate three to five times as high as those of normal mothers. About half of cases of eclampsia that occur in multiparous women are preceded by hypertension. When eclampsia complicates previous hypertension, the fetal mortality rate approximates 50%.

The prognosis of mild preeclampsia is good with bed rest and sodium restriction, but if the condition progresses with increase of weight, edema, proteinuria, and hypertension, termination of pregnancy should be instituted promptly before convulsions occur. In primiparous women with eclampsia, there is no increased incidence of permanent hypertension (Chesley, 1976).

Multiparous women who survive eclampsia have a worse prognosis and an incidence of cardiovascular deaths almost three times the expected number. Perhaps "gestational" hypertension (without proteinuria) is a sign of latent essential hypertension. Convulsions may lead to cerebral hemorrhage, pulmonary edema, aortic dissection, and adrenal hemorrhage or necrosis. Interruption of pregnancy in severe preeclampsia usually prevents convulsive eclampsia. Treatment of convulsions permits cesarean section, reducing the maternal and fetal mortality rate. Patients with a history of severe preeclampsia or eclampsia should be discouraged from becoming pregnant again.

REFERENCES

American Heart Association Committee on Rheumatic Fever, Endocarditis, and Kawasaki Disease: Prevention of Bacterial endocarditis. JAMA 1990;264:2919.

Arias F, Mancilla-Jimenez R: Hepatic fibrinogen in preeclampsia: Immunofluorescent evidence. N Engl J Med 1976;295:578.

Becker RM: Intracardiac surgery in pregnant women. Ann Thorac Surg 1983;36:453.

Ben Ismail M et al: Cardiac valve prostheses, anticoagulation, and pregnancy. Br Heart J 1986;55:101.

Bortolotti U et al: Pregnancy in patients with a porcine valve bioprosthesis. Am J Cardiol 1982;50:1051.

Brown MA et al: Fluid volumes in pregnancy-induced hypertension. J Hypertens 1992;10:61.

Chesley LC: Severe rheumatic cardiac disease and pregnancy: The ultimate prognosis. Am J Obstet Gynecol 1980;136:552.

Chesley LC, Annitto JE, Cosgrove RA: The remote prognosis of eclamptic women: Sixth period report. Am J Obstet Gynecol 1976;124:446.

Cockburn J et al: Final report of study on hypertension during pregnancy: The effects of specific treatment of the growth and development of the children. Lancet 1982;1:647.

Cole P et al: Longitudinal changes in left ventricular architecture and function in peripartum cardiomyopathy. Am J Cardiol 1987;60:871.

Collins R, Yusuf S, Peto R: Overview of randomized trials of diuretics in pregnancy. Br Med J 1985;290:17.

Collins R et al: Pharmacological prevention and treatment of hypertensive disorders in pregnancy. In: Chalmers I, Enkin M, Keirse MJNC (editors). *Effec-*

tive Care in Pregnancy and Childbirth. Vol 1: *Pregnancy.* Oxford Univ Press, 1989.

Cunningham FG, Lindheimer MD: Hypertension in pregnancy. (Current Concepts.) N Engl J Med 1992;326:927.

Dicke JM: Cardiovascular drugs in pregnancy. In: *Principles of Medical Therapy in Pregnancy.* Gleicher N et al (editors). Plenum, 1985.

Ehrlich EN, Nolten WE, Lindheimer MD: Mineralocorticoids and the regulation of sodium metabolism in normal and hypertensive pregnancy: A review. Clin Exp Hypertens 1980;2:803.

Elkayam U, Gleicher N: Cardiac problems in pregnancy: 1. Maternal aspects: The approach to the pregnant patient with heart disease. JAMA 1984;251:2838.

Elkayam U, Gleicher N (editors): *Cardiac Problems in Pregnancy: Diagnosis and Management of Maternal and Fetal Disease,* 2nd ed. Liss, 1990.

Elliott DL et al: Medical illness and pregnancy: An annotated bibliography of recent literature. Ann Intern Med 1983;99:83.

Fitzgerald DJ et al: Decreased prostacyclin biosynthesis preceding the clinical manifestation of pregnancy-induced hypertension. Circulation 1987;75:956.

Gleicher N et al: Eisenmenger's syndrome and pregnancy. Obstet Gynecol Surv 1979;34:721.

Graves SW: The possible role of digitalis-like factors in pregnancy-induced hypertension. Hypertension 1987;10(Suppl):I-84.

Hall JG, Pauli RM, Wilson KM: Maternal and fetal sequelae of anticoagulation during pregnancy. Am J Med 1980;68:122.

Handin RI: Thromboembolic complications of pregnancy and oral contraceptives. Prog Cardiovasc Dis 1974;16:395.

Iturbe-Alessio I et al: Risks of anticoagulant therapy in pregnant women with artificial heart valves. N Engl J Med 1986;315:1390.

Lindheimer MD, Katz AI: Hypertension in pregnancy. N Engl J Med 1985;313:675.

Lindheimer MD, Katz AI: Pathophysiology of pre-eclampsia. Annu Rev Med 1981;32:273.

Lynch CM et al: Use of antibiotics during pregnancy. Clin Pharm 1991;43:1365.

Lowe SA, Rubin PC: The pharmacologic management of hypertension in pregnancy. J Hypertens 1992;10:201.

The Medical Letter on Drugs and Therapeutics: Drugs in pregnancy. Med Lett Drugs Ther 1987;29:61.

Metcalfe J, McAnulty JH, Ueland K: *Burwell and Metcalfe's Heart Disease and Pregnancy: Physiology and Management,* 2nd ed. Little, Brown, 1986.

Noble MIM: The contribution of blood momentum to left ventricular ejection in the dog. Circ Res 1968;23: 663.

Oakley GDG et al: Management of pregnancy in patients with hypertrophic cardiomyopathy. Br Med J 1979;1: 1749.

O'Connell JB et al: Peripartum cardiomyopathy: Clinical, hemodynamic, histologic and prognostic characteristics. J Am Coll Cardiol 1986;8:52.

Page EW: *The Hypertensive Disorders of Pregnancy.* Thomas, 1953.

Palacios IF et al: Percutaneous mitral balloon valvotomy during pregnancy in a patient with severe mitral stenosis. Cathet Cardiovasc Diagn 1988;15:109.

Pedersen EB et al: Preeclampsia: A state of prostaglandin deficiency? Urinary prostaglandin excretion, the renin-aldosterone system, and circulating catecholamines in preeclampsia. Hypertension 1983;5:105.

Petrucco OM et al: Immunofluorescent studies in renal biopsies in pre-eclampsia. Br Med J 1974;1:473.

Pettifor JM, Benson R: Congenital malformations associated with the administration of oral anticoagulants during pregnancy. J Pediatr 1975;86:459.

Phippard AF et al: Circulatory adaptation to pregnancy: serial studies of haemodynamics, blood volume, renin and aldosterone in the baboon *(Papio hamadyas).* J Hypertens 1986;4:773.

Pitts JA, Crosby WM, Basta LL: Eisenmenger's syndrome in pregnancy: Does heparin prophylaxis im-prove the maternal mortality rate? Am Heart J 1977;93:321.

Pritchard JA, Pritchard SA: Standardized treatment of 154 consecutive cases of eclampsia. Am J Obstet Gynecol 1975;123:543.

Remuzzi G et al: Prevention and treatment of pregnancy-associated hypertension: What have we learned in the last 10 years? Am J Kidney Dis 1991;18:285.

Rosa FW et al: Neonatal anuria with maternal angiotensin-converting enzyme inhibition. Obstet Gynecol 1989;74:371.

Rotmensch HH, Elkayam U, Frishman W: Antiarrhythmic drug therapy during pregnancy. Ann Intern Med 1983;98:487.

Rubin PC (editor): *Hypertension in Pregnancy.* Vol 10 of: *Handbook of Hypertension.* Birkenhager WH, Reid JL (editors). Elsevier, 1988.

Rubin PC et al: Placebo-controlled trial of atenolol in treatment of pregnancy-associated hypertension. Lancet 1983;1:431.

The safety of antimicrobial drugs in pregnancy. Med Lett Drugs Ther 1987;29:61.

Selzer A: Management of pregnant patients with valvular heart disease. Primary Cardiol (Feb) 1981;7:127.

Shapiro EP et al: Safety of labor and delivery in women with mitral valve prolapse. Am Heart J 1985;56:806.

Sullivan JM, Ramanathan KB: Management of medical problems in pregnancy: Severe cardiac disease. N Engl J Med 1985;313:304.

Svensson A: Hypertension in pregnancy: State of the art lecture. J Hypertens 1985;3(Suppl 3):S395.

Thomsen JK et al: Atrial natriuretic peptide concentrations in preeclampsia. Br Med J 1987;294:1508.

Wallenburg HC et al: Low-dose aspirin prevents pregnancy-induced hypertension and preeclampsia in angiotensin-sensitive primigravidae. Lancet 1986;1:1.

Whittemore R, Hobbins JC, Engle MA: Pregnancy and its outcome in women with and without surgical treatment of congenital heart disease. Am J Cardiol 1982;50:641.

Wooley CF, Sparks EH: Congenital heart disease, heritable cardiovascular disease, and pregnancy. Prog Cardiovasc Dis 1992;35:41.

Working Group: National High Blood Pressure Education Program Working Group Report on High Blood Pressure in Pregnancy. Am J Obstet Gynecol 1990;163 (5 Pt 1):1689.

Preoperative assessment of the cardiac patient for noncardiac surgery is a frequent responsibility of the internist or cardiologist. The object of the consultation is not to "clear" the patient for surgery or to share responsibility with the surgeon if there is a medical complication associated with the surgery.

The most important function of the preoperative assessment is to define any cardiac problems the patient may have and assess the risks they may impose during anesthesia and surgery. The anesthesiologist will be most interested in obtaining a list of all drugs the patient is taking and the possible drug-drug interactions that could occur.

Postponing a scheduled operation creates serious problems for the patient, the surgeon, and the anesthesiologist and upsets the operating room schedule. Postponement should be recommended only if something can be done during the postponement that will reduce the surgical risk. Postponement therefore implies further diagnostic tests or therapy that will improve the patient's ability to handle the stresses of anesthesia and surgery.

Finally, it is inappropriate for the internist to presume to advise the anesthesiologist that hypoxia and hypotension should be avoided.

RISKS OF ANESTHESIA & SURGERY

The risks to any surgical patient include both anesthetic and surgical complications, many of which are preventable. Unexpected hemorrhage, acidosis, impaired ventilation, hypercapnia, decreased systemic vascular resistance, decreased cardiac contractility and conduction, cardiac arrhythmias (with or without increased release of catecholamines), and hypotension with or without a decreased blood volume (such as may occur from hemorrhage)—all interfere with cardiovascular function. Some anesthetic agents such as cyclopropane increase adrenergic activity to the cardiovascular system, whereas others such as halothane reduce cardiovascular sympathetic tone. Anesthetic agents decrease the force of cardiac contraction and may decrease cardiac output. Release of catecholamines may induce arrhythmia or hypertension. Drugs that inhibit the sympathetic nervous system may induce hypotension and reduced systemic flow

that impair coronary perfusion, especially in patients with preexisting coronary atherosclerotic lesions. Muscle-relaxing drugs may induce bradycardia and release large amounts of potassium from injured muscles following trauma.

Each hazard producing respiratory or cardiac problems poses a greater risk in patients who have underlying cardiac disease. Cardiac arrest with ventricular fibrillation is the most feared event and is principally due to excessive blood loss, hypotension, accidental administration of potassium or its release by muscle-relaxing drugs, airway obstruction as a result of laryngeal spasm or aspiration of gastric contents, difficulty in intubation at the onset of the surgical procedure, or hypoxemia and acidosis secondary to impaired ventilation. These complications can be minimized by preoperative evaluation and by prophylactic continuous monitoring of cardiovascular variables (eg, arterial pressure, ECG) and intermittent evaluation of blood gases. Preoperative placement of an endocardial right ventricular pacemaker should be done in patients who have symptomatic sick sinus syndrome with bradycardia, Stokes-Adams attacks, or bifascicular block with episodes of dizziness or syncope. Meticulous anesthetic and surgical technique combined with prompt recognition and treatment of any complication that may arise decreases the hazard to the patient. Postoperative sodium and water retention may occur, causing disturbances in fluid and electrolyte balance.

URGENT VERSUS ELECTIVE SURGERY

Because of the increased hazard of general surgery in the cardiac patient, especially in those with coronary heart disease, the physician must answer certain questions to ascertain when the risks of surgery exceed the risks of the underlying disease and when the reverse is true. Key questions that must be answered are the following: (1) Is the operation urgent or elective? (2) If elective, does the patient have cardiac disease? (3) What is the risk of the underlying surgical disease if surgery is not performed? (4) What additional risk does the heart disease impose on the surgical procedure? (5) Is the surgical diagnosis correct, or could the symptoms, such as abdominal pain, be a manifestation of cardiac disease and not a surgical disease? (6) Can anything be done in term of risk stratification or therapy which would reduce the risk of surgery?

URGENT SURGERY

Urgent operations must be done regardless of the underlying cardiac disease and include conditions that threaten life or limb, eg, gross hemorrhage, strangulated hernia, perforation of the bowel or gallbladder, acute bowel obstruction, proximal aortic dissection, ruptured aortic aneurysm, and arterial embolism. The presence of heart disease does not mean that the patient will not tolerate the surgical procedure; one should not withhold a lifesaving procedure merely because of the presence of heart disease but should identify and reverse any reversible cardiac risk factor.

CARDIAC CONDITIONS MASQUERADING AS SURGICAL ILLNESSES

Gastrointestinal symptoms, including acute abdominal pain, may so dominate the clinical picture that heart disease is not recognized or, if recognized, is not thought to be responsible for the symptoms. Early evidence of cardiac failure is often overlooked because it is overshadowed by the gastrointestinal symptoms. The most common causes of diagnostic confusion are the following:

(1) Angina pectoris or myocardial infarction presenting with predominant epigastric pain.

(2) Fairly abrupt right heart failure presenting with right upper quadrant pain simulating gallbladder disease. This is particularly apt to occur in patients with tight mitral valve stenosis who develop atrial fibrillation or in patients with mild right heart failure following exercise.

(3) Slowly developing right heart failure, which may present with nonspecific gastrointestinal symptoms of anorexia, nausea, a sensation of heaviness and fullness after meals, and perhaps vomiting. These lead to weight loss and may seem to justify a diagnosis of carcinoma of the upper gastrointestinal tract. If there are no murmurs, the diagnosis of heart disease is often missed.

(4) Pulmonary infarction presenting as jaundice, leading to a diagnosis of biliary tract disease.

(5) Right heart failure or constrictive pericarditis presenting as ascites.

(6) Dysphagia, which may be the presenting symptom in a variety of heart diseases, eg, mitral stenosis with large left atrium, pericarditis, aortic aneurysm, aortic dissection, or anomalies of the aortic arch.

(7) Acute rheumatic fever, which may present with acute abdominal pain, especially in children.

(8) Acute abdominal pain, which may result from acute myocardial infarction or emboli to the splenic, renal, or mesenteric arteries in infective endocarditis or atrial fibrillation. Surgical treatment may be required secondarily if gangrene of the bowel occurs.

(9) Nausea and vomiting, which may occur in cardiac failure, especially as a result of digitalis therapy.

Space does not permit a discussion of the differential diagnosis of these conditions, but one should search for positive diagnostic evidence of heart disease: (1) a history of angina pectoris, dyspnea on effort, orthopnea, or previous ventricular arrhythmias or atrial fibrillation or flutter. (2) Cardiac enlargement with a left or right ventricular heave, with or without characteristic murmurs. (3) Evidence of right heart failure, with increased venous pressure, enlarged and tender liver, and edema or ascites. Orthopnea, decreased vital capacity, and rales and gallop rhythm may be present in left ventricular failure. (4) Signs of myocardial necrosis with fever, tachycardia, or enzyme changes. (5) Typical serial electrocardiographic changes of ischemia, infarction, hypertrophy, pericarditis, etc. (6) Echocardiographic evidence of cardiac abnormality, as in (5). (7) Radiologic evidence of cardiac enlargement or pulmonary venous congestion.

Considering the possibility of heart disease during the diagnostic process often leads to a better examination and appropriate therapy.

PREOPERATIVE EVALUATION OF THE SURGICAL PATIENT WITH KNOWN OR SUSPECTED CARDIOVASCULAR DISEASE

A thorough history and physical examination combined with a resting ECG and chest x-ray— and, in selected patients, noninvasive procedures such as two-dimensional echocardiography and nuclear angiography—are sufficient to diagnose most cardiac diseases. Twelve- to 24-hour monitoring of the ECG may be required if the patient has unexplained symptoms of dizziness, syncope, weakness, chest pain, or palpitations in order to determine the presence of cardiac arrhythmias, heart block, or ischemic ST depression.

See Special Precautions (below) for a discussion of drugs the patient might be taking and that might influence the general state of health or the outcome of operation.

RECOGNITION OF HEART DISEASE

The presence of heart disease is recognized on the basis of symptoms, significant murmurs, an enlarged heart, electrocardiographic or echocardiographic abnormality, evidence of cardiac failure, hypertension, conduction defects, atrial fibrillation or flutter, or ventricular arrhythmias. A history of angina pectoris or previous myocardial infarction, Stokes-Adams attacks, cardiac failure, intermittent claudication, or cerebral ischemic attacks may alert the physician to the possibility of cardiac disease. A history of antihypertensive treatment or treatment for cardiac failure may be obtained.

A baseline ECG is advisable in patients over 40 years of age to interpret postoperative changes. An ECG may also show evidence of digitalis therapy, electrolyte disturbances, conduction defects, or arrhythmias. In general, a stable abnormality on the ECG in the absence of cardiac failure or a change in the pattern of angina pectoris indicates that the patient will probably tolerate surgery almost as well as a normal individual. Such a patient with a healed previous myocardial infarction has an added mortality risk of about 3–5%.

The most important contraindications to elective surgery are recent onset angina pectoris, a crescendo change in the pattern of angina pectoris in recent weeks or months, unstable angina, acute myocardial infarction, myocardial infarction within the preceding 3 months, severe aortic stenosis, a high degree of atrioventricular block, untreated cardiac failure, and severe hypertension.

A multifactorial index providing point scores for various predictors of cardiac risk has been used to estimate the additional risk following major noncardiac surgery. These include age over 70 years, recent myocardial infarction, raised venous pressure, S_3 gallop, multiple premature beats, hypoxemia, hypokalemia, elevated serum creatinine, and aortic stenosis. The weighted index serves as a basis for predicting the probability of postoperative cardiac complications and for fashioning guidelines for managing and assessing patients requiring major surgery (Goldman, 1983).

Detsky (1986) has modified Goldman's cardiac risk index to assess patients undergoing noncardiac surgery. More than a third of severe complications occurred in patients with the lowest preoperative index scores. Care must therefore be taken not to rely exclusively on these statistical indexes. As always, clinical judgment is required.

A prospective study found that the only independent predictor of perioperative complications was the ability of the patient to exercise preoperatively (Gerson, 1985).

Thallium redistribution indicating myocardial ischemia greatly increased the odds of a serious cardiac event in patients who had peripheral vascular repair (Leppo, 1987). The management of postoperative complications such as arrhythmias, conduction disturbances, myocardial ischemia, cardiac failure, and hypotension is discussed by Wohlgelernter (1984).

SPECIFIC DISEASE PROBLEMS

1. CORONARY HEART DISEASE

The usual patient seen for preoperative evaluation is an older individual with possible coronary heart disease. The patient may be at high risk for coronary disease because of factors such as age, hypertension, smoking history, diabetes, lipid abnormalities, or peripheral vascular disease—or may have known coronary artery disease, as manifested by a history of angina pectoris or previous myocardial infarction. There is strong evidence that excessive risk related to acute myocardial infarction disappears after 3–6 months.

The most important feature preoperatively is assessment of the stability of the patient's disease. If it is determined that the patient probably has coronary disease but that exercise tolerance is good in that there is no difficulty climbing two flights of stairs, that the patient has no angina or only stable infrequent angina, and that there is no evidence of congestive heart failure, the patient can probably tolerate the added stress of anesthesia and surgery. In the presence of known coronary artery disease, the operative mortality rate is increased about threefold.

If, on the other hand, the patient has had a change in anginal pattern, with increasing severity or duration of angina; if there is unprovoked angina or angina at rest; or if there is evidence of decreased ventricular function or failure—in all such cases the patient clearly needs assessment for the possibility of revascularization, and this should be done before any other elective surgery.

If the patient is unable to give a history of normal exercise tolerance or is unable to exercise because of neurologic, orthopedic, or peripheral vascular disease, it cannot be assumed that the patient will accommodate the oxygen demands of general anesthesia and surgery. Under these circumstances, exercise testing (if the patient can walk) or dipyridamole-thallium or sestamibi perfusion scanning may be advisable.

The value of risk-stratifying patients at high risk for coronary disease or those who have known coronary disease but appear to be stable prior to undergoing noncardiac surgery is still controversial. The type of noncardiac surgery most likely to be associated with an ischemic event at or after operation is that involving the aorta or major abdominal and extremity arteries.

In a study from the Cleveland Clinic in which patients undergoing peripheral vascular surgery over a 4-year period were analyzed, of about 1000 patients, one-third of whom had abdominal aortic aneurysmectomy, myocardial infarction occurred in 3.8% and was the leading cause of death, accounting for about half the postoperative deaths. Followed for 8–11 years postoperatively 47% of these survivors died, 44% with myocardial infarction. Subsequent evaluation of patients from the same institution who were found to have ischemia and were vascularized prior to peripheral vascular surgery shows a better survival rate both perioperatively and in late follow-up. This experience has led the Cleveland Clinic group to advocate routine coronary angiography prior to peripheral vascular surgery (Hertzer, 1984).

A less invasive approach advocated by Boucher et al uses dipyridamole-thallium or stress testing to risk-stratify patients prior to peripheral vascular surgery. These and other investigators (Boucher, 1985; Leppo 1987; Hendel, 1990) have shown that redistribution defects on thallium-dipyridamole studies were sensitive in predicting subsequent ischemic events. However, the specificity was not high in that many patients with redistribution defects did not have ischemic events. Eagle (1989) showed that specificity could be improved by adding to clinical predictors, including Q waves on electrocardiography, a history of angina, a history of ventricular ectopy requiring treatment, diabetes requiring therapy, and age over 70 years to the dipyridamole-thallium data. Risk stratification of cardiac risk by dipyridamole-thallium scintigraphy has been used in the preoperative evaluation of patients prior to nonvascular surgery with similar findings (Coley, 1992).

Treadmill testing with electrocardiographic changes, 24-hour electrocardiographic monitoring for silent ischemia, and two-dimensional transesophageal echocardiography during surgery have all been used to diagnose ischemic events that may be silent. In general, these studies show that intraoperative and postoperative silent ischemia identifies patients at high risk for subsequent ischemic events.

However, not all studies suggest that preoperative screening is helpful. In a prospective study, 60 patients undergoing vascular surgery were examined preoperatively with dipyridamole-thallium scintigraphy, intraoperatively by continuous 12-lead electrocardiography and transesophageal echocardiography, and postoperatively by continuous electrocardiography. In 37% of the patients there were perfusion defects; in 30% the defects persisted after redistribution; and 33% showed no defects. There was no association between redistribution defects and adverse cardiac outcomes and none between intraoperative ischemia and preoperative redistribution defects (Mangano, 1991). Another study showed that when compared with predictive clinical data and two-lead electrocardiographic monitoring, little additional information about risk for perioperative ischemic outcomes was obtained by monitoring with continuous 12-lead electrocardiography or intraoperative transesophageal echocardiography (Eisenberg, 1992).

Finally, at the Mayo Clinic, preoperative risk stratification by dipyridamole-thallium and exercise testing was performed in patients prior to vascular surgery. If there was a strongly positive dipyridamole-thallium or treadmill test or if the patients had unstable angina or cardiac class III or class IV angina, coronary arteriography followed by myocardial revascularization was performed. Late survival statistics showed that patients with coronary artery disease had a lower survival rate than an age-matched population regardless of the management of the coronary artery disease. In the older patients, survival of those with coronary artery disease was similar whether or not myocardial revascularization was done. It thus appeared that there was no survival advantage in the selective use of coronary artery bypass grafting. It is also not clear whether clinical indices would help improve the predictive outcome of dipyridamole-thallium scanning.

This subject is therefore still controversial. It is our policy to risk-stratify only when we cannot tell from the history what the patient's exercise capacity and state of symptomatology is by the history alone. In patients who are having major aortic surgery, who have a history of coronary disease or are at high risk of having coronary disease, at present we are risk stratifying by exercise treadmill testing or thallium-sestamibi perfusion scanning. If exercise can't be done, perfusion scanning after dipyridamole-thallium is performed.

Emergency surgery must often be done despite a recent myocardial infarction, but the mortality rate is high. Important but not lifesaving surgery is best delayed at least 3 weeks if possible. Purely elective surgery should be postponed for 3–6 months whenever possible.

In patients with known coronary heart disease, the added risk of a new myocardial infarction, as indicated previously, decreases as the time interval following the previous myocardial infarction lengthens. It averages about 20% if general surgery is performed within the first 3 months after an acute myocardial infarction, decreases to 3–5% if it is delayed for at least 6 months, and is about 10% between 3 and 6 months (Steen, 1978).

The diagnosis of a new myocardial infarction during or following operations is often difficult; myocardial infarction may occur at rest during the perioperative period without anginal pain because of medication for postsurgical pain and the relative diagnostic unreliability of postoperative serum enzymes except for MB (myocardial band) creatine phosphokinase isoenzymes. Transesophageal echocardiography for intraoperative demonstration of myocardial ischemia and left ventricular function was found to be specific; the findings were encouraging, though there were technical problems requiring further evaluation (Shiveley, 1986). The mortality rate is about 30% if a new infarct occurs during or after surgery. A new myocardial infarction is more common with operations on the chest and upper abdomen than in those involving the pelvis or lower abdomen and is more apt to occur on the second or third postoperative day than on the day of operation. For this reason, postoperative patients with known or suspected coronary heart disease should be monitored by daily ECGs and MB creatine phosphokinase isoenzyme determinations in order to determine whether a new infarction has occurred. Older individuals without known coronary heart disease may have flattening of the T waves in the left ventricular leads postoperatively but rarely have deep inversions of the T wave, ischemic ST depression, or new Q waves. Development of the last three suggests myocardial ischemia or infarction.

Ventricular arrhythmias (see below) are more common during and following surgery when coronary heart disease is present; if the patient is known to have angina pectoris, continuous monitoring of the ECG is recommended, and the physician should pay careful attention to the possible development of hypoxia, hypotension, and acidosis. If the patient has severe atherosclerosis elsewhere (eg, aortoiliac) and borderline left ventricular function or a history of heart failure, a flow-directed catheter should be introduced preoperatively to allow intermittent measurements of pulmonary artery diastolic (wedge) pressure, cardiac output, and blood gases. An attempt is made during surgery to keep the parameters related to myocardial oxygen demand—heart rate, systolic blood pressure, and cardiac output (see below)—within 20% of preoperative values.

In addition, other advances in intraoperative monitoring such as transesophageal echocardiography have been developed where the immediate cessation of myocardial wall motion occurs with ischemia. Intraoperative use of vasoactive and inotropic drugs together with newer anesthesia techniques all may influence operative outcome.

In general, we keep patients with coronary disease on their anti-ischemic regimen before and after surgery. Intraoperatively, we recommend intravenous nitroglycerin or beta-blockers.

As noted previously, any indication of an acute change in the preoperative condition, such as unstable angina, means that elective surgery should be postponed, usually for at least 3 months or until revascularization has been accomplished.

2. HYPERTENSION

Patients with uncomplicated chronic hypertension, even with left ventricular hypertrophy and an abnormal ECG, tolerate surgery without a significantly increased mortality rate if there are no evidences of coronary heart disease or cardiac failure and if renal function is normal. Antihypertensive medication should be continued until the time of surgery, and the anesthesiologist should be alerted to the medications used and informed about any difficulties noted in preoperative control of blood pressure. If medications are stopped earlier, there may be wide fluctuations in blood pressure during surgery (Pickering, 1983). If diuretics have been given, the body potassium must be replenished preoperatively. Volume depletion in these patients may require fluid therapy.

3. ARRHYTHMIAS

Chronic atrial fibrillation with a well-controlled ventricular rate does not increase the risk of surgery, nor does an asymptomatic isolated right or left bundle branch block. Bifascicular block in asymptomatic patients does not require prophylactic pacing but does require close observation. Second- or third-degree atrioventricular block is a warning sign, especially if associated with left or right ventricular conduction defects; a transvenous electrode catheter should be inserted into the right ventricle before the surgical procedure and the patient monitored, with a pacemaker available in case ventricular standstill occurs. Infrequent atrial or ventricular premature beats usually do not require special treatment. Monitoring of the ECG during anesthesia and surgery has shown that ventricular arrhythmias are infrequent unless there is underlying left ventricular disease or unless catecholamine release is excessive as a result of ventilatory problems.

If ventricular premature beats preoperatively are frequent and from multiple foci, or if they occur in salvos, correct management is debatable. Many currently believe no antiarrhythmic therapy is needed if the arrhythmia is not associated with ischemia and left ventricular function is normal. Others believe surgery can be delayed and treatment for premature beats instituted as discussed in Chapter 15, especially if the arrhythmia is occurring in a patient with underlying cardiac disease. If the clinical situation is more urgent, or if it is considered unsatisfactory to delay surgery for 2–3 days to obtain the effect from oral drugs, lidocaine, 2% solution (20 mg/mL), 50–100 mg intravenously, followed by an intravenous infusion of 1–2 mg/min, will usually quickly abolish the premature beats.

If the premature beats are unifocal and infrequent, they should not be treated with antiarrhythmic drugs but monitored by continuous electrocardiography. If salvos of ventricular beats or complex arrhythmias develop, intravenous lidocaine should be used. Elderly patients undergoing thoracotomy for cardiac or pulmonary surgery have a high incidence of atrial fibrillation. There is evidence that this incidence is reduced if the patient is given digoxin preoperatively, and some authorities recommend that precaution.

4. VALVULAR HEART DISEASE

Severe aortic stenosis, tight mitral stenosis, and severe coronary ostial involvement due to syphilitic aortitis are the three major "valvular" conditions in which general surgery presents a considerably increased hazard. An aortic systolic murmur not associated with evidence of severe aortic valvular disease or significant left ventricular hypertrophy does not increase the mortality rate. Mitral insufficiency is usually tolerated well, but tight mitral stenosis, especially if the patient has sinus rhythm, may result in acute pulmonary edema if the patient abruptly develops atrial fibrillation during surgery. Patients with severe mitral stenosis or severe symptomatic aortic stenosis should be considered for valve surgery prior to the noncardiac elective surgery. Balloon valvuloplasty could be an alternative temporizing approach (Roth, 1989). Patients who are functional class III or class IV with mitral or aortic regurgitation should also be considered for valve surgery prior to cardiac surgery.

5. CONGENITAL HEART DISEASE

In the absence of cardiac failure, ventricular septal defect and atrial septal defect usually pose no particular problems or extra hazard. Pulmonary hypertension with Eisenmenger's syndrome carries a significantly increased mortality risk, and surgery should be performed only upon urgent indications. Patients with coarctation of the aorta and patent ductus arteriosus should have their congenital lesions repaired before undergoing elective general surgical procedures. Mild pulmonary stenosis is not a contraindication to elective surgery, but severe pulmonary stenosis is a contraindication because of the hazard of acute right heart failure and a reversed shunt through the foramen ovale or a small atrial septal defect. Patients with tetralogy of Fallot or other cyanotic congenital cardiac lesions are relatively poor surgical risks because of the polycythemia and because of the possibility of contraction of the infundibulum of the right ventricle, with resulting decrease in pulmonary blood flow.

6. CARDIAC FAILURE

Patients with mild cardiac failure whose symptoms and signs are controlled with digitalis and diuretics have only a slightly increased risk from general surgery provided ordinary activity does not cause symptoms. As the functional class worsens, the mortality rate increases, irrespective of the nature of the underlying cardiac disease which has caused the congestive failure. Patients who have dyspnea even when walking on level ground; orthopnea or nocturnal dyspnea; and signs of cardiac failure such as gallop rhythm, increased venous pressure, and rales are at a significantly increased risk, and surgery should be delayed if possible. Cardiac failure should be treated adequately before surgery. It is desirable to have the pa-

tient's condition stabilized for at least a month before surgery and to avoid digitalis toxicity and potassium depletion by diuretics. Diuretics and digitalis can then be withheld for a day before surgery. Digitalization of a patient with cardiac hypertrophy but no heart failure is unwise because of the hazard of digitalis toxicity, including arrhythmias. Although digitalis has a positive inotropic action even in normal hearts, clinical evidence of benefit from the drug has not been demonstrated when it has been given to patients with hypertrophy but no failure. If there is a question about whether or not heart failure is present preoperatively, a period of bed rest and restricted dietary sodium may be adequate treatment.

MANAGEMENT OF KNOWN CARDIAC DISEASE PRIOR TO GENERAL SURGERY

If the preoperative assessment reveals known cardiac disease or severe hypertension, especially in the presence of acute symptoms, anemia, or unstable state, serious ventricular arrhythmias, heart block or cardiac failure, these conditions should be managed before the surgical procedure is undertaken. The treatment of any cardiac condition discovered in the preoperative evaluation should be along the lines of treatment discussed elsewhere in this book and should not differ substantially in the patient with an elective surgical condition from treatment of a nonsurgical patient. Careful judgment is required in patients with more urgent surgical conditions, and delay in surgery for as long as possible may be indicated until the cardiac status is somewhat improved. If the surgical condition is urgent, the ability of the physician to treat the cardiac problem may be limited, and surgical treatment must take precedence even though the risk is considerably enhanced.

If the patient has severe valvular or coronary heart disease correctable by cardiac surgery, or if there are transient cerebral ischemic attacks proved by aortogram to be due to significant carotid stenosis, surgical treatment of the correctable lesion should precede elective general surgery in order to avoid pulmonary edema, cardiac arrest, or hemiplegia, which may follow the increased demands and variable blood pressure resulting from anesthesia and surgery. In such cases, carotid occlusive disease should usually be treated first unless the cardiac lesion is life-threatening. Fortunately, unexpected severe cardiac disease is uncommon in the patient scheduled for elective surgery, so the psychologic and other disturbances incident to cancellation of scheduled operations are reduced.

Middle-aged or elderly patients suspected of having heart disease should be evaluated for a few days before scheduled surgery to allow effective diagnosis and management of any cardiac problem that is unexpectedly elicited. If uncontrolled atrial fibrillation, congestive heart failure, or progressive angina is found, the patient should be hospitalized for more intensive evaluation and therapy.

SPECIAL PRECAUTIONS

In addition to conducting a preoperative surgical evaluation for any heart condition that should be managed before elective cardiac or other surgery, the physician should take special precautions if patients are receiving general treatment that may require modification because of the intended surgery. As a rule, anticoagulants should be stopped 2–3 days before surgery and resumed about 3 days postoperatively. If it is deemed necessary to maintain anticoagulation as long as possible, the patient can be converted to heparin intravenously, which can be stopped 6 hours before surgery and restarted 18–24 hours after surgery. Patients who have had intensive or prolonged corticosteroid treatment, even if it has been stopped for several months, should be identified, and supplementary corticosteroids should be administered (up to the equivalent of 200–300 mg of hydrocortisone per day perioperatively and for several days postoperatively). Patients receiving long-acting insulin for diabetes mellitus should be given regular insulin, and frequent analyses of urine, blood sugar, and ketones should be performed. Any hypersensitivity to drugs, especially antibiotics, should be determined so that patients will not receive them inadvertently.

The administration of sodium-containing fluids should be carefully controlled during the preoperative, intraoperative, and postoperative periods because of the known sodium and water retention that follows general surgical operations. Sodium retention is probably due to hemodynamic and perhaps hormonal influences on the nephron. Water retention is due to increased secretion of antidiuretic hormone (ADH) and not to increased aldosterone levels or decreased glomerular filtration rate. Sodium retention occurring postoperatively or arising from the use of intravenous sodium-containing fluids may precipitate pulmonary edema, and the speed and volume of the infused fluid should be regulated with this hazard in mind. If there is preoperative anemia or extensive blood loss during surgery, packed red cells rather than whole blood should be given slowly, and the patient should be supine and closely watched. If dyspnea, rales, or raised jugular venous pressure appears, the patient should be placed in the Fowler position to decrease the pulmonary blood volume and the infusion slowed or stopped.

MONITORING IN THE PRESENCE OF SEVERE CARDIAC DISEASE

If urgent surgery is required in the patient with severe coronary disease, aortic stenosis, mitral stenosis, or atrioventricular block; if extensive surgery is required in patients with borderline cardiac reserve; or if the multifactorial risk index is high, the patient should be monitored directly by a Swan-Ganz catheter. If it is difficult to evaluate the physiologic status in elderly patients thought to be of high risk, preoperative invasive assessment should be considered (Del Guercio, 1980), but this should not be a routine practice. Noninvasive clinical, echocardiographic, and radionuclide studies usually suffice.

In the management of high-risk patients during major noncardiac abdominothoracic surgery, invasive monitoring results in treatment that decreases morbidity and mortality rates. High-risk patients include those who have had a recent acute myocardial infarction and those with poor left ventricular function and congestive heart failure. Monitoring of heart rate, arterial pressure, pulmonary artery wedge pressure, and cardiac output and keeping these variables to within 20% of the preanesthetic values has resulted in considerably fewer reinfarctions in patients who have had major surgery following a prior myocardial infarction. The incidence of reinfarction fell from 7.9% (28/364) in the years 1973–1976 to 1.9% (14/733) in the years 1977–1982, primarily as a result of invasive monitoring. In the period 0–3 months postinfarction, the incidence of reinfarction fell from 36% in the earlier years to 5.7% in the later years. In the period 4–6 months postinfarction, the rate fell from 26% to 2.3% (Rao, 1983). Many anesthesiologists believe that high risk patients can be monitored during surgery just as effectively with continuous transesophageal echocardiography.

Invasive monitoring during surgery is also indicated for patients in the Goldman class IV cardiac risk index and those undergoing abdominal or thoracic aneurysmectomy.

A temporary transvenous right ventricular pacemaker should be inserted when indicated to allow prompt institution of pacing in the event complete heart block develops. Emergency cardiac drugs and facilities for defibrillation should be readily available.

The choice and details of anesthesia are best left to the anesthesiologist, who must be alerted to any possible problems that might occur and informed of any medications the patient has taken even if they have recently been discontinued, such as digitalis, diuretics, antihypertensive agents, corticosteroids, insulin, propranolol, anticoagulants, or tricyclic antidepressants.

REFERENCES

Abraham SA et al: Coronary risk of noncardiac surgery. Prog Cardiovasc Dis 1991;34:205.

Berkoff HA, Levine RL: Management of the vascular patient with multisystem atherosclerosis. Prog Cardiovasc Dis 1987;29:347.

Boucher CA et al: Determination of cardiac risk by dipyridamole-thallium imaging before peripheral vascular surgery. N Engl J Med 1985;312:389.

Coley CM et al: Usefulness of dipyridamole-thallium scanning for preoperative evaluation of cardiac risks for nonvascular surgery. Am J Cardiol 1992;69:1280.

Consensus Conference of the National Institutes of Health: Prevention of venous thrombosis and pulmonary embolism. JAMA 1986;256:744.

Del Guercio LRM, Cohn JD: Monitoring operative risk in the elderly. JAMA 1980;243:1350.

Detsky AS et al: Cardiac assessment for patients undergoing noncardiac surgery: A multifactorial clinical risk index. Arch Intern Med 1986;146:2131.

Eagle KA et al: Combining clinical and thallium data optimizes preoperative assessment of cardiac risk before major vascular surgery. Ann Intern Med 1989;110:859.

Eisenberg MJ et al: Monitoring for myocardial ischemia during noncardiac surgery. JAMA 1992;268:210.

Gerson MC et al: Cardiac prognosis in noncardiac geriatric surgery. Ann Intern Med 1985;103:832.

Goldman L: Cardiac risks and complications of noncardiac surgery. Ann Intern Med 1983;98:504.

Hendel RC et al: Prognostic value of dipyridamole-thallium subgroups for evaluation of ischaemic heart disease.

Hertzer NR et al: Coronary artery disease in peripheral vascular patients: A classification of 1000 coronary angiograms and results of surgical management. Ann Surg 1984;199:223.

Katholi RE, Nolan SP, McGuire LB: The management of anticoagulation during noncardiac operations in patients with prosthetic heart valves: A prospective study. Am Heart J 1978;96:163.

Katz JD et al: Pulmonary artery flow-guided catheters in the perioperative period: Indications and complications. 1977;237:2832.

Leppo J et al: Noninvasive evaluation of cardiac risk before elective vascular surgery. J Am Coll Cardiol 1987;9:269.

Mangano DT et al: Association of perioperative myocardial ischemia with cardiac morbidity and mortality in men undergoing noncardiac surgery. N Engl J Med 1990;323;1781.

Mangano DT et al: Dipyridamole-thallium-201 scintigraphy as a preoperative screening test: A reexamination of its predictive potential. Circulation 1991;84:493.

O'Keefe JH et al: Risk of noncardiac surgical procedures in patients with aortic stenosis. Mayo Clin Proc 1989;64:400.

Pastore JO et al: The risk of advanced heart block in surgical patients with right bundle branch block and left axis deviation. Circulation 1978;57:677.

Pettigrew RA, Hill GL: Indicators of surgical risk and clinical judgment. Br J Surg 1986;73:47.

Pickering TG: Anesthesia and surgery for the hypertensive patient. Cardiovasc Rev Rep 1983;4:1569.

Rao TL, Jacobs KH, El-Etr AA: Reinfarction following anesthesia in patients with myocardial infarction. Anesthesiology 1983;59:499.

Reigel MM et al: Late survival in abdominal aortic aneurysm patients: The role of selective myocardial revascularization on the basis of clinical symptoms. J Vasc Surg 1987;5:222.

Rogers MC: Anesthetic management of patients with heart disease. Mod Concepts Cardiovasc Dis 1983;52:29.

Roth RB, Palacios IF, Block PC: Percutaneous aortic balloon valvuloplasty: Its role in the management of patients with aortic stenosis requiring major noncardiac surgery. J Am Coll Cardiol 1989;13:1039.

Shiveley BK, Schiller NB: Transesophageal echocardiography in the intraoperative detection of myocardial ischemia and infarction. Echocardiography 1986;3:001.

Smith JS et al: Intraoperative detection of myocardial ischemia in high-risk patients: Electrocardiography versus two-dimensional transesophageal echocardiography. Circulation 1985;72:1015.

Steen PA, Tinker JH, Tarhan S: Myocardial reinfarction after anesthesia and surgery. JAMA 1978;239:2566.

Wohlgelernter D, Cohen LS: Common cardiovascular problems after general surgery. Cardiovasc Med 1984;9:763.

Zeldin RA: Assessing cardiac risk in patients who undergo noncardiac surgical procedures. Can J Surg 1984;27:402.

Index

Note: Page numbers followed by t and f indicate tables and figures, respectively.